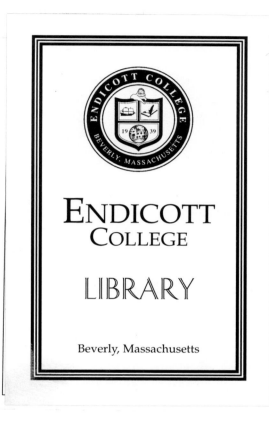

Health psychology is a rapidly expanding discipline at the interface of psychology and clinical medicine. This important work collates international and interdisciplinary expertise to form a unique encyclopaedic handbook to this field which will be valuable for both medical practitioners and psychologists from trainee to professional level. Intended primarily as a reference text, it is expected that readers will seek out particular chapters for particular purposes. To facilitate this, chapters have been alphabetically organized with extensive cross-referencing. The first of three parts introduces the non-specialist reader to broad areas of psychology relevant to the practice of medicine. The second and third follow behavioural factors in relation to practice through to an analysis of specific medical conditions. Coverage is broad with extensive referencing – an invaluable resource to all those with an interest in health issues, promotion and care.

Cambridge Handbook of Psychology, Health and Medicine

Cambridge Handbook of Psychology, Health and Medicine

EDITED BY

ANDREW BAUM
University of Pittsburgh, USA

STANTON NEWMAN
University College and Middlesex School of Medicine, London, UK

JOHN WEINMAN
United Medical and Dental Schools of Guy's and St Thomas's, London, UK

ROBERT WEST
St George's Hospital Medical School, London, UK

CHRIS McMANUS
St Mary's Hospital Medical School, London, UK

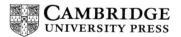

CAMBRIDGE
UNIVERSITY PRESS

PUBLISHED BY THE PRESS SYNDICATE OF THE UNIVERSITY OF CAMBRIDGE

The Pitt Building, Trumpington Street, Cambridge CB2 1RP, United Kingdom

CAMBRIDGE UNIVERSITY PRESS

The Edinburgh Building, Cambridge CB2 2RU, United Kingdom

40 West 20th Street, New York, NY 10011–4211, USA

10 Stamford Road, Oakleigh, Melbourne 3166, Australia

First published 1997

Printed in the United Kingdom at the University Press, Cambridge

Typeset in Ehrhardt MT 9/12 pt

*A catalogue record for this book is available from
the British Library*

Library of Congress Cataloguing in Publication data

Cambridge handbook of psychology, health, and medicine / edited by Andrew Baum . . .
   [et al.].
      p.   cm.
   Includes index.
   ISBN 0 521 43073 9 (hardcover). ISBN 0 521 43686 9 (pbk.)
   1. Medicine and psychology. I. Baum, Andrew.
   [DNLM: 1. Psychology, Medical – handbooks. 2. Behavioral Medicine – handbooks.
   WB 39 C178 1997]
R726.5.C354 1997
616′.001′9–dc21.
DNLM/DLC   96—44596 CIP
for Library of Congress

ISBN 0 521 43073 9 hardback
ISBN 0 521 43686 9 paperback

Every effort has been made in preparing this book to provide accurate and up-to-date
information which is in accord with accepted standards and practice at the time of publication.
Nevertheless, the authors, editors and publishers can make no warranties that the information
contained herein is totally free from error, not least because clinical standards are constantly
changing through research and regulation. The authors, editors and publisher therefore
disclaim all liability for direct or consequential damages resulting from the use of material
contained in this book. The reader is strongly advised to pay careful attention to information
provided by the manufacturer of any drugs or equipment that they plan to use.

CONTENTS

Section 2: Psychological assessment and intervention

Section 3: Health-care practice

CONTRIBUTORS

Leif E. Aarø, Research Centre for Health Promotion and Department of Psychosocial Science, University of Bergen, Oistereinsgate 3, N-5007 Bergen, Norway

Beth Alder, Department of Epidemiology and Public Health, University of Dundee, Ninewells Hospital and Medical School, Dundee DD1 9SY, UK

John Allen, Psychology Department, City University, School of Social Science, Northampton Square, London EC1V 0HB, UK

Ruth Allen, Department of Oncology, UCLMS, 3rd Floor Bland Sutton Institute, Middlesex Hospital, 48 Riding House Street, London W1P 7PL, UK

Barbara L. Andersen, Department of Psychology, 1885 Neil Avenue, The Ohio State University, Columbus, OH 43210–1222, USA

John Archer, Department of Psychology, University of Central Lancashire, Preston PR1 2HE, UK

Michael Argyle, Department of Experimental Psychology, Oxford University, South Parks Road, Oxford OX1 3UD, UK

Ana M. Arroyo, Department of Psychology, Indiana University, Bloomington, IN 47405, USA

Heather Ashton, School of Neurosciences, Division of Psychiatry, The Royal Victoria Infirmary, Queen Victoria Road, Newcastle upon Tyne NE1 4LP, UK

Peter Ayton, Psychology Department, The City University, Northampton Square, London EC1 V 0HB, UK

Elizabeth Bachen, Center for AID Prevention Studies, University of California at San Francisco, 74 New Montgomery Street, Suite 600, San Francisco, CA 94105, USA

Albert Bandura, Psychology Department, Stanford University, Stanford, CA 943052310, USA

Andrew Baum, 3600 Forbes Avenue, Suite 405, Pittsburgh, PA 15213, USA

Paul Bennett, Gwent Psychology Services, and Department of Psychology, University of Bristol, UK

Yael Benyamini, Institute for Health, Rutgers, The State University of New Jersey, 30 College Avenue, PO Box 5062, New Brunswick, NJ 08903–5062, USA

John W. Berry, Department of Psychology, Queen's University, Kingston K7L 3N6, Canada

Maurice Bloch, Riverview Hospital, Port Coquitlam, British Columbia, IG4 Canada

Robert Bor, Psychology Department, City University, Northampton Square, London EC1V 0HV, UK

Ron Borland, Centre for Behavioural Research in Cancer, Anti-Cancer Council of Victoria, 1 Rathdowne Street, Carlton South, Victoria 3053, Australia

Peter Bower, University of Manchester, NPCRDC, 5th Floor, Williamson Building, Oxford Road, Manchester M13 9PL, UK

Clare Bradley, Department of Psychology, Royal Holloway College, London University, Egham, Surrey TW20 0EX, UK

Kelly J. Brown, Department of Medical and Clinical Psychology, USUHS, 4301 Jones Bridge Road, Bethesda, MD 20814–4799, USA

Kevin Browne, School of Psychology, University of Birmingham, Edgbaston B15 2TT, UK

Michael H. Bruch, Academic Department of Psychiatry, Middlesex Hospital Medical School, Wolfson Building, London W1P 8AA, UK

Denise Brunt, Psychology Department, Victoria University of Technology, PO Box 14428, MMC, Melbourne, Victoria 3000, Australia

Deanna Buick, Department of Psychiatry and Behavioural Science, University of Auckland School of Medicine, Private Bag, Auckland, New Zealand

Elizabeth Burrin, Psychology Department, St George's Hospital Medical School, Cranmer Terrace, London SW17 0RE, UK

Nina Butler, Unit of Health Psychology, Department of Psychiatry and Behavioural Sciences, University College London Medical School, Wolfson Building, Riding House Street, London W1N 8AA, UK

Timothy P. Carmody, VA Hospital, 4159 Clement Street, San Francisco, CA 94121, USA

Douglas Carroll, School of Sport and Exercise Sciences, University of Birmingham, Birmingham B15 2TT, UK

Denise Charman, Department of Psychology, Victoria University, PO Box 14428, MCMC, Melbourne 8001, Victoria, Australia

Chris Code, Cumberland College of Health Sciences, The University of Sydney, East Street (PO Box 170), Lidcombe, NSW 2141, Australia

Sheldon Cohen, Department of Psychology, Carnegie-Mellon University, Pittsburgh, PA 15213–3890, USA

Colin Coles, Institute of Health and Community Studies, Bournemouth University, Royal London House, Christchurch Road, Bournemouth BH1 3LT, UK

Thomas L. Creer, Ohio University, Athens, Ohio 45701, USA

Ilana Crome, North Staffordshire Combined Health Care, Substance Abuse Unit, Ward 93, City General Hospital, Stoke-on-Trent ST4 6QG, UK

Peggy Dalton, 20 Cleveland Avenue, London W4, UK

George Davey Smith, Department of Social Medicine, University of Bristol, Bristol BS8 2PR, UK

Hilton Davis, Bloomfield Clinic, Guy's Hospital, London Bridge, London SE1 9RT, UK

Gerald C. Davison, Department of Psychology, University of Southern California, University Park, Los Angeles, CA 90089, USA

Kathryn P. Davison, Southern Methodist University, Dallas, Texas, USA

David De L. Horne, Department of Psychology, University of Melbourne, c/o Royal Victoria Hospital, 9th Floor, Charles Connibere Building, Parkville, Victoria 3052, Australia

Jennifer Devlen, 11655 Old Mill Road, Shippensburg, PA 17257, USA

Ingrid Doherty, Community Support Team, West Lambeth Community Care (NHS) Trust, Tooting Bec Hospital, Church Lane, London SW17 8BL, UK

Simon Dupont, Clinical Psychology Department, Guy's Hospital, Three Tuns House, London Bridge, London SE1 9RT, UK

Louise Earll, Department of Health Psychology, Gloucester Royal Hospital, Great Western Road, Gloucester GL1 3NN, UK

Robert J. Edelmann, Department of Psychology, University of Surrey, Guildford, Surrey GU2 5XH, UK

Christine Eiser, Department of Psychology, University of Exeter, Exeter EX4 4GQ, UK

J. Richard Eiser, Department of Psychology, University of Exeter, Exeter EX4 4GQ, UK

James Elander, Institute of Psychiatry, MRC Child Psychiatry Unit, De Crespigny Park, London SE5 8AF, UK

Bjorn Ellertsen, Department of Biological and Medical Psychology, University of Bergen, Arstadveien 21, N-5009, Bergen, Norway

Sandra A. Elliott, University of Greenwich School of Social Sciences, Avery Hill Road, London SE9 2UG, UK

Ruth Epstein, Ferens Institute, Middlesex Hospital, Mortimer Street, London W1N 8AA, UK

Chris Evans, Department of General Psychiatry, St George's Hospital Medical School, Cranmer Terrace, London SW17 0RE, UK

Olga Evans, Department of Psychology, St George's Hospital Medical School, London SW17 0RE, UK

Michael W. Eysenck, St George's Hospital Medical School, Royal Holloway College, London University, Egham, Surrey TW20 0EX, UK

Lesley Fallowfield, Academic Unit of Psychology, The London Hospital Medical College, Alexandra Wing, Turner Street, London E1 2AD, UK

Rosalie E. Ferner, Neurology Department, Guy's Hospital, London Bridge, London SE1 9RT, UK

Jenny Firth-Cozens, Department of Psychology, University of Leeds, Leeds LS2 9JT, UK

Baruch Fischhoff, Department of Social and Decision Sciences, Carnegie Mellon University, Pittsburgh, PA 15213–3890, USA

Ray Fitzpatrick, Nuffield College, Oxford OX1 1NF, UK

Robert G. Frank, College of Health Professions, University of Florida, Health Sciences Center, Gainesville, Florida, USA

Irene H. Frieze, Department of Psychology, University of Pittsburgh, PA 15260, USA

Elaine Funnell, Psychology Department, Royal Holloway College, London University, Egham, Surrey TW20 0EX, UK

Adrian Furnham, Department of Psychology, University College London, Gower Street, London WC16BT, UK

Sheryle J. Gallant, The University of Kansas, 426 Fraser Hall, Lawrence, KA 66045–2160, USA

Robert J. Gatchel, Department of Psychiatry, University of Texas Southwestern Medical Center, 5323 Harry Himes Boulevard, Dallas, TX 75235–9044, USA

Russell E. Glasgow, Oregon Research Institute, 1899 Willamette Street, Eugene, OR 97401, USA

Claire Glasscoe, Children and Families Consultative Service, West London Health Care NHS Trust, Windmill Lodge, Uxbridge Road, Middlesex UB1 3EU, UK

Deanna M. Golden-Kreutz, Department of Psychology, 1885 Neil Avenue, The Ohio State University, Columbus, OH 43210–1228, USA

Michael Gossop, National Addiction Centre, Institute of Psychiatry, DeCrespigny Park, London SE5 8AF, UK

Thomas Green, Child Care and Development Group, Cambridge University, Free School Lane, Cambridge CB2 3RF, UK

Mary Banks Gregerson, Family Therapy Institute of Alexandria, 220 South Washington Street, Alexandria, VA 22314–22315, USA

Neil E. Grunberg, Department of Medica and Clinical Psychology, USUHS, 4301 Jones Bridge Road, Bethesda, MD 20814–4799, USA

Peter Hajek, Academic Department of Psychiatry, the London Hospital Medical College, Alexandra Wing, 3rd Floor, Turner Street, London E1 2AD, UK

Tirril Harris, Department of Social Policy, Royal Holloway College, London University, 11 Bedford Square, London WC1B 3RA, UK

Siobhan Hart, Essex Rivers Health Care Trust, Essex County Hospital, Lexden Road, Colchester CO3 3NB, UK

Nigel Harvey, Department of Psychology, University College London, Gower Street, London WC1E, UK

Trudy Havermans, Hoevehei 15, 5508 TK Veldhoven, The Netherlands

Michael Heap, Department of Psychiatry, University of Sheffield, 15 Claremont Crescent, Sheffield S10 2TA, UK

Barbara Hedge, Department of Psychological Medicine, William Harvey House, St Bartholomew's Hospital, London EC1A 7BE, UK

Kenneth Heller, Department of Psychology, Indiana University, Bloomington, IN 47405, USA

Peter G. Hepper, School of Psychology, Queen's University of Belfast, Belfast BT7 1NN, UK

Michael Herbert, International Medical College, Kuala Lumpur, 21 Jalan Selangor, 46050 Petaling Jaya, Selangor Darui Ehsan, Malaysia

Jenny Hewison, Department of Psychology, The University of Leeds, Leeds LS2 9JT, UK

George Higgins, Counseling Center, Trinity College, Hartford, CT 06106–3187, USA

Kenneth A. Holroyd, Ohio University, Athens, OH 45701, USA

Diane B. Howieson, Department of Psychology, Department of Veterans Affairs, Medical Center, 3710 South West Veterans Hospital Road, Portland, OR 97207, USA

Michael R. Hufford, Department of Psychology, University of Pittsburgh, PA 15260, USA

Gerry Humphris, Department of Clinical Psychology, University of Liverpool, Whelan Building, PO Box 147, Liverpool L69 3BX, UK

A. Jackie Hunter, Neurology Research, SmithKline Beecham Pharmaceuticals, New Frontiers Science Park, Third Avenue, Harlow, Essex CM19 5AW, UK

Myra S. Hunter, Unit of Psychology, UMDS at Guy's Campus, London Bridge, University of London, London SE1 9RT, UK

Staffan Hygge, National Swedish Institute for Building Research, Box 785, S-801 29 Gävle, Sweden

Marjan Jahanshahi, MRC Human Movement and Balance Unit, Institute of Neurology, Queen's Square, London WC1N 3BG, UK

Jean E. Johnson, School of Nursing, University of Rochester, 601 Elmwood Avenue, Rochester, NY 14642, USA

Derek W. Johnston, Department of Psychology, University of St Andrews, Fife KY16 9JU, UK

Marie Johnston, Department of Psychology, University of St Andrews, St Andrews, Fife KY16 9JU, UK

David Jones, Psychology Department, Birkbeck College, University of London, Malet Street, London WC1E 7HX, UK

Ad A. Kaptein, Medical Psychiatry, Department of Psychiatry, University of Leiden, PO Box 1251, 2340 BG Oegstgeest, The Netherlands

Stanislav V. Kasl, Division of Epidemiology and Public Health, Yale University, 60 College Street, New Haven, CT 06510, USA

Joel Katz, Department of Psychology, Toronto Hospital/ General Division, 200 Elizabeth Street, CW2–306 Toronto, Canada M5G 2C4 BG

Francis J. Keefe, Duke University Medical Center, Box 3159, Durham, NC 27710, USA

Tony Kendrick, Division of General Practice, St George's Hospital Medical School, Cranmer Terrace, London SW17 0RE, UK

Paul Kennedy, Department of Clinical Psychology, Stoke Mandeville Hospital, The National Spinal Injuries Centre, Aylesbury, Bucks HP21 8AL, UK

Christie M. King, Department of Psychology, Indiana University, Bloomington, IN 47405, USA

L. Cousino Klein, Department of Medical and Clinical Psychology, USUHS, 4301 Jones Bridge Road, Bethesda, MD 20814–4799, USA

Hallgrim Kløve, Department of Clinical Neuropsychology, University of Bergen, Arstadveien 21, N-5009 Bergen, Norway

Gerjo Kok, Department of Health Education, University of Limburg, PO Box 616, 6200 MD Maastricht, The Netherlands

Willem J. Kop, Department of Psychology, USUHS, F. Edward Herbert School of Medicine, 4301 Jones Bridge Road, Bethesda, MD 20814–4799, USA

David S. Krantz, Medical Psychology, F. Edward Herbert School of Medicine, 4301 Jones Bridge Road, Bethesda, MD 20814–4799, USA

David Lester, Center for the Study of Suicide, RR41, 5 Stonegate Court, Blackwood, NJ 08012, USA

Naomi Lester, Department of Psychology, University of North Florida, 4567 St John's Bluff Road, South Jacksonville, FL 32224–26645, USA

Elaine A. Leventhal, Department of Medicine, Robert Wood Johnson Medical School, State University of New Jersey, USA

Howard Leventhal, Rutgers, The State University, Institute of Health, Healthcare and Aging, 30 College Avenue, New Brunswick, NJ 08903–5063, USA

Vivien J. Lewis, Psychology Consultancy, RSH Shelton, Bicton Heath, Shropshire SY3 3DN, UK

Philip Ley, University of Sydney, Australia

Robert R. McCrae, Personality Stress and Coping Section, Gerontology Research Center, 4940 Eastern Avenue, Baltimore, MD 21224, USA

Hannah M. McGee, Department of Psychology, Royal College of Surgeons in Ireland Medical School, 123 St Stephen's Green, Dublin 2, Ireland

Maureen C. McHugh, Women's Studies, Indiana University of Pennsylvania, 350 Sutton Hall, Indiana, PA 15705–1087, USA

Lawrence McKenna, Clinical Psychology Department, York Clinic, UMDS at Guy's Campus, University of London, London Bridge, London SE19RT, UK

Jill Macleod Clark, Department of Nursing Studies, School of Life, Medical and Health Sciences, Cornwall House Annexe, King's College, Waterloo Road, London SE1 8TX, UK

Peter Maguire, CRC Psychological Medicine Group, University of Manchester, Stanley House, Wilmslow Road, Withington, Manchester M20 9BX, UK

Antony Manstead, Department of Social Psychology, University of Amsterdam, Roetersstraat 15, 1018 WB Amsterdam, The Netherlands

Ivana Marková, University of Stirling, Stirling FK9 4LA, UK

Anna L. Marsland, Behavioral Psychology Laboratory, University of Pittsburgh, PA 15260, USA

Christina Maslach, University of California at Berkeley, Berkeley, CA 94720, USA

Donald Meichenbaum, Department of Psychology, University of Waterloo, Ontario N2L 3G1, Canada

Ronald Melzack, McGill University, Stewart Biological Sciences Building, 1205 Dr Penfield Avenue, Montreal, Quebec H3A 1B1, Canada

Susan Michie, Psychology and Genetics Research Group, UMDS at Guy's Campus, University of London, London Bridge, London SE1 9RT, UK

Keith Millar, Behavioural Sciences Group, University of Glasgow, 4 Lilybank Gardens, Glasgow G12 8QQ, UK

John Mollon, The Psychological Laboratory, University, Downing Street, Cambridge CB2 3EB, UK

Rudolph H. Moos, VA Medical Center, Stanford University School of Medicine, 3801 Miranda Avenue (152), Palo Alto, CA 94304, USA

Stephen Morley, Division of Psychiatry and Behavioural Sciences, University of Leeds, 15 Hyde Terrace, Leeds LS2 9LT, UK

Carol A. Morse, Faculty of Nursing, Primary Health Care Practice, Royal Melbourne Institute of Technology, Plenty Road, Bundoora 3083, Victoria, Australia

Rona Moss-Morris, School of Medicine, Department of Psychiatry, the University of Auckland, Private Bag, Auckland, New Zealand

Colin Murray Parkes, High Mart, 21 South Road, Chorleywood, Hertfordshire WD3 5AS, UK

Stanton Newman, Unit of Health Psychology, Department of Psychiatry and Behavioural Sciences, University College London Medical School, Wolfson Building, Riding House Street, London W1N 8AA, UK

David K.B. Nias, Department of Psychological Medicine, St Bartholomew's Hospital Medical College, London EC1A 7BA, UK

Mary K. O'Brien, Allegheny University of the Health Science, Division of Medical Education, 2900 Queen Lane, PA 19129, USA

Neville Owen, Department of Community Medicine, University of Adelaide, PO Box 498, Adelaide 500, Australia

R. Glynn Owens, Department of Psychology, University of Auckland (Tamaki Campus), Private Bag 92019, Auckland, New Zealand

Shirley Pearce, School of Health Policy and Practice Unit, University of East Anglia, Norwich NR4 7TJ, UK

Keith Petrie, Department of Psychiatry, School of Medicine, University of Auckland, Private Bag, Auckland, New Zealand

Alan D. Pickering, Psychology Department, St George's Hospital Medical School, Cranmer Terrace, London SW17 0RE, UK

T. John Pimm, Rayner's Hedge, Croft Road, Aylesbury Buckinghamshire HP21 7RD, UK

Deborah E. Polk, Department of Psychology, Indiana University, Bloomington, IN 47405, USA

Sally Porter, Division of Addictive Behaviours, St George's Hospital Medical School, Cranmer Terrace, London SW17 0RE, UK

Graham Powell, Department of Psychology, University of Surrey, Guildford, Surrey GU2 5XH, UK

Jane Powell, Psychology Department, Goldsmith's College, New Cross, London SE14 6NW, UK

Michael Preece, Nutrition, Metabolism, Endocrinolgy & Dermatology Unit, The Institute of Child Health, 30 Guilford Street, London WC1N 3JH, UK

[xv]

Linda Pring, Psychology Department, Goldsmiths' College, New Cross, London SE14 6NW, UK

Lyn Quine, Centre for Research in Health Behaviour, University of Kent, Canterbury, Kent CT2 7LS, UK

Colette Ray, Department of Human Sciences, Brunel University, Uxbridge, Middlesex UB8 3PH, UK

Shuli Reich, Elderly Care Unit, St Thomas' Hospital, Lambeth Palace Road, London SE1 7EH, UK

Philip H. Richardson, Academic Department of Psychiatry, St Thomas' Hospital. Lambeth Palace Road, London SE1 7EH, UK

Alan J. Riley, Human Sexuality Unit, St George's Hospital, Medical School, London, UK

Lucy Rink, 2 Camp View, Wimbledon, London SW19 4UL, UK

Deborah Rosenblatt, Psychology Department, Reading University, 3 Earley Gate, Whiteknights, Reading RG6 2AL, UK

Irwin M. Rosenstock, Department of Health Behavior and Health Education, School of Public Health, University of Michigan, USA

Rachel Rosser, Academic Department of Psychiatry, UCMSM, Wolfson Building, Riding House Street, London W1N 8AA, UK

Gene Rowe, Psychology Department, University of Surrey, UK

Nichola Rumsey, Department of Psychology, Applied Sciences, University of the West of England, St Matthias Campus, Fishponds, Bristol BS16 2JP, UK

Michael A. Sayette, Psychology Department University of Pittsburgh, 604 Old Engineering Hall, Pittsburgh, PA 15260, USA

Graham Scambler, Unit of Sociology, Department of Psychiatry and Behavioural Sciences, UCMSM, Wolfson Building, Riding House Street, London W1N 8AA, UK

Jeanne A. Schaefer, Center for health Care Evaluation, Department of Veterans Affairs and Stanford University Medical Centers, Palo Alto, CA 94304, USA

Lothar R. Schmidt, Fachbetreich 1- Psychologie, University of Trier, Postfach 3825, 5500 Trier, Germany

S. Shahidullah, School of Psychology, The Queen's University of Belfast, Belfast BT7 1NN, UK

Peter Slade, Department of Clinical Psychology, New Medical School, Liverpool University, PO Box 147, Ashton Street, Liverpool L69 3BX, UK

Pauline Slade, Department of Psychology, University of Sheffield, PO Box 603, Western Bank, Sheffield S10 2UR, UK

Marjorie Smith, Thomas Coram Research Unit, Institute of Education, 27/28 Woburn Square, London WC1H 0AA, UK

Maurice Smith, Thomas Coram Research Unit, Institute of Education, 27/28 Woburn Square, London WC1H 0AA, UK

Stacie Spencer, University of Pittsburgh, PA 15260, USA

Susan H. Spence, University of Queensland, Queensland 4072, Australia

Annette L.Stanton, Department of Psychology, University of Kansas, Lawrence, KS66045–2160, USA

Andrew Steptoe, Department of Psychology, St George's Hospital Medical School, Cranmer Terrace, London SW17 ORE, UK

Robert J. Sternberg, Yale University, PO Box 208205, New Haven, CT 06520, USA

Stephanie V. Stone, Gerontology Research Center, National Institute on Aging, NIH, Baltimore, MD 21224, USA

Victor J. Strecher, Department of Health Behavior and Health Education, University of North Carolina, 312 Rosenau Hall, Chapel Hill, NC 27599–7400, USA

Jan Stygall, Academic Department of Psychiatry and Behavioural Sciences, UCMSM, Wolfson Building, Riding House Street, London WC1N 8AA, UK

Valerie Sutherland, 7 Rozelle Avenue, Newton Mearns, Glasgow G77 6SY, UK

Stephen Sutton, ICRF Health Behaviour Unit, Department of Epidemiology and Public Health, University College London, Brook House, 2–16 Torrington Place, London WC1E 6BT, UK

Sven Svebak, Department of Biological and Medical Psychology, Division of Somatic Psychology, University of Bergen, Arstadveien 21, N-5009 Bergen, Norway

Emma Taylor, Unit of Psychology, UMDS at Guy's Campus, University of London, London Bridge, London SE1 9RT, UK

Christine M. Temple, University of Essex, Wivenhoe Park, Colchester, Essex CO4 3SQ, UK

James R. Terborg, Oregon Research Institute, 1899 Willamette Street, Eugene, OR 97401, USA

Nicky Thomas, Department of Nursing Studies, School of Life, Medical and Health Sciences, Cornwall House Annexe, King's College, Waterloo Road, London SE1 8TX, UK

Natalie Timberlake, Academic Department of Psychiatry, UCMSM, Wolfson Building, Riding House Street, London W1N 8AA, UK

Dennis C. Turk, Department of Anesthesiology, University of Washington, Washington 98195, USA

Jeremy Turk, Section of Child and Adolescent Psychiatry, St George's Hospital Medical School, Cranmer Terrace, London SW17 0RE, UK

Jane M. Ussher, Department of Psychology, University College London, Gower Street, London WC1E 6BT, UK

Charles Vincent, Department of Psychology, University College, London, UK

Philip Vita, University of Sydney, Sydney, Australia

Jane Volans, Department of Clinical Psychology, Oxleas NHS Trust, Bostall House, Goldie Leigh Hospital, Lodge Hill, Abbey Wood, London SE2 0AY, UK

Kenneth A. Wallston, School of Nursing, Vanderbilt University, Nashville, TN 37205, USA

Tony Ward, Research Centre, University of Luton, 24 Crawley Green Road, Luton, Bedfordshire, UK

Jane Wardle, University of London Health Behaviour Unit, Department of Epidemiology and Public Health, 1–19 Torrington Place, London WC1E 6BT, UK

John Weinman, Unit of Psychology, UMDS at Guy's Campus, University of London, London Bridge, London SE1 9RT, UK

Robert West, Department of Psychology, St George's Medical School, Cranmer Terrace, London SW17 0RE, UK

Thomas Ashby Wills, Albert Einstein College of Medicine, 1300 Morris Park Avenue, Room 1301B, Department of Epidemiology and Social Medicine, The Bronx, NY 10461–1924, USA

Barbara A. Wilson, University Rehabilitation Unit, Southampton General Hospital, Tremona Road, Southampton SO9 4XY, UK

George Wright, Strathclyde Business School, University of Strathclyde, 199 Cathedral Street, Glasgow G4 0QU, UK

Stephen Wright, Department of Medical Psychology, Hadley House, Leicester General Hospital, Gwendolen Road, Leicester LE5 4PW, UK

Lucy Yardley, Department of Psychology, University College London, Gower Street, London WC1E 6BT, UK

PREFACE

Health psychology is a rapidly growing field, with an impact on many aspects of medical training, practice and research. Although there are some very good textbooks and handbooks of health psychology available, these are directed primarily at psychologists working in health-related areas. There has been a need for a comprehensive reference text suitable for medical practitioners who wish to be appraised of ways in which psychology can help them in their work. Such a book should also be useful in undergraduate and postgraduate medical education.

This book is intended as a comprehensive handbook for medical practitioners and health professionals, and for psychologists who work with health professionals. It should also be of interest to undergraduates undertaking psychology, medicine and other health related courses, and to postgraduate students on MSc and PhD courses.

The book is in three parts.

Part I: Psychological foundations provides an overview of important areas of psychology relevant to medicine, suitable for those readers who have not studied psychology professionally, or for those who wish to refresh, broaden or update their knowledge.

Part II: Psychology, health and illness is in three sections and reviews the main theories and findings in psychology as applied to medicine, covering psychological effects of illness, psychological influences on health and illness, psychological methods of assessment and intervention and psychological factors associated with the practice of health care.

Part III: Medical topics examines psychological theories and findings relevant to particular medical conditions, investigations, treatments and prophylaxes.

It will be apparent that the decision to place some chapters in Part III rather than in Part II is a matter of judgement. In general, the decision was made on whether the topic appeared to cut across a range of illnesses or treatments. However, if the reader cannot find a topic in Part III, he or she is quite likely to find material relevant to it in Part II.

This is primarily a reference text and therefore it is expected that readers will seek out particular chapters for particular purposes. For this reason the chapters within each section are arranged alphabetically and the titles phrased in encyclopaedic language. Inevitably there is some overlap between chapters dealing with related topics because each chapter is self-contained and we have tried to keep to a minimum the need for movement back and forth between entries.

Clinical practitioners will probably wish to use the book by looking up entries in Part III that are of interest, gaining further background information or clarification of concepts from Parts I and II as necessary. Teachers will probably focus mostly on chapters in Part I and II as basic reading for courses on psychology as applied to medicine, using material from Part II as supplementary reading to show how basic principles can be applied.

Although we have attempted to make the book as comprehensive as possible, it would be unrealistic to imagine that a single text could encompass the whole field adequately. It must also be the case that there are topics that have not been addressed at all. However, we have tried to make the coverage as broad as possible, and keep such gaps to a minimum. For added depth of coverage, the extensive reference lists should be an invaluable resource.

This book has been a long time in the gestation and the editors are deeply indebted to the contributors for their efforts in producing what we believe are some very fine chapters and for their patience. We believe that the effort has been worthwhile and that the result has been worth waiting for. We hope that the contributors and the readers will agree.

Special thanks are due to Joy Searle for secretarial assistance and to Jocelyn Foster of Cambridge University Press for continued support and help throughout.

Andy Baum

Stanton Newman

John Weinman

Robert West

Chris McManus

PART I: **Psychological foundations**

This part provides a brief introduction to some general psychological topics that are useful in understanding the material in the remainder of the book. Clearly, it is no substitute for an introductory psychology textbook, but the material is chosen and presented so as to be of use to readers interested in the application of psychology to medicine.

Attitudes and beliefs
Child development
Conditioning and learning
Intelligence

Judgement and decision-making
Memory
Personality
Psychoimmunology

Psychopharmacology
Psychophysiology
Skilled performance
Social interaction

Attitudes and beliefs

JOHN RICHARD EISER

Department of Psychology,
University of Exeter, UK

There are many different reasons for studying people's attitudes and beliefs. Opinion pollsters may wish to measure public opinion on various issues, and politicians may look at their findings so as to assess the popularity or unpopularity of various policies. Health promoters are typically more concerned with the extent to which people are attracted to different kinds of behaviour (e.g. exercise, diet, smoking and drinking) and particularly with what people believe the consequences of such behaviour to be. In this context, it is often assumed that unhealthy behaviour arises from a lack of relevant factual knowledge and hence that better communication of 'the facts' will lead to improvements in behaviour. When such improvements fail to occur, it is often people's attitudes (rather than their material circumstances) that get the blame.

Social psychology takes a rather different approach. Attitudes and beliefs are studied in their own right, as indicators of how people make sense of their experience, and so there is as much concern with their antecedents as with their effects. In other words, if we are to say how attitudes may influence behaviour, we need to know how attitudes are acquired in the first place, how they are sustained over time, and how they may be modified in response to various forms of persuasion. The distinction between attitudes on the one hand and beliefs on the other need not detain us long. Strictly, we might wish to reserve the term 'belief' for claims that could be settled as true or false as matters of fact, whereas 'attitude' may refer to judgements of value or preference which go beyond mere factual evidence. In practice, this distinction can be hard to draw. Most of the beliefs we study (e.g. 'Smoking can seriously damage your health') have clear evaluative implications, and many expressions of attitude (e.g. 'I regard smoking as an unhealthy habit') are only one step away syntactically from a factual claim about what is the case. Sometimes attitudes can be considered as more general and beliefs as more specific, but we can also have specific attitudes and general beliefs. Psychologically, what matters most is how strongly such thoughts and feelings (be they 'attitudes' or 'beliefs') are held.

ATTITUDE MEASUREMENT

The main emphases of attitude research have shifted considerably within the history of modern psychology (Eagly & Chaiken, 1993). For the first half of this century, the main concern was with devising valid and reliable quantitative measures of people's attitudes on a variety of social issues. The hope was that attitudes could be measured, in much the same way as personality traits, by standardized instruments that would survive over time and across cultures. Such measurements were intended to locate individuals on an underlying 'attitude continuum' of approval–disapproval of a given object, issue or policy. Attitude thus was regarded as a continuum of affect or

evaluation (e.g. how much you approve or disapprove of abortion). People's reasons for approving or disapproving (of abortion, or whatever) were not part of the measurement exercise. As a result of this work, we nowadays have few qualms about quantifying people's attitudes. However, although we have standard procedures for scale construction, we have few, if any, standard scales. Most measuring instruments (typically self-completion questionnaires) generalize rather poorly from the cultural context in which they have been developed. Attitude scale construction is definitely a made-to-measure business.

ATTITUDE ORGANIZATION

Whereas attitude measurement research was not especially concerned with how different attitudes relate to one another, considerable work during the 1950s and 1960s explored the notion that we organize our separate attitudes together into 'consistent' structures. There are several variations on this theme of 'cognitive consistency'. Heider's (1946) theory of 'cognitive balance' dealt primarily with the idea that we are motivated to agree with people we like and to disagree with those we dislike. This idea was modified and extended by various authors. Osgood and Tannenbaum's (1955) principle of 'congruity' makes quantitative predictions of the amount of attitude change following supportive or unsupportive communications about an issue from a liked or disliked communicator. Rosenberg's (1960) theory of 'affective–cognitive consistency' proposes that we make our (affective) evaluations of some object consistent with our (cognitive) beliefs or expectations concerning it: for instance, if we expect smoking to cause lung cancer (obviously a bad effect) we will evaluate it negatively. These theories derive support from evidence that attitudes are more stable and resistant to change when they involve clear-cut evaluations with which our friends agree, than when they are more ambivalent or open to challenge by other people.

COGNITIVE DISSONANCE

The most influential application of the notion of cognitive consistency was Festinger's (1957) theory of 'cognitive dissonance'. Its main difference from the other theories mentioned is that it deals with the attitudes we hold about our own behaviour, including how we attempt to justify such behaviour and its consequences for ourselves and others. In particular, it predicts that, under certain circumstances, we may re-evaluate our attitudes so as to make them more consistent (less 'dissonant') with our present or past behaviour. This leads to the interesting conclusion that we may bring our attitudes into line with our behaviour, and not simply behave in accordance with our prior attitudes. What makes dissonance theory really stand out, however, are predictions concerning the effects on attitude of different kinds of rewards and incentives.

Suppose we somehow find ourselves acting in a way which is incompatible with what we took to be our true attitudes, feelings or moral standards – we find that we have deceived or hurt a friend, or publicly defended a viewpoint which is contrary to our own. The distress we quite probably feel under such circumstances is what Festinger means by 'dissonance'. According to Festinger, this feeling motivates us to re-appraise our attitudes and behaviour so that this dissonance 'resolved'. Dissonance can be resolved by a number of means, but particularly by either finding excuses for our behaviour (so that we can see it as not really reflecting our true feelings) or by changing our attitudes (so that we come to believe that we really felt this way all along). What excuse might there be? One excuse (which was manipulated in many well-known experiments) could be that we received a large payment or reward. In other words, being highly paid for doing something incompatible with one's prior attitudes removes (or reduces) the dissonance and hence the motivation for attitude change. On the other hand, being paid very little for acting in this way would mean that we could not think of the payment as an excuse, so to resolve dissonance we might change our reports of our attitude so that it was now consistent with our behaviour. Crudely, if you pay people a little for doing something they don't really want to do, they'll say they enjoy it more than if you pay them a lot. High rewards lead to less attitude change than low rewards.

That at least is the hypothesis. In practice, the data show that such effects occur only under certain limiting conditions. One of the most important requirements is that people feel that they have chosen freely to act in a manner contrary to their prior attitudes. What matters is not just that one has acted in a way that may produce bad consequences, but that one decided voluntarily to do so. It is also important that any such bad consequences were foreseeable (even if not actually foreseen) at the time of one's decision. In other words, if one can be held responsible for one's action and its consequences, high rewards can produce less attitude change. However, if the unwanted consequences of one's behaviour could not have been anticipated, and particularly if one feels one had no choice over whether or not to behave that way, the opposite effect is typically found: higher rewards lead to more attitude change (in the direction of more consistency with the behaviour) than do lower rewards. So there can be psychological arguments in favour of better pay after all!

Although some of these complexities may seem to undercut the generality of dissonance theory, some broad implications for health and behaviour are still valid. The term 'dissonance' has sometimes been used by applied research to refer to where people admit to fears or regrets about their own behaviour – as when smokers acknowledge that they are damaging their health. This usage is misleading. Knowing that one's behaviour can have unwanted consequences does not, by itself, constitute dissonance, that is a motivation for attitude and/or behaviour change. Dissonance depends on the feeling that (a) such unwanted consequences are not adequately offset by compensatory benefits; and/or (b) something could and should be done to avoid these effects. Smokers who regard their smoking as highly pleasurable, and/or feel themselves to be so addicted that they have no choice about whether to continue, cannot strictly be said to be experiencing dissonance (Eiser, 1982). More broadly, convincing people of the negative health consequences of their behaviour is not necessarily going to persuade them to give up their habits if they regard these habits as sufficiently pleasurable in themselves and beyond their personal competence or will-power to change.

ATTITUDE–BEHAVIOUR RELATIONSHIP

The relationship between attitude and behaviour change has been studied from other perspectives than that of dissonance theory. Especially influential has been the application of 'expectancy-value' models to the prediction of behaviour. Such models assume (very much along the lines of affective-cognitive consistency) that our preferences reflect our expectancies about possible consequences of our behaviour, weighted by the values we attach to those consequences. (Quantitative tests of this assumption involve multiplying expectancies and values for specific consequences together, and then summing the products; thus, this approach has much in common with economic techniques such as cost–benefit analysis.) Foremost within this tradition has been the work of Ajzen and Fishbein (e.g. 1980). The problem they first sought to address was the common failure, in the published literature, of standard measures of social attitudes to predict specific behaviours. Their explanation for this was that many previous studies had failed to match their measures of attitude closely enough to the behaviours being considered. For instance, while general attitude measures may predict general behavioural predispositions, in order to predict a specific form of action, one needs a specific measure of attitude. Moreover, this specific measure must concern the person's attitude towards the act itself, rather than simply towards the topic as a whole. In other words, the focus is on how the person would regard his or her own performance of the act, in a specific context and, where relevant, towards specific target people. For example, the distinction is between asking 'Do you approve of giving money to the poor?' and 'Do you want to give money now to this beggar sitting here?'

Ajzen and Fishbein's 'Theory of Reasoned Action' (TRA) formalizes these notions as follows. First, the main task of the theory is conceived of as predicting, not behaviour *per se*, but 'behavioural intention'. Not unreasonably, they argue that there can be any number of reasons why people fail to do what they sincerely intend to do, which may have nothing to do with the attitudes they hold. None the less, they offer evidence that people's intentions, suitably measured, are frequently good predictors of their actual behaviour. Behavioural intention is seen to depend on the combined effect of two classes of variables – 'attitude (towards the act)' and 'subjective norm' – which may differ in their relative importance. Attitude, in its turn, is dependent on the summative effect of 'evaluative beliefs' (i.e. expectancy-values) concerning the probability of desired or undesired consequences. Subjective norm refers to the individual's overall judgement of whether other people would or would not approve of his or her performance of that act. The judgement is assumed to depend on beliefs about the potential approval of specific others, weighted by the individual's motivation to comply with their view (i.e. another kind of sum-of-products calculation).

HEALTH BELIEFS

When the (somewhat stringent) measurement requirements of this model are fully met, this model generates remarkably good behavioural predictions. None the less, expectancy-value notions can be found in a number of other approaches. Becker's (1974) 'Health Belief Model' (HBM) has been widely used by social medicine researchers. Despite its name, this model incorporates a number of predictor variables, such as demographic and personality characteristics, which have little directly to do with beliefs. Its main appeal is that it offers headings for classes of variables, which may combine to influence a particular form of health behaviour. These include the individual's health motivation, that is how much he or she cares about being healthy, perceived threats to health, and 'cues to action', which include both general calculations of the costs and benefits of taking a course of action, expectancies for success, and situationally specific 'triggers' and 'barriers'. These last concepts are some of the most interesting, in that they can help address the question of why change does or does not occur on a specific occasion (e.g. when a patient decides to consult a doctor), even though more general motivational factors may have been in place for some time. Thus, a colleague's heart attack may be the 'trigger' for a middle-aged man to arrange to have his blood-pressure checked, but a clash with a business meeting the 'barrier' which makes him miss his appointment at the surgery. The ability of the model to embrace a wide variety of such concepts, though, is its weakness as well as its strength. Almost anything that could be reasonably expected to influence health behaviour can be found or placed under one of the model's headings or another. The HBM is thus a valuable *aide-memoire* for anyone considering what kinds of variables should be incorporated into a piece of social medicine research. On the other hand, the HBM provides no explicit statement of the psychological processes (such as motivation, learning, memory and the encoding of information), which will determine how these different variables combine to influence a particular decision. This makes it difficult to identify distinctive predictions of the HBM compared with other models. Whereas the TRA is rather sparse in its description of relevant variables, but specific in its assumptions of how these variables interrelate, the HBM is rich in content but loose in structure.

BEYOND EXPECTANCY – VALUE MODELS

But does the TRA adequately encapsulate the relevant psychological processes? There are grounds for supposing that some important elements are missing. One problem is that the TRA predicts behavioural intentions at just one point in time, and so says nothing about stability of behaviour over time. In fact, where tests of the TRA have been extended to incorporate a longitudinal aspect, present behaviour can be shown to be highly predictable from past behaviour, over and above the effect of present attitudes (Bentler & Speckart, 1979). This is especially pertinent to health applications, where we are typically concerned with the relevance of attitudes to longstanding behavioural habits. Further, when such habits are especially longstanding and stable, we may ask whether the individual will be able to change them anyway. Ajzen and Fishbein insist that the TRA should only predict behaviour where this is mediated by intention, and they make no claims to be able to predict behaviour which is beyond 'volitional control'. The prime example could be addictive behaviours, such as cigarette smoking and other forms of drug use. Smokers who regard themselves as addicted may say that they would like to quit if they could do so easily, and would see great benefits in doing so, but may not make the attempt as they are convinced it would fail.

A number of researchers have therefore extended this approach to incorporate notions of people's expectancies that their attempts at behavioural change (or, in other contexts, some medical treatment) will actually succeed. Becker included 'expectancy of success' as a predictor in the HBM. Eiser & Sutton (1977) demonstrated that smokers' intentions to quit were more directly predictable from their 'confidence' that they would succeed in the attempt than from how much they expected quitting (if achieved) to benefit their health. Bandura's (1977) notion of 'self-efficacy' has been applied to many different kinds of health behaviour, the central hypothesis being that people's motivation to undertake difficult tasks depends on their confidence in their own ability to succeed or bring about desired outcomes. More recently, Ajzen (1991) has modified the TRA and renamed it the 'Theory of Planned Behaviour', the added ingredient being that of 'perceived behavioural control'.

A more general difficulty with all expectancy-value models, however, is in specifying which values and expectancies an individual will take into account (Eiser & van der Pligt, 1988). Ajzen and Fishbein (1980) proposed that attitudes (i.e. global evaluations) should be based on only a limited subset of 'salient' or personally relevant beliefs. Unfortunately, they offer no theoretical account of what might make one belief more salient to a given individual than another. Other research, however, suggests that a person's attitude may help direct his or her attention selectively towards particular aspects or arguments, so that what one sees as salient depends on one's attitude rather than (or as well as) vice versa. Thus, Fazio (1990) proposes that attitudes 'guide' behaviour by a number of processes, including by influencing people's selective definitions of situations and events. This leads us to look at attitudes, not simply as evaluative reactions, but as ways of organizing knowledge and interpreting events. To understand how attitudes motivate behaviour, we need to understand how they shape the processing of information.

ATTITUDE CHANGE

Interest in the relationship between attitudes and information-processing has its roots in one of the most longstanding areas of attitude research – that of persuasion and attitude change. The classic programme of research at Yale University during the 1950s followed a framework much influenced by experimental research on learning and behaviour change. Attitude was seen as a response which could vary in magnitude as a function of stimulus and contextual factors – the content of a persuasive message and characteristics of the communicator – as well as being moderated by personal attributes and experience of the individual receiving the message. Thus, many studies were concerned with identifying whether some individuals were more easily influenced than others, whether greater credibility, status and/or attractiveness enhanced communicators' persuasiveness, whether one-sided or two-sided messages were more effective, and so on.

FEAR AROUSAL AND APPRAISAL

One particular question from this period aroused special interest, to become an area of research with a life of its own. This was whether messages which arouse fear are more or less effective than those

[5]

which do not. The relevance of this to health and medicine should be obvious, since many health messages contain potentially frightening warnings about the dangers of not complying with medical advice. Indeed, the study that started everything in this field used a medical example – how much high school students reported compliance with recommendations for more effective toothbrushing after receiving messages which illustrated the negative consequences of improper dental hygiene in more or less gruesome detail (Janis & Feshbach, 1953). The finding was that least compliance was shown by the group receiving the most gruesome (fear-arousing) message.

There followed a long and lively debate concerning both the exact form of the relationship between fear-arousal and attitude change and its theoretical explanation. The earliest assumptions were that fear constitutes a drive or motivator, which people try to remove by changing their behaviour (as when a rat moves to another part of a cage to avoid an electric shock in early animal learning experiments), but that excessive levels of fear were assumed to be counter-productive. However, not all studies that claimed to test this 'fear-drive' theory contained independent measures of the level of fear or controlled systematically for the effects of other variables (Sutton, 1982). In particular, the effectiveness of a communication seems to depend to a great extent on what specific recommendations for behavioural change are offered. Subsequent research therefore has paid increasing attention to the cognitive and emotional processes in which people engage when presented with threatening information.

'Protection Motivation Theory' (Rogers, 1975; Rippetoe & Rogers, 1987) combines notions of fear-appraisal with an expectancy-value account of attitude–behaviour relations. The motivation to protect oneself is a function of two kinds of 'appraisal processes'. 'Threat appraisal' depends on expectancies of the severity of any threat and one's personal vulnerability, whereas 'coping appraisal' involves judgements of one's own ability to undertake protective action and of the likely effectiveness of that action.

According to Janis and Mann (1977), the provision of information about any potential threat or danger can lead people to experience conflict over what decision should be made. They address the question of what decision-making styles or strategies people may adopt to resolve or escape from such feelings of danger. The strategies employed are hypothesized to depend on how the risk information is appraised. This approach makes many interesting predictions about how people's reactions to threat evolve over time, since (e.g. defensive) reactions that allow one to avoid experiencing conflict in the short term may leave one cognitive and behaviourally unprepared as more serious dangers accumulate. It also underlines the very important point that, as far as communicating (e.g. health)

information is concerned, you can take a horse to water but not necessarily be able to make it drink. People may be more or less motivated to think through the information presented to them and adapt their behaviour accordingly.

ATTITUDES AND INFORMATION PROCESSING

The question of how people think through the information presented to them is central to the most influential contemporary approach to attitude change and persuasion. Petty and Cacioppo's (1986) 'Elaboration-likelihood model' (ELM) is built around the notion that a target person's cognitive responses to persuasion are all important. In particular, persuasion is hypothesized to depend on an interaction between the strength or cogency of a message and the extent to which the individual engages in elaborated thought about the message's content. If a message is strong, it will produce more change the more the individual thinks about it and its implications. If a message is inherently weak, it will produce more change if the target person attends less closely to it. This relates to a distinction between what are termed 'central' and 'peripheral' routes to persuasion – the former depending on analysis of the argument, the latter on less logical cues and associations (e.g. liking for the communicator). Much of the empirical research is concerned with situational and motivational factors which may increase the likelihood that the target person will engage in elaborated thought about the message. For instance, feeling personally involved in the issue should increase the likelihood of elaborated processing. Applying this to health communications, making people motivated to think more closely about a health issue carries with it the need to design communications so that they are more informative and coherent.

The interrelationships between information processing, evaluative and motivational processes are at least as important to contemporary attitude theory as they ever have been. Traditional research regarded attitude as a quasi-perceptual response to social issues and events, which could be quantified as some point on an underlying evaluative continuum. From this perspective, attitude change was interpreted as a shift along this continuum. Nowadays many of the classic questions are being reinterpreted within a new conceptual framework, involving notions of how information is organized in memory and how readily it can be accessed for subsequent judgements and decisions. Within this framework, what is important is not so much the location of an attitude as a point on a continuum, but rather the strength of association between attitude objects, evaluations and related memories (Fazio, 1990). What remains true is that the study of attitudes and beliefs is vital to social psychology's claims to practical usefulness on the one hand and its theoretical integrity on the other.

REFERENCES

Ajzen, I. (1991). The theory of planned behavior. *Organizational Behavior and Decision Processes*, **50**, 1–33.

Ajzen, I. & Fishbein, M. (1980). *Understanding attitudes and predicting social behavior.* Englewood Cliffs, NJ: Prentice-Hall.

Bandura, A. (1977). Self-efficacy: toward a unifying theory of behavioral change. *Psychological Review*, **84**, 191–215.

Becker, M.H. (Ed.) (1974). The health belief model and personal health behavior. *Health Education Monographs*, **2**, 324–473.

Bentler, P.M. & Speckart, G. (1979). Models of attitude-behavior relations. *Psychological Review*, **86**, 452–64.

Eagly, A.H. & Chaiken, S. (1993). *The psychology of attitudes.* Orlando, FL: Harcourt Brace, Jovanovich.

Eiser, J.R. (1982). Addiction as attribution: cognitive processes in giving up smoking. In J.R. Eiser (Ed.). *Social psychology and behavioral medicine*, pp. 281–99. Chichester: Wiley.

Eiser, J.R. & Sutton, S.R. (1977). Smoking as a subjectively rational choice. *Addictive Behaviors*, **2**, 129–134.

Eiser, J.R. & van der Pligt, J. (1988). *Attitudes and decisions.* London: Routledge.

Fazio, R.H. (1990). Multiple processes by

which attitudes guide behavior: the MODE model as an integrative framework. In M.P. Zanna (Ed.). *Advances in experimental social psychology*, Vol. 23, pp. 75–109.

Festinger, L. (1957). *A theory of cognitive dissonance.* Evanston, IL: Row, Peterson.

Heider, F. (1946). Attitudes and cognitive organization. *Journal of Psychology*, **21**, 107–12.

Janis, I.L. & Feshbach, S. (1953). Effects of fear-arousing communications. *Journal of Abnormal and Social Psychology*, **48**, 78–92.

Janis, I.L. & Mann, L. (1977). *Decision making: a psychological analysis of conflict, choice, and commitment.* New York: Free Press.

Osgood, C.E. & Tannenbaum, P.H. (1955). The principle of congruity in the prediction of attitude change. *Psychological Review*, **62**, 42–55.

Petty, R.E. & Cacioppo, J.T. (1986). The elaboration likelihood model of persuasion. In L. Berkowitz (Ed.). *Advances in experimental social psychology*, vol. 19, pp. 123–205. New York: Academic Press.

Rippetoe, P.A. & Rogers, R.W. (1987). Effects of components of protection-motivation theory on adaptive and maladaptive coping with a health threat. *Journal of Personality and Social Psychology*, **52**, 596–604.

Rogers, R.W. (1975). A protection motivation theory of fear appeals and attitude change. *Journal of Psychology*, **91**, 93–114.

Rosenberg, M.J. (1960). An analysis of affective-cognitive consistency. In C.I. Hovland & M.J. Rosenberg (Eds.). *Attitude organization and change: an analysis of consistency among attitude components*, pp. 15–64. New Haven, CT: Yale University Press.

Sutton, S.R. (1982). Fear-arousing communications: a critical examination of theory and research. In J.R. Eiser (Ed.). *Social psychology and behavioral medicine*, pp. 303–37. Chichester: Wiley.

Child development

DAVID JONES

Department of Psychology, Birkbeck College, University of London, UK

Child development can be defined as the study of how children develop and change. The topic is a major subarea of lifespan developmental psychology which seeks to evaluate continuity and change in both behaviour and psychological processes from conception to maturity and on into old age. For convenience, childhood is often taken as starting at birth, but an awareness of development from conception to delivery and of the possible short and longer-term effects of prenatal influences is an essential prerequisite for studying children. Most textbooks on child development include an account of adolescence as a separate developmental subperiod whilst recognizing the difficulty of establishing clear and universally acceptable criteria for marking the transitions from childhood to adolescence and from adolescence to adulthood.

The study of childhood has provided both a seedbed and a battleground for the development and testing of many aspects of psychological theory. In addition, observing children and designing experimental measures of their abilities has yielded important information on how best to provide care and education. Much of the research effort has been concerned with attempts to resolve the nature versus nurture controversy. The newborn infant is the closest we can get to a being with intact nervous system structure but very little experience of interacting with the environment. The problem for any attempts at theoretical interpretation is the need to take account of changes attributable to growth and maturation. By studying very young infants it is possible to make inferences about the degree of innate capacity they are likely to possess for processing their environment. It is important to recognize that the development of structure from its earliest stages is influenced by interaction with the physical and social world.

Some important issues in the study of development are whether or not there are sensitive periods during which the child is able to benefit most from appropriate stimulation and possibly even more importantly whether the effects of low levels of stimulation or even deprivation can be reversed. These questions arise when the field of study is at the level of basic psychological processes and when it involves apparently more complicated topics in the development of personality and social functioning.

A brief consideration of the methods which have been used to study children shows that there has been a greater reliance on both naturalistic and controlled observation than is the case in other areas of psychology. Early methods included detailed diary descriptions of the development of individual children for short periods of their lifespan. Darwin's record of the infancy of one of his own children is a good example of this technique. Time sampling was developed as a method for collecting normative data on a wide range of behaviours, e.g. the frequency of nail-biting in the classroom by six-year olds or the presence of stop consonants in the babbling of nine-month olds. With the ready availability of video recording techniques it has become possible to increase the reliability of such observational methods and measure concordance between different observers. The method of event sampling was used to provide a more systematic view of complete units of behaviour or social interactions between children such as quarrels. Trait ratings by parents, teachers and others were used, and continue to be used, in attempts to quantify and monitor change in a wide range of characteristics such as anxiety, friendliness and aggression.

The choice between longitudinal and cross-sectional methods for studying children depends upon the nature of the problem being researched, the acceptable time scale for the study and the availability of resources. Longitudinal study provides data on the same children on repeated occasions over months or even years. Subjects serve as their own controls but investigators must exert great care to avoid influencing the children or their carers. Disadvantages of longitudinal methods lie in their cost, controlling for subject drop–out and the need to obtain independent estimates of changes like parental practices, educational standards and diet. Cross-sectional methods give immediate comparisons between groups of children of different ages. Careful matching of groups is essential but even then variations in the development of individual children will not be detected. Sequential-cohort methods provide a powerful way of estimating environmental influences and changes in several age groups in a relatively short time (Schaie, 1965). Retrospective methods have been used to explore the early histories of children with problem behaviours, e.g. hyperactivity or delinquency, but such findings must be treated with caution when normative data on the development of children with similar background factors is not available.

There have been a number of attempts to develop theories of development. An issue which keeps coming up is whether there are discrete stages. Are these stages hierarchical in the sense that they must be passed through in a fixed sequence? Can any of the stages be missed out? To what extent are they related to age? Freud's psychoanalytic theory is the best known example of a stage theory of personality development from infancy to adolescence (Freud, 1937). Erikson (1963) described a sequence of psychosocial stages which takes account of changes throughout the lifespan including old age. Piaget developed a stage theory to account for cognitive development (Piaget & Inhelder, 1969). In contrast, learning theory and social learning theories place less emphasis on stages although they do allow for maturation.

In the space available it will only be possible to introduce a few of the areas of child psychology which have been actively researched in recent years. Examples of textbooks which give more detailed accounts are Mussen *et al.* (1990), Vasta, Haith and Miller (1992) and Shaffer (1993). Among the many journals devoted to the subject are *Child Development*, *Developmental Psychology*, *British Journal of Developmental Psychology*, *Journal of Child Psychology and Psychiatry* and *Journal of Experimental Child Psychology*.

INFANCY
By any standards the birth process is a significant life event. Even for babies who experience a normal delivery and whose mothers do not receive medication immediately before or during the birth, there is an element of ordeal. They are subjected to compression and pushing for several hours or more and must emerge from a fluid-filled environment which provided support, nutrition, oxygen and a constant temperature. In the new environment the immediate challenge is to establish and maintain respiration. The newborn must adjust to lack of body support except from hard surfaces, and to variations in air temperature. Soon they must respond to offers of food. For those who experience delivery complications there may be additional pressures and pulling especially of the head. Brackbill (1979) and others have suggested that anaesthetics and other medication given to the mother before the birth are likely to get into the infant's circulatory system and may influence functioning for some hours or even days after delivery. The term neonate is sometimes

used for babies, born at full term, for the first month after birth. Status at birth can be evaluated using the Apgar Scale which takes account of the quality of such things as respiration and reflexes (Apgar *et al.*, 1958). The Neonatal Behavioral Assessment Scale (NBAS) gives a more detailed assessment of the young baby's functioning and allows monitoring of change over the early days (Brazelton, 1973).

Premature and low birthweight infants may need special care. There is evidence that taken as a group, premature infants appear to be more vulnerable than full-term babies for later difficulties in areas such as language acquisition and school attainments. However, these differences do not hold if premature infants from underprivileged backgrounds are removed from the sample.

Neonates possess a range of innate reflexes. One of the most highly organized is the rooting reflex which occurs in response to light tactile stimulation of the cheek or mouth region. The head turns slightly in the direction of the stimulation and the mouth opens to engulf the object. Once the nipple or other object is in the mouth, the baby will suck and any fluid obtained will be swallowed. Newborns spend much of their time asleep. Even when their eyes are open they are not always responsive to stimulation, so assessment of their perceptual and cognitive abilities is only possible when they are in an alert state. They rapidly pass into a state of active crying when they are unresponsive to experimental tasks (Prechtl, 1977).

PERCEPTION IN INFANCY
There is little doubt that the visual system of neonates is less efficient than that of adults. The eye is smaller so the focal length is shorter. Visual accommodation, or the ability to focus, is poor in the first weeks after birth but it improves rapidly by six months of age. It has been suggested that the neonate focuses best on objects around 20 cm away, which might be quite good for looking at a face when being held. In the early weeks the eyes do not move in unison, so binocular disparity cannot be used as a cue for depth perception.

The immaturity of the baby's motor system and the lack of language have made it necessary to assess perception by measuring changes in other kinds of response systems. For example, Fantz, Ordy and Udelf (1962) used optokinetic nystagmus (OKN) to estimate visual acuity. Babies in common with adults show OKN as an involuntary reflex when vertical stripes are moved across the field of vision. There is a slow phase in which the eye follows the stripe and then a fast phase when it jumps back in the opposite direction. When the stripes are made progressively narrower, they will eventually appear as a uniform colour and the nystagmus ceases. Defining acuity in terms of the angle subtended at the eye by stripes of a given width, it was shown that some infants under one month of age responded to 20 minutes of arc.

Many studies have followed the pioneering work of Fantz in using spontaneous visual preference to assess perceptual ability. Using a relatively simple viewing chamber, it is possible to observe the baby's looking behaviour by monitoring the reflection of the stimuli on the eye. The method has been used to estimate acuity by pairing stripes of different widths with neutral grey of the same overall level of reflectance. Babies prefer to look at the stripes. From around 2 months of age, a preference was found for curved lines rather than straight lines.

Similarly, it has been shown that babies prefer to look at complex patterns rather than simple ones and that, by around 3 months of age, they prefer to look at a schematic face in preference to a jumbled face of similar complexity.

The visual preference technique has also been used to study the effects of repeated exposure and novelty. Babies over 2 months of age show a preference for novelty after quite a small number of exposures. This demonstrates that some representation of the repeated stimulus must become established for habituation to take place and for the baby to be able to demonstrate a preference. The rate of habituation may be an early indication of later intelligence levels.

Gibson and Walk (1961) described the use of an apparent visual cliff to test the presence of depth perception. Babies were placed on the central platform of a glass covered table with checkerboard patterns observable through the glass on shallow and deep sides. The majority of infants above 6 months of age would not venture on to the deep side when called by their mothers. The limitation of the study is that the babies needed to be old enough to crawl. Other workers have shown that babies as young as 2 months show a heart rate change when held over the deep side, but not the shallow side, so early awareness of depth cues is likely.

There is good evidence that the foetus is responsive to sounds well before birth. Auditory acuity may be reduced for a day or so after birth because fluid in the middle ear takes a little while to dry out. Studies using habituation of heart rate to a repeated stimulus followed by measurement of the response to a novel stimulus indicate that some babies have good discrimination for frequency in the first few days after birth. Young babies have also been shown to adjust the pattern of their non-nutritive sucking to listen to their own mothers' voices in preference to strangers' voices (DeCasper & Fifer, 1980). The indications are that babies can recognize their own mothers' voices at birth.

Compelling evidence for innate capacities in the nervous system comes from the observation that infants as young as 4 weeks appear to have categorical perception for some speech sounds, even before they produce these sounds themselves. They are able to discriminate between pairs of phonemes on the basis of differences in such characteristics as voice onset time or place of articulation (Eimas, 1985). Furthermore, babies are able to discriminate contrasts used in languages different from the one spoken by their carers, although they may subsequently lose the ability to make these discriminations.

Other studies have demonstrated that babies in the first few weeks after birth can discriminate odours and tastes. Also, they quickly acquire the ability to integrate information from different senses. On balance it seems that, despite their immaturity, neonates have considerable perceptual abilities and that these improve rapidly in the early months (Bremner, 1988).

COGNITION

The study of cognitive development has been greatly influenced by the pioneering work of Piaget. With a background training in biology and a knowledge of mathematics and logic, he was both a structuralist and a stage theorist. He set out to explain how structures developed through interaction with the environment.

Taking the model of evolutionary biology he tried to show that, in cognitive development, existing structures take on new functions and sometimes existing functions are taken on and performed differently by new structures. The unit of structure is the scheme which goes through adaptation. Adaptation depends upon the relative balance at any time between the processes of assimilation and accommodation. In assimilation the scheme needs to take in aspects of the environment, as in the example of the grasping scheme in the 4 month-old infant which has its origins in the innate grasping reflex. The infant is able to pick up, or assimilate, small blocks or grasp at noses, but slender objects remain a problem. In accommodation the scheme itself changes to meet the demands of the environment. The grasping scheme accommodates and the infant has a finer degree of eye–hand control, which is now ready to benefit from further handling of small objects. Schemes can be representations of objects and actions.

Piaget described a sequence of stages which children pass through as they achieve changes in their cognitive structures. From birth to around 18 months to 2 years of age, children are said to be in the Sensorimotor Period. During this period they acquire representations as evidenced by the gradual development of object permanence. They start by reaching for partially covered objects and later will search for hidden objects or things which have dropped from sight. By the end of infancy they can watch a ball roll behind a chair and show that they expect to find it on the other side, simple but impressive evidence of some form of internalization.

The Preoperational Period covers the approximate age range from 2 to 7 years. Here, the child shows evidence of using symbolic representation but is egocentric in the sense of lacking in awareness that the perceptions and viewpoints of others may be different from one's own. Donaldson (1978) and others have challenged Piaget's interpretation of egocentricity and have demonstrated that pre-school children's performance is likely to be influenced by the precise form of the verbal instructions they are given. Piaget also found that preoperational children have difficulty with tasks involving transitive inference, although in this case others have shown that performance improved for children given over-training on the original comparisons.

Perhaps the most famous of Piaget's experiments on children is his work on conservation, in particular the conservation of liquid and number. Centration or the tendency to focus on a perceptual aspect of the problem rather than the whole experience is given as an explanation for failure. Critics have argued that conservation skills in preoperational children can be improved by identity training for objects and substances.

In the Concrete Operational Period which typically covers the age range 7 to 11 years, children acquire an understanding of classification. They can perform class-inclusion problems, conserve and use number systems. Finally from 11 years onwards, many children reach the Formal Operational Period. At this level they use combinatorial thinking and are aware of the hypothetical. Flavell (1963) provides a complete summary of Piaget's descriptions of the logical structures which subsume both levels of operational thinking. The most frequent criticism of Piaget is that he may have underestimated children's abilities in his account of the first two cognitive stages.

Other approaches to cognitive development have focused on changes in information processing capacity and attentional strategies with age and training. There are developmental changes in metamemory which is children's awareness of their own memory processes (Flavell, 1985). Knowledge about memory begins as early as the preschool period and increases rapidly in the age range 7–11 years. Traditional intelligence tests have long sought to measure the association between age, memory, attention and processing skills.

PERSONALITY AND SOCIAL DEVELOPMENT

Whilst it may not be appropriate to claim that personality characteristics can be identified in young infants, the work of Thomas, Chess and Birch (1968) indicates that it is possible to classify infants according to temperament, based on behaviours such as their feeding patterns and reactions to changes in routine. Easy babies (40%) were those who showed regular patterns and adapt easily, slow-to-warm-up babies (15%) had a low activity level and adapt slowly and difficult babies (10%) had irregular patterns, adapt slowly and react with intensity.

Studies of the smiling response indicate that most babies smile in response to social stimulation by 6–8 weeks of age. Evidence that this is almost certainly an innate reaction, which is modified by experience, comes from the observation that blind infants also start smiling at an early age but the smile remains wan and does not develop in the same way as in sighted infants. By 12–16 weeks of age, babies show selective social smiling and no longer respond to strangers. Home-reared infants have been reported to smile earlier and more frequently than institution-reared infants.

There is some dispute over whether skin-to-skin contact between mother and baby in the early hours after birth facilitates bonding. On balance it would appear that, although this is a highly pleasurable experience for mothers, the vast majority of those deprived of the opportunity will bond effectively to their babies.

Recently, there has been a considerable resurgence of interest in the style of attachment between the young child and the mother. Bowlby (1969) discussed attachment in terms of control systems theory. He drew attention to the evolutionary significance of attachment as a process designed to increase chances of survival by ensuring proximity to the mother. From around 8 months of age, babies become aware of the strange and unfamiliar and react to separation by crying and other forms of protest which are signalling behaviours and sometimes by following or active searching.

Ainsworth has devised the strange situation as a means for measuring the security of attachment of infants aged between 12 and 18 months of age. The procedure involves cumulative stress with the infant experiencing two brief separations from the mother and interactions with a stranger in an unfamiliar room. Security of attachment is assessed from the infant's behaviour in the second reunion. About 65% of infants tested were classified as securely attached. Whether or not they were distressed by the separation they greeted the mother in some way on reunion. Two types of insecurely attached infants were described. Avoidant infants (20%) tended to ignore the mother rather than seek interaction on reunion and resistant or ambivalent infants (10–15%) mingled contact seeking with angry and rejecting behaviour (Ainsworth et al., 1978).

Bowlby's view that the child's representation of his or her relationship with the primary carer is a prototype for subsequent relationships has greatly influenced theorizing in both child psychology and child psychiatry (Holmes, 1993). Insecure infants as assessed by the strange situation appear to be more at risk to develop later emotional disturbances. There is evidence that the same distribution of attachment styles occurs in adult populations, and that the attachment style of mothers assessed before the birth of their babies is predictive of the later behaviour of the babies in the strange situation (Fonagy et al., 1994).

LANGUAGE DEVELOPMENT

Most babies begin using recognizable words between 10 and 15 months of age. The early one-word utterances often refer to concrete objects used or seen in specific situations such as a toy duck at bath time. A little later in development the child may overgeneralize in the use of the word, for example referring to any moving four-legged animal as 'dog'. It is noticeable that adults adopt a higher pitch of voice when speaking to babies and use short, semantically simple, utterances. This pattern of communication, sometimes referred to as 'motherese', often serves to amplify ongoing activities which already have the child's attention (Snow & Ferguson, 1977).

One-word sentences and many two-word combinations may take the form of telegraphic speech. The listener needs to be aware of the context to infer meaning. An inability to make two-word combinations by the age of 2 years is an indication of likely language delay. Between the ages of 2 and 5 years, children have an enormous growth in vocabulary. They also acquire many rules of the grammar of the language they are learning and an awareness of how to use speech to communicate, sometimes called the pragmatics of communication. Most children show amusing evidence that they are acquiring grammatical rules when they misapply them, e.g. 'two foots' and 'he hitted me'. Whilst many aspects of language depend on learning and observation, the very speed of language acquisition supports the theory of a species specific language acquisition device which is able to respond to whatever language the child is exposed to. Chomsky (1965) described the development of a transformational grammar or set of rules linking the surface structure of the specific language and the child's deep structure of knowledge about language.

More cognitive approaches have emphasized the importance of children's knowledge of the world as a basis for their own use of language (Bruner, 1983). There has also been considerable debate on the extent to which language influences thought. The strongest form of linguistic determination as expressed in the Sapir–Whorf Hypothesis holds that language determines perception and thought. The example frequently quoted is that the Eskimos' ability to discriminate between different sorts of snow is facilitated by having a number of words to describe it. In contrast, Vygotsky (1934) took the view that language and thought have separate origins. The primary function of language is seen as communication.

DEVELOPMENT OF SEX ROLE BEHAVIOUR

Adults respond in different ways to boys and girls from the first days after birth. Boys are referred to as stronger than girls and, in western cultures, girls are picked up sooner than boys when they cry. Boys are given more physical stimulation than girls, especially by fathers, and girls tend to receive more verbal stimulation than boys. Handling patterns and reinforcement of what is considered to be gender-appropriate toy play become even more stereotypical when the child reaches pre-school. At school, both teachers and other children tend to show disapproval of boys who play games regarded as feminine.

By the age of 3 years, children are usually showing preferences for playmates of the same sex and gender identity at the level of awareness of being a boy or girl is present. Gender stability in the sense of the child knowing what gender he or she will be as an adult comes a year or so later, followed by an awareness that gender is unlikely to change.

Social learning theory explanations emphasize the importance of imitating adult role behaviour. The choice of model is influenced by gender awareness and a preference for the stereotype that is 'like self', but it has been suggested that this choice is more likely to be modified for girls if they perceive adult males to have more power than adult females.

Some years ago there was evidence in the literature of cognitive differences between the sexes with boys showing slight advantages in mean scores on mathematical skills and spatial abilities and girls showing an advantage on verbal skills (Maccoby & Jacklin, 1974). More recent studies indicate smaller differences and the likelihood that the pattern of abilities is influenced by environmental factors.

AGGRESSIVE BEHAVIOUR AND MORAL AWARENESS

Pre-school children show less inhibition of aggressive behaviour than older children. At a cognitive level they are less aware of the likely consequences of their action and assessment of intentionality to injury is far from easy. Sadly, experimental studies indicate that children of most ages show a tendency to imitate aggressive acts performed by adult models, especially if the models are not punished. There is also considerable evidence that aggressive acts performed on films and television both increase arousal in children and in some cases are copied in real-life situations.

Moral awareness in children is linked to cognitive development and is not necessarily related to moral behaviour. Kohlberg (1984) has devised an elaborate stage model of the development of moral awareness based on analyses of children's responses to moral dilemmas facing characters in stories. In the two stages of Preconventional morality the child views morality in terms of external rules or obtaining rewards. At the level of Conventional morality, there is an awareness of social order and rules seem to be followed to maintain the approval of others. Finally, in the stages of Post-conventional morality, which not all adolescents will reach, there is a reliance on principles and individual conscience.

ADOLESCENCE

Some authorities see the onset of puberty, typically some time between 11 and 14 years of age, as the point of change to adolescence. On average girls reach puberty about 2 years ahead of boys, but there are considerable variations for both sexes. Typically there is a preadolescent growth spurt and puberty is accompanied by the gradual acquisition of secondary sexual characteristics. In many cases the physical and growth changes themselves and fears about normality based on comparisons with others in the peer group give rise to stress. Other adolescents may be troubled by intense emotional feelings associated with their emerging sexuality.

Cognitive changes and the attainment of formal operational thought often result in sudden concerns over moral and social issues and an unwillingness to compromise. Throughout these transitions the adolescent is typically economically dependent on the family and often under pressures to conform at school. It is not surprising that many have labelled adolescence as a period of turmoil. Erikson (1968) has referred to the adolescent's act of becoming aware of the inner self as the beginning of the identity crisis. He suggested that the individual needs time to experiment with roles before fitting in to adult society, a psychosocial moratorium. Identification with the parents weakens and identification with peer groups may assume importance.

The ending of adolescence and the transition to adulthood is more complex than the attainment of physical maturity. It is also marked by social and legal conventions (Coleman, 1980).

CONCLUDING REMARKS

Recent emphasis is upon studying the child in the context of the family and viewing the family itself as a system passing through a sequence of developmental stages. Parental practices, sibling relationships, social class and culture are all seen as powerful influences on the child. Nevertheless it is important not to construe development in terms of linear causality. The environment and the family act on the child but they in turn are modified by the child. Cross-cultural studies provide an opportunity to unravel further some of the complexities of child development.

REFERENCES

Ainsworth, M.D.S., Blehar, M., Waters, E. & Wal, S. (1978). *Strange situation behavior of one-year-olds. Its relation to mother–infant interaction in the first year and to qualitative differences in the infant–mother attachment relationships.* Hillsdale, N.J.: Erlbaum.

Apgar, V., Holaday, D.A., James, L.S., Weisbrot, I.M. & Bemen, C. (1958). Evaluation of the newborn infant – second report. *Journal of the American Medical Association,* 168, 1985–8.

Bowlby, J. (1969). *Attachment and loss: Vol.1 Attachment.* New York: Basic Books.

Brackbill, Y. (1979). Obstetrical medication and infant behaviour. In Osofsky, J.D. (Ed.). *Handbook of infant development,* pp.76–125. New York: Wiley.

Brazelton, T.B. (1973). *Neonatal behavioral assessment scale.* Philadelphia: Lippincott.

Bremner, J.G. (1988). *Infancy.* Oxford: Basic Blackwell Ltd.

Bruner, J. (1983). *Child's talk: learning to use language.* New York: Norton.

Chomsky, N. (1965). *Aspects of the theory of syntax.* Cambridge, MA: MIT Press.

Coleman, J.C. (1980). *The nature of adolescence.* London: Metheun.

DeCasper, A. & Fifer, W. (1980). Newborns prefer their mothers' voices. *Science,* 208, 1174–6.

Donaldson, M. (1978). *Children's minds.* London: Fontana Press.

Eimas, P.D. (1985). The perception of speech in early infancy. *Scientific American,* 252, 46–52.

Erikson, E.H. (1963). *Childhood and society* 2nd edn. New York: Norton.

Erikson, E.H. (1968). *Identity, youth and crisis.* New York: Norton.

Fantz, R.L., Ordy, J.M. & Udelf, M.S. (1962). Maturation of pattern vision in infants during the first six months. *Journal of Comparative and Physiological Psychology,* 55, 907–17.

Flavell, J.H. (1963). *The developmental psychology of Jean Piaget.* London: D. Van Nostrand Co.

Flavell, J.H. (1985). *Cognitive development.* 2nd edn. Engelwood Cliffs, NJ: Prentice-Hall.

Child development

Fonagy, P., Steele, M., Steele, A.H. & Target, M. (1994). *Journal of Child Psychology and Psychiatry.* 35, 231–57.

Freud, S. (1937). *New introductory lectures in psycho-analysis* (2nd edn.). London: Hogarth Press and The Institute of Psycho-Analysis.

Gibson, E.J. & Walk, R.D. (1961). A comparative and analytical study of visual depth perception. *Psychological Monographs*, 75, 2–34.

Holmes, J. (1993). *John Bowlby and attachment theory.* London: Routledge.

Kohlberg, L. (1984). *The psychology of moral development: the nature and validity of moral stages.* San Fransisco: Harper and Row.

Maccoby, E.E. & Jacklin, C.N. (1974). *The psychology of sex differences.* Stanford, CA: Stanford University Press.

Mussen, P.H., Conger, J.J., Kagan, J. & Huston, A.C. (1990). *Child development and personality* (7th edn.). New York: Harper & Row.

Piaget, J., & Inhelder, B. (1969). *The psychology of the child.* New York: Basic Books.

Prechtl, H.F.R. (1977). *The neurological examination of the full-term newborn infant.* London: Heinemann.

Schaie, K.W. (1965). A general model for the study of developmental problems. *Psychological Bulletin*, 64, 91–107.

Shaffer, D.R. (1993). *Developmental psychology: childhood and adolescence* (3rd ed.). Pacific Grove, California: Brooks Grove Publishing Company.

Snow, C.E. & Ferguson, C. (1977). *Talking to children: language input and acquisition.* Cambridge: Cambridge University Press.

Thomas, A., Chess. S. & Birch, H. (1968). *Temperament and behavior disorders in children.* New York: New York University Press.

Vasta, R., Haith, M.M. & Miller, S.A. (1992). *Child psychology: the modern science.* Canada: John Wiley & Sons.

Vygotsky, L.S. (1934). *Thought and language.* Cambridge, Mass: MIT Press.

Conditioning and learning

ALAN DAVID PICKERING

Department of Psychology, St George's Hospital Medical School, London, UK

In many areas of psychology, important concepts are given labels drawn from everyday language. This is not always helpful to the individual who is trying to come to grips with the subject, and it is therefore particularly important to begin with the definitions of key terms. Learning has at least two important usages in psychology. The first refers to observed changes in behaviour which have resulted from a previous experience, or experiences. For example, I may observe that my cat always runs into the kitchen when she hears the squeaky sound of the old can-opener which I use to open her cans of cat food. I can safely assume that, at one time, a squeaky can-opener produced no response at all and therefore may attribute the change in behaviour to learning acquired over the many hundreds of occasions when the squeak of the can-opener was associated with the subsequent arrival of cat food in her dish. The first use of learning thus refers to a change between a starting-state (no response) and an end-state (immediate rushing into the kitchen). The second, related, use of the term concerns the acquisition of the behaviour between the starting-, and end-, states. Successive changes in the acquired behaviour may be considered as a function of the number of learning experiences; that is, in terms of the number of learning trials. These definitions thus distinguish learning from the memory of an event or fact which is the awareness of having experienced that event or fact in the past. Of course, learning will often, but not always, be accompanied by memories of the learning experiences.

It is fair, although something of a simplification, to say that the majority of research on learning has been conducted using laboratory animals (principally rats, monkeys and pigeons) while memory research is conducted with human subjects. The chapter on Memory emphasizes the way psychologists have subdivided memory into various subsystems. With the above definitions, the notion of animal memory is quite problematic; although we may observe a change in the animal's behaviour as a result of past experiences, could we ever know that the animal had memories of (i.e. was aware of) those past experiences? A human being, by contrast, can use language to demonstrate an awareness that a particular event or fact has been experienced previously. These definitions also mean that memory without awareness (usually now referred to as implicit memory, see the chapter on Memory for details) is also a contradiction in terms; it should be viewed as a kind of learning.

CLASSICAL CONDITIONING: BASIC PROPERTIES

Within the study of animal learning, many will be aware of the pioneering work of the Russian, Ivan Pavlov, who discovered a basic learning process which is referred to as classical or Pavlovian conditioning. His experiments with dogs (e.g. Pavlov, 1927) revealed that these animals could learn an association between one event (e.g. a bell) and another (e.g. the subsequent delivery of food); this learning is similar to my cat's ability to associate the squeak of the can-opener with food. Pavlov's explanation began with an innate reflex, 'hard-wired' in the dog's brain; for example, the release of saliva at the sight and smell of food. He termed the food an unconditioned stimulus (UCS) because it unconditionally produced the reflex, or unconditioned response (UCR), of salivation. However, the repeated pairing of the UCS with another stimulus (e.g. a bell) led to the bell alone being able to produce the salivation response. Pavlov termed the bell a conditioned stimulus (CS) because its ability to produce salivation (the conditioned response, CR) was conditional upon having been paired previously with the food. Pavlov regarded the CS as becoming neurally-linked to the existing salivation reflex thus substituting for the UCS. He referred to this idea as stimulus substitution. It should also be noted that classical conditioning involves the learning of an association between two stimuli (the CS and the UCS), and hence is sometimes referred to as S-S learning.

Classical conditioning can be demonstrated under a variety of temporal arrangements between the CS and the UCS. The strongest classical conditioning is found when the start of the CS precedes the UCS in time but both stimuli terminate at the same point in time (called delay conditioning). Fairly good conditioning can be obtained when the CS occurs first and also terminates just before the start of the UCS (this is called trace conditioning because some kind of memory trace for the CS is needed in order for it still to be 'in mind' when the UCS subsequently occurs). In trace conditioning, the success of the learning usually deteriorates markedly with increases in the temporal gap between the end of the CS and the start of the UCS. Some learning, although often it is quite weak, occurs in simultaneous conditioning, when the CS and UCS begin and terminate together. It is quite common to interpret the above evidence in terms of the predictive nature of classical conditioning. Such a view assumes that the learning mechanism of classical conditioning has evolved in order that the organism may use associations between events to predict future important occurrences. UCSs (food, water, an opportunity for sex, etc.) represent important future occurrences and so it would be useful to predict them via associated, previously unimportant, stimuli such as smells, sights and sounds. A system which has evolved to allow CSs to predict UCSs would naturally lead to better learning when CSs occur shortly before UCSs, rather than simultaneously, as described above. The predictive nature of classical conditioning is also emphasized in the Rescorla – Wagner theory described below.

One demonstrates conditioning by showing that the CS elicits a CR. A CR is demonstrated if the CS, on its own, is able to elicit the response normally produced by a UCS; Pavlov's dogs salivated in response to the bell only. It is natural to consider what would happen to this CR when the CS is repeatedly presented without continuing to be paired with the UCS. Pavlov explored this himself and found that as the CS is presented alone, the amount of conditioned responding decreases. This process was termed extinction of classical conditioning. Pavlov made a number of interesting discoveries about extinction which are still not well understood today. If CS presentation is carried out for long enough he found that the CR would eventually disappear altogether. However, on testing the same animal some days later, the CS would usually no longer be fully extinguished: some conditioned responding would be evident. Pavlov referred to this as spontaneous recovery.

Spontaneous recovery may be important in behaviour therapy. These forms of psychological treatment, for disorders such as anxiety, addictions, phobias, obsessions and compulsions, are based on the theory of basic learning mechanisms such as classical conditioning. The disorder is often viewed, in simple terms, as the product of unwanted (classically conditioned) learning. The treatment may be viewed, again in simplistic terms, as an attempt to extinguish the maladaptive learning. However, a problem for behaviour ther-

apy is that the unwanted behaviour, successfully extinguished during treatment, often shows a tendency to recur later in the patient's daily life. Spontaneous recovery may be partly responsible for this effect and so, clearly, a better understanding of the mechanisms of spontaneous recovery could be of great value in improving the success of behaviour therapy.

Further important questions about classical conditioning concern the kinds of stimuli which can serve as CSs for a given UCS and which can serve as UCSs for a given CS. In answer to the first question, it appears that a very wide range of CSs can enter into an association with a given UCS. It appears likely, however, that each organism may have evolved such that certain CSs may form associations with a particular UCS more readily than other CSs. This phenomenon is described as preparedness: evolution has prepared some stimuli to be more easily conditioned to a UCS than others. For example, it may be easy to associate a particular taste (as a CS) with the subsequent UCS of nausea and vomiting. This learning, being both quite commonplace and potentially useful to the organism, may have evolved to be more efficient than the formation of associations between, for example, a sound and subsequent nausea. Preparedness could offer an explanation for the finding that certain types of phobia (namely spider and snake phobia) are much more common than others, a finding echoed across almost all the cultures of the world. This simple idea is to this day, however, surprisingly complex and controversial (Davey, 1995).

In response to the second question raised above, one might reiterate that typical UCSs are stimuli of significance to the organism such as food, water, opportunities for sex, and so on. In fact, many UCSs are precisely the same stimuli which serve as reinforcers in instrumental conditioning described below. In fact, this observation is an important reminder that, although described separately in textbooks, classical and instrumental conditioning processes will often both occur in any learning situation. This can explain the great difficulty which psychologists have had in devising procedures which represent examples of 'pure' classical or 'pure' instrumental conditioning (Gray, 1975).

Another observation about the nature of UCSs is important. A logical extension of Pavlov's idea of stimulus substitution was that, after pairing with a UCS, a CS comes to 'stand for' the UCS itself. If this were true, then the CS should be able to act as a UCS for other CSs in the same way as the original UCS. Pavlov confirmed this prediction by experiments. He used a buzzer as a CS and obtained strong conditioned salivation to the buzzer alone. He then paired the buzzer with a visual stimulus (a black square) ten times, using delay conditioning, and found that the black square alone produced a weak but reliable conditioned response, even though the black square had never been paired with food. Pavlov referred to this as an example of higher-order (specifically secondary) conditioning. We shall see that this observation will play an important role in understanding instrumental conditioning.

THE RESCORLA – WAGNER THEORY OF CLASSICAL CONDITIONING

A wide variety of phenomena have been documented in classical conditioning experiments. A major theory, which can account for many of these phenomena, was developed by Rescorla and Wagner (1972). I shall refer to this account, henceforth, as the RW theory.

Since its original proposal, it has undergone some minor modifications but remains today the most complete and widely accepted theory of classical conditioning. In recent years, interest in the RW theory has increased because it has been shown to be formally similar to the highly influential connectionist, or neural network, accounts of human learning (Shanks, 1991). We shall return to this similarity after describing the basic details of the RW theory.

The central concept of the RW theory is the strength of the learned association between the CS and the UCS. This associative strength is considered to vary from zero (no learning) up to a maximum value (usually denoted λ) beyond which associative strength can increase no further. The RW theory provides an account for the degree of learning, in terms of the change in associative strength, between CSs and a UCS, and it has the advantage of being able to predict the relative degrees of learning for several CSs presented simultaneously in association with a common UCS. In the RW theory, the degree of learning between a particular CS and a UCS on a particular learning trial is proportional to the difference between two quantities. The first is the maximum possible total associative strength which the UCS can sustain (i.e. λ) and the second is the total current associative strength summed across all the CSs present in the current learning trial. The RW theory deals with extinction by proposing that the associative strength between a particular CS and UCS is reduced whenever the CS is presented without the associated UCS. The degree of reduction is again proportional to the total current associative strength for the absent UCS, summed across all the CSs present on the extinction trial.

We have already seen that a simple way of thinking about classical conditioning is to consider the CSs as predicting the future occurrence of the UCS. We can extend this viewpoint to cover the RW theory. If there are several CSs present which are associated with a particular UCS, then the total of their current associative strengths gives the degree to which the UCS is predicted by the CSs present. When the UCS is very well predicted (the total associative strength is close to the maximum possible, λ) then little further learning occurs. However, when CS is relatively poorly predicted, learning occurs rapidly and the degree of learning is proportional to the discrepancy between the current level of prediction and the maximum associative strength possible. In the case of extinction, prior learning means that there is a degree of associative strength between the CSs and the UCS, and so the UCS is to some extent predicted. When the expected UCS fails to occur, the associative strength between the CSs and the UCS decreases in proportion to the degree to which the UCS was predicted when extinction began. Thus, when the original conditioning is strong extinction will initially proceed rapidly. The RW theory does not have a ready explanation for why spontaneous recovery should occur, and it still represents a major puzzle for conditioning theory (Bouton, 1993).

One important conditioning phenomenon which is very simply explained by the RW theory is blocking (Kamin, 1968). In blocking experiments there are several learning phases. In phase 1, subjects are trained, by the repeated pairing of the stimuli concerned, to associate one CS (denoted CS-A) with a UCS. In phase 2, subjects are trained with further stimulus pairings, this time between a compound stimulus and the same UCS that was used in phase 1. The compound stimulus is formed by the simultaneous presentation of

two CSs (CS-A and CS-B), one of which (CS-A) was used in phase 1. A third and final phase assesses the degree of learning formed between stimulus B and the UCS during the compound stimulus training of phase 2. The blocking procedure is summarized in Fig. 1. The blocking phenomenon is so named because there is a failure to learn anything about the association between CS-B and the UCS during the compound training phase; the learning has been blocked by the prior learning of an association between CS-A and the UCS. This phenomenon is demonstrated in comparison with the control procedure in which subjects do not receive training of an association between CS-A and the UCS in phase 1; these subjects display some learning of the association between CS-B and the UCS which was acquired during the compound training phase.

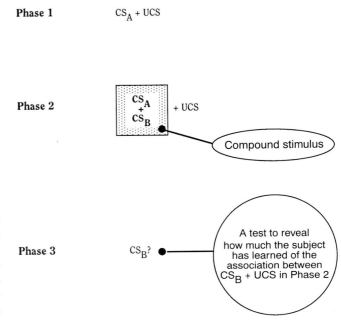

Fig. 1. The three phases of a typical blocking task are depicted. In phases 1 and 2 the subject has a number of learning trials in which they are trained that stimuli X and Y are associated (denoted by X+Y). Phase 3 is a test (denoted by a ?) of the learning acquired for a particular stimulus as a result of the training in phases 1 and 2. The Figure depicts the blocking task for an experimental subject. A control subject differs in phase 1: the control subject may not receive phase 1 at all, or will experience the same stimuli as the experimental subject in phase 1 (CS-A and the UCS), although these stimuli will not be associated with one another.

The RW theory provides a neat and simple explanation for blocking effects. When CS-A and the UCS are associated during phase 1 training, associative strength develops between CS-A and the UCS. This means that when CS-A is subsequently presented the UCS is to some extent predicted and expected. If training in phase 1 is reasonably extensive, then the degree of associative strength may approach the maximum value possible for that UCS. In the compound stimulus training of phase 2 CS-A is presented as part of the compound and so the UCS will be expected and predicted, due to the prior learning. This will reduce the rate at which associative strength will be accrued for any other stimuli present along with CS-A. CS-B will therefore be prevented from acquiring associative strength for the UCS to the extent that the UCS is predicted by the other component of the compound stimulus (CS-A).

It may appear that understanding the subtle details of animal learning experiments, such as blocking, is likely to have little importance for understanding human behaviour. In a striking recent experiment, acutely ill schizophrenic subjects failed to show blocking on a human analogue of the procedure typically used with animals (Jones, Hemsley & Gray, 1992). This result is particularly interesting as more chronic schizophrenic patients, who had been stabilized on their neuroleptic (dopamine-blocking) medication, showed a largely normal pattern of blocking. Moreover, blocking in animals is known to be affected by the administration of the dopamine-releasing drug amphetamine, and by lesions to the hippocampus (see Jones *et al.*, 1992, for details). Blocking may therefore be a powerful tool for attempting to understand the psychological and neurobiological features of schizophrenia, as the dominant neurochemical hypotheses of schizophrenia stresses the role of brain dopamine overactivity (Carlsson, 1987) and the primary site of neuroanatomical abnormalities in schizophrenics is thought to involve the hippocampal region (see Gray *et al.*, 1991, for details).

There are other reasons to feel that a detailed understanding of classical conditioning processes may illuminate human behaviour. We have already noted that many currently popular connectionist models of human cognition bear close resemblance to the RW theory sketched above. Specifically, the computer program at the heart of these connectionist models learns via association, and does so in proportion to a critical difference between parameters. This difference is exactly analogous to the difference measure controlling learning in the RW theory (the difference between current levels of associative strength and the possible maximum). In light of this similarity, any aspects of human cognition which may be successfully explained by a connectionist model using the 'difference' learning rule, can also be modelled by the RW theory. Given the widespread view that connectionist accounts may be a major step forward in understanding human cognition (Schneider, 1987), the same may apply to the RW theory and to classical conditioning phenomena in general.

Shanks' (1991) studies took the above ideas further by showing that a number of classical conditioning phenomena, each explicable in terms of the RW theory, can also be demonstrated in a complex human learning task. In his studies, the subjects had to learn the relationships between fictitious medical diseases and fictitious symptoms. In one study, an effect equivalent to blocking was demonstrated in the subjects' learning.

Subjects were trained, over ten repetitions, to diagnose that patients with both symptoms A and B had disease D1. Intermixed with these trials were ten others in which patients had symptom B only but no diagnosable illness. This combination of trials was described as the contingent condition, because disease D1 was contingent upon the presence of symptom A. RW theory would predict that subject would learn this predictive association between symptom A and disease D1. Intermixed with the trials comprising the contingent condition were two other sets of ten trials each. In these subjects were trained either that patients with symptoms C and D had disease D2 or that patients with symptom D alone also had disease D2. These latter two sets were referred to as the non-

contingent condition because disease D2 was not contingent on the presence of symptom C. RW theory would predict that subjects would not associate symptom C with disease D2 because this would be blocked by the reliable association between symptom D and disease D2. In a test phase, these predictions were borne out. Subjects were asked to rate 'how strongly on a 0–100 scale' they associated each symptom with each disease. Subjects gave significantly higher ratings for the association between symptom A and disease D1 (average = 62.3, based on three sets of contingent and non-contingent conditions) than for that between symptom C and disease D2 (average = 41.8). Several other, more complex, features of animal conditioning were also demonstrated in the human learning performance.

The RW theory has a number of limitations. These cannot be reviewed here due to a lack of space. In summary, there appear to be a small number of classical conditioning phenomena which cannot be easily accommodated within the basic theory (Grossberg, 1982; Pearce, 1994, for details). These findings can largely be accommodated by modifications to the basic theory.

INSTRUMENTAL CONDITIONING: BASIC PROPERTIES

An alternative type of animal learning has also been intensively studied during this century, namely instrumental conditioning. This form of learning, also widely known as operant learning, was the major focus of inquiry for the Behaviourist school in psychology. Behaviourism flourished during the first half of this century, in the United States especially, under the guidance of J.B. Watson and B.F. Skinner in particular. The basis of instrumental conditioning was to consider the consequences of an action and, most importantly, the effect of those consequences upon the probability that the action would be repeated in future. If a child touches a hot pan on a cooker the consequence of the action of touching is a sharp burning pain on the hand. The child is unlikely to touch any pan on a cooker again; more formally we could say that the probability of the touching response has decreased as a result of the (very rapid) learning. The learning is also said to have been reinforced by the aversive pain stimulus, which may therefore be described as a reinforcer. The pain stimulus (S) causes the response (R) probability to decrease (−), and so the reinforcer is described as an S^{R-}. The sequence of events in instrumental conditioning involves a response followed by a stimulus and so instrumental conditioning is sometimes described as R–S learning.

Some reinforcing stimuli, such as food, water and sex, are appetitive; the animal desires these stimuli and will actively seek them out. In instrumental conditioning situations, the probability of repetition of any action which produces such a reinforcing stimulus is likely to increase and so the stimulus is described as an S^{R+}. The standard apparatus of operant learning, the Skinner box, exploits the reinforcing properties of appetitive stimuli. The rat in this cage will eventually, by accident, depress a lever on one wall of the cage. This lever triggers the release of a food pellet into a tray. The rat rapidly learns the relationship between depressing the lever and the delivery of food so that the probability of lever-pressing when in the cage rises dramatically.

There are a variety of different operant learning situations which have been studied; these are achieved by arranging for the response

Table 1. *R denotes response and p(R) denotes the probability of the response. The cases in which p(R) increases, are sometimes collectively known as reinforcement; the cases where p(R) decreases as punishment (see note [3] below). S^{R+} are appetitive stimuli (e.g. food) sometimes called positive reinforcers. S^{R-} are aversive stimuli (e.g. pain) sometimes called negative reinforcers.*

p(R) afterwards	Situation	Name describing reinforcement	Name describing behaviour produced
Increases	R is followed by onset of S^{R+}	Reward, also known as positive reinforcement	Approach
Increases	R is followed by offset of S^{R-}	Negative reinforcement	Escape or active avoidance[a]
Decreases	R is followed by offset of S^{R+}	Time out, also known as response cost	Extinction[b]
Decreases	R is followed by onset of S^{R-}	Punishment[c]	Passive avoidance

[a]The situation described in the table is escape, active avoidance would be the situation in which a response was followed by the non-occurrence of an expected punishment.

[b]This is a different sense of the term from extinction in classical conditioning.

[c]Here punishment is a type of reinforcement caused by a negative reinforcer (S^{R-}) following a response.

under study to be followed by the offset or onset of either an S^{R+} or an S^{R-}. These variations in procedure are outlined in Table 1 where the terminology appropriate to each situation is also given.

REINFORCEMENT, DRIVES, AND THE DEVELOPMENT OF TWO-PROCESS THEORY

We have described some of the terminology of operant learning without elaborating on the possible mechanisms underlying the phenomena. Above, we emphasized that a reinforcer is a stimulus which, if presented following a response, has the consequence of altering the probability of future emission of that response. Radical behaviourists argued that (operant) learning could not occur without reinforcement. We shall briefly note exceptions to this later on, but first will explore the nature of reinforcement in more detail.

The concept of reinforcement is intimately tied to the notion of drive. Although different conceptions of drive can be distinguished (Gray, 1975) drive has been most widely viewed (since Hull, 1952) as a kind of energizer of goal-directed behaviour. There may be several kinds of specific drive (e.g. hunger, thirst, sexual drive) each of which may build up when the animal is deprived of appropriate stimuli (food, water, etc.). When these appropriate stimuli are subsequently available, the animal's response is energized, i.e. emitted with greater probability and more vigorously than if no deprivation had occurred. However, such effects of drive seem to occur only for goal-directed behaviour. Goal-directed behaviour is seen when an animal changes its behaviour, in response to environmental changes, to attain the same end point (the goal). For example, we might interpose a clear screen between an animal and food, and the screen can be raised by depressing a lever. The animal may learn to depress the lever to raise the screen in order to access the goal (food). The

animal would then be learning a goal-directed behaviour. Goal-direction appears to be a characteristic of the learned behaviours which can be energized by depriving the animal of a specific drive stimulus (e.g. food).

Two influential claims have been made about the relationship between drive and reinforcement. First, it has been claimed that drive is necessary for reinforcement, and secondly, that reinforcement consists in the reduction of drive. The second proposal (which entails the first) makes intuitive sense when drives are viewed as biological 'needs'; in other words, seeing the drive for food as existing to protect the animal from any biological damage caused by prolonged lack of food. The behaviour of a hungry animal would then be expected to be particularly reinforceable by food if this reduced the animal's drive for food. However, this intuitively simple notion of drives as needs is inadequate. Hungry animals will learn a maze (i.e. exhibit goal-directed behaviour) for saccharin which, although sweet, has no nutritional value. This is the first kind of observation which can challenge the view of drives as biological needs. Worse is to come, as the above experiments do suggest that some drive reduction may be occurring. After eating saccharin, rats eat less saccharin when offered it subsequently. Interestingly, this satiation effect extends to other types of food such as milk or solids (Miller, 1955). So the 'reduction in drive', putatively responsible for the reduction in subsequent food consumption, is actually doing nothing for the biological needs of the animal; in fact, it acts to continue nutritional deprivation while nutritional needs increase.

Drives are therefore not a direct manifestation of biological needs. However, it is still worth considering the view that drives, whatever they are, may need to be reduced and that drive-reduction may be the substrate of reinforcement. Unfortunately, the drive-reduction view of reinforcement has been strongly refuted by the experimental data when considered *in toto* (Gray, 1975, pp. 142–7), particularly in experiments addressing the issue of satiation. We do not have space to review this evidence, but one can think of several commonsense examples which also appear problematic for a drive reduction theory. Sexual arousal would appear to be a state of increased sexual drive and yet human beings often engage in goal-directed behaviour with the express purpose of feeling sexually aroused and thus increasing drive (often at a time quite distant from the opportunity to engage in sexual behaviour). Similarly, after eating a small amount of food, one's hunger appears initially to increase; by drive-reduction theory one should avoid eating if this initially produced an increase in drive. In summary, we can see that we appear often to be reinforced by drive-induction as opposed to drive-reduction.

It must be stressed that drives are obviously of importance for reinforcement: one cannot train a well-fed rat to learn a new behaviour if the relevant responses are reinforced with food. However, the concept of drive has not clarified our understanding of reinforcement mechanisms.

Reinforcement has also been viewed as resulting from the action of a positive feedback loop: this idea is simply the suggestion that some behaviours, such as drinking, may sustain and strengthen themselves. Consider an animal drinking. If drinking were interrupted, at a point prior to satiation, then the self-sustaining, positive feedback aspects of drinking (should they exist) would also be interrupted. When the animal is subsequently given a chance to drink, drinking should thus resume at a slower rate than that observed at the point of interruption. This has been observed experimentally in doves (McFarland & McFarland, 1968), over delays long enough to rule out the contribution of a delayed satiation effect of water subsequently reaching the stomach.

There is a further major puzzle with reinforcement: a positive feedback account can explain how a reinforcer can maintain the level of a response which has already been produced. However, it does not explain how a reinforcer can cause an organism to learn that a new response sequence will be followed by that reinforcer, given that the reinforcer must act after the whole response sequence has already been executed. The full response sequence may initially occur by accident, but how can the subsequent reinforcer act 'backwards in time' to allow learning? The goal-directed nature of operant behaviour suggests that, at the time that the response sequence is about to be made, the organism has a mental representation of the future consequences of the possible courses of action open to it. These mental representations of future reinforcements can be thought of as expectancies and they provide the so-called incentive motivation for the operant behaviour. The puzzle is to explain how such expectancies may be learned. The predictive view of classical conditioning can also be viewed as an account of the development of expectancies and so one might turn to classical conditioning to provide an account of incentive motivation. Such accounts of operant behaviour are often described as representing a two-process theory, so-called because important roles are ascribed to both instrumental and classical conditioning processes.

In fact, the two-process account of incentive motivation draws specifically on the occurrence, noted earlier, of higher-order classical conditioning. The ideas can be illustrated by reference to a classic study by Butter and Thomas (1958). In their experiment three groups of rats were used. A control group was repeatedly presented with the audible click of the liquid dispenser in their cage which occurred without consequence. The experimental groups also heard their dispenser click, but it was always followed by the delivery of some sucrose solution, in one of two different concentrations (8% and 24%). In a subsequent stage of the experiment, the rats were in cage with a lever. When the lever was depressed, this produced the same click as that produced by the liquid dispenser in the earlier stage of the experiment. The rats in the experimental group pressed the lever more than the control animals. The animals in this study therefore appeared to be prepared to 'work' for a secondary reinforcer (whose properties were formed solely by classical conditioning), in much the same way as rats will learn to press a lever for a natural primary reinforcer such as a sugar solution itself. The money with which most of us are paid for our occupations is a good example of a secondary reinforcer; the value of money is ultimately based on its association with primary reinforcers such as food and drink.

The similarity of the effects of primary and secondary reinforcers was made very clearly by comparison of the two experimental groups in the Butter and Thomas study. It was already known that rats given 24% sucrose solution for pressing a lever learn the relationship between lever-pressing and sucrose reward faster, and respond more vigorously, than rats given an 8% solution.

The rats who had formed a classically conditioned association between 24% sucrose and the click in the Butter and Thomas study pressed the lever (which produced only the secondarily reinforcing click) at a significantly higher rate than the rats which had been trained with the click and 8% sucrose. The incentive motivation was clearly higher for the 24% sucrose group even though the same click was produced by the lever-pressing response. The click, of course, differed in what it signalled to the animals; those which had previously been trained that the click was followed by concentrated sucrose solution had a different expectation from those rats which had been trained to associate the click with dilute sucrose solution.

The interpretations just given offer a mechanism by which whole response sequences can be reinforced by an event at the end of the sequence. The final part of the response sequence will result in a number of neutral stimuli including visual and auditory consequences, plus bodily sensations associated with the response itself. These stimuli enter into classical conditioning with the primary reinforcing stimulus (e.g. food) resulting from the response sequence. The neutral stimuli thus acquire secondary reinforcing properties by this mechanism and therefore may act as reinforcers themselves for the penultimate part of the response sequence. By repeating this chaining process, the value of the terminal reinforcement can be passed back through the whole response sequence so that the organism can be motivated to execute the initial part of the sequence. This is a two-process theory account of approach behaviour under positive reinforcement. There are a number of further complications which arise in regard to the other scenarios, particularly passive and active avoidance, depicted in Table 1. Although there is not space to go into this here, the topic is treated in detail in Gray's (1975) book.

To close, we must return to the question of whether operant learning can occur without reinforcement. The role of expectancies, which has just been stressed, suggests that an organism will change its behaviour if it expects reinforcement to occur even without the experience of reinforcement itself. Such a view is also consistent with the influential social learning theory proposed by Bandura and others (e.g. Bandura, 1977) as an extension of the animal learning theories just described. As the name suggests this theory is concerned with how individuals learn in a social context. Often such learning involves an observer who learns from a model executing a particular piece of behaviour. The observer can learn to reproduce the observed behaviour although it is the model who may be reinforced for the original behaviour. The observational experience may, of course, allow the observer to develop an expectancy that a certain kind of reinforcement follows the action being observed. Social learning theory has been influential in areas such as the learning of stereotypical gender roles where observational learning may be particularly important. Imagine that a young boy observes his father being reinforced by his mother for fixing the broken washing machine; the boy may learn that these 'male' behaviours are worth adopting because of the reinforcements which are expected to result from them. Once again, these phenomena illustrate the importance of basic simple learning processes for complex human behaviour in the real world.

REFERENCES

Bandura, A. (1977). *Social learning theory*. Englewood Cliffs, NJ: Prentice-Hall.

Bouton, M.E. (1993). Context, time, and memory retrieval in the interference paradigms of Pavlovian learning. *Psychological Bulletin*, 114, 80–99.

Butter, C.M. & Thomas, D.R. (1958). Secondary reinforcement as a function of the amount of primary reinforcement. *Journal of Comparative and Physiological Psychology*, 51, 346–8.

Carlsson, A. (1987). The dopamine hypothesis of schizophrenia 20 years later. In H. Hafner, W.F. Gattaz & W. Janzarik (Eds.). *Search for the causes of schizophrenia*, pp. 223–235. Berlin: Springer-Verlag.

Davey, G. (1995). Preparedness and phobias: specific evolved associations or a generalised expectancy bias? *Behavioral and Brain Sciences*, 18, 289–325.

Gray, J.A. (1975). *Elements of a two-process theory of learning*. London: Academic Press.

Gray, J.A., Feldon, J., Rawlins, J.N.P.,

Hemsley, D.R. & Smith, A.D. (1991). The neuropsychology of schizophrenia. *Behavioral and Brain Sciences*, 14, 1–84.

Grossberg, S. (1982). processing of expected and unexpected events during conditioning and attention: a psychophysiological theory. *Psychological Review*, 89, 529–72.

Hull, C.L. (1952). *A behaviour system*. New Haven, CT: Yale University Press.

Jones, S.H., Hemsley, D.R. & Gray, J.A. (1992). Loss of the Kamin blocking effect in acute but not chronic schizophrenics. *Biological Psychiatry*, 32, 739–55.

Kamin, L.J. (1968). Predictability, surprise, attention and conditioning. In B.A. Campbell & R.M. Clark (Eds.). *Punishment and aversive behaviour*, pp. 279–96. New York: Appleton-Century-Crofts.

McFarland, D.J. & McFarland, F.J. (1968). Dynamic analysis of an avian drinking response. *Medical and Biological Engineering*, 6, 659–68.

Miller, N.E. (1955). Shortcomings of food consumption as a measure of hunger.

Annals of the New York Academy of Science, 63, 141–3.

Pavlov, I.P. (1927). *Conditioned reflexes* [trans. G.V. Anrep]. London: Oxford University Press.

Pearce, J.M. (1994). Similarity and discrimination: a selective review and a connectionist model. *Psychological Review*, 101, 587–607.

Rescorla, R.A. & Wagner, A.R. (1972). A theory of Pavlovian conditioning: variations in the effectiveness of reinforcement and nonreinforcement. In A.H. Black & W.F. Prokasy (Eds.). *Classical conditioning II: Current theory and research*, pp. 64–99. New York: Appleton-Century-Crofts.

Shanks, D.R. (1991). Categorisation by a connectionist network. *Journal of Experimental Psychology: Learning, Memory, and Cognition*, 17, 434–43.

Schneider, W. (1987). Connectionism: is it a paradigm shift for psychology? *Behavioral Research Methods, Instruments, and Computing*, 19, 73–83.

Intelligence

ROBERT J. STERNBERG

Department of Psychology, Yale University, New Haven, USA

Intelligence is the ability to adapt flexibly and effectively to the environment. Although theorists of intelligence might disagree as to the exact details of how intelligence should be defined, most of them would accept the general idea of this definition.

Intelligence is important. Without it, we would quickly become extinct as a species, and with substantially less of it, we would be no different from any other species of animal. In order to understand one of the main things that distinguishes us as a species, we need to understand intelligence.

In this chapter, we will consider three of the many questions that might be asked about intelligence. First, what is it? Secondly, how, if at all, can it be measured? Thirdly, to what extent is it heritable, and to what extent environmentally determined? And, if environment plays some role, can people increase their intelligence? These questions are now addressed in turn.

WHAT IS INTELLIGENCE?

Theorists of intelligence do not agree about much, and strangely enough, they probably agree least as to what intelligence is, beyond the ability to adapt flexibly to the environment. Let's consider some of the alternative views.

Intelligence as factors of mind

One of the earliest views of intelligence, going back to the beginning of the century, is that intelligence can be understood in terms of hypothetical mental entities called 'factors'. These factors are alleged to be the sources of the individual differences we observe in people's performance in school, on the job, and even in their social interactions. Factors are identified by giving people various tests of their mental functioning, and then applying a statistical technique called 'factor analysis', which identifies the hypothetical underlying constructs, or factors.

How many factors of the mind are there, and what is the nature of these factors? The various theories of abilities cover a wide range.

Charles Spearman (1923) proposed that there is just one important factor, general intelligence or general ability (sometimes called g), which permeates performance in all intellectual tasks. There are also specific factors relevant to individual tasks, but in Spearman's theory, they are not very important. Spearman was not sure of what the general factor was, but he suggested it might be what he referred to as 'mental energy'.

Thurstone (1938) suggested that there are, in fact, seven important factors, not just one. He identified these factors as verbal comprehension (as measured by vocabulary or reading comprehension), number (arithmetic operations), space (visualizing relations between objects in space), verbal fluency (generating words), perceptual speed (rapidly recognizing simple visual patterns), memory (remembering names or numbers of objects), inductive reasoning (seeing patterns).

As if seven factors were not enough, Guilford (1967) first proposed 120 factors, and later (Guilford, 1982) proposed 150 factors, obtained by crossing different mental processes, contents, and products. The problem with this theory is that it proposed so many different abilities, it was hard to measure them separately, much less to remember them!

Other factorial models have also been proposed. Cattell (1971), for example, has suggested a hierarchical model of intelligence, and other theorists have suggested even more complicated forms in which factors may relate. But all of these theories have in common the notion that people differ in some basic abilities, which can be identified by the use of the statistical technique of factor analysis.

Intelligence as mental processes

An alternative view has conceived of intelligence as a set of mental processes. From this point of view, as people think, they execute a set of mental operations, and these operations plus the system that generates them constitute the bases of intelligence. Many followers of this viewpoint liken the mind to a computer.

Process theorists differ in how complex they believe these processes to be. Some theorists, like Jensen (1982), have proposed that very simple processes underlie intelligence. In a typical experiment, he will measure these processes in terms of the time it takes a person to see one of several lights flash and then press a button under that light, and not under one of the others. Earl Hunt (1978) has looked at processes that are just slightly more complex, such as those involved in recognizing that 'A' and 'a', despite their difference in physical appearance, represent the same letter. Sternberg (1977) looked at still more complex processes, such as those involved in solving an analogy of the form A : B :: C : D (e.g. lawyer is to client as doctor is to patient). And Newell and Simon (1972) looked at even more complex processes, such as those involved in playing chess or solving complex logic problems.

Although these theorists have differed in the level of processing they have investigated, they have had in common the notion that, to understand the nature of human abilities, we need to understand the mental processes that underlie them.

Intelligence as a biological entity

Some psychologists have proposed that factor and process theorists miss the essence of abilities, which in their view are biologically based. These psychologists try to understand abilities in terms of the functioning of the brain.

Several approaches have yielded interesting insights about the relation between abilities and the brain. Vernon and Mori (1992) have collected evidence suggesting that abilities may be related to the speed of conduction of neural impulses. Eysenck (1982) has proposed an alternative view, namely, that abilities are related to accuracy of conduction of neural impulses. Haier and his colleagues (1992) have done PET scans of brains of people while they solve tasks, and have found that more able people exert less mental effort to solve complex tasks than do less able people. There also seem to

be relations between measured abilities and patterns of evoked potentials (e.g. Schafer, 1982).

Some scientists have been more interested in qualitative than in quantitative differences. For example, Levy (1974) has found that the left hemisphere of the brain generally tends to be more analytic in its processing of information, whereas the right hemisphere tends to be more holistic. Moreover, it has been known for some time that, in the majority of people, processing of language occurs in the left hemisphere of the brain.

Some psychologists interested in the biological approach to abilities have not studied the brain directly. For example, Piaget (1972) proposed a theory based on biological ideas, but never studied the brain directly. Piaget suggested a series of stages through which children pass as they develop mentally, and argued that each stage of mental development builds on earlier ones.

Not everyone who pursues a biological approach to abilities is reductionist. Some psychologists view biological measures as just one kind of measure among others that help elucidate the phenomenon of human abilities. From this point of view, for example, biological measures can elucidate cognitive processing, just as cognitive processing can help elucidate biological functioning.

Intelligence as a cultural construction

The next point of view we shall consider is that of human intelligence as cultural constructions. Some psychologists have suggested that cultures create their notions of what intelligence is (e.g. Laboratory of Comparative Human Cognition, 1982). On this view, the nature of intelligence can differ from one culture to another. What one culture considers essential to intelligence, such as speed of functioning, might be considered inessential in a second culture, or even stupid in a third. We know from cross-cultural research that different societies have different conceptions of intelligence (Berry, 1984). And their performance on tests will be influenced by their conception. For example, members of a culture that does not emphasize speed of processing will have trouble understanding why they should think quickly on an intelligence test. On this view, any attempt to understand intelligence as occurring solely inside the head will miss the differences in conceptions of intelligence across cultures.

Intelligence as a system

Some recent theorists have tried to view intelligence as a complex system. For example, Gardner (1983) has suggested that intelligence is not a unitary construct, but rather that there are multiple intelligences, namely, linguistic, logical – mathematical, spatial, musical, bodily – kinesthetic, interpersonal, and intrapersonal. Sternberg (1985) has suggested that there are three aspects of intelligence, namely, analytic, synthetic – creative, and practical ones. On these views, most conventional conceptions of intelligence are too narrow, and thus deal with only a small portion of intelligence as a whole. In particular, on these views, measures of intelligence fail to measure the whole of intelligence as a psychological construct.

THE MEASUREMENT OF INTELLIGENCE

Historically, there are two traditions in the measurement of intelligence. The first tradition, dating back to Galton (1883), consists of psychophysical measures, such as of strength, visual acuity, pain sensitivity, and the like. This tradition has not met with much enthusiasm in the present century. The other approach, dating back to Binet and Simon (1908), uses various judgement tasks to measure intelligence. Such tasks include recognizing absurdities in pictures and in verbal statements, defining words, completing number series, visualizing what objects would look like if they were cut in certain ways with scissors, and the like. This tradition has had much more acceptance.

Although there are a number of tests of intelligence in use today, the two most widely used are the Stanford–Binet Intelligence Scale and the Wechsler Intelligence Scales. Both tests are available for people varying in ages, ranging from early childhood to adult.

The current versions of the test yield an overall score, an intelligence quotient (IQ), for which the average score is 100 and the standard deviation, 15 (Wechsler) or 16 (Stanford–Binet), meaning that roughly two-thirds of scores fall within plus or minus one standard deviation of the mean. The tests also yield subscores. For example, on the Wechsler tests, one obtains a total score as well as verbal and performance test scores.

IQs were once computed by dividing a construct called 'mental age' by chronological (physical) age, and then multiplying by 100. Mental age was supposed to represent a person's mental level of functioning. Because of conceptual as well as statistical problems with the mental-age construct, however, this construct is rarely used today. Rather, IQs are computed on the basis of scores that measure how unusual a person's performance is vis-à-vis the performance of others.

HERITABILITY AND MODIFIABILITY OF INTELLIGENCE

Is intelligence a result of heredity or environment? A multitude of studies have addressed this issue (for a review see Sternberg & Grigorenko, 1997). The consensus of almost all researchers is that both heredity and environment play important parts in intelligence. A variety of kinds of studies have been done to assess just what these parts are. Some studies look at identical twins separated at birth; others look at IQ levels in relatives of varying degrees of genetic proximity; still other studies look at just two groups: identical versus fraternal twins. The general consensus of these studies seems to be that the heritability of intelligence is about 0.5, meaning that half of the population variation in intelligence is due to hereditary factors,

and the rest is not. It is important to realize that this statistic does not mean that half of intelligence is due to heredity. We wouldn't even know what such a statement means. There is also some recent evidence that the heritability of intelligence increases with age, meaning that people's IQs as adults are more predictable from the IQs of their parents than are the people's IQs when they are children.

Although intelligence appears to be partly heritable, it is almost certainly modifiable. There is no contradiction here. Height is highly heritable, much more so than intelligence, but it is also environmentally modifiable. For example, average heights have increased over recent years in many counties.

A number of programmes have been devised to help people increase their intelligence (e.g. Feuerstein, 1980). Psychologists disagree as to the effectiveness of particular programs, but most psychologists believe that modification of abilities is possible in at least some degree. The best way in which to achieve such modification is a matter of debate.

To summarize, intelligence is the ability to adapt flexibly and effectively to the environment. Although there are different theories of intelligence, all have in common their attempt to understand just how people adapt. A number of measures of intelligence have been proposed. Although the measures differ somewhat, all show fairly high correlations, meaning that they seem to measure relatively similar abilities. New attempts to understand and measure intelligence are generally taking a broader view, according to which the conventional tests measure just a small fraction of the full range of human intelligence.

ACKNOWLEDGEMENTS

Research for this chapter was supported under the Javits Act Program (Grant R206RG50001) as administered by the Office of Educational Research and Improvement (OERI), US Department of Education. Grantees undertaking such projects are encouraged to express freely their professional judgement. This chapter therefore, does not necessarily represent positions or policies of the Government, and no official endorsement should be inferred.

I would like to thank the Office of Educational Research and Improvement for supporting my work and research on human intelligence.

REFERENCES

Berry, J.W. (1984). Towards a universal psychology of cognitive competence. In P.S. Fry (Ed.). *Changing conception of intelligence and intellectual functioning*, pp. 35–61. Amsterdam: North Holland.

Binet, A. & Simon, T. (1908). Méthodes nouvelles pour le diagnostic du niveau intellectuel des anormaux. *L'Année psychologique*, 11, 245–336.

Cattell, R.B. (1971). *Abilities: their structure, growth, and action*. Boston: Houghton Mifflin.

Eysenck, H.J. (1982). *A model for intelligence*. Berlin: Springer.

Feuerstein, R. (1980). *Instrumental enrichment: an intervention program for cognitive modifiability*. Baltimore: University Park Press.

Galton, F. (1883). *Inquiry into human faculty and its development*. London: Macmillan.

Gardner, H. (1983). *Frames of mind: the theory of multiple intelligence*. New York: Basic Books.

Guilford, J.P. (1967). *The nature of intelligence*. New York: Mc Graw-Hill.

Guilford, J.P. (1982). Cognitive psychology's ambiguities: some suggested remedies. *Psychological Review*, 89, 48–59.

Haier, R.J., Siegel, B., Tang, C., Abel, L. & Buchsbaum, M.S. (1992). Intelligence and changes in regional cerebral glucose metabolic rate following learning. *Intelligence*. 16, 415–26.

Hunt, E.B. (1978). Mechanics of verbal ability. *Psychological Review*, 85, 109–30.

Jensen, A.R. (1982). Reaction time and psychometric g. In H.J. Eysenck (Ed.) *A model for intelligence*. Heidelberg: Springer-Verlag.

Laboratory of Comparative Human Cognition (1982). Culture and intelligence. In R.J. Sternberg (Ed.) *Handbook of human intelligence*, pp. 642–719. Cambridge University Press.

Levy, J. (1974). Psychobiological implications of bilateral asymmetry. In S. Dimond & S. Beaumond (Eds.). *Hemispheric function in the human brain*, pp. 121–83. New York: Halsted.

Newell, A. & Simon, H.A. (1972). *Human problem solving*. Englewood Cliffs, NJ: Prentice-Hall.

Piaget, J. (1972). *The psychology of intelligence*. Totowa, NJ: Littlefield, Adams.

Schafer, E.W.P. (1982). Neural adaptability: a biological determinant of behavioral intelligence. *International Journal of Neuroscience*, 17, 183–91.

Spearman, C. (1923). *The nature of 'intelligence' and the principles of cognition*. London: Macmillan.

Sternberg, R.J. (1977). *Intelligence, information processing, and analogical reasoning: The componential analysis of human abilities*. Hillsdale, NJ: Erlbaum.

Sternberg, R.J. (1985). *Beyond IQ: A triarchic theory of human intelligence*. New York:

Cambridge University Press.

Stemberg, R.J. & Grigorenko, E.L. (1997). *Intelligence, heredity and environment*. New York: Cambridge University Press.

Thurstone, L.L. (1938). *Primary mental abilities*. Chicago: University of Chicago Press.

Vernon, P.A. & Mori, M. (1992). Intelligence, reaction times, and peripheral nerve conduction velocity. *Intelligence*, 16, 273–88.

Judgement and decision-making

GENE ROWE

University of Surrey, Psychology Department, UK

GEORGE WRIGHT

The School of Business and Economic Studies, Leeds University, UK

PETER AYTON

City University, London. Psychology Department, UK

INTRODUCTION

Decision-making is a mental process by which a person (or indeed, a group or organization) identifies a choice or judgement to be made, gathers and evaluates information about alternatives, and selects from amongst these (e.g. Carroll & Johnson, 1990). In many cases, researchers and writers do not differentiate decision-making from judgement, although the latter concept may be seen as a specific and important component of the decision-making process, that differs from choice. In particular, judgement is an inferential cognitive process by which an individual draws conclusions about an unknown quantity or quality on the basis of available information; it is a kind of comparison or matching task, in the sense that a single alternative or attribute is matched to a response scale label (e.g. on a rating scale). By contrast, a choice task involves comparisons of, and selection among, a number of alternatives. The reader should not be alarmed by the interchangeability of the various terms in this chapter, or in many articles in this field: the essence of this research realm is simply understanding and assessing the adequacy of a number of human cognitive activities that may broadly be called decisions.

The following example from Bakwin (1945) practically demonstrates the kind of issues that are of concern to researchers in this field, and why the topic is important to medical practitioners, amongst others. In this study, a panel of three physicians were recruited to screen 389 schoolboys, of whom 45% were recommended for the surgical removal of their tonsils. A second panel of a different three physicians, however, when asked to assess the need for tonsillectomies in the cleared 215 boys, suggested that 46% of these would require surgery too. Furthermore, a third panel of physicians, who considered the 116 boys who had been twice cleared, recommended that 44% of these would also need tonsillectomies! Clearly the quality of the decision-making of the physicians

here was not all that it could have been, and had action been taken on their advice, the result would have been a waste of time and money, and not a little pain!

The questions which arise from Bakwin's study are numerous. Considering that the physicians must have undergone similar training, their lack of consistency of advice is surprising, although the proportions recommended for surgery by successive panels suggests that the physicians were making consistent relative judgements, but were insensitive about aspects of the absolute nature of tonsils. Was their training inappropriate? Does the misdiagnosis of the need for tonsillectomies reflect a more general human inability or an inherently difficult task? Are these results unique, or are they reflective of common trends in other medical tasks, other experts or other disciplines? If decision-making is poor, is it possible to ameliorate or improve it, and if so, how? Consideration of these issues form the basis of this chapter.

CLASSICAL DECISION THEORY

Interest and research in decision making has its roots in classical economic theory (e.g. von Neumann and Morgenstern, 1944), being introduced into the field of cognitive psychology in the 1950s in the form of the Subjective Expected Utility theory, or SEU (e.g. Edwards, 1954). The SEU theory or model assumes that decision-makers follow a highly rational procedure for making a decision, with decisions relying upon the combination of two independent types of information: subjective probabilities attached to the occurrence of events, and subjective values (utilities) attached to the outcomes of those events. The details of the theory are best made clear by a simple example.

Suppose an individual has to make a decision concerning whether or not to take his umbrella to work. The individual is faced with two alternatives, namely, 'take umbrella' or 'leave umbrella'. Clearly, a number of events may arise that will influence the individual's choice, most particularly, whether or not it will rain. If the individual leaves his umbrella and it rains, then he will get wet (an outcome with negative (subjective) utility) but if it does not rain, then the outcome may be said to have positive utility, in that the individual does not have to carry the umbrella around all day. Conversely, if the individual takes his umbrella and it rains, then the outcome may be seen to be of positive utility (or at least, non-negative utility) although the absence of rain may make carrying the umbrella an annoyance. SEU theory suggests that the individual will attempt to maximize his (subjective) expected utility, by assessing the probability of rain and the utilities of the various outcomes, such as getting wet, or carrying an unused umbrella. By summing the product of probability and utility for each event/outcome within a particular alternative, a value may be derived for each alternative.

In our hypothetical example, assume the individual rates the probability of rain as 0.6 (or 60%) and consequently, that of 'no rain' as 0.4 (40%). The individual rates, subjectively, the four events as follows: get wet (−2), stay dry without umbrella (+2), stay dry with umbrella (+1), and stay dry but carry umbrella (−1). The SEU formula therefore gives the following results:

Alternative 1 (take umbrella) = (0.6 × 1) + (0.4 × −1) = 0.2

Alternative 2 (leave umbrella) = (0.6 × −2) + (0.4 × 2) = −0.4

Here, theory suggests that the individual will take the umbrella, since the subjective expected utility for this is higher than that for leaving the umbrella behind.

Although in the above example the utility and probability values have been noted as though simply voiced by the hypothetical individual (a direct method which is often used) other methods have been developed for their elicitation because of difficulties with the direct approach (e.g. people dislike giving extreme values; estimates elicited as odds or straightforward probabilities often differ, etc.). One method frequently used is that of the reference wager. In the case of utilities, an example of this method might involve offering an individual the choice between, say, a certain £500, and a wager in which they would win either £1000 or nothing. The individual would be required to indicate the probability of winning the wager that would make them indifferent between the two choices. If the individual quoted a 0.7 or 70% value, then the expected utility of the wager would be computed as: (0.7 × 1000) + (0.3 × 0) = 700. That is, relative to the utilities of £1000 or nothing, the wager is given a utility of 700, and since the wager's utility is 700, and the individual is indifferent between the wager and £500, it follows that £500 must have associated with it a utility of 700. This specific result indicates that the individual's utility for money is risk adverse in the sense that the certainty of £500 is seen as equivalent to the expectation, in monetary value, of £700.

The basic normative prescription that individuals should combine information according to the SEU formula, follows from a set of relatively uncontroversial first principles, or axioms, concerning the behaviour of the decision-maker. These include: that the decision maker has a consistent set of preferences, of which they are aware; that they know all available alternatives; and that they have access to information concerning the consequences of selecting each alternative. See Goodwin and Wright (1991) for a full discussion of the axioms and their acceptability.

PROBLEMS WITH CLASSICAL THEORY: BOUNDED RATIONALITY

Research throughout the 1950s and 1960s, however, soon began to call into question the descriptive validity of the classical model of decision-making. Much of this research sought to show that people do not make decisions according to the SEU formulation, although doubt was often cast upon such demonstrations because of the lack, in this field, of an appropriate error theory. Error theories are concerned with the accuracy of measurement instruments; they dictate the amount of trust one can place in the reading of an apparatus, as when stating that a thermometer is accurate to within plus or minus one degree centigrade. Unfortunately, techniques for eliciting utilities and probabilities from decision makers lack the precision of the instruments of the natural sciences. One example of this measurement difficulty was alluded to above, namely, that different subjective probabilities tend to be gained from subjects according to whether they are asked to express their uncertainty in terms of odds or direct probabilities. People also tend to show inconsistencies in expressing such uncertainties under apparently similar circumstances. In the case of utilities, such an inconsistency could be interpreted as being due to either a change in a subject's utility occurring between measurements, or due to the imprecision of the utility instrument.

Evidence against the descriptive status of SEU, however, has continued to accumulate, with experiments demonstrating that people tend to behave in manners at odds to various of the SEU axioms. For example, evidence has shown that people sometimes infringe the transitivity axiom (which states that, in assessing the utilities of three events, 'a', 'b' and 'c', if an individual prefers 'a' to 'b', and 'b' to 'c', then they should prefer 'a' to 'c'), and also the independence axiom (that is, that a preference of one choice over another should not be affected by the presence or absence of a third choice option). Other evidence suggests that people generally do not utilize probabilities very well and do not behave coherently according to the laws of probability, for example, in being supra-additive (i.e. in assessing the probabilities of a set of mutually exclusive and exhaustive events, they sum probabilities to greater than one). A good review on the arguments against (and for) SEU has been provided by Slovic, Fischhoff and Lichtenstein (1977).

One of the earliest and most influential critics of SEU was Herbert Simon (e.g. 1945). In the economic literature, he argued against the so-called economic man characterized by the classic decision making theories, an entity who uses his thorough insight of all possible alternatives to rationally choose the best of these, and postulated the administrative man, who possesses only a limited knowledge of possible alternatives, and is able to evaluate only a few of these simultaneously. The key concept behind the administrative man was Simon's idea of bounded rationality, that human decision-makers look at the world with a simplified model of reality and exhibit satisficing rather than *maximizing* behaviour, i.e. choosing the alternative which gives just enough satisfaction for their level of aspiration, rather than seeking further for a best alternative. At the heart of the idea of bounded rationality is the recognition that humans possess certain cognitive limitations in terms of attention, processing capacity, and so on, that prevent them (in many cases) from following behaviour which is optimal according to logically derived models. From this viewpoint, SEU at best provides a normative or prescriptive model of how decisions ought to be made, rather than how they actually are made.

HEURISTICS AND BIASES

The idea of cognitive limitation implicit in the concept of bounded rationality is an important one. Much research, particularly from the 1970s to the present time, has been concerned with understanding exactly what these limitations are, and how they affect or characterize typical patterns of human decision making. The most significant recent contributors have been Tversky and Kahneman. In several highly influential papers (e.g. Tversky & Kahneman, 1974) they reported the results of a number of studies (mainly) involving the assessment of probabilities, in which they identified patterns of behaviour which they labelled heuristics; specifically, the heuristics of availability, representativeness and anchoring and adjustment. In many cases these heuristics, or rules of thumb, may lead to accurate probability assessment or good decisions (hence, a form of 'rationality' within constraints), although Tversky and Kahneman's research also showed how they might result in systematic *biases*. Because of the large amount of research that has followed, the heuristics, and associated potential biases, will be briefly described.

The representativeness heuristic concerns the extent to which one event or variable is representative, or resembles, another. That is, many probabilistic questions with which people are concerned are of the form: what is the probability that event A belongs to class B? and what is the probability that event A originates from process B? According to Tversky and Kahneman, individuals' answers to such questions will depend upon the degree to which A and B are similar, or resemble one another. For example, when asked to choose one of several occupations as that most likely for 'Steve, who is very shy and withdrawn, invariably helpful, but with little interest in people or the world of reality . . . (he is) meek and tidy . . . with a need for order and structure and a passion for detail', subjects tend to select 'librarian' (as opposed to, for example, an engineer), because of the high degree to which the individual description (A) is representative of the stereotype of a librarian (B). This heuristic, though often useful, may also lead to a number of systematic biases, which include (a) insensitivity to prior probability of outcomes (i.e. base rates); (b) insensitivity to sample size (conservatism); (c) misconceptions of chance (e.g. gambler's fallacy); (d) insensitivity to predictability (i.e. the degree to which the reliability of descriptions allow accurate prediction); (e) the illusion of validity (unwarranted confidence in the apparently good fit between predicted outcome and input information); and (f) misconceptions of regression (typically, observed regression to the mean is something which is almost negatively related to resemblance). (For further details of these biases, the reader is referred to the original article.)

Availability concerns situations in which people assess the frequency of a class, or the probability of an event, by the ease with which instances or occurrences are called to mind (e.g. in assessing the likelihood of lung cancer, a person might recall instances among family and friends). According to Tversky and Kahneman, this heuristic may often be valid for judging the frequency or probability of an event, since instances of frequent events are typically easier to recall than instances of less-frequent events. However, because availability may be affected by factors other than frequency this may lead to predictable biases, which include: (a) biases due to retrievability of instances (instances may be recalled easier for reasons other than frequency, such as due to familiarity, saliency, or recency); (b) biases due to the effectiveness of a search set (e.g. words starting with 'r' are easier to search for than those ending in 'r', so the former may be assessed as more frequent); (c) biases of imaginability (e.g. imagining lots of dangers may lead to a biased view of how dangerous a project really is); and (d) illusory correlation (certain characteristics are more easily/ readily associated with others, creating illusory correlations even when they do not exist).

The anchoring and adjustment heuristic describes a process by which people make an estimate by starting from a certain value, or anchor, and then adjusting this value to yield a final answer. This initial value may be either given, or produced as the result of a partial calculation, in either case, adjustment is usually insufficient, and final answers are biased towards the initial value. Tversky and Kahneman suggest that this process might explain biases in the evaluation of conjunctive and disjunctive events (i.e. events whose probability depend upon either the occurrence or otherwise of other, 'simpler' probabilistic events), due to inappropriate anchoring on the simpler probability values, with overestimation of the former and underestimation of the latter. They also suggest that this heuristic might account for other observed phenomena, such as the insufficient adjustment of the range of a subjective probability distribution from the anchor of a single initial best guess.

Tversky and Kahneman's work appeared to tie in with, and potentially explain, a large number of the growing list of examples of poor human judgement and decision-making. We have previously noted some of these, such as incoherence with the laws of probability, such as the laws of additivity and intersection. Other frequently demonstrated biases include those of overconfidence (i.e. when judges express a greater certainty in the occurrence or correctness of a judgement than is subsequently shown to be inappropriate in terms of calibration), and the hindsight bias (in which the predictability of a prior event is overestimated). Although the adequacy of the above heuristics to account for and explain such biases has been a matter of some debate, many researchers use (and have used) a heuristic framework to explain their results (for review, see Wright & Ayton, 1994).

Another major line of research has considered the inadequacy of human judgement and decision-making according to more objective performance criteria, rather than in comparison to the prescriptions of normative theories like SEU, or the laws of probability theory. Much of this work has stemmed from that of Meehl (1954), who summarized approximately 20 studies in which the clinical predictions of trained experts were compared to statistical predictions in the form of linear models, these being derived through regression analysis on the same information on which the experts themselves based their predictions (usually test scores or biographical facts). In all of these studies the statistical method was as accurate as, or more so than, clinical judgement. Subsequent research has supported and extended these findings (e.g. Dawes & Corrigan, 1974). In particular, research has shown that improper linear models, which use expert predictions *per se* as the modelled criterion variable, also tend to have higher external validity than the judges themselves. Explanations of this phenomenon, known as bootstrapping, centre upon the ability of statistical models to counter human inconsistency and unreliability in judgement (with reliability being a necessary, though not necessarily sufficient condition for validity). Other explanations centre upon a human inability to appropriately combine and weight the importance of predictor variables (i.e. to combine large amounts of information in an appropriate mathematical manner). See Bunn and Wright (1991) for a fuller discussion of the issue.

The key point which emerges from the above research is that human judgement and decision making can be of low validity, being typically characterized by unreliability, a lack of mental capacity to deal with complex problems, and the existence of simplistic strategies or heuristics that may lead to systematic and predictable errors. Indeed, on the basis of such research findings, a number of researchers have suggested that man may be an 'intellectual cripple', whose intuitive judgments and decisions violate many of the fundamental principles of optimal behavior. Other researchers, however, have argued that the question of the quality of human judgement has not been settled and it is to these studies we turn next.

THE NATURE OF BIAS: ILLUSORY, METHODOLOGICAL OR REAL?

One counter-view is that the pervasiveness of bias is exaggerated. Christensen–Szalanski and Beach (1984), for example, have suggested that the evidence for poor judgement is not quite so compelling as a scan of the literature would lead one to believe. They reviewed more than 3500 abstracts of articles published on judgement and reasoning between 1972 and 1981, and found that of these, only 84 (or 2.4%) were actual empirical studies, of which 47 obtained poor performance compared to 37 which found good performance (i.e. a ratio of 1.3 to 1). Examining the Social Science Citation Index, however, they found that poor performance results were cited, on average, six times as often as those of good performance, an effect they termed the Citation Bias. From this perspective, bias may exist, but it is not as endemic as often made out.

Other criticisms even question the results of those studies which have shown bias and faulty judgement. For example, Beach, Christensen–Szalanski and Barnes (1987) have suggested that much of the apparent poor performance of subjects in judgemental tasks may be due to subjects framing problems differently to experimenters, and hence effectively working on a different task to that intended, with dispute also arising as to whose frame (subject or experimenter) is the most appropriate. Indeed, Cohen (1979) conducted a major critique on the derogatory view of the human decision-maker along these latter lines, arguing that supposedly normative models (such as SEU) may not be as optimal for making real-world judgements and decisions as is commonly accepted, and that supposed biases may actually reflect logical approaches to situations that are more complex than those found in laboratory tasks set by psychologists.

Following from the above criticisms, the main concern of a number of researchers about the work in this area focuses upon its ecological validity or the extent to which research conditions are analogous and applicable to workaday conditions and tasks. A number of authors have noted that many of the most widely cited studies have used subjects who are undergraduate students completing paper and pencil tasks or abstract word problems, the generalizability of which are questionable. In particular, arguments against generalizability have referred to the static nature of laboratory tasks (as opposed to the dynamic nature of those in the real-world); the real-world utility of so-called biases; and findings that judgemental problems may sometimes be overcome by rephrasing or altering problems or by concretizing them, such as by having subjects actually experience frequencies, rather than simply assessing figures (e.g. for discussions see Beach, Christensen–Szalanski and Barnes, 1987).

Indeed, there has been a growing trend towards more ecologically-valid studies, considering judgement and decision making by 'people who care in situations that matter', viz professional experts. Results from these studies, however, have been somewhat equivocal on the question of judgemental quality. Although, evidence for good judgement has come from a number of studies, such as on weather forecasters, bridge players, and bankers predicting future interest rates, others have found evidence of poor judgement and identifiable biases, in estates agents valuing houses, court judges giving sentences, and physicians overestimating the risk of certain diseases, etc. (for reviews see Bolger & Wright, 1992).

One suggestion to account for the equivocality of these more-ecological studies has been forwarded by Bolger and Wright (1992), who propose that the potential for making unbiased judgements depends as much on situational factors related to the task domain as upon any personal characteristics of the judge. They predict that experts will only be able to develop an unbiased expertise when certain situational requirements hold, namely, when the task allows accurate, relevant and objective data upon which the expert's decisions may be based; when there is the possibility of the experts expressing their judgements in a coherent and quantifiable manner, and when the task allows rapid and meaningful feedback about the accuracy of experts' judgements. Arguably, many real-world situations do not provide these ideal circumstances, and the biases deriving from misapplications of heuristics or the use of natural judgement strategies, and from our limited mental capabilities, are likely to arise.

CONCLUSION: CONTENDING WITH BIAS

Accepting bias and unreliability to exist in decision making (more widely) and judgement (more specifically), a number of approaches have been developed to pre-empt or ameliorate their impact. Decision analysis uses classical decision theory to help individuals (and groups) analyse difficult problems, by eliciting simple probabilities and utilities and then doing the complex mathematical combinations, according to the laws of probability and dictates of expected utility theory, for them (e.g. see Goodwin & Wright, 1991). Similarly, statistical techniques such as linear modelling restrict human input to the identification of appropriate predictor variables and their sign (i.e. whether they are positively or negatively related to the criterion variable being judged), but then mathematically combine and weight these in place of the individual, while also reducing the impact of inconsistent human behaviour. In essence, these approaches allow the human judge or decision-maker to supply whatever input they are able, but then replaces them at those tasks at which they have typically been shown to be poor (e.g. see Kleinmuntz, 1990 for review).

Difficulties arise, however, in the practical application of techniques like linear modelling. For example there is often, in organizations, a lack of appropriate model-building skills; an absence of awareness that judgemental difficulties may exist and are amenable to cure, and a lack of will to surrender important organizational decisions and judgements to such techniques (a phenomenon which Dawes (e.g. 1988) has attributed to organizational resistance and cognitive conceit). Nevertheless, at present such approaches seem the best available for dealing with poor judgemental performance:

other procedures aimed at debiasing the individual, such as by simply alerting them to the cause of poor judgements or decisions, have generally been shown to have little impact (e.g. Fischhoff, 1982). However, much more research needs to be conducted on the debiasing of individuals over a wider range of biases, as well as on determining the contingency of bias, that is, where and when it might be expected to occur, and where good judgement might reasonably be expected.

REFERENCES

Bakwin, H. (1945). Pseudoxia pediatrica. *New England Journal of Medicine*, **232**, 691–7.

Beach, L.R., Christensen-Szalanski, J.J.J. & Barnes, V. (1987). Assessing human judgment: has it been done, can it be done, should it be done?. In G. Wright and P. Ayton (Eds.). *Judgmental forecasting*, Chichester: Wiley.

Bolger, F. & Wright, G. (1992). Reliability and validity in expert judgment. In G. Wright and F. Bolger (Eds.). *Expertise and decision support*, New York: Plenum.

Bunn, D. & Wright, G. (1991). Interaction of judgemental and statistical forecasting methods: Issues and analysis. *Management Science*, **37**, 501–18.

Carroll, J.S. & Johnson, E.J. (1990). *Decision research: a field guide*. Newbury Park, CA.: Sage.

Christensen-Szalanski, J.J.J. & Beach, L.R. (1984). The citation bias: fad and fashion in the judgment and decision literature. *American Psychologist*, **39**, 75–8.

Cohen, L.J. (1979). On the psychology of prediction: Whose is the fallacy? *Cognition*, **7**, 385–407.

Dawes, R. (1988). *Rational choice in an uncertain world*. San Diego: Harcourt Brace, Jovanovich.

Dawes, R.M. & Corrigan, B. (1974). Linear models in decision making. *Psychological Bulletin*, **81**, 95–106.

Edwards, W. (1954). The theory of decision making. *Psychological Bulletin*, **51**, 380–417.

Fischhoff, B. (1982). Debiasing. In D. Kahneman, P. Slovic and A. Tversky (Eds.). *Judgement under uncertainty: heuristics and biases*, Cambridge: Cambridge University Press.

Goodwin, P. & Wright, G. (1991). *Decision analysis for management judgment*, Chichester: Wiley.

Kleinmuntz, B. (1990). Why we still use our heads instead of formulas: towards an integrative approach. *Psychological Bulletin*, **107**, 296–310.

Meehl, P.E. (1954). *Clinical versus statistical prediction: a theoretical analysis and a review of the evidence*. Minneapolis: University of Minnesota Press.

Simon, H.A. (1945). *Administrative behavior*. New York: Macmillan.

Slovic, P. & Fischhoff, B. (1977). On the psychology of experimental surprises. *Journal of Experimental Psychology: Human Perception and Performance*, **3**, 544–51.

Slovic, P., Fischhoff, B. & Lichtenstein, S. (1977). Behavioral decision theory. *Annual Review of Psychology*, **28**, 1–39.

Tversky, A. & Kahneman, D. (1974). 'Judgment under uncertainty: heuristics and biases'. *Science*, **185**, 1124–31.

von Neumann, J. & Morgenstern, D. (1944). *Theory of games and economic behavior*. New York: Wiley.

Wright, G. & Ayton, P. (1994). *Subjective probability*. Chichester and New York: Wiley.

Memory

MICHAEL W. EYSENCK
Royal Holloway, University of London, UK

INTRODUCTION

The simplest possible way of conceptualizing memory would be to assume that there is a single, unified memory system that is involved in all our activities. That seems implausible at a commonsensical level because of the enormous variety of disparate ways in which memory is used. We remember a new telephone number for the few seconds it takes to dial it, we remember important details of our own past, we possess much general knowledge about the world, we perhaps know how to perform motor skills such as piano playing or riding a bicycle, and so on. It is reasonable to assume that a number of different interacting memory systems are involved in handling this variety.

The notion that there is an important distinction between a short-term memory store and a long-term memory store goes back a very long way. One of clearest conceptions was offered by James (1890). He drew a distinction between primary memory and secondary memory. Primary memory refers to information forming part of the psychological present, in the sense that it remains the focus of attention after it has been perceived. In contrast, secondary memory refers to information forming part of the psychological past, meaning that the information has left conscious awareness.

It is now almost universally accepted that the distinction between short-term memory and long-term memory is an important one, so there is no need to discuss the evidence in detail. However, it is worth mentioning briefly what is perhaps the strongest evidence in favour of the distinction. Most amnesic patients have essentially intact short-term memory in spite of having severely impaired long-term memory, but a few brain-damaged patients exhibit the opposite pattern of impaired short-term memory coupled with almost normal long-term memory (for a review, see Eysenck & Keane, 1990). These findings indicate convincingly that there are at least partially separate short-term and long-term memory systems occupying somewhat different areas within the brain.

During the 1960s, several multi-store models were proposed. All of these models (e.g. Atkinson & Shiffrin, 1968) had, at their centre, separate short-term and long-term memory stores. None of these models has stood the test of time, in large measure because they were grossly over-simplified. In particular, it was assumed that there is a unitary short-term store and a unitary long-term store. So far as short-term memory is concerned, there is now reasonable agreement that the unitary short-term store should be replaced by a working memory system. According to Baddeley's (1986) working memory model, working memory consists of three major components: a central executive, which is an attention-like system; an articulatory loop system, which is involved in rehearsing and storing information in a speech-based form; and a visuo-spatial sketch pad, which is specialized for spatial and/or visual coding.

One piece of evidence indicating the value of a multi-component approach was reported by Baddeley (1979). He discovered that articulatory suppression (i.e. repeatedly saying something simple such as 'the the the') had no effect on processing time or comprehension on a reading task. This finding is somewhat mysterious from the viewpoint of a unified short-term memory system, but is readily explained in terms of the working memory model. According to that model, articulatory suppression utilizes the resources of the articulatory loop, whereas reading comprehension uses primarily the resources of the central executive. It is because the two tasks (i.e. reading and articulating) do not compete for the same limited processing resources that they can be combined without disruption to performance.

So far as long-term memory is concerned, there is almost complete agreement that it no longer makes sense to think in terms of a unitary long-term store. However, there is markedly less agreement on the number and nature of systems operating in long-term memory.

For most practical purposes, long-term memory is considerably more importance than short-term memory. In research terms, too, long-term memory has attracted far more interest than short-term memory. Accordingly, the rest of this chapter will be concerned with long-term memory and with the applicability of the findings to practical and medical issues.

COMPONENTS OF LONG-TERM MEMORY

Episodic and semantic memory

An influential attempt to sub-divide long-term memory into two major components was made by Tulving (1972), who drew a distinction between episodic memory and semantic memory. Episodic memory is sometimes known as autobiographical memory, because it is concerned with personal memories for events or episodes. There is usually at least partial ability to remember where and when

any given event occurred. In contrast, semantic memory is concerned with the general knowledge that we possess about the world. According to Tulving (1972), 'It is a mental thesaurus, organized knowledge a person possesses about words and other verbal symbols, their meanings and referents, about relations among them, and about rules, formulas, and algorithms for the manipulation of these symbols, concepts, and relations' (p. 386).

Episodic and semantic memory obviously differ in terms of the content of the information stored in them. However, that is not, in and of itself, sufficient evidence to support the existence of two separate memory systems. There is less compelling evidence that episodic and semantic memory differ in terms of the processes involved. In addition, all the evidence suggests that episodic and semantic memory are strongly interdependent in their functioning. For example, remembering your last summer holiday would usually be regarded as involving episodic memory. However, thinking about planes, cars, hotels, tents, beaches, and so on involves substantial reliance on semantic memory.

Tulving (1990) reported some interesting findings that appear to strengthen the view that there are major differences between episodic and semantic memory. Regional cerebral bloodflow patterns were obtained while subjects focused on episodic or semantic memories. The key result was that rather different regions of the cortex were most active in the two memory conditions: the anterior (frontal and temporal) regions of the cortex were relatively more activated during episodic recollection, whereas the posterior (parietal and temporal) regions of the cortex were relatively more activated during semantic recollection. These findings provide evidence that different areas of the brain are implicated in episodic and semantic memory.

In sum, the distinction between episodic and semantic memory is an important one. However, the evidence has so far failed to indicate that there are two separate long-term memory systems as was originally proposed by Tulving (1972).

Declarative and procedural knowledge

Cohen and Squire (1980) proposed that long-term memory is divided into separate declarative and procedural systems. In general terms, declarative knowledge corresponds to knowing that (e.g. knowing that San Francisco is in California), and encompasses both episodic and semantic memory. Procedural knowledge, on the other hand, corresponds to knowing how, and is concerned with the ability to behave in a skilled fashion in the absence of conscious recollection. Common examples of procedural knowledge are knowing how to ride a bicycle and knowing how to play tennis.

As we will see later in the chapter, the strongest empirical support for the distinction has come from research on amnesic patients. There is good evidence that amnesic patients are generally very poor at new declarative learning, but they are virtually normal at new procedural learning. This evidence indicates that long-term memory is subdivided in approximately the way proposed by Cohen and Squire (1980). However, it should be noted that a complicating factor is that many skills involve a mixture of both kinds of knowledge. As Eysenck and Keane (1990) pointed out, while golfing skills would appear to be procedural, it is nevertheless the case that most golfers make use of declarative knowledge (e.g. 'Hit through the ball') while playing golf.

RETRIEVAL FROM LONG-TERM MEMORY

Recall and recognition

We all know from personal experience that it is often easier to retrieve information from long-term memory when the information has to be recognized than when it has to be recalled. For example, you may not be able to recall an acquaintance's name, but as soon as someone mentions the name, you remember immediately that you did actually have that person's name stored away in long-term memory.

Tulving has made a substantial contribution to our understanding of how information is retrieved from long-term memory. He assumes that there are various basic similarities between recall and recognition, and he assumes that both conform to his encoding specificity principle: 'The probability of successful retrieval of the target item is a monotonically increasing function of informational overlap between the information present at retrieval and the information stored in memory' (Tulving, 1979, p. 408). In other words, the success of recall and recognition both depend on the similarity between the information stored in memory and the information available at the time of the recall or recognition test.

According to the encoding specificity principle, recognition memory is better than recall because the informational overlap is typically greater with recognition (because the to-be-remembered item is physically present) than with recall (where the to-be-remembered item is not physically present). However, it follows from the encoding specificity principle that recall could be superior to recognition if the informational overlap were greater on the recall test than on the recognition test, and this surprising finding has been obtained several times. For example, Muter (1978) presented his subjects with people's names (e.g. Doyle, Ferguson, Thomas) and asked them to recognize those people who were famous before 1950. After this recognition test, they were given a test of cued recall (e.g. author of the Sherlock Holmes stories: Sir Arthur Conan _____; Welsh poet: Dylan _____). Subjects recognized only 29% of the names but recalled 42% of them. Presumably the greater amount of relevant information provided at recall than on the recognition test enabled recall to surpass recognition memory.

Tulving's encoding specificity principle has been one of the most influential theoretical notions in memory research. However, two limitations with it need to be mentioned. First, while the central focus of the principle is on 'informational overlap' between what is in long-term memory and what is presented at retrieval, it is seldom, if ever, possible to measure this informational overlap in a direct fashion. This clearly reduces the testability of Tulving's theory. Secondly, Tulving assumed that retrieval operates in a very simple and direct fashion on the basis of informational overlap. This may be a reasonable assumption in some situations, but is clearly not so in others. For example, take the situation in which someone endeavours to answer a question such as, 'What did you do in the evening six days ago?'. There is overwhelming introspective evidence that people answer such questions by using various problem-solving strategies; they are certainly not answered by simply assessing the informational overlap between the question and stored information.

There is increased acceptance of the view that retrieval from memory often operates in a relatively flexible fashion. Thus, recognition memory can occur either directly on the basis of familiarity or indirectly on the basis of a search through long-term memory for relevant information. In similar fashion, recall can occur either in a very direct and immediate fashion or it can occur after strategic or problem-solving activities. The details of these various forms of retrieval are discussed at length by Eysenck and Keane (1990). Some of the relevant issues are dealt with in the next section.

Retrieval without conscious recollection

Traditional tests of retrieval from memory such as recall and recognition involve giving subjects explicit instructions to remember information that was presented previously. In recent years there has been much interest in the possibility that information can be retrieved from long-term memory in the absence of such instructions. A distinction between these two kinds of retrieval was drawn by Graf and Schachter (1985): 'Implicit memory is revealed when performance on a task is facilitated in the absence of conscious recollection; explicit memory is revealed when performance on a task requires conscious recollection of previous experiences' (p. 501).

In order to illustrate how implicit memory can be tested, we will consider a study by Tulving, Schachter and Stark (1982). In the first phase of their experiment, they asked their subjects to learn a list of long words, each of which is encountered relatively rarely in everyday life (e.g. toboggan). They were subsequently presented with word fragments (e.g. _ O _ O _ GA_), and instructed to fill in each blank so as to form a word. The subjects were not told this, but half of the solutions corresponded to words from the list that had been presented during the first phase of the experiment.

The main finding was that the subjects were generally more successful in finding a word to complete those word fragments where the word had previously been presented. This finding is commonly referred to as the repetition priming effect. It can be regarded as a measure of implicit memory, in that it indisputably reflects the existence of relevant long-term memories and subjects were not given instructions to recollect past experiences. However, it has to be admitted that the subjects might have realized that some of the solutions corresponded to list words, and so engaged in active and conscious recollection of those list words. However, there was a further finding that tends to argue against that possibility. Subjects were also given the explicit test of recognition memory. If the fragment–completion task and the recognition–memory test were both simply measures of explicit memory, then it would be expected that words that were recognized would be more likely to be associated with successful fragment completion than words that were not recognized. In fact, however, the size of the repetition priming effect was no greater for recognized words than for unrecognized words, suggesting that quite different processes were involved in the two tasks.

There have been numerous demonstrations of implicit memory (for a review, see Eysenck & Keane, 1995), and these demonstrations have involved a large number of different tasks. One of the most commonly used tasks is perceptual identification, in which subjects attempt to identify words which are displayed visually for very brief periods of time. There is a priming effect, in that words that have been seen previously are associated with better performance on the perceptual identification task (e.g. Jacoby, 1983).

There have been a number of attempts to provide a theoretical framework within which to understand explicit and implicit memory. One of the most influential approaches was developed by Roediger (1990). He distinguished between data-driven processes, which are those initiated directly by presented stimuli, and conceptually driven processes, which are those initiated by the individual. The major assumption of the theory is that performance on memory tasks will be better when the processing required on the memory task (data-driven or conceptually driven) matches the processing that was used at the time of learning than when there is a mismatch between processing at learning and at test. The relevance of this theory to the explicit/implicit distinction is that Roediger (1990) assumed that data-driven processes are typically involved in implicit memory, whereas conceptually driven processes are generally involved in explicit memory.

There is reasonable evidence (reviewed by Eysenck & Keane, 1995) that memory performance is better when there is a match between the processes used at learning and at test than when there is a mismatch. In other words, if the learning task involves data-driven processing, then performance will be better when the memory task also involves data-driven processing, and similarly for conceptually driven learning tasks (e.g. Jacoby, 1983). However, it is becoming increasingly clear that most learning and memory tasks involve a combination of data-driven and conceptually driven processes, and it is typically very difficult to assess the precise involvement of each type of processing.

AMNESIA AND LONG-TERM MEMORY

Many of the issues that have been discussed in this chapter have been clarified by the study of amnesic patients. In general terms, it has been found that the study of amnesic patients very often provides a good test-bed for existing theories of long-term memory. Consider, for example, the issue of whether there are two or more long-term memory systems. If it were found that amnesic patients showed an impaired ability to acquire certain kinds of long-term memories but an intact ability to acquire other kinds of long-term memories, then it would be a reasonable inference that long-term memory does not consist of a single, unified system.

In fact, there is strong evidence that amnesic patients exhibit normal rates of learning for many skills. First, most amnesic patients can acquire a range of motor skills as rapidly as normals; the skills examined include dressmaking, billiards, mirror drawing, and jigsaw completions. Secondly, amnesic patients exhibit a variety of priming effects. A priming effect occurs when the processing of a stimulus is facilitated the second time the stimulus is presented compared to the first even when there is an absence of conscious awareness that the stimulus has been presented previously. We have already seen an example of a priming effect (Tulving *et al.*, 1982).

Priming effects in amnesics were investigated by Graf, Squire and Mandler (1984). A word list was presented, and was followed by a memory test. Four different memory tests were used, but only the word-completion test assessed priming. On this test, subjects were given three-letter word fragments, and were told to write down the first word they could think of that started with those three letters. Priming was assessed by the extent to which the word completions corresponded to words from the list that had been presented. Amnesic patients performed as well as controls on this test, even though they performed significantly worse than controls on all of the other tests used (free recall; recognition; cued recall).

This study by Graf *et al.* (1984) can be related to the distinction between explicit and implicit memory that was discussed earlier. In essence, the findings suggest that amnesic patients have a severe deficit in explicit memory (since free recall, cued recall, and recognition memory all depend on conscious recollection), but they do not have a deficit in implicit memory. The fact that amnesic patients often show normal rates of learning on motor tasks is also consistent with that viewpoint if one assumes that motor skills do not rely on conscious recollection.

Schachter (1987) advocated precisely the theoretical position suggested in the previous paragraph. However, he also pointed out that implicit and explicit memory 'are descriptive concepts that are primarily concerned with a person's psychological experience at the time of retrieval' (p. 501). One way of moving from description to explanation would be to apply Roediger's (1990) theory about data-driven and conceptually driven processes to amnesic patients. This has been done by Blaxton (1992). She used Roediger's general approach to argue that amnesic patients should perform well when data-driven processes are used at learning and at test, but they should perform poorly when conceptually driven processes are required. The findings were generally in line with prediction. However, the amnesic patients did better on implicit memory tests than on explicit memory tests even when an attempt was made to hold constant the involvement of data-driven and conceptually driven processes. This indicates that the distinction between data-driven and conceptually driven processes cannot account for all of the findings.

Memory systems

Probably the most adequate theoretical approach is the one advocated by Squire, Knowlton and Musen (1993). They assumed that there is a memory system centred in the hippocampus, medial temporal lobes, and the diencephalon. This memory system is concerned primarily with declarative knowledge or explicit memory, and it is this brain system which is damaged in amnesic patients. Squire *et al.* argued that Korsakoff patients often also suffer damage to the frontal lobes, and they suggested that damage to the frontal lobes causes impairment to the ability to remember when events or episodes occurred. In general terms, it seems preferable to relate the problems of amnesics to identifiable brain structures as Squire *et al.* (1993) have done rather than to argue simply that amnesic patients have problems with conceptually driven processing (Blaxton, 1992).

There has been relatively little progress in terms of identifying the brain structures underlying procedural knowledge or implicit memory. This is only to be expected given that implicit memory involves a wide range of disparate skills and processes. However, there is some evidence that patients suffering from Huntington's disease (which is known to affect the basal ganglia) experience great difficulty in acquiring motor skills in spite of having normal recognition memory (Heindel, Butters & Salmon, 1988). It will be for future research to clarify the issue of the number and nature of procedural memory systems.

VALUE OF THE MEMORY SYSTEMS

In sum, research on normals and on amnesic patients has provided convincing evidence that there are at least two major memory systems, one of which is concerned with explicit memory and declarative knowledge and the other of which is concerned with implicit memory and procedural knowledge. Since that has been established, it is of interest to address the issue as to why it is that humans are equipped with these two rather separate memory systems. A provisional answer, emphasizing the special characteristics of each system, has been provided by Squire et al. (1993):

> One system involves limbic/diencephalic structures, which in concert with neocortex provides the basis for conscious recollections. This system is fast, phylogenetically recent, and specialized for one-trial learning.
> ... The system is fallible in the sense that it is sensitive to interference and prone to retrieval failure. It is also precious, giving rise to the capacity for personal autobiography and the possibility of cultural evolution.
> Other kinds of memory have also been identified. ... Such memories can be acquired, stored, and retrieved without the participation of the limbic/diencephalon brain system. These forms of memory are phylogenetically early, they are reliable and consistent, and they provide for myriad, nonconscious ways of responding to the world ... they create much of the mystery of human experience (pp. 485–486).

REFERENCES

Atkinson, R.C. & Shiffrin, R.M. (1968). Human memory: A proposed system and its control processes. In K.W. Spence & J.T. Spence (Eds.). *The psychology of learning and motivation, Vol. 2*. London: Academic Press.

Baddeley, A.D. (1979). Working memory and reading. In P.A. Kolers, M.E. Wrolstadf & H. Bouma (Eds.). *Processing of visible language*. New York: Plenum.

Baddeley, A.D. (1986). *Working memory*. Oxford: Oxford University Press.

Blaxton, T.A. (1992). Dissociations among memory measures in memory-impaired subjects: evidence for a processing account of memory. *Memory & Cognition*. 20, 549–62.

Cohen, N.J. & Squire, L.R. (1980). Preserved learning and retention of pattern-analyzing skill in amnesia using perceptual learning. *Cortex*, 17, 273–8.

Eysenck, M.W. & Keane, M.T. (1995). *Cognitive psychology: a student's handbook*. London: Lawrence Erlbaum Associates Ltd.

Eysenck, M.W. & Keane, M.T. (in press). *Cognitive psychology: a student's handbook*. 2nd edn. London: Lawrence Erlbaum Associates Ltd.

Graf, P. & Schachter, D.L. (1985). Implicit and explicit memory for new associations in normal and amnesic subjects. *Journal of Experimental Psychology: Learning, Memory, and Cognition*, 11, 501–18.

Graf, P., Squire, L.R. & Mandler, G. (1984). The information that amnesic patients do not forget. *Journal of Experimental Psychology: Learning, Memory, and Cognition*, 10, 164–78.

Heindel, W.C., Butters, N. & Salmon, D.P. (1988). Impaired learning of a motor skill in patients with Huntington's disease. *Behavioral Neuroscience*, 102, 141–7.

Jacoby, L.L. (1983). Remembering the data: analyzing interactive processes in reading. *Journal of Verbal Learning and Verbal Behavior*, 22, 485–508.

James, W. (1890). *Principles of psychology*. New York: Holt.

Muter, P. (1978). Recognition failure of recallable words in semantic memory. *Memory and Cognition*, 6, 9–12.

Roediger, H.L. III (1990). Implicit memory: retention without remembering. *American Psychologist*, 45, 1043–56.

Schachter, D.L. (1987). Implicit memory: history and current status. *Journal of Experimental Psychology: Learning, Memory, and Cognition*, 13, 501–18.

Squire, L.R., Knowlton, B. & Musen, G. (1993). The structure and organisation of memory. *Annual Review of Psychology*, 44, 453–95.

Tulving, E. (1972). Episodic and semantic memory. In E. Tulving & W. Donaldson (Eds.). *Organisation of memory*. London: Academic Press.

Tulving, E. (1979). Relation between encoding specificity and levels of processing. In L.S. Cermak & F.I.M. Craik (Eds.). *Levels of processing in human memory*. Hillsdale, NJ: Lawrence Erlbaum Associates Ltd.

Tulving, E. (1990). Memory: performance, knowledge, and experience. *European Journal of Cognitive Psychology*, 1, 3–26.

Tulving, E., Schachter, D.L. & Stark, H.A. (1982). Priming effects in word-fragment completion are independent of recognition memory. *Journal of Experimental Psychology: Learning, Memory, and Cognition*, 8, 336–42.

Personality

ROBERT R. McCRAE
and
STEPHANIE V. STONE
Gerontology Research Center, National Institute on Aging, NIH Baltimore, USA

Although the term personality is widely used by laypersons as well as psychologists, it has no universally accepted meaning. Different schools of psychology use it in widely different ways, and personality psychologists continue to debate the proper scope and limits of their discipline. In this chapter, personality refers to features of the individual that are enduring, pervasive, and distinctive; an accurate description of personality tells us what the person is really like.

The beginning of the twentieth century was marked by radical challenges to the view long held by scholars and laypersons alike that human beings were rational creatures with propensities, abilities, and beliefs that guided their conduct. For psychoanalysts, the essence of the person was instead to be found in unconscious and often irrational processes that secretly shaped thoughts, feelings, and relationships. For behaviourists, the person was an empty organism, a collection of learned responses defined by a history of reinforcements from the environment. Contemporary research has led to a rejection of both these radical positions by most contemporary personality psychologists, who once again view the person in terms of characteristic dispositions or traits and goal-directed behaviour.

But the similarity of folk and scientific conceptions of personality should not lead the reader to assume that personality psychology is nothing but common-sense. It is only common sense to believe that old age leads to depression and social withdrawal, that raising the standard of living will make everyone happier, that parental discipline is the most important determinant of character. But none of these beliefs happens to be true (McCrae & Costa, 1990). It is particularly important to view common-sense beliefs about psychological effects on physical health with some scepticism.

Trait psychology has become the dominant paradigm for the study of personality, and the remainder of this chapter will focus on current conceptions of individual differences and some of their broad implications for health and medicine. For a discussion of alternative approaches to personality, consult McAdams (1990) or Pervin (1993).

THE NATURE OF TRAITS

Personality traits can be defined as 'dimensions of individual differences in tendencies to show consistent patterns of thoughts, feelings, and actions' (McCrae & Costa, 1990, p. 23). One patient, for example, may be friendly and talkative and eager to communicate with the physician, whereas another may be reserved and volunteer little information. In part, these behavioural differences may be due to past experience with physicians who encouraged or discouraged a personal relationship. But, in part, they are also likely to reflect pervasive characteristics of the patient, individual differences in the personality dimension of extraversion. Extraverts tend to be sociable, energetic, and enthusiastic whether they are at home, at work, at a party, or in the hospital.

The definition calls attention to several important aspects of traits. The word dimension implies a continuous distribution of traits in the population. Although it is convenient to talk about 'introverts' and 'extraverts', in fact most people have an intermediate level of extraversion. All personality traits approximate a normal, bell-shaped distribution. The word tendencies highlights the fact that trait influences are probabilistic: even the most well-adjusted person is occasionally anxious or depressed; even the most conscientious person occasionally fails to complete a task. As a consequence, personality traits usually cannot be inferred from a single behavior or a single interaction; instead, personality assessment requires the search for consistent patterns across many times and situations. Personality traits cut across the academic distinctions between cognitive, affective, and behavioural domains; they are inferred not merely from overt behaviour, as habits would be, but

also from patterns of thoughts and feelings. One implication of this fact is that the individual, who is privy to his or her inner experiences, is often the best source of information on personality.

THE STRUCTURE OF TRAITS

The English language has well over 4000 adjectives to describe personality traits, and personality psychologists have developed hundreds of scales to measure traits they considered important. For decades, the sheer number of traits made systematic research difficult. If a researcher wished to discover the traits associated with, say, hypertension or arthritis, which should be measured? Short of assessing all 4000, research was bound to be hit-or-miss. When different researchers chose to measure different traits, how could their results be compared?

If all 4000 words referred to completely different traits, there would be no easy solution to those problems. But, in fact, there is great redundancy among trait terms and formal psychological constructs. The terms assertive, bossy, controlling, dominant and exacting all refer to similar, if not identical, attributes. These similarities can be used to organize a trait taxonomy.

Factor analysis has been the chief tool in investigating personality structure. A group of individuals complete measures of a number of different traits, and their scores are intercorrelated. Factor analysis provides a way to identify dimensions of traits that covary with each other and that are relatively independent of other dimensions of traits. For example, people who score high on measures of orderliness tend also to score high on measures of dutifulness and punctuality, and people who score high on imaginativeness also tend to score high on measures of curiosity and artistic interests.

In the past decade it has become clear that personality traits can be described in terms of five very broad dimensions of personality. Table 1 lists some of the adjectives and personality questionnaire scales that define each dimension. These five dimensions should be thought of as constituting the highest level of a hierarchy; within each of the five it is possible and sometimes important to make distinctions. Anxiety and depression, for example, are both definers of neuroticism, and people who are anxious are frequently depressed as well. But the two traits are also distinguishable both conceptually and empirically, and psychotherapists often find that distinction very important.

PERSONALITY ASSESSMENT

Unlike blood pressure or temperature, personality traits cannot be directly measured. Instead, they must be inferred from actions and reactions in a variety of circumstances. Traits are often masked by temporary moods or states (for example, those related to acute illness) and overpowered by environmental pressures: extraverts do not laugh heartily at funerals. Behaviour may be ambiguous: is a smile genuine or ironic?; and people are often highly motivated to dissemble their true feelings or beliefs. Because of all these factors, accurate personality assessment is difficult and challenging.

Contemporary assessment draws on two strengths: the perceptiveness of lay observers, and the principles of psychometrics. Difficult as it may be to understand people, it is also vital to everyday social interaction. As a result, all human beings to a greater or lesser extent develop the ability to interpret what people do and say in trait terms. They learn a large vocabulary of trait names, recall and integrate patterns of behaviours, make allowances for situational effects, and draw inferences about motivations. Most people have no difficulty in deciding whether an acquaintance is kind or cruel, lazy or hardworking, liberal or conservative.

In fact, the real danger comes from the ease with which inferences about personality are made. It is apparently possible to judge with some degree of accuracy how introverted or extraverted a stranger is after only a few seconds of observation, but equally facile judgements about the other four dimensions show little accuracy (Borkenau & Liebler, 1995). First impressions are powerful but often misleading bases of personality judgements.

In consequence, personality psychologists have developed standardized instruments for quantifying personality judgements and a series of procedures for evaluating the quality of information obtained from these instruments. The most common approach is the personality questionnaire (such as the Minnesota Multiphasic Personality Inventory, the Eysenck Personality Questionnaire, or the NEO Personality Inventory), in which respondents are asked whether or how well each of a series of statements describes them. Another self-report approach asks respondents to check off adjectives that characterize them. Because self-reports may be deliberately or defensively distorted, an important alternative is the use of informant reports or observer ratings.

Personality assessment instruments can be evaluated in terms of internal consistency (the extent to which respondents give similar answers to similar questions), retest reliability (the extent to which respondents give similar answers on two different occasions), and validity (the extent to which scores can be corroborated by independent sources of information). Initial evaluations of instruments can suggest refinements in the items that lead to better versions of the test. Although personality traits are complex psychological phenomena that will probably never be measured with the precision of height or weight, contemporary personality measures show sufficient accuracy to be important guides to understanding the person.

Development and life course of personality

One of the most surprising findings of recent years has come from studies of the behaviour genetics of personality. Monozogotic twins, whether raised together or apart, strongly resemble each other in personality. Children who are raised in the same family but who are biologicality unrelated (adoptee studies) show little or no resemblance in personality. The conclusion seems to be that personality traits are more influenced by heredity than by child-rearing practices (Plomin & Daniels, 1987), a finding that both psychoanalysts and behaviourists would have difficulty explaining.

Developmentalists have known for years that certain temperamental traits, like activity level and distress-proneness, appear to be biologically based, and these temperaments are clearly linked to the two dimensions of extraversion and neuroticism. But imaginativeness and intellectual curiosity, aspects of Openness, and diligence and dutifulness, aspects of Conscientiousness, also seem to be influenced by genetics. The evidence is less consistent and clear for traits in the domain of Agreeableness, but several studies point to a genetic component there, too.

This does not mean that the individual's personality is fixed at infancy, and that adult character can be read from infant behaviour. There are many changes from infancy through adolescence, and

personality changes continue through the decade of the 20s. From college to middle age, both men and women tend to become less emotional and excitable, and more altruistic and organized. These declines in neuroticism and extraversion and increases in agreeableness and conscientiousness seem to summarize much of what is meant by 'maturity'.

After age 30, personality changes little. There are small declines in activity and excitement seeking over a period of many years, but few other changes are consistently seen. In particular, old age is not marked by increasing depression, social withdrawal, conservativism, or crankiness. Figure 1 provides some representative data. Observer ratings on the NEO Personality Inventory were obtained from 157 raters of 54 men and 37 women (some individuals had more than one rater) in 1983 and again in 1990. On the first occasion, the rated subjects ranged in age from 31 to 81. Figure 1 shows mean values expressed as T-scores. Although there is a statistically significant increase in Conscientiousness over the 7-year interval, it is trivial in magnitude. None of the other domains shows any reliable change at all. Mean levels of personality traits are stable.

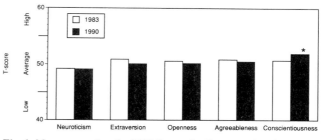

Fig. 1. Mean peer ratings for NEO Personality Inventory domains on two occasions; $N = 157$. Adapted from Costa & McCrae, 1992b. *Longitudinal change significant at $p < .05$.

Personality is also stable in another sense: Individual differences are preserved. That is, those individuals who score highest on a personality trait at one time also tend to score highest at a later time, even over intervals of 30 years (Costa & McCrae, 1992b). People who are well adjusted, imaginative, and persistent at age 30 are likely to be well adjusted, imaginative, and persistent at age 80. This fact is crucial to an understanding of adult development; it means that people's basic tendencies are highly predictable over long periods of time. One implication is that people can plan rationally for their own future by taking into account their current values, motivations, and interests. Another implication is that, once adequately assessed, personality trait information will retain its utility. Like sex, race, and education, personality traits might be considered basic background information that could be included in an individual's medical record.

Personality traits are not immutable, but in the absence of deliberate psychological or psychiatric interventions, they change very little. One important exception to this generalization is found in the case of dementing disorders. Researchers have documented progressive changes in rated personality (notably increased neuroticism and decreased conscientiousness) in individuals with Alzheimer's disease (Siegler et al., 1991). Given the normative stability of personality, any marked change in personality traits may signal the need for medical evaluation.

THE FIVE FACTORS AND THEIR RELEVANCE TO MEDICAL PRACTICE

Historically, personality traits were of interest to physicians chiefly because they were thought to predispose individuals to particular diseases. Different personality patterns were believed to be contributing causes to hypertension, ulcer, asthma, and other so-called psychosomatic disorders. Today, there are major research efforts under way examining psychoneuroimmunology (O'Leary, 1990) and links between hostility and cardiovascular disease (Dembroski *et al.*, 1989). But, most of the classical psychosomatic theories have not been supported by empirical research, and many others are the subject of ongoing controversy. It is not clear to what extent personality traits directly influence biochemical processes, but there is no doubt that they influence the ways patients perceive illness, interact with health-care providers, and comply with medical advice. At this level, personality psychology is of clear relevance to medicine.

Health-care professionals treat patients, not diseases, and in recent years they have been sensitized to the importance of taking into account patient differences in gender, age, race, education, and ethnicity. Differences in personality cut across all these categories, and they too make a difference in the way health care is perceived and utilized. In this section we discuss the five major personality factors in greater detail and suggest ways in which a knowledge of personality traits might help health care providers.

Neuroticism

Modern psychiatric nomenclature no longer recognizes a category of neuroses, but personality psychologists still use the term Neuroticism to describe a basic dimension of personality (see Table 1 for some alternative labels). Individuals who score high on this dimension are prone to experience a wide variety of negative emotions, such as fear, shame and guilt. External stressors and internal drives often overwhelm them, leading them to feel helpless and act impulsively. They are prone to unrealistic thinking and have a poor self-image. Low scorers on this dimension are calm and hardy, resilient in the face of stress.

Although neuroticism, even at very high levels, is a dimension of normal personality rather than a psychiatric disorder, it is associated with increased risk for a wide variety of psychiatric disorders. Most of the scales used to measure psychiatric maladjustment are strongly related to neuroticism, and patients in psychotherapy typically score high on this dimension.

Neuroticism is also related to somatic distress. Individuals who are chronically anxious and depressed make more somatic complaints, perhaps because they are more sensitive to minor aches and pains, or more prone to interpret physiological sensations as signs of illness, or more likely to remember or report symptoms. At an extreme level, this is recognizable as hypochondriasis, but even moderate levels of Neuroticism are associated with moderate increases in somatic complaints.

This phenomenon complicates medical diagnosis, which depends heavily on patient reports of medical history and symptoms. If the patient is very high in Neuroticism, he or she may exag-

Table 1. *Examples of Adjectives and questionnaire scales defining the five factors*

Factor name	Definers	
	Adjectives	Scales
Neuroticism	Anxious	Anxiety
(or Negative	Self-pitying	Angry hostility
affectivity	Tense	Depression
vs.	Touchy	Self-consciousness
emotional	Unstable	Impulsiveness
stability)	Worrying	Vulnerability
Extraversion	Active	Warmth
(or Surgency,	Assertive	Gregariousness
dominance	Energetic	Assertiveness
vs.	Enthusiastic	Activity
introversion)	Outgoing	Excitement seeking
	Talkative	Positive emotions
Openness to experience	Artistic	Fantasy
(or intellect,	Curious	Aesthetics
culture	Imaginative	Feelings
vs.	Insightful	Actions
conventionality)	Original	Ideas
	Wide interests	Values
Agreeableness	Appreciative	Trust
(or Love,	Forgiving	Straightforwardness
friendly	Generous	Altruism
compliance	Kind	Compliance
vs.	Sympathetic	Modesty
antagonism)	Trusting	Tender-mindedness
Conscientiousness	Efficient	Competence
(or dependability,	Organized	Order
will to achieve	Planful	Dutifulness
vs.	Reliable	Achievement striving
undirectedness)	Responsible	Self-discipline
	Thorough	Deliberation

Note: Scales are facet scales from the Revised NEO Personality Inventory. Adapted from McCrae & John, 1992.

gerate medical problem, whereas if the patient is very low, he or she may minimize symptoms and fail to seek appropriate care. It would be naive for a physician to assume that all self-reports are perfectly accurate accounts of medical status; yet self-reports cannot be ignored even when they come from very maladjusted individuals – after all, even hypochondriacs get sick. Standing on neuroticism is one of many factors that the health-care professional should take into account when evaluating a patient's somatic complaints.

Does neuroticism actually cause disease? Certainly acute emotional reactions have physiological consequences, and individuals high in Neuroticism have more frequent distressing emotional reactions. It would be reasonable to believe that the long-term effect of these physiological disturbances would include organic disease. However, a number of large-scale studies have failed to show any link between neuroticism and mortality or morbidity from cancer or coronary disease. In most cases, it appears that neuroticism is more strongly related to subjective perceptions of health than it is to objective health status (Costa & McCrae, 1987).

Extraversion

Extraversion includes both interpersonal and temperamental aspects. Interpersonally, extraverts are warm and friendly, enjoying conversation and having close personal relationships; they also enjoy the sheer social stimulation of crowds of strangers. Extraverts are assertive and easily take on leadership roles. Temperamentally, extraverts are characterized by need for excitement, high levels of energy and activity, and cheerful optimism; they laugh easily. Introverts, although they may have perfectly adequate social skills, prefer to avoid crowds and tend to be serious in mood and measured in their pace of activity. Contrary to popular belief, introverts are not necessarily introspective or deep thinkers, nor are extraverts necessarily well adjusted.

The characteristics that define extraversion are readily observed, and this dimension is the one which is most easily noticed by the health-care provider. Most obviously, extraverts are talkative. This fact is of particular significance in view of the fact that 'talk is the main ingredient in medical care' (Roter & Hall, 1992, p. 3). How much and what is said in a medical interview depends upon many factors (Beisecker & Beisecker, 1990), including the physician's willingness to listen, but the patient's extraversion plays a key role. In particular, physicians may need to make extra efforts to elicit information from very introverted patients, who are less likely to volunteer it.

The health care provider's own level of extraversion is also an important determinant of patient/provider interactions. Mechanic (1978) has suggested that family practitioners may be more sociable than internists, and their interactions with patients will be correspondingly more warm and personal. This will be especially appreciated by extraverted patients; introverts may prefer to maintain their distance and focus attention on the medical problem.

Openness to experience

Individuals who are open to experience prefer novelty, variety, and ambiguity in many aspects of life. They are imaginative and creative, with an active fantasy life, and they are responsive to beauty in art and nature. They are keenly aware of their own inner states, including emotional ambivalence. Open men and women are innovative and willing to try new approaches, and they have a high degree of intellectual curiosity. They are liberal and unconventional in their political and social views. Closed individuals, by contrast, are conservative, conventional, and down-to-earth: they prefer symmetry and simplicity and tend toward black-and-white thinking. They are reluctant to change either their behaviours or their views. Open individuals tend to be somewhat better educated than closed individuals, but Openness should not be confused with intelligence.

The experience of clinical psychologists (Miller, 1991) suggests that differences along this dimension are likely to be particularly important determinants of the patient's view of therapy. Closed patients are likely to prefer conventional medical treatment; they will tend to assume that doctors are the authorities and believe what they are told. Open patients may be less compliant: they may want more information than is normally provided, asking for second opinions and perhaps even researching the topic themselves. They are more willing to consider innovative and non-traditional therapies, and it seems likely that they make disproportionate use of altern-

ative medicine. Acupuncture, aroma therapy, and hypnosis are more appealing to open than to closed patients.

Agreeableness

Like extraversion, agreeableness is primarily an interpersonal dimension. Agreeable people are prosocial. They trust others and are themselves candid and straightforward; they try to help others and are sympathetic in attitudes. Antagonistic people are more self-centred, suspicious, and devious. They may be arrogant and quarrelsome. Although agreeableness is socially desirable and agreeable people are more popular with their peers, there are also advantages to being disagreeable. Antagonistic individuals are competitive and proud of their tough-mindedness; they see agreeable people as weak and gullible.

In a number of recent studies, individuals who are rude, condescending, and quarrelsome, that is, low in agreeableness, have been shown to be at higher risk for developing coronary heart disease (Dembroski et al., 1989). Antagonistic hostility has thus been identified as the 'toxic component' of the Type A Behaviour Pattern. The mechanisms that underlie the association of antagonism with heart disease are not yet fully understood, nor is it clear that levels of agreeableness can be changed by interventions. Physicians with highly antagonistic patients might emphasize control of other risk factors such as smoking and hypertension.

Antagonistic patients present another problem for health-care providers: they are mistrustful, demanding, and manipulative. Physicians not surprisingly find such patients unlikeable, and such patients are frequently dissatisfied with their medical treatment (Roter & Hall, 1992). Extremely agreeable patients are well liked and generally satisfied, but may be too compliant for their own good, they are unlikely to adopt the consumerist perspective that some patient advocates recommend.

Conscientiousness

The final dimension of the five-factor model is Conscientiousness, a cluster of traits that encompass both self-restraint (order, dutifulness, and deliberation) and active pursuit of goals. High scorers on measures of this dimension are hardworking, persistent, and highly motivated; low scorers are easy-going and somewhat disorganized, and lack a clear direction in their life. At best, highly conscientious people are purposeful and effective; at worst, they are driven to perfectionism and neglect their personal life for the sake of their work.

Booth-Kewley and Vickers (1994) have shown that Conscientiousness is intimately related to health promotion. Conscientiousness scores on the NEO-PI were found to be predictive of wellness behaviours (e.g. exercise, taking vitamins), accident control (e.g. learning first aid), and low traffic risk-taking. Conscientious people have the self-discipline and prudence to follow the advice that public service announcements offer. Perhaps as a consequence, at least one study has reported that more conscientious individuals live longer (Friedman et al., 1993).

Conscientious people are presumably also the most likely to adhere faithfully to prescribed medical regimens (Christensen & Smith, 1995). Patients who are very low in conscientiousness present a problem to the health care system. Regimens that are distasteful or that require organization or effort are likely to be abandoned. Ideally, treatments would be designed to take into account the patient's level of conscientiousness. For example, a rigorous exercise programme might be best for a high scorer, whereas a more passive drug therapy might be more realistic for a low scorer. Where patient efforts are essential, health-care providers should make special efforts to motivate the patient low in conscientiousness.

ASSESSING PERSONALITY IN MEDICAL PRACTICE

It should be clear that knowledge of a patient's personality can be of considerable value in medical practice. But physicians and nurses are not trained as personality assessors, nor is there time at each medical visit for the completion and scoring of validated personality questionnaires. How, in practical terms, can a health-care provider make use of personality information?

The first answer is that he or she can develop an appreciation of individual differences. There is no single right or wrong way to interpret a patient's symptom reports, or interact with the patient, or prescribe treatment. Different individuals respond best to different approaches. Good clinicians recognize this implicitly and act accordingly; an explicit understanding of the nature, structure, and stability of personality traits may facilitate tailoring medical practice to the individual. Further information on the traits in the five-factor model are provided in McCrae and Costa (1990), McCrae and John (1992), and Costa and McCrae (1992a, b).

A second answer would be that brief interviews for assessing personality could be developed to be used by physicians, much as the mini-mental status exam is used to assess cognitive status. No such instrument currently exists, and it is likely that it would be useful only for very gross screening. Physicians might also be trained to use brief self-report measures of the five-factor model.

A third possibility is that personality data could be included in the patient's medical record. Standardized inventories administered and interpreted by trained psychologists could be summarized in terms of standing on each of the five factors. For most adults, a single administration, like a single blood typing, would provide information that could be used for many years. Including information on personality traits in a medical record raises ethical issues about the individual's privacy and the use of psychological information by non-psychologists that are beyond the scope of this chapter, but if they can be satisfactorily addressed, the potential benefits for medical practice are large.

ACKNOWLEDGEMENT
We thank Francis Caprio, MD, Vanderbilt University Medical Center, for valuable comments on these issues.

REFERENCES

Beisecker, A.E. & Beisecker, T.D. (1990). Patient information-seeking behaviors when communicating with doctors. *Medical Care*, **28**, 19–28.

Booth-Kewley, S. & Vickers, R.R., Jr. (1994). Associations between major domains of personality and health behavior. *Journal of Personality*, **62**, 281–98.

Borkenau, P. & Liebler, A. (1995). Observable attributes as manifestations and cues of personality and intelligence. *Journal of Personality*, **63**, 1–25.

Christensen, A.J. & Smith, T.W. (1995). Personality and patient adherence: correlates of the five-factor model in renal dialysis. *Journal of Behavioral Medicine*, **18**, 305–13.

Costa, P.T., Jr. & McCrae, R.R. (1987). Neuroticism, somatic complaints, and disease: is the bark worse than the bite? *Journal of Personality*, **55**, 299–316.

Costa, P.T., Jr. & McCrae, R.R. (1992a). *Revised NEO Personality Inventory (NEO-PI-R) and NEO Five-Factor Inventory (NEO-FFI) professional manual.* Odessa, FL: Psychological Assessment Resources, Inc.

Costa, P.T., Jr. & McCrae, R.R. (1992b). Trait psychology comes of age. In T.B. Sonderegger (Ed.). *Nebraska Symposium on Motivation: Psychology and Aging*, pp. 169–204. Lincoln, NE: University of Nebraska Press.

Dembroski, T.M., MacDougall, J.M., Costa, P.T., Jr. & Grandits, G. (1989). Components of hostility as predictors of sudden death and myocardial infarction in the Multiple Risk Factor Intervention Trial. *Psychosomatic Medicine*, **51**, 514–22.

Friedman, H.S., Tucker, J.S., Tomlinson-Keasey, C., Schwartz, J.E., Wingard, D.L. & Criqui, M.H. (1993). Does childhood personality predict longevity? *Journal of Personality and Social Psychology*, **65**, 176–85.

McAdams, D.P. (1990). *The person: An introduction to personality psychology.* San Diego, CA: Harcourt Brace Jovanovich.

McCrae, R.R. & Costa, P.T., Jr. (1990). *Personality in adulthood.* New York: Guilford.

McCrae, R.R. & John, O.P. (1992). An introduction to the five-factor model and its applications. *Journal of Personality*, **60**, 175–215.

Mechanic, D. (1978). *Medical sociology.* 2nd edn. New York: Free Press.

Miller, T. (1991). The psychotherapeutic utility of the five-factor model of personality: a clinician's experience. *Journal of Personality Assessment*, **57**, 415–33.

O'Leary, A. (1990). Stress, emotion, and human immune function. *Psychological Bulletin*, **108**, 363–82.

Pervin, L.A. (1993). *Personality: Theory and research.* 6th edn. New York: Wiley.

Plomin, R. & Daniels, D. (1987). Why are children in the same family so different from one another? *Behavioral and Brain Sciences*, **10**, 1–16.

Roter, D.L. & Hall, J.A. (1992). *Doctors talking with patients/patients talking with doctors: improving communication in medical visits.* Westport, CT: Auburn House.

Siegler, I.C., Welsh, K.A., Dawson, D.V., Fillenbaum, G.G., Earl, N.L., Kaplan, E.B. & Clark, C.M. (1991). Ratings of personality change in patients being evaluated for memory disorders. *Alzheimer Disease and Associated Disorders*, **5**, 240–50.

Psychoimmunology

ELIZABETH BACHEN
Center for AIDS Prevention Studies, University of California, San Francisco, USA

SHELDON COHEN
Department of Psychology, Carnegie Mellon University, USA

ANNA L. MARSLAND
Behavioral Physiology Laboratory, University of Pittsburgh, USA

PSYCHOLOGICAL STRESS AND THE IMMUNE SYSTEM IN HUMANS

Stressful life events have been linked to a range of immune-related disorders, including autoimmune diseases, infectious diseases, and cancer (Cohen & Williamson, 1991; Grant *et al.*, 1989; Jensen, 1987). One means by which stress may lead to increased susceptibility to these diseases is by altering the function of the immune system. This hypothesis is one of the central concerns of the growing field of psychoneuroimmunology (PNI), which attempts to elucidate the relations between psychosocial factors, nervous, endocrine and immune systems, and health.

How stress influences the immune system is not entirely clear. One possibility is that stress alters immune responses through the adoption of coping behaviours, such as smoking or drinking alcohol, that are known to compromise immunity (Kiecolt-Glaser & Glaser, 1988). Alternatively, stress may directly influence immune function through the activation of neuroendocrine pathways that lead to the release of various hormones and neurotransmitters, such as cortisol and catecholamines. Direct anatomical links exist between the nervous and immune systems, as evidenced by sympathetic innervation to lymphoid organs, such as the thymus and spleen (Livnat *et al.*, 1985). Immune cells, which migrate between the lymphoid organs and peripheral bloodstream, have also been shown to have receptors for numerous hormones and neurotransmitters that are produced and secreted during stress, suggesting that these substances play a role in altering cell function.

MEASUREMENTS OF IMMUNOCOMPETENCE

The function of the immune system is to identify and destroy foreign or non-self materials. Such non-self materials include invading foreign agents (or antigens), such as bacteria or viruses or altered host cells such as tumour or infected cells. The immune system is complex and is composed of natural barriers, such as skin and mucous, immune organs, and immune cells. In PNI research, the most commonly measured component of the immune system is the immune cells, which collectively work together to mount a response against non-self materials. As a group, such cells are known as white blood cells (WBCs) or leukocytes. While there are many types of leukocytes, each with distinct functions, such cells are interdependent and perform their functions in an orchestrated fashion to achieve immunocompetence. Table 1 lists the different types of immune cells and their primary functions.

Assessments of immune cells fall into two categories, quantifying the number of cells in circulation and assessing their function *in vitro*. An overview of the immunological assessments commonly used in PNI research is presented in Table 2.

Table 1. *Cells of the Immune system*

Cell type	Function
White blood cells (WBC)	Respond to antigens; include lymphocytes and phagocytes
Lymphocytes	Subset of WBCs that include T- and B-lymphocytes, and NK cells; functions described below
T-helper lymphocytes	Enhance immune responses by stimulating T-cell replication and activating antibody production by B-lymphocytes
T-suppressor lymphocytes	Inhibit immune responses
T-cytotoxic lymphocytes	Destroy virus-, parasite-, and tumour-infected cells; reject transplanted tissue
B-lymphocytes	Produce antibodies
NK cells	Destroy virally infected and tumour cells
Phagocytes	Subset of WBCs that include basophils, eosinophils, neutrophils, monocytes and macrophages; ingest and destroy antigens

In enumerative assays, investigators quantify specific populations of immune cells in the peripheral bloodstream. Typically, these cells include: (i) T-helper lymphocytes (designated CD4), which enhance immune responses through the release of substances promoting the replication and activation of other immune cells; (ii) T-suppressor cells (designated CD8), which down-regulate or suppress immune responses; (iii) T-cytotoxic lymphocytes (also designated CD8), which destroy antigens and play an important role in immune reactions against intracellular parasites and viruses, tumour cells, and tissue transplants; (iv) B lymphocytes (designated CD19), which produce antibodies, proteins that destroy bacteria and prevent viruses from penetrating host cells; (v) natural killer (NK) cells, that destroy certain tumour and virally infected cells; and (vi) phagocytes, such as monocytes and macrophages, which injest and degrade foreign matter and initiate T-lymphocyte activity.

In enumerative assays, the various populations of immune cells are identified and counted by staining the unique surface molecules of each cell type with specific fluorescent reagents. Using this technique, one can quanitify the percentages or absolute numbers of T-lymphocytes (and their subsets), B-lymphocytes, macrophages, and NK cells from the peripheral circulation. In addition, the ratio

Table 2. *Immune assessments commonly used in PNI studies*

Measure	What it tells us
Numbers or percentages of WBC populations (lymphocytes and phagocytes)	Composition of WBC populations in the peripheral bloodstream
Lymphocyte proliferation	Ability of lymphocytes to divide in response to a stimulating mitogen, such as PHA, Con A, or PWM *in vitro*
Natural killer cell activity	Ability of natural killer cells to destroy tumour cells *in vitro*
Lymphokine and interleukin production	Ability of activated lymphocytes and monocytes to produce and release molecules that serve as regulating signals between immune cells *in vitro*
Antibody levels	Amount of antibody production in response to an antigen *in vitro*

of T-helper to T-suppressor/cytotoxic cells, which is used as an index of immune status, may be determined. Although the interpretation of quantitative immune cell changes in the circulation during stress is not entirely clear, it is likely that such alterations reflect the redistribution of immune cells between the peripheral blood and lymphoid organs (O'Leary, 1990). Migratory shifts in lymphocyte populations may influence immunocompetence by determining whether lymphocytes will encounter an environmental antigen in a particular location in a timely fashion (Ottaway & Husband, 1992).

In addition to quantitative assessments, functional assessments of immunity can be made using a variety of *in vitro* assays. One of the most fundamental functions of immune cells is to divide, or proliferate in response to antigens. In proliferation assays, lymphocytes are exposed, *in vitro*, to chemicals or plant extracts that stimulate cell division. These stimulants are called mitogens. The most commonly used mitogens in PNI research are phytohaemagglutinin (PHA) and Concavalin A (Con A) which stimulate the division of T-cells, and Pokeweed mitogen which stimulates division of both T- and B-cells.

The ability of NK cells to destroy tumours by rupturing their membranes (cell lysis) can also be assessed *in vitro*. In the chromium-release assay, NK cells are incubated with tumour cells that contain a radioactive substance, such as radioactive-labelled chromium. Natural killer cell activity is reflected by the extent of tumour cell lysis, which in turn, is determined by the amount of radioactivity released from the lysed cells into the culture medium.

Other functional assays are designed to measure levels of antibodies in saliva or serum. Antibodies are specialized proteins that carry out a number of immune functions and they are produced by B cells in response to antigens. Greater antibody response is usually interpreted as better immunocompetence. However, elevated antibody levels to latent viruses, such as herpesviruses may reflect a weakened ability of the immune system to keep such viruses from becoming active. Therefore, higher antibody levels to latent viruses are often interpreted as indicating *poorer* immunocompetence (Kiecolt-Glaser & Glaser, 1987).

Finally, *in vitro* functional assays are also used to measure sub-

stances produced and secreted by lymphoyctes and monocytes, called cytokines. In these assays, immune cells are first activated by mitogens, such as PHA or Con A. After incubation, the cell mixture is exposed to labelled antibody that attaches to the specific cytokine in question. The quantity of cytokine secreted by these cells is then determined by the degree of binding between the specific cytokine and labelled antibody.

PSYCHOLOGICAL STRESS AND IMMUNITY

A growing literature in both humans and animals supports associations between immunological changes and psychological and physical forms of stress (for extensive reviews involving humans, see Herbert & Cohen, 1993; O'Leary, 1990). Changes in the immune system have been found to accompany exercise, exams, confronting a phobic stressor, bereavement and divorce, occupational stress, unemployment, and the ongoing uncertainty associated with living near Three Mile Island (TMI) several years after the nuclear accident.

Perhaps the most commonly examined stressors in relation to immunological status have been examinations. Indeed, several indices of immunosuppression have been observed among medical students during final exams. Compared to test-free periods, students undergoing exams have shown decrements in lymphocyte response to mitogenic stimulation, reduced NK cell activity, alterations in T-cell populations, increased plasma levels of circulating antibodies, and decreased cytokine production (Kennedy, Kiecolt-Glaser & Glaser, 1988; Glaser *et al.*, 1986). Increased levels of circulating antibodies to Epstein–Barr and other herpesviruses have also been observed during examination periods, indicating, perhaps, the reactivation of latent virus by either direct neuroendocrine influences or weakened immunocompetence. In some cases, the most extreme immunological changes were found to occur in subsets of students with the highest levels of overall life stress, loneliness, or tendency to ruminate about stressful events during the examination period (Kiecolt-Glaser *et al.*, 1984; Workman & La Viá, 1987).

The loss of an intimate relationship from either death or divorce has also been associated with altered immunity, including suppression of lymphocyte responses to mitogenic stimulation, reduced NK cell activity, and changes in T-cell subpopulations. Early investigations found lowered mitogenic lymphocyte proliferation in bereaved subjects following the loss of a spouse, as compared to both non-bereaved controls (Bartrop *et al.*, 1977) and the pre-bereavement period (Schleifer *et al.*, 1983). Subsequent findings indicated that the degree of immune change among bereaved persons was related to the severity of depressive response before and after the loss (Irwin *et al.*, 1987).

Separation and divorce have similarly been associated with immune alterations. Kiecolt-Glaser, Glaser, and colleagues found that recently separated or divorced women demonstrated lower percentages of circulating NK and T-helper cells, decreased proliferative responses to PHA and Con A, and higher antibodies to Epstein–Barr virus than a comparison group of married persons (cited in Kennedy, Kiecolt-Glaser & Glaser, 1988). Similar findings were reported in a subsequent investigation comparing separated or divorced men to matched married controls. As in the previous study, separated or divorced men had higher antibody levels to latent viruses (here, Epstein–Barr virus and herpes simplex virus).

T-lymphocyte populations, however, did not differ between the two groups. Finally, both studies showed that, for married couples, poorer marital quality was related to higher levels of distress, loneliness, and latent virus antibody response (cited in Kennedy, Kiecolt-Glaser, & Glaser, 1988).

Immunological changes accompany other prolonged stressors, as well, such as long-term unemployment, occupational stress, caregiving for a terminally ill patient, and residing near a damaged nuclear power plant. In an examination of the immune-related effects of caregiving for a family member with Alzheimer's Disease, Kiecolt-Glaser and colleagues found that caregivers exhibited lower percentages of total lymphocytes and T-helper cell subsets, and higher antibody titres to Epstein–Barr virus (Kiecolt-Glaser et al., 1987).

Heightened distress and higher latent antibody levels were also observed in TMI residents more than 6 years after the nuclear accident, as compared to demographically comparable controls (McKinnon et al., 1989). Living near TMI was also associated with enumerative immune alterations, including higher numbers of circulating neutrophils, and lower numbers of B lymphocytes, T-suppressor/cytotoxic lymphocytes, and NK cells (McKinnon et al., 1989).

Both job stress and long-term unemployment have been linked to lowered lymphocyte reactivity to PHA (Arnetz et al., 1987; Dorian et al., 1985). In one study, immunological function was found to remain depressed throughout the study interval, despite the inclusion of a psychosocial intervention programme designed to assist the unemployed (Arnetz et al., 1987).

Taken together, most studies involving stress and immunity indicate that psychological stressors are associated with changes in immune cell numbers and functions (Herbert & Cohen, 1993). The most consistent alterations include reduced NK cell activity and lymphocyte proliferation to PHA and Con A, and increased antibody levels to latent herpesviruses. Decreases in percentages or absolute numbers of circulating B cells, T cells, T-helper cells, T-suppressor/cytotoxic cells, and NK cells are also frequently reported stress-related immune responses. Moreover, such alterations may persist (i.e. fail to habituate) with prolonged stressor exposure. However, because the aforementioned studies document *correlational* relations between stress and immunity, causal interpretations cannot be made. Even if stress, itself, does lead to changes in the immune system, it is not clear whether this occurs because stress influences health behaviours or neuroendocrine parameters. Few investigations have examined relationships between health practices or neuroendocrine factors and immune alterations during stress (Herbert & Cohen, 1993). Whereas extreme modifications in health practices result in altered immunity, it is not yet clear if more modest changes similarly influence the immune system. Although few PNI investigations with humans measure concomitant changes in hormonal or catecholamine levels, the small number of naturalistic studies that have included neuroendocrine variables suggest that the sympathetic nervous system may play a significant role in stress-induced immune alterations (e.g. McKinnon et al., 1989).

SHORT-TERM LABORATORY STRESSORS AND IMMUNITY

While associations between naturally occurring stressors and alterations in immune function are well documented, only recently have investigators utilized controlled, experimental studies to examine stress–immune interactions. Experimental manipulations where subjects are randomly assigned to stressor exposure or non-exposure (i.e. control groups) are required for clarifying causal interpretations about stress-immune relations. Experimental studies are also useful for the investigation of potential neuroendocrine mechanisms associated with immunological changes during stress, since they eliminate other potential influences, such as changes in health behaviours.

There are now several studies demonstrating immunological alterations following exposure to standardized laboratory stressors, including challenging computer tasks, mental arithmetic, electrical shocks, loud noise, unsolvable puzzles, graphic films depicting combat surgery, marital discussions involving conflict, and interviews eliciting the recollection of positive and negative experiences and mood states (for a recent review, see Kiecolt-Glaser et al., 1992). Exposure to these tasks has been shown to evoke a variety of enumerative immune changes; the most consistent findings include increases in the numbers of circulating NK cells and T-suppressor/cytotoxic lymphocytes, and a decrease in the ratio of T-helper to T-suppressor cells (primarily as a function of augmented T-suppressor lymphocytes, rather than altered T-helper cells) (Bachen et al., 1992; Brosschot et al., 1992; Naliboff et al., 1991). Most of these studies failed to demonstrate significant stress-induced changes in numbers of total T-lymphocytes, T-helper lymphocytes, or B cells (Brosschot et al., 1992; Manuck et al., 1991; Naliboff et al., 1991).

In studies examining changes in percentages of lymphocyte subsets, rather than absolute numbers, findings are mixed. Some investigations have shown significant shifts in the proportions of circulating immune cells (Naliboff et al., 1991), whereas others have failed to detect such changes (Knapp et al., 1992; Sieber et al., 1992; Weisse et al., 1990).

Changes in functional measures of immunity, including diminished lymphocyte mitogenesis (Bachen et al., 1992; Knapp et al., 1992; Manuck et al., 1991; Weisse et al., 1990; Zakowski et al., 1992) and altered NK cell activity (Naliboff et al., 1991, Sieber et al., 1992) also occur following exposure to brief psychological stress. The specific effects of acute stress on NK cell activity are less clear, and studies have demonstrated increases as well as decreases in this parameter (Naliboff et al., 1991; Sieber et al., 1992). It is possible that the different task characteristics employed by these experiments may have accounted for the discrepant findings. Naliboff et al. (1991) observed increases in NK cell activity following active attempts to perform a mental arithmetic task, whereas Sieber et al. (1992) found reduced NK cell activity following passive exposure to uncontrollable bursts of loud noise. Because active coping strategies frequently accompany sympathetic arousal, it is possible that enhanced sympathetic activation associated with effortful attempts to perform well on mental arithmetic may have resulted in the increased NK cell activity observed by Naliboff et al.; indeed, the infusion of catecholamines have previously been shown to elicit increases in NK cell activity in humans (Buske-Kirschbaum et al., 1992).

The appearance of immunological changes in response to acute psychological stress is rapid, occurring as early as 5 minutes from stressor onset (Herbert et al., 1994). Increases in NK cell and T-suppressor/cytotoxic lymphocytes return to baseline levels by 15 minutes after stressor termination (Brosschot et al., 1992). The immediate effects of short-term stressors may not necessarily reflect longer-term changes seen during exposure to naturalistic stressors, which are of more chronic duration. Whereas acute stressors elicit immediate elevations in NK and T-suppressor/cytotoxic cell numbers, naturalistic stressors tend to be associated with reductions in these cell types (Herbert & Cohen, 1993). The reasons for these discrepancies are not yet clear, but may reflect complex differences in the hormonal environment surrounding immune cells (Herbert & Cohen, 1993). Interestingly, long-term sympathetic activation, induced by the drug terbutaline, results in a similar reduction of circulating T-suppressor/cytotoxic lymphocytes and NK cells in humans (Maisel et al., 1990).

In contrast to quantitative alterations, reductions in lymphocyte proliferation persist up to at least 90 minutes after stressor termination (Weisse et al., 1990; Zakowski et al., 1992). With respect to NK cell activity, decreases persist as much as 72 hours after the exposure to laboratory stress (Sieber et al., 1992). As the authors note, it is not yet known if these changes represent a sustained decrease in NK cell function or a conditioned response elicited by a return to the laboratory setting.

The aforementioned studies also suggest that immune changes elicited by short-term mental stress may be modulated by sympathetic activation. First, the rapid appearance of lymphocytic changes during mental stress makes it unlikely that other, slower-responding hormones (e.g. cortisol) are contributing to the effects. Indeed, two studies found immune alterations in the absence of concomitant cortisol responses to the stressors (Manuck et al., 1991). Zakowski et al. (1992) reported enhanced cortisol levels following exposure to a stressful film, but found that proliferative reductions preceded the cortisol response by 30 minutes. Secondly, infusion of catecholamines invoke functional and enumerative immune alterations that are similar to those seen during acute mental stress (van Tits et al., 1990). Finally, only those subjects with the most pronounced sympathetic activation in response to laboratory stressors display suppression of mitogenic stimulated lymphocyte proliferation (Manuck et al., 1991; Zakowski et al., 1992).

Laboratory manipulations of mood states are similarly associated with increased sympathetic arousal and altered immune function. Knapp et al. (1992) reported that decreased proliferation during interviews eliciting negative mood states were related to increases in heart rate ($r = .56$). In addition, the tendency for NK cell activity to rise was also associated with increases in heart rate ($r = .51$), as well as systolic blood pressure ($r = .49$). Interestingly, Knapp et al. (1992) observed decreases in lymphocyte proliferation during the induction of both positive and negative mood states; such findings are consistent with a catecholamine-mediated hypothesis, since both positive and negative emotions have been linked to elevations in urinary levels of catecholamines (Levi, 1972).

Overall, experimental studies indicate that psychological stressors of a short-term nature elicit reliable and transient alterations in immune cell numbers and function. While functional immune changes following acute stress are similar to those accompanying chronic naturalistic stress, the direction of quantitative changes in some lymphocyte subpopulations differ in the two forms of stress. Whereas increases in NK cell and T-suppressor/cytotoxic lymphocytes are typically seen following laboratory stressors, decreases in these cell types occur during chronic stress. Studies assessing indices of sympathetic activity through cardiovascular and catecholamine responses to stress offer compelling evidence for the role of the sympathetic nervous system in at least some of these immune modifications.

IMPLICATIONS

Stressors of various types do induce a wide range of immunological alterations in humans. It is through such changes in immune system functioning that stressors may ultimately be linked to subsequent disease. Before these firm conclusions can be reached, however, several remaining gaps in our knowledge of stress–immune–disease relationships must be empirically addressed. One of the foremost gaps concerns the clinical significance of observed immunological alterations. It is not yet clear that either the nature or magnitude of immunological change found in PNI research bears any relevance to increased disease susceptibility. Indeed, immune responses of stressed persons generally fall within normal ranges (Rabin et al., 1989). Furthermore, the immune system is complex and one or even several measures of immune function may not provide an adequate representation of host resistance (Palmblad, 1981). Finally, stress-related changes in immune parameters may not be linked to disease in a straightforward manner. For instance, a decrease in one parameter could result in an increased risk for one type of disease (i.e. acute viral infections), but decreased risk for another (i.e. autoimmune disease) (Irwin, Daniels & Weiner, 1987).

It is also possible that a number of other variables, such as age and genetic factors, interact with stress exposure and immune response to determine health outcomes. It is well known, for instance, that ageing, itself, is associated with a decline in immune function, as indicated by decreases in the proliferative response to mitogens, natural killer cell activity, antibody production, and phagocytic activity (for a discussion, see Scapagnini, 1992). Stress-related immune alterations may have more important consequences for individuals with already compromised immune systems, such as the elderly or those with autoimmune disorders or HIV-infection (Kiecolt-Glaser & Glaser, 1987).

Over the last 20 years, PNI research has made great strides in establishing links between psychological stressors and altered functioning in the immune system. This remains one of the most promising pathways through which stress may alter host resistance to disease onset or exacerbation. Carefully designed prospective studies, measuring all three aspects of the stress–immune–disease model are needed to more fully understand these associations.

REFERENCES

Arnetz, B.B., Wasserman, J., Petrini, B., Brenner, S.O., Levi, L., Eneroth, P., Salovaara, H., Hjelm, R., Salovaara, L., Theorell, T. & Petterson, I.L. (1987). Immune function in unemployed women. *Psychosomatic Medicine*, **49**, 3–12.

Bachen, E.A., Manuck, S.B., Marsland, A.L., Cohen, S., Malkoff, S.B., Muldoon, M.F. & Rabin, B.S. (1992). Lymphocyte subset and cellular immune responses to a brief experimental stressor. *Psychosomatic Medicine*, **54**, 673–9.

Bartrop, R., Lazarus, L., Luckhurst, E., Kiloh, L.G. & Penny, R. (1977). Depressed lymphocyte function after bereavement. *Lancet*, i, 834–6.

Brosschot, J.F., Benschop, R.J., Godaert, G.L., DeSmet, M.B.M., Olff, M.,

Heijnen, C.J. & Balieux, R.E. (1992). Effects of experimental psychological stress on distribution and function of peripheral blood cells. *Psychosomatic Medicine*, **54**, 394–406.

Buske-Kirschbaum, A., Kirschbaum, C., Stierle, H., Lehnert, H. & Hellhammer, D. (1992). Conditioned increase of natural killer cell activity (NKCA) in humans. *Psychosomatic Medicine*, **54**, 123–32.

Cohen, S. & Williamson, G.M. (1991). Stress and infectious disease in humans. *Psychological Bulletin*, **109**, 5–24.

Dorian, B., Garfinkel, P., Keystone, E., Gorczyinski, R. Darby, P. & Garner, D. (1985). Occupational stress and immunity. *Psychosomatic Medicine*, **47**, 77. (Abstract).

Glaser, R., Rice, J., Speicher, C.E., Stout, J.C. & Kiecolt-Glaser, J.K. (1986). Stress depresses interferon production by leukocytes concomitant with a decrease in natural killer cell activity. *Behavioral Neuroscience*, **100**, 675–8.

Grant, I., Brown, G.W., Harris, T., McDonald, W.I., Patterson, T. & Trimble, M.R. (1989). Severely threatening events and marked life difficulties preceding onset or exacerbation of multiple sclerosis. *Journal of Neurology, Neurosurgery, and Psychiatry*, **52**, 8–13.

Herbert, T.B. & Cohen, S. (1993). Stress and immunity in humans: A meta-analytic review. *Psychosomatic Medicine*, **55**, 364–79.

Herbert, T.B., Cohen, S., Marsland, A.L., Bachen, E.A., Rabin, B.S., Muldoon, M.F. & Manuck, S.B. (1994). Cardiovascular reactivity and the course of immune response to an acute psychological stressor. *Psychosomatic Medicine*, **56**, 337–44.

Irwin, M., Daniels, M. & Weiner, H. (1987). Immune and neuroendocrine changes during bereavement. *Psychiatric Clinics of North America*, **10**, 449–65.

Irwin, M., Daniels, M., Smith, T.L., Bloom, E. & Weiner, H. (1987). Impaired natural killer cell activity during bereavement. *Brain, Behavior, and Immunity*, **1**, 98–104.

Jensen, M.R. (1987). Psychobiological factors predicting the course of breast cancer. *Journal of Personality*, **55**, 317–42.

Kennedy, S., Kiecolt-Glaser, J.K. & Glaser, R. (1988). Immunological consequences of acute and chronic stressors: Mediating role of interpersonal relationships. *British Journal of Medical Psychology*, **61**, 77–85.

Kiecolt-Glaser, J.K. & Glaser, R. (1987). Psychosocial moderators of immune function. *Annals of Behavioral Medicine*, **9**, 16–20.

Kiecolt-Glaser, J.K. & Glaser, R. (1988). Methodological issues in behavioral immunology research with humans. *Brain, Behavior, and Immunity*, **2**, 67–78.

Kiecolt-Glaser, J.K., Garner, W., Speicher, C., Penn, G.M., Holliday, J. & Glaser, R. (1984). Psychosocial modifiers of immunocompetence in medical students. *Psychosomatic Medicine*, **46**, 7–14.

Kiecolt-Glaser, J.K., Glaser, R., Shuttleworth, E., Dyer, C., Ogrocki, P. & Speicher, C.E. (1987). Chronic stress and immunity in family caregivers of Alzheimer's disease victims. *Psychosomatic Medicine*, **49**, 523–35.

Kiecolt-Glaser, J.K., Cacioppo, J.T., Malarkey, W.B., & Glaser, R. (1992). Acute psychological stressors and short-term immune changes: what, why, for whom, and what extent? *Psychosomatic Medicine*, **54**, 680–5.

Knapp, P.H., Levy, E.M., Giorgi, R.G., Black, P.H., Fox, B.H. & Heeren, T.C. (1992). Short-term immunological effects of induced emotion. *Psychosomatic Medicine*, **54**, 133–48.

Levi, L. (1972). Sympathoadrenomedullary responses to pleasant and 'unpleasant' psychosocial stimuli. *Acta Medica Scandinavia*, **528**, (Suppl.), 55–73.

Livnat, S., Felten, S.Y., Carlson, S.L., Bellinger, D.L. & Felten, D.L. (1985). Involvement of peripheral and central catecholamine systems in neural–immune interactions. *Journal of Neuroimmunology*, **10**, 5–30.

Maisel, A.S., Knowlton, K.U., Fowler, P., Reardon, A., Ziegler, M.G., Motulsky, H.J., Insel, P.A. & Michel, M.C. (1990). Adrenergic control of circulating lymphocyte subpopulations. Effects of congestive heart failure, dynamic exercise, and terbutaline treatment. *Journal of Clinical Investigation*, **85**, 462–7.

McKinnon, W., Weisse, C.S., Reynolds, C.P., Bowles, C.A. & Baum, A. (1989). Chronic stress, leukocyte subpopulations, and humoral response to latent viruses. *Health Psychology*, **8**, 389–402.

Manuck, S.B., Cohen, S., Rabin, B.S., Muldoon, M.F. & Bachen, E.A. (1991). Individual differences in cellular immune response to stress. *Psychological Science*, **2**, 111–15.

Naliboff, B.D., Benton, D., Solomon, G.F., Morley, J.E., Fahey, J.L. Bloom, E.T., Makinodan, T. & Gilmore, S.L. (1991). Immunological changes in young and old adults during brief laboratory stress. *Psychosomatic Medicine*, **53**, 121–32.

O'Leary, A. (1990). Stress, emotion, and human immune function. *Psychological Bulletin*, **108**, 363–82.

Ottaway, C.A. & Husband, A.J. (1992). Central nervous system influences on lymphocyte migration. *Brain, Behavior, and Immunity*, **6**, 97–116.

Palmblad, J. (1981). Stress and immunologic competence: studies in humans. In R. Ader (Ed.). *Psychoneuroimmunology*, pp. 229–257. New York: Academic Press.

Rabin, B.S., Cohen, S., Ganguli, R., Lysle, D.T. & Cunnick, J.E. (1989). Bidirectional interaction between the central nervous system and immune system. *Critical Reviews in Immunology*, **9**, 279–312.

Scapagnini, U. (1992). Psychoneuroendocrinoimmunology: the basis for a novel therapeutic approach in aging. *Psychoneuroendocrinology*, **17**, 411–20.

Schleifer, S.J., Keller, S.E., Camerino, M., Thornton, J.C. & Stein, M. (1983). Suppression of lymphocyte stimulation following bereavement. *Journal of American Medical Association*, **250**, 374–7.

Sieber, W.J., Rodin, J., Larson, L., Ortega, S. & Cummings, N. (1992). Modulation of human natural killer cell activity by exposure to uncontrollable stress. *Brain, Behavior, and Immunity*, **6**, 141–56.

van Tits, L.J.H., Michel, M.C., Grosse-Wide, H., Happel, M., Eigler, F.W., Soliman, A. & Brodde, O.E. (1990). Catecholamines increase lymphocyte beta-2 adrenergic receptors via a beta-2 adrenergic, spleen-dependent process. *American Journal of Physiology*, **258**, E191–202.

Weisse, C.S., Pato, C.N., McAllister, C.G., Littman, R., Breier, A., Paul, S.M. & Baum, A. (1990). Differential effects of controllable and uncontrollable acute stress on lymphocyte proliferation and leukocyte percentages in humans. *Brain, Behavior, and Immunity*, **4**, 339–51.

Workman, E.A. & La Viá, M.F. (1987). Immunological effects of psychological stressors: a review of the literature. *International Journal of Psychosomatics*, **34**, 35–40.

Zakowski, S.G., McAllister, C.G., Deal, M. & Baum, A. (1992). Stress, reactivity, and immune function in healthy men. *Health Psychology*, **11**, 223–32.

Psychopharmacology

A.JACKIE HUNTER

SmithKline Beecham Pharmaceuticals, Harlow,
Essex, UK

Psychopharmacology is the study of the effects of drugs on psychological functioning. As the initial studies with new classes of compound are in the main carried out in animals prior to studies in people, psychopharmacology is also commonly referred to as the study of the effects of drugs on behaviour. The reason that chemicals can have such profound effects on behaviour is due to the fact that the nerve cells in the brain (neurones) communicate with one another via chemicals called neurotransmitters. Chemicals that intervene at some point in this process of neurotransmission are capable of altering the subsequent behaviour of neurones and neural networks downstream, ultimately causing a change in the behaviour of the animal or person. An understanding of psychopharmacology is important in health psychology for a number of reasons. Perhaps the most important is that, despite many advances in our knowledge in the past two decades, the boundaries between normal and abnormal mental functioning remain unclear. For example, to what extent are the mechanisms involved in mediating normal anxiety involved in mediating the abnormal levels of anxiety in patients? Secondly, it is also important that those involved in treating patients who are receiving medication understand the actions of that medication. Finally, an appreciation of the methods used to study the effects of such drugs can help both in evaluating the potential strengths and weaknesses of current therapies and in assessing the potential of newer therapeutic approaches. The focus of this chapter will be on the effects of drugs on neuronal activity but there is increasing evidence that the glia, the so-called support cells of the nervous system, are also capable of releasing and responding to transmitters. Good introductory references to the subject are provided by Strange (1992), Cooper, Bloom and Roth (1991), Fischbach (1992) and Spiegel (1989). Those readers more interested in the preclinical aspects of psychopharmacology are referred to Sahgal (1993) and Van Haaran (1993).

HOW NEURONES COMMUNICATE

Figure 1 shows a simplified neurone communicating with another neurone, although in real life such a neurone would make and receive many thousands of such connections with other neurones. The synapse is the specialized area where contact occurs and consists of a nerve terminal or presynaptic membrane (the transmitting portion of the synapse), the synaptic cleft (the gap across which the neurotransmitter has to travel) and the postsynaptic membrane of the receiving cell which contains specialized receptors for the neurotransmitters released from the presynaptic membrane. From the diagram overleaf it is obvious that the synapse is specialized for one-way traffic and, whilst neurotransmitter receptors are usually present in low density on the presynaptic terminal to provide a mechanism for regulating release, neurotransmitter release itself can only occur from the presynaptic terminal due to the presence of storage vesicles for the transmitter. When a neurone is excited, a wave of electrical depolarization (the inside of neurone is negatively charged relative to the exterior) called an action potential passes down the axon. When this action potential reaches the nerve terminal (presynaptic membrane) it causes neurotransmitter release into the synaptic cleft. The transmitter diffuses across the cleft and reaches receptors as shown in Figure 1. The transmitter then binds to the receptor and changes the conformation of that receptor which elicits a response. This process is called transduction. Broadly speaking the receptors involved in this process fall into two main superfamilies: those coupled to ion channels and those coupled to G-proteins.

Activation of a receptor coupled to an ion channel will alter the permeability of that channel to ions such as calcium, sodium, chloride or potassium depending on the specificity of the channel. For example the $GABA_A$ receptor is coupled to a chloride channel. The structure of the $GABA_A$ receptor is similar to other ion channel linked receptors and it consists of five subunits that are glycosylated integral membrane proteins. Multiple isoforms of these subunits can exist with differing distribution in various brain areas as demonstrated by *in situ* hybridization studies. These subunits combine to form an oligomeric array with a central pore which forms the ion channel and the receptor binding site and various additional binding sites for regulatory molecules. The activity of the $GABA_A$ receptor can be modulated by benzodiazepines (e.g. Valium), steroids and barbiturates. Other examples of ion channel linked receptors are the $5-HT_3$ subtype of the serotonergic receptor and the nicotinic acetylcholine receptor. Ion channel linked receptors will produce a much faster initial response than those linked to G proteins.

Activation of a receptor coupled to a G-protein causes cleavage of a high energy phosphate bond from guanosine triphosphate which sets in train a cascade of biochemical events within the postsynaptic neurone. These secondary effects may be due to the activation of second messengers such as adenylate cyclase and phospholipase C. The latter activates second messengers which are capable of regulating ion channels via phosphorylation and so G-protein linked receptors are capable of indirectly regulating responsiveness of ion channels. The dopamine receptors upon which neuroleptic drugs such as haloperidol ('Haldol') act are coupled to G-proteins as are muscarinic cholinergic receptors.

Once the transmitter has effected a response, it dissociates from the receptor and is then either broken down in the synaptic cleft, as in the case of acetylcholine, or taken back up into the presynaptic terminal for storage and release or breakdown as in the case of dopamine. Release of neurotransmitter can be reduced by stimulation of

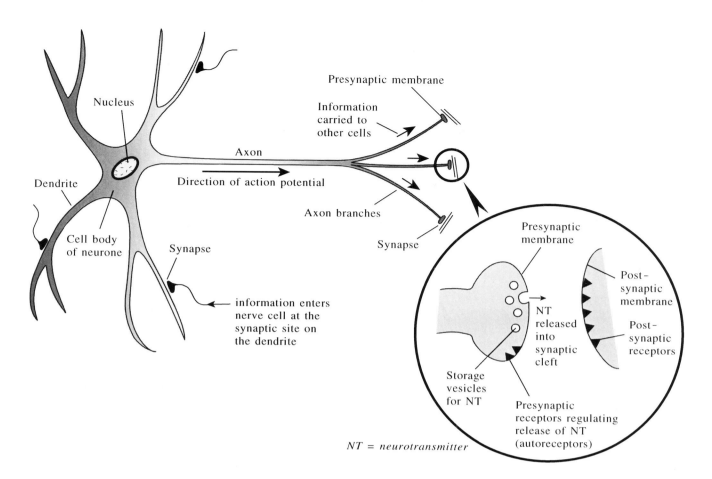

Fig. 1. Simplified diagram of neurone with an enlargement of a synapse.

Table 1. *Major neurotransmitters in brain*

Neurotransmitter	Existing subtypes[a]	Main behavioural effects
Adrenalin (Ad)/ Noradrenalin (NAd)	α_1, α_2, β_{1-3}	Sleep, arousal, depression
Dopamine (DA)	D_{1-5}	Motor behaviour, psychosis, reward
Acetylcholine (Ach)	Nicotnic Muscarinic M_{1-5}	Cognition, attention, motor behaviour
Serotonin (5HT)	$5HT_{1-7}$	Anxiety, depression, sleep, emesis
γ-aminobutyric acid (GABA)	$GABA_A$, $GABA_B$	Anxiety, seizure, cognition
Glutamate	NMDA, Kainate, AMPA Metabotropic ($mGluR_{1-8}$)	Neurodegeneration anxiety, cognition, pain

[a] These subtypes may be further divided, e.g. $5-HT_2$ receptors comprise a family of receptors: $5-HT_{2A,2B \text{ and } 2C}$; α_1 receptors comprise $\alpha_{1A, 1B, 1C}$ and $_{1D}$. Full details of all subtypes can be found in *TIPS Receptor and Ion Nomenclature Supplement*, 1994.

presynaptic autoreceptors. This acts as a feedback control mechanism on neurotransmitter release and antagonism of these receptors increases neurotransmitter release.

Prolonged stimulation of the postsynaptic or presynaptic receptors can lead to a phenomenon called receptor desensitization. This occurs very rapidly and is defined as the loss of responsiveness to an agonist following a strong stimulation. This may represent an acute means of preventing over-stimulation at the synaptic level and involves a conformational switch in the receptor protein. Of more relevance clinically is the phenomenon of receptor down-regulation which occurs with chronic agonist challenge. Studies in animals have demonstrated that prolonged treatment with agonists can alter the density of receptors at the cell surface. Conversely prolonged administration of an antagonist can cause an increase in receptors at the cell surface (receptor up-regulation). These phenomena may be very important in explaining why tolerance to some drugs occurs and why other drugs such as antidepressants may take some weeks to reach maximum therapeutic benefit.

A list of the major neurotransmitters in the brain and some of their known roles in behaviour is given in Table 1 but it should be remembered that more than 40 peptide and non-peptide neurotransmitters have been identified since the first neurotransmitter was discovered in 1921. Another important concept is the fact that chemically defined pathways exist in the brain which are in effect subdivisions of the neuroanatomically defined pathways clearly joining one structure to another. This is important because some diseases cause lesions of specific neurotransmitter pathways. The best known of these pathways is probably the dopaminergic pathway between the substantia nigra and striatum which degenerates in Parkinson's disease. This results in the profound disruption of motor function seen in Parkinsonian patients. Other diseases, such as Alzheimer's disease, may ultimately affect a number of different neurotransmitter systems.

HOW CAN WE INTERVENE IN NEUROTRANSMISSION?

There are many points at which intervention in neurotransmission is possible. At the level of the postsynaptic receptor a drug which binds to the receptor and causes the same conformational change, and hence effects, as the normal neurotransmitter is an agonist at that receptor. A drug which binds to the receptor and does not produce the same effects as the normal neurotransmitter, thereby blocking the effects of the endogenous neurotransmitter is called an antagonist. Thus a post synaptic agonist will enhance neurotransmission and an antagonist decrease it.

Neurotransmission may also be enhanced by prolonging the presence of the neurotransmitter within the synaptic cleft either by stopping breakdown of the neurotransmitter or by blocking reuptake into the presynaptic terminal. The tricyclic antidepressants which were, for many years, the mainstay of antidepressant therapy were thought to be effective by virtue of their blockade of the reuptake of noradrenalin and serotonin, although they possessed many other effects as well (e.g. cholinergic antagonism). The selective serotonin reuptake inhibitors (SSRIs) such as paroxetine, which are also prescribed for depression, act, as their name suggests, by specifically blocking the reuptake of serotonin. Acetylcholinesterase inhibitors, on the other hand, increase levels of acetylcholine in the synapse by stopping breakdown of the neurotransmitter by acetylcholinesterase. Other means of altering activity include enhancement of synthesis of the transmitter by increasing the levels of precursor, e.g. administration of L-dopa to Parkinsonian patients to elevate brain dopamine levels, or by inhibiting breakdown of the neurotransmitter within the presynaptic terminal. Monoamine oxidase inhibitors increase concentrations of serotonin, noradrenalin and dopamine by inhibiting the intracellular enzyme, monoamine oxidase, which is responsible for the breakdown of these transmitters in the terminal.

More recently, as our understanding of receptors has increased, we have been able to use the fact that different subtypes of receptors exist to target specific receptors subtypes (see Table 1) which will hopefully reduce the side-effects of many current medications and improve efficacy. This increase in ability to define different subtypes of receptors has resulted from two major areas of research. One is the advances made in molecular biology which have enabled the cloning and expression of different receptor subtypes. Such cloning studies have demonstrated that there are many more subtypes of receptors for a number of neurotransmitters than had hitherto been suspected on the basis of pharmacological studies, the dopamine receptor is a classic example (see below). The second is the advances in biochemical pharmacology which have enabled the detailed analyses of ligand binding and functional responses in isolated tissues and membranes.

HOW IS PSYCHOPHARMACOLOGY USED TO DEVELOP THERAPEUTICALLY USEFUL AGENTS?

The process for delineating the role of a particular neurotransmitter system in disease relies on the pooling of clinical and preclinical information. Clinical studies of patients both during life and at postmortem can provide evidence that a particular neurotransmitter system is disrupted in a particular disorder. At postmortem the level of activity of the neurotransmitter system can be monitored by studying levels in the brain of metabolites, the neurotransmitter itself or the activity of enzymes that are rate limiting in the synthesis or breakdown of the neurotransmitter. The density of the receptors for that neurotransmitter can be measured in various brain regions of interest. The advent of non-invasive imaging technology has also meant that the activity of brain regions in patients with and without medication can be examined. Positron emission tomography (PET) and single photon emission computerized tomography (SPECT) are the two most commonly employed methods of functional imaging. PET studies can use labelled carbon, nitrogen or oxygen to study changes in cerebral blood flow, cerebral brain energy metabolism and protein synthesis. Thus regional changes in activity in these parameters during normal activity can be compared in volunteers and patients. For example, reductions in blood flow to the frontal cortex have been noted in schizophrenic patients. PET is much more costly than SPECT, but SPECT can be used to study cerebral blood flow. In some cases, where ligands of suitable radioactivity are available, PET or SPECT studies can be performed to look at the activity of particular neurotransmitter systems in the living human brain, e.g. dopamine D_1 and D_2 receptor activation. For such clinical studies of 'brain neurochemistry' to be meaningful they must be carried out on a well defined group of patients. This has proved particularly difficult in the areas of schizophrenia and depression and although more consistent diagnostic criteria are being applied, some of the conflicting evidence for neurochemical changes may be the result of heterogeneity in patient groupings.

Data from clinical studies is then complemented by work in animals. Where possible animal models of various disorders are used. Perhaps the area where animal models have been most successful is anxiety. Although there is no consensus about the aetiology of anxiety, a number of studies suggest that anxiety is an exacerbation of a normal response. Thus animal tests for anxiolytic drugs have relied on studying normal fearful behaviour in animals. In the past, tests such as conflict tests have been used. An example of such a conflict is that experienced by a thirsty rat when it receives a very mild shock when it drinks from a spout. An anxiolytic drug will increase responding, in this case drinking, under these conditions. These tests have proved extremely predictive of anxiolytic actions in man. In recent years there has been a move towards more ethologically based tasks. These include the elevated plus maze and social interaction tests. The plus maze consists of an elevated X-shaped maze with two opposing arms open and the other two opposing arms enclosed by high walls. Initially mice and rats naturally prefer to remain in the enclosed arms rather than explore the open arms. Giving anxiolytic drugs increases the time the animals spend on the open arms compared to that observed in untreated animals. In the social interaction test, two unfamiliar animals are placed together and allowed to explore each other. The effect seen with an anxiolytic drug is an increase in the amount of time the two animals spend in close contact. Unfortunately some classes of compound have shown marked effects on these ethological tests and weak effects on conflict tests of anxiety. These compounds have also been shown to be less effective as anxiolytics in man.

A second area where reasonable animal models exist is that of drug withdrawal. Chronic treatment of mice with ethanol will produce symptoms of withdrawal when the ethanol is removed, e.g. seizures. However, for many psychological disorders, e.g. depression and schizophrenia, no good animal models of the disease or its symptomatology exist. Animal studies in these cases are used to confirm the activity and brain penetration of compounds with a defined mechanism of action, e.g. antagonism of a particular type of neurotransmitter receptor, where clinical studies have implicated this receptor in the disease.

Two examples will be used to illustrate how preclinical and clinical studies have combined to elucidate the role of neurotransmitters and in particular specific receptors for those neurotransmitters in disease. These are the role of the cholinergic system in Alzheimer's dementia and the role of dopamine in schizophrenia.

THE ROLE OF THE CHOLINERGIC SYSTEM IN ALZHEIMER'S DEMENTIA

Alzheimer's dementia is a progressive neurodegeneration of the cortex and limbic system, initially resulting in memory loss but subsequently progressing to much more profound changes in personality and consciousness. The disease at present can only be confirmed at postmortem by the presence in the brain of characteristic neurofibrillary tangles and senile plaques containing amyloid deposits. The first neurochemical studies on Alzheimer's disease patients showed a profound and consistent loss of markers for the cholinergic system such as decreased levels of the synthetic enzyme, choline acetyl transferase (ChAT) and reductions in levels of the enzyme which breaks down acetylcholine in the synapse, acetylcholinesterase (AChE). Reductions in these markers in the cerebral cortex were also shown to correlate with the degree of cognitive impairment. Acetylcholine acts on two types of receptors, nicotinic receptors and muscarinic receptors. Anyone who smokes, or who has smoked, will be aware of the effects of stimulating nicotinic receptors with exogenous nicotine, increased physiological arousal and gastric motility, for example. Stimulation of muscarinic receptors results in a different pattern of effects, namely tremor, bradycardia, hypothermia and increased salivation and lacrimation. However levels of muscarinic receptors are not consistently reduced in Alzheimer's disease and interest has focused on the ascending basal forebrain cholinergic systems which supply the hippocampus and cortex, areas known to be involved in learning and memory. Studies carried out by Drachman and colleagues in the 1970s and 1980s had demonstrated that scopolamine, a muscarinic receptor antagonist, when given to people, causes an impairment in memory (Drachman et al., 1980) and this finding has been confirmed by numerous other investigators. Thus all the evidence pointed to an important role for the cholinergic system in memory and learning but further work was needed in animals to pinpoint the nature of the involvement of the cholinergic system in learning and memory.

There are two main approaches that have been traditionally used in preclinical studies, first the use of pharmacological agents selective for different muscarinic receptor subtypes and secondly the lesioning of specific brain areas to try to mimic the deficits seen in the disease states. Although currently there is no animal model of Alzheimer's disease, we can study learning and memory in animals and examine the effects of drug administration and lesioning on the performance of learning and memory tests.

Lesion experiments in animals have revealed that both the septal-hippocampal and basal forebrain cholinergic systems play an important role in learning and memory. For example, lesions of the cholinergic cell bodies in the septum, which supply the cholinergic input to the hippocampus, result in impairments in performance on spatial learning tasks. These spatial tasks include the Morris water maze and radial arm maze. The Morris water maze consists of a large circular pool filled with water made opaque by the addition of a latex compound (synthetic asses' milk!). Hidden just under the surface of the water is a small platform or island. On successive trials the rat is placed in the water and learns quite quickly to find the island using cues around the pool to navigate. The radial arm maze consists of eight or more arms radiating from a central hub rather like spokes on a wheel. The maze is elevated above the floor so the rats have an incentive to stay on the arms which are usually not enclosed to any great extent. At the end of each arm is a food reward in a shallow dip so the animal cannot see the food. Obviously the best strategy for the rat is to visit each arm only once. Over a period of days, normal animals learn the task to a high degree of accuracy.

Cholinergic lesions also produce deficits in working memory tests such as delayed non-match or match to sample. The delayed match to sample test is similar to tests used in humans. For rodents, choices are usually limited. The animal is presented with a stimulus (a lever, or light) and then given a choice between the previously presented stimulus and a new stimulus. In the matching condition the animal has to respond to the previously presented stimulus. The converse is true in the non-matching condition. With primates a large number of stimuli can be presented on the choice portion of the test. This type of test has obvious parallels in computerized tests of memory in humans such as the CANTAB test. The forebrain cholinergic systems terminate in areas which have been shown by autoradiography to possess a high density of muscarinic cholinergic receptors. This, coupled with the finding that the muscarinic antagonists scopolamine and atropine produce deficits in learning and memory in animals and man, suggests that the cholinergic system is important for memory and learning and that the key receptors are of the muscarinic receptor subtype rather than the nicotinic.

Work with human cloned receptors has identified at least five subtypes of muscarinic receptor (m1–5) which, coupled with previous pharmacological studies, primarily using isolated tissues, has enabled the development of compounds selective for these various receptor subtypes. It is believed that M_1 receptors mediate cognitive effects whereas M_2 receptors appear to be important in mediating other effects such as tremor. Thus a compound preferentially active on M_1 receptors might be expected to be cognitive enhancing without showing the side effects seen with non-selective compounds such as oxotremorine and arecoline. Presynaptic M_3 receptors are also present and regulate acetylcholine release so another way of increasing cholinergic activity might be to develop an antagonist for the presysnaptic M_3 receptor which would cause an increase in acetylcholine release, i.e. block the negative feedback on release

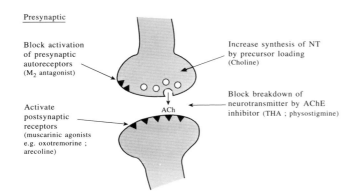

Presynaptic

Block activation
of presynaptic
autoreceptors
(M₂ antagonist)

Increase synthesis of NT
by precursor loading
(Choline)

Activate
postsynaptic
receptors
(muscarinic agonists
e.g. oxotremorine ;
arecoline)

Block breakdown of
neurotransmitter by AChE
inhibitor (THA ; physostigmine)

ACh

Fig. 2. Ways of increasing cholinergic muscarinic neurotransmission.

which acetylcholine in the synaptic cleft causes via stimulation of these presysnaptic autoreceptors. This is shown diagrammatically in Fig. 2.

Cholinesterase inhibitors have also demonstrated some benefit in Alzheimer's disease by increasing the availability of acetylcholine at the synapse (Figure 2), although early studies using physostigmine were inconclusive probably due to the short half-life of the drug. Indeed the only compound currently approved by the Food and Drug Administration (FDA) in the USA for this disease is tetrahydroaminoacridine (THA), a cholinesterase inhibitor with good bioavailability and duration of action. It is not the ideal drug, however, as it has activity at other receptors and causes elevation of liver enzymes. It is only active in a narrow dose range before side-effects become apparent, requiring dose titration for patients. Additionally it is only active in a certain percentage of patients, whether this is due to a true lack of response to cholinesterase therapy or to the fact that side-effects are too marked in these patients has not been answered.

THE ROLE OF THE DOPAMINE SYSTEM IN SCHIZOPHRENIA

Although psychological, social and structural explanations for schizophrenia exist, the most widely accepted theory for the aetiology of schizophrenia is the dopamine theory. This states that excessive levels of dopamine are responsible for the induction of psychotic/schizophrenic symptoms. Much of the evidence for this comes from reports that drugs which increase dopamine function such as amphetamine (which increases dopamine release and inhibits reuptake) exacerbate psychotic symptoms in patients and mimics them in normal individuals. Although there is evidence that other neurotransmitters such as neurotensin and serotonin may play a role in central dopaminergic function, most work has concentrated on the development of dopamine antagonists as neuroleptics/antipsychotic agents. Examples of older style antipsychotics are chlorpromazine, trifluoperazine and haloperidol and the introduction of these drugs in the 1950s produced a profound decrease in the number of schizophrenic patients requiring hospitalization. The mode of action of these drugs is to block central dopaminergic receptors. Blockade of central dopamine receptors in animals results in a number of behavioural effects, e.g. catalepsy, as dopamine receptors are present not only in the areas of the brain thought to be involved in psychosis (limbic system; cortex) but also in areas

responsible for homeostasis (hypothalamus; pituitary) and motor control (striatum). Therefore it was not surprising that in people these drugs were capable of producing a number of side-effects, especially after prolonged use. The most debilitating of these are the extrapyramidal side-effects due to blockade of the dopamine receptors in the nigrostriatal system. These side-effects can be divided into dystonias, akathesias, tardive dyskinesia, Parkinsonism and tremors.

Until the 1990s only two types of dopamine receptor had been identified, D_1 and D_2 and it was thought that the antipsychotic activity of the neuroleptics was related to their potency at blocking D_2 receptors. However, there were a number of discrepancies between the occupancy of D_2 receptors by the drug and antipsychosis. PET studies have shown that antipsychotics rapidly block D^2 receptors in the brain, yet the antipsychotic effects can take several weeks to reach maximum efficacy. Recently, gene cloning studies have demonstrated that there are further subtypes of dopamine receptors, the D_1 and D_5 receptors belong to the D_1-like superfamily, and the D_2, D_3 and D_4 receptors belong to the D_2 superfamily. The roles of these subtypes is not clear but they offer the possibility that compounds selective for the various D_2 subtypes may be of benefit in schizophrenia as the receptors have different distributions within the brain. The D_3 receptor, for example, is expressed at relatively high levels in the limbic system, lower levels in the striatum and is absent in the pituitary. Unlike the Alzheimer's disease area, work mapping the distribution and levels of these new receptor subtypes has occurred relatively recently and any changes observed may be due to the medication that such patients may have been taking. Most neuroleptic drugs do not show any selectivity for the various members of the D_2 receptor family. Another problem is that, until recently, most animal models were designed to predict the antischizophrenic activity of D_2 compounds. In this instance, animal studies can only be used for an assessment of the brain penetration and the side-effect potential of a compound. More recently, sophisticated paradigms based on human findings have been employed. These include prepulse inhibition and latent inhibition (Braff & Geyer, 1990, Solomon *et al.*, 1981). However, until truly selective compounds are synthesized, the role of the D_3 and, indeed, the D_4 receptor in both animal and human behaviour remains to be assessed.

The so-called atypical neuroleptics developed in the late 1980s, such as clozapine and risperidone, have been reported to produce less extrapyramidal side-effects. The reasons for this lack of side-effect potential are not known but are thought by some to be related to the antagonistic action of these atypical compounds at serotonergic receptors.

FUTURE DIRECTIONS

Although much has been achieved in psychopharmacology in the last 30 years, there are still major unmet needs in the treatment of neurodegenerative and psychiatric disorders. Studies utilising more selective drugs may ultimately improve diagnosis and patient classification in heterogeneous groups of patients such as depressives and schizophrenics. Currently, much of our efforts are based on alleviation of symptoms but in the neurodegenerative disorders it may be possible in future to envisage pharmacological treatments which may also halt disease progression.

REFERENCES

Braff, D.L. & Geyer, M.A. (1990). Sensorimotor gating and schizophrenia. Human and animal studies. *Archive General Psychiatry*, 47, 181–8.

Cooper, J.R., Bloom, F.E. & Roth R.H. (1991). *The biochemical basis of neuropharmacology*. Oxford: Oxford University Press.

Drachman, D.A., Noffsugar, D., Sahakian, B.J., Kurdziel, S. & Fleming, P. (1980). Aging, memory and the cholinergic system: a study of dichotic listening. *Neurobiology of Aging*, 1, 39–43.

Fischbach, G.D. (1992). Mind and brain. *Scientific American*, 267 (3), 24–33.

Sahgal, A., ed. (1993). Behavioural neuroscience. A practical approach, vols I & II. Oxford: IRL Press.

Solomon, P.R., Crider, A., Winkelman, J.W., Turi, A., Kamer, R.M. & Kaplan, L.J. (1981). Disrupted latent inhibition with chronic amphetamine or haloperidol-induced supersensitivity: relationship to schizophrenic attention disorder. *Biological Psychiatry*, 16, 519–37.

Spiegel, R. (1989). *Psychopharmacology: an introduction*. Chichester: John Wiley.

Strange, P.G. (1992). *Brain biochemistry and brain disorders*. Oxford: Oxford University Press.

TIPS (1994). *TIPS Receptor and ion channel nomenclature Suppl.*. Oxford: Elsevier Science Ltd.

Van Haaran, F. (1993). *Methods in behavioural pharmacology*. Oxford: Elsevier Science Ltd.

Psychophysiology

ROBERT J. GATCHEL

Department of Psychiatry, University of Texas
Southwestern Medical Center at Dallas, USA

Any introductory psychology textbook is certain to review the history of the 'mind–body' controversy. Are experiences purely mental, purely physical, or an interaction of the physical and the mental? As I have recently reviewed elsewhere, the perception of the nature of this relationship has changed over the ages (Gatchel, 1993). Also, as will be discussed, most professionals today take the position that the mind and body are not separate entities, but are part of an interacting 'whole'. Psychophysiology is a field that has developed effective research methods for examining such interactions.

A HISTORICAL OVERVIEW OF MIND–BODY PERSPECTIVES

The ancient Greeks emphasized the interaction of physical or biological factors with the personality or psychological state of an individual. Thus, the ancient Greek physician Hippocrates proposed one of the earliest temperamental theories of personality. He suggested that four bodily fluids, called humours, were responsible for personality or temperament, as well as physical or mental illness. This model emphasized how physical or biological factors can interact with, and affect, the personality or psychological state of an individual.

This traditional view of the interrelationship between mind and body, however, lost favour in the seventeenth century with the advent of physical medicine during the Renaissance period. The belief that the mind (or the soul) could influence the body came to be regarded as unscientific. The understanding of the mind and soul was regulated to religion and philosophy, whereas understanding of the body was considered to be in the separate realm of physical medicine. A biomedical reductionism view was advanced during this time in which it was viewed that the body could be explained by its own mechanisms. This gradually led to the belief that concepts such as the mind or soul were not needed to explain physical functioning or behaviour. Revolutions of knowledge in the simultaneously evolving sciences of physics, anatomy, and physiology were all based on the principles of objective, scientific investigation. Physical mechanisms could be so investigated; mental or spiritual ones could not. This new mechanistic approach to the study of human behaviour also, unfortunately, fostered a dualistic viewpoint that mind and body function separately and independently. Before this point in time, society's physicians, who functioned in the multiple roles of philosopher, teacher, priest, and healer, had approached the understanding of mind–body interactions in a more holistic, integrated way.

The individual who is usually credited with developing and popularizing this dualistic viewpoint was the seventeenth century French philosopher, René Descartes. Descartes argued that the mind or soul was a separate entity, parallel to, and incapable of, affecting physical matter or somatic processes in any direct way. This viewpoint, which came to be known as cartesian dualism of mind and body, became the predominant philosophical basis for medicine. Even though Descartes suggested that the mind and body could interact, with the pineal gland located in the midbrain being the vital connection between the mind and the body, his basic tenet of dualism moved the newly independent field of medicine away from a holistic approach of psycho-physical interactions and toward the mechanistic pathophysiological approach that has dominated the field of western medicine until relatively recently. The discovery in the nineteenth century that microorganisms caused certain diseases further reinforced the acceptance of this dualistic viewpoint. In the new scientific era of medicine, mechanical laws and physiological principles became the only acceptable basis for explaining disease.

With the emergence of psychiatry and psychology during the mid-nineteenth century, however, strict dualism began to be

Psychophysiology

questioned. Physicians such as Sigmund Freud became quite influential in stressing the interaction of psychological and physical factors in various disorders. Although the emphasis at this time was still on the role that the body, microorganisms, and biological factors had in determining illness, the field of medicine gradually became aware of other significant influences. Indeed, the concept of psychogenesis (i.e. the belief that psychological factors can affect bodily processes) gradually re-emerged. The twentieth century evidenced a great deal of re-emergence and growth in an integrated, holistic approach to health and illness, especially because of the advent of modern psychiatry and psychology. The principal arena for this integration has traditionally been the field developed within psychiatry called psychosomatic medicine. The basic belief of psychosomatic medicine was that social and psychological factors are important in the etiology, development, and maintenance of many illnesses, as well as in the treatment of these illnesses.

THE EMERGENCE OF PSYCHOPHYSIOLOGY

Psychophysiology is an outgrowth of the field of psychosomatic medicine. One influential early figure in this area was Harold G. Wolff. Wolff's publication in 1953 of his work *Stress and disease* made significant contributions to the field. He emphasized a rigorous scientific approach to the simultaneous measure of both psychological and physiological factors. In a well-known experimental study of gastric functioning in a fistula patient, 'Tom', Wolf and Wolff (1947) systematically evaluated changes in gastric secretion and motor activity under different emotional conditions. In the aggressive emotional states of anger and resentment, Tom displayed an increase of gastric secretion and motor activity; the emotional states of fright and depression, on the other hand, lead to corresponding decreases in gastric functioning. Studies such as these began to move the field towards a more integrated approach to the study of psychological and physical characteristics. Actually, his approach became known as the psychophysiological approach because of its objective and quantifiable method of studying psychophysiological interactions. Wolff's work remains of interest today, as does that of several other pioneering researchers (see Alexander, 1950; Graham, 1972), who were important in linking physiological and psychological realms of inquiry and in demonstrating how emotional factors influence functioning by organ systems.

The area of psychophysiological research started to emerge during the 1950s and provided basic evidence of the relationships between psychological and physiological responses. At this point in time, psychologists, who were more well grounded in experimental methodology and analysis than psychiatrists, began to make major contributions to the field. In an early classic experiment conducted by a psychologist, Ax (1953) designed a study which induced emotion in a laboratory setting. A major problem encountered in the study of emotion is that it is extremely difficult to realistically elicit various emotions in a laboratory situation. However, Ax was quite creative in producing 'realistic' and powerful emotion-producing situations. In this study, male subjects were recruited for a study of 'hypertension'. Upon entering the laboratory, a number of physiological recording electrodes were attached to subjects by the experimenter. The subjects were also informed by this experimenter that the regular polygraph equipment operator was ill and that another operator was filling in for him on this day. After a brief rest period during which physiological measurements were recorded, the temporary equipment operator shouted from the next room that there was some trouble with the recordings. This prompted the experimenter to go into the next room and switch places with the operator. The equipment operator, upon entering the room where the subject was seated, then proceeded to act in an obnoxious, criticizing manner and informed the subject sarcastically that the problems encountered were probably the subject's fault. He continued to verbally abuse the subject during the next 5 minutes for not cooperating or for even the slightest movement that could affect the physiological recordings. During this time period, physiological responses were monitored. The experimenter subsequently returned to the room and apologized for the operator's 'rude' behavior. This staged situation appeared quite effective in inducing anger, with subjects openly verbalizing their anger. Subsequently, another rest period was introduced before the induction of the fear condition (it should be noted that for half of the subjects, the order was reversed with fear followed by anger).

In the fear condition, a shock which gradually increased in intensity was administered to the subject's finger until he complained, at which time the experimenter acted very alarmed and concerned, frantically moving around the room, and cautioning the subject that he must remain perfectly still for his own good. Sparks from the equipment also began to fly around the room. This contrived threat of accidental electrocution potential continued for 5 minutes, and produced quite a bit of fear in the subject. Once again, physiological responding was recorded throughout this period.

Results of this study clearly showed different patterns of physiological responding associated with these two emotional states. The anger pattern appeared to be related to what would be produced by the biochemical action of the 'stress' hormone noradrenaline (norepinephrine); the fear pattern appeared to be related to the action of adrenaline (epinephrine). Thus, specific physiological response patterns paralleled emotional responding.

Obviously, the ethical concern of deceiving subjects in such a drastic manner would make conducting a study such as this quite difficult to justify today. However, there have been other more recent studies using different methodologies (e.g. having subjects read different affect-laden material; having subjects visualize different emotional situations). These studies have again demonstrated unique physiological response patterns associated with different emotional states (see Gatchel & Barnes, 1989).

Studies such as these clearly demonstrated the close interaction of psychological or emotional states and physiological states. Indeed, in light of such findings, most professionals today take the position that mind and body are not separate entities. A change in emotional state will be accompanied by a change in physiological response, and a change in physiological functioning will frequently be accompanied by alterations and emotional affect. Indeed, as Lipowski (1977, page 234) notes, in order to understand comprehensively health and disease, it is important to study people as 'individual mind–body complexes easily interacting with the social and physical environment in which they are embodied'. The research methods of psychophysiology allow one to systematically evaluate such interactions.

WHAT IS PSYCHOPHYSIOLOGY?

The word psychophysiology itself indicates a relationship between mental events (psyche) and related bodily changes (physiology). It is the scientific study of the relationship or role of the many physiological processes in behavior and both conscious and unconscious experience. The various behavioural situations that may be studied can range from basic emotional responses such as anger or fear, to conditioning and learning phenomena, and to higher cognitive processes such as information processing and thinking. Because these states are accompanied by physiological responses, changes in sweat gland secretion, muscle tension, heart and respiratory rates, brain waves, and so on, the evaluation of physiological responses is a valuable assessment procedure. The field itself is best defined by a certain set of scientific methods. It typically involves the careful measurement of human physiology under various psychological conditions. These physiological changes can be non-invasively recorded on a polygraph by electrodes fastened to the individual's skin. A polygraph is simply an electronic device that allows one to amplify or increase the size of bioelectric signals so that they can be visually observed and measured; it records physiological activity. Nearly all the organ systems of the body generate bioelectric signals that can be recorded in this way. Special amplifiers have been developed to measure specific physiological responses and various aspects of the electrical signals generated. Commercially available polygraphs are designed to eliminate the potential risk of shock hazard to a subject. Researchers, though, must always remain alert to any potential shock hazards created by interfacing with other experimental equipment.

With the significant advances in the field of biomedical engineering, we have greatly expanded our ability to measure minute physiological responses in living organisms by primarily noninvasive means. This allows us to carefully evaluate complex biological processes underlying human behaviour and experience. For the uninitiated, Hassett (1978) published the *Primer of psychophysiology* which initially provided valuable basic information for the interested novice in psychophysiology. For the more advanced researcher, there have been a number of texts and handbooks on methods in psychophysiology published over the years (e.g. Brown, 1967; Venables & Martin, 1967; Greenfield & Sternbach, 1972; Ackles, Jennings & Cole, 1988; Cacioppo & Tassinary, 1990).

PHYSIOLOGICAL RESPONSE SYSTEMS

Commonly recorded physiological events such as heart rate, blood pressure, sweat glands or electrodermal activity (the galvanic skin response or GSR), and skin temperature are controlled by the autonomic nervous system (ANS). The ANS, sometimes referred to as the visceral or vegetative system, modulates the activity of the internal organs, glands, heart, and all the smooth muscles of the body. It regulates the body's internal environment. Its activities are usually involuntary and automatic, and they most often occur without our conscious awareness. It is not true, however, that the ANS is totally exempt from voluntary control. With biofeedback training, people can gain some control over autonomic response (see Part II of this Handbook).

The ANS is divided into a sympathetic nervous system (SNS) and a parasympathetic nervous system (PNS). The SNS mobilizes emergency responses that prepare the organism for sudden activity or stress. For example, the heart beats faster and increases the amount of blood pumped with each heart beat; the arteries supplying the large muscles dilate so that more blood reaches those muscles; and the pupils dilate to facilitate perception. The PNS is usually dominant during states of quiescence such as sleep, when cardiovascular activity and other physiological functions are reduced and metabolism slows down. Both branches of the ANS, however, are always active; even during an emergency stress reaction, when the sympathetic system dominates, the parasympathetic system is not completely inactive. Psychophysiologists have mapped out methods for determining the relative level of activity of the SNS and PNS during different states.

Two other commonly recorded physiological measures, striate (voluntary) muscle activity (recorded by the electromyogram or EMG) and cortical or brain-wave activity (recorded by the electroencephalogram or EEG), reflect the actions of the central nervous system (CNS). The CNS, which consists of the brain and spinal cord, controls voluntary behaviours such as walking and thinking.

During the past decade, with the advent of sensitive biochemical assay measurement technology, neurohormonal measures, such as the catecholamines, adrenaline and noradrenaline, have also become a part of the repertoire of psychophysiologists in recording the body's responses to different psychological states and environmental events. The adrenal glands, controlled by the ANS, are part of the neuroendocrine system and generally serve as a complementary system to the nervous system in regulating bodily function. The neuroendocrine system is made up of several glands that secrete hormones directly into the circulating bloodstream, and includes the adrenals, the pituitary, thyroid, and the reproductive organs.

Finally, measures of immune system functioning are also being used more in psychophysiology research. Unlike many of the systems already discussed, the wide array of immune organs and cells are not primarily concerned with signalling the body to work in special ways or with transporting nutrients. Rather, the immune system is responsible for providing a defense against pathogens and 'foreign' agents, particles and substances that do not 'belong' in the body. Bacteria, viruses, abnormal cells, transplant tissue, and allergens are all subject to attack by the immune system. The immune system, in turn, can be affected by a number of factors, including psychological stress (Gatchel, Baum & Krantz, 1989). As such, it has become another important psychophysiological marker to use in research studies.

Table 1 provides a summary of the various psychophysiological responses that can be reliably recorded. It should also be noted that, once a physiological response is recorded, another important determination to be made is the measurement unit to be used for quantification purposes. For example, is the measurement of inter-beat interval the most sensitive index for evaluating transient, phasic changes in heart rate? Is average heart rate the best unit of measurement for gauging tonic or baseline levels? The major professional psychophysiology research society in the United States, the Society for Psychophysiological Research, regularly publishes recording and measurement guidelines that allow a researcher to select the best, scientifically agreed-upon measures.

Table 1. *Commonly used measures in psychophysiology*

System	Response	Measures
Central nervous system	Brian activity	Electroencephalogram (EEG) measure of brain wave activity
		Cortical evoked potential (CEP)
		Cortical slow wave Activity (Contingent negative variation)
		P300 wave of CEP
	Muscular activity	Electromyogram (EMG) measure of muscle activity
		Electrooculogram (EOG) measure of eye movements
	Respiration	Respiration rate and amplitude
Autonomic nervous system	Cardiovascular	Heart rate
		Systolic and diastolic blood pressure
		Skin temperature
		Blood flow/volume
	Sweat gland (Electrodermal activity)	GSR:
		Skin conductance
		Skin resistance
	Digestive system	Gastric motility
	Visual system	Pupil dilation/ constriction
		Eye blink
	Sexual response	Penile tumescence
		Vaginal blood flow
Neuroendocrine system	Adrenal medullary activity	Catecholamines
	Adrenal cortex activity	Corticosteroids
Immune system	Lymphocyte (white blood cell) activity	T-cells
		B-cells
		Natural killer cells

the correlations or associations among physiological responses under particular conditions tend to be sometimes low (e.g. Gatchel, 1988).

The multidimensional nature of arousal

There is also the issue of situational response stereotypy. This refers to the fact that slight changes in the situational characteristics may produce different patterns of physiological responding. Thus, two 'stress situations' might not produce the same pattern of physiological responding. For example, if there is more of an active coping capability in one situation (a subject's performance on a reaction time task can lead to electric shock avoidance) versus a more passive acceptance of the stress situation (escape or avoidance of electric shock by the subject is not possible), different physiological response patterns will be produced (e.g. Obrist, *et al.*, 1978).

Indeed, a classic paper by Lacey (1967) challenged the validity of the unidimensional view of arousal which suggested that along a single continuum of arousal, any psychophysiological variable was interchangeable with any other. Rather, Lacey proposed a multidimensional view in which there may often be low correlations among measures in certain situations. In a reaction time experiment demonstrating this, Lacey used a paradigm in which a warning light came on a few seconds before a target light to which the subject was to press a button as quickly as possible. Heart rate and sweat gland activity were measured continuously throughout the experiment. Results demonstrated that, as would be expected, sweat gland activity (a measure of arousal) increased. However, there was a concurrent beat-by-beat heart rate deceleration during the warning stimulus–target–stimulus interval. Heart rate acceleration would be expected during states of arousal produced by reaction time performance. Lacey labelled this phenomenon directional fractionation. The simultaneous occurrence of sweat gland activity increases and heart rate decreases run counter to a simple unidimensional view of arousal, and supported a multidimensional view. Lacey also demonstrated various other compelling results that supported this multidimensional view: cardiovascular response increases were sometimes associated with cortical deactivation; under certain drug conditions, EEG and behavioural arousal can become dissociated; psychophysiological measures often do not systematically covary with one another.

KEY ISSUES IN PSYCHOPHYSIOLOGY

Individual differences

One major problem usually encountered in psychophysiological measurement is the presence of individual differences in physiological reactivity. It has been consistently demonstrated that people do not show identical physiological responses to the same stimuli or situation. This is referred to as individual response stereotypy. The system that responds most actively to a given stimulus can differ greatly from subject to subject. One person may be an 'EMG responder' who demonstrates a great increase in muscular activity under stress (let us say) but little increase in heart rate. Another individual may be a 'heart rate responder' who responds to the same situation with a great acceleration of heart rate but little EMG increase. Such differences account for the common finding that

Law of initial values

The law of initial values was first proposed by Wilder (1957) to account for the fact that the true magnitude or size of a particular physiological response measure to a stimulus or situation is often affected by the prestimulus level of that response system being measured. That is to say, if the prestimulus level is high, then the smaller will be the expected increase in the physiological response to the given stimulus because of a ceiling effect; in contrast, if the prestimulus level is low, then a larger response would be produced because of the greater potential 'upward' range available. Although not all psychophysiological response measures are affected by the law of initial values, investigators need to be alert to its possible influence when evaluating psychophysiological response measures. Statistical adjustments will need to be considered before analysing the data if such effects are present.

The issue of interpretation

Another key issue associated with psychophysiological assessment is interpretation. Many investigators became interested in the use of physiological measures for assessment because they hoped such measures would directly reflect a person's psychological state. However, this is not necessarily true. One cannot assume that a single measure of physiological functioning will have a simple and direct relationship to a particular psychological construct such as anxiety or arousal. Almost all physiological responses can be elicited by a great many internal and external stimuli. For example, a stressful situation will produce an increase in heart rate, but so will sexual arousal. Thus, it is sometimes difficult for researchers to know the psychological significance of a single physiological response. Taking a multidimensional view of arousal, researchers now are more careful to map out specific psychophysiological patterns associated with specific psychological constructs or states.

One widely applied psychophysiological method which produced a rapidly growing and thriving industry in the United States was the 'lie detector' test. In this interrogation method, an individual is asked various questions while a number of his or her autonomic responses are monitored on a polygraph. The traditional polygraph test recorded three channels of physiological data. One channel recorded GSR or sweat gland activity, a second, the plethysmographic channel, usually recorded changes in the upper arm blood volume, from which heart rate and pulse volume changes could be determined, and the third channel recorded respiration which was monitored from an expandable belt placed around the subject's chest. Additional channels are also sometimes used. In evaluating a lie detector test, the examiner usually assesses whether autonomic response disturbances associated with the answers given by an individual to a set of critical questions are more magnified or persistent than responses associated with irrelevant and emotionally controlled questions. A global evaluation is made. A traditional problem with the lie detector test is that the examiner must interpret the results (although computer-analysed techniques are now being developed).

One of the basic assumptions on which the lie detector test is based is that physiological measures can be used as a direct measure of some internal psychological state. However, as Lang (1971) has noted, this is an example of indicant fallacy. There is no evidence to indicate that there is a unique pattern of autonomic responses that emerges when an individual is deliberately lying, but does not when that person is answering truthfully. There are well-documented individual differences in physiological response tendencies that argue against the possibility of there being a specific 'lying' response. Indeed, early reviews by individuals such as Lykken (1974), after surveying the relevant literature, indicated that there was no well-replicated empirical evidence demonstrating the test's absolute validity. A more recent review by a US Congressional Committee through the Office of Technology Assessment came to a similar conclusion (1983). This lack of proven validity, unfortunately, has not prevented the widespread use of the procedure by individuals who pedal it commercially as though it were an entirely effective and error-free technique. This view also naively assumes an overly simplistic view of psychophysiological responding.

It should also be pointed out that autonomic responses are usually used in the lie detector test because they are viewed as involuntary responses that an individual cannot 'fake' or control. However, as noted earlier, it has been empirically demonstrated that individuals can learn voluntarily to control autonomic responses through the use of biofeedback training procedures. It is therefore conceivable that an individual who has acquired voluntary control over physiological responses could 'beat' the lie detector procedure.

CONCLUSIONS

Psychophysiology involves the investigation of the interaction of physiology and human behavior/experience. It provides a powerful assessment tool to better understand these complexities, with studies ranging from the evaluation of basic emotional responses such as anger and fear to higher cognitive processes such as thinking. Expertise in a number of different areas, though, is required in this field: an understanding of biomedical electronic recording technology, ranging from the electrodes to be used to the amplification/distortion characteristics of the recording devices; an understanding of the basic physiology of the responses to be recorded; an understanding of basic measurement unit and analysis issues; an understanding of other key issues in the field such as individual and situational response stereotypy, the law of initial values, and interpretation complexities. All of the above, in addition to a firm background in basic research methodology, are needed for the serious researcher in psychophysiology. Moreover, this is an ever-changing field. The researcher needs to keep abreast of new developments in biomedical engineering technology, as well as our ever-expanding knowledge of basic physiological processes. With advances in both areas, we will be able to continue delineating the important psychophysiological mechanisms that can significantly lead to a better understanding of human behaviour and experience.

REFERENCES

Ackles, P.I., Jennings, J.R. & Coles, N.C.H., Eds. (1988). *Advances in psychophysiology. 3.* London: Jessica Kingsley Publishers, 1988.

Alexander, F. (1950). *Psychosomatic medicine: its principles and applications.* New York, NY: Norton.

Ax, A.R. (1953). The physiological differentiation between fear and anger in humans. *Psychosomatic Medicine*, **15**, 433–42.

Brown, C.C. (1967). *Methods in psychophysiology.* Baltimore, MD: Waverly Press.

Cacioppo, J.T. & Tassinary, L.G. (1990). *Principles of psychophysiology: physical, social, and inferential elements.* New York, NY: Cambridge University Press.

Gatchel, R.J. (1988). Clinical effectiveness of biofeedback in reducing anxiety. In H. Wagner (Ed.). *Social psychophysiology: theory and clinical applications.* London: Wiley,

Gatchel, R.J. (1993). Psychophysiological disorders: past and present perspectives. In R.J. Gatchel & E.B. Blanchard (Eds.). *Psychophysiological disorders: research in clinical applications.* Washington, DC: American Psychological Association Press.

Gatchel, R.J. & Barnes, D. (1989). Physiological self-control and emotion. In H.L. Wagner & A.S. Manstead (Eds.). *Handbook of social psychophysiology.* Chichester: John Wiley & Sons, Ltd.

Psychophysiology

Gatchel, R.J., Baum, A. & Krantz, D.S. (1989). *An introduction to health psychology.* New York, NY: McGraw-Hill.

Graham, D.T. (1972). Psychosomatic medicine. In N.S. Greenfield & A. Sternbach (Eds.). *Handbook of psychophysiology.* New York, NY: Holt, Reinhardt, and Winston.

Greenfield, N.S. & Sternbach, R.A. (1972). *Handbook of psychophysiology.* New York, NY: Holt, Reinhardt, and Winston.

Hassett, J. (1978). *A primer of psychophysiology.* San Francisco, CA: W.H. Freeman.

Lacey, J.I. (1967). Somatic response patterning in stress: some revisions of activation theory. In M.H. Appley & R. Trumbull (Eds.). *Psychological stress.* New York, NY: McGraw-Hill.

Lang, P.J. (1971). The application of psychophysiological methods to the study of psychotherapy and behavior modification. In A.E. Bergin and S.L. Garfield (Eds.). *Handbook of psychotherapy and behavior change: an empirical analysis.* New York: Wiley.

Lipowski, Z.J. (1977). Psychosomatic medicine in the 70's: an overview. *American Journal of Psychiatry,* **134**, 233–43.

Lykken, D.T. (1974). Psychology and the lie detector industry. *American Psychologist,* **29**, 725–39.

Obrist, P.A., Gabelein, C.J., Teller, E.S., *et al.* (1978). The relationship among heart rate, carotid, dP/dT and blood pressure in humans as a function of the type of stress. *Psychophysiology,* **15**, 102–15.

Scientific validity of polygraph testing (1983). a Research review and evaluation – a technical memorandum (Washington, DC: US Congress, Office of Technology Assessment, OTA-TM-H-15).

Venables, P.H. & Martin, P.H. (1967). *Manual of psychophysiological methods.* Amsterdam: North Holland Publishing Company.

Wilder, J. (1957). The law of initial values in neurology and psychiatry. *Journal of Nervous and Mental Disease,* **125**, 73–86.

Wolff, H.G. (1953). *Stress and disease.* Springfield, IL: Charles C. Thomas.

Wolf, S. & Wolff, H.G. (1947). *Human gastric function: an experimental study of a man and his stomach.* New York, NY: Oxford University Press.

Skilled performance

NIGEL HARVEY

*Department of Psychology, University College
London, UK*

Ryle (1949) distinguished 'knowing how' from 'knowing that'. Psychologists have referred to the former type of knowledge as procedural and to the latter as declarative. This distinction is not merely philosophical: amnesic patients have difficulty retrieving declarative knowledge but can still retrieve and acquire procedural knowledge (Cohen & Squire, 1980).

A simple definition of skilled performance is that it is the use of procedural knowledge that has been acquired through practice. This is not to deny that declarative knowledge is not also needed in tasks to ensure that performance leads to the desired outcome: a surgeon skilled at wielding a scalpel still needs a knowledge of anatomy and accurate information about the patient.

Other definitions emphasize the attributes of highly skilled performers. For Schmidt (1991, p. 5) 'skills generally involve achieving some well-defined environmental goal by maximizing the achievement certainty, minimizing the physical and mental energy costs of performance, and minimizing the time used'.

There are two ways of classifying motor skills. The first involves distinguishing closed skills from open skills. The former are performed in a predictable environment and include activities such as typewriting and handwriting; the latter are carried out in an unpredictable context and include activities such as playing hockey. The second classification distinguishes discrete skills that involve single actions (e.g. hitting a golf ball) from continuous skills that involve ongoing modulation of movement (e.g. steering a car).

My aim here is to provide a brief overview of work on skill. I shall restrict myself to covering five important topics. These are the execution, planning, self-assessment, training and transfer of skilled performance. Readers who discover that they require more comprehensive reviews of these issues should refer to Rosenbaum (1991) and Schmidt (1991). The second of these texts provides a useful conceptual framework that I shall employ as a basis for discussion. It is shown in Fig. 1.

There are two main parts to this framework. The planning system includes stimulus identification, response selection and response programming. Responses comprise an overlapping sequence of movements that is specified in a motor programme. The execution system receives and executes this programme. This involves passing information via the spinal cord to instruct muscles to contract to produce the movements specified in the programme. In addition to the planning and execution systems, there is a reference that defines response correctness and a comparator that matches the response that is produced with this reference. The return of information from the periphery and environment to the comparator is response-produced feedback. This is shown with light lines in Fig. 1. It enables the performer to determine whether the planned response had the desired effect and, if not, to make the appropriate planning modifications. There are also various movement feedback loops to ensure that each movement specified by the motor programme is made as planned. These are indicated with bold lines in Fig. 1. They return information from the periphery to earlier stages of the execution process: they form parts of the long-loop and spinal reflex systems.

EXECUTION

Once the response selection system has determined the response that is required (e.g. a successful pole-vault or golf swing), the response programming system selects a motor programme, perhaps

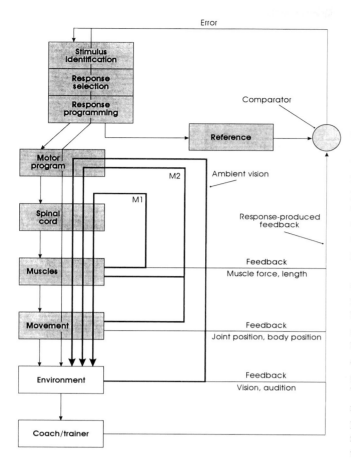

Fig. 1. A conceptual framework for understanding skilled performance based on Schmidt (1991). (Adapted from Schmidt, R.A. 1991.) *Motor learning and performance: from principles to practice*, pp. 130, Champaign, IL: Human Kinetics Publ. Reprinted by permission. © R.A. Schmidt,

ruption to the planned movement than the spinal reflex. Furthermore the degree of compensation is under some voluntary control. In some situations (e.g. skiing over bumps), it is more appropriate to yield to unexpected perturbation than in others. Voluntary setting of the long-loop reflexes prior to execution of the motor program allows for this.

The remaining movement feedback loop shown in Fig. 1 carries ambient visual information back from the environment to the motor programme. Schmidt (1991) contrasts this type of visual information with focal vision. The latter arrives from the centre of the visual field, is degraded by low illumination, reaches awareness and is primarily concerned with object perception. Ambient vision, on the other hand, arrives from the whole of the visual field, is not degraded by low illumination, does not reach awareness and is generally concerned with location of the performer within the environment.

Ambient vision is important in the visual control of balance. It can also specify how long it will take for an approaching object to make contact with the performer (Lee & Young, 1985). This is because the performer's retinal image of an approaching object dilates as the object closes in on him or her. The rate of dilation can be used to derive an optical variable (*tau*) that specifies time-to-contact. A value for this variable can be inserted into the motor programme as a parameter by the planning system prior to execution. When ambient vision shows that this value has been reached, the next part of the programme is executed without the need for the planning system to intervene. For example, the planning system might have parameterized a catching response programme to ensure that the grasping phase of the action is initiated when tau reaches a particular value. If the planning system has chosen the parameter value correctly, the catch will be successful. If it has not done so, the catch will fail. Hence, like other movement feedback loops, ambient vision ensures that movements are produced as planned.

PLANNING

The movement feedback loops can ensure that movements are produced as planned but they can provide no guarantee that the planned movement is appropriate for reaching the outcome that is required. Response-produced feedback is needed for this.

To learn a skill, people must learn two things. First, they must learn to identify and parameterize a motor programme that will produce the responses that are associated with the outcomes that they desire. Secondly, they must learn what response-produced feedback is associated with these responses (i.e. appropriate references). Adams' (1971) closed-loop theory of skill acquisition deals with acquisition of both types of information. In his model, the motor programme is a simple one. It is called the 'memory trace' and is responsible for initiating all movements. It is also used for terminating those that are rapid and open-loop. The reference for feedback is called the 'perceptual trace' and is a representation of the central tendency of the past feedback states that have been associated with responses that have produced appropriate outcomes. Whenever the performer receives information that outcomes are of this type, both perceptual and memory traces are strengthened.

Adams suggests that the perceptual trace can be used in two different ways. When movements are slow and under closed-loop control, feedback information coming from the ongoing movement is continually compared with the reference that the perceptual trace

tailors it to the particular circumstances by inserting appropriate parameters into it, sets an appropriate reference, loads the programme into the execution system and starts it going. Once initiated, the programme is executed without reference to response-produced feedback. However, the various movement feedback loops may be used to ensure that each component of the programme is produced as specified. When are they used in this way?

Use of even the shortest feedback loops shown in Fig. 1 takes time. If no feedback is used (e.g. because movements are very fast), control is said to be open-loop. There has been much debate in the literature about whether this mode of control is ever used. If feedback is used, control is termed closed-loop. This mode of control allows compensation to be made for unexpected perturbations to the effectors. The longer loops shown in Fig. 1 enable this compensation to be more flexible. The spinal reflex (labelled M1 in Fig. 1) starts 30–50 ms after the perturbation: muscle spindles register the change and send information to the spinal level to ensure that the muscles eliminate the mismatch between their specified and their actual contraction. This reflex allows (non-conscious) compensation for unexpected loading of limbs but does not appear to be subject to any significant degree of voluntary control.

The long-loop reflex (labelled M2 in Fig. 1) starts 50–80 ms after any perturbation. It appears capable of coping with more severe dis-

provides. Action is terminated once a match is obtained. This has an important consequence: because a match has been obtained, people cannot perceive an error in their own movement. When movements are rapid and open-loop, the system operates differently. Feedback associated with the finished movement is compared with the reference provided by the perceptual trace. The larger the difference, the greater is the error that is perceived in the movement.

Adams' (1971) theory was modified by Schmidt (1975). Some modification was necessary because the original theory specified that two separate memories must be retained for every outcome that a skill may be required to produce. Also, it implied that the production of each outcome must be learned separately: practice in producing one outcome does not transfer to producing another. Thus, for example, the actions of hitting a golf ball 50 yards and 100 yards would require separate memory traces and separate perceptual traces and acquiring these internal representations would not benefit a golfer who wished to hit a ball over a distance of 75 yards.

At the heart of Schmidt's (1975) model lies the concept of a generalized motor programme. A single programme is responsible for producing a whole class of actions (e.g. golf swings). The planning system parameterizes it to ensure that the action that is executed produces the required outcome (e.g. 15 foot putt) under the prevailing conditions (e.g. wet grass). Through practice, performers learn rules that enable them to identify the parameters appropriate for any give occasion. These rules are obtained by a mental process akin to statistical regression. They are of two main types. The recall schema is used to identify appropriate muscle parameters (e.g. specifying force) given a required outcome and a set of environmental conditions. The recognition schema enables the performer to identify the response-produced feedback to be expected when a particular outcome is produced under a particular set of environmental conditions. Hence the recall and recognition schema enable the appropriate programme to be executed and the reference for it to be set appropriately. Clearly then, the role that these schemata have within Schmidt's theory are similar to those that the memory trace and the perceptual trace have within Adams' theory. However, there is an important difference. Schmidt's schemata enable all possible outcomes (including novel ones) to be produced on the basis of just two internal representations.

Some implications of the two theories are also different. According to Adams' model, people only learn skills by producing correct responses: perceptual and motor traces are not strengthened when incorrect responses are made. Within Schmidt's theory, however, incorrect responses produce additional data points to be entered into the mental regression process that identifies and strengthens the recall and recognition schemata. As a consequence, responses that do not produce the outcomes that are required still contribute to skill acquisition.

Schmidt's theory makes a clear and distinctive prediction. We have seen that the recall and recognition schemata are extracted by a mental process analogous to statistical regression. Rules obtained by this type of procedure are stronger (i.e. make better predictions) when the ranges of the variables entered into the regression are larger. Within the context of Schmidt's theory, this implies that people will perform better after experience with a wider range of outcomes and conditions: a golfer who has experience at hitting the ball over many different distances will be better at hitting it over some novel distance than other golfers who have previously hit the ball the same number of times over a single distance (or over a few very similar distances). Shapiro and Schmidt (1982) reviewed many experiments that were designed to test this prediction. They concluded that those using children as subjects obtained reasonably good support for it whereas those using adults as subjects obtained evidence that was more equivocal. They argued that adults may have already developed schemata for the relatively simple tasks employed in the experiments through day-to-day experience outside the laboratory.

The domain of Schmidt's theory is broader than that of Adams. Because the schemata take contextual conditions into account the theory can account for performance in *open* as well as in closed skills. However, both theories are restricted to providing explanations for performance of discrete skills. They need to be elaborated if they are also to account for performance of continuous skills. One common feature of such skills is that good performance requires response not to the stimulus configuration currently on display but to an anticipation of the stimulus configuration that will be present by the time that the response has its effect. In other words, motor programmes must be parameterized on the basis of predictions about future features of the stimulus display. There is still some debate about how such predictions are made (Harvey, 1988) but Pew (1974) has shown how they could be incorporated into a model similar to the one proposed by Schmidt (1975).

Schmidt's theory of skill acquisition has been subject to some updating (e.g. Schmidt, 1991) but has not been superseded. Updating became necessary because the original theory did not explicitly account for certain phenomena that have recently come to light. Prominent among these is the 'contextual interference effect'. When skill practice includes attempts to produce a number of different outcomes, practice at each outcome can be grouped together in a block of trials (blocked practice) or else randomly intermixed with practice at reaching other outcomes (random practice). Shea and Morgan (1979) gave random or blocked practice on two versions of a task and then examined how well people performed on a novel third version. Performance improvement in the first stage of the experiment was faster with blocked practice but transfer to the new version of the task in the second stage of the experiment was greater after random practice. How can conditions that degrade practice produce more learning?

One possibility derives from the fact that re-parameterization of the motor programme is more likely to be required before each trial in the random practice condition. This impairs practice performance itself but gives performers experience in a process (i.e. re-parameterization of the motor programme) that is necessary for the transfer task. In contrast, people in the blocked practice condition have no need to re-parameterize the motor programme during the practice stage: all they need to do is to re-execute the programme that they have already parameterized. Performance during practice benefits from this. However, because they have not had experience at re-parameterizing the programme, they are at a disadvantage during the transfer stage.

In Schmidt's theory, skill learning depends on a mental process analogous to statistical regression. There are many ways in which this could be accomplished. However, it seems unlikely that people permanently store the independent data points pertaining to each and every previous performance and recalculate the regression each time an additional performance of the skill adds another point to the database. It seems more likely that the data points provided by each performance are used to update the existing regression and are then discarded. Updating of this sort can be interpreted as a filtering (Harvey, 1988) or optimization process. As such, it could be accomplished by a connectionist system (e.g. a neural network). This has been recognized in some of the most recent theoretical work on skill acquisition (e.g. Jordan, 1990).

Schmidt's cognitive approach to skilled performance has been contrasted with one developed by ecological psychologists (e.g. Turvey, 1990). Their model differs from Schmidt's in certain ways. First, the motor programme loaded into the execution system by the planning system is not seen as a sequence of separate instructions. Instead, it is more akin to a mathematical function: like a differential equation, it encodes, as a global unit, the complete time course of a particular type of movement (e.g. walking). Different parameterizations of the function produce different versions of the movement (e.g. strolling; marching). Second, ecological psychologists argue that response-produced feedback has no role to play during execution of a movement. However, movement feedback may still be important: during execution, ambient visual information can act on the function responsible for producing the movement (e.g. Lee & Young, 1985).

In the past, the debate between cognitive and ecological psychologists about the nature of skilled performance has been quite intense (e.g. Meijer & Roth, 1988). Increasingly, however, the difference between the two approaches appears to be one of emphasis. Ecological psychologists are primarily interested in how our patterns of movement are adapted by evolution to fit our ecology. Cognitive psychologists focus on how they are adapted by learning to cope with demands from the environment that are too novel or idiosyncratic to have evoked an evolutionary response.

SELF-ASSESSMENT
When considering the self-assessment of skilled performance, we need to address two issues (Harvey, 1994). The first concerns how well people's confidence in their performance *reflects* their actual performance and how well changes in their confidence *reflect* changes in their performance. The second concerns whether their confidence *influences* their performance.

Does confidence reflect performance? Many experiments have shown that people do become more confident as practice improves their level of skill. However, this does not necessarily indicate that they can assess how well they will perform or have performed in a task: when experience at a task does not produce improvement in performance, it still increases confidence. Thus confidence may increase because people expect that practice will improve their performance.

Other work has shown that people tend to overestimate their probability of success and underestimate their probability of failure in skilled tasks. Overconfidence such as this may have serious consequences. For example, it may contribute to causing traffic accidents. However, people do not appear to continually assess the riskiness of their behaviour while driving (Wagenaar, 1992). Instead, they seem to have developed risk-taking habits. In other words, they habitually perform in a way that is consistent with some probability

of having an accident and, when asked, they underestimate that probability. Again, it may be that people think that experience at driving has improved their performance more than it actually has done.

As the contextual interference effect (Shea & Morgan, 1979) demonstrates, difficult conditions during practice may speed up learning. Thus deciding to adopt a high risk approach to a skill (e.g. skiing down a black run) has both advantages (faster learning) and disadvantages (higher probability of accidents). This suggests that a higher level of risk should be selected during learning than after learning has finished. However, the higher level of risk that is appropriate during learning may be maintained either because it has become a maladaptive habit or because people wrongly expect additional experience to produce more learning.

Does confidence influence performance? Work on levels of aspiration suggests that it does. In the absence of externally set rewards, people generally choose a version of the task that they feel gives them a 50% chance of success. However, the level selected by any one individual depends on his or her personality. Many experiments have been performed to determine the personality variables that are important. Curiosity and fear of failure are two that appear to be involved (Sorrentino, Hewitt & Raso-Knott, 1992).

How does level of aspiration affect performance? Work on goal-setting (e.g. Locke & Latham, 1990) suggests that those who select more difficult tasks will perform better but still fail more often. To clarify this apparently paradoxical statement, consider a high-jumper. With the bar set at 1.70 metres, she jumps an average of 1.74 and clears the bar on 90% of attempts. However, with the bar set higher at 1.80 metres, she jumps an average of 1.78 metres but clears the bar on 50% of attempts. Thus, her performance measured in terms of the height that she jumps is better than before but she fails to reach the task criterion (i.e. clearing the bar) as often.

This goal-setting effect provides managers with a useful tool to increase productivity of their workforce. During 'performance assessment', they encourage employees to work towards difficult but not totally unrealistic goals. As long as the goals are accepted, productivity will increase. Of course, the goal themselves will rarely be reached and the workforce may find this frustrating and stressful. Managers have to decide whether the short-term productivity gains to be obtained by manipulating employees via goal-setting outweigh any long-term problems caused by stress. This decision is not an easy one to make because there is little research to base it on: most studies of goal-setting have been short-term and have measured productivity but not work-related stress.

TRAINING
How should one go about increasing skill levels in other people? This is a complex topic and is currently under-researched by psychologists. Training techniques can be divided into 'on-job' methods that take place during the time that people are performing the skill (e.g. provision of knowledge of results; guidance) and 'off-job' methods that take place at other times (e.g. lectures). In what follows, I shall focus on on-job methods of training.

Knowledge of results (KR) is a type of response-produced feedback that informs performers of the effectiveness of their responses. It is usually given in verbal form and is additional to the response-produced information that performers can expect to receive automatically when performing the skill. It is often provided by a trainer or coach. In practical situations, this costs money: training managers have an interest in knowing the optimal amount of KR to provide in order to produce maximum financial return.

Early work produced a number of findings of potential importance in practical learning situations. First, the length of time between the response and KR provision does not matter much. However, it should not be filled with other motor activity because this can interfere with memory of the feedback that was required (i.e. the reference). Secondly, the length of time between providing KR and the next response should be sufficient to allow people to process the feedback information. Thirdly, it helps to make KR as precise as possible. However, more precise KR may take longer to process and therefore may require a slightly longer delay before the next response is made. Fourthly, the absolute number of times that KR is given is a better predictor of skill level than the ratio of the number of times it is given to the number of times it is not given. In other words, skill level after ten trials with KR on every trial will be similar to that after 100 trials with KR on every tenth trial. Fifthly, performance level will drop if KR is withdrawn and this effect will be greater early in learning.

This last finding forced researchers to recognize the importance of distinguishing the effect of KR on performance (e.g. it may affect arousal or provide an incentive to greater effort) from its effect on learning. Once KR is withdrawn, its effect on performance vanishes to leave only its effect on learning. It is, of course, its effect on learning that is important for those devising training schemes. Recently, early findings about the effects of frequency of KR (mentioned fourthly in the above list) have been re-assessed in the light of this distinction between the effects of KR on learning and performance. Experiments have shown that although performance during training is better when KR is provided on every trial than on, say, half the trials, performance after KR-withdrawal is better when KR has been provided less frequently during training.

Other manipulations have also been found to influence KR's effects on performance and learning differentially. For example, the effects of providing KR after every trial (immediate KR) have been compared with the effects of providing information about each set of, say, ten trials after the last trial in the set (summary KR). During training, performance was better with the immediate KR but, after KR withdrawal, post-training performance was better when training had involved summary KR. This finding begs a question: how many trials should be summarized? One experiment showed better learning when five trials were summarized than when either one trial (i.e. immediate KR) or 10 trials were summarized. However, the optimum number of trials in a summary appears to depend on task complexity: fewer trials should be summarized when the task is complex. Presumably, working memory capacity is the limiting factor here.

Relatively infrequent KR and summary KR appear to stop trainees becoming over-dependent on trainers. They force people to attempt to associate information in KR with response-produced feedback information that is intrinsic to the task. Other techniques are also used in attempts to prevent over-dependence on KR. One approach is to start with a relatively high frequency of KR at the beginning of training and then to reduce this frequency gradually over the training period. This fading of KR

does appear to produce better learning than continued high frequency KR.

Unlike KR, guidance is provided before performance. If it were perfect, it would produce learning with no errors. In practical situations, it is a useful technique when errors must be avoided during training. It can be classified into physical guidance (moving someone's limbs) and restrictive guidance (preventing them from moving in certain ways). In addition, observational learning (showing someone what to do) can be regarded as visual guidance and instruction (telling someone what to do) can be regarded as verbal guidance. In general, guidance appears to have a strong effect on performance during training but little effect after training has finished. In other words, people become dependent on the guidance and fail to perform the mental processing that would enable them to carry out the task autonomously. It seems best to limit guidance to very early stages of practice and to the acquisition of dangerous skills.

TRANSFER

Does previous training on one skill help or hinder performance on another skill that has not been previously trained? Generally speaking, it rarely provides hindrance and, if the two skills are similar, it may provide a little help. In other words, motor transfer tends to be small but positive.

Transfer will be higher if the two skills are similar. But what is meant by similarity here? It does not refer to procedures that have the same function. For example, in certain types of task analysis, overall performance is divided into functional components. Driving a car can be divided into starting the engine, operating the vehicle and stopping the engine. Operating the vehicle can be divided into leaving the parking space, cruising and parking. Cruising can then be further divided into smaller components and so on. Hierarchical task analysis such as this may be useful for training purposes because there is some evidence that learning a complex task in parts is easier than learning it as a whole. However, it is of no use for making predictions about transfer of skill. There is no reason to suppose that learning to park a car will help you to dock an oil tanker.

For the purposes of predicting transfer, skills are regarded as more similar when they have more ability requirements in common. What is known about motor abilities? Pioneering factor analytic work by Fleishman and his colleagues (e.g. Fleishman & Bartlett, 1969) has demonstrated that there is no such thing as a general motor ability (analogous to a general factor in intelligence). Instead, there appear to be many specific motor abilities, such as finger dexterity, multi-limb co-ordination, speed of movement, stamina, explosive strength and so on. Schmidt (1991) estimates that there are between 20 and 50 such abilities but others have argued that there are many more. By correlating performance on a skill with tests of these individual motor abilities, it is possible to determine the ability requirements of the skill.

Transfer tends to be small for two reasons. First, even those pairs of skills that appear to be similar often require different combinations of abilities. Second, practice at a task reduces the proportion of variance that can be explained by the motor abilities identified by Fleishman and, therefore, increases the proportion of variance that is specific to that task alone. This means that proportionately less of a highly practised skill is available for transfer.

British Government agencies responsible for industrial training strategy (e.g. the erstwhile Manpower Services Commission and the National Council for Vocational Qualifications) emphasize the need to train people in core skills and transferable skills. It would be nice if such skills existed: people who have them and who have lost a job in one industry would be able to perform a similar job in another industry with minimal re-training. Unfortunately, such skills do not exist in the motor domain and they may not exist in other domains.

Training agencies do not appear to be aware of this. For example, the Manpower Services Commission specified manual competence as a core skill but, as we have seen, there is no evidence for a general motor ability of this sort. Furthermore, both the Manpower Services Commission and the National Council for Vocational Qualifications define job similarity on the basis of the number of shared functional components that are revealed by task analysis: skills are deemed transferable across jobs if the jobs share these components. In fact, as we have seen, the jobs must require common abilities for transfer to occur. In practice, this rarely happens to any significant extent: it is certainly not guaranteed by a task analysis that shows that they share functional components. Thus any agency that directs unemployed people only towards potential jobs that share functional components with their previous jobs is placing unnecessary limits on their prospects (Annett & Sparrow, 1985).

Many social, political and economic factors must contribute to the formulation of a successful industrial training policy. But, however optimally these factors are set, the policy will fail if it is not based on a realistic model of human nature. To develop such a model, it is more important to take account of the scientific knowledge produced by psychologists than to be swayed by the wishful thinking of manpower planners.

REFERENCES

Adams, J.A. (1971) A closed-loop theory of motor learning. *Journal of Motor Behaviour*, 3, 111–49.

Annett, J. and Sparrow, J. (1985). Transfer of training: a review of research and practical implications. *Programmed Learning and Educational Technology*, 22, 116–24.

Cohen, N.J. & Squire, L.R. (1980). Preserved learning and retention of pattern-analysing skills in amnesia: dissociation of knowing how from know that. *Science*, 210, 207–10.

Fleishman, E.A. & Bartlett, C.J. (1969). Human abilities. *Annual Review of Psychology*, 20, 344–80.

Harvey, N. (1988). The psychology of action: current controversies. In G. Claxton (Ed.) *Growth points in cognition*. London: Routledge.

Harvey, N. (1994). Relations between confidence and skilled performance. In G. Wright & P. Ayton (Eds.). *Subjective probability*. New York: Wiley.

Jordan, M.I. (1990). Motor learning and the degrees of freedom problem. In M. Jeannerod (Ed.). *Attention and Performance 13*. Hillsdale, NJ: Erlbaum.

Lee, D.N. & Young, D.S. (1985). Visual timing of interceptive action. In D. Ingle, M. Jeannerod & D.N. Lee (Eds.). *Brain mechanisms and spatial vision*. Dordrecht: Martinus Nijhoff.

Locke, E.A. & Latham, G.P. (1990). *A theory of goal setting and task performance*. Englewood Cliffs, NJ: Prentice-Hall.

Meijer, O.G. & Roth, K. (1988). *Complex movement behaviour: The 'motor-action' controversy*. Amsterdam: North-Holland.

Pew, R.W. (1974). Human perceptual-motor performance. In B.H. Kantowitz (Ed.). *Human information processing: tutorials in performance and cognition*. Hillsdale, NJ: Erlbaum.

Rosenbaum, D.A (1991) *Human motor control*. New York: Academic Press.

Ryle, G. (1949). *The concept of mind*. London: Hutchinson.

Schmidt, R.A. (1975). A schema theory of discrete motor skill learning. *Psychological Review*, 82, 225–80.

Schmidt, R.A. (1991). *Motor learning and performance: from principles to practice*. Champaign, IL: Human Kinetics.

Shapiro, D.C. & Schmidt, R.A. (1982). The schema theory: recent evidence and developmental implications. In J.A.S Kelso & J.E. Clark (Eds.). *The development of motor control and co-ordination*. New York: Wiley.

Shea, J.B. & Morgan, R.L. (1979). Contextual interference effects on the acquisition, retention and transfer of a motor skill. *Journal of Experimental Psychology: Human Learning and Memory*, 5, 179–87.

Sorrentino, R.M., Hewitt, E.C. & Raso-Knott, P.A. (1992). Risk-taking in games of chance and skill: informational and affective influences on choice behaviour. *Journal of Social and Personality Psychology*, 62, 522–33.

Turvey, M.T. (1990). Coordination. *American Psychologist*, 45, 938–53.

Wagenaar, W.A. (1992). Risk taking and accident causation. In J.F. Yates (Ed.). *Risk-taking behaviour*. New York: Wiley.

Social interaction

ADRIAN FURNHAM

Department of Psychology, University College
London, UK

Whilst some believe that all psychology is social, it is social psychologists who have the nature of social interaction at the heart of their discipline. Social psychology is concerned with the relationship between the individual and society particularly those medicated by face-to-face interaction with others.

Social psychologists regard their discipline as an attempt to understand how the thoughts, feelings and behaviour of individuals are influenced by the actual, imagined and implied presence of others.

Like all sections of psychology the scientific study of social interaction has a long past but a short history. Textbooks appeared in the first decade of this century. The first study in this area is attributed to Triplett (1898) who noted that racing cyclists rode faster when competing with each other than when simply competing against the clock. He proposed a theory of social facilitation which looked at the effects of an audience on performance and later tested it in the laboratory.

Social psychology has been at one and the same time empirical and ideological reflecting the early influence of Comte. It has seen its task at one and the same time to socialize psychological research (and stress the role of social forces) but to individualize sociology (and stress the role of individual differences).

Social behaviour is shaped by various factors including the behaviour and characteristics of other persons; social cognition or attitudes, beliefs and memories, ecological variables including the direct and indirect influences of the physical environmental; the sociocultural or moral context in which social interaction occurs, and finally aspects of our biological nature relevant to social behaviour.

Over the years, the range of topics considered by social psychologists has grown considerably. The following topics give some idea of the breadth of the scientific study of social interaction.

1. How are stereotypes formed? How can they be changed?
2. How does alcohol affect human social behaviour?
3. Does our present mood affect our evaluations of others or the information about them that we later remember?
4. What are the causes of shyness? Do individuals sometimes use this behaviour as a means of protecting their self-image?
5. Does exposure to pornography contribute to the occurrence of sexual assaults and related crimes?
6. How do people react when they feel they have been treated unfairly?
7. Do males and females differ in their performance of various tasks?
8. How do intimate relationships form, develop, and sometimes dissolve?
9. Why do some individuals behave consistently across a wide range of social situations, while others seem to change their behaviour (and even their personalities) as they move from one setting to another?
10. Why do individuals tend to take credit for favourable outcomes but tend to blame others for unfavourable ones?
11. When jury members are told to disregard information they have previously received, can they really do so?
12. Why are the members of large crowds often willing to engage in actions they would never perform as individuals?
13. How do people communicate non-verbally?
14. What effect does loud noise or bad smells have on people's social behaviour?
15. How are lay people's theories of social interaction different from psychologists' theories.

The following list covers the topics currently researched by social psychologists: aggression; attitudes and attitude change; attribution (perceiving the causes of others' behaviour); bargaining and coalition formation; conformity and compliance; cross-cultural research; crowding and interpersonal distance; equality (fairness in our relations with others); environmental issues; group processes (leadership, group decision-making, etc); helping behaviour; law and crime-related research; non-verbal communication; person perception (first-impressions, etc.); self-disclosure and self-presentation; sex roles and sex differences; social cognition (how we process, store, and remember information about others); social influence; social development.

Rather than develop a specific or unique grand theory, social psychologists have borrowed, stolen or adapted theoretical concepts from other branches of psychology as well as other disciplines. Six 'grand' theories have influence the study of social interactions.

Psychoanalysis

This is a theory of personality structure and development that explains social behaviour in terms of the level of personality development and the unconscious forces at work within the personality of individuals. Experiences during childhood are considered to be strong determinants of adult social behaviour.

Role theory

This seeks to explain social behaviour through an analysis of roles, role obligations, role expectations, and role conflicts. A role is a socially defined pattern of behaviour that accompanies a particular position within a social context.

Stimulus-response or learning theories

These study the associations between specific stimuli, responses and reinforcements. These approaches assume that complex social behaviour can be understood as a chain of simple responses, and that the consequences of a social behaviour are highly influential in determining whether similar behaviours will occur in the future.

Gestalt theory

This holds that social behaviour cannot be properly understood if it is separated, analysed and reduced to specific responses. The whole is greater than the sum of its parts is the basic level of Gestalt psychology. More recently developed cognitive theories share some of these same assumptions, although they do not necessarily accept all of the Gestalt principles. *Phenomenological* approaches assume that understanding a person's perceptions of their world is more important in explaining the person's social behaviour than is an objective description of the environment.

Field theory

This assumes that social behaviour is always a function of both the person and the environment at a specific point in time. Although less specific than some of the other theories, the general concept of person/situation interaction is an important one.

Differences among theories will lead the student of social interaction to examine certain aspects of that behaviour and to disregard others. The factors that help determine what kind of questions a given theory will generate include: the belief in historical versus contemporary causation; the importance of internal versus situation factors; the unit of analysis that is studied; and the assumption about human nature on which the theory is founded. In spite of the variation among theories, they serve as a guide to the investigator who is seeking explanations for human behaviour.

The very complexity of social behaviour means that social psychologists use many methods to study social interaction. A description of the major methods gives one a good idea of how and what social psychologists study.

Social psychologists are eclectic in their research methodology. To some extent, pragmatic and ethical issues dictate which method is used, though often it is the preferences and training of the researcher. Ideally, the research question should dictate which method is used, and often this is the case. Each method has its advantages and disadvantages.

LABORATORY EXPERIMENT

It is possible to measure social behaviour in a lab, such as how non-verbal communication works, the effects of group vs individual problem-solving, etc. The social behavioural researcher's aim is to test the effects of one or more independent variables on one or more dependent variables. Independent variables in an experiment are those factors that are controlled or arranged by the experimenter and may often be considered the cause of behaviour. Dependent variables refer to those behaviours of the subject that are observed or recorded by the experimenter.

Characteristic of the laboratory experiment is the investigator's ability to control the independent and dependent variables. Indeed, this aspect of control is one of the most important features of the laboratory experiment. Through this control, numerous extraneous variables could be eliminated.

In addition to control, the laboratory experiment also offers another important advantage: the ability to assign subjects randomly to conditions. In order for an investigator to draw conclusions regarding cause and effect, he or she must be sure that the pattern of results was not due to some systematic difference in the groups being compared. On average, randomization ensures an equality of subject characteristics across the various experimental conditions. One other characteristic of the laboratory experiment should be mentioned: the manipulation check. Although experimenters are able to control the independent variable, it is still important for them to be sure that the subject in the experiment perceives the manipulation as it is intended. The advantages of the laboratory experiment as a means of acquiring knowledge have been largely summarized above. Principal among these is the ability of the experimenter to control the independent variables and to randomly assign subjects to conditions. The two capabilities provide some basis for conclusions regarding cause and effect. Furthermore, the laboratory allows the investigator to 'sort out' factors, to simplify the more complex events of the natural world by breaking them down into their component parts. Although the laboratory experiment has some considerable advantages in terms of its ability to isolate and control variables, it has some substantial disadvantages as well. In recent years, these disadvantages have become the topic of considerable debate. Four of the major issues of concern have been the possible irrelevance of the laboratory setting; the reactions of subjects to the laboratory setting; the possible influence of experimenters on their results, and deception and ethics.

The issue of relevance concerns the artificiality of the laboratory setting and the fact that many of the situations created in the laboratory bear little direct relationship to the situations a person encounters in real organizational life. Aronson and Carlsmith (1968) have argued for the distinction between experimental realism and mundane realism. They contend that, in the laboratory, one can devise situations that have impact and that evoke valid psychological processes (experimental realism), even if the situation itself does not look like the real world (mundane realism). Yet, it remains true that many laboratory tasks seem suspiciously artificial and their external validity has not been demonstrated. External validity refers to the 'generalizability' of research findings to other populations, treatment variables, and measurement variables.

A second criticism of the laboratory experiment focuses on the reactions of subjects to the laboratory setting. These reactions may involve demand characteristics and evaluation apprehension. The first term refers to the fact that the experimental setting may evoke certain demands, that is, expectations on the part of subjects to act in the way that they think the experimenter would wish.

Evaluation apprehension refers to the concerns that a subject has about being observed and judged while in the laboratory setting. Because subjects come to a laboratory experiment knowing that the investigator is interested in some aspect of their behaviour, they may try to present themselves in a favourable light.

A third criticism of the laboratory experiment concerns experimenter expectancies (Rosenthal, 1966). It has been shown in a variety of situations that an experimenter knowing the hypothesis of the study, can unknowingly influence the results of the study.

The influence of these experimenter expectancies can be controlled to a large extent. For example, many experiments involve instructions that have been tape recorded in advance, thus assuring constancy in experimenter approach to all subjects. Other techniques include the use of a 'blind' experimenter, wherein the individual conducting the experiment is not informed of the experimental hypotheses and thus is less likely to exert a systematic bias on the results.

A fourth problem concerns the ethics of laboratory research, particularly when deception is involved. In order to ensure subjects are naive or unaware about the point of the study (and to reduce demand characteristics and evaluation apprehension), they are often deceived. Although they are fully debriefed afterwards the ethical problems must be faced.

Theories of social behaviour can be tested in laboratories: that is in controlled settings, though this remains fairly limited.

FIELD EXPERIMENT

In contrast to the laboratory experiment, the setting of the field experiment is a natural one and the subjects are not generally aware that they are subjects in an experiment. Rather than contriving an artificial situation in a laboratory, the investigator who uses a field experiment to test a hypothesis is looking at behaviour in its natural setting.

Like the laboratory experiment, in the field experiment the experimenter has control of the independent variables and the random assignment of subjects to conditions.

The advantages of the field experiment are that, by focusing on behaviour in a natural setting, the experimenter can be much more certain of the external validity of his or her findings. Furthermore, because subjects are generally unaware of their status as subjects, the problems of reactivity and the subjects' desire to be seen in a positive light are eliminated. In addition, because control over the independent variable and principles of randomization are maintained, the field experiment allows the same possibilities for conclusions about cause and effect as does the laboratory experiment.

Although the field experiment may seem to ideally combine the application of the strict rules of experimentation with the realism of natural behaviour settings, it too has some disadvantages. These disadvantages relate to the nature of the independent variable, the nature of the dependent variable, the ethics of the experiment, and the practical difficulties involved.

Because the experimenter is working in a complex natural setting where many events may be occurring simultaneously, the independent variable in the study must be quite obvious to the potential subject. Subtle manipulations of a variable may simply go unnoticed. The experimental independent variable is, in effect, competing with all of the other stimuli present in the setting.

The dependent variable in a field experiment needs to be selected carefully. The experimenters must be able to readily observe and reliably judge the dependent-variable behaviour. An additional problem in field experimentation concerns ethics. Is it reasonable for the investigator to involve individuals in an experiment without their knowledge or permission? Finally, the field experiment often poses practical problems. In contrast to the investigator in the laboratory, the investigator in the field has no control over the majority of events in the environment; unexpected events may reduce or destroy the effectiveness of the manipulation.

QUASI-EXPERIMENTAL RESEARCH

The defining characteristics of quasi-experimental research are that the investigator does not have full experimental control over the independent variables but does have extensive control over how, when, and for whom the dependent variable is measured (Campbell & Stanley, 1966). Generally, these experiments involve behaviour in a natural setting and focus on the effect of intervention in a system of ongoing behaviour.

In other cases, the intervention may be a natural disaster, such as flood, earthquake or tornado. Power blackouts could serve as the independent variable in a study of reactions to stressful events; or the introduction of new laws. The experimenter would have no control over the independent variable, but he or she could carefully select a set of dependent variables to measure the effect of the phenomena.

One unique advantage of quasi-experimental research conducted in a natural setting is that it allows for the study of very strong variables that cannot be manipulated or controlled by the experimenter. Often, quasi-experimental research deals with policy decisions that have consequences for very large numbers of people. The broad impact of such decisions gives considerable weight to the external validity of the study, in a manner that can rarely be matched in the more limited laboratory or field experiment.

Because the investigator has no control over the primary independent variable in quasi-experimental research it is always possible that other uncontrolled variables are affecting the dependent-variable behaviour. Random assignment of subjects to conditions can rarely be assumed in the quasi-experimental design, either. Often such research must literally be done 'on the run'. Furthermore, the arbitrariness of events in the quasi-experimental world precludes the experimenter's ability to vary factors according to any theoretical model. Intensity of a stressful event, for example, might

be an important variable in predicting the nature of response to stress. None the less, it is clearly impossible for the experimenter to control such a variable, and hence the levels of intensity would need to be accepted as they naturally occurred.

FIELD STUDY

Most field studies are characterized by their in-depth consideration of a limited group of people. The investigator in this setting plays a more reactive role than in the field experiment. Rather than manipulate some aspect of the environment and observe the changes that occur, the investigator in the field study records as much information as possible about the characteristics of that situation without altering the situation in any substantial way. Most often, people in the environment are aware of the investigator's presence and the general purpose of the investigation. Many times the investigator is a participant observer, i.e. is, someone actively engaged in the activities of the group, while at the same time maintaining records of the group members' behaviours.

Observation is the key element of the field-study method. Considerable time must be devoted in advance to familiarizing oneself with the environment and becoming aware of the kinds of behaviours that are most likely to occur. Then, one must decide which types of behaviour are to be recorded.

Once categories of behaviour are selected for observation, the investigator must devise specific methods of recording the desired information. Finally, the observer must conduct a series of preliminary investigations to determine the reliability of the measures. In other words, it must be demonstrated that a series of different observers watching the same event and using the methods chosen to record observations will code the behaviour in the same way. Without such reliability, a coding system merely reflects one observer's biases and cannot be used as a basis for scientific statement.

The major advantage lies in its realism. The focus of the study is on events as they normally occur in a real-life setting. Furthermore, because most field studies take place over an extended period of time, they provide information about the sequence and development of behaviours that cannot be gained in the one-shot observation typical of field and laboratory experiments. Additionally, the duration of the field study generally allows for the collection of several different types of dependent measures.

Although well-conducted field studies furnish a wealth of data, the lack of control in such settings can be a problem. Because there is no controlled independent variable, it is difficult to form conclusions regarding cause and effect. Although there are some statistical techniques to assist in making causal conclusions, the process is a more difficult one than in the controlled experimental design. A second potential problem in the field study is the subjects' awareness of the investigator's observations. When subjects are aware of being observed, their behaviour may be reactive, that is, influenced by the process of observation. Most experienced observers believe, however, that in a long-term field study the subjects become indifferent to the observer's presence, though the problem remains a serious one in briefer studies.

ARCHIVAL RESEARCH

Archival research refers to the analysis of any existing records that have been produced or maintained by persons or organizations other than the experimenter. In other words, the original reason for collecting the records was not a social psychological experiment. Newspaper reports and government records of airplane fatalities are two forms of archival data. Other sources of material include books and magazines, folk stories of preliterate societies, personal letters, and speeches by public figures.

First, it allows the investigator to test hypotheses over a wider range of time and societies than would otherwise be possible. Many records date back for centuries, a period of time that cannot be examined today using the other methods we have discussed. Demonstrating the validity of a hypothesis in a number of different cultures and historical periods, instead of being restricted to a specific group in the present time and place, gives us considerable confidence in the validity of that hypothesis as a test of human behaviour in general.

A second advantage of the archival method is that it uses unobtrusive measures: measures that did not cause reactivity in the participants at the time they were collected. Because the information used in archival research was originally collected for some other purpose, there is little or no chance that demand characteristics or evaluation apprehension will be problems for the present investigator.

Although experimenters doing research did not collect the data personally and thus are spared some problems in terms of reactivity, they may encounter some difficulties in terms of data availability. Frequently, a researcher will not be able to locate the kind of data needed to test a hypothesis. Not being able to design the dependent measures, the investigator is left at the mercy of those who collected the data. Sometimes, of course, creativity and ingenuity will help the investigator to locate the kinds of data needed; in other cases, however, missing or inaccurate records will prevent an adequate experimental test. Even if the material is available, it is sometimes difficult to categorize it in the way necessary to answer the research question. Such procedures are time consuming, although the development of computer programs has provided a welcome assist in some instances.

SIMULATION AND ROLE PLAYING

Although the range of simulation studies is considerable, the aim of each is to imitate some aspect of a real-world situation in order to gain more understanding of people's psychological processes. Subjects in these studies are typically asked to role play: to adopt a part and act as if they were in the real situation. In advance of their participation, the subjects are fully informed about the situation and are asked to develop their part to the best of their ability.

The success of simulation or role-play study depends heavily on the degree of involvement that the experimental setting can engender. If the subjects get deeply involved in the setting, then the simulation may well approximate the real-life conditions that it intends to match. Furthermore, because participants are fully informed of the purposes of the study in advance, they basically take on the role of co-investigators, a role that is both ethically and humanistically more satisfying in many respects than the more typical experimental subject role in which the subject is unaware of many of the experimenter's intentions. An additional advantage of the simulation is that it may allow the investigator to study in the laboratory phenomena and situations that are difficult to study in the real world.

In spite of their advantages, simulation and role playing are two of the most controversial methods in the social psychological repertoire. Critics of the method claim that when one asks subjects to act as if they are in a certain role, the subjects will do only what they think they *might* do and not necessarily what they *would* do in the real situation.

In addition, the problems of experimental demands and evaluation apprehension, discussed earlier in relation to laboratory experiments, are even more serious when the subject is fully informed of purposes of the study. On the other hand, proponents of role playing argue that, to some degree, the participant in an experiment is always playing a role in real life, whether it is the general role of subject or a more specific role defined by the investigator.

SURVEYS AND INTERVIEWS

Although many other methods in social psychology make use of questionnaires as part of their procedures, survey and interview methods rely solely on this type of information. In both cases, the investigator defines an area for research and designs a set of questions that will elicit the beliefs, attitudes, and self-reported experiences of the respondent in relation to the research topic.

Designing a good questionnaire is deceptive. Some considerations that enter into the design include the wording of questions, the provision of sufficient responses, and the format of the questionnaire itself. Considerable pretesting is necessary to ensure that the questions are objective, unbiased, understandable to the average respondent, and specific enough to elicit the desired information.

When the questionnaire is being presented by an interviewer, additional precautions against biasing the responses are necessary. The issue of experimenter bias, discussed earlier in relation to laboratory experiments, can be a problem in the interview method if the interviewer consciously or unconsciously encourages some responses and discourages or seems uninterested in others. Thus, interviewers must be carefully trained to standardize the delivery of questions to respondents. In addition, the interview method requires some skills on the part of the interviewer in developing rapport, so that the respondent will be willing to answer questions in a straightforward and honest manner. Interviews are notoriously unreliable if not conducted by highly trained personnel.

In both questionnaire surveys and interviews, the investigator must be concerned with sampling procedures. A major advantage of both survey questionnaires and interviews is that they allow the investigator to formulate the issues of concern very specifically. Rather than devising a situation to elicit desired behaviour or finding a natural situation in which to observe that behaviour, constructors of questionnaires directly question people about the behaviour or area under investigation.

Survey questionnaires are easier and more economical to use than interview procedures. In addition, they provide a greater anonymity for the respondent, which is important in the case of sensitive or personal issues. Face-to-face interviews, on the other hand, allow the interviewer to gather additional information from observation. Furthermore, the interviewer can clarify questions that may be confusing to the respondent and assure that the person intended to answer the questions is indeed the person responding.

Perhaps the major difficulty with self-report data, whether from interviews or surveys, is the issue of accuracy. Other topics may lead

Table 1. *Summary assessment of ten selection tests by five criteria*

	Validity	Cost	Practicality	Generality	Legality
Interviews	Low	Medium/high	High	High	Untested
References	Moderate	Very low	High	High	A few doubts
Peer ratings	High	Very low	Very limited	Military only	Untested
Biodata	High	Medium	High	High	Some doubts
Ability tests	High	Low	High	High	Major doubts
Personality tests	Low	Low	Fair	?White-collar	Untested
Assessment centre	High	Very high	Fair	Fairly high	No problems
Work sample	High	High	High	Blue-collar only	No problems
Job knowledge test	High	Low	High	Blue-collar only	Some doubts
Education	Low	Low	High	High	Major doubts

to embellishments by the respondent, who attempts to appear favourably.

As suggested earlier, survey questionnaires and interviews also have opposite sets of weaknesses. The survey questionnaire gives the investigator less control over the situation and cannot assure the conditions under which the questionnaire is being administered, who is answering it, and whether the respondent fully understands the questions. For its part, the interview is more costly, more time consuming, and is more susceptible to examiner bias.

In summary, questionnaire and interview methods allow the investigator to ask directly about the issues of concern. Particularly in the case of questionnaires, very large-scale studies are possible,

thus allowing greater generalizability of the results. Both methods, however, rely on the accuracy and honesty of the respondent and depend on self-reports of behaviour rather than observations of the behaviour itself.

To a large extent the research question dictates the methodology. But there are other important considerations like reliability and validity. Further, other methods may be used, not for research but for specific OB purposes. There are, for instance, a number of methods one could use to select people for a job. Cook (1990) lists ten methods and five criteria (Table 1). Though not all would agree with this analysis, it provides a useful map for the social behaviour researcher.

REFERENCES

Aronson, E. & Carlsmith, J. (1968). Experimentation in social psychology. In G. Ludzey & E. Aronson (Eds.). *Handbook of social psychology*, vol 2. Reading, Mass: Addison-Wesley.

Campbell, S. & Stanley, J. (1966). *Experimental and quasi-experimental designs for research*. Chicago: Rand-McNally.

Cook, M. (1990). *Personal selection and productivity*. Chichester: Wiley

Rosenthal, R. (1966). *Experimenter effects on behavioural research*. New York: Appleton-Crofts.

Triplett, N. (1898). The dynamogenic factors in pacemaking and competition. *American Journal of Psychology*, 9, 507–35.

PART II: Psychology, health and illness

SECTION 1: **Psychological aspects of health and illness**

This Part aims to provide in an easily digestible form a comprehensive picture of the general issues covered by health psychology. The first Section, Psychological aspects of health and illness, covers psychological and social factors that may influence or be influenced by illness. In some cases the same psychological factor may both contribute to and result from ill health. The second Section, Psychological assessment and intervention, covers the range of approaches used to assess the psychological impact of illnesses and psychological constructs that may contribute to illness as well as psychological approaches to prevention and treatment. The third Section, Health care practice, examines the psychology of the health care professional and his or her interaction with patients. It includes chapters on the impact of the job on the health care professional as well as factors that influence his or her effectiveness.

Adolescent lifestyle
Adoption
Architecture and health
Attributions and health
Childhood influences on health
Children's perceptions of illness and death
Coping with bereavement
Coping with chronic illness
Coping with chronic pain
Coping with death and dying
Coping with stressful medical
    procedures
Cultural and ethnic factors in health
Emotional expression and health

Family influences on health
Gender issues and women's health
Health belief model
Health-related behaviours: common
    factors
Hospitalization in adults
Hospitalization in children
Hospitalization in the elderly
Lay beliefs about health and illness
Life-events and health
Noise: effects on health
Old age and health behaviour
Pain: a multidimensional perspective
Perceived control and health behaviour

Physical activity and health
Risk perception and health behaviour
Self-efficacy and health behaviour
Sexual behaviour
Sleep, circadian rhythms and health
Social support and health
Socioeconomic status and health
Stress and disease
Theory of planned behaviour
Transtheoretical model of behaviour change
Type A behaviour, hostility and coronary artery
    disease
Unemployment and health
Weight control

Adolescent lifestyle

LEIF EDVARD AARØ

Research Centre for Health Promotion and
Department of Psychosocial Science, University of
Bergen, Norway

DEFINITIONS
According to Elliott (1993):

'a lifestyle has been defined as a distinctive mode of living that is defined by a set of expressive, patterned behaviors of individuals occurring with some consistency over a period of time. The lifestyle construct is not intended to capture the totality of a person's behavior, but rather to reflect that complex subset of diverse behaviors that is relatively stable and predictable.'

In order to characterize a person' lifestyle, the behaviours in question have to be observable, and we are referring to behaviours over which the individual has some degree of control. A lifestyle means that there are combinations of behaviour or behavioural domains that occur consistently. Health-related lifestyles refers to patterns of health-related behaviours.

When defining 'adolescence', several criteria are relevant, for instance, secondary sex characteristics, cognitive abilities, social criteria, or simply age (Crockett & Petersen, 1993). According to a recent definition (Adams, Gullotta & Markstrom-Adams, 1994), adolescence covers the age-groups 11–20, and it is distinguished between early adolescence (11–14), middle adolescence (15–17) and late adolescence (18–20). During this period of life, through a complex interplay between biological, physiological, psychological, social and cultural factors, health-related behaviours are shaped.

HEALTH BEHAVIOUR CHANGE DURING ADOLESCENCE
During adolescence a number of health compromising behaviours emerge. When entering adolescence, children are normally spontaneously physically active, and use of tobacco, alcohol or other addictive substances hardly exists. When leaving adolescence, a substantial proportion are physically inactive, and use of addictive substances is common. The sexual debut usually takes place during adolescence, and being sexually active without adequate protection against unwanted pregnancies, venereal disease and HIV represents a serious threat to health and wellbeing. According to Elliott (Elliott, Huizinga & Menard, 1989; Elliott & Morse, 1989), 50% or more of all adolescents, who will engage in delinquent behaviour, do so by the age of 12. For alcohol use, half of all adolescent users begin using by age 14, for marijuana use, by age 16, for sexual involvement and hard drug use, by age 17, and for driving while under the influence, by age 18. According to a report from the international study on Health Behaviour in School-Aged Children, the recruitment of smokers accelerates during the age interval between 13 and 15 (King & Coles, 1992).

It must be kept in mind, however, that most young people never become regular smokers, heavy drinkers or drug addicts, and a large proportion of young adults are physically active. During adolescence, the basis for a life-long health-enhancing lifestyle can be established.

A CROSS-CULTURAL PERSPECTIVE
In the developing world, health compromising lifestyles are gradually becoming a threat to health among young people. Eide and Acuda (1995) have shown that cultural influences from the industrialized countries introduce forms of alcohol use which is less well regulated by rituals and social norms than the traditional beverages. Young people with a 'western' cultural orientation have alcohol preferences which are different from those with a more traditional cultural orientation, and their consumption is higher. Similar cultural processes of cultural influence may operate on a variety of health behaviours, and the introduction of a 'modern' lifestyle may lead to a gradual increase in the diseases which are typical for industrialized countries.

DIMENSIONS OF HEALTH BEHAVIOURS
A number of studies have examined to what extent health behaviours are intercorrelated, and to what extent these correlations reflect underlying clusters or dimensions. Analyses from the international study on Health Behaviour in School-Aged Children indicate two such underlying dimensions: (a) addictive and risk taking behaviours and (b) health enhancing behaviours (Nutbeam, Aarø & Wold, 1991; Aarø, Laberg & Wold, 1995). The correlation between the factors is negative and varies between .40 and .50.

The addictive and risk taking dimension corresponds well with Jessor's 'problem behaviours' (Jessor & Jessor, 1977; Jessor, 1984). According to Jessor, a number of health related behaviours reflect a 'syndrome', or an underlying tendency to behave defiantly and unconventionally. He includes such behaviours as use of alcohol, marijuana and tobacco, and he maintains that these are associated with a higher likelihood of involvement in other types of risk behaviour, such as precocious sexual activity, aggression, and delinquency. Jessor claims that, for these behaviours, the pattern of associations with a number of personality and social environmental correlates is essentially the very same.

The health-enhancing behaviours forming the second factor include physical activity, consumption of healthy food, oral hygiene, use of seat belts, and use of vitamins. In order to explain why these behaviours actually correlate, the diffusion of innovation processes which have been described by Rogers and Shoemaker (1971) and

Rogers (1987) have to be taken into account. If we assume that health education reaches and influences health behaviours in certain individuals and certain groups to a larger extent than other individuals and other groups, correlations between health-enhancing behaviours emerge (Aarø, Laberg & Wold, 1995).

Intercorrelations and clusters of intercorrelations imply that health behaviours do not exist as separate and independent domains, and thereby indicate the usefulness of the notion of 'lifestyles'. Furthermore, it may be argued that such intercorrelations indicate similarities in the processes underlying different health behaviours. Intercorrelations between health behaviours imply overlap in target groups across behavioural risk factors, and support the notion of a more integrated and holistic approach to health promotion among adolescents.

PERSONALITY CORRELATES

Although the major determinants of health-related lifestyles must be traced in the social environment of young people, some personality characteristics have been shown to be consistently associated with 'problem behaviours'. Jessor claims that in the personality system, the main characteristics of proneness to problem behaviour include lower value on academic achievement and lower expectations for academic achievements (Jessor, 1984). This has been confirmed in more recent studies (Nutbeam Aarø & Catford, 1988; Nutbeam et al., 1993). In one study, the sensation-seeking personality trait (Zuckerman, 1979) has been shown to correlate with such problem behaviours as smoking, alcohol consumption, number of lifetime sex partners and experience of casual sex (Kraft & Rise, 1994).

ATTITUDES AND SOCIAL NORMS

Among theories on environmental predictors of behaviours some choose to focus on aspects of the perceived environment (Fishbein & Ajzen, 1975; Ajzen, 1988) while other theories explicitly take objective environmental conditions into account (Jessor & Jessor, 1977; Jessor, 1984; Jessor, Donovan & Costa, 1991). The expectancy-value theories, which belong to the former category, hypothesize that behaviours can be predicted via behavioural intentions. Behavioural intentions are formed by such factors as personal attitudes towards the relevant behaviour and perceived social norms. Perceived behavioural control, a concept which comes very close to Bandura's concept 'self-efficacy' has been included among the predictors in the Theory of Planned Behaviour (Ajzen, 1988).

Expectancy-value theory claims that attitudes can be predicted by behavioural beliefs and by the evaluation of such beliefs. To the extent that we believe that a certain behaviour will produce certain negative outcomes, and to the extent that these are regarded as important to avoid, negative attitudes to the actual behaviour are likely to follow.

Perceived social norms can similarly be predicted by a combination of others' expectations as we perceive them, and by our motivation to comply.

As far as the prediction of health behaviours in young people is concerned, there is reason to assume that long-term consequences in terms of increased risk of disease or death play a moderate role in predicting health behaviours. Short-term consequences are corres-

pondingly important. There is also reason to believe that environmental factors are more influential during adolescence than later in life. In the field of smoking behaviour it has been shown that while correlations between variables measuring epidemiological knowledge on one hand and behaviours on the other are generally low (Aarø, Wold, Kannas, & Rimpela" 1986), environmental factors are convincingly strong predictors of behaviour (Aarø, Haukes & Berglund, 1981).

One study has shown that alcohol use of parents as perceived by offsprings predicts offspring's use of alcohol more strongly than the alcohol use as reported by the parents (Aas, Jakobsen & Anderssen, 1996)

Alcohol expectancies are hypothesized to be a major factor in predicting alcohol use among adolescents, and an instrument for the measurement of such expectancies has been developed (Christiansen, Goldman & Inn, 1982; Christiansen & Goldman, 1983). A review of the literature has concluded that alcohol expectancies are correlated with use of alcohol (Goldman, 1989).

Rather than assuming that such factors as expectancies and attitudes are pure predictors while behaviours are outcomes, we must suppose that there is an ongoing and continuous process of reciprocal determinism (Bandura, 1977, 1986). Experiences with alcohol are likely to change our expectations and attitudes, and simultaneously these factors may influence future intentions, decisions and practices regarding use of alcohol.

DEMOGRAPHIC CONDITIONS AND SOCIETAL CONTEXT

Health-compromising lifestyles are, to a large extent, a product of the modern world. Physical inactivity is fostered by modern means of transportation and by passive exposure to TV channels and videos. Widespread use of addictive substances may reflect alienation and a weakening of social norms and the deterioration of social networks. Broken families and family problems may lead to a weakening of parental control over food habits and sleeping habits. The change in health behaviours does not take place at the same speed and simultaneously in all groups. In the industrialized countries the use of tobacco first became widespread among high status groups. Presently, high status groups have reduced their use of tobacco substantially. Low status groups are falling behind, and in many countries the prevalence of regular smokers in low status segments of the population is four to five times higher than among those belonging to high status segments.

Similar processes can be observed across behaviours. Belonging to high status groups means that you are more likely to be physically active, to eat healthy food, to be a non-smoker and to wear seat belts (Aarø, 1987). Since health behaviours of adolescents are closely related to those of their parents, similar socioeconomic inequalities may exist for adolescents as well. The correlation between school alienation and use of addictive substances, which consistently has been shown (Nutbeam et al., 1988, 1993), indicates that a socioeconomic gradient exists also for adolescents. The prevalence of smoking and drinking is considerably higher than average among adolescents who do not plan to have a higher education. When parents' occupations are rated as having lower socioeconomic status, adolescents report to be less physically active than others (Wold, 1989).

Researchers have concluded that health-related behaviours to some extent carry over from one generation to the next (Ketterlinus, Lamb & Nitz, 1994), and that a process of social reproduction of socioeconomic inequalities in lifestyles can be demonstrated (Wold, 1989).

Health behaviours are also influenced by such factors as advertising, legislation (including bans on advertising), price, and availability. Increasing the price of tobacco products leads to a decrease in consumption, and this decrease is higher for adolescents than for adults. Among adults the price elasticity is probably close to -0.5 (Townsend, 1992; US Department of Health and Human Services, 1992; Godfrey & Maynard, 1988). A price elasticity of -0.5 means that increasing the price by 10% leads to a 5% reduction in the consumption. The price elasticity is particularly high among young people. In one study (Warner, 1986) it was shown to be -1.40 among 12–17 year-olds. It is reasonable to assume that, in order to make the healthy choice the easiest choice, the prices of healthy products should be kept low.

The effects of tobacco advertising and the effects of banning such advertising has been debated. Finland and Norway were among the first countries to adopt a total ban on tobacco sales promotion, and these two countries are sometimes referred to as illustrations that such legislation has been successful. Tobacco industry spokesmen interpret available evidence in the opposite way. A report from 1993 concludes that the few scientifically valid reports available today give both theoretical and empirical evidence for a causal relationship between advertising and use of tobacco, and it is likely that 'the dynamic tobacco market represented by children and adolescents' is the main target of tobacco sales promotion (Rimpelä, Aarø & Rimpelä, 1993). It follows that effectively enforced bans of advertising contribute to reducing smoking among adolescents.

STABILITY AND CHANGE

The effects of health compromising behaviours can be short term as well as long term. Drunk driving increases the risk of dramatic and fatal accidents. Daily smoking may lead to coronary heart disease and lung cancer, but these effects usually are visible only after many years. The importance of promoting healthy lifestyles among adolescents therefore, to some extent, depends on the stability of such behaviours. Jessor and associates (1991) have studied the stability of problem behaviours from adolescence to adulthood, and conclude that there is considerable stability and continuity in that change. They conclude that 'the adolescent is parent of the young adult'. Consequently the promotion of healthy lifestyles among young people is important not only because of its short-term impact on health and disease, but also because of its consequences for health behaviours later in life.

CONCLUDING REMARKS

To describe adolescent health-related lifestyles and its correlates and predictors is like putting together a puzzle. As far as smoking, use of alcohol and use of other addictive substances in concerned, a considerable amount of research has been carried out. There is considerable less behavioural research on use of seat belts and other use of safety equipment, oral hygiene, healthy food habits and physical activity. The picture is therefore more detailed on the problem behaviour side, and less complete on the health enhancing behaviour side. New publications continuously add new pieces to the picture, and the picture itself gradually changes under the technological, societal and cultural changes which take place.

REFERENCES

Aarø, L.E. (1987). Health behaviours and socioeconomic status. A survey among the adult population in Norway. Doctoral thesis. Bergen: University of Bergen.

Aarø, L.E., Haukes, A. & Berglund, E.-L. (1981). Smoking among Norwegian school-children 1975–1980. II. The influence of the social environment. *Scandinavian Journal of Psychology*, 22, 297–309.

Aarø, L.E., Wold, B., Kannas, L. & Rimpelä, M. (1986). Health behaviour in schoolchildren. A WHO cross national survey. A presentation of philosophy, methods and selected results of the First Survey. *Health Promotion*, 1, 17–33.

Aarø, L.E., Laberg, J.C. & Wold, B. (1995). Health behaviours among adolescents: towards a hypothesis of two dimensions. *Health Education Research*, 10, 83–93.

Aas, H., Jakobsen, R. & Anderssen, N. (1995). Predicting 13 year olds' drinking using parents' self-reported alcohol use and restrictiveness compared with offspring's perception. *Scandinavian Journal of Psychology*, 37, 113–20.

Adams, G.R., Gullotta, T.P. & Markstrom-Adams, C. (1994). *Adolescent life experiences*. 3rd edition. Pacific Grove, California: Brooks/Cole Publishing Company.

Ajzen, I. (1988). *Attitudes, personality, and behavior*. Buckingham: Open University Press.

Bandura, A. (1977). *Social learning theory*. Englewood Cliffs, New Jersey: Prentice-Hall.

Bandura, A. (1986). *Social foundations of thought and action. A social cognitive theory*. Englewood Cliffs, New Jersey: Prentice-Hall.

Christiansen, B.A., Goldman, M.S. & Inn, A. (1982). Development of alcohol-related expectancies in adolescents: separating pharmacological from social learning influences. *Journal of Consulting and Clinical Psychology*, 50, 336–44.

Christiansen, B.A. & Goldman, M.S. (1983). Alcohol-related expectancies versus demographic/background variables in the prediction of adolescent drinking. *Journal of Consulting and Clinical Psychology*, 51, 249–57.

Crockett, L.J. & Petersen, A.C. (1993). Adolescent development: health risks and opportunities for health promotion. In Millstein, S.G., Petersen, A.C. & Nightingale, E.O. (Eds). *Promoting the health of adolescents. New directions for the twenty-first century*. New York: Oxford University Press. pp. 13–37.

Eide, A. & Acuda, S.W. (1996). Cultural orientation and adolescents' alcohol use in Zimbabwe. *Addiction* 91, 807–14.

Elliott, D.S. (1993). Health enhancing and health-compromising lifestyles. In Millstein, S., Petersen, A.C. & Nightingale, E.O. (Eds.). *Promoting the health of adolescents. New directions for the twenty-first century*. New York, Oxford: Oxford University Press, pp. 119–145.

Elliott, D.S. & Morse, B.J. (1989). Delinquency and drug use as risk factors in teenage sexual activity. *Youth and Society*, 21, 21–60.

Elliott, D.S., Huizinga, D. & Menard, S.

(1989). *Multiple problem youth: delinquency, substance use and mental health problems.* New York: Springer Verlag.

Fishbein, M. & Ajzen, I. (1975). *Belief, attitude, intention, and behavior: an introduction to theory and research.* Reading, Massachusetts: Addison-Wesley.

Godfrey, C. & Maynard, A. (1988). Economic aspects of tobacco use and taxation policy. *British Medical Journal, 297,* 339–97.

Goldman, M.S. (1989). Alcohol expectancies as cognitive-behavioral psychology: theory and practice. In Løberg, T., Miller, W.R., Nathan, P.E. & Marlatt, G.A. (Eds.). *Addictive behaviors: prevention and early intervention.* Amsterdam: Swets & Zeitlinger, pp. 11–30.

Jessor, R. (1984). Adolescent development and behavioral health. In Matarazzo J.D., Weiss, S.M., Herd, J.A., Miller, N.E. & Weiss, S.M. (Eds.) *Behavioral health: A handbook of health enhancement and disease prevention.* New York: Wiley, pp. 69–90.

Jessor, R. & Jessor, S.L. (1977). *Problem behavior and psychosocial development: a longitudinal study of youth.* New York: Academic Press.

Jessor, R., Donovan, J.E. & Costa, F.M. (1991). *Beyond adolescence. Problem behavior and young adult development.* New York: Cambridge University Press.

Ketterlinus, R.D., Lamb, M.E. Nitz, K.A. (1994). Adolescent nonsexual and sex-related problem behaviors: Their

prevalence, consequences, and co-occurrence. In Ketterlinus, R.D. & Lamb, M.E. (Eds.). *Adolescent problem behaviors. Issues and research.* Hillsdale: New Jersey: Lawrence Erlbaum Associates.

King, A.J.C. & Coles, B. (1992). *The health of Canada's youth. Views and behaviours of 11-, 13- and 15-year olds from 11 countries.* Ottawa: Health and Welfare Canada.

Kraft, P. & Rise, J. (1994). The relationship between sensation seeking and smoking, alcohol consumption and sexual behavior among Norwegian adolescents. *Health Education Research, 9,* 193–200.

Nutbeam, D., Aarø, L.E. & Catford, J. (1988) Understanding children's health behaviour: The implications for health promotion for young people. *Social Science and Medicine, 29,* 317–25.

Nutbeam, D., Aarø, L.E. & Wold, B. (1991). The lifestyle concept and health education with young people. Results from a WHO international survey. *World Health Statistics Quarterly, 44,* 55–61.

Nutbeam, D., Smith, C., Moore, L. & Bauman, A. (1993). Warning! Schools can damage your health: alienation from school and its impact on health behaviour. *Journal of Paediatrics and Child Health, 29,* 25–30.

Rimpelä, M.K., Aarø, L.E. & Rimpelä, A.H. (1993). The effects of tobacco sales promotion on initiation of smoking. *Scandinavian Journal of Social Medicine,* Suppl. 49, 1–23.

Rogers, E.M. & Shoemaker, F.F. (1971). *Communication of innovations. A cross-cultural approach.* New York: The Free Press.

Rogers, E.M. (1987). The diffusion of innovations perspective. In Weinstein, N.D. (Ed) *Taking care. Understanding and encouraging self-protective behavior.* Cambridge: Cambridge University Press.

Townsend, J. (1992). Reducing smoking through price and other means. *Proceedings of the UK Presidency Seminar.* pp. 75–88, London: Department of Health.

US Department of Health and Human Services (1992). *Strategies to control tobacco use in the United States: a blueprint for public health action in the 1990's.* Bethesda, Maryland: National Institutes of Health, National Cancer Institute.

Warner, K.E. (1986). Smoking and health implications of a change in the Federal cigarette excise tax. *Journal of the American Medical Association, 255,* 1028–32.

Wold, B. (1989). Lifestyles and physical activity. A theoretical and empirical analysis of socialization among children and adolescents. Doctoral thesis. Bergen: University of Bergen, Research Center for Health Promotion.

Zuckerman, M. (1979). *Sensation seeking. Beyond the optimal level of arousal.* London: Lawrence Erlbaum Associates.

Adoption

SUSAN MICHIE

Psychology and Genetics Research Group, United Medical and Dental Schools, Guy's Campus, London, UK

There is now a greater variety of adoptive parents and adopted children than the historically typical pattern of white, middle-class infertile parents adopting infants. With fewer babies available for adoption, adopted children are more likely to be older, have special needs and be from a different country or ethnic group than their adoptive parents. The range of social backgrounds and family compositions of adoptive parents is also widening. The particular features of each adoptive family are likely to be important in considering the psychological aspects of the adoption process. There are, however, certain issues that all adopted children and their families face.

PSYCHOLOGICAL IDENTITY

Research into adopted children's adaptation to their losses suggest that it is usually not until adolescence that such losses may cause

problems (Schechter & Bertocci, 1990). The adolescent questions and develops an autonomous identity as he or she becomes more independent and separate from the family and home. The questions 'who am I, and where am I going?' raise the questions 'who made me, and where did I come from?' It is at such time that a lack of knowledge about the birth family and a loss of 'connectedness' to a genealogical line may become acutely felt.

There are two schools of thought in considering the situation of adopted children who desire more knowledge about their birth family. One is that they are 'genealogically bewildered', experiencing confusion and uncertainty that undermines their security and mental health (Sants, 1964). Curiosity about birth parents has also been seen as a sign of psychological stress or poor adoptive experience (Triseliotis, 1973). These views are based on clinical impressions, rather than on empirical studies of non-clinical populations.

The other view is that the desire for more information is a normal process of separating from one's parents, which helps in the rational aim of creating a social identity (Haimes, 1987). Haimes' study of 45 adoptees found that those who wanted to trace their birth parents were well adjusted and were motivated by curiosity rather than by crisis or pathology. Their motivation was to discover their life story in order to compile a complete and consistent biography for themselves.

In one of the few controlled research studies using normative populations of adopted and non-adopted adolescents, Stein and Hoopes (1985) found that adoptees did not show more problems of identity or adjustment. One of their conclusions was that adoptive parents need to be made aware that their adolescent's interest in information about his or her origins is a normal manifestation of the process of identity consolidation.

Identity problems and low self-esteem amongst adolescent adoptees have been found to be associated with unfavourable reports about birth parents (Frisk, 1964). Adoptees took the reports to be proof of their biological parents' inferiority and, hence, their own genetic inferiority. This may be compounded by a perception in adoptees that their adoptive parents would have preferred children sharing their own genes, rather than those of other, unknown people.

STRESS AND COPING

There is evidence that adopted children may be at increased risk for various psychological and academic problems (see Brodzinsky, 1990). Various explanations have been put forward, all acknowledging the role that stress plays in the adoption process for both children and parents. Stress is caused by disruptions in early life, by losses of attachment figures and familiar environments, and by change, even when that change is for the better.

Children who are adopted face several losses: their birth family and previous environment; access to their family history, and hence cultural and genealogical heritage; 'status loss' associated with being different; and loss of stability in their relationship with their adoptive parents.

Some of these are similar to the losses experienced by non-adopted children following family disruption and life transitions; some are unique to the experience of being adopted.

Children's awareness and adaptation to these losses change with age. By about eight years of age, as children's understanding develops and they are able to reflect on their unknown past and their unknown birth parents, their initially positive response to being adopted becomes one of ambivalence (Singer, Brodzinsky & Braff, 1982).

Clinical experience suggests that most adopted children appear to cope quite well with the losses, stresses and demands of adoptive family life. Those with high self-esteem and a sense of their own control and efficacy are best able to adjust. The child's sense of trust in others and commitment to the adoptive family are also helpful. This will be influenced by the quality of parenting and family life and by the openness and sensitivity with which adoption issues are discussed.

As the adoption process is becoming more open and more geared towards meeting the psychological needs of adoptees and their families, it may be that the problems of adjustment and identity documented in the past are decreasing. To answer this question, and questions about how best to prepare for, and support, the adoption process, we need more research of non-clinical, community samples with adequate control groups.

REFERENCES

Brodzinsky, D.M. A stress and coping model of adoption adjustment. In D.M. Brodzinsky, and M.D. Schechter (Eds.). *The psychology of adoption*, Oxford: Oxford University Press.

Frisk, M. (1964). Identity problems and confused conceptions of the genetic ego in adopted children during adolescence. *Acta Paediatrica Psychiatrica*, **31**, 6–12.

Haimes, E. (1987). 'Now I know who I really am.' Identity change and redefinitions of the self in adoption. In T. Honess, and K. Yardley (Eds.). *Self and identity*. London: Routledge Kegan and Paul.

Sants, H.J. (1964). Genealogical bewilderment in children with substitute parents. *British Journal of Medical Psychology*, **37**, 133–41.

Schechter, M.D. and Bertocci, D. (1990). The meaning of the search. In D.M. Brodzinsky, & M.D. Schechter (Eds.). *The psychology of adoption*, Oxford: Oxford University Press.

Singer, L.M., Brodzinsky, D.M. & Braff, A.M. (1982). Children's belief about adoption: a developmental study. *Journal of Applied Development Psychology*, **3**, 285–94.

Stein, L.M. & Hoopes, J.L. (1985). *Identity formation in the adopted adolescent*. New York: Child Welfare League of America.

Triseliotis, J. (1973). *In search of origins*. London: Routledge and Kegan Paul.

Adoption

Architecture and health

STACIE SPENCER
and
ANDREW BAUM
University of Pittsburgh, USA

Architecture can be considered in many ways, as art or aesthetic stimuli, as an expression of societal pride or aspiration, and as a way of structuring interior and exterior spaces to facilitate their use by human occupants. This latter function of architectural design has strong but modifiable effects on social behavior and users' mood and productivity and, to some extent, design features also affect health and well-being. Too often, however, these important sources of influence are ignored or not recognized, despite repeated demonstrations of these effects. While much remains to be done, research has identified several architectural features that appear to be associated with mood and health. Design characteristics or the way space is structured, presence or absence of windows, and illumination all appear to affect people. For some features, the relationship to health is indirect (e.g. small, crowded work spaces may result in stress that may in turn affect health) while for other features the relationship to health is more direct (e.g. eye strain from poor lighting, illness from exposure to fumes).

The structural design or arrangement of space imposes restrictions on behaviour. Doorways determine our access to a room and room dimensions restrict the kinds of behaviours that can take place inside a room. As a result, one of the most important goals when designing a building is to match the built environment with the needs of the individuals for whom the environment is designed. However, even under the best conditions, primary uses of a building may change and interior changes must be made to meet the current purposes. Flexibility may therefore supersede many desirable design characteristics, which may have negative effects on use. Regardless, among its effects, the interior design of space has an impact on the perception of density and crowding, can impose excess interaction or isolation and has been associated with arousal and stress (cf. Baum & Paulus, 1987).

Three inter-related variables are important considerations in the design of space because of the potential for indirect influences on mood and health. These variables are the perception of density, privacy and control. Density is the ratio of the number of individuals within a space to the actual size of that space and is thus an expression of physical properties of the setting (Baum & Koman, 1976; Stokols, 1972). Density can increase when the absolute amounts of available space decrease, and such changes in spatial density reflects the negative effects of decreasing space. For example, as density increases, people may have to work harder to maintain privacy (Altman, 1975). As the number of people increases, regardless of how much space is available, social overload and stress are also likely. This focus on social density reflects the subjective experience of frequent or unwanted interaction and is often not easy to change (Baum & Valins, 1979). The high social density environment may threaten the control an individual tries to maintain over privacy and regulation of social interactions. If density increases because the amount of available space decreases, stress associated with exposure to high social density environments where there is little privacy or control over social interaction can lead to negative health outcomes (Paulus, McCain, & Cox, 1978).

A series of studies done in the 1970s investigated the impact of architecturally determined differences in social density on behaviour in college dormitories. Long-corridor type dormitories in which a large number of individuals were required to share a hallway, bathroom, and lounge also required residents to interact with many individuals, often with people they disliked and/or did not know very well. Further, many interactions occurred at inconvenient times (Baum & Valins, 1977). In comparison, suite-type dormitories structurally determined smaller groups and reduced the number of required interactions when using shared spaces (usually three to five suite-mates) (Baum & Valins, 1977). Residents of corridor dorms reported that they felt more crowded than did suite residents, despite living on halls with comparable densities and total numbers of residents. Associated with this, corridor residents exhibited lower thresholds for crowding and avoided social interaction outside of the dormitory (Baum & Valins, 1977), reported lower feelings of control in shared spaces, were less likely to know how hallmates felt about them, and were less willing to share information about themselves with other people living on the floor (Baum & Valins, 1977; Baum, Harpin, & Valins, 1975). In comparison to suite residents, long-corridor residents were more competitive and reactive, and appeared to be more motivated to regulate social contacts in the first few weeks of dormitory residence. However, in as few as seven weeks, behaviour changed and residents became more withdrawn and exhibited symptoms of helplessness (Baum, Aiello, Calesnick, 1978). The effects of crowding were strong enough to generalize to non-dormitory settings (Baum & Valins, 1977).

High social density and loss of control have also been associated with self-report, behavioural, and biochemical indices of stress. In studies of prison inmates, death rates and rates of psychiatric commitments were higher in years when prison population was higher (Paulus *et al.*, 1975). Paulus *et al.* (1975) also found that inmates living under high social density conditions had higher blood pressure. In another study of prison inmates, perceived crowding was associated with urinary catecholamine levels (Schaeffer *et al.*, 1988). Residents of low density cells (private cells) reported less crowding and exhibited lower urinary catecholamine levels than did residents of high density cells (open-dormitories). Residents of high density cells that had been modified to reduce social density (cubicles within a dormitory) exhibited catecholamine levels comparable to the private-cell inmates. However, these inmates had the highest number of health complaints (Schaeffer *et al.*, 1988).

These studies suggest that design of residential space has far-ranging effects on residents and should be considered when designing new buildings. In the case of pre-existing buildings, modifications can be made to reduce the stress of crowding. Studies have shown that partitioning space can accommodate increases in spatial density without increasing effective social density (Desor, 1972). These changes should be aimed at increasing the perception of control over regulation of social experiences and supporting local control of shared spaces. Cubicles within dormitory-style prison housing increased regulatory control and were associated with catecholamine levels similar to that of private-cell inmates (Schaeffer *et al.*, 1988). Similarly, an architectural intervention, in which a long-corridor dormitory hall was bisected, resulted in greater confidence in residents' control over social interactions in the dormitory, less residential and non-residential social withdrawal, and less crowding stress compared to the non-bisected long-corridor residents (Baum & Davis, 1980).

These findings have implications for the design of other spaces in which large numbers of individuals must share areas and/or work together. For example, in work environments it is often too costly to provide private offices for every employee. Simply filling a large room with desks would not be a good alternative because of resulting noise as well as in efficiency and decreased regulatory control over social interaction. Such a design would likely decrease productivity, increase stress levels, and increase the likelihood of negative health outcomes. Use of modular cubicles or other methods of breaking space up would provide the structure for increasing control over local spaces and productivity and prevent increases in distress associated with crowding.

Other architectural features also have important influences on behaviour and health. Windows and illumination appear to be particularly important factors. As with the interior design of space, each of these features has an impact on perceptions and behaviours that may affect health. Windows are so important to individuals that the assignment to an office with a window is tied directly to office hierarchies. Big promotions often include a move to an office with a window. The importance of windowed offices is also demonstrated by findings indicating that people in windowless offices report less job satisfaction, less interest in their jobs, and are less positive about the physical work conditions (e.g. appearance, light, temperature) (Finnegan & Solomon, 1981). People in windowless offices also use more visual materials (typically of nature scenes) than do occupants of windowed spaces to decorate their environments (Heerwagen & Orians, 1986). While there is little argument about whether windows are a desired feature, they are expensive, energy inefficient, and are limited to exterior walls. In large office buildings, some windowless offices are inevitable. The reductions or changes in the views people have, the positive ambience of the setting, and other effects of having or not having windows appear to affect mood and health in dramatic ways.

For example, research suggests that windows are important in recovery from surgery and in intensive care units. Ulrich (1983, 1984) argues that natural views are associated with positive emotional states which may play a role in the reduction of stressful thoughts and recovery from surgery. In a study with patients recovering from a cholecystectomy procedure, Ulrich compared post-cholecystectomy patients who had a window view of trees to patients who had a window view of a brick wall. In comparison to the wall-view patients, patients with a natural view had fewer post-surgical complications, took fewer moderate and high doses and more weak doses of pain medication, were described by nurses as demonstrating fewer negative characteristics (e.g. upset and crying, needs much encouragement), and stayed in the hospital for less time postsurgery. In a different study, Keep, James and Inman (1980) found that intensive care patients in windowless units had less accurate memories of the length of their stays and were less well oriented during their hospitalization than intensive care patients in windowed units.

Windows are also related to illumination; they provide natural lighting and the extent and nature of illumination are important features of design on many different levels. The kind of illumination (incandescent, fluorescent), the brightness of illumination, and the spectral range of the illumination, are all important characteristics of light and govern their effects on mood and behaviour. The cool-white fluorescent lights used in public places are economical, energy efficient, and maintenance free, but these lights produce only partial spectrum light waves and lack the spectrum of natural sunlight (Sperry, 1984). In comparison to exposure to full spectrum lights, exposure to cool white fluorescent lights for as little as four hours has been associated with increased lethargy, visual fatigue, and decreased visual acuity (Maas, Jayson & Kleiber, 1974). This is important in settings such as libraries and offices, where the majority of work is visual (Sperry, 1984). Over days and weeks, the cumulative effects of repeated exposure to cool white fluorescent lighting may result in job stress, chronic fatigue, and poor vision. The use of lighting which includes the full spectrum may be preferable.

Architectural features such as the design of space, the presence of windows, and illumination affect social behaviour, mood, and productivity, and appear to be associated with health. While these features are important to consider during the design of space, they are sometimes easy to modify in existing space. Partitions can be used to decrease social density while allowing increases in spatial density. Window views can be designed to include natural scenes and, where a window looks onto another building or in offices in which a window does not exist, murals can be used to simulate natural scenes. Interior lighting can be chosen to maximize the full spectrum of available light. Research and intervention in the design or redesign of space with these features in mind will provide further evidence of the impact of the design of interior spaces and will provide new insights into the complex but important interactions of behavioural, biological, and environmental variables in determining health and well-being.

REFERENCES

Altman, I. (1975). *The environment and social behavior*. Monterey, CA: Brooks/Cole.

Baum, A. & Davis, G.E. (1980). Reducing the stress of high-density living: an architectural intervention. *Journal of Personality and Social Psychology*, **38**, 471–81.

Baum, A. & Koman, S. (1976). Differential response to anticipated crowding: psychological effects of social and spatial density. *Journal of Personality and Social Psychology*, **34**, 526–36.

Baum, A. & Paulus, P.B. (1987). Crowding. In D. Stokols & I. Altman (Eds.). *Handbook of environmental psychology*. New York: Wiley.

Baum, A. & Valins, S. (1977). *Architecture and social behavior: psychological studies of social density*. Hillsdale, NJ: Erlbaum.

Baum, A. & Valins, S. (1979). Architectural mediation of residential density and control: crowding and the regulation of social contact. *Advances in Experimental Social Psychology*, **12**, 131–75.

Baum, A., Harpin, R.E. & Valins, S. (1975). The role of group phenomena in the experience of crowding. *Environment and Behavior*, **7**, 185–98.

Baum, A., Aiello, J.R. & Calesnick, L.E. (1978). Crowding and personal control: social density and the development of learned helplessness. *Journal of Personality and Social Psychology*, **36**, 1000–11.

Desor, J.A. (1972). Toward a psychological theory of crowding. *Journal of Personality and Social Psychology*, **21**, 79–83.

Finnegan, M.C. & Solomon, L.Z. (1981). Work attitudes in windowed vs. windowless environments. *Journal of Social Psychology*, **115**, 291–2.

Heerwagen, J.H. & Orians, G.H. (1986). Adaptations to windowlessness: a study of the use of visual decor in windowed and windowless offices. *Environment and Behavior*, **18**, 623–39.

Keep, P., James, J. & Inman, M. (1980). Windows in the intensive therapy unit. *Anaesthesia*, **35**, 257–62.

Maas, J.B., Jayson, J.K. & Kleiber, D.A. (1974). Effects of spectral difference in illumination on fatigue. *Journal of Applied Psychology*, **59**, 524–6.

Paulus, P., McCain, G. & Cox, V. (1978). Death rates, psychiatric commitments, blood pressure and perceived crowding as a function of institutional crowding. *Environmental Psychology and Non-Verbal Behavior*, **3**, 107–16.

Paulus, P., Cox, V., McCain, G. & Chandler, J. (1975). Some effects of crowding in a prison environment. *Journal of Applied Social Psychology*, **5**, 86–91.

Schaeffer, M.A., Baum, A., Paulus, P.B. & Gaes, G.G. (1988). Architecturally mediated effects of social density in prison. *Environment and Behavior*, **20**, 3–19.

Sperry, L. (1984). Health promotion and wellness medicine in the workplace: programs, promises, and problems. *Individual Psychology: Journal of Adlerian Theory, Research and Practice*, **40**, 401–11.

Stokols, D. (1972). On the distinction between density and crowding: some implications for future research. *Psychological Review*, **79**, 275–7.

Ulrich, R.S. (1983). Aesthetic and affective response to natural environment. *Human Behavior and Environment: Advances in Theory and Research*, **6**, 85–125.

Ulrich, R.S. (1984). View through a window may influence recovery from surgery. *Science*, **224**, 420–1.

Attributions and health

YAEL BENYAMINI
Institute For Health, Rutgers, The State University of New Jersey, USA

ELAINE A. LEVENTHAL
Department of Medicine Robert Wood Johnson Medical School, State University of New Jersey, USA

HOWARD LEVENTHAL
Institute for Health Rutgers, State University Of New Jersey, USA

People are often motivated to determine the causes of events: the more unexpected and disruptive the event, the more likely is the individual to ask, 'Why did this happen?' (Weiner, 1985). As the symptoms and diagnosis of illness are often unexpected and disruptive and may have threatening implications, we can expect health threats to stimulate preoccupation with questions of cause. As social psychologists suggested decades ago (Heider, 1958), causal, i.e. attributional, thinking can clarify the meaning of an event and define its long-term implications. In this brief article we will address the following four questions about the attributional facet of common-sense psychology: (i) Do illnesses (symptoms and diagnoses) stimulate causal thinking, i.e. attributions, and when are these attributions most likely to be made? (ii) What kinds of attributions do people make? (iii) What are the behavioural consequences of these attribu-

tions for management of and adjustment to illness? (iv) Do attributions have long-term effects on health?

Unfortunately, a straightforward review of results for each of these questions would be difficult to complete and difficult to follow as there is considerable disagreement among published findings. We decided to begin, therefore, by addressing a prior question: 'Where do attributions fit within the context of common-sense reasoning and adjustment to anticipated and current health threats?' The answer to this question assumes that the meaning of an attribution, hence its consequences, will differ as a function of the context, i.e. disease model, in which it is made. Thus, we hope to provide a framework which will transform inconsistencies into an orderly set of moderated effects.

[72]

A MODEL FOR UNDERSTANDING ATTRIBUTIONS

If attributions are important for clarifying meaning (Jones, 1990), it is critical to define the structure and content of the behavioural system within which attributions are made. Our 'common-sense model of self regulation in response to health threats' (Leventhal, Meyer & Nerenz, 1980; Leventhal, Diefenbach & Leventhal, 1992; Leventhal & Benyamini, this volume), provides such a framework. The constituents of the behavioural system as defined by this and similar models, are the representation of an illness/threat, a set of procedures for threat-illness management, and criteria for evaluating outcomes. Thus, the implication or meaning of an attribution will vary depending upon the question it addresses, i.e. is it an attribution about a symptom, e.g. is the symptom a manifestation of a particular disease or of some non-disease process; is it an attribution about the cause of a disease, e.g. a virus, genetic factor, etc.; is it an attribution about the coping procedures for disease management, e.g. who is responsible for performing the procedure, self or doctor; or is it an attribution about the outcome of a treatment procedure, e.g. did the symptoms/disease go away because of the treatment or fade on its own?

Both explicit memory (current experience based upon recall of similarity and/or differences to prior events) and implicit memory (automatic response sans awareness of prior event) participate in the construction of each of the three components. For example, the concrete symptoms of a disorder such as pain, and bleeding, can elicit automatic procedures for threat management without the actor comparing the current symptom to consciously recalled, prior symptoms. By contrast, the disease label is more likely to be the source of more elaborate, planned procedures, where the decision to adopt one or another act is made on the basis of recall of its prior suitability for threat control.

As diseases are differentiated by biology and culture, the content of the system will vary by disease, i.e. different diseases have different models. For example, the concrete experience and abstract meaning of illness representations will differ for hypertension, breast cancer and the common cold; hypertension is believed to be accompanied by heart pounding, warm face and headaches though it is actually asymptomatic (Meyer, Leventhal & Gutmann, 1985); breast cancer can produce discolouration of the breast and palpable lumps, and the common cold is accompanied by stuffed noses, headaches, sneezing and coughing. Abstract, cultural concepts of methods for controlling these diseases and their likely success also differ, e.g. surgery is appropriate for cancer but not the cold, and cultural expectations for the success of control (cure) is clearly poorer for breast cancer than for hypertension or the common cold. Finally, the facet of the representation that is salient at a given point in time, e.g. its symptoms or consequences, will reflect the history of the specific disease episode, e.g. is the episode at its beginning with only vague manifestations, or has it progressed to diagnosis, treatment, or recovery and rehabilitation (Alonzo, 1980; Safer et al., 1979), and it will reflect the illness history of the individual, e.g. is this the first or one of several chronic conditions. The motivation for question asking, the type of question asked, the attribution that is made and its consequences, will vary as a function of these factors. With this understood, we can proceed to address our questions.

ATTRIBUTIONS IN RESPONSE TO ILLNESS THREATS: ARE THEY MADE?

Our self-regulation model suggests that questions are more likely to be asked and causal attributions formed at some points within a disease episode than at others, e.g. when trying to identify the nature of a symptom than when considering the consequences of a diagnosis or treatment, and for some rather than for all diseases, e.g. a life-threatening cancer in contrast to an innocuous cold. Surprisingly, relatively little data is available regarding this question. The reasons for the deficit are twofold. First, as we have suggested, attributions can be of many types ranging from attributions of symptoms to disease, of diseases to causes, and of responsibility for the performance and success of procedures for disease management. Secondly, when focusing on one or another of these questions, investigators have typically used direct questions to determine the type of attributions being made rather than using open-ended approaches to find out whether they are being made at all. Thus, we will attend to the question, 'Are attributions made?', as we address the different types of questions that patients can raise from the common-sense framework of self-regulation.

ATTRIBUTIONS: TYPES AND CONSEQUENCES

Attributions of symptoms

Do women later diagnosed with cancer ask questions about the source of their symptoms early in the disease process? In a retrospective study of women diagnosed with cancer, Cacioppo et al. (1986) report that their subjects were clearly motivated to find explanations for uncertain physiological signs and symptoms, and that the strength of this motivation was related to the salience and the perceived personal consequences of these bodily reactions. As symptoms do not advertise their underlying disease cause, people are far from accurate in self-diagnoses. In addition, their evaluations of the perceived symptoms tend to be hedonically biased, many subjects in the Cacioppo et al. study found it much easier to accept a non-threatening explanation for unexpected symptoms and stopped searching for further explanations.

The tendency to attribute symptoms to non-disease sources is particularly noticeable in the early stages of illness episodes when symptoms are ambiguous. Thus, when the symptoms of a disease are mild and slow to develop, they can be interpreted as 'normal' or unavoidable signs of aging rather than as signs of disease (Kart, 1981; Prohaska et al., 1987). In a similar vein, ambiguous symptoms whose onset is associated with recent life stresses, e.g. examination, family quarrels, etc., are likely to be attributed to stress rather than illness (Baumann et al., 1989; Cameron, Leventhal & Leventhal, 1995). Both interpretations lead to delays in seeking professional care.

A disease attribution is no assurance, however, of appropriate action. Studies find mis-attribution due to both the inherent ambiguity of symptoms, e.g. cardiovascular symptoms can be confused with symptoms of gastrointestinal disorders, and to fear-motivated defensiveness. While defensiveness seems more likely to occur for life-threatening diseases, its frequency varies with the type of disease. For example, data suggest that defensive avoidance is more likely for many cancers than for heart attacks; as while both sets may be susceptible to 'safe' alternative interpretations, the symptoms of cancer are usually slower to develop, less disruptive of daily function, and therefore, easier to misinterpret (Cacioppo *et al.*, 1986). Attributions to the 'wrong' disease generate wrong meanings and inappropriate procedures for self management. An interesting example of both misinterpretation and changing interpretation was reported by Matthews *et al.* (1983) in their study of delay in care seeking following the onset of coronary symptoms by type A and type B males; the type A delayed longer than did type Bs while symptoms were vague during the early phase of an attack, but were quicker to seek care once it became clear they were having a coronary.

Attributions of disease cause

It is often assumed that people will attempt to probe the cause of their illness once it is diagnosed and the meaning of symptoms clarified (Rodin, 1978). Taylor, Lichtman and Wood (1984) interviewed women who have been diagnosed with breast cancer and found that 95% of them had a causal attribution for their cancer. Similarly, only one of 29 subjects paralysed as a result of serious accidents did not come up with an hypothesis respecting its cause (Bulman & Wortman, 1977). In their review of the literature, Turnquist, Harvey and Andersen (1988) report that 69 to 95% of individuals make causal attributions for their illness, and that the frequency of causal reporting is usually higher the more severe the diagnosis (e.g. cancer) and the longer the time since diagnosis. Although patients do not always report explicit causes for their illness, they view cause as one of the most important pieces of information from their physician at diagnosis (Greenberg *et al.*, 1984).

These findings clearly indicate that people generate hypotheses about the causes of their illness, but they do not address whether they do so without being prompted. Two studies that asked chronically ill patients (with arthritis, diabetes, hypertension or soon after a myocardial infarction) if they have ever thought why this has happened to them, found that roughly half of the sample had said that they had not (Lowery, Jacobsen & McCauley, 1987; Lowery *et al.*, 1992). These findings question the validity of the assumption that causal search is universally initiated under the conditions of unexpectedness, uncertainty and threat that are posed by illness, at least for diseases other than cancer. For cancer, attributions may serve a function in promoting the belief that recurrence can be prevented; but for arthritis, hypertension or diabetes, recurrence is not the issue, and for myocardial infarction, soon after the event it is recovery and not recurrence that troubles people. When taking into account the low utility in holding attributions for these diseases, it is not surprising that studies have found lower preoccupation with causes in these cases.

Studies have also examined the strength and perceived importance of causal attributions for disease, and found that patients with severe conditions and patients perceiving the outcome of their treatment to be a failure seem to hold their attributions with less conviction (Turnquist *et al.*, 1988). This also seems to have an adaptive value. As health status changes, people change their illness model to include causes that show more promise in terms of current and future management of the illness threat. Being highly committed to any specific cause sets a higher price on such changes.

Rules for causal attribution

Efforts have been made to identify the rules guiding the attributional process. Examples from studies of social cognition include factors such as the observer actor bias, i.e. actors identify environmental factors as the causes for their actions while observers attribute these actions to the personal characteristics of the actor (Jones & Davis, 1965), and self-serving biases such as attributing failure to environmental factors and success to characteristics of the self (Fiske & Taylor, 1991). Rules identified in disease attributions include the symmetry rule (Leventhal *et al.*, 1992), or the need to find labels for symptoms, and symptoms for labels; the stress-illness rule, or the tendency to attribute symptoms to stress in the presence of stressors (Cameron *et al.*, 1995); and the age-illness rule (Leventhal *et al.*, 1992).

As is the case with determining if people make attributions spontaneously, the method of questioning is a source of difficulty for identifying mental rules. A wide variety of methods have been used to assess attributions in prior studies, and each may create its own biases. For example, closed-ended methods included Q-sort of possible causes, attribution of percentage of blame to different factors, ratings of importance of different internal and external causes, and more. Open-ended questions also varied, especially in their focus on 'what caused your illness?', on 'why me?' or even more specifically on why me 'instead of someone else'. By focusing on the specifics of the disease, the first approach may generate information on rules that are disease specific, while the second may elicit thoughts and comparisons that generate rules relevant to one's life situation and disease development. And, as patients become more knowledgeable over time regarding the causes of their disease, their answers may increasingly come to reflect medical and cultural views based on what they heard from their physician and other sources rather than reflecting their own thoughts and mental operations.

There are some indications that patients who have little medical knowledge follow very simple causal rules in addressing attributional issues, such as 'causes should be temporally and spatially close to effects', and 'causes should resemble effects' (Taylor, 1982). These rules are especially in error for chronic diseases such as cancer that have lengthy developmental histories. Most studies have paid little attention to variations in the content of attributions associated with differences in socioeconomic status (Pill & Stott, 1982) and ethnic group membership. For example, minority respondents are more likely to view serious chronic illnesses as uncontrollable, because of the fatalistic themes sometimes present in their culture (Landrine and Klonoff, 1994). Thus, the questions asked about illness, and the rules of inference observed in subjects from these social backgrounds, will reflect orientations general to the culture rather than rules specific to the person.

Attributions of responsibility

It is important to distinguish attributions of causes of the event from attributions of success or failure in controlling it, and to recognize that internal attributions, i.e. to self, in contrast to external ones, can lead to quite different outcomes depending upon the model of the underlying condition. For example, Brown *et al.* (1991) found that diabetic children who held themselves responsible for symptomatic episodes when their diabetes was out of control were in better metabolic control than children attributing such episodes to external factors. Thus, self-control was superior to external control. By contrast, Ogden and Wardle (1990) found poorer adherence to diets among those moderately overweight women who attributed adherence failures to internal, i.e. self, factors. The seeming contradiction in outcome reflects fundamental differences in the models of the underlying conditions. Whereas the cause of diabetes in children is perceived as external, it is a disease that one must act to control, the cultural view of overweight is that it is caused by failure of control in the actor, a perception that is contrary to medical findings (Garner & Wooley, 1991). Thus, holding the self responsible for failure episodes, an internal attribution, by diabetic children, implies temporary deficits in self-regulation rather than chronic deficiencies in self-control, the inference for failure episodes among the overweight.

That differences in models of treatment and disease can alter the meaning of an internal attribution is supported by data from the participants in the Hypertension Prevention Trial (Jeffery, French & Schmid, 1990). They found that participants assigned to weight-loss groups were significantly more likely to blame themselves for adherence failures than participants assigned to a non-weight-loss intervention, e.g. reduced sodium group, though there was no relationship between these attributions and health outcomes. Thus, even though it is presumed to be more difficult to adhere to diets for reducing sodium and increasing potassium than to diet for reductions in caloric intake, failure in the latter may lead to self-blame as dieting to reduce caloric intake can be perceived as a weight loss issue that requires self-efficacy skills that have been proven to be deficient by the very presence of the hypertensive disorder.

Attributions and adjustment to illness

Two hypotheses have been tested respecting the relationship of attributions to adjustment. The first is that adjustment is better when attributions are made than when they are not made, and the second is that adjustment is better if attributions are made to self rather than to others. Data on the first is inconsistent, several studies showing more depression, anxiety and feelings of helplessness among patients failing to make causal attributions for their conditions (Affleck et al. 1987; Lowery, Jacobsen & Murphy, 1983, Lowery & Jacobsen, 1985; DuCette & Keane, 1984), others showing lower levels of anxiety in the presence of denial and the absence of causal search (Lowery et al., 1992). These inconsistencies appear to be resolvable if, as suggested in our discussion of the common-sense framework, we postulate that different aspects of a disease problem may be salient at different points in time. Thus, three days after a myocardial infarction (Lowery et al., 1992) and soon after the occurrence of an accident (van den Bout et al., 1988), the absence of causal search is related to lower levels of anxiety, while later in time the presence of causal attributions is related to lower levels of anxiety (Affleck, et al., 1987; Lowery et al., 1983, Lowery & Jacobsen, 1985). As Suls and Fletcher (1985) suggest, engaging in causal search soon after an event may be maladaptive, though causal search at later time points plays a positive role by providing the meanings needed to motivate risk reduction and avoidance of recurrence.

Data on the second question, i.e. the relationship of self-other attributions to adjustment, is also inconsistent. Turnquist et al.

(1988) concluded in their review that attributions to 'others' tend to relate to poorer outcomes, and attributions to 'self' fail to relate clearly to either a beneficial or a detrimental outcome. The inconsistent findings for internal attributions could be due to at least two sets of factors. First, the distinction between internal and external cause has been coded in different ways by different investigators, and the meaning of an internal attribution could be different depending upon whether it is an attribution for the initial cause of illness or an attribution of responsibility for managing oneself in relation to treatment or rehabilitation. If internal attribution is for self-management, it will be equivalent to the perception of internal control which is usually coupled with events that are controllable in contrast to external control, which is usually attributed to events that are uncontrollable. Several findings are consistent with this reasoning, e.g. Taylor et al. (1984) found that attributions of cancer patients for the disease were mostly unrelated to adjustment, while belief in control of treatment and rehabilitation by self and medical experts were both independently associated with better adjustment; DuCette and Keane (1984) found that patients were better adjusted if they had attributed their post-thoracic surgical performance to their own effort or to care from the staff; and Gilutz et al. (1991) found that thoughts of self 'limits and strengths' were positively associated with rehabilitation 6 months post MI, while a cluster of thoughts about 'fate and luck' were predictive of poor rehabilitation. It seems, therefore, that attributing the onset of an illness to an uncontrollable event, as opposed to personal responsibility due to 'bad habits', and attributing responsibility for treatment and rehabilitation to controllable, mostly internal though sometimes external factors, is the combination that results in the least emotional distress and the most optimistic view of the future health status.

Secondly, many of the studies of illness attributions were cross-sectional or at best retrospective. Thus, a note of caution is in order as reports of negative correlations of emotional distress with factors such as preoccupation with 'why me?', the absence of causal attributions, and/or the presence of a specific type of attribution, may only reflect distress in the face of deteriorating health. As health deteriorates, individuals may shift from internal attributions to attributions that are external and unstable that reflect the realities of loss of control over the disease process. Lowery and Jacobsen (1985) have suggested that this shift, along with reduced conviction about any specific causal factor, was characteristic of chronically ill patients whose disease was no longer under control, with actual loss of control generating causal beliefs that are least emotionally upsetting, i.e. to factors implying that the failure to control the disease was unavoidable. Indeed, Lowery et al. (1992) suggested most recently that patients may oscillate between preoccupation and ignoring of causes, focusing on causes as they attempt to come to terms with illness and retreating to denial when anxiety levels are too high, and both the focus of attention and the rate of fluctuation may vary as a function of where they are in the disease and coping process. Given the capricious nature of chronic, life threatening diseases, the most effective way of minimizing distress produced by disconfirmation of expectations may be to consider alternative explanations and not commit strongly to any of them.

Finally, it is essential to recognize that attributions and adjustment are likely to vary with different illnesses. Accident victims are faced with an irreversible disaster resulting from a one-time mistake; cancer patients are dealing with long treatments accompanied by fear of recurrence; the prognosis for breast cancer is far more optimistic than that for lung cancer; MI survivors experienced a serious trauma with a brief recovery period and lingering fear of recurrence; daily, lifetime coping is the concern for arthritics and diabetics, recurrence is not. If attributions affect adjustment via their impact on control, it is clear that attributions and control will have different meanings in each of these contexts, as perceived control can be helpful only when it can contribute to positive outcomes. When the disease prognosis is extremely unfavourable, e.g., for lung cancer, an internal attribution can induce control but control will have no effect on adjustment (Berckman & Austin, 1993).

ATTRIBUTIONS AND LONG-TERM EFFECTS ON HEALTH

Individual differences in the types of attributions people form may be a function of more stable, dispositional tendencies, namely, attributional styles. Research has focused mainly on the pessimistic attributional style, or the tendency to perceive negative events as caused by internal, stable and global factors. This attributional style is considered to be characteristic of learned helplessness (Abramson, Seligman & Teasdale, 1978) and has been found to be related to depression (for reviews see Sweeney, Anderson & Bailey, 1986; Robins, 1988; but see also Cochran & Hammen, 1985 for an alternative view) and to be a risk factor for illness, as Peterson, Seligman and Vaillant (1988) have found in a 35-year longitudinal study. A possible mediator for this effect may be the effect of pessimistic explanatory style on immune functions: Kamen-Siegel et al. (1991) found this style to be related to lowered immunocompetence, controlling for current health status and depressive mood, and other possible mediators.

Another dispositional difference that may be related to health outcomes was reported by Strube (1985), who found more internal, stable and global attributions for positive than for negative outcomes for all respondents, but this self-serving bias was more characteristic of Type As than Type Bs.

CONCLUSIONS

Attributions are important for the person forming them and for investigators of health and illness behaviours if they help us to predict and to understand the determinants of these behaviours and their consequences for treating and adjusting to disease. In the attribution literature, internal attributions have often been linked with control, and therefore usually expected to be associated with more favourable outcomes, whereas external attributions have been linked with depression, illness and overall poorer adjustment. The majority of studies of attributional processes, however, are cross-sectional, involve a short time-frame, are about interpersonal perception and academic performance, and are conducted in laboratory settings with subjects who are not deeply involved in a problem eliciting high levels of emotional distress. Both subjects' performance and experimenters' theorizing have been constrained by these factors, resulting in a social–psychological view of attributions that does not necessarily capture the critical dimensions required for understanding attributions in the domain of health and illness. Studies in this domain can reveal, however, the multiple meanings that can be assigned to attributions and their varied consequences. Thus, we should view the study of attributions in the health area as an opportunity for developing a more comprehensive and deeper view of the determinants of human behaviour rather than viewing it as a less interesting area of applied research. (See 'Lay beliefs about health and illness' and 'Effects of hospitalization in adults', 'Perceived control and health behaviour.')

ACKNOWLEDGEMENT

Preparation was supported by Grants AG 03501 and AG 12072 from the National Institute on Aging.

REFERENCES

Abramson, L.Y., Seligman, M.E.P. & Teasdale, J.D. (1978). Learned helplessness in humans: Critique and reformulation. *Journal of Abnormal Psychology*, 87, 49–74.

Affleck, G., Pfeiffer, C, Tennen, H. & Fifield, J. (1987). Attributional processes in rheumatoid arthritis patients. *Arthritis and Rheumatism*, 30, 927–31.

Alonzo, A.A. (1980). Acute illness behavior: a conceptual elaboration and specification. *Social Science and Medicine*, 14, 515–25.

Baumann, L., Cameron, L.D., Zimmerman, R. & Leventhal, H. (1989). Illness representations and matching labels with symptoms. *Health Psychology*, 8, 449–69.

Berckman, K.L. & Austin, J.K. (1993). Causal attribution, perceived control, and adjustment in patients with lung cancer. *Oncology Nursing Forum*, 20, 23–30.

Brown, R.T., Kaslow, N.J., Sansbury, L.,

Meacham, L. & Culler, F.L. (1991). Internalizing and externalizing symptoms and attributional style in youth with diabetes. *Journal of the American Academy of Child and Adolescent Psychiatry*, 30, 921–5.

Bulman, R.J. & Wortman, C.B. (1977). Attributions of blame and coping in the 'real world': severe accident victims react to their lot. *Journal of Personality and Social Psychology*, 35, 351–63.

Cacioppo, J.T., Andersen, B.L., Turnquist, D.C. & Petty, R.E. (1986). Psychophysiological comparison processes: interpreting cancer symptoms. In: B. Andersen (Ed.). *Women with cancer: psychological perspectives*. New York: Springer-Verlag.

Cameron, L., Leventhal, E.A. & Leventhal, H. (1995). Seeking medical care in response to symptoms and life stress. *Psychosomatic Medicine*, 57, 37–47.

Cochran, S.D. & Hammen, C.L. (1985).

Perceptions of stressful life events and depression: a test of attributional models. *Journal of Personality and Social Psychology*, 48, 1562–71.

DuCette, J. & Keane, A. (1984). 'Why me?': an attributional analysis of a major illness. *Research in Nursing and Health*, 7, 257–64.

Fiske, S.T. & Taylor, S.E. (1991). *Social cognition*. 2nd ed. New York: McGraw-Hill.

Garner, D.M. & Wooley, S.C. (1991). Confronting the failure of behavioral and dietary treatment for obesity. *Clinical Psychology Review*, 11, 729–80.

Gilutz, H., Bar-On, D., Billing, E., Rehnquist, N. & Cristal, N. (1991). The relationship between causal attribution and rehabilitation in patients after their first myocardial infarction: a cross-cultural study. *European Heart Journal*, 12, 883–8.

Greenberg, L.W., Jewett, L.S., Gluck, R.S., Champion, L.A.A., Leiken, S.L.,

Altieri, M.F. & Lipnick, R.N. (1984). Giving information for a life-threatening diagnosis. *American Journal of Diseases of Children*, **138**, 649–53.

Heider, F. (1958). *The psychology of interpersonal relations.* New York: John Wiley & Sons.

Jeffery, R.W., French, S.A. & Schmid, T.L. (1990). Attributions for dietary failures: problems reported by participants in the hypertension prevention trial. *Health Psychology*, **9**, 315–29.

Jones, E.E. (1990). *Interpersonal perception.* New York: W.H. Freeman & Company.

Jones, E.E. & Davis, K.S. (1965). From acts to dispositions: the attribution process in person perception. In L. Berlowitz (Ed.). *Advances in experimental social psychology*, vol. 2. pp. 219–266. New York: Academic Press.

Kamen-Siegel, L., Rodin, J., Seligman, M.E. & Dwyer, J. (1991). Explanatory style and cell-mediated immunity in elderly men and women. *Health Psychology*, **10**, 229–35.

Kart, C. (1981). Experiencing symptoms: attributions and misattributions of illness among the aged. In M. Haug (Ed.). *Elderly patients and their doctors.* pp. 70–78. New York: Springer.

Landrine, H. & Klonoff, E.A. (1994). Cultural diversity in causal attributions for illness: the role of the supernatural. *Journal of Behavioral Medicine*, **17**, 181–93.

Leventhal, H., Meyer, D. & Nerenz, D. (1980). The common sense representation of illness danger. In S. Rachman (Ed.). *Contributions to medical psychology*, Vol. II, pp. 7–30. New York: Pergamon Press.

Leventhal, H., Diefenbach, M. & Leventhal, E.A. (1992). Illness cognition: using common sense to understand treatment adherence and affect cognition interactions. *Cognitive Therapy and Research*, **16**, 143–63.

Lowery, B.J. & Jacobsen, B.S. (1985). Attributional analysis of chronic illness outcomes. *Nursing Research*, **34**, 82–8.

Lowery, B.J., Jacobsen B.S. & Murphy, B.B. (1983). An exploratory investigation of causal thinking of arthritics. *Nursing Research*, **32**, 157–62.

Lowery, B.J., Jacobsen B.S. & McCauley, K. (1987). On the prevalence of causal search in illness situations. *Nursing Research*, **36**, 88–93.

Lowery, B.J., Jacobsen, B.S., Cera, M.A., McIndoe, D., Kleman, M. & Menapace, F. (1992). Attention versus avoidance: attributional search and denial after myocardial infarction. *Heart and Lung*, **21**, 523–8.

Matthews, K.A., Seigel, J.M., Kuller, L.H., Thompson, M. & Varat, M. (1983). Determinants of decisions to seek medical treatment by patients with acute myocardial infarction symptoms. *Journal of Personality and Social Psychology*, **44**, 1144–56.

Meyer, D., Leventhal, H. & Gutmann, M. (1985). Common-sense models of illness: the example of hypertension. *Health Psychology*, **4**, 115–35.

Ogden, J. & Wardle, J. (1990). Control of eating and attributional style. *British Journal of Clinical Psychology*, **29**, 445–6.

Peterson, C., Seligman, M.E.P. & Vaillant, G.E. (1988). Pessimistic explanatory style is a risk factor for physical illness: a thirty-five-year longitudinal study. *Journal of Personality and Social Psychology*, **55**, 23–7.

Pill, R. & Stott, N.C.H. (1982). Concepts of illness causation and responsibility: some preliminary data from a sample of working class mothers. *Social Science and Medicine*, **16**, 43–52.

Prohaska, T.R., Keller, M.L., Leventhal, E.A. & Leventhal, H. (1987). Impact of symptoms and aging attribution on emotions and coping. *Health Psychology*, **6**, 495–514.

Robins, C.J. (1988). Attributions and depression: why is the literature so inconsistent? *Journal of Personality and Social Psychology*, **54**, 880–9.

Rodin, J. (1978). Somatophysics and attribution. *Personality and Social Psychology Bulletin*, **4**, 531–40.

Safer, M., Tharps, Q., Jackson, T. & Leventhal, H. (1979). Determinants of three stages of delay in seeking care at a medical clinic. *Medical Care*, **17**, 11–29.

Strube, M.J. (1985). Attributional style and the type A coronary-prone behavior pattern. *Journal of Personality and Social Psychology*, **49**, 500–9.

Suls, J. & Fletcher, B. (1985). The relative efficacy of avoidant and non-avoidant coping strategies: a meta analysis. *Health Psychology*, **4**, 249–88.

Sweeney, P.D., Anderson, K. & Bailey, S. (1986). Attributional style in depression: a meta-analytic review. *Journal of Personality and Social Psychology*, **50**, 974–91.

Taylor, S. (1982). Social cognition and health. *Personality and Social Psychology Bulletin*, **8**, 549–62.

Taylor, S., Lichtman, R.R. & Wood, J. (1984). Attributions, beliefs about control, and adjustment to breast cancer. *Journal of Personality and Social Psychology*, **46**, 489–502.

Turnquist, D.C., Harvey, J.H. & Andersen, B.L. (1988). Attributions and adjustment to life-threatening illness. *British Journal of Clinical Psychology*, **27**, 55–65.

van den Bout, J., van Son-Schoones, N., Schipper, J. & Groffen, C. (1988). Attributional cognitions, coping behavior, and self-esteem in inpatients with severe spinal cord injuries. *Journal of Clinical Psychology*, **44**, 17–22.

Weiner, B. (1985). 'Spontaneous' causal thinking. *Psychological Bulletin*, **97**, 74–84.

Childhood influences on health

CHRISTINE EISER

Department of Psychology, University of Exeter, UK

INTRODUCTION

Patterns of disease in childhood have changed substantially during the course of this century. Improvements in sanitation and housing and the introduction of major inoculation programmes have resulted in much improved general health and the eradication of some diseases. There remain, however, serious threats to child health in the form of chronic or life-threatening conditions for which there is no cure. In addition, the health of today's children is undermined by a number of essentially preventable problems. These include poor diet, health risk behaviours, such as tobacco, alcohol and illegal drug use, and early and unprotected sexual activity.

Children can be affected indirectly through the behaviour of others. Before birth, maternal health is influential, and in extreme cases, the health of the foetus can be jeopardized through maternal smoking, drinking or drug abuse. The health of young children can be harmed through passive smoking, especially where there is a history of respiratory problems. However, it is during later childhood and adolescence that individuals become more directly responsible for their own health, through their own decisions as to whether to adopt health-promoting behaviours (such as regular exercise) or health risk behaviours such as substance abuse.

ADOLESCENTS

The extent of the problem is reflected in statistics which point to the fact that health risk behaviours are the major cause of mortality and morbidity in adolescents (Irwin & Millstein, 1986). More than half of known cases of morbidity and mortality in adolescents can be accounted for by preventable risk behaviours, including sexual activity, substance abuse and motor accidents.

Why do adolescents engage in risky behaviours?

Three hypotheses have been put forward to account for adolescent risky behaviour:

(i) Changes in hormone levels are directly responsible for behavioural changes and risk-taking; this model suggests that those with earlier physical maturation are at greater risk than those who develop later;

(ii) Changes in adolescent physical appearance influence people to behave differently; thus the social context is seen to be influential; and

(iii) Risk-taking is influenced directly by sociodemographic factors; for example, children of alcoholics are more likely to have drink problems themselves.

Interest in adolescent risk-taking is generally justified on two grounds. First, such behaviours can have a direct and immediate effect on current health. Secondly, patterns of risk-taking during adolescence are thought to be predictive of adult behaviour. Since it is difficult to change adult behaviour (for example, to persuade adults to stop smoking or eat more sensibly) it is felt important to focus attention on the prevention of risky behaviours during adolescence. Research often focuses on particular risk behaviours, such as smoking. In practice, there is considerable overlap in that individuals who engage in one form of risk behaviour tend to be more inclined also to experiment with others.

THE EXTENT OF THE PROBLEM

Surveys of school children indicate that as many as 80% have had their first drink by 13 years of age, and only 10% were abstinent by 17 years of age. Young people tend to report that they have their first drink at home, and preference for drinking with friends does not emerge till 15 years (Plant & Plant, 1992). Although the legal age for buying alcohol in public houses is 18, 25% of boys and 15% of girls drink there. Swadi (1988) surveyed 3333 adolescents in London about drug and substance use. Results suggested that one in five had tried solvents or drugs, one in 12 were repeated users, and one in 20 had tried hard drugs. Two-thirds reported that they had used alcohol, and one in nine described themselves as frequent or heavy users. One in five smoked cigarettes regularly. Smoking was more common among girls, though other drug and alcohol use did not differ between the sexes.

Surveys by the OPCS (1986) indicate some reduction in alcohol consumption in recent years especially among young men. Many adolescents experience low-level adverse consequences as a result of drinking, and a proportion experience more serious consequences associated with serious, sometimes fatal accidents. Some 5% of all convictions for drinking occur in 14–17 year-olds.

Heavy adolescent drinking can be associated with other risk behaviours, including tobacco and illegal drug use. Eating disorders were found in 30% of young women with alcohol problems; a significant relationship has also been reported between alcohol intoxication and bulimia. Alcohol abuse has been linked with poor school performance, school-based problem behaviour, truancy, unemployment and delinquency. Adolescents are more likely to have casual sex and less likely to use condoms when under the influence of alcohol, thereby increasing the risk of HIV infection.

Sexual activity is seen to be a problem independently of the relationship with alcohol use. The mean age for first intercourse has decreased over the years, while the number of partners for both adolescent males and females has increased. Adolescent pregnancy is associated with health risks for the mother as well as increased risk of stillbirths, lower birthweight and reduced health in the foetus and neonate.

Healthy eating in young children is considered important, both for the child's current health as well as for the implications for health in later life. Obesity, dietary deficiencies and excesses, dental caries and iron and protein deficiency are frequently cited as common current health problems today (Gortmaker *et al.*, 1993). In addition, obesity has been linked with poor academic and psychosocial functioning.

THE LONG-TERM CONSEQUENCES

There is no simple association between the extent to which adolescents engage in risky behaviours and their long-term health and behaviour. For example, only low levels of association have been reported between adolescent drinking and alcohol use 10 years later. Peak alcohol consumption occurs around 20 years of age and may be related to living circumstances; excess drinking appears to be self-limiting and reduces with marriage and again with the birth of children.

One concern is that young people who adopt one risky behaviour subsequently become more vulnerable to engage in other risks. Yamaguchi and Kandel (1984) followed a group of 16 year-olds over a 9-year period. They describe a sequence of drug use from legal drugs (cigarettes or alcohol) through to marijuana and illegal drugs. Cigarette smoking was an important early risk factor for women, but less so for men. The major risk for initiation into tobacco, alcohol and marijuana use was over by 20 years, and for other illicit drugs by 21 years. Those who have not experimented with drugs by 21 years of age are unlikely to do so.

However, children's dietary attitudes and behaviour are viewed as risk factors for later development of heart disease and hypertension (Harsha *et al.*, 1987). Gortmaker *et al.* (1993) followed a large nationally representative sample of young people between 16 and 24 years of age. Women who were overweight completed fewer years of high school education, were less likely to be married, and had lower personal incomes than women who were not overweight. Men who were overweight were also less likely to marry. Gortmaker *et al.* concluded that the social and economic consequences of overweight were greater than the disadvantages of chronic physical conditions, suggesting that discrimination may limit opportunities for the overweight as much as the health disadvantage itself.

While much attention has been focused on the long-term negative consequences of behaviours adopted during childhood for adult health, less has been directed to understanding the link between healthy behaviours established in childhood, which might be associated with more positive adult health. There are indications that adults who exercise regularly also participated in school-based sports, suggesting that patterns of health-enhancing behaviour, specifically participation in sports, are laid down during childhood (Armstrong, 1989).

FACTORS WHICH INFLUENCE HEALTH RISK BEHAVIOURS

Personality

Adolescents at risk for substance abuse are frequently seen to be rebellious, antisocial and alienated from traditional socializing institutions such as school and family. A number of longitudinal studies point to rebelliousness, aggressiveness and poor school performance as predictors of subsequent substance abuse. Jessor and Jessor (1977) suggest that adolescent substance use represents an age-graded problem behaviour that is acceptable in adults but not in children. This model of 'deviance proneness' suggests that adolescent health risk behaviours are part of a larger syndrome of behaviour problems. However, given the relatively high incidence of risk behaviours during adolescence, some have argued that experimentation must be seen as part of normal development rather than indicative of deviance. Chassin, Presson and Sherman (1989) present some evidence that adolescents who engage in substance use are more creative and genuinely autonomous compared with those who do not experiment.

The family

A major task of adolescence is seen to be the attainment of close links within the family, while also achieving a degree of personal autonomy. Attachment to parents does appear to be a key factor in determining adolescent health behaviour. Turner *et al.* (1993) found that adolescents who were treated autonomously by their parents were less likely to initiate sexual intercourse, while those who were emotionally detached from their parents were more likely to fight and use substances. In turn, those who were emotionally detached tended to come from families with low levels of cohesion and acceptance. Closeness to parents was related to less drug use and choice of friends who are not drug-users.

INTERVENTIONS

Available evidence points to some continuities between healthy behaviour during childhood and adult health behaviour, especially with regard to smoking and eating habits. It is not inevitable that young people who drink or take drugs will continue to do so during adult life. However, in that it is very difficult to change unhealthy behaviours once they are established, much attention has been given to encouraging appropriate behaviour among the young.

Such educational programmes have not always met with approval. There have been substantial fears that education of this kind will result in more permissive attitudes and consequently increased incidences of experimentation. Education may encourage drug use or sexual activity by removing anxieties and overcoming prejudices which operated to limit risky behaviour.

In comparison with the number of educational programmes developed, there has been less interest in evaluations. In part, this reflects the difficulties involved in assessing the success of programmes which are directed at young children, where the aim is to reduce consumption among young adults. In terms of behavioural success, it would be necessary to wait many years before it was apparent that any programme was successful in these terms. Researchers are often therefore forced to rely on identifying changes in knowledge and attitudes.

A number of theoretical approaches have formed the basis of intervention programmes (Bruvold & Rundall, 1988). A broad distinction can be made between the Rational model (Ajzen & Fishbein, 1980); and social skills or life skills approaches (Jessor & Jessor, 1977). Approaches based on rational models try to influence behaviour by increasing factual knowledge; socially orientated programmes try to influence behaviour by enabling individuals to implement that knowledge in social contexts. A common argument against the traditional rational approach to health education is that social norms, environmental contingencies and motivations to enhance self-esteem are more important than knowledge about possible health consequences. Despite this, programmes based on the rational model tend to be fairly successful in increasing knowledge (Bruvold & Rundall, 1988) but achieve less in terms of changing attitudes or influencing behaviour. Both short- and longer-term success has been reported for school-based smoking programmes, though effects have been mixed for similar approaches to alcohol education. Programmes concerned with sexuality have reported parallel findings; it is relatively easy to increase knowledge, but attitudes are more resistant to change. Adolescents, and older adults, are characterized by 'unrealistic optimism'; they assume that their own chances of contracting HIV infection through unprotected sex, or lung cancer through smoking are less, than the risks for the rest of the population (Weinstein, 1987).

There are practical disadvantages associated with 'life-skills' approaches. They involve a large amount of curriculum time and are therefore increasingly difficult to fit in with other educational requirements. They are heavily dependent on the skills of the teacher. Evaluations which have been conducted have tended to be based in schools with white middle-class samples; thus it is not clear how well the approach would work for the populations most at risk. The effects of attrition are likely to be particularly great for these vulnerable groups.

CONCLUSIONS

Educational programmes need to encourage a sensible attitude to risk behaviours, encouraging drivers to abstain, for example, rather than advocating general abstinence. Education also needs to be targeted more directly at individuals who are clearly at risk, for example, children whose parents drink or smoke. The single most important message from all this work, however, is that the health of a population is inextricably linked with the health of its youth. Both health-enhancing and health-damaging behaviours have their roots in childhood. Consequently, health education is not only important for children's current health, but also has implications for their health as adults, and of their children.

REFERENCES

Ajzen, I. & Fishbein, M. (1980). *Understanding attitudes and predicting behavior.* Englewood Cliffs, NJ: Prentice Hall.

Armstrong, N. (1989). *Children's physical activity patterns and coronary heart disease. In Coronary Prevention Group, should the prevention of heart disease begin in childhood?* pp. 37–44. London: Coronary Prevention Group.

Bruvold, W.H. & Rundall, T.G. (1988). A meta-analysis and theoretical review of school based tobacco and alcohol intervention programs *Psychology and Health 2*, 53–78.

Chassin, L., Presson, C.C. & Sherman, S.J. (1989). 'Constructive' vs. 'destructive' deviance in adolescent health-related behaviours. *Journal of Youth and Adolescence*, 18, 245–62.

Gortmaker, S.L., Must, A., Perrin, J., Sobol, A. & Dietz, W.H. (1993). Social and economic consequences of overweight in adolescence and young adulthood. *The New England Journal of Medicine*, 329, 1008–12.

Harsha, D.W., Smoak, C.G., Nicklas, T.A., Webber, L.S. & Berenson, G.S. (1987). Cardiovascular risk factors from birth to 7 years: the Bogolusa Heart study. *Pediatrics*, 80, (Suppl) 779–83.

Irwin, C.E. & Millstein, S.G. (1986). Biopsychosocial correlates of risk taking behaviors during adolescence: can the physician intervene? *Journal of Adolescent Health Care*, 7, 82S–96S.

Jessor, R. & Jessor, S.L. (1977). *Problem behavior and psychosocial development: a longitudinal study of youth*, New York: Wiley.

OPCS, Office of Population Censuses and Surveys (1986). *Adolescent drinking.*

Plant, M.A. & Plant, M.L. (1992). *Risk-takers: alcohol, drugs, sex and youth.* London: Tavistock, Routledge.

Swadi, H. (1988). Drug and substance use among 3,333 London adolescents. *British Journal of Addiction*, 83, 935–42.

Turner, R.A., Irwin, C.E., Tschann, J.M. & Millstein, S.G. (1993). Autonomy, relatedness, and the initiation of health risk behaviors in early adolescence. *Health Psychology*, 12, 200–8.

Weinstein, N.D. (1987). Unrealistic optimism about susceptibility to health problems: conclusions from a community-wide sample. *American Journal of Public Health*, 5, 481–500.

Yamaguchi, R.A. & Kandel, D.B. (1984). Patterns of drug use from adolescence to young adulthood; II Sequences of progression. *American Journal of Public Health*, 74, 668–72.

Children's perceptions of illness and death

CHRISTINE EISER

Department of Psychology, University of Exeter, Devon, UK

THE POTENTIAL APPLICATIONS

While initially of interest for theoretical reasons, this literature has expanded rapidly because of its apparent relevance to applied and clinical work. Many children need to understand the reasons for illness and death at some time during their lives. First, such a need may arise through their own illness. Children who contract chronic or life-threatening conditions need to understand why they need treatment. Depending on their age, many are encouraged to accept personal responsibility for aspects of their own treatment, including the need in diabetes to self-inject insulin or in cystic fibrosis, to manage their own physiotherapy. While death from diabetes is rare in children, it is less so from cystic fibrosis. To work with, and help, a child who is dying, it is first important to understand the meaning of death in a child's world. Secondly, the need may arise through the illness or possible death of a parent. In these circumstances, families need help to communicate and children should be helped to express their fears. Thirdly, children may become aware of illness through interactions with friends. Treatments can affect the physical appearance of a child, or may be associated with irritability or aggression. In these instances, children need to understand the reasons for changes in behaviour or physical appearance of their friends. Explanations for these changes are considered critical in order to promote empathy with the sick child, reduce the incidence of teasing and facilitate as normal a lifestyle for the sick child as possible. Peers who are well informed and understanding can help a sick child by encouraging participation in self care activities. La Greca (1990), for example, found that peers were generally very supportive and instrumental in ensuring that adolescents with diabetes adhered to treatment demands, especially with regard to diet. Fourthly, understanding of illness, and especially the relationship between personal behaviour and subsequent risk has received considerable attention, particularly with regard to AIDS (Sigelman *et al.*, 1993).

DEVELOPMENTAL CHANGES IN UNDERSTANDING OF ILLNESS

The cognitive developmental approach

Age-related changes in children's conceptions of illness and death have been amply documented; what is more in question is the theoretical rationale for these changes. Traditionally, explanations have been made within the context of Piaget's theory of cognitive development. From this perspective, there are indications that children in the prelogical phase (2–7 years) hold beliefs about illness which are superstitious, circular and non-differentiated. Thus, asked why children get colds, Bibace and Walsh (1981) quote the following examples: 'from kissing old ladies' 'they just do'. The belief that illness (and its treatment) is a form of punishment develops naturally from adult admonitions 'if you don't come in out of the cold, you will be ill'. During the concrete operational phase (7–11 years), children's reasoning becomes more specific; they acknowledge a limited number of causal factors in precipitating different illnesses. During the formal operational phase (age 11 onwards), understanding of illness is enhanced by formal biological education. Children understand the cause of illness in biological terms. For some, these biological explanations are later refined as the relation between biological and psychological health is understood.

A parallel framework has been used to account for children's understanding of death and dying. During the prelogical phase, children believe that death can be avoided or reversed, and have difficulty understanding the finality and irreversibility of death. Children in this stage may see themselves to be responsible for another's death. In the following concrete operational phase, children come to realize the reality of death and, towards the end of this stage, that they themselves or their family will die eventually (Jewett, 1982).

Much work was initially based on children's concepts of common conditions, including colds (Bibace & Walsh, 1981). More recently, the emphasis has shifted toward more serious disease, especially cancer and AIDS. Given the widespread concern about AIDS and implication that young people are particularly at risk, much recent work has focused on adolescents' understanding of AIDS and beliefs about risk factors. There is evidence that children know a good deal about risks associated with sexual contact and sharing drug needles, but are confused about other risk factors, including kissing and blood donation (Brown, Nassau & Barone 1990).

Variables which influence the course of understanding

One frequent criticism of the cognitive developmental framework is that considerable variability occurs in the specific ages at which children express particular beliefs about illness or death. Much variability has been attributed to social and cultural factors. In addition, experience itself plays some role. Experience of a particular illness may enhance children's understanding, at least of that condition (Perrin, Sayer & Willett, 1991). However, for both sick and healthy children (Sigelman *et al.*, 1993) knowledge of one disease does not predict knowledge of another. Experience may also limit understanding, perhaps through increasing awareness of personal vulnerability, resulting in denial of the potential seriousness of the situation. Family environment, social support and previous experience with death influence children's understanding and acceptance of death (Kubler-Ross, 1983).

This point is particularly clear from work which has assessed the responses of well children to the death of a sibling. Children who were more involved throughout the period, especially where the child was nursed at home rather than in hospital, fared better than those who were kept away from the dying child (Lauer *et al.*, 1983).

THE STRUCTURAL ORGANIZATION OF KNOWLEDGE OF ILLNESS

While accepting the overall changes in understanding of illness and death which occur during childhood, there have been many criticisms of the theoretical perspective adopted. Similar behaviours may be cited as evidence for different operational functioning. For example, the idea that all illnesses are caused by infection is attributed to preoperational functioning by some authors but to concrete operational functioning by others (Kister & Patterson, 1980). The procedure in many studies is to infer the child's level of cognitive functioning through performance on a single Piagetian task (e.g conservation or perspective-taking). Yet, there are generally low correlations between these tasks, limiting the reliability of any one task as a general indicator of development. Finally, categorizing children's thought in terms of specific operations implies a rigidity about children's cognition and that understanding of concepts beyond a particular stage would be impossible. This rigidity is seen to be very much a limitation to the theory (Eiser, 1989).

An alternative approach stresses that it is the organization of knowledge which determines children's beliefs. Development involves both the acquisition of knowledge and reorganization of that knowledge. Thus, Carey (1985) suggested that younger children think about illness in terms of what they know about people and human behaviour. Illness is defined by adults; you must be ill because you are sent to bed. With increasing sophistication, children understand that symptoms define illness, not adult behaviour. In some support of this hypothesis, Hergenrather and Rabinowitz (1991) found that, when younger children were asked to sort pictures showing various causes, treatments and symptoms of illness, they based their decisions on general knowledge rather than illness-specific dimensions. Older children used illness-specific information to guide their judgements. When asked how you knew if you were ill, younger children reported that they used behavioural cues (take your temperature or go to bed); older children relied on changes in symptoms (you have a sore throat).

The view that development is driven by experience suggests that the kinds of inferences children make about disease are based on the kinds of information to which they are most frequently exposed.

Young children are most often exposed to information about common illnesses such as colds, and therefore they assume that all illnesses are contagious and readily transmitted through casual contact (Kister & Patterson, 1980). Sigelman *et al.* (1993) argues that this may be changing, as children are increasingly exposed to information about serious disease such as cancer and AIDS. In the future, it is likely that these diseases will act as a model for children to understand illness more generally. In her own work, Sigelman *et al.* (1993) compared children's understanding of three diseases; colds, cancer and AIDS. The youngest children (aged 9 years) were able to make some distinctions between the diseases. However, they used their knowledge that colds are contagious to guide their views about other diseases; thus they assumed that risk factors for colds also constituted risk factors for cancer. While children appeared relatively well informed about risk factors for a disease, they were less informed about non-risk factors.

IMPLICATIONS FOR INTERVENTIONS AND PREVENTIVE PROGRAMMES

Any programme designed to educate children about illness needs to take into account developmental changes in conceptual understanding of disease. 'We should take our cues from the child, to tell the child what he or she wants to know, on his or her terms. The issue is not whether to tell but rather when to tell, why you are telling, and who should do the telling' (Bluebond-Langer, 1989).

School-based programmes have been partially successful in improving children's knowledge of illness and encouraging empathy and consideration towards sick or disabled classmates (Treiber, Schramm & Mabe, 1986). However, the effects of these programmes appear to be short-lived, and much follow-up work is essential. Programmes to improve knowledge in children with chronic disease have also had limited success. It is possible to improve knowledge of the condition, but more difficult for the child to translate this knowledge into routine behaviour. The limitation seems to be in the focus on illness from a cognitive perspective. Social and cultural beliefs underlie the acquisition of knowledge and impose restrictions on how readily knowledge is translated into related behaviour. Future interventions need to provide a more integrated programme of the cognitive and social influences on children's knowledge of and attitudes towards illness. (See also 'Effects of hospitalization on children.')

REFERENCES

Bibace, R. & Walsh, M.E. (Eds.) (1981). *Children's conceptions of health, illness and bodily functions.* San Francisco: Jossey-Bass.

Bluebond-Langer, M. (1989). Worlds of dying children and their well siblings. *Death Studies*, **13**, 1–16.

Brown, L.K., Nassau, J.H. & Barone, V.J. (1990). Differences in AIDS knowledge and attitudes by grade level. *Journal of School Health*, **60**, 270–5.

Carey, S. (1985). *Conceptual change in childhood.* Massachusetts: MIT Press.

Eiser, C. (1989). Children's concepts of illness: towards an alternative to the 'stage' approach. *Psychology and Health*, **3**, 93–101.

Hergenrather, J.R. & Rabinowitz, M.R. (1991). Age-related differences in the organization of children's knowledge of illness. *Developmental Psychology*, **27**, 952–9.

Jewett, C.L. (1982). *Helping children cope with separation and loss* Harvard, Ma: Harvard Common Press.

Kister, M.C & Patterson, C.J. (1980). Children's conceptions of the causes of illness: understanding use of contagion and use of imminent justice. *Child Development.* **51**, 839–46.

Kubler-Ross, E. (1983). *On children and death.* New York: Macmillan.

La Greca, A. (1990). Social consequences of

pediatric conditions: a fertile area for future investigation and intervention? *Journal of Pediatric Psychology*, **15**, 285–307.

Lauer, M., Mulhern, R., Wallskig, J. & Camitta, B. (1983). A comparison study of parental adaptation following a child's death at home or in hospital. *Pediatrics.* **71**, 107–11.

Parmalee, A. H. (1986). Children's illnesses: their beneficial effects on behavioural development. *Child Development*, **57**, 1–10.

Perrin, E.C., Sayer, A.G. & Willett, J.B. (1991). Sticks and stones may break my bones . . . . Reasoning about illness causality and body functioning in children who have a chronic illness. *Pediatrics*, **88**, 608–19.

Sigelman, C., Maddock, A., Epstein, J. & Carpenter, W. (1993). Age differences in

understanding of disease causality: AIDS, colds and cancer. *Child Development*, **64**, 272–84.

Treiber, F.A., Schramm, L. & Mabe, P.A.

(1986). Children's knowledge and concerns toward a peer with cancer. A Workshop intervention. *Child Psychiatry and Human Development*, **16**, 249–60.

Coping with bereavement

JOHN ARCHER

Department of Psychology, University of Central Lancashire, Preston, UK

Bereavement refers to the death of someone with whom a person had a close relationship. Sometimes, it is used to refer to the emotional, cognitive and motivational reactions which are experienced, but a more usual convention is to refer to these as grief. Similar reactions occur after other personally important losses, such as a home or a job, or a bodily part or function.

Mortality is increased by bereavement and this 'loss effect' is more pronounced for men than for women. The causes of death include heart disease, cancer, various forms of violent deaths including suicide, and cirrhosis of the liver. Changes in immunomodulation (in particular lower natural killer cell activity) have been demonstrated following bereavement, and are associated with depression (see Stroebe, Stroebe & Hansson, 1993).

Freud (1917) described grief as an active process ('grief work') of seeking to rid oneself of mental ties to the deceased. The view that confronting thoughts and feelings about the deceased is necessary for readjustment is widely accepted to this day, but recent research indicates that confronting rather than suppressing grief does not necessarily facilitate adjustment (Stroebe & Stroebe, 1991). Another widely held view about readjustment following bereavement is that it proceeds through stages or phases (e.g. Bowlby, 1980). Although this seeks to capture the dynamic nature of grief, longitudinal studies indicate that, with the exception of the initial responses, grief reactions are intermingled and wax and wane under the influence of internal and external influences (see Stroebe, Stroebe & Hansson, 1993).

Grief reactions (see Parkes, 1972/1986) are complex, but can be considered as four inter-related processes. The first two are versions of the separation reactions which form widespread reactions to losses, both temporary and permanent, among children and among social birds and mammals. One of these can be viewed as resulting from continued attachment to the deceased. It involves active dis-

tress and preoccupation with the deceased and the loss, together with the urge to search and to seek reunification in thought and deed: the bereaved person may, for example, feel drawn to places and people associated with the deceased, and may feel his/her presence nearby or internally. The emotions accompanying this separation reaction are anxiety, and periodic outbreaks of anger or self-blame. A second, more passive, separation reaction involves a feeling of hopelessness and a depressed mood: this can be viewed as a recognition of the futility of continuing the attachment.

A third process involves ways of mitigating or regulating the psychological distress. Initial reactions of numbness and disbelief may persist in some cases, but longer-term strategies tend to involve avoidance, distraction or a pretence that the deceased is nearby. Experimental evidence indicates that avoidance has physiological costs, that suppressed thoughts become reinstated later together with the mood which accompanied them, and that distraction can facilitate adjustment.

Interspersed with these three processes is a gradual change in the person's identity and self-definition, which involves acceptance of the loss and its implications. People who cannot accept the loss and continue to ask 'Why?' typically show poor adjustment. Overall, there is enormous individual variation in both the initial level of distress to the same sort of bereavement and in the time taken to return to the level of well-being experienced beforehand. Some of this variation can be understood in terms of causal attributions and coping strategies, but other important considerations include whether the loss was expected or sudden, whether it involved additional traumas (as in the case of murder or suicide), the relationship with the deceased and the personal characteristics and social circumstances of the bereaved: for example, confiding in others is associated with less preoccupation with the loss, and with fewer health-related problems (Pennebaker, 1988).

REFERENCES

Bowlby, J. (1980). *Attachment and loss. Volume 3, Loss: sadness and depression.* London: The Hogarth Press & Institute of Psychoanalysis. (Penguin edition, 1981).

Freud, S. (1917). *Mourning and Melancholia.* Reprinted in: J. Strachey (trans. & ed.), *Standard edition of complete psychological works of Sigmund Freud*, vol. 14, pp. 239–

260. London: Hogarth Press & Institute of Psychoanalysis (1957).

Parkes, C.M. (1972/1986). *Bereavement: studies of grief in adult life.* London & New York: Tavistock. (Penguin editions, 1975 & 1986).

Pennebaker, J.W. (1988). Confiding traumatic experiences and health. In S. Fisher & J. Reason (Eds.). *Handbook of life stress,*

cognition and health, pp. 669–682. Chichester & New York: Wiley.

Stroebe, M.S. & Stroebe, W. (1991). Does 'grief work' work? *Journal of Consulting and Clinical Psychology*, **59**, 479–82.

Stroebe, M.S., Stroebe, W. & Hansson, R.O. (Eds.) (1993). *Handbook of bereavement: theory, research and intervention.* New York: Cambridge University Press.

Coping with chronic illness

KEITH PETRIE

and

RONA MOSS-MORRIS

Department of Psychiatry and Behavioural Science, The University of Auckland School of Medicine, New Zealand

THE INCREASE IN CHRONIC ILLNESS

At the beginning of this century infectious disease dominated the health lives of individuals. Diseases such as tuberculosis, pneumonia, and influenza were the leading causes of death and resulted in high rates of infant mortality and a low life expectancy. Changes in living conditions, the development of antibiotics, and other advances in medicine have turned many previously deadly infectious diseases into treatable conditions and some have almost disappeared completely. As the rate of infectious disease has declined, and life expectancy increased, there has been a corresponding rise in the number of people suffering a chronic illness at some time during their life. Now at the end of the twentieth century, diseases such as cancer, heart disease, arthritis, diabetes, hypertension, and AIDS are part of the daily lives of large numbers of people. These illnesses bring with them considerable difficulties in adjustment and coping.

ADJUSTMENTS REQUIRED

The initial psychological adjustments following the diagnosis of a chronic disease generally involve issues related to a loss of function. Individuals at the stage of diagnosis confront the reality that their state of health has inexorably changed and the integrity and function of their body has been limited in some way. The speed that individuals confront this loss can be strongly influenced by the nature of the illness. With some chronic illnesses, such as heart disease which is diagnosed following a myocardial infarction, awareness of the presence of the disease is usually sudden. In other chronic illnesses, such as arthritis, the patient may be aware of disease long before a formal diagnosis is made.

Dealing with the on-going demands of a chronic illness often requires the learning of new skills and adjustments to daily lifestyle. Moos and Schaefer (1984) identified a set of illness-related tasks that face the individual dealing with a chronic illness. These comprise adjusting to the symptoms and incapacities brought by the illness, dealing with and learning any special treatment required, and maintaining adequate relationships with health-care providers. Many illnesses, such as insulin-dependent diabetes and end-stage renal disease, require patients to learn specific techniques for controlling symptoms, such as dialysis in the case of renal disease. Furthermore, an active awareness and monitoring of bodily function may be necessary in diseases like diabetes, to avoid medical crises.

Relationships with health-care staff can be a major source of difficulty in the management of chronic illness. The issue of patient autonomy versus independence from health-care professionals is

often an on-going problem in long-term treatment programmes. While increasing patient participation in the management of chronic illness by promoting greater involvement in the medical interview has shown to result in improved health care outcomes and quality of life in a diabetic sample (Greenfield *et al.*, 1988), more work needs to be done in this complex area to determine which behaviours in medical encounters are critical in fostering participation.

Managing the emotional and social consequences of chronic illness is another major area where individuals face adjustment. Physical illness generally results in an increase in levels of negative affect and higher rates of depression, suicidal behaviour, and distress have been found in chronic illness populations (e.g. Whitlock, 1986). The restriction in social and other previously pleasurable activities is often an outcome of living with a chronic illness. This change, along with the emotional demands of integrating a new view of the self that includes the chronic illness, results in difficulties in affect regulation and an increased risk of adjustment and emotional disturbances (Cassileth *et al.*, 1984). Clinicians need to be aware of the high risk of depression in chronic illness populations and the fact that these difficulties commonly extend to distress in the patient's family and wider social network.

It is important to note, however, that not all the emotional consequences of chronic illness are negative. The few studies that have investigated positive outcomes report that individuals have found an increased value in close relationships, greater meaning in day-to-day activities, and a greater compassion towards others with difficulties (e.g. Laerum *et al.*, 1987).

THE COPING PROCESS

How well patients adjust to chronic illness can be explained in part by their individual coping responses. Coping is the cognitive, behavioural, and emotional ways that people manage stressful situations. Coping has been previously conceptualized by researchers as a trait which is stable across situations, or alternatively, as a process that is strongly influenced by situational factors. However, Lazarus and Folkman's (1984) transactional model has had the largest impact on the current conceptualization of coping with chronic illness. This model sees the patient's coping response being determined by both their appraisal of the degree of threat posed by an illness, and the resources seen as being available to help them cope in the situation. Coping responses in this model are divided into emotion-focused and problem-focused strategies. The function of problem-focused coping is to actively alter the stressful situation in some way, while emotion-focused coping is directed at regulating the patient's emotional response to a stressor.

Each response can be potentially adaptive or maladaptive depending on the situation. Some emotion-focused strategies show positive benefits across illnesses. Reframing the illness in a positive light, acceptance of the disease, and utilizing social support appear to be adaptive coping strategies across many chronic illnesses. Other emotion-focused strategies such as disengaging from the situation by giving up or avoiding thinking about the illness have generally been related to increased distress and disability (Carver et al., 1993; Dunkel-Schetter et al., 1992; Felton, Revenson & Hinrichsen, 1984). Problem-focused strategies, which in theory should have a greater adaptive potential, have frequently failed to demonstrate a strong relationship to outcome in chronic illness. However, seeking information about the illness and planning seem to be two strategies that do have the most consistent relationship with positive outcomes (Felton et al., 1984). These strategies seem to have the greatest effect when the stressor is appraised by the patient as controllable (Folkman et al., 1993). The lack of a strong relationship between problem-focused strategies and positive outcomes in chronic illness may be due to a mismatch between situations that are not amenable to change or control and the use of problem-focused strategies by the individual. In such circumstances emotion-focused strategies may be more useful, and recently interventions have been developed for patients with chronic illness to more accurately match the coping strategy to the characteristics of the situation.

INFLUENCES ON COPING

The severity and nature of the disease does not seem to have a consistent relationship to patient coping and adjustment to chronic illness. However, the coping process is strongly affected by both psychological and social influences. An important new line of research has begun to investigate the role of the patient's own subjective understanding of their illness as a key factor in directing coping strategies and influencing adjustment. Individuals seem to organize their representations of illnesses around five major cognitive components: identity, which is composed of the label and symptoms of the disease; cause; personal ideas about aetiology; time line, how long they believe the illness will last; consequences, expected effects and outcome of the illness; and cure/control, how one recovers from or controls the illness (Lau & Hartman, 1983; Leventhal, Meyer & Nerenz, 1980). Leventhal has proposed that cognitive illness representations direct coping strategies and emotional responses to an illness in a parallel process that feeds back again to influence the patient's own illness model. For example, a patient who attributes her hypertension to stress caused by work and who subsequently gives up her job only to find that this has made no difference to her level of blood pressure, may revise her view of the cause of her hypertension. It seems that particular illness models may be associated with more functional coping strategies (Moss-Morris, Petrie & Weinman, 1996), and that illness representations may have a critical role in influencing adjustment to a range of common chronic illnesses such as heart disease, cancer, and diabetes (Weinman et al., 1996).

Social and partner support also plays an important role in adjustment to chronic illness. A number of studies have shown social support to be related to better disease outcomes and psychological adjustment in a variety of illnesses. A large follow-up study of chronically ill patients found social support was beneficial for health over time and this effect was strongest in older patients (Sherbourne et al., 1992). Social support has been associated with better metabolic control in diabetes patients (Marteau, Bloch & Baum, 1987), as well as improved outcome in breast cancer (Waxler-Morrison et al., 1991), kidney failure (Dimond, 1979), and heart disease (Ruberman et al., 1984; Wiklund et al., 1988). However, sometimes support can be too intrusive and people can be deluged with help or conflicting advice causing negative effects on the outcome of chronic illness (e.g. Garrity, 1973).

It is not clear what exact benefits accrue from social support in the context of chronic illness. The improved adherence to treatment and better health habits associated with higher levels of social support are likely to be important factors. The role of family and friends noticing changes in the patient's health that need attention may also reduce treatment delay if the illness worsens and the patient needs medical assistance. It seems that patients' perceptions of what actions are helpful is influenced by the social role of the provider. Esteem and emotional support are seen as most helpful when it comes from spouses or family (Dakof & Taylor, 1990). Some researchers have suggested that the benefits of social support may not, in fact, derive from its positive aspects but rather from the absence of upsetting or conflictual relationships that interfere with successful function (Coyne & Bolger, 1990).

As well as the critical role of illness perceptions and social support, there is evidence that a number of individual difference variables also influence the coping process. The age of the person, their educational background, and personality traits such as optimism can act to influence coping with chronic illness (Carver et al., 1993; Felton et al., 1984). Factors related to the disease itself in terms of its stage, physical characteristics, and symptomotology are also important. It is apparent that each chronic illness is made up of a large number of stressors, and patients may apply different coping responses to each of these illness-related problems (Cohen et al., 1986).

COPING INTERVENTIONS

A number of successful intervention strategies have recently been developed for patients suffering from chronic illness. These programmes vary in their focus from being strictly information based to teaching specific skills that help address problems faced by the patient. Treatment programmes also differ in terms of the degree to which they have been theoretically derived from the coping literature. A new intervention called the Coping Effectiveness Training Programme (Chesney & Folkman, 1994) focuses both on the way patients appraise the stressors associated with their illness and the strategies used to deal with them. An important emphasis in this programme is promoting the match between appraisals and coping strategies. When situations are appraised as uncontrollable, emotion-focused strategies are encouraged, while problem-focused strategies are advocated for the controllable aspects of the illness. Rather than just providing social support, patients are also educated on how to access appropriate social support networks in the wider community. In men infected with HIV, Coping Effectiveness Training increased positive reframing and planning and reduced reliance on disengagement strategies which resulted in improved levels of psychological well-being (Chesney & Folkman, 1994).

[85]

Another coping skills training programme which included structured sessions on stress management, communication, and problem-solving has been shown to be more effective than supportive group therapy. A comparative study of the two methods with a small group of cancer patients found that patients undergoing the coping programme demonstrated significantly greater well-being and functioning (Telch & Telch, 1986).

There is some recent evidence that interventions designed to improve coping with chronic illness can also have positive health benefits. The most well-known study in this area was conducted by Spiegel *et al.* (1989) who found that metastatic breast cancer patients randomly assigned to a one-year group coping intervention programme lived on average twice as long as controls. This unstructured intervention programme consisted of a number of components including emotional expression, discussion of improved coping strategies, extracting meaning from the illness experience, as well as learning self-hypnosis for pain control. Following on from this study, Fawzy and his collaborators showed that malignant melanoma patients who had undergone a six-week coping intervention that enhanced active problem-orientated coping, were less likely to have a recurrence or to have died of their cancer when compared with a control group (Fawzy *et al.*, 1993). A comparison of the groups at six months post intervention demonstrated that the intervention had decreased distress, increased use of active coping skills, and improved immune functioning (Fawzy *et al.*, 1990).

While the results from intervention studies provide impressive support for developing coping skills as a treatment, it is difficult to separate the non-specific factors that occur in these group interventions from the specific effects of enhancing coping skills. These group treatment programmes incorporate other aspects such as psychological support and education with the teaching of coping strategies, and further research needs to be done to ascertain the specific benefits of coping training. Intervention studies are a valuable method of testing the coping skills model and they provide a useful way of investigating coping processes over time.

Coping with chronic illness has become an important area for research and intervention in health psychology because of the large numbers of individuals suffering from such diseases. The diagnosis of a chronic illness typically brings with it a number of complex problems, emotional difficulties, and changes in lifestyle. The patient's own understanding of the illness and the levels of appropriate social support available to them are key factors in promoting successful long-term coping. Interventions that develop coping strategies and improve the match between the use of problem-focused or emotion-focused strategies with the characteristics of the situation seem to provide a promising avenue to improve the quality of life for patients living with a chronic illness. (See also 'Coping with chronic pain', 'Effects of hospitalization in adults', 'Emotional expression and health', Group therapy, 'Lay beliefs about health and illness', 'Relaxation training'.)

REFERENCES

Carver, C.S., Pozo, C., Harris, S.D., Noriega, V., Scheier, M.F., Rodinson, D.S., Ketcham, A.S., Moffat, F. & Clark, K.C. (1993). How coping mediates the effect of optimism on distress: a study of women with early stage breast cancer. *Journal of Personality and Social Psychology*, 65, 375–90.

Cassileth, B.R., Lusk, E.J., Strouse, T.B., Miller, D.S., Brown, L.L., Cross, P.A. & Tenaglia, A.N. (1984). Psychosocial status in chronic illness: a comparative analysis of six diagnostic groups. *New England Journal of Medicine*, 311, 506–11.

Chesney, M.A. & Folkman, S. (1994). Psychological impact of HIV disease and implications for intervention. *Psychiatric Clinics of North America*, 17, 163–82.

Cohen, F., Reese, L.B., Kaplan, G.A. & Roggio, R.E. (1986). Coping with the stresses of arthritis. In R.W. Moskowitz & M.R. Haug (Eds). *Arthritis in the elderly*. New York: Springer.

Coyne, J.C. & Bolger, N. (1990). Doing without social support as an explanatory concept. *Journal of Social and Clinical Psychology*, 9, 148–58.

Dakof, G.A. & Taylor, S.E. (1990). Victims perceptions of social support: what is helpful from whom? *Journal of Personality and Social Psychology*, 58, 80–9.

Dimond, M. (1979). Social support and adaptation to chronic illness: the case of maintenance hemodialysis. *Research in Nursing and Health*, 2, 101–8.

Dunkel-Schetter, C., Feinstein, L.G., Taylor, S.E. & Falke, R.L. (1992). Patterns of coping with cancer. *Health Psychology*, 11, 79–87.

Fawzy, F.I., Cousins, N., Fawzy, N.W., Elastoff, R. & Morton, D.L. (1990). A structured intervention for cancer patients. I Changes over time in methods of coping and affective disturbance. *Archives of General Psychiatry*, 47, 720–5.

Fawzy, F.I., Fawzy, N.W., Hyun, C.S., Elastoff, R., Guthrie, D., Fahey, J.L. & Morton, D.L. (1993). Malignant melanoma: effects of an early structured psychiatric intervention, coping, and affective state on recurrence and survival 6 years later. *Archives of General Psychiatry*, 50, 681–9.

Felton, B.J., Revenson, T.A. & Hinrichsen, G.A. (1984). Stress and coping in the explanation of psychological adjustment among chronically ill adults. *Social Science and Medicine*, 18, 889–98.

Folkman, S., Chesney, M., Pollack, L. & Coates, T. (1993). Stress, control, and depressive mood in human immunodeficiency virus-positive and -negative gay men in San Francisco. *The Journal of Nervous and Mental Disease*, 181, 409–16.

Garrity, T.F. (1973). Vocational adjustment after first myocardial infarction: comparative assessment of several variables suggested in the literature. *Social Science and Medicine*, 7, 705–17.

Greenfield, S., Kaplan, S.H., Ware, J.E., Yano, E.M. & Frank, H.J.L. (1988). Patients' participation in medical care: effects on blood sugar control and quality of life in diabetes. *Journal of General Internal Medicine*, 3, 448–57.

Laerum, E., Johnson, N., Smith, P. & Larsen, S. (1987). Can myocardial infarction induce positive changes in family relationships? *Family Practice*, 4, 302–5.

Lau, R.R. & Hartman, K.A. (1983). Common-sense representations of common illnesses. *Health Psychology*, 2, 167–85.

Lazarus, R.S. & Folkman, S. (1984). *Stress, appraisal, and coping*. New York: Springer.

Leventhal, H., Meyer, D. & Nerenz, D. (1980). The common-sense representations of illness danger. In S. Rachman (Ed.). Medical psychology 2. pp. 7–30. New York: Guilford Press.

Marteau, T.M., Bloch, S. & Baum, J.D. (1987). Family life and diabetic control. *Journal of Child Psychology and Psychiatry*, 28, 823–33.

Moos, R.H. & Schaefer, J.A. (1984). The crisis of physical illness: An overview and conceptual approach. In R. Moos (Ed.). Coping with physical illness 2: new perspectives. New York: Plenum.

Moss-Morris, R., Petrie, K.J. & Weinman, J. (1996). Functioning in chronic fatigue syndromes: do illness perceptions play a regulatory role? *British Journal of Clinical Psychology*, **1**, 15–25.

Ruberman, W., Weinblatt, E., Goldberg, J.D. & Chaudhary, B.S. (1984). Psychosocial influences on mortality after myocardial infarction. *New England of Medicine*, **311**, 522–59.

Sherbourne, C.D., Meredith, L.S., Rogers, W. & Ware, J.E. (1992). Social support and stressful life events: age differences in their effects on health-related quality of life among the chronically ill. *Quality of Life Research*, **1**, 235–46.

Spiegel, D., Bloom, J.R., Kraemer, H.C. &

Gottheil, E. (1989). Effect of psychosocial treatment on survival of patients with metastatic breast cancer. *Lancet*, 888–91.

Telch, C.F. & Telch, M.J. (1986). Group coping skills instruction and supportive group therapy for cancer patients: a comparison of strategies. *Journal of Consulting and Clinical Psychology*, **54**, 802–8.

Waxler-Morrison, N. Hislop, T.G., Mears, B. & Can, L. (1991). The effects of social relationships on survival with women with breast cancer: a prospective study. *Social Science and Medicine*, **33**, 177–83.

Weinman, J., Petrie, K.J., Moss-Morris,

R.E. & Horne, R. (1996). The illness perception questionnaire: a new method for assessing the cognitive representation of disease. *Psychology and Health*, **11**, 431–45.

Whitlock, F.A. (1986). Suicide and physical illness. In A. Roy (ed.). *Suicide*, pp. 151–170. Baltimore: Williams & Wilkins.

Wiklund, I., Oden, A., Sanne, H., Ulvenstam, G., Wilhelmsson, C. & Wilhemsen, L. (1988). Prognostic importance of somatic and psychosocial variables after a first myocardial infarction. *American Journal of Epidemiology*, **128**, 786–95.

Coping with chronic pain

NAOMI LESTER
and
FRANCIS J. KEEFE

Department of Psychology, University of North Florida,
Duke University Medical Center
South Jacksonville, USA

A large proportion of the general population experiences pain on a daily basis (Von Korff *et al.*, 1988). Individuals vary greatly in their ability to cope with such daily pain. Some individuals cope well and are able to live a relatively full life despite having severe and persistent pain. Other individuals cope poorly and become physically and psychologically disabled by pain.

In the past 15 years, psychologists have begun to systematically analyse the importance of coping in understanding persistent pain. Evidence suggests that coping may be more important in explaining the adjustment to chronic pain than medical variables such as evidence of underlying tissue pathology (Keefe *et al.*, 1987).

The purpose of this chapter is to provide a brief overview of the status of research on coping with chronic pain. The chapter describes and evaluates the three basic approaches currently used to conceptualize and assess pain coping.

PAIN COPING: MODELS AND ASSESSMENT METHODS

Coping with pain can be generally conceptualized as thoughts and behaviours that serve to manage or decrease pain and the distress caused by pain (Jensen *et al.*, 1991). Within this basic framework, researchers have formulated three models of pain coping: the problem–emotion focused coping model, the active–passive coping model, and the cognitive–behavioural coping model. Each of these models has a theoretical and empirical basis and a specific assessment instrument to which it is tied.

The Problem–Emotion Focused Coping Model

Folkman and Lazarus developed a coping model that categorizes coping strategies as either problem focused or emotion focused (Lazarus & Folkman, 1984). Problem-focused coping efforts include behaviours that are designed to alter the individual's relationship to the stressor, e.g. making a plan of action and following it. Emotion-focused coping includes efforts designed to alter one's internal reactions to a stressors, e.g. the use of calming self-statements.

Although the problem–emotion focused model had its roots in stress research, the model can be extended to an analysis of coping in chronic pain patients (Parker *et al.*, 1988). For example, a chronic low back pain patient faced with the choice of engaging in an activity known to cause pain (say sitting in a movie theatre), may well use a problem-focused coping strategy, such as having a friend rent a videotape. Alternatively, the same patient might use an emotion-focused strategy such as thinking about a future pleasant activity to control their disappointment about missing the movie.

To measure problem- and emotion-focused coping efforts, Folkman and Lazarus developed a 42 item self-report instrument, the Ways of Coping Checklist (WCCL) (Folkman & Lazarus, 1980). The WCCL asks individuals to rate how they have coped with a recent stressful experience. In studies of chronic pain, respondents are specifically asked to list a stressor associated with their pain (e.g. pain experiences, loss of job, inability to do daily activities). Respondents then rate the extent to which they use each coping strategy on the questionnaire. Ratings are made either on a yes/no basis or using a 4 point scale on which 0 = never used and 3 = regularly used.

Responses on the WCCL are summed to yield one problem-focused subscale and four emotion-focused coping subscales. The problem-focused subscale measures specific actions individuals take

Table 1. *Items from the Ways of Coping Checklist*

Coping subscale	Items
Problem-focused coping	Concentrated on something good that could come out of the whole thing
	Made a plan of action and followed it
Seeking social support	Talked to someone to find out about the situation
	Asked someone for advice and followed it
Wishful-thinking	Hoped a miracle would happen
	Wished I could change what happened
Self-blame	Realized that I brought the problem on myself
	Blamed myself
Avoidance	Went on as if nothing had happened
	Tried to forget the whole thing

Table 2. *Items from the Vanderbilt Pain Management Inventory*

Coping subscale	Items
Active coping	Engaging in physical exercise or physical therapy
	Clearing your mind of bothersome thoughts or worries
Passive coping	Restricting or cancelling your social activities
	Taking medication for the purposes of immediate pain relief

to cope with the stressor. The four emotion-focused subscales measure steps individuals take to deal with the emotional aspects of the stressor and include seeking social support, wishful-thinking, self-blame, and avoidance. Table 1 lists typical items included on each of the subscales of the WCCL.

Several studies have evaluated the utility of the problem–emotion–focused coping model in understanding pain in osteoarthritis and rheumatoid arthritis patients (e.g. Turner, Clancy & Vitaliano, 1987; Parker *et al.*, 1988). These studies have found that arthritis patients who rely on wishful thinking, and to a lesser extent, on blame and avoidance coping strategies, experience more depression and greater physical disability than those who use fewer of these emotion-focused types of coping.

Turner and her colleagues (1987) used the WCCL to analyse coping in 85 patients suffering from low back pain. Patients completed the WCCL by identifying a stressor from a list of 14 stressful situations such as problems with family, work or health. Of the patients 43% identified their back pain as a major stressor. Patients who reported pain as their primary stressor used less problem-focused coping and seeking social support. In addition, for all patients self blame was negatively associated with pain.

Comment

The problem–emotion focused coping model has two major advantages for understanding chronic pain coping. First, research has demonstrated that this coping model is valid not only for pain but for a wide range of stressful conditions (Lazarus & Folkman, 1984). Use of this model, thus enables pain researchers to link their research to other recent studies in the coping literature. Secondly, the questionnaire instrument used to assess problem–emotion focused coping, the WCCL, is an established instrument that meets reasonable psychometric standards. Thirdly, the WCCL assesses a broad selection of coping strategies. Because of its breadth and utility for measuring both pain coping and coping with other stressors, the WCCL may be used to compare the ways an individual copes with pain and with the ways that they cope with other stressors.

The Active–Passive Coping Model

Another way to conceptualize pain coping is along an active–passive

dimension (Brown & Nicassio, 1987). According to this model, patients faced with pain either may take: (i) an active coping approach in which they purposely engage in adaptive behaviours designed to manage their pain, or (ii) a passive and maladaptive approach in which they withdraw and give up instrumental control over pain. Examples of active coping include engaging in muscle strengthening exercises or ignoring pain. Examples of passive coping include taking medications and resting in bed.

Brown and Nicassio developed the Vanderbilt Pain Management Inventory (VPMI) (Brown & Nicassio, 1987) to measure the degree to which individuals' use active and passive strategies to cope with chronic pain. The VPMI is an 18-item questionnaire on which respondents are asked to rate the frequency they use specific active and passive coping strategies to cope with moderate to high levels of pain. Ratings of frequency of use of these strategies are made on a 1 to 5 scale on which 1 = never do when in pain, and 5 = very frequently do when in pain. Table 2 lists typical items drawn for the two scales of the VPMI: Active Coping and Passive Coping.

The VPMI has been used primarily in studies of arthritis patients. In one study, Brown and Nicassio (1987) investigated the relationships between coping, pain, functional impairment, and depression in rheumatoid arthritis patients. Over 300 patients completed the questionnaire and provided information on their pain, depressive symptoms, and the extent to which pain caused functional disability and interfered with daily activities. Results indicated that patients who frequently used active coping strategies had lower levels of pain, functional disability, and depression. Patients who primarily relied on passive coping strategies, in contrast, reported more pain, functional disability, and depression.

Comment

The active/passive coping model is appealing because it is simple and straightforward. Treatment efforts based on this model seek to increase active, adaptive coping and decrease maladaptive, passive coping. The questionnaire instrument developed from this model (the VPMI) is a very brief instrument that enables one to quickly and reliably categorize a patients' coping strategies. One limitation of this model is that some of the strategies that are labelled as passive (e.g. taking medication) require an active effort on the part of patients (Keefe *et al.*, 1992).

The Cognitive–Behavioural Model of Pain Coping

The cognitive-behavioural model maintains that two processes are important in understanding chronic pain coping: (i) the specific cognitive and behavioural coping strategies patients used to deal with pain, and (ii) the perceived effectiveness of those strategies

Table 3. *Items from the Coping Strategies Questionnaire*

Coping Subscale	Items
Diverting attention	I try to think of something pleasant
	I count numbers in my head or run a song through my mind
Reinterpreting pain sensations	I don't think of it as pain but rather as a dull or warm feeling
	I imagine that the pain is outside my body
Coping self-statements	I tell myself to be brave and carry on despite the pain
	I tell myself that I can overcome the pain
Ignoring pain sensations	I don't pay any attention to the pain
	I go on as it nothing happened
Praying or hoping	I pray to God that it won't last long
	I have faith in doctors that some day there will be a cure for my pain
Catastrophizing	It's awful and I feel that it overwhelms me
	I worry all the time about whether it will end
Increasing behavioural activity	I do something I enjoy, such as watching TV or listening to music
	I do something active, like household chores or projects

(Rosenstiel & Keefe, 1983; Jensen *et al.*, 1991). This model served as the conceptual basis for the most widely used pain coping instrument, the Coping Strategies Questionnaire (CSQ) (Rosenstiel & Keefe, 1983).

The CSQ is a 44-item instrument that assesses the frequency that patients use cognitive and behavioural strategies and the degree to which patients perceive themselves as able to use these strategies to control and decrease pain. The CSQ has six cognitive coping subscales and one behavioural coping subscale, each of which has six items. Patients rate the degree to which they use each coping strategy on a 7-point scale on which 0 = never, and 6 = always. The CSQ cognitive subscales include diverting attention, reinterpreting pain sensations, coping self statements, ignoring pain sensations, praying or hoping, and catastrophizing. The CSQ behavioural subscale is increasing behavioural activities. At the end of the CSQ, respondents are asked to rate how much control they feel they have over pain and how much they are able to decrease pain using their coping strategies. These ratings are made on a 7-point scale on which 0 = no control/cannot decrease it at all to 6 = complete control/can decrease it completely. Table 3 lists items from each subscale.

The CSQ has been used in many studies of chronic pain coping (for recent reviews of this literature see Jensen *et al.*, 1991 and Keefe *et al.*, 1992). Typically, higher-order factor analysis is used to reduce CSQ data and the resulting factors are then correlated with various indices of pain and adjustment. The first study to use the CSQ was carried out with a sample of 61 low back pain patients (Rosenstiel & Keefe, 1983). This study found that the CSQ subscales were internally reliable and identified three factors that explained a large proportion of variance in responses on the CSQ: (i) Cognitive Coping and Suppression, (ii) Helplessness, and (iii)

Diverting Attention or Praying. High scores on these coping factors were related to poor adjustment to chronic pain. High scores on the Helplessness factor were related to higher levels of depression and anxiety. Patients scoring high on the Diverting Attention or Praying factor had higher levels of pain and functional impairment. High scores on the Cognitive Coping and Suppression factor were related to higher levels of functional impairment. These findings regarding coping are particularly noteworthy because they were obtained after controlling for variables known to influence pain and disability in chronic low back pain patients (e.g. duration of pain, disability/compensation status, number of prior operations, tendency to somaticize).

The CSQ has been used with a wide variety of chronic pain populations (e.g. Lawson *et al.*, 1990). Factor analysis of CSQ responses suggest that there are three basic factors evident in most chronic pain populations. Lawson *et al.* (1990), for example, carried out a confirmatory factor analysis of the CSQ using data from five different chronic pain patient samples (total $N = 620$ patients). They identified three factors: (i) Conscious Cognitive Coping (with high loadings on ignoring pain and coping self statements), (ii) Self-Efficacy Beliefs (with high loadings on ability to control and decrease pain), and (iii) Pain Avoidance (with high loadings on diverting attention and praying or hoping).

The CSQ has been used in a number of recent studies of arthritis patients. In our early research on osteoarthritis patients having persistent knee pain, we carried out a factor analysis that identified two basic factors on the CSQ: (i) Pain Control and Rational Thinking (with high positive loadings on ability to control and decrease pain, and negative loadings on catastrophizing) and (ii) Coping Attempts (with high loadings on most of the remaining CSQ subscales) (Keefe *et al.*, 1987). Regression analyses revealed that high scores on the Pain Control and Rational Thinking factor were clearly related to pain (Keefe *et al.*, 1987). Even after controlling for pain severity, this coping factor was a much stronger predictor of physical and psychological disability than medical variables thought to affect osteoarthritic knee pain (e.g. X-ray ratings of disease severity and obesity status) (Keefe *et al.*, 1987). Studies carried out by Parker and colleagues (1989) and in our own lab have found similar results in rheumatoid arthritis patients.

Comment

The cognitive–behavioural model of coping has had a major impact on chronic pain assessment and treatment. The CSQ is now widely used in clinical pain assessment and in programmatic research examining the efficacy of cognitive behavioural interventions. The CSQ measures a variety of pain coping strategies as well as identifying a patient's sense of efficacy for controlling pain. This emphasis on both coping and the appraisal of pain controllability fits well with theories of stress coping and provides additional information for the clinicians who are designing programmes to help patients cope more effectively.

CONCLUSIONS

Although the studies reviewed above differ in terms of their models and assessment methods, their results support two basic conclusions. First, coping efforts which focus on thinking rationally about pain and taking concrete cognitive and behavioural steps to control

[89]

pain seem to be the most effective methods for managing chronic pain. Secondly, coping efforts which lead the individual to withdraw or become passive when dealing with pain appear to be ineffective.

Recent studies have shown that chronic pain patients can learn to increase their use of adaptive coping efforts and decrease their use of maladaptive coping efforts. We recently reported, for example, that osteoarthritis patients who increased their scores on the Pain Control and Rational Thinking factor of the CSQ over the course of a pain-coping skills training programme had much lower levels of physical disability and much better long-term outcomes (Keefe *et al.*, 1990).

Additional research is needed to advance our understanding of chronic pain coping (Keefe *et al.*, 1992; Keefe & Van Horn, 1993). Research in this area is currently exploring the usefulness of new assessment methods such as daily coping diaries. Daily diaries ask patients to record daily stressors, pain and the methods they use to cope with pain. Using this methodology, pain coping can be studied prospectively. This approach also reduces problems with recall bias of information about pain and coping. Another new strategy for studying pain coping is the structured patient interview (Keefe & Van Horn, 1993). During such an interview, patients are asked to describe, in detail, situations where they have increased pain and the thoughts and behaviours they engage in when coping with pain.

Having patients describe how they cope, using their own words, may provide a greater understanding of the variety of methods individuals use when coping with pain.

One promising area for future research is examining the relationships between pain and coping over longer periods of time. Many studies assess coping only once or follow people for several months. Some coping methods may not affect adjustment in the short term, but may contribute to disease progression and quality of life over the course of many years. In addition, the ways that individuals cope with pain episodes early in life may shape how they cope with persistent pain later in life. Understanding the associations between reactions to early pain experiences and later pain coping may lead to the identification of a subgroup of individuals who, because of lack of early success in coping with pain, may be at risk for poorer adjustment in the face of chronic pain conditions such as arthritis.

In summary, in the past decade, much has been learned about how individuals cope with persistent pain. New methods for assessing coping have been developed and refined. These methods have already increased our understanding of pain and have led to the development of new interventions designed to enhance individuals' ability to cope with chronic pain. (See also 'Coping with chronic illness', 'Pain management', 'Pain perception', 'Placebo', 'Relaxation training'.)

REFERENCES

Brown, G.K. & Nicassio, P.M. (1987). The development of a questionnaire for the assessment of active and passive coping strategies for chronic pain patients, *Pain*, 31, 53–65.

Folkman, S. & Lazarus, R.S. (1980). An analysis of coping in a middle-aged community sample. *Journal of Health and Social Behavior*, 21, 219–39.

Jensen, M.P., Turner, J.A., Romano, J.M. & Karoly, P. (1991). Coping with chronic pain: a critical review of the literature. *Pain*, 249–83.

Keefe, F.J., Caldwell, D.S., Queen, K.T., Gil, K.M., Martinez, S. Crisson, J.E., Ogden, W. & Nunley, J. (1987). Pain coping strategies in osteoarthritis patients. *Journal of Consulting and Clinical Psychology*, 55, 208–12.

Keefe, F.J., Caldwell, D.S., Williams, D.A., Gil, K.M., Mitchell, D., Robertson, C., Martinez, S., Nunley, J., Beckham, J.C., Crisson, J.E. & Helms, M. (1990). Pain coping skills training in the management of osteoarthritic knee pain: follow-up results. *Behavior Therapy*, 21, 435–48.

Keefe, F.J., Salley, A. & Lefebvre, J.C. (1992). Coping with pain: conceptual concerns and future directions. *Pain*, 51, 131–4.

Keefe, F.J. & Van Horn, Y. (1993). Cognitive behavioral treatment of rheumatoid arthrits pain: understanding and enhancing maintenance of treatment gains. *Arthritis Care and Research*, 6, 213–22.

Lawson, K., Reesor, K.A., Keefe, F.J. & Turner, J. (1990). Dimensions of pain-related cognitive coping: cross-validation of the factor structure of the Coping Strategy Questionnaire, *Pain*, 43, 195–204.

Lazarus, R.S. & Folkman, S. (1984). *Stress, appraisal and coping*. New York: Springer Publishing Co.

Parker, J., McRae, C., Smarr, K., Beck, N., Frank, R., Anderson, S. & Walker, S. (1988). Coping strategies in rheumatoid arthritis, *Journal of Rheumatology*, 15, 1376–83.

Parker, J.C., Smarr, K.L., Buescher, K.L., Phillips, L.R., Frank, R.G., Beck, N.C., Anderson, S.K. & Walker, S.E. (1989). Pain control and rational thinking. *Arthritis and Rheumatism*, 32, 984–90.

Rosenstiel, A.K. & Keefe, F.J. (1983). The use of coping strategies in chronic low back pain patients: relationships to patient characteristics and current adjustment. *Pain*, 17, 34–44.

Turner, J.A., Clancy, S. & Vitaliano, P.P. (1987). Relationships of stress appraisal and coping to chronic low back pain. *Behavior Therapy and Research*, 25, 281–8.

Von Korff, M.R., Dworkin, S.F., Le Resche, L.L. & Kruger, A. (1988). An epidemiologic comparison of pain complaints. *Pain*, 32, 173–83.

Coping with death and dying

COLIN MURRAY PARKES
Chorleywood, Hertfordshire, UK

Death is, perhaps, the ultimate test which we face as patients, relatives and members of the caring professions. All of us have to cope with it and, no matter how experienced we become, the coping is seldom easy. Death is often a loss but it can also be a time of peaceful transition. It may represent failure or success, ending or beginning, disaster or triumph. We may try to improve our ways of caring but, whatever the circumstances, death must never become routine.

In recent years, the psychological care of the dying and the bereaved has improved greatly, largely thanks to the work of the Hospices and the various organizations, such as Cruse – Bereavement Care, that provide counselling to the bereaved. Hospices have always seen the unit of care as being the family, which includes the patient, rather than the patient with the family as an optional extra to be taken on if we have time.

The field is a large one and it will not be possible, in the space available here, to give more than an outline of some of the major issues or to review the scientific and clinical research which underlies the theory and practice which I shall describe. The interested reader will find this type of information in Dickenson and Johnson (1993), Jacobs (1993) and my own book (Parkes, 1996). A more detailed examination of the theory and practice of the counselling of dying patients and their families is given by Parkes, Relf and Couldrick (1996).

When people are coming close to death, the professionals may have little or no control over what is happening. Scientific medicine can help us to mitigate some of the pains of dying but, with all our knowledge, 100% of our patients will still die. Despite this, patients and their families continue to turn to us for help. To a large extent, we have replaced priests as the recognised authorities on death, a change of role with which most of us feel uncomfortable.

Death is a social event, it affects the lives of many people. In this circle of people, the patients are the centre of care as long as they are alive; but their troubles will soon be over, those of the family may just be beginning.

Whether or not we think of death as a transition for the patient, it is certainly a transition for the family. Their lives will never be the same again. Death tips the survivors into new situations, new roles, new dangers and new opportunities. They are often forced to learn new ways of coping at a time when overwhelming grief makes it hard for them to cope with old responsibilities, let alone new ones.

The traditional training of doctors and nurses does little to prepare us for the challenges of terminal and bereavement care. We are so preoccupied with saving life that we are at a loss to know what to do when life cannot be saved. Some of us deal with the problem by denying its existence; we insist on fighting for a cure until the bitter end. Sadly, the weapons that we employ too often impair the quality of the life that is left; the end, when it comes, is truly bitter.

Others acknowledge to themselves that the patient is dying but attempt to conceal it from the patient. If they succeed, the patient may die in 'blissful' ignorance, but they often fail. As the disease progresses, the patient looks in the mirror and realizes that somebody is lying. At a time when they most need to trust their medical attendants, they realize that they have been deceived. In either case, the family who survive are denied the opportunity to say 'Goodbye', and to conclude any unfinished psychological business with the patient.

Of course, it is not only the professional staff who find it hard to cope with people who are dying; friends, workmates and family members are equally at a loss and they may deal with their own feelings of inadequacy by putting pressure on us to continue treatment long after it can do good or to collude with them in concealing the true situation from the patient. 'You won't tell him he's dying, will you doctor? It would kill him if he found out.' While such remarks may occasionally be justified, they are more likely to reflect the informant's own inability to cope with the truth rather than that of the patient.

In all our work with terminally ill patients and their families, we must consider three psychological problems that complicate the psychosocial transitions which they face. These are fear, grief and resistance to change.

THE PROBLEM OF FEAR

Fear is the natural response to any threat to our own life or to the lives of those we love. It has important biological functions in preparing our minds and bodies to fight or to flee. Our entire autonomic nervous system exists to support these ends. Among the many consequences of fear are hyperalertness to further dangers, increased muscular tension, increased cardiac rate and inhibition of digestive and other inessential vegetative functions. In the types of emergency that arose in the environment of evolution, these reactions ensured our survival, but they are seldom of much use to us today.

It would be highly inappropriate for a cancer patient who has been told the nature of his diagnosis to run away or to hit out at the doctor, yet he may have an impulse to do both things. The hyperalertness produced by fear may cause fearful people to imagine additional dangers where none exists. It may also impair their ability to pay attention to anything but the danger itself. If increased muscle tension goes on for long, the muscles begin to fatigue and to ache; such symptoms may themselves be misinterpreted as signs of cancer or whatever disease it is that the person dreads. Similarly, cardiac hyperactivity is often misinterpreted as a sign of heart disease, thereby increasing fear and setting up a vicious circle of escalating fear and symptoms.

All of us have our own ways of coping when we are afraid. Some of us become aggressive, seeking someone or something to blame in the hope that we can rectify the situation. Thus some patients, faced with worsening symptoms, respond by blaming them on the treatment. It is easier to fight a doctor than a cancer. Others use alcohol or other drugs in an attempt to find 'Dutch courage', a habit which can give short-term relief but may cause fresh problems in the long run.

The logical response to danger is to seek help and, if doctors have failed to cure an illness, we should not be surprised or angry if the patient seeks for a cure from unorthodox practitioners. But, cure is not the only thing that people need. Comfort of the non-verbal kind, that a mother can give to a frightened child, is just as welcome to the frightened adult and just as effective in reducing fear. Nurses, who are touching patients all the time, know how powerful a touch of the hand can be. Doctors are often bad at touching, avoiding physical contact with their patients as if the patient's fear might be infectious, which, of course, it is.

When somebody is dying, it is not only the patient who is likely to be afraid, it is everybody around them. This can produce another kind of vicious circle when frightened patients see their fear reflected in the eyes of the people around them. Although most healthy people, asked where they would want to die, will say, 'At home', the level of anxiety which sometimes surrounds a person who is dying at home often gives good reason to admit them to a hospital or hospice. As one person who had been admitted to a hospice said, 'It's safe to die here'!

Since most people are afraid of dying, we tend to assume that we know why a dying person is afraid. It is tempting to say, 'I understand'. The truth is, none of us can know another's fear and many of the fears of terminally ill patients have nothing to do with death. Time and again patients have said to me, 'It's not being dead that frightens me, doctor, it's dying.' Most people in our society have not seen anybody die. Their image of death comes from the horror comics and other dramatic and often horrific portrayals of death, which sell newspapers and the like. When people learn about real deaths, it is often the deaths that have been badly handled that get talked about. To many people 'death' means 'agony' and it may come as a surprise to them to learn that, with proper care, pain need not be a problem.

THE PROBLEM OF GRIEF

Grief is the normal reaction to any major loss and is not confined to bereavement. Illnesses such as cancers and AIDS tend to progress in steps. At each setback the patient is faced with another cluster of losses. Initially, the loss of security and body parts affected by the disease constitute the major losses but, in later stages of the illness, increasing disability may cause loss of mobility, occupation, and an increasing range of physical functions. In the last phase, the patient faces the prospect of losing life itself and all the attachments that go with it.

Each new loss will tend to evoke intense feelings of pining and yearning for the object that is lost. The person experiences a strong need to cry aloud and to search for ways of retaining some or all of the lost object. A woman may intensely miss the breast that she has lost and find some solace in a good prosthesis or in reconstructive surgery. A man may long to return to work and surprise his work-

mates by arriving at his place of work despite severe debility. Patients in a hospital regularly pine to go home, and many will do so despite the problems that this may cause to their families.

It is important not to confuse normal grief with clinical depression. Grief is transient and, even within an hour or so, people who allow themselves to express grief will usually begin to feel better. Depression, by contrast, is lasting and undermines sufferers, preventing them from doing the very things that would get them out of the slough of depression. The slowing down of thought and movement, and the feelings of worthlessness which characterize clinical depression, contrast with the restlessness and pining of the grieving person. Other symptoms of depression, anorexia, loss of weight and early morning waking, also occur as part of grieving (particularly if the grief is caused by a debilitating illness).

Diagnosis is important because clinical depression requires, and will usually respond to, treatment with antidepressant medication. Given this help, people who are grieving and depressed often find that, as the depression gets better, they can grieve more easily.

RESISTANCE TO CHANGE

More problematic is the tendency to deny the reality of the diagnosis, or prognosis, or to avoid facing the implications of this. Many patients make it clear that they do not want to be told about their illness. This is most likely to happen if the doctors are themselves uncertain or are giving conflicting messages. Family members too may find it hard to accept the fact that a loved person's lifespan is very limited and may be more resistant to facing reality than the patient.

Denial is a defence against overwhelming anxiety, and may enable people to adjust more gradually to the massive changes that threaten their internal world. It is a basic assumption in the minds of most people that we know where we stand. This rather trite statement covers a major but under-rated fact that we can only relate to the world around us because we possess an internal model of that world by which we recognize the world that we meet and plan our behaviour accordingly. This applies at the level of everyday habits (getting up in the morning, walking across the room, laying two places for breakfast etc.) and at the deeper level of finding meaning and direction in life (wanting to get up in the morning, eat breakfast, etc.).

Major losses render obsolete large sections of our internal world and require a process of restructuring at both levels of functioning. For a while, people who are faced with a discrepancy between the world that is, and the world that should be (on the basis of our experience up to now), continue to operate the old obsolete mode which is, after all, the only model they have. The amputee leaps out of bed and finds himself sprawling on the floor, the widow lays the table for two. Even more common are the habits of thought which lead into blind alleys ('When I get better, I shall go back to work' or 'I must ask my husband about that').

Each time we are brought up short by a discrepancy of this kind, we suffer another pang of grief, intense, painful pining for what we have lost. This forces us to take stock and to begin the long and difficult process of revising our assumptive world. This takes time and it takes even longer for us to revise the basic assumptions that give meaning to life, e.g. that we can find new sources of self-esteem without having to go to work each day, that life in a wheelchair can be quite tolerable or that a widow is not condemned to perpetual mourning.

Because we rely on the possession of an accurate internal model of the world to cope with the world and to keep us safe, we feel, and are, extremely vulnerable whenever we are faced with major discrepancies of this kind. More than at any other time, we need the understanding and protection of people close to us; small wonder that patients and family members grow closer to each other at times of threat and that many people would rather be at home than in a strange or impersonal hospital ward. For those without families, the support of doctors and nurses may be invaluable, but such patients may cling to the security of their home as if this were the only safe place in the world.

The psychosocial transition faced by the dying patient may be more frightening but is usually less complex than the transition faced by the patient's spouse. Having faced the facts of the illness, the patient has not got to learn new ways of coping, acceptance brings its own rewards and the patient will often find that family and other carers are happy to take over responsibility for managing the affairs which previously caused anxiety and stress in the patient's life. 'Don't you worry, we'll look after things now', can be very reassuring to someone who has never previously had the opportunity to 'let go'. Perhaps, because of this, patients who face their illness, and accept that there is nothing more to be done, often enter a peaceful state and achieve a relatively happy conclusion to their lives. They seem to come through the process of grieving more quickly and completely than their spouses who have to discover a new identity and who will often continue to grieve for years to come.

INFLUENCING THE TRANSITION

The process of revising one's internal world is made easier if the issues are clear and if there is someone nearby who will keep us safe during the period of vulnerability. It follows that members of the caring professions can do a great deal to help people through these psychosocial transitions. Accurate information is essential to planning; hence the reaction of relief that is expressed by many patients when they are told they have cancer. It is easier to cope with the worst than to live in a state of planlessness.

Much has been written about the patient's right to know the truth about an illness, but we must also respect their right to monitor the amount of new and painful information that they can cope with at any given time. It is just as wrong to tell people too much, too soon, as it is to tell them to little, too late. The patient who refuses to give consent to major surgery may just need a little time to call on the support of his family before changing his mind. If we respond by threatening him with the dire consequences of his refusal, this may increase his anxiety and delay the final decision.

Similarly, we need to recognize that it takes time to break bad news. To impart the information to a person that they have cancer or AIDS is to inflict a major psychological trauma. No surgeon would think of operating without booking an operating theatre and setting aside sufficient time to do the job properly. The same should apply to all important communication between professional carers and the families we serve.

We need to know whose lives are going to be affected by the information we possess, to decide who should be invited to meet us and where the meeting should take place. This means that someone must draw a genogram, a family tree which identifies each relevant person in the patient's family. Having identified the key people, we must decide who is the best person to talk with them and whether they should be seen together or separately. (Some are so overprotective of each other that they will never ask questions that might cause distress unless they are seen on their own.)

People will remember, for the rest of their lives, the details of the occasions when important news was broken. Even the pictures on the wall are important, and there is a world of difference between the doctor who adopts a relaxed and supportive attitude in a pleasant home-like atmosphere and the busy, impersonal consultant who breaks bad news in a public ward, or in the sterile environment of a treatment room. The placing of chairs at the same level, and at an angle to each other so that human contact is possible and there are no desks or other barriers between us, helps to create the conditions in which communication is possible.

Before telling people what we think they need to know, we should find out what they already know or think they know about the situation and what are their priorities. If they use words like 'cancer' or 'death', we should check out that these words mean the same to them as they do to us. 'There are many kinds of cancer, what does the word mean to you?', 'Have you seen anyone die? How do you view death?' will often reveal considerable ignorance and open the door to positive reassurance and explanation. Too often, doctors fail to invite questions and miss the opportunity to help people with the issues that are concerning them most.

Members of the primary care team are in a position to provide continuity of care throughout the illness and bereavement, and are particularly important sources of support. They are likely to be familiar with the social context in which the illness has arisen, to know the family members who are most at risk of adjustment problems and to have a relationship of trust with them that will enable the team to see them through this turning point in their lives. The fact that the primary care team are providing long-term care means that they will often have more time and opportunities to help the family to work things out than other caregivers.

Eventually the time may come when further active treatment aimed at curing symptoms will cause more problems than it solves. From now on, we shall be more concerned with palliation than with cure and the need for psychosocial care will be greater than ever. The question will arise whether to refer the patient to a hospice or specialist home care team. Hospices have focused attention on the need for improved symptom control at the end of life. Although St Christopher's Hospice in Sydenham, the first of the modern style of hospice, was initially restricted to in-patients, the home care which is now provided by most hospices was not long to follow. More recently, support teams have been set up in many hospitals to enable some of the methods of care which have been developed in hospices to be provided in general hospitals, and most hospitals and primary care teams are now able to relieve pain and other distressing symptoms in the later stages of cancer. Less easy to provide is the psychosocial care, which not only relieves the mental suffering of the patient but can help those members of the family whose lives must change, because of the death, to achieve a smooth and satisfactory transition. It is a criticism of existing services in the United

Kingdom that the excellent psychosocial and spiritual care that is provided by many (but not all) hospices is not more widely available, and is limited to the final phase of life.

Finally we must recognize that the care of the dying can be stressful for the professionals as well as those for whom they care. A good staff support system is essential and should include the recognition that, if it is all right for patients and their families to cry when they grieve, it should be all right for us too. The 'stiff upper lip' which makes it so hard to help some patients and family members is even more of a problem in doctors.

REFERENCES

Dickenson, D. & Johnson, M. (1993). *Death, dying and bereavement*. London: Open University and Sage.

Jacobs, S. (1993). *Pathologic grief: maladaptation to loss*. Washington, DC & London: Amer. Psychiat. Pr.

Parkes, C.M. (1996). *Bereavement: studies of grief in adult life*. 3rd edn. London: Tavistock/Routledge, NY: Pelican, Harmondsworth and International Universities Press.

Parkes, C.M., Relf, M. & Couldrick, A. (1996). *Counselling in terminal care and bereavement* London: British Psychological Society.

Coping with stressful medical procedures

YAEL BENYAMINI

and

HOWARD LEVENTHAL

Institute for Health and Department of Psychology, Rutgers, The State University of New Jersey, New Brunswick, USA

There are vast differences in the amount of stress associated with different medical procedures. Surgery, chemotherapy, and radiation treatment for cancers are likely to define the high end of the stress dimension, and blood drawing and vaccination, the low end. Diagnostic tests such as endoscopy and colonoscopy will likely be in the middle ground. Studies describing the level of stress over major surgical episodes have found that distress and anxiety rise as the day of surgery nears, peaks following recovery from anaesthesia and declines gradually in the week to 10 days till discharge (Johnston, 1980). Substantial individual differences in level of distress are reported by patients during the same treatment procedure, e.g. reported number and severity of side-effects during breast cancer chemotherapy ranges from zero to a high of 12 out of 17 items (fatigue, nausea, vomiting, etc.; Love *et al.*, 1989); similar differences have been found for reports of anxiety (Manne *et al.*, 1994). Anxiety and distress also change with the repetition of a treatment, e.g. reductions in anxiety and distress over cycles of cancer chemotherapy (Nerenz *et al.*, 1986), reflecting increasing familiarity with the procedure and habituation of emotional responses, increases reflecting unexpected and unmanageable experiences that create uncertainty and stimulate anxiety, and classical conditioning of nausea and anxiety over treatment trials (Andrykowski, 1990; Leventhal *et al.*, 1988).

These, and other such findings, indicate that the level of stress and anxiety observed during a threatening medical treatment depends upon the meaning the individual assigns to it, the availability of resources to manage it, and the outcome of efforts at self-management. Thus, pain, distress, and anxiety are not solely proportional to the amount of tissue injury and pain associated with a noxious, medical procedure. For example, a colonoscopy performed as part of an annual check-up will be less threatening and less stressful than one conducted to determine whether bleeding is due to a recurrent cancer. The significance of this point was clear in the seminal study by Egbert *et al.* (1964), demonstrating that preparatory information could greatly minimize the distress of surgical treatment. The observation that situational factors and information can alter meaning and moderate the level of anxiety and distress during invasive treatments, made clear that it was inappropriate to attribute the florid symptomatology frequently observed both prior to, and after, surgery to individual differences in psychopathology; such attributions blame the patient and ignore the contribution of meaning and coping responses to stress reactions (Janis & Leventhal, 1967).

COPING WITH STRESS AS A PROBLEM-SOLVING PROCESS

The vast individual differences and temporal changes in stress response, and the benefits of informational preparation on adaptation to noxious medical treatments, made clear that adaptation to stressful medical treatments should be conceptualized as a self-regulation process. In this framework, the patient is conceptualized as an active problem-solver who either attends to, or avoids attending to, disease and treatment relevant cues, assigns meaning to and responds emotionally to these cues (Cioffi, 1991), copes both with the objective environment (as it is perceived) and his emotional reactions, and appraises the outcome of coping responses. The self-regulation process is extended in time and varies in breadth, ranging from short-term issues such as managing postoperative pain to long term issues such as re-establishing life patterns and minimizing dysfunctions while learning to live with an incurable disease. One consequence of this variation has been ambiguity in the use of the term, 'coping'. It is used to refer both to the activity of the problem-solving system and to the specific overt and covert actions used to manage stressful procedures and their associated emotional reactions.

The ambiguity has led investigators to propose hierarchical models that differentiate among different levels of the coping process (Krohne, 1993; Leventhal, Suls & Leventhal, 1993). General behavioural strategies such as risk aversion and energy conservation (Leventhal, Leventhal & Schaefer, 1991) define the upper levels, strategies such as monitoring and blunting for regulating emotional responses define the middle level (Miller, 1987), and a host of specific coping procedures, such as taking an aspirin and/or seeking medical care to manage somatic symptoms, define the most concrete level of coping. Attention to the effects of personality factors, e.g. trait anxiety, optimism, etc., on both the selection of coping responses and distress during treatment, has deflected attention from the role of contextual factors on distress, although the latter may have the greater influence on both the selection and effectiveness of specific coping responses. It is likely, for example, that personality will have less effect on experienced threat, and the choice and efficacy of coping responses, than factors such as the structure of the medical system, e.g. cystoscopy as an outpatient versus as an inpatient, the disease for which a procedure is undertaken, e.g. X-ray for an annual check-up versus suspected cancer, the cultural meaning of a procedure, the availability of social support during it, and prior experiences that generate situational specific expectancies. Be this as it may, the study of personality factors and coping styles has succeeded in generating information on the ways in which an individual may choose to manage or self-regulate the problem-solving system, in addition to coping with or managing the 'objective' treatment procedure and disease.

COMPONENTS OF SELF-REGULATION

Parallel processing

Data from descriptive studies of coping and experimental studies of preparation for stressful treatments show that individuals facing threatening treatments have two parallel and potentially conflicting tasks: Management of the external setting and management of thoughts and emotions (Leventhal, 1970; Lazarus & Launier, 1977). The separation of problem and emotion management appears in factor analyses of coping checklists which typically generate a factor for problem-focused behaviours, and multiple factors for the self-regulation of emotion (Folkman & Lazarus, 1985; Endler & Parker, 1990). A similar division emerged in experimental studies examining emotional reactions and coping responses to fear-provoking messages that gave specific recommendations for the prevention of life-threatening diseases (Leventhal, 1970).

Given the variety of ways that one might attempt to solve a problem, it is surprising that nearly all factorial studies identify only a single factor for problem-focused coping. The various factors for coping with emotion range from efforts to reduce or control affect,

e.g. mental control tactics such as distraction, thinking positive thoughts, reinterpreting situational cues, and physical control tactics such as substance use and eating, to expressive reactions that appear to amplify emotional distress, e.g, catastrophizing. The use of amplifying tactics such as catastrophizing may reflect a prior history in which expression of affect communicated the need for, and was rewarded by, social comforting, though little is known about the origins of this or other procedures.

Representation, coping, and appraisal

The management of treatment procedures involves factors from three sets of variables: the representation of the illness and treatment and the emotional responses accompanying them, procedures (actions) for coping, and outcome appraisals (Leventhal, Diefenbach & Leventhal, 1992). The representation of an illness, i.e. its cause, controllability, consequences, time-line (acute vs chronic) and identity (symptoms and label), helps to define the meaning and appropriateness of treatment procedures. For example, surgical removal of the breast is a sensible, and possibly the only reasonable treatment, given the common-sense representation of breast cancer as an alien, palpable lump that is potentially uncontrollable and life threatening once it spreads. Thus, the representation shapes the selection and outcome expectations for available coping procedures. As meaning is situational specific and dynamic, representations will change leading to changes in coping behaviours (Leventhal, Leventhal & Schaefer, 1991).

The importance of the combination of response (coping) and representation factors for the management of distress during medical procedures, and the separation of problem and emotion management, is evident in experimental studies of patient preparation. For example, Johnson and Leventhal (1974) prepared patients for a gastric endoscopy by giving half of the patients information about what they would feel during the procedure (sensory information), and half general information about the procedure. Half of each group was given information on coping responses, e.g. breathing and swallowing to facilitate throat anaesthetization and later tube passage. The sensory message reduced affective distress, as expected, but it was the combination of sensory and coping information that both lessened distress and allowed patients to exert control over the rate of swallowing the endoscopic tube. Baron and Logan (1993) replicated the basic effect, i.e. the combination of sensation monitoring and coping procedures reducing distress during endodontic treatment, and deepened our understanding of coping (action) by showing that distress is heightened when felt control is low only for patients who feel a need for control; patients who report having little control during this treatment do not report more pain and distress if they do not feel the need for control. Baron and Logan's approach could deepen our understanding of the selection of tactics for emotional control, as it is possible that the absence of felt need for, and felt ability to control emotion account for the use of expressive rather than control orientated procedures.

Individual differences in coping style

As individuals differ in the strategies and tactics they bring to stressful situations, it has been suggested that preparatory information may increase rather than reduce emotional distress during medical procedures (Langer, Janis & Wolfer, 1975). Miller (1987) has measured and contrasted two coping styles: monitoring or attending to noxious stimuli, and blunting or avoiding noxious cues. Patients disposed toward 'blunting' prefer to avoid threat cues and appear less distressed when allowed to do so. Patients disposed to 'monitor', on the other hand, prefer information to ignorance, though on some occasions, they report more distress and anxiety when information is provided. That sensory information reduces distress while individuals assessed as 'monitors' are more distressed with information, is somewhat puzzling unless one recognizes that 'monitors' may be of two types: some may attend to sensory cues to guide adaptation, and others may attend to their emotional reactions and catastrophize.

Timing of coping

The typical checklist used to assess coping (Did you do X, Y, Z, etc. when you were treated for cancer?) assumes that coping is consistent over the duration of a disease and/or treatment episode. This expectation is unreasonable as any medical problem consists of a sequence of changing episodes, and every episode consists of an unfolding series of differentiable experiences. The patient's place in time in the unfolding of a disease and set of treatments will affect the salience of different features of the illness representation. At the initial stage of diagnosis, a patient may be concerned with the causes of a disease and prevention, the focus shifting to duration, consequences and choice of treatment postdiagnosis. Shiloh, Larom and Ben-Rafael (1991) found that women viewed fertility treatments in terms of the currently used procedure when they were in treatment, while fertile controls viewed fertility treatments in relation to causes of infertility and the guilt caused by it.

Data show that different coping tactics may contribute to distress reduction in different phases of treatment. A study examining pain and distress during childbirth as a function of prior attendance at Lamaze classes and receipt of instructions to monitor or distract from the sensory experiences of labour contractions (Leventhal et al., 1989) found two different effects of prior preparation. Class attendance generated a sense of familiarity and security that reduced anxiety and anticipatory distress soon after admission to the labour suite: instructions by the physician to monitor the sensations of contractions had no effect at this time. But, monitoring instructions produced substantial reductions in pain and anger during the second, and most stressful stage of labour (delivery of the neonate), especially for the women who had attended Lamaze classes and were trained in coping (breathing and pushing). The control group given distraction instructions reported higher levels of pain and anger. The findings contradict the popular belief that distraction is the most effective way of dealing with painful procedures, and show that labour and delivery, as is true for other treatments, can be differentiated into stages which require different problem-based coping strategies.

Disagreement about the relative merits of monitoring and distraction as ways of coping with noxious treatments, led Suls and Fletcher (1985) to conduct a meta-analysis which examined the relative efficacy of these procedures at different points in time. As hypothesized, they found that distraction is superior to monitoring for relatively brief stressors, while monitoring has the advantage when adaptation requires prolonged self-management. Adaptation in the latter case clearly benefits from the accumulation of information needed to resolve ongoing medical problems.

FINAL ISSUES

Measurement

It would appear that the changing dynamics of illness and treatment create major difficulties for measurement if general questions are used to assess coping. As Stone et al. (1991) indicate, it is not clear what is measured even with situation-specific coping questionnaires: respondents may be referring to different stages in a stressful episode and to different aspects of a coping tactic (duration, frequency, usefulness, effort). But when Manne et al. (1994) used situational specific questions to assess coping with chemotherapy, contrary to their hypothesis, they did not find different correlates of distress any more than did studies taking a more general approach to coping assessment. They point out, however, that an individual may answer with respect to the disease or to different aspects of treatment (side-effects; limitations of daily activities, etc.) even when asked to concentrate on chemotherapy, making it difficult to study coping responses that are specific to this stressor for different patients. It may also be that the same general *strategies* influence coping at all stages of disease and treatment though different *tactics* stem from those strategies at different time points.

Social versus individual control

Carver and Scheier's (1981) analysis of coping procedures generated both a problem-focused and an emotion-focused factor for social support. That both problem and emotion control can be mediated by contact with others, is suggested by Kulik and Mahler's (1987) finding that preoperative coronary-bypass patients were less anxious prior to their operations, and recovered faster after the operation, if their room-mates were postoperative patients rather than patients who were also awaiting surgery. Interestingly, the similarity in the type of the operation had no effect on these outcomes. They suggest several mechanisms that may account for these effects: lower anxiety levels exhibited by the postoperative patient and his/her visitors; reassurance through concrete evidence that someone has 'made it through'; and exchange of sensory information and specific coping instructions. All of these may increase a person's feeling of control and enable him to direct his coping efforts more effectively. A concrete role model of a recovering person may enable the patient to view himself not only from the 'inside', which may intensify anxiety and fear before the procedure, but from the 'outside', envisioning himself in the same role, looking and feeling better from day to day. Both upward and downward social comparison can provide valuable information and modelling for managing stressful treatments (Taylor, 1983).

Synergism of problem and emotion control

Pigeonholing individuals and responses as problem or emotion focused ignores the integral quality of problem and emotion-focused coping; i.e. that virtually any coping response can function to manage a problem and to reduce affect, and the same individual will pursue both objectives when in a stressful setting. Thus, the effective problem-focused response reduces threat and emotion, and the effective emotion-focused response reduces emotion to facilitate problem solving. The success of the problem-based efforts is dependent upon parallel success in emotion control. When emotion control fails, and distress exceeds a certain criterion or dose level, further problem-focused coping may prove ineffective until the individual focuses on system management, so that the external information does not overwhelm the system and cause breakdown. As problem-focused coping can be costly in time and energy, especially with prolonged or repeated exposure to stressful procedures, an individual may develop a more deliberate and balanced alternation between problem-focused activity and the relief-time needed to replenish resources.

The theoretical framework of representation and coping with medical procedures sets the guidelines for planning interventions. Any intervention must interact with the ongoing process of constructing representations of the situation, planning and managing coping resources and setting appraisal rules and criteria. The intervention must take into account the highly uncertain nature of the situation. Uncertainty creates special demands both as a problem and as a source of anxiety and distress. The intervention must focus upon adaptation to the specific problem in the context in which it is encountered, and deal both with controlling the problem itself and with the emotional distress which it produces. The context is both problem specific and person specific, rendering it impractical to apply any intervention universally for patients undergoing a specific procedure. This specificity is responsible for failure to find simple effects of personality on distress. Personality factors, such as beliefs in control, have quite different effects on distress depending upon the time point in the disease history, e.g., beliefs in control associated with higher levels of distress upon the recurrence of a life threatening condition (Christiansen et al., 1991). Thus, interventions have to be adapted not only to answer the needs of the individual but to match the needs of the individual at a given point in time. Moreover a successful intervention should aim at both the procedure and its after-effects, resulting both in an enhanced ability to cope with the procedure and in better, more rapid recovery from it.

AKNOWLEDGEMENT

Preparation was supported by Grants AG03501 and AG12072 from the National Insititute on Aging.

REFERENCES

Andrykowski, M.A. (1990). The role of anxiety in the development of anticipatory nausea in cancer chemotherapy: a review and synthesis. *Psychosomatic Medicine*, **52**, 458–75.

Baron, R.S. & Logan, H. (1993). Desired control, felt control, and dental pain. *Motivation and Emotion*, **17**, 181–204.

Carver, C.S. & Scheier, M.F. (1981). *Attention and self-regulation: a control-theory approach to human behavior.* New York: Springer-Verlag.

Christiansen, A.J., Turner, C.W., Smith, T.W., Holman, J.M. & Gregory, M.C. (1991). Health locus of control and depression in end-stage renal disease. *Journal of Consulting and Clinical Psychology*, **59**, 419–24.

Cioffi, D. (1991). Beyond attentional strategies: a cognitive–perceptual model of somatic interpretation. *Psychological Bulletin*, **109**, 25–41.

Egbert, L.D., Battit, G.E., Welch, C.E. & Bartlett, M.K. (1964). Reduction of post operative pain by encouragement and instruction of patients. *New England Journal of Medicine*, **270**, 852–7.

Endler, N.S. & Parker, J.D.A. (1990). Multidimensional assessment of coping: a critical evaluation. *Journal of Personality and Social Psychology*, **58**, 844–54.

Folkman, S. & Lazarus, R.S. (1985). If it changes it must be a process: study of emotion and coping during three stages of a college examination. *Journal of Personality and Social Psychology*, **48**, 150–70.

Janis, I.L. & Leventhal, H. (1967). Human reactions to stress. In E. Borgatta & W. Lambert (Eds.). *Handbook of personality theory and research*, pp. 1041–1085. Chicago: Rand McNally.

Johnson, J.E. & Leventhal, H. (1974). Effects of accurate expectations and behavioral instructions on reactions during a noxious medical examination. *Journal of Personality and Social Psychology*, **29**, 710–18.

Johnston, M. (1980). Anxiety in surgical patients. *Psychological Medicine*, **10**, 145–52.

Krohne, H.W. (1993). In H.W. Krohne (Ed.). *Attention and avoidance: strategies in coping with aversiveness* pp.3–15. Seattle, WA: Hogrefe.

Kulik, J.A. & Mahler H.I.M. (1987). Effects of preoperative roommate assignment on preoperative anxiety and recovery from coronary-bypass surgery. *Health Psychology*, **6**, 525–43.

Langer, E.J., Janis, I.L. & Wolfer, J.A. (1975). Reduction of psychological stress in surgical patients. *Journal of Experimental Social Psychology*, **11**, 155–65.

Lazarus, R.S. & Launier, R. (1977). Stress-related transactions between person and environment. In L.A. Pervin & M. Lewis (Eds.). *Perspectives in interactional psychology*. New York: Plenum.

Leventhal, H., Easterling, D., Nerenz, D. & Love, R. (1988). The role of motion sickness in predicting anticipatory nausea. *Journal of Behavioral Medicine*, **11**, 117–30.

Leventhal, E.A., Leventhal H., Shacham, S. & Easterling, D.V. (1989). Active coping reduces reports of pain from childbirth. *Journal of Consulting and Clinical Psychology*, **57**, 365–71.

Leventhal, H., Leventhal, E.A. & Schaefer, P. (1991). Vigilant coping and health behavior: A life span problem. In M. Ory & R. Abeles (Eds.). *Aging. health, and behavior*, pp. 109–140. Baltimore: Johns Hopkin.

Leventhal, H. Diefenbach, M. & Leventhal, E.A. (1992). Illness cognition: using common sense to understand treatment adherence and affect cognition interactions. *Cognitive Therapy and Research*, **16**, 143–63.

Leventhal, E.A., Suls, J. & Leventhal, H. (1993). Hierarchical analysis of coping: evidence from life-span studies. In H.W. Krohne (Ed.). *Attention and avoidance: strategies in coping with aversiveness* pp. 71–99. Seattle, WA: Hogrefe.

Leventhal, H. (1970). Findings and theory in the study of fear communications. *Advances in Experimental Social Psychology*, **5**, 119–86.

Love, R.R., Leventhal, H., Easterling, D. & Nerenz, D. (1989). Side effects and emotional distress during cancer chemotherapy. *Cancer*, **63**, 604–12.

Manne, S.L., Sabbioni, M., Bovbjerg, D.H., Jacobsen, P.B., Taylor, K.I. & Redd, W.H. (1994). Coping with chemotherapy for breast cancer. *Journal of Behavioral Medicine*, **17**, 41–55.

Miller, S. (1987). Monitoring and blunting: validation of a questionnaire to assess styles of information seeking under threat. *Journal of Personality and Social Psychology*, **52**, 345–53.

Nerenz, D.R., Leventhal, H., Easterling, D.V. & Love, R.R. (1986). Anxiety and drug taste as predictors of anticipatory nausea in cancer chemotherapy. *Journal of Clinical Oncology*, **4**, 224–33.

Shiloh, S., Larom, S. & Ben-Raphael, Z. (1991). The meaning of treatments for infertility: cognitive determinants and structure. *Journal of Applied Social Psychology*, **21**, 855–74.

Stone, A.A, Greenberg, M.A., Kennedy-Moore, E. & Newman, M.G. (1991). Self-report, situation-specific coping questionnaires: what are they measuring? *Journal of Personality and Social Psychology*, **61**, 648–58.

Suls, J. & Fletcher, B. (1985). The relative efficacy of avoidant and non-avoidant coping strategies: a meta-analysis. *Health Psychology*, **4**, 249–88.

Taylor, S.E. (1983). Adjustment to threatening events: a theory of cognitive adaptation. *American Psychologist*, **38**, 1161–73.

Cultural and ethnic factors in health

JOHN W. BERRY

Department of Psychology, and School of Rehabilitation Therapy, Kinston, Canada

INTRODUCTION

Understanding how cultural and ethnic factors relate to health is very much an interdisciplinary enterprise: anthropology, biology, economics, history, medicine, nursing, psychiatry, psychology, rehabilitation and sociology have all participated in the study and application of their own concepts and findings to health. The focus of this chapter, however, will be on the contributions of anthropology ('medical anthropology': see e.g. Foster & Anderson, 1978, Helman, 1990), psychiatry ('transcultural psychiatry': see e.g. Kleinman, 1980; Murphy, 1981; Yap, 1974) and psychology ('cross-cultural psychology': see, e.g. Dasen, Berry & Sartorius, 1988). In particular, because of the placement of this chapter in a Section on 'Psychology, health and illness', and the background of the author, the approach will be from the perspective of cross-cultural health psychology (Berry, 1997.

The field of cross-cultural health psychology can be divided into two related domains. The earlier, and more established, domain is the study of how cultural factors influence various aspects of health. This enterprise has taken place around the globe, driven by the need to understand individual and community health in the context of the indigenous cultures of the people being examined and served. The second, more recent and very active, domain is the study of the health of individuals and groups as they settle into, and adapt to, new cultural circumstances, as a result of their migration, and the persistence of their original cultures in the form of ethnicity. This enterprise has taken place in culturally plural societies where there is a need to understand and better serve an increasingly diverse population. This separation into work across cultures (internationally) and with ethnic groups within societies is a common one in the field of cross-cultural psychology more generally (Berry *et al.*, 1992). Despite this division, it is a common position that the methods, theories and findings derived from the international enterprise should inform the domestic enterprise. That is, immigrants and members of ethnic communities should be understood and served in culturally informed ways, and not simply categorized and treated as 'minorities'.

CULTURAL DOMAIN

The broad, international and comparative work linking culture and health has been carried out by medical anthropology, transcultural psychiatry and cross-cultural health psychology. Much of this work has resulted from the collaboration of medical, social and behavioural scientists. The field is thus inherently an interdisciplinary one, and is concerned with all aspects of health: physical, social and psychological.

Three orientations

In this large and complex body of work, three theoretical orientations can be discerned: absolutism, relativism and universalism (Berry *et al.*, 1992).

The absolutist position is one that assumes that human phenomena are basically the same (qualitatively) in all cultures: 'honesty' is 'honesty' and 'depression' is 'depression', no matter where one observes it. From the absolutist perspective, culture is thought to play little or no role in either the meaning or display of human characteristics. Assessments of such characteristics are made using standard instruments (perhaps with linguistic translation) and interpretations are made easily, without alternative culturally based views taken into account.

In sharp contrast, the relativist approach is rooted in anthropology, and assumes that all human behaviour is culturally patterned. It seeks to avoid ethnocentrism by trying to understand people 'in their own terms'. Explanation of human diversity is sought in the cultural context in which people have developed. Assessments are typically carried out employing the values and meanings a cultural group gives to a phenomenon. Comparisons are judged to be problematic and ethnocentric, and are thus virtually never made.

A third perspective, one that lies somewhat between the two positions, is that of universalism. Here it is assumed that basic human characteristics are common to all members of the species (i.e. constituting a set of biological givens), and that culture influences the development and display of them (i.e. culture plays different variations on these underlying themes). Assessments are based on the presumed underlying process, but measures are developed in culturally meaningful versions. Comparisons are made cautiously, employing a wide variety of methodological principles and safeguards, and interpretations of similarities and differences are attempted that take alternative culturally based meanings into account.

Table 1. *Eight areas of interest in the relationship between culture and individual health*

Level of analysis	Categories of health phenomena			
	Cognitive	Affective	Behavioural	Social
Community (cultural)	Conceptions and definitions	Norms and values	Practices and customs	Roles and institutions
Individual (psychological)	Beliefs and knowledge	Attitudes	Behaviours	Interpersonal relationships

Intersection of Culture and Health

Perhaps the most comprehensive exposition of the way in which culture can influence health and disease was presented by Murphy (1982). He proposed that cultural factors can affect the following aspects: definition, recognition, symptomatology, prevalence, and response (by society or healer).

Numerous studies have shown that the very concepts of health and disease are defined differently across cultures; this basic link between culture and health was recognized early (Polgar, 1962) and has continued up to the present time (Helman, 1985, 1990, Ch. 2). The concept of health has recently undergone rapid change in international thought, witness the WHO emphases on the existence of (positive) wellbeing, and not only on the absence of (negative) disease or disability. Of special interest here is the existence of 'culture-bound syndromes' that appear to be unique to one (or a few) cultures (Simons & Hughes, 1985).

Recognition of some condition as healthy or as a disease is also linked to culture. Some activities such as trance are recognized as important curing (health-seeking) mechanisms in some cultures, but may be classified as psychiatric disorder in others (Ward, 1989). Similarly, the expression of a condition through the exhibition of various symptoms has also been linked to cultural norms (Zola, 1966). For example, it is claimed by many (e.g. Kleinman, 1982; Kirmayer, 1984) that psychological problems are expressed somatically in some cultures (e.g. Chinese) more than in other cultures.

Prevalence studies across cultures have produced very clear evidence that disease and disability are highly variable. From heart disease (Marmot & Syme, 1976) (Prener *et al.*, 1991), to schizophrenia (Murphy, 1982), cultural factors such as traditional diets, substance abuse, and social relationships within the family all contribute to the prevalence of disease.

The response by society generally (and within society, by the healer) to ill health also varies across cultures. Acceptance or rejection of persons with particular diseases (such as leprosy or AIDS) has changed over time, and differs between cultures. Healing practices, based on variations in medicines and beliefs about causation have wide variation in the treatment of both physical and psychological disorder (Murphy, 1981; Yap, 1974).

An attempt has been made to link culture to health, drawing upon some established conceptual distinctions in the behaviourial sciences by Berry (1989). In Table 1 are four categories of health phenomena, and two levels of analyses (community and individual). Crossing the two dimensions produces eight areas in which information can be sought during the study of links between culture and individual health. The community level of work typically involves ethnographic methods, and yields a general characterization of shared health conceptions, values, practices and institutions in a society.

The individual level of work involves the psychological study of a sample of individuals from the society, and yields information about individual differences (and similarities), which can lead to inferences about the psychological underpinings of individual health beliefs, attitudes, behaviours, and relationships.

The reason for taking cultural level health phenomena into account is so that the broad context for the development and display of individual health phenomena can be established; without an understanding of this background context, attempts to deal with individuals and their health problems may well be useless, even harmful. The reason for considering individual level phenomena is that not all persons hold the same beliefs or attitudes, nor do they engage in the same behaviours and relationships; without an understanding of their individual variations from the general community situation, harm may well, again, be inflicted.

Examples of work in the eight areas of interest are common in the research and professional literature. At the cultural level, as we have already seen in relation to Murphy's ideas, the way in which a cultural group defines what is health and what is not, can vary substantially from group to group. These collective cognitive phenomena include shared conceptions, and categories, as well as definitions of health and disease. At the individual level, health beliefs and knowledge, while influenced by the cultural conceptions, can also vary from person to person. Beliefs about what causes an illness or disability, or about how much control one has over it (both getting it and curing it) shows variation across individuals and cultures (Berry *et al.*, 1994). For example, in one community, the general belief is that if pregnant women eat too much (or even 'normally') there will be insufficient room for the foetus to develop; hence, undereating is common, and prenatal malnutrition results, with an associated increase in infant disability. However, there are variations across individuals in this belief, with education, status and participation in public health programmes making a difference.

With respect to affective phenomena, the value placed on health is known to vary from culture to culture, and within cultures across subgroups. For example, Judaic Law prescribes that health is given by God, and it is the responsibility of the individual to sustain it; the value placed on good health is thus a shared belief among practising Jews. However, there is significant variation in the acceptance of this value across three Jewish groups; Orthodox Jews have the highest value, Reformed Jews have a lower value, and Secular Jews have an even lower value on health (Dayan, 1993). And, within the three groups, there are further variations according to a number of personal and demographic factors.

Health practices and behaviours also vary across cultures and individuals. For example, with respect to nutrition (Dasen & Super, 1988), what is classified as suitable food, and who can eat it are matters of cultural practice. Many high protein 'foods' are not placed in the food category (e.g. grubs, brains) and avoided, while in other

[99]

cultures they are an important part of the diet. Within these general cultural practices, however, individuals vary in what they can eat, depending on age, status or food factors related to clan membership. The social organization of health activities into instructions, and the allocation of roles (e.g. healer, patient) is also known to vary across cultures. In some cultures, religious or gender issues affect the role of healer (e.g. only those with certain spiritual qualities, or only males, may become a healer), while in others, the high cost of medical or other health professional training limits the roles to the wealthy. In some cultures, health services are widely available and fully integrated into the fabric of community life (e.g. Averasturi, 1988) while in others, doctors and hospitals are remote, mysterious and alien to most of the population. In the former case, individual patient–healer relationships may be collegial, in which a partnership is established to regain health, while in the latter, the relationship is likely to be hierarchical, involving the use of authority and compliance.

Psychosocial Factors

A second approach to understanding individual health in a broader context has been through the conceptualization and measurement of psychosocial factors (WHO, 1992). While these factors are not usually seen as 'cultural', a case can be made that all known psychosocial factors are also cultural factors, in the sense that they vary substantially across cultures. Hence they have to be treated as cultural variables, and be understood in terms of local cultural beliefs, values and behaviours. This position was advocated early (WHO, 1982):

> psychosocial factors have been increasingly recognized as key factors in the success of health and social actions. If actions are to be effective in the prevention of diseases and in the promotion of health and well being, they must be based on an understanding of culture, tradition, beliefs and patterns of family interaction (p. 4).

Most of these psychosocial factors (WHO, 1992) are known to vary across cultures. For example, the psychosocial factor of specific behaviour patterns (such as the Type A/Type B distinction, or 'burn out') is probably more prevalent in western industrial cultures. Similarly, the influence of life style (including a diet of 'fast foods'), is also likely to be a factor in some societies and not in others. A third psychosocial factor, that of problems of person–environment fit is obviously linked to culture (as a fundamental 'environment'). In particular, the acculturation problems of immigrants and refugees are identified by WHO; these, we will be considering in detail later in the 'ethnic' section.

Three of the psychosocial factors refer to excessive stress (relating to close social relations, to the work place, and to broader sociated settings). Problems with family and friends are likely to vary according to family organization and type (monogamous/polygamous; endogamous/exogamous; nuclear/extended; matrilineal/patrilineal; matrilocal/patrilocal, etc.). Since these are core contrasts in the ethnographic literature, the type and extent of such problems will likely be linked to their cultural variations. Similarly, the work place (the hunt, the garden, the pasture, the factory, the office, the unemployment line), and broader social conditions (poverty, war, famine, imprisonment, being the victim of crime or racism) all plausibly vary from culture to culture.

Finally, in the WHO list of psychosocial factors, are health hazards and protective factors that are present in one's social environment, including: on the one hand, malnutrition, unsafe settings where accidents are likely to occur, and iatrogenic factors; and, on the other, social support and health promotion programmes.

The degree of cultural variation in the psychosocial factors is plausibly very high, but as yet the extent is not known. It is proposed that such cultural variations be the focus of concerted research.

ETHNIC DOMAIN

When we focus on the health of culturally distinct groups and individuals who live in culturally plural societies, we are dealing with the ethnic domain. By 'ethnic' is meant those phenomena that are derived from fully independent cultures; ethnic groups operate with an evolving culture that flows from their original heritage culture, in interaction with the culture of the larger (dominant) society.

Approach to Ethnicity

While ethnic groups are not full-scale or independent cultural groups, it is a working belief of cross-cultural psychology that all the methodological, theoretical and substantive lessons learned from working with cultural groups in the international enterprise should inform our work with ethnic groups. That is, we need to know about both their community health conceptions, values, practices and institutions, and about how these are distributed as health beliefs, attitudes, behaviours and interpersonal relationships among individual members of the ethnic groups.

Put another way, we are not dealing with 'minorities' that are simply deviant from some 'mainstream', but with communities that deserve to have their health, and health needs, understood just as well as any other cultural community. In this sense, work on health in the ethnic domain does not differ in principle from work in the cultural domain. However, there is now an important new element, that of contact and possibly conflict, between cultural groups; this is the case in a number of respects: first, the health phenomena of ethnic individuals may be quite different from those of the larger society, and create misunderstanding, confusion and conflict between the two groups; secondly, these conflicts may themselves generate health problems; and thirdly, the health services of the larger society may not be sufficiently informed, or sensitive, to enable them to deal with either the health problems that are linked to the heritage of the ethnic group, or those that have their roots in the conflict between the two groups in contact. Since the first of these issues is very similar to the discussion of the cultural domain, it will not be pursued further here. However, there is one important difference: when a health professional does not understand an individual's health needs while practising in another country, at least the individual may have recourse to an indigenous health system; when this lack of understanding occurs with respect to an ethnic individual, there may no longer be such an alternative service of health support. The second and third issues can be considered using the notions of acculturative stress, and multicultural health.

Acculturative Stress

In the literature on the health and well-being of ethnic groups and individuals, there was an earlier assumption that the experience of culture contact and change will always be stressful, and lead to loss of health status. As is the case for other forms of stress (as one psychosocial factor), this assumption is no longer supported; to understand why there are variable outcomes to culture contact, the notions of acculturation and acculturation strategies need to be introduced.

Acculturation was first identified as a cultural level phenomenon by anthropologists (e.g. Redfield, Linton & Herskovits, 1936) who defined it as culture change resulting from contact between two autonomous cultural groups. Acculturation is also an individual level phenomenon, requiring individual members of both the larger society and immigrants to work out new forms of relationships in their daily lives. This idea was introduced by Graves (1967), who has proposed the notion of 'psychological acculturation' to refer to these new behaviours and strategies. One of the findings of subsequent research in this area is that there are vast individual differences in how people attempt to deal with acculturative change (termed 'acculturation strategies'). These strategies have three aspects: their preferences ('acculturation attitudes'; Berry *et al.*, 1989); how much change they actually undergo ('behavioural shifts'; Berry, 1980); and how much of a problem these changes are for them (the phenomenon of 'acculturative stress'; see Berry *et al.*, 1987).

Perhaps the most useful way to identify the various orientations individuals may have toward acculturation is to note that two issues predominate in the daily life of most acculturating individuals. One pertains to the maintenance and development of one's ethnic distinctiveness in society, deciding whether or not one's own cultural identity and customs are of value and should be retained. The other issue involves the desirability of interethnic contact, deciding whether relations with other groups in the lager society are of value and should be sought. These two issues are essentially questions of values, and may be responded to on a continuous scale, from positive to negative. For conceptual purposes, however, they can be treated as dichotomous ('yes' and 'no') preferences, thus generating a fourfold model. Each cell in this fourfold classification is considered to be an acculturation strategy or option available to individuals and to groups in plural societies, towards which individuals may hold attitudes; these are assimilation, integration, separation, and marginalization.

When the first question is answered 'no' and the second is answered 'yes', the assimilation option is defined, namely, relinquishing one's cultural identity and moving into the larger society. This can take place by way of absorption of a non-dominant group into an established dominant group, as in the 'melting pot' concept.

The integration option (answering 'yes' to both questions) implies the maintenance of the cultural integrity of the group, as well as the movement by the group to become an integral part of a larger societal framework. In this case, there is a large number of distinguishable ethnic groups, all co-operating within a larger social system, resulting in the 'mosaic' concept.

When there are no relations desired with the larger society, and this is accompanied by a wish to maintain ethnic identity and tradition, another option is defined. Depending upon which group (the dominant or non-dominant) controls the situation, this option may take the form either of segregation or separation. When the pattern is imposed by the dominant group, classic segregation to 'keep people in their place' appears. On the other hand, the maintenance

of a traditional way of life outside full participation in the lager society may derive from a group's desire to lead an independent existence, as in the case of separatist movements. In these terms, segregation and separation differ primarily with respect to which group or groups have the power to determine the outcome.

Finally, there is an option (answering 'no' to both questions) that is difficult to define precisely, possibly because it is accompanied by a good deal of collective and individual confusion and anxiety. It is characterized by striking out against the larger society and by feelings of alienation, loss of identity, and by acculturative stress. This option is marginalization, in which groups lose cultural and psychological contact with both their traditional culture and the larger society.

Inconsistencies and conflicts between various acculturation strategies are one of many sources of difficulty for acculturating individuals. Generally, when acculturation experiences cause problems for acculturating individuals, we observe the phenomenon of acculturative stress. In an overview of this area of research (Berry *et al.*, 1987), it was argued that stress may arise, but it is not inevitable. Or as Beiser *et al.* (1988) have phrased it: migrant status is a mental health risk factor; but risk is not destiny.

There are three concepts involved in understanding the appearance of acculturative stress. First, acculturation occurs in a particular situation (e.g. ethnic community), and individuals participate in and experience these changes to varying degrees; thus, individual acculturation experience may vary from a great deal to rather little. Secondly, stressors may result from this varying experience of acculturation; for some people, acculturative changes may all be in the form of stressors, while for others, they may be benign or even seen as opportunities. And thirdly, varying levels of acculturative stress and health problems may become manifest as a result of one's inability to cope with acculturation experience and stressors.

Results of studies of acculturative stress have varied widely in the level of difficulties found in acculturating groups and individuals. Early views were that culture contact and change inevitably led to acculturative stress; however, current views (Berry, 1992) are that stress is linked to acculturation in a probabilistic way, and the level of stress experienced will depend on a number of factors, such host society prejudice, coping resources and strategies, education, acculturation strategies and national policies dealing with the issue of cultural diversity.

Research in a number of countries has typically revealed variations in, but sometimes no greater acculturative stress or mental health problems among ethnic groups than in the general population (Beiser *et al.*, 1988). However, stress is usually lower when: integration is being sought (but is highest for marginalization); migration was voluntary (i.e. for immigrants) rather than forced (i.e. for refugees); there is a functioning social support group (i.e. an ethnic community willing to assist during the settlement process); and when tolerance for diversity and ethnic attitudes in the larger society are positive (Berry, 1992).

In summary, the health outcomes for acculturating individuals are highly variable, and depend on a variety of factors that are under the control of policy makers. Stress, with resultant poor health, can be avoided if certain steps are taken. One of these, to which we now turn, is the development of a pluralistic health care system, one that is knowledgeable about, and sensitive to the health needs of ethnic groups and individuals.

Multicultural Health

Essentially, the area of multicultural health involves research and action directed toward improving the level of understanding and quality of services available to ethnic groups and individuals who now live in culturally plural societies (Beiser *et al.*, 1988).

The research component is driven by the work in the cultural domain, and on acculturative stress, and should result in better understanding of the health, and health needs of ethnic groups. To many observers, it is obvious why this research should be undertaken: it is unethical to presume to provide health service to people one does not understand; it is inequitable to train health service providers to know the needs of only part of the population; and it is unjust (especially in countries with a tax-supported health system) to allocate all of the resources to assist only some of the people.

The action component is directed towards changing the health institutions of the larger society, and the beliefs, attitudes, behaviours and relationships of members of the larger society with respect to these issues. That is, the same framework employed earlier to outline areas of interest in the relationship between culture and health can guide the actions that are required.

To provide one example (from Canada), there is a national organization that promotes the need for multicultural health, with active member organizations in every Province. It advocates curriculum change, in all health education programmes, to more fully portray the role of culture and ethnicity in health; it provides in-service workshops on issues of ethnocentrism and racism, and on the special needs of immigrants and refugees; and it promotes awareness in the ethnic communities of their rights to health, and how to gain access to better health care.

Many of these and related activities are supported by governments, in recognition of the value, not only of pluralism, but of healthy pluralism. Experience in many countries suggests that diverse populations can be denied basic services such as health only to a certain extent, and only for a limited period, before social pathologies become manifest, and the health status of all deteriorate further.

CONCLUSIONS

This chapter has ranged widely over a number of disciplines, across and within cultures, and from research to action advocacy. Despite this diversity, there is a set of core ideas: cultures vary in their understanding and treatment of health; individuals also vary both across and within cultures; this dual variation needs to be taken into account whether working internationally, or with ethnic groups domestically.

It is well understood that health and disease are complex phenomena, and that they are multidetermined. This chapter has necessarily added to this complexity by focusing on the role of cultural and ethnic factors, but it also has attempted to present a systematic account of their relationships, along with what we already know, and what we should, but do not yet know and do. (See also 'Gender issues and health' and 'Lay beliefs about health and illness.')

ACKNOWLEDGEMENT

This chapter was prepared while the author was a Visiting Scholar at the Research Centre for Health Promotion, and Department of Psychosocial Science, University of Bergen, Norway.

REFERENCES

Averasturi, L. (1988). Psychosocial factors in health: the Cuban model. In P. Dasen, J.W. Berry & N. Sartorius (Eds.). *Health and cross-cultural psychology: towards applications*. London: Sage.

Beiser, M., Barwick, C., Berry, J.W. et al. (1988). *After the door has been opened: report of taskforce on mental health issues affecting immigrants and refugees*. Ottawa: Health and Welfare and Multiculturalism and Citizenship.

Berry, J.W. (1980). Social and cultural change. In H.C. Triandis & R. Brislin (Eds). *Handbook of cross-cultural psychology, Vol 5, Social*. Boston: Allyn & Bacon.

Berry, J.W. (1989). The role of cross-cultural psychology in understanding community-based health. In M. Peat (Ed.). *Community-based rehabilitation: science and practice*. Kingston: Queen's University School of Rehabilitation Therapy.

Berry, J.W. (1992). Acculturation and adaptation in a new society. *International Migration*, 30, 69–85.

Berry, J.W. (1997). Immigration, acculturation and adaptation. Cross-cultural health *Applied Psychology* (in press).

Berry, J.W., Kim, U., Minde, T. & Mok, D.

(1987). Comparative studies of acculturative stress. *International Migration Review*, 21, 491–511.

Berry, J.W., Kim, U., Power, S., Young, M. & Bujaki, M. (1989). Acculturation attitudes in plural societies. *Applied Psychology*, 38, 185–206.

Berry, J.W., Poortinga, Y.H., Segall, M.H. & Dasen, P. (1992). *Cross-cultural Psychology: research and applications*. New York: Cambridge University Press.

Berry, J.W., Dalal, A., Pande, N. et al. (1994). *Disability beliefs, attitudes and behaviours across cultures*. Report from International Center for the Advancement of Community Based Rehabilitation. Kingston: Queen's University.

Dasen, P. & Super, C. (1988). The usefulness of a cross-cultural approach in studies of malnutrition and psychological development. In P. Dasen, J.W. Berry & N. Sartorius (Eds). *Health and cross-cultural psychology: towards applications*. London: Sage.

Dasen, P.R., Berry, J.W. & Sartorius, N. (Eds.). (1988). *Health and cross-cultural psychology: towards applications*. London: Sage.

Dayan, J. (1993). Health values, beliefs and behaviours of Orthodox, Reformed and Secular Jews. Unpublished MA thesis, Queen's University at Kingston.

Foster, G. & Anderson, B. (1978). *Medical anthropology*. New York: Wiley.

Graves, T. (1967). Psychological acculturation in a triethnic community. *Southwestern Journal of Anthropology*, 23, 337–50.

Helman, C. (1985). Psyche, soma and society: the social construction of psychosomatic disorders. *Culture, Medicine and Psychiatry*, 9, 1–26.

Helman, C. (1990). *Culture, health and illness*. London: Wright.

Kirmayer, L. (1984). Culture, affect and somatization. *Transcultural Psychiatric Research Review*, 21, 139–58; 237–62.

Kleinman, A. (1980). *Patients and healers in the context of culture*. Berkeley: University of California Press.

Kleinman, A. (1982). Neurasthenia and depression: a study of somatization and culture in China. *Culture, Medicine and Psychiatry*, 6, 117–90.

Marmot, M. & Syme, S.L. (1976). Acculturation and coronary heart disease in Japanese Americans. *American Journal of Epidemiology*, 104, 225–47.

Murphy, H.B.M. (1981). *Comparative psychiatry*. Berlin: Springer-Verlag.

Murphy, H.B.M. (1982). Culture and Schizophrenia. In I. Al-Issa (Ed.). *Culture and Psychopathology*. Baltimore: University Park Press.

Polgar, S. (1962). Health and human behaviour: areas of common interest to the social and medical sciences. *Current Anthropology*, **2**, 159–205.

Prener, A., Hojgaard-Nielson, N., Storm, H. & Hart Hansen, J.P. (1991). *Cancer in Greenland: 1953–1985*. Acta Pathologica,

Microbiologica et Immunologica Scandinavica, 99, Suppl. 20.

Redfield, R., Linton, R. & Herskovits, M.J. (1936). Memorandum on the study of acculturation. *American Anthropologist*, **38**, 149–52.

Simons, R. & Hughes, C. (Eds.). (1985). *The culture-bound syndromes*. Dordrecht: Reidel.

Stonequist, E. (1937). *The marginal man*. New York: Scribner.

Ward, C. (Ed.). (1989). *Altered states of consciousness and mental health*. London: Sage.

WHO (1982). *Medium term programme*. Geneva: WHO.

WHO (1992). *The ICD-10 Classification of mental and behaviourial disorders: clinical descriptions and diagnostic guidelines*. Geneva: WHO.

Yap, P.M. (1974). *Comparative psychiatry*. Toronto: University of Toronto Press.

Zola, I. (1966). Culture and symptoms: an analysis of patients' presenting symptoms. *American Sociological Review*, **31**, 615–30.

Emotional expression and health

KATHRYN P. DAVISON
Department of Psychology,
Southern Methodist University,
Dallas, Texas, USA

KEITH J. PETRIE
Department of Psychiatry and
Behavioural Science, University of
Auckland Medical School,
New Zealand

The experience and expression of emotion represent potent and fundamental aspects of the individual's social life. Within the social context, the individual is both a sender and receiver of emotional communication through verbal and non-verbal channels. Unexpressed jealousy, advertised joy, thinly veiled anger and overt disgust represent just a few examples of the grades and varieties of emotional display that colour social relations on a daily basis. There are obviously large individual differences in the experience and reporting of emotion, and it may be that individual strategies for regulating emotional expression have effects on health. This chapter reviews the measurement issues involved in identifying emotional expression and summarizes the recent findings in the both short-term laboratory investigations and longer-term studies of emotional experience and health.

CAPTURING EMOTIONAL EXPRESSION

Emotion represents one of the most intriguing and yet elusive aspects of personality and social dynamics. The experience of emotion is fleeting and its public manifestations are limited by the regulation processes of the individual. Valid measurement of the emotional experience is subject to the vagaries of timing and by individual differences in reporting. Conceptualizations of individual sensitivity to emotional experience have classically distinguished between the 'repressor' on the one extreme, considered to have a heightened recognition threshold for anxiety-producing stimuli and the 'sensitizer' on the other extreme, whose sensitivity to emotion is high (Byrne, 1961; Weinberger, Schwartz & Davidson, 1979). Questionnaire measures of these constructs include Byrne's Repression-

Sensitization Scale (1961), the Self-Concealment Scale (Larson & Chastain, 1990), and the contrast of scores on the Taylor Manifest Anxiety and Marlowe-Crowne Social Desirability Scales (Weinberger, 1990). A slightly different approach has been used by King and Emmons (1990), who compared and contrasted scores on self-reports of emotional expressiveness (EEQ) with those of ambivalence over emotional expression (AEQ).

Convincing arguments have been made, outlining the pitfalls of relying solely on questionnaire measures to measure psychological styles and mental health (e.g. Shedler, Mayman & Manis, 1993), so it has been incumbent upon researchers to assess the range of emotional experience and expressiveness across a number of verbal and non-verbal channels. Social psychophysiologists have been successful in identifying nervous system correlates of particular emotions and emotional expression (Ekman, Levenson & Friesen, 1983). One effective strategy based on this approach has been to identify a repressive style through self-reports of low distress with autonomic measures that show indications of increased anxiety or stress such as skin conductance and heart rate (Pennebaker & Chew, 1985; Sackheim & Gur, 1979). Other approaches to the measurement of expression or expressiveness have included judges' ratings of facial and vocal characteristics of videotaped interviews; analysis of language usage that features emotionally relevant words; and objective signals of emotion such as crying, blushing, and smiling or laughing.

A third approach to the evaluation of emotional expression and its effects is through manipulations designed to induce emotional states in the subjects. These strategies include the use of method-trained actors imagining hypothetical situations, the induction of emotion under hypnosis, requests that subjects recall or write about emotionally potent aspects of their personal histories, and other procedures that mimic the psychotherapeutic process and inherently involve emotional expression.

Research into the effects of emotional expression and health has a brief history and draws on a wide range of methodologies. In the next section we first discuss emotion and the body from a relatively microscopic perspective: that is, measurable effects of laboratory-induced states occurring over a period of minutes or seconds. We then shift to the broader perspective of emotional expression and its links with health, disease, and mortality.

SHORT-TERM INVESTIGATIONS OF EMOTIONAL EXPRESSION AND HEALTH

The evidence that distinct emotions are accompanied by distinct autonomic patterns, and that extensive communication occurs between the nervous and immune systems points to the potentially instrumental role of the emotions in health processes. However, few published studies have investigated the effect of emotional experience on immune function. Knapp *et al.* (1992) asked healthy volunteers to recall and re-experience disturbing emotional experiences under conditions of cardiovascular, video, and immunological monitoring via catheterization. They reported that the induction of negative mood was associated with poorer lymphocyte response to challenge particularly related to the experience of anxiety. They also reported that brief increases in Natural Killer Cell Activity were associated with the experience of sadness. Futterman *et al.* (1992) observed no significant differences from before, to during, induction of emotional state using method-trained actors, except a slight trend towards greater circulation of NK cells during the negative emotion period. The authors concluded that small subject numbers and the lack of personal memory might have contributed to the lack of direction of the findings. Overall, these findings suggest that even relatively brief experiences of emotion can modestly affect the trafficking and functional quality of immune cells, and that the immune system's relationship to psychological states is not unidimensional.

The effects of expressed versus unexpressed emotion are somewhat less clearcut. A simple way to conceptualize emotional expression is to divide it between those who do express emotions and those who do not. The problem, however, lies in understanding the experience of the group who are not expressing emotion: is it because of some strategy of suppression or inhibition, or for some other reason such as not experiencing a particular emotion? Drawing conclusions based on non-behaviour is a risky business.

To address this problem, Weinberger *et al.* (1979) divided subjects according to their scores on the Taylor Manifest Anxiety Scale and the Marlowe-Crowne Social Desirability Scale, with those reporting low anxiety but high levels of defensiveness classified as 'repressors', and those reporting low anxiety and low levels of defensiveness as true low-anxious. Those who scored high on anxiety were classified as either high-anxious or defensive high-anxious, according to their levels of defensiveness. Those subjects classified as repressors exhibited higher levels of autonomic activity in the form of resting EMG activity and skin conductance. The same findings were offered by Sackheim and Gur (1979), who reported that they found an inverse relationship between self-reports of disturbance and physiological activity, particularly skin conductance.

Individuals who employ a repressive coping style have also been found to have slower learning times regarding the use of provocative material, slower reaction times to emotion-relevant stimuli, and impoverished access to emotionally relevant memories, suggesting that a general strategy of blunting unpleasant thoughts and feelings is indeed occurring, whether consciously or unconsciously (for a review see Barger, 1995).

Labott *et al.* (1990) examined effects of either inhibiting or expressing laughter or weeping in subjects who watched humorous or sad films. The humorous film resulted in higher levels of the antibody IgA, regardless of expressive condition; while the sad film resulted in lower levels of IgA only for those who overtly wept. Thus, immune effects of emotional expression appear to also vary according to the type or valence of emotion.

Short-term studies of the physiology of emotional expression are largely based on the premise that longer-term, chronic experiences of such states would contribute in a meaningful way to the pathogenesis and/or progression of disease. As yet, there are very few investigations that have examined both short-term physiology and their relationship to long-term health outcomes. Such comprehensive approaches would supply valuable information about the generalizability of laboratory studies of emotion.

BROADER INVESTIGATIONS OF EXPRESSION AND HEALTH

It is useful to bear in mind that different motivating factors may underlie levels of emotional expressiveness, and that such factors may impact on health in different ways. For example, individual differences such as shyness and extroversion may mediate expressiveness differently from event-driven motivations like shame or embarrassment surrounding the experience of rape, incest, war, or unethical conduct. Other motives include environmental considerations such as professionalism, interpersonal attitudes like suspicious defensiveness, and value systems that discount emotional experience. Insufficient work has been done in this area to adequately assess the distinct roles of these factors in health processes, and certainly the factors are not mutually exclusive; but some studies have fruitfully examined these relationships. Jerome Kagan and his colleagues have investigated a number of aspects of individuals classified as extremely shy. Observations of children who are socially and behaviourally inhibited have revealed that this group shows a greater autonomic reactivity to stress than others, as well as a significantly greater incidence of allergic rhinitis (Bell *et al.*, 1990). Social anxiety was also a significant factor in the follow-up findings of the Harvard Mastery Study, a 35-year longitudinal investigation of psychological and physical factors predicting health and illness (Russek *et al.*, 1990).

The repressive coping style, which appears to involve a more unconscious level of emotional inhibition, has most frequently been associated with the onset and progression of cancer (Gross, 1989). A number of studies have found that a repressive personality style was significantly associated with poorer NK cell activity, the index of immune function most directly implicated in the surveillance and destruction of tumours (Levy *et al.*, 1985), a diagnosis of malignancy (Greer & Morris, 1975), a poorer disease prognosis (Jensen, 1987), and death from cancer (Pettingale *et al.*, 1985).

Schwartz (1983, 1990) has advanced a model of repression and disregulation based on general systems theory and cybernetics that integrates findings from biofeedback, neuroendocrinology, and psychology. In brief, the theory asserts that disattention to signals of distress results in physical disregulation due to cortical overriding of immunoregulatory homeostatic mechanisms. Temoshok (1987) has proposed a model of the cancer prone individual based on a constellation of psychological traits that seemed to be consistent with a diagnosis of cancer and poor disease prognosis. She identified this 'Type C' personality as having three central characteristics, namely: stoicism, a difficulty in expressing emotions, and an attitude of resignation or helplessness/hopelessness. The findings overall have been mixed, leading researchers as a whole to treat the notion of the repression-cancer link with some scepticism (Anderson, Kiecolt-Glaser & Glaser, 1994).

If repression and inhibition are associated with increased vulnerability to illness, it stands to reason that measures to induce openness and emotional expression would serve to enhance health. It is now well known that a number of psychologically stressful events are associated with poorer immune function and increased incidence of illness (Kennedy, Kiecolt-Glaser & Glaser, 1988). Moreover, there is also evidence that events which are difficult to discuss with others, such as sexual abuse, may have more pervasive health effects than other difficulties (Golding et al., 1988; Pennebaker & Susman, 1988).

Over the past decade, James Pennebaker and colleagues have operationalized a kind of confessional setting, in which subjects are ushered to a small private room and asked to write about the most upsetting event of their entire lives. The procedure is repeated over three or four consecutive days for periods of approximately 20 minutes. More recent investigations have employed a computerized system of autonomic recording as subjects type their stories at a computer terminal. Pennebaker and Beall (1986) found that subjects who wrote their thoughts and feelings about upsetting events showed reduced health centre visits over the follow-up period compared to subjects who wrote in thoughts-only and feelings-only conditions. Pennebaker, Kiecolt-Glaser and Glaser (1988) found that those who wrote about upsetting events exhibited better immune function and fewer health centre visits over follow up than did subjects who wrote about trivial topics. Based on these and other findings, Pennebaker (1989) developed a theory of inhibition and disease that posited that inhibition requires autonomic work (evidenced in higher skin conductance levels) and thus constitutes an ongoing stressor, depleting the body's resources for resisting illness.

Other laboratories since then have employed a number of different variations on this basic theme and different measures of health and immune function, and the results have been strikingly similar. Esterling, Antoni, Kumar, and Schneiderman (1990) reported poorer cellular control of a latent virus (Epstein–Barr) in those subjects judged to be repressing disclosure of negative affect in a study that required discussion of emotional material. Similar findings were reported in a more recent replication of that study (Esterling et al., 1994). Moreover, Petrie et al. (1995) found decreased skin conductance levels over the course of writing and improved response to a hepatitis B vaccination programme following emotional disclosure.

It is likely that future work will be directed towards elucidating links between specific aspects of self-expression and physiological correlates. In an attempt to identify linguistic and autonomic pre-

dictors of health and health enhancement, Pennebaker has begun to employ methods of recording various autonomic channels as subjects type about their upsetting memories, and the essays are, in turn, subjected to a detailed programme of linguistic and content categorization (Pennebaker & Uhlmann, 1994; Francis & Pennebaker, 1994).

Evidence supporting the health benefits of self-disclosure has received an explosion of attention in light of recently reported findings indicating that group therapy, which consisted mostly of self-disclosure, resulted in increased life expectancy for a group of metastatic breast cancer patients randomly assigned to condition (Spiegel et al., 1989). In addition, use of an early structured psychiatric intervention was found to have beneficial effects for prognosis of a group of melanoma patients (Fawzy et al., 1993). Meaningful self-disclosure has also been described as central to a non-surgical approach for reversing coronary artery disease in patients whose conditions precluded bypass or other surgical interventions (Ornish et al., 1990). Thus, longer-term interventions that feature emotional expression have demonstrated physical benefits, but is not possible from the studies to date to separate the non-specific effects of the group process from the specific results of emotional disclosure.

CONCLUSIONS

In this chapter we have attempted to highlight the central issues in the measurement and impact of emotional expression on health, and a number of pressing questions emerge from a review of the data. For instance, what is the relationship of self-reports of particular emotional states and expression of such states within the social context of the individual? Many of us would anonymously report the experience of anger in the workplace; but few overtly express such emotions, especially to superiors. Future research will also need to clarify more carefully distinctions between emotion experienced and emotion expressed, and the relative levels of each (overall emotionality). Is it high hostility that drives coronary plaque formation, or is it hostility that must remain silent, or is it the difference between the two that really contributes to disease? And, can researchers feel confident of the validity of subjects' self-reports? Unconscious associations may contribute to illness in ways that neither researchers nor subjects appreciate (Epstein, 1994).

Even more troublesome is the question of specificity. If certain psychological states are associated with certain physiological substrates, how do they manifest in illness? It would be simplistic to assume that particular emotions issued in specific disease patterns. As many have pointed out, rarely is one emotion experienced in a vacuum, so more realistically emotional states come in clusters that represent situational coping or personality attitudes. This issue also underscores the difficulty of inducing emotional states and drawing conclusions based on single inductions. Future studies would do well to induce one emotion from a variety of hypothetical situations to test for reliability. It is useful to bear in mind that emotions may not constitute psychosomatic causal factors, but in reality may be symptoms of larger predicaments or challenges that may contribute to health status over time. The field is new, so gaping holes in findings are more the rule than the exception. A greater understanding of the effect of emotional expression on health will be enhanced by future studies that incorporate both short- and long-term measures in their design. (See also 'Coping with chronic illness'.)

Andersen, B.L., Kiecolt-Glaser, J.K. & Glaser, R. (1994). A biobehavioral model of cancer stress and disease course. *American Psychologist*, **49**, 389–404.

Barger, S.D. (1995). *The repressive coping style: a review.* Manuscript submitted for publication.

Bell, I.R., Janoski, M.L., Kagan, J. & King, D.S. (1990). Is allergic rhinitis more frequent in young adults with extreme shyness? *Psychosomatic Medicine*, **52**, 517–25.

Byrne, D. (1961). The repression-sensitization scale: Rationale, reliability, and validity. *Journal of Personality*, **29**, 334–49.

Ekman, P., Levenson, R.W. & Friesen, W.V. (1983). Autonomic nervous system activity distinguishes among emotions. *Science*, **221**, 1208–10.

Epstein, S. (1994). Integration of the cognitive and the psychodynamic unconscious. *American Psychologist*, **49**, 709–24.

Esterling, B.A., Antoni, M.H., Fletcher, M.A., Margulies, S. & Scheiderman, N. (1994). Emotional disclosure through writing or speaking modulates latent Epstein–Barr virus antibody titers. *Journal of Consulting and Clinical Psychology*, **62**, 130–40.

Esterling, B.A., Antoni, M., Kumar, M. & Schneiderman, N. (1990). Emotional repression, stress disclosure responses, and Epstein–Barr viral capsid antigen titers. *Psychosomatic Medicine*, **52**, 397–410.

Fawzy, F.I., Fawzy, N.W., Hyun, C.S., Gutherie, D., Fahey, J.L. & Morton, D. (1993). Malignant melanoma: Effects of an early structured psychiatric intervention, coping, and affective state on recurrence and survival six years later. *Archives of General Psychiatry*, **50**, 681–9.

Francis, M.E. & Pennebaker, J.W. (1994). *LIWC: Linguistic inquiry and word count.* Manuscript submitted for publication.

Futterman, A.D., Kemeny, M.E., Shapiro, D., Polonsky, W. & Fahey, J.L. (1992). Immunological variability associated with experimentally induced positive and negative affective states. *Psychological Medicine*, **22**, 231–8.

Golding, J.M., Stein, Siegel, Burnam, M.A. & Sorenson, S.B. (1988). Sexual assault and the use of health and mental health services. *American Journal of Community Psychology*, **16**, 625–44.

Greer, S. & Morris, T. (1975). Psychological attributes of women who develop breast cancer: a controlled study. *Journal of Psychosomatic Research*, **19**, 147–53.

Gross, J. (1989). Emotional expression in cancer onset and progression. *Social Science and Medicine*, **28**, 1239–48.

Jensen, M.R. (1987). Psychobiological factors predicting the course of breast cancer. *Journal of Personality*, **55**, 317–42.

Kennedy, S., Kiecolt-Glaser, R. & Glaser, R. (1988). Immunological consequences of acute and chronic interpersonal stressors: mediating role of interpersonal relationships. *British Journal of Medical Psychology*, **61**, 77–85.

King, L.A. & Emmons, R.A. (1990). Conflict over emotional expression: psychological and physical correlates. *Journal of Personality and Social Psychology*, **58**, 864–77.

Knapp, P.H., Levy, E.M., Giorgi, R.G., Black, P.H., Fox, B.H. & Heeren, T.C. (1992). Short-term immunological effects of induced emotion. *Psychosomatic Medicine*, **54**, 133–48.

Labott, S.M., Ahleman, S., Wolever, M.E. & Martin, R.B. (1990). The physiological and psychological effects of the expression and inhibition of emotion. *Behavioral Medicine*, **16**, 182–9.

Larson, D.G. & Chastain, R.L. (1990). Self-concealment: conceptualization, measurement, and health implication. 439–55.

Levy, S.M., Herberman, R.B., Maluish, A.M., Schlien, B. & Lippman, M. (1985). Prognostic risk assessment in primary breast cancer by behavioral and immunological parameters. *Health Psychology*, **4**, 99–113.

Ornish, D., Brwon, S.E., Scherwitz, L.W., Billings, J.H., Armsrong, W.T., Ports, T.A., McClanahan, S.M., Kirkeide, R.L., Brand, R.J. & Gould, K. (1990). Can lifestyle changes reverse coronary artery disease? The lifestyle heart trial. *Lancet*, **336**, 129–33.

Pennebaker, J.W. (1989). Confession, inhibition, and disease. In L. Berkowitz (Ed.). *Advances in experimental social psychology*, Vol. 22, pp. 211–244. New York: Academic Press.

Pennebaker, J.W. & Beall, S.K. (1986). Confronting a traumatic event: toward an understanding of inhibition and disease. *Journal of Abnormal Psychology*, **95**, 274–81.

Pennebaker, J.W. & Chew, C.H. (1985). Behavioral inhibition and electrodermal activity during deception. *Journal of Personality and Social Psychology*, **49**, 1427–33.

Pennebaker, J.W. & Susman, J.R. (1988). Disclosure of traumas and psychosomatic processes. *Social Science and Medicine*, **26**, 327–32.

Pennebaker, J.W. & Uhlmann, C. (1994). Direct linking of autonomic activity with typed text: the CARMEN machine.

Behavior Research Methods, Instruments and Computers, **26**, 28–31.

Pennebaker, J.W., Kiecolt-Glaser, J. & Glaser, R. (1988). Disclosure of traumas and immune function: health implications for psychotherapy. *Journal of Consulting and Clinical Psychology*, **56**, 239–45.

Petrie, K.J., Booth, R.J., Pennebaker, J.W., Davison, K.P. & Thomas, M.G. (1995). Disclosure of trauma and immune response to a hepatitis B vaccination program. *Journal of Consulting and Clinical Psychology*, **63**, 787–92.

Pettingale, K.W., Morris, T., Greer, S. & Haybittle, J.L. (1985). Mental attitudes to cancer: an additional prognostic factor. *The Lancet*, 750.

Russek, L.G., King, S.H., Russek, S.J. & Russek, H.I. (1990). The Harvard mastery of stress study 35-year follow-up: prognostic significance of patterns of psychophysiological arousal. *Psychosomatic Medicine*, **52**, 271–85.

Sackheim, H.A. & Gur, R.C. (1979). Self-deception, other-deception, and self-reported pathology. *Journal of Consulting and Clinical Psychology*, **47**, 213–15.

Schwartz, G.E. (1983). Disregulation theory and disease: applications to the repression/cerebral disconnection/cardiovascular disorder hypothesis. *International Review of Applied Psychology*, **32**, 95–118.

Schwartz, G.E. (1990). Psychobiology of repression and health: a systems approach. In J.L. Singer (Ed.). *Repression and dissociation*, pp. 405–434. Chicago: University of Chicago Press.

Shedler, J., Mayman, M. & Manis, M. (1993). The illusion of mental health. *American Psychologist*, **48**, 1117–31.

Spiegel, D., Bloom, H.C., Kraemer, J.R. & Gottheil, E. (1989). Effect of psychosocial treatment on survival of patients with metastatic breast cancer. *The Lancet*, 888–901.

Temoshok, L. (1987). Personality, coping style, emotion, and cancer: towards and integrative model. *Cancer Surveys*, **6**, 545–67.

Weinberger, D.A. (1990). The construct validity of the repressive coping style. In J.L. Singer (Ed.). *Repression and dissociation: implications for personality theory, psychopathology and health*, pp.337–385. Chicago: University of Chicago Press.

Weinberger, D., Schwartz, G. & Davidson, R. (1979). Low-anxious, high-anxious, and repressive coping styles: psychometric patterns and behavioral and physiological responses to stress. *Journal of Abnormal Psychology*, **88**, 369–80.

SECTION 1: Psychological aspects of health and illness

Family influences on health

JENNY HEWISON

Department of Psychology, University of Leeds,
UK

Some kinds of families are much more healthy than others; and there is a clear pattern in the distribution of health and illness across families. Health gradients are found when families are classified by social class, i.e. according to the occupation of the 'head of household', with lower social class being associated with worse health. Classification by education produces a similar picture. The health of all family members is affected. Since occupation and education have few direct effects on health, at least in developed countries, it is accepted that these variables are markers for differences in the way that people in different kinds of families live their lives. These differences reflect economic and social constraints on families as well as individual attitudes and choices.

Families are an important medium, perhaps the most important medium, through which social and demographic factors exert their influence on the health of individuals. Other entries discuss the effects on health of socioeconomic deprivation, or of specific factors such as unemployment, or membership of certain minority ethnic groups. Family influences on health cannot be understood in isolation from wider forces which shape the structure of families, constrain behaviour, and exert pressure upon family members to think and behave in certain ways.

The relative importance of social and individual factors in determining behaviour continues to be debated. It is well known, for example, that risk factors such as smoking, acknowledged as having a role in the causation of many diseases, are more common in families with less education and/or lower social class. There has been a regrettable tendency to emphasize either those working class families that smoke, or those that do not, i.e. the power of social influences, or the reality of individual choice. It is regrettable that psychology as an academic discipline has been almost entirely identified with the second of these positions; and more regrettable still that that has carried with it the implication of a certain kind of political philosophy, which has limited the influence of psychology within the caring professions. Recent calls for research (Carroll, Bennett & Davey Smith, 1993; Williams, 1990) into the social patterning of individual choices and behaviour is welcome but long overdue.

Part of understanding family influences on health is about understanding the distribution of risk factors across families. Such risk factors only tell part of the story, however. In studies of Whitehall civil servants, men in lower grade occupations still had worse health even after adjustments had been made for smoking, diet, exercise, and so on. The second Whitehall study (Marmot *et al.*, 1991) gathered more data on psychological factors, and found that potentially important influences on ill-health such as stress, personal control and social support were unequally distributed across grades, and may have contributed to the health gradients observed.

Workplace factors are important, but families are an important source of both stress and support in individuals' lives. Changes in family composition are important life events. The death of a parent, spouse or child is a major stressor, as is divorce or a child leaving home. Such changes affect the psychological and physical well-being of rich and poor alike. Even so, social gradients cannot be forgotten. Unemployment and inadequate income, for example, are related to marital dissatisfaction and to divorce. From whatever cause, stress and depression in one family member can have effects on others, so the cumulative influence on family health can be considerable.

As well as providing stressors, families can be a source of psychological as well as practical support for individuals coping with stress. Sufferers from chronic illness, for example, derive psychological and possibly physical benefit from social support (Henderson & Brown, 1988). Its absence may be associated with ill-health either indirectly, via an increase in unhealthy behaviours such as smoking or excess drinking, or directly via physiological mechanisms, which are as yet poorly understood.

Social and economic factors influence the way in which family structures change over time, and hence the family's capacity to generate stress and provide support. There are fewer large families, fewer extended families living under the same roof, more single parent families, more stepmothers and stepfathers, and more elderly people, many of whom live alone. The resources available to families have changed. Although many have seen an increase in their standard of living, there has been an increase too in the proportion of babies born to families on means-tested benefits. Families also change their behaviour, e.g. more women now combine child-rearing with paid work. The net effect of all these forces is different for different members of the family: men who are married or living with a partner, for example, have a lower mortality rate than men of the same age living alone, but the association is much less strong for women.

Relationships within families may also be important in mediating other subtle influences on health. Life expectancy is higher in countries with a more equitable income distribution, and it has been suggested that, at least in developed countries, health may be influenced by relative as well as absolute living standards (Wilkinson, 1992). The topic has not yet been researched, but it seems at least plausible that stress derived from drawing unfavourable comparisons with the circumstances of others could be either amplified or reduced by the response of family members.

It must be emphasized that this entry refers to family influences on health in affluent countries. In developing countries, economic concerns may be paramount. Except in the worst circumstances, however, it is still often found that mothers' education has an effect on infant mortality that is independent of family income, in part via its effect on the mother's child-rearing practices.

When seeking to explain favourable or unfavourable outcomes in later childhood or beyond, developmental psychologists now insist on the need to look at the interaction of early adversity with a child's subsequent rearing environment. A number of family influences on health may profitably be viewed within this framework (Bradley & Casey, 1992).

Low birthweight is associated with increased perinatal and infant mortality, and with a number of adverse health outcomes such as an increased risk of cerebral palsy, seizure and sensory disorders, and respiratory problems. It is more common in lower social class groups, and contributes to observed gradients in mortality and morbidity (Woodroffe et al., 1993). Known risk factors such as smoking and younger maternal age contribute to these excess risks, but do not explain them completely. Recent work on the foetal and infant origins of adult cardiovascular disease has suggested that poor infant health and growth are also associated with a decreased life expectancy among children who survive into adulthood (Barker, 1991). In understanding these adverse outcomes, however, it must be remembered that continuity of disadvantage is the rule rather than the exception. A woman who is pregnant in conditions of social adversity is unlikely to escape them after the baby is born. Further, an interaction between medical and social factors occurs, in that mothers who are most likely to have vulnerable babies are least likely to have the psychological, social and economic resources necessary to achieve satisfactory developmental and health outcomes. The health risks associated with disadvantage accumulate throughout life.

One of the most important of all family influences on health is smoking (Pless, 1994). In pregnant women, smoking is associated with greatly increased levels of mortality and morbidity in the foetus. Parental smoking is associated with more respiratory illness in childhood, which is, in turn, associated with chronic obstructive airways disease and cancer in adulthood. Raised levels of sudden infant death syndrome, asthma, hearing disorders, short stature and hospital admissions can all be attributed to parental smoking; and smokers' materials are the most frequent cause of fatal home fires. Risk factors are passed across generations, because children are more likely to become active smokers if their parents smoke. The decision to smoke, like many other health-related decisions, is not a simple matter of individual choice. Smoking can be a method of coping with stress, for example, so the family influences on health can work both ways. Family relationships or responsibilities can lead to stress, which can lead to smoking; but smoking damages the health of all the members of a family.

By comparison with the effects of smoking, the bottle-feeding of babies confers relatively few health disadvantages on children in developed countries, mainly because good sanitation means bottle-feeds can be made with clean water. The relationship between behaviour and health outcome, in other words, is different in different physical circumstances. Possible interaction effects of this kind need to be borne in mind when claims are made for the importance of behavioural factors in determining health outcome.

Family influences on diet and weight are not straightforward. Eating habits established within the family during childhood tend to influence behaviour in adult life. However, most obese adolescents and young adults were not obese as children. Drawing conclusions about cause and effect within families is made more difficult by the strong overall trend over time: the proportion of young people who are overweight has increased considerably in the last few years (Woodroffe et al., 1993).

Between 1 and 19 years of age, injuries are the largest single cause of death. Deaths from unintentional injury have a steeper social gradient than any other cause of death in childhood (Pless, 1994). Attempts have been made to reduce children's exposure to risk: by legislation, e.g. the introduction of child-resistant containers, and by environmental modification, e.g. traffic calming. Guidance to parents on children's abilities, e.g. judging the speed of a car, is seen as one part of a wider preventive strategy, which recognizes that it can be made easier or harder for families to keep their children safe.

More generally, the attitude of families towards risk-taking by their younger members has links with beliefs about the nature of adolescence, autonomy and responsibility. Cross-cultural comparisons are useful here. A study of young people's health found that parents brought up in Asian or Middle Eastern countries emphasized responsibility rather than autonomy in their adolescents, and placed many more restrictions on what young people were allowed to do (Brannen et al., 1994). The behaviour of particular families cannot be separated from wider cultural and religious pressures, but the overall consequences were clear: far fewer Asian young people engaged in 'risky' behaviour (smoking, drinking alcohol, taking drugs) than their white indigenous counterparts.

As well as influencing whether their members engage in risky behaviours, families are also involved in decisions about the use of preventive health services, such as the immunization of children. Social inequalities in the uptake of these services are well documented. Psychological models have not so far been very successful in explaining why patterns of service use vary. Health-related attitudes and beliefs have a modest role to play; but the uptake of preventive health care is also heavily influenced by more mundane factors, such as whether letters are personalized, reminders are sent, and so on. A recent intervention study designed to improve overall uptake succeeded in its aim, but found that inequalities between affluent and deprived areas had persisted or even become wider (Reading et al., 1994). Essentially, poorer families had not been able, for whatever reason, to take advantage of improvements in the service. Perhaps their priorities lay elsewhere. The study illustrates a general point. The UK's failure to reduce health inequalities in the last few decades has mainly happened because the health of poorer people has not improved as much as the health of the affluent. Improving overall service standards cannot be relied upon to reduce inequalities; if this is desired, it must be a policy goal in its own right, and it must begin by seeking to understand the priorities, and the reasons for those priorities, of families who currently have a poor uptake of preventive health services.

Most of the care which family members need when they become ill is provided by others in the family. The decision to seek professional advice is often made after consulting members of the family. For common childhood illnesses, the perceived severity of the condition is the main factor increasing the likelihood of consultation; but at any given level of severity, social and individual factors can shift the balance one way or the other (Wyke & Hewison, 1991). Concepts of health differ between social groups (Blaxter, 1990): families which assume children will have coughs most of the time are less likely to consult a GP about these and other childhood ailments. Other factors, such as parents' employment, which might be thought to present problems regarding access to a GP, apparently have little effect (Hewison & Dowswell, 1994). At a more individual level, a family in which one child has asthma, for example, will be more likely to consult a GP about respiratory problems in other children.

A GP is more likely to refer an unresolved but non-urgent health problem to secondary care if the sufferer or family members actively seek a referral. Parents' decision to seek treatment may be influenced by grandparents' reactions, e.g. to the fact that a child still wets the bed, or has prominent ears. The reaction of all these people will play a part in whether further treatment is sought, a fact which it is sometimes hard for health professionals to accept.

Families in which complaining about health is frowned upon may deter their members from seeking help even for serious conditions. Examples are known of people who suffered the symptoms of a heart attack for some time before finally acknowledging that they needed help. In other cases, family members are the ones to encourage help-seeking, against active resistance by the sufferer. This balance of forces in the relationships between family members is important in diverse health fields. In work on chronic pain, the concept of solicitousness has proved valuable (Flor, Kerns & Turk, 1987). Showing care and concern when people are in pain is desirable; but solicitousness can go too far, and effectively reward people for treating themselves as invalids, with undesirable health consequences. Sometimes the health of one family member is used to justify aspects of family functioning that will eventually prove counterproductive, e.g. diabetes in a young person used to maintain dependence on parents. A 'systems' approach to family functioning can help identify competing interests, and form the basis of therapeutic intervention if required.

When the health of one family member deteriorates, another member often becomes a 'carer'. Receiving care obviously benefits the sufferer (from stroke, arthritis, Alzheimer's disease, or whatever); but providing care over a long period can have effects on the health of the carer. Women are especially likely to be overloaded by responsibilities, since they may simultaneously be caring for children and older members of the family. Social support and other psychological factors are important in maintaining the well-being of carers.

More needs to be known about the place of families in the network of influences linking social and economic factors to psychological variables, and to health outcomes for individuals. Intervention strategies which target family influences on health but ignore social and economic influences on families are unlikely to succeed. (See also 'Socioeconomic status and health', 'Social support and health'.

REFERENCES

Barker, D.J.P. (1991). The foetal and infant origins of inequalities in health in Britain. *Journal of Public Health Medicine*, 13, 64–8.

Blaxter, M. (1990). *Health and lifestyles.* London: Tavistock/Routledge.

Bradley, R.H. & Casey, P.H. (1992). Family environment and behavioural development of low-birthweight children. *Developmental Medicine and Child Neurology*, 34, 822–32.

Brannen, J., Dodd, K., Oakley, A. & Storey, P. (1994). *Young people, health and family life.* Milton Keynes: Open University Press.

Carroll, D., Bennett, P. & Davey Smith, G. (1993). Socio–economic health inequalities: their origins and implications. *Psychology and Health*, 8, 295–316.

Flor, H., Kerns, R.D. & Turk, D.C. (1987). The role of spouse reinforcement, perceived pain, and activity levels of chronic pain patients. *Journal of Psychosomatic Research*, 31, 251–9.

Hewison, J. & Dowswell, T. (1994). *Child health care and the working mother.* London: Chapman & Hall.

Henderson, A.S. & Brown, G.W. (1988). Social support: the hypothesis and the evidence. In A.S. Henderson & G.W. Brown (Eds.). *Handbook of social psychiatry.* Amsterdam: Elsevier Scientific Publications.

Marmot, M.G., Davey Smith, G., Stansfeld, D., Patel, C., North, F., Head, J., White, I., Brunner, E. & Feeney, A. (1991). Health inequalities among British civil servants: the Whitehall II study. *Lancet*, 337, 1387–92.

Pless, I.B. (Ed.) (1994). *The epidemiology of childhood disorders.* Oxford: Oxford University Press.

Reading, R., Colver, A., Openshaw, S. & Jarvis, S. (1994). Do interventions that improve immunisation uptake also reduce social inequalities in uptake? *British Medical Journal*, 308, 1142–4.

Wilkinson, R.G. (1992). Income distribution and life expectancy. *British Medical Journal*, 304, 165–8.

Williams, D.R. (1990). Socioeconomic differentials in health: a review and redirection. *Social Psychology Quarterly*, 53, 81–99.

Woodroffe, C., Glickman, M., Barker, M. & Power, C. (1993). *Children, teenagers and health: the key data.* Milton Keynes: Open University Press.

Wyke, S. & Hewison, J. (Eds.). (1991). *Child health matters.* Milton Keynes: Open University Press.

Gender issues and women's health

JANE M. USSHER

Women's Health Research Unit, Psychology
Department, University College London, UK

INTRODUCTION

The issue of gender differences in health and illness has, until relatively recently, been marginalized or ignored by the majority of researchers and clinicians working in the field of health and medicine. If differential rates of diagnosis or treatment between men and women are acknowledged, the traditional stance has been to adopt a simple sex differences approach: assuming that biological factors account for this imbalance. However, whilst the preponderance of women patients in fields such as obstetrics or gynaecology can be simply explained by biological differences between men and women, there are other areas in which women predominate, or clearly outnumber men, where simple biological aetiological theories have been contested, such as in the field of mental health. This has led to a growing body of research suggesting that we should be focusing on gender issues; the influence of social and cultural factors on women and men's behaviour and subjective experience, and the influence of the current social constructions of masculinity and femininity on health and illness. This does not lead to a denial of biological factors, but suggests that psychosocial and cultural explanations must be given equal weight in understanding differential patterns of health and illness between men and women. In this chapter, the field of mental health will be used as an example to explain the implications of this approach. However, it is important to note that these arguments have been utilized in health areas where men predominate, such as in the field of coronary heart disease, or in attempts to explain sex differences in life expectancy; topics covered elsewhere in this volume.

GENDER DIFFERENCES IN CHILDHOOD DISORDERS

There are clear gender differences in the occurrence, diagnosis and treatment of a range of mental health problems from infancy through to late adulthood. Prior to the age of eight, boys predominate in a range of behavioural and psychological disorders, including bedwetting/soiling, feeding and appetite problems, sleep problems, over activity and restlessness. Throughout childhood, boys outnumber girls in reading and writing difficulties, autism, hyperactivity and antisocial problems, the latter continuing as a predominantly male problem through to adult life. Conversely, From the age of eight through to adulthood, girls and women predominate in the presentation and diagnosis of neurotic problems, particularly depression, anxiety and eating disorders.

Aetiological theories of childhood mental health and behavioural problems predominantly focus on issues other than gender. Whilst differential rates of diagnosis between boys and girls are acknowledged in discussions of incidence and prevalence, in the main, research and clinical intervention has concentrated on non-gender specific aetiological theories for childhood problems. These include factors such as teratogens or perinatal trauma, parental attachment, separation and hospital admission, family discord and divorce, maternal depression, bereavement, school effects, social deprivation and social class, temperament, or cognitive differences, such as absence of theory of mind as an explanation for autism (Rutter & Hersov, 1985). Any analysis of differential patterns of problems between boys and girls invariably attributes them to biological differences between the male and female foetus, infant or child, which are said to produce developmental differences between boys and girls, making boys more vulnerable to difficulties in the early years. However, psychological interpretations of gender imbalances have been adopted in some areas. For example, it is recognized that the persistence of childhood problems is associated with maturational delay in cognitive ability, in boys, and conversely with higher intelligence in girls. The explanation for this is that boys' cognitive delays result in difficulties with peer groups and a general vulnerability to stress; whereas conversely girls' higher intelligence results in a greater internalization of problems and increased likelihood of identification with a depressed mother. However, to date, there has been a paucity of research investigating these and other gender differences in childhood disorders. In contrast, there is now a wide body of research examining gender differences in adult mental health.

GENDER DIFFERENCES IN ADULT MENTAL HEALTH

Incidence and prevalence

Since the early nineteenth century when statistics were first kept, women have outnumbered men in the diagnosis and referral for treatment of mental health problems (Showalter, 1987). For example, the statistics on psychiatric inpatient care in England published in 1986, recorded 83 865 men and 113 386 women per hundred thousand admitted for psychiatric care in 1986. This gender imbalance is also reflected in primary care treatments. Women are more likely to be referred to a psychologist, psychiatrist or therapist than men, at a rate of 4 : 1–12 : 1, depending on the sample studied (Briscoe, 1982), and are twice as likely to be prescribed psychotropic medication (Ashton, 1991).

However, women do not outnumber men in every psychiatric category. For example, taking the 1986 hospital statistics, 4978 men compared to 10 291 women were treated for neurotic disorders (which includes anxiety, eating disorders, neurotic depression and phobias), and 11 740 men as compared to 23 469 women treated for depressive disorders. However, 8301 men compared to 3508 women were treated for alcohol dependence syndrome, and 1382 men compared to 806 women for drug dependency. Researchers also consistently report that men are more likely to be diagnosed as suffering from 'irresponsible and antisocial conduct', or personality disorders than women (Briscoe, 1982). So, it is in the neurotic or affective disorders that women predominate.

Other forms of epidemiological research reinforce these findings. Community surveys, in which assessments are made of psychological distress in men and women living in the community who are, as yet, unknown to mental health professionals, show that women are more likely to report psychological distress, and particularly depression, than men.

It has been suggested that women are more likely to report symptomatology than men, particularly in the case of psychological distress (Cooperstock, 1976), and therefore that community surveys and referrals for treatment reflect this reporting bias, rather than differential rates of problem occurrence. However, others contest this finding, claiming that 'women are no more likely than men to articulate their symptoms' (Gove, 1979). These disagreements reflect the fact that many conflicting aetiological theories have been developed to explain gender differences in mental health, with two major distinctions between those who accept the existence of a gender difference in the occurrence of mental health problems, and subsequently propose a range of psychological and biological explanations to account for it, and those who argue that the difference is an artefact of labelling and gender-biased diagnosis, with women more likely to be pathologized than men.

Labelling theory

A number of critics have argued that gender differences in mental health statistics can be accounted for by gender biases in labelling and diagnosis of problems. One piece of evidence is from studies demonstrating that women are more likely to be given a psychological diagnosis for a non-specific problem, whereas a man will receive a physical diagnosis (Penfold & Walker, 1984). This may lead to overdiagnosis of neurotic disorders in women, and underdiagnosis in men, and conversely to problems such as alcohol or drug dependency being ignored or overlooked in women.

It has also been shown that cultural stereotypes of femininity and masculinity are accepted and internalized by mental health professionals of various disciplines, and are used in the evaluation and diagnosis of problems. A number of research studies have demonstrated that clinicians classify similar traits as being characteristic of both femininity and mental illness: traits such as 'more submissive, less independent, less adventurous, more easily influenced, less aggressive, less competitive, more excitable in minor crises, having their feelings more easily hurt, more conceited about their appearance, (and) less objective' (Broverman et al., 1970). At the same time, there is evidence that 'unfeminine' behaviour such as violence, anger or aggression is seen as a sign of pathology in women, but not in men. Thus women are potentially pathologized for behaviour which is at odds with stereotypes of femininity, yet femininity itself is also pathologized (Chesler, 1972).

However, labelling theory cannot account for all of the gender differences observed. It has been criticized for appearing to dismiss the reality of women's distress, suggesting that mental health problems do not exist, but are merely a process of inaccurate labelling.

Bio-medical explanations

The predominant biomedical interpretation of gender differences in mental health problems attributes the imbalance to female hormones and reproduction, associating it with premenstrual syndrome (PMS), postnatal depression (PND) and the menopause. Within a strictly biological model, this has led to the view that hormonal or biochemical changes associated with the menstrual cycle, the perinatal period, and the menopause account for many psychological and physical problems reported by women, and hence can largely account for women's preponderance in mental health statistics.

However, the notion of a simple causal relationship between hormones and reproductive syndromes has been severely criticized (Ussher, 1989), as there is no clear evidence for a simple biological substrate for psychological, physical or behavioural problems associated with reproduction. Many of the psychological symptoms attributed to PMS, PND or the menopause have been explained within a psychosocial model (see below), which posits that psychological and social factors are associated with many mental health problems. For example, premenstrual symptomatology has been found to be associated with stress, or with cognitive-personality variables, such as the differential attribution of negative moods to menstruation and positive moods to life events, as a result of the negative stereotyped expectations associated with the menstrual cycle. There is no agreement in the medical literature about the hormonal or biochemical causes of PMS, with high placebo responses in the majority of placebo-controlled treatment trials, and in many cases researchers finding that the placebo is equal to, or more effective than, the active treatment. Similarly, many of the symptoms of postnatal depression have been attributed to the social and psychological consequences of childbirth and childcare, rather than to simple imbalances in hormones, or have been explained within models used to understand depression at any other time in the life cycle, be they biological, cognitive–behavioural or psychodynamic, which are not tied to female hormones. Equally, a number of large-scale epidemiological studies have demonstrated that only a small number of physical symptoms, namely hot flushes, vaginal dryness and night sweats, can be clearly associated with the hormonal changes taking place during the menopause. Psychological symptoms, such as depression or anxiety, have been explained within a psychosocial model, and it has been consistently reported that depression and anxiety are no greater during the menopausal period than they are at any other stage in the life-cycle (see entries on PMS, PND and the menopause in this volume).

Psychosocial explanations

Many psychological and social factors have been posited to account for women's health problems, and in particular mental health problems. The importance of psychological and social factors is evidenced by the fact that not all women, but only specific social groups, are at high risk of diagnosis and treatment for mental health problems.

Economic factors, such as poverty and economic powerlessness are known to be a major risk factor for a range of physical and psychological problems (Russo, 1990). World Health Organization Statistics collected over successive decades provide evidence for women's relative poverty: even in the developed world where many women are educated and qualified to take up employment equal to that of men, women earn significantly less than their male counterparts, and are significantly more likely to be without any independent income. This leads to powerlessness and economic dependence, factors associated with mental health problems. Powerlessness has also been posited as an explanation for the finding that women in traditional marital relationships, where they do not work outside the home and are responsible for the full burden of domestic and childcare, are at higher risk of mental health problems than single women, women in more egalitarian relationships, or women in paid employment.

The traditional caring role of women has, in itself, been seen as a major precipitator of mental health problems, as caring for young children, for elderly relatives, or for a dependant spouse are major risk factors for depression. Women predominate in caring roles throughout the life span. They still shoulder the major responsibility for childcare and for housework even when both partners are working, with national surveys reporting that 95% of women do all of the housework and childcare even though 70% are in outside employment (Social Trends, HMSO, 1994). It has thus been estimated that women have 15 hours less leisure time than men in an average week. Women also shoulder the responsibility for care of the sick and elderly: a caring role which has also been associated with mental health problems due to social isolation, deteriorating personal relationships, financial hardship and the emotional and physical burden of caring. That gender rather than sex differences account for mental health problems associated with the caring role is attested by the fact that men who take responsibility for full-time childcare or caring for the sick or elderly are also at high risk of experiencing depression or anxiety disorders.

Sexual violence and childhood sexual abuse have also been posited as major factors in the aetiology of mental health problems. It is estimated that 70% of women have experienced sexual harassment; that between 1 in 4 and 1 in 10 women have experienced rape; and that between 1 in ten and 3 in 10 girls have been sexually abused as children. Accurate statistics are impossible to obtain in this area because of the fact that few women or children report the abuse, and official statistics are recognized to be only the tip of the iceberg. It is now widely acknowledged that sexual violence is a major precipitator of a range of mental health problems in childhood, adolescence and adulthood, with surveys of survivors of abuse reporting significantly higher rates of problems than is found in non-abused populations. Rates of between 40% and 70% of history sexual abuse and violence have also found in many clinical populations, including eating disorders, depression and anxiety, gynaecological complaints, and sexual problems. Yet, it has been argued that rape and sexual abuse are merely the extreme end of a continuum of objectification and sexism facing all women, which is a major factor in the development of mental health problems across the lifespan (Chesler, 1993).

CONCLUSION

The field of mental health is one where there are clear gender differences between men and women in the presentation and treatment of problems. A number of unidimensional theories have been put forward to explain these gender differences. However, the research evidence clearly suggests that multifactorial models which acknowledge an interaction between biological, psychological and social factors are most appropriate. This results in a movement away from a simple sex differences approach, and suggests that aetiological theories and clinical intervention must acknowledge the importance of psychological, social and cultural factors, as well as biology, without privileging one above the other. The implication of this is that prevention and intervention must focus on the social and psychological as well as on the biomedical aspects of illness (Ussher & Nicolson, 1992).

REFERENCES

Ashton, H. (1991). Psychotropic drug prescribing for women. *British Journal of Psychiatry*, **158**, 30–5.

Briscoe, M. (1982). Sex differences in psychological wellbeing. *Psychological Medicine*, Monographs, Suppl. 1.

Broverman, K., Broverman, D., Clarkson, F., Rosenkrantz, P. & Vogel, S. (1970). Sex role stereotypes and clinical judgements of mental health. *Journal of Consulting and Clinical Psychology*, **34**, 1–7.

Chesler, P. (1993). *Women and madness*. New York: Doubleday.

Cooperstock, R. (1976). Women and psychotropic drugs. In MacLennan, A. (ed.). *Women: their use of alcohol and other legal drugs*. Toronto: Addiction Resarch Foundation.

Gove, W. (1979). Sex differences in the epidemiology of mental illness: evidence and explanations. In Gomberg, E. & Franks, V. (eds.) *Gender and disordered behaviour*. New York: Brunner/Mazel.

Penfold, S. & Walker, G. (1984). *Women and the psychiatric paradox*. Milton Keynes: Open University Press.

Russo, N.F. (1990). Forging priorities for women's mental health. *American Psychologist*, **45**, 368–73.

Rutter, M & Hersov, L. (1985). *Child and adolescent Psychiatry: modern approaches*. London: Blackwell. Basil.

Showalter, E. (1987). *The female malady*. London: Virago.

Ussher, J.M. (1989). *The psychology of the female body*. London: Routledge.

Ussher, J.M. (1991). *Women's madness: misogyny or mental illness?* London: Harvester Wheatsheaf.

Ussher, J.M. & Nicolson, P. (1992). *Gender issues in clinical psychology*. London: Routledge.

The health belief model

VICTOR J. STRECHER
*Department of Health Behavior and
Health Education, School of Public
Health, University of North
Carolina, USA*

IRWIN M. ROSENSTOCK
*Department of Health Behavior and
Health Education, School of Public
Health, University of Michigan,
USA*

ORIGINS OF THE MODEL

Over the past four decades, the Health Belief Model (HBM) has been one of the most widely used psychosocial approaches to explaining health-related behaviour. Initially developed in an effort to explain the widespread failure of people to participate in programmes to prevent or to detect disease (Hochbaum, 1958; Rosenstock, 1960, 1966, 1974), the HBM was later extended to apply to people's responses to symptoms (Kirscht, 1974) and to their behaviour in response to diagnosed illness, particularly compliance with medical regimens (Becker, 1974).

The HBM is based on value-expectancy concepts. When value-expectancy concepts were gradually reformulated in the context of health-related behaviour the translations were as follows: (i) the desire to avoid illness or to get well (value); and (ii) the belief that a specific health action available to a person would prevent (or ameliorate) illness (expectation). The expectancy was further delineated in terms of the individual's estimate of personal susceptibility to, and severity of, an illness, and of the likelihood of being able to reduce that threat through personal action.

The development of the Health Belief Model grew out of real concerns with the limited success of various programmes of the Public Health Service in the 1950s. One such early example was the failure of large numbers of eligible adults to participate in tuberculosis screening programmes provided at no charge, in mobile X-ray units conveniently located in various neighbourhoods. The concern of the programme operators was with explaining people's behaviour by illuminating those factors that were facilitating or inhibiting positive responses.

Beginning in 1952, Hochbaum (1958) studied probability samples of more than 1200 adults in three cities that had conducted recent TB screening programme in mobile X-ray units. He assessed their 'readiness' to obtain X-rays, which included their beliefs that they were susceptible to tuberculosis and their beliefs in the personal benefits of early detection. Perceived susceptibility to tuberculosis itself comprised two elements, first, the respondents' beliefs about whether contracting tuberculosis was a realistic (not merely a mathematical) possibility for them personally; and secondly the extent to which they accepted the fact that one may have tuberculosis in the absence of all symptoms.

The measure of perceived personal benefits of early detection also included two elements: whether respondents believed that X-rays could detect tuberculosis prior to the appearance of symptoms and whether they believed that early detection and treatment would improve the prognosis. For the group of persons that exhibited both beliefs, that is, belief in their own susceptibility to tuberculosis and the belief that overall benefits would accrue from early detection, 82 % had had at least one voluntary chest X-ray during a specified period preceding the interview. Of the group exhibiting neither of these beliefs, only 21 % had obtained a voluntary X-ray during the criterion period. In short, four out of five people who exhibited both beliefs (susceptibility and benefits) took the predicted action, while four of five people who accepted neither of the beliefs had not taken the action. Hochbaum thus demonstrated with considerable precision that a particular action to screen for a disease was strongly associated with the two interacting variables: perceived susceptibility and perceived benefits.

Hochbaum also thought that the readiness to take action (perceived susceptibility and perceived benefits) could only be potentiated by other factors, particularly by 'cues' to instigate action, such as bodily events, or by environmental events, such as media publicity. He did not, however, study the role of cues empirically. Indeed, while the concept of cues as a trigger mechanism is appealing, it has been most difficult to study in explanatory surveys; a cue can be as fleeting as a sneeze, or the barely conscious perception of a poster.

COMPONENTS OF THE HBM

Since Hochbaum's survey in the 1950s, investigations have helped to expand and clarify the model, extending it beyond screening behaviours to include all preventive actions to illness behaviours and to sick-role behaviour (see summaries in Rosenstock, 1974; Kirscht, 1974; Becker, 1974; Becker & Maiman, 1980; Janz & Becker, 1984). In general, it is now believed that individuals will take action to ward off, to screen for, or to control ill-health conditions if they regard themselves as susceptible to the condition; if they believe it to have potentially serious consequences; if they believe that a course of action available to them would be beneficial in reducing either their susceptibility to, or the severity of, the condition; and if they believe that the anticipated barriers to (or costs of) taking the action are outweighed by its benefits. The following definitions and commentary specify the key variables in greater detail:

Perceived susceptibility

This dimension refers to one's subjective perception of the risk of contracting a health condition. In the case of medically established illness, the dimension has been reformulated to include acceptance of the diagnosis, personal estimates of resusceptibility, and susceptibility to illness in general.

[113]

Perceived severity

Feelings concerning the seriousness of contracting an illness or of leaving it untreated include evaluations of both medical and clinical consequences (for example, death, disability, and pain) and possible social consequences (such as effects of the conditions on work, family life and social relations). We have come to label the combination of susceptibility and severity as 'perceived threat.'

Perceived benefits

While acceptance of personal susceptibility to a condition also believed to be serious (perceived threat) produces a force leading to behaviour, the particular course of action that will be taken depends upon beliefs regarding the effectiveness of the various available actions in reducing the disease threat, termed the perceived benefits of taking health action. Thus, an individual exhibiting an optimal level of beliefs in susceptibility and severity would not be expected to accept any recommended health action unless that action was perceived as potentially efficacious.

Perceived barriers

The potential negative aspects of a particular health action, or perceived barriers, may act as impediments to undertaking the recommended behaviour. A kind of non-conscious, cost – benefit analysis occurs wherein the individual weighs the action's expected effectiveness against perceptions that it may be expensive, dangerous (having negative side-effects or iatrogenic outcomes), unpleasant (painful, difficult, upsetting), inconvenient, time-consuming, and so forth.

Thus, 'The combined levels of susceptibility and severity provided the energy or force to act and the perception of benefits (less barriers) provide a preferred path of action.' (Rosenstock, 1974, p. 332)

Cues to Action

In various early formulations of the HBM, the concept of cues which trigger action were discussed and may ultimately prove to be important, but they have not been systematically studied.

Other Variables

Diverse demographic, sociopsychological, and structural variables may affect the individual's perceptions and thus indirectly influence health-related behaviour. Specifically, sociodemographic factors, particularly educational attainment, are believed to have an indirect effect on behaviour by influencing the perception of susceptibility, severity, benefits, and barriers.

Self-efficacy

In 1977, Bandura introduced the concept of self-efficacy, or efficacy expectation, as distinct from outcome expectation (Bandura, 1977a, b, 1986), which we believe must be added to the HBM in order to increase its explanatory power (Rosenstock, Strecher and Becker, 1988) and to become a more useful tool for the practitioner. Outcome expectation, defined as a person's estimate that a given behaviour will lead to certain outcomes, is quite similar to the 'perceived threat' and 'perceived benefits' of the HBM. Self-efficacy is defined as 'the conviction that one can successfully execute the behaviour required to produce the outcome'. (Bandura, 1977a, p.79).

It is not difficult to see why self-efficacy was never explicitly incorporated into early formulations of the HBM. The original focus of the early model was on circumscribed prevenative actions, usually of a one-shot nature, such as accepting a screening test or an immunization, actions which generally were simple behaviours for most people to perform. Since it is likely that most prospective members of target groups for those programme had adequate self-efficacy for performing those simple behaviours, that dimension was not even recognized.

The situation is vastly different, however, in working with lifestyle behaviours requiring long-term changes. The problems involved in modifying lifelong habits concerning eating, drinking, exercising, smoking and sexual practices are obviously far more difficult to surmount than are those for accepting a one-time immunization or a screening test. It requires a good deal of confidence that one can, in fact, alter such lifestyles before successful change is possible. Thus, for behaviour change to succeed, people must (as the original HBM theorizes) feel threatened by their current behavioural patterns, (perceived susceptibility and severity), and believe that change of a specific kind will be beneficial by resulting in a valued outcome at acceptable cost, but they must also feel themselves competent (self-efficacious) to implement that change. A growing body of literature supports the importance of self-efficacy in helping to account for initiation and maintenance of behavioural change, (Bandura, 1977b; Bandura, 1986; Marlatt & Gordon, 1985; Strecher et al. 1986).

As a convenient way of summarizing the Health Belief Model components, we may subsume the key variables under three categories, which are summarized in Fig.1.

EVIDENCE FOR AND AGAINST THE MODEL

In 1974, Health Education Monographs devoted an entire issue to 'The Health Belief Model and Personal Health Behavior' (Becker 1974). That monograph summarized findings from research on the HBM to understand why individuals did, or did not, engage in a wide variety of health-related actions; the monograph provided considerable support for the model in explaining behaviour pertinent to prevention and behaviour in response to symptoms or to diagnosed disease.

During the decade following publication of the monograph, the HBM continued to be a major organizing framework for explaining and predicting acceptance of health and medical care recommendations. Accordingly, an updated critical review was made of HBM studies conducted between 1974 and 1984, which also combined the new results with earlier findings to permit an overall assessment of the model's performance (Janz and Becker, 1984). Space limitations do not permit more than a brief summary of the findings of the detailed reviews of 1974 and 1984; the interested reader should consult those sources for details.

Included in the 1984 review were such prevenative health and screening behaviours as influenza inoculations, practice of breast self-examination, and attendance at screening programmes for Tay-Sachs carrier status, high blood pressure, seat-belt use, exercise, nutrition, smoking, visits to physicians for check-ups, and fear of being apprehended while under the influence of alcohol. Sick-role behaviours included compliance with anti-hypertensive regimens, diabetic regimens, end-stage renal disease regimens, medication

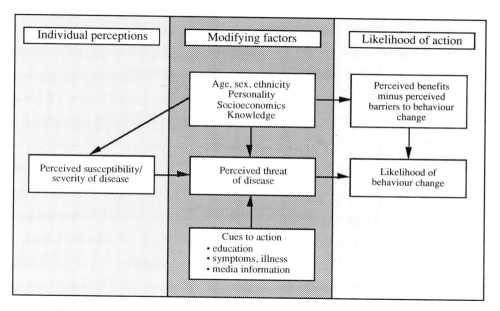

Fig. 1. Health belief model.

regimens for parents to give their children with otitis media, weight loss regimens, and medication regimens for parents to give to asthmatic children. Summary results provide substantial empirical support for the HBM, with findings from prospective studies at least as favourable as those obtained from retrospective research.

'Perceived barriers' was the most powerful single predictor of the HBM dimensions across all studies and behaviours. While both 'perceived susceptibility' and 'perceived benefits' were important overall, 'perceived susceptibility' was a stronger predictor of preventative health behaviour than sick-role behaviour while the reverse was true for 'perceived benefits'. Overall, 'perceived severity' was the least powerful predictor; however, this dimension was strongly related to sick-role behaviour.

One thing that strikes the authors in their review of HBM studies is the lack of data examining the HBM as a whole model. Researchers generally fail to examine how individuals with various combinations of health beliefs were more or less likely to change health-related behaviours. One would predict, for example, perceptions of susceptibility and severity to be associated largely with an intention to take action, similar to the predicted functions of attitudes in the Theory of Reasoned Action (Ajzen & Fishbein, 1980). In the AIDS area, for example, we agree with Catania and colleagues' (1990) theoretical analysis that, for individuals who objectively exhibit high risk behaviours, perceived susceptibility is a factor required before commitment to changing these risky behaviours can occur. The HBM goes on to hypothesize that those committed to taking action would then assess the benefits of taking a recommended health action, and the barriers to taking the action. If the benefits outweigh the barriers, the individual would be more likely to take the recommended health action.

Unfortunately, almost none the research examining the Health Belief Model analyses the constructs in this manner. The vast majority of HBM-related research analyse the constructs separately. Analyses that essentially throw all health belief constructs into a multiple regression model do not test the HBM in the manner we

are advising here. One would hypothesize, for example, that among those with high perceived threat, perceptions of benefits and barriers would be more predictive of behaviour change. Appropriate tests of this hypothesis would require analyses of subgroups (for example, testing the effects of benefits and barriers only for those with high perceived threat) or multivariate analyses involving a carefully constructed series of interaction terms.

RECOMMENDATIONS TO RESEARCHERS AND JOURNAL REVIEWERS

We offer the following recommendations for researchers and reviewers of manuscripts submitted for publication that examine Health Belief Model variables:

(i) Test the Health Belief Model as a model, or at minimum, as a combination of constructs, not as a collection of equally weighted variables operating simultaneously. It makes little sense to throw health belief variables into a multivariate analysis, selecting the 'strongest swimmers', and claiming that these are the factors on which to intervene. We offer the following hypotheses as a starting point for testing the Health Belief Model as a model:

(a) Perceived threat is a sequential function of perceived severity and perceived susceptibility. A heightened state of severity is required before perceived susceptibility becomes a powerful predictor. Perceived susceptibility, under the state of high perceived severity, will be a stronger predictor of intention to engage in health-related behaviours than it will be a predictor of actual engagement in health-related behaviours.

(b) Perceived benefits and barriers will be stronger predictors of behaviour change when perceived threat is high than when it is low. Under conditions of low perceived threat, benefits of, and barriers to, engaging in health-related behaviour will not be salient. The only exception to this may be when certain benefits of the recommended behaviour are perceived to be high, perceived threat may not need to be high.

(c) Self-efficacy, a factor now included in the Health Belief Model, will be a strong predictor of many health-related behaviours. Self-efficacy will be a particularly strong predictor of behaviours that require significant skills to perform.

(d) Cues-to-action will have a greater influence on behaviour in situations where perceived threat is great. The cue-to-action construct is a little-studied phenomenon: we know little about what cues to action exist or of their relative impact.

(ii) Specify the measures used to study belief constructs in publications. We suspect that an important reason for variance in results between studies is because of large variations in the specific measures used. When the actual questions were included in the chapter or could be uncovered in some manner, a disconcertingly large proportion did not appear to be good indicators of HBM constructs.

(iii) Researchers should delay aggregating items measuring benefits, barriers, and cue-to-action into general constructs; such items are often unrelated to one another, and have low inter-item correlations. To the practitioner charged with creating programmes that will contain health messages, analysis of single items can often offer more relevant information than a general grouped construct.

(iv) Include a behavioural anchor when measuring perceived susceptibility. For example, a behaviourally anchored question for AIDS-preventative behaviour would ask, '*If you do not practise safer sex*, how likely are you to become infected with the AIDS virus?' as opposed to, 'How likely are you to become infected with the AIDS virus?'. The reader is referred to recent research by Ronis (1992), which finds strong evidence for the importance of asking susceptibility questions that are conditional on action or inaction.

IMPLICATIONS FOR PRACTICE

This chapter has described both strengths and limitations in the HBM as formulated to date. It is hoped that future theory building or theory testing research will direct efforts more towards strengthening the Model where it is weak than towards repeating what has already been established. More work is needed on experimental interventions to modify health beliefs and health behaviour than on surveys to reconfirm already established correlations. More work is also needed to specify and measure factors that need to be added to the Model to increase its predictive power. The addition of self-efficacy to the traditional HBM should improve explanation and prediction, particularly in the area of lifestyle practices.

It is timely for professionals who are attempting to influence health-related behaviours to make use of the health belief variables, including self-efficacy in their programme planning, both in needs assessment and in programme strategies. Programmes to deal with a health problem should be based, in part, on knowledge of how many, and which members of, a target population feel susceptible to a particular health-related outcome, believe the health-related outcome to constitute a serious health problem, and believe that the threat of having the health-related outcome could be reduced by changing their behaviour at an acceptable psychological cost. Moreover, health professionals should also assess the extent to which clients possess adequate self-efficacy to carry out the prescribed action(s), sometimes over a long period of time.

The collection of data on health beliefs, along with other data pertinent to the group or community setting, permits the planning of more effective programmes than would otherwise be possible. Interventions can then be targeted to the specific needs identified by such an assessment. This is true whether dealing with the problems of individual patients, with groups of clients or with entire communities. In planning programmes to influence the behaviour of large groups of people for long periods of time, the role of the HBM (including self-efficacy) must be considered in context. Permanent changes in behaviour can rarely be wrought solely by direct attacks on belief systems. Even more, where the behaviour of large groups is the target, interventions at societal levels (for example, social networks, work organizations, the physical environment, the legislature) along with interventions at the individual level will likely prove more effective than single-level interventions. Yet, we should never lose sight of the fact that a crucial station on the road to improved health is in the beliefs and behaviour of each of a series of individuals. (See also Health-related behaviours: common factors', 'Old age and health behaviour', 'Perceived control and health behaviour', 'Physical activity and health', 'Risk perception and health behaviour'.)

REFERENCES

Ajzen, I. & Fishbein, M. (1980). Understanding attitudes and predicting behavior. Englewood Cliffs, NJ: Prentice Hall.

Bandura, A. (1977a). *Social learning theory*. Englewood Cliffs, NJ: Prentice-Hall.

Bandura, A. (1977b). Self-efficacy: toward a unifying theory of behavior change. *Psychological Review*, **84**, 191–215.

Bandura, A. (1986). *Social foundations of thought and action*. Englewood Cliffs, NJ: Prentice-Hall.

Becker, M.H. (Ed.). (1974). The health belief model and personal health behavior. *Health Education Monographs*, **2**, 324–473.

Becker, M.H. & Maiman, L.A. (1980). Strategies for enhancing patient compliance. *Journal of Community Health*, **6**, 113–35.

Cantania, T., Kegeles, J. & Coates, T. (1990). Towards an understanding of risk behavior: an AIDS risk reduction model (AARM). *Health Education Quarterly*, **17**, 53–72.

Hochbaum, G.M. (1958). *Public participation in medical screening programs: a sociopsychological study*. (Public Health Service, PHS Publication 572). Washington, DC: US Government Printing Office.

Janz, N.K. & Becker, M.H. (1984). The health belief model: a decade later. *Health Education Quarterly*, **11**, 1–47.

Kirscht, J.P. (1974). The health belief model and illness behavior. *Health Education Monographs*, **2**, 387–408.

Marlatt, G.A. & Gordon, J.R. (Eds.). (1985). *Relapse prevention*. New York: Guilford Press.

Ronis, D. (1992). Conditional health threats: health beliefs, decisions, and behaviors among adults. *Health Psychology*, **11**, 127–34.

Rosenstock, I.M. (1960). What research in motivation suggests for public health. *American Journal of Public Health*, **50**, 295–301.

Rosenstock, I.M. (1966). Why people use health services. *Milbank Memorial Fund Quarterly*, **44**, 94–124.

Rosenstock, I.M. (1974). Historical origins of the health belief model. *Health Education Monographs*, **2**, 328–35.

Rosenstock, I.M., Strecher, V.J. & Becker, M.H. (1988). Social learning theory and the health belief model. *Health Education Quarterly*, **15**, 175–83.

Strecher, V.J., DeVellis, B.M., Becker, M.H. & Rosenstock, I.M. (1986). The role of self-efficacy in achieving health behavior change. *Health Education Quarterly*, **13**, 73–92.

Health-related behaviours: common factors

TIMOTHY P. CARMODY

San Francisco VA Medical Center,
University of California, USA

INTRODUCTION

Any behaviour that affects health, either positively or negatively, can be considered to be a health-related behaviour. It is difficult to imagine any activity or behaviour that does not affect our health in some way, either directly or indirectly.

Commonly, lists of health-related behaviours include such behaviour patterns as diet, exercise, smoking, alcohol use, safety practices, and participation in health screening exams such as testing for cholesterol levels, breast and prostate cancer. However, there are many other behaviours that affect health, which are less obvious to the general public. For example, the way that a person expresses anger may be associated with the development or acceleration of coronary heart disease (CAD) and neoplasms in some individuals (e.g. Eysenck, 1988). Similarly, engaging in a pleasurable activity can be health related when such behaviour helps an individual to manage pain, stress, or depressed mood.

Some health-related behaviours (e.g. health screening, diet modification, smoking cessation, drug abuse, or safe sex practices) have such an impact on the health of entire populations that they become the focus of public health education campaigns aimed at promoting health and preventing disease in school, work, and community settings. Such health education campaigns are aimed either at healthy people to promote health maintenance and disease prevention or at individuals who are already afflicted with certain illnesses or diseases in order to enhance the quality of their lives, reduce level of disability, delay death, or prevent further deterioration.

To determine the need for, and effectiveness of, such health education campaigns, public health assessment and surveillance surveys have been developed to monitor health-related behaviours or lifestyle patterns in representative samples. For instance, Walker, Sechrist and Pender (1987) developed the Health-Promoting Lifestyle Profile (HPLP) which assesses six dimensions of health-related behaviours: self-actualization, health responsibility, exercise, nutrition, interpersonal support, and stress management. Likewise, Sugarman *et al.* (1992) recently described the Behavioral Risk Factor Surveillance System, a data set based on telephone surveys conducted by state departments of public health in co-ordination with the Center for Disease Control (CDC) to assess progress toward the health objectives for the United States.

In this chapter, common dimensions shared by health-related behaviours will first be reviewed. Psychosocial factors will then be described that are common to health-related behaviours in terms of their initiation, maintenance, and modification. Finally, various theoretical models that have been applied to health-related behavior research will be discussed.

COMMON DIMENSIONS OF HEALTH-RELATED BEHAVIOURS

Health-related behaviours can be described in terms of several dimensions, including duration, frequency, and manner of impact on health (i.e. positive versus negative; direct versus indirect; immediate versus long term). Some health-related behaviours are single actions that occur at a certain point in time and usually involve only one primary decision. Participating in a health-screening exam (e.g. mammography, cholesterol, etc.) is an example of this type of health-related behaviour. Other health-related behaviours continue over an extended period of time in the context of long-term habits or patterns of behaviour that involve many decisions. Smoking, physical exercise, dietary patterns, Type A behaviour are examples of these behaviours.

Health-related behaviours that affect health in a positive way are sometimes referred to as health-protective behaviours. Examples of health-protective behaviours include eating a low-fat diet, engaging in regular physical exercise, using sunscreen, wearing seat belts, and engaging in safe sex practices (e.g. wearing condoms). Likewise, some health behaviours have a negative or deleterious effect on health (e.g. eating a high-fat diet, sedentary lifestyle, substance abuse, and stress-inducing behaviours). Still other health-related behaviours can have both a positive and negative impact on our health. For instance, dietary restraint can facilitate weight loss, but also can result in a restraint–disinhibition pattern of problematic 'yo–yo' dieting and weight fluctuation associated with health risk (Herman & Polivy, 1980; Lowe, 1993).

Behaviour can influence health either directly or indirectly. Some health-related behaviours have a direct impact on physical health. Cigarette smoking is an example of this kind of health-risk behaviour (US Public Health Services, 1990). Other behaviours have an *indirect* impact on health by way of their association with other behaviours or lifestyle patterns, which have a direct impact on health. For instance, according to one theory, hostility increases coronary risk because of its association with other coronary-risk behaviours such as smoking (Scherwitz & Rugulies, 1992; Smith & Christensen, 1992).

Health-related behaviours also vary in terms of the timing of their impact on health. Some behaviours have an immediate impact on health (e.g. accidentally cutting a finger with a knife); others have a long-term effect (e.g. high-fat diet), and still other actions have both immediate and long-term impact on health (e.g. cigarette smoking, dietary restraint, use of sunscreen, regular physical exercise).

Another common feature of health-related behaviours is that they interact. For example, it is well known that alcohol, smoking, and coffee consumption are inter-related (Carmody *et al.*, 1985; Istvan & Matarazzo, 1984). Most of the empirical research has shown a robust association between smoking and alcohol use, and between smoking and coffee consumption. However, there is a dearth of research investigating the co-occurrence of all three of these behaviours (Istvan & Matarazzo, 1984). Similarly, health-protective behaviours can interact with health-risk behaviours. For instance, exercise may provide a healthy substitute for smoking. Some health-related behaviours may become cues for other behaviours (e.g. a cocktail and a cigarette). In some cases, stopping one health-related behaviour may even lead to the onset of another (e.g. quitting smoking leading temporarily to overeating).

COMMON DETERMINANTS OF HEALTH-RELATED BEHAVIOURS

Common psychosocial and environmental factors are involved in the development and modification of health-related behaviours. The psychosocial determinants of health-related behaviours include cognitive factors (i.e. attitudes, beliefs, intentions), soci-cultural variables (influences of family, friends, health-care providers), environmental factors (e.g. stressful events), and individual differences (e.g. hardiness, optimism, locus of control) involved in learning and decision-making processes.

These psychosocial determinants can be categorized in terms of their chronological proximity to a particular health behaviour. Determinants that are more distant from the health-related behaviour might include biological vulnerabilities, developmental characteristics, early learning history, and other cognitive, social, and background variables. More immediate psychosocial precipitants that cue or trigger particular health behaviours can also include cognitive, social, or environmental factors.

The initiation, maintenance, and modification of long-term health-related behaviours often involve classical (respondent) conditioning, operant and social learning factors such as stimulus control, modelling, positive reinforcement, and punishment (Skinner, 1953). Classical conditioning has been shown to be involved in the development of addictive behaviours (e.g. Niaura *et al.* 1988) and dietary behaviour patterns (e.g. Rozin, 1984). As learned behaviours,

health-related behaviours have cues and consequences that influence the occurrence of these behaviours. According to operant learning theory, immediate consequences tend to exert a more powerful influence on behavior than long-term consequences (Skinner, 1953). Research has shown that the most effective methods for changing health-related behaviours are based on the principles of respondent and operant learning (Bandura, 1986). These include: self-monitoring, goal specification, stimulus control, self-reinforcement, and behavioural rehearsal.

Health-related behaviours also have various cognitive determinants. Some of the cognitive factors thought to be involved in the initiation, maintenance, and modification of various health-related behaviours include attributions, expectations, intentions, attitudes, and core beliefs. Attitudes have been conceptualized as including both cognitive and affective components. Intentions are usually considered to be the most immediate influence on behaviour as people make rational use of information available to them (Ajzen & Fishbein, 1980). Beliefs and attributions about the determinants of health and expectations about one's ability to control health play important roles in the learning and decision-making processes involved in the development and modification of health-related behaviours (Bandura, 1986). Expectations about one's ability to accomplish certain behaviours (i.e. self-efficacy expectations) are thought to be important determinants of health-related behaviour. Self-efficacy has been studied in relation to several health-related behaviours, including diet, smoking, alcohol use, weight control, and physical exercise (i.e. Bandura, 1982).

Health-related behaviours have also been studied from a personality or individual difference perspective. For example, optimism has been positively associated with health-protective behaviours (Scheier & Carver, 1987). Likewise, hardiness (Funk, 1992; Kobasa, 1979), which has been conceptualized as involving challenge, commitment, and control, has been shown to be positively associated with health. Both of these individual difference variables have been investigated in relation to their buffering effects on stress. Other individual differences that have been studied in relation to health include: Type A behaviour pattern (Friedman, 1992; Matthews, 1982), health-protection motivation (Prentice-Dunn & Rogers, 1986), dispositional sense of coherence (Antonovsky, 1990), sensation-seeking (Zuckerman, Buschbaum & Murphy, 1980), introversion–extraversion (Eysenck, 1970), and health locus of control (Strickland, 1989). These individual differences involve patterns of behaviour that are themselves health related. Likewise, personality traits may have a moderating effect on other lifestyle risk factors (e.g. Denollet, 1993). The relationships between personality, behaviour and health are complex and largely remain to be elucidated in future multifactorial and longitudinal research.

Health-related behaviours are also influenced by social factors. For example, peer pressure is a primary factor leading to onset of smoking behaviour in adolescents (Mills & Noyes, 1984). Social support can be an important factor in the development and modification of all forms of addictive behaviours. Social factors can play a role in maintenance of health-risk behaviours (e.g. specific forms of substance abuse) as well as health-protective behaviours (e.g. Kaplan & Toshima, 1990). For example, social support has been shown to be an important factor in smoking cessation and the prevention of smoking relapse (Carmody, 1990). Since social skills can be helpful in eliciting and maintaining social support, such behaviours can also be viewed as health related.

Stress has been shown to have a direct impact on the autonomic nervous, neuroendocrine, cardiovascular, and immune systems (Selye, 1980). Stress is also associated with health-related behaviours. The manner in which an individual copes with stressful situations can be considered to be health-related behaviour (Lazarus & Folkman, 1984). Stress can also have an indirect effect on health by disrupting health-protective lifestyle patterns. For instance, adolescents who are in more distress are more likely to experiment with addictive drugs and develop chemical dependencies (Mills & Noyes, 1984). Similarly, depression has been associated with difficulty in quitting cigarette smoking (Carmody, 1990). In fact, stress is the most commonly reported trigger for relapse among chemical-dependent individuals (Marlatt & Gordon, 1985).

Environmental determinants of health-related behaviours include all aspects of an individual's physical surroundings and life circumstances, including exposure to information available on electronic and printed media and proximity to health care and health education resources. Socioeconomic status (SES) has generally been regarded as an important determinant of health-related behaviours and overall health status. For example, health-risk factors such as obesity and cigarette smoking tend to be more prevalent among individuals from lower socioeconomic backgrounds (US Public Health Services, 1988). The mechanisms involved in determining the association between SES and health are yet to be elucidated (Adler et al. 1994). Legal, economic, and regulatory factors also influence health-related behaviours. For instance, in California and elsewhere in the United States, health economists (e.g. Glanz, 1993) are examining the impact of various taxation and other regulatory practices on exposure to environmental tobacco smoke (ETS).

THEORIES OF HEALTH-RELATED BEHAVIOURS

Numerous theories of motivation, learning, and decision-making have been applied to the study of health-related behaviours. These theories have been helpful in guiding research aimed at enhancing our understanding health-related behaviours and developing more effective behaviours-change strategies. However, behavioural scientists have only just begun to apply their theories and methods of studying human behaviour to the field of health promotion.

The most widely researched theories of health-related behaviour include: the health belief model (e.g. Kirscht, 1988), subjective expected utility theory (e.g. Sutton, 1982), conflict theory of decisional balance (Janis & Mann, 1968; Velicer et al., 1985), protection-motivation theory (e.g. Prentice-Dunn & Rogers, 1986), and theory of reasoned action (e.g. Ajzen & Fishbein, 1980). Each of these theories emphasizes the role of beliefs regarding the health consequences of particular behaviours as determinants of health-related decision-making and behaviour. The influence of significant others is also acknowledged as a source of information about subjective norms. These theories are based on the notion that people are rational and typically engage in a process of weighing the pros and cons of engaging in any behaviours that affect their health. Traditionally, they have emphasized perceptions of risk but not beliefs about non-risk issues such as self-esteem which also influence decision-making regarding health-related behaviours (Weinstein, 1993).

Most of these theories of health-related decision-making aim toward predicting a single decision (Weinstein, 1993). In contrast, dynamic models assume that the adoption of health behaviours is a dynamic process involving more than one decision rule and usually consisting of several steps or stages (e.g. Prochaska & DiClemente, 1984). An example of such a dynamic model is the transtheoretical stages of change model (Prochaska & DiClemente, 1984) which includes the following stages in the modification of any health-related behaviour: precontemplation (not thinking about change), contemplation (thinking about change in the next six months), action (overt change), and maintenance (continued change beyond six months). According to this model, specific behaviour-change processes and decision rules tend to be associated with different stages. This transtheoretical model of change has been applied to a variety of addictive behaviours (e.g. smoking, compulsive eating, alcohol use) as well as health-protective behaviours (e.g. weight control, physical exercise) (e.g. Prochaska, et al., 1988).

Recently, Prochaska et al. (1994) studied the stages of change and decisional balance variables in relation to 12 health-related behaviours: smoking cessation, quitting cocaine, weight control, high-fat diets, adolescent delinquent behaviours, safe sex, condom use, sunscreen use, radon gas exposure, physical exercise, mammography screening, and physicians' preventive practices with smokers. Their results supported the applicability of the transtheoretical model of change (Prochaska & DiClemente, 1984) and demonstrated commonalities in terms of the stages of change and decisional balance factors across these 12 health-related behaviours.

Beliefs about risks associated with certain health-damaging behaviours may not necessarily be associated with the absence of those health-risk behaviours. In a recent survey of health behaviours in young adults in eight countries throughout Europe (Steptoe & Wardle, 1992), the results showed that respondents who engaged in more drinking and smoking behaviour were just as much aware of the negative consequences of these health-damaging behaviours as people who did not engage in these addictive behaviours. Across the countries surveyed in this study, few relationships were observed between health-risk behaviours and risk awareness. However, beliefs about the positive effects of health-protective behaviours (e.g. eating a low-fat diet) were strongly associated with the prevalence of those positive health behaviours.

Since compliance with medical regimen involves behaviour that impacts health, theories of compliance have been useful in furthering our understanding of the psychosocial and environmental determinants of health-related behaviours. Leventhal and Cameron (1987) summarized five theories of compliance which focused on biomedical, behavioural, communication, decision-making, and self-regulatory factors. They advocated for an integration of these theories in compliance research that addresses the patient's history of illness, perceptions, coping strategies, and habitual versus reasoned determinants of behaviour change.

SUMMARY AND CONCLUSIONS

Most of our behaviour is health related in the sense that most of our actions affect our health, either directly or indirectly. Some behaviours have multiple effects on our health, some positive and some negative. Common psychosocial and environmental factors influence the learning and decision-making processes involved in the initiation, maintenance, and modification of health-related behaviours. These include cognitive, sociocultural, environmental, and individual difference factors.

Long-term patterns of health-related behaviours usually involve various respondent conditioning and operant learning factors that influence multiple decision-making processes. Moreover, health-related behaviours often interact both in terms of their impact on lifestyle and health. These behaviours evolve in a dynamic process that involves many decisions and multiple cognitive, social, and environmental determinants. Different sets of psychosocial determinants may be critical at different stages in the development and modification of a particular health-related behaviour.

Several theories of learning and decision-making have been applied to the investigation of the psychosocial and environmental determinants of health-related behaviours. Most of these theories have focused on motivational, learning, cognitive, social, and environmental influences on decision-making processes. Theories of health-related behaviours share several common elements that are assumed to affect the decision-making process, including perceived susceptibility, fear arousal, social influences, perceived barriers and benefits, and self-efficacy expectations. These psychosocial constructs provide potential theoretical frameworks for studying the psychosocial determinants of health-related behaviours and designing more effective public health interventions aimed at promoting health-protective behaviours and eliminating health-risk behaviours.

Nevertheless, behavioural scientists have only just begun to apply their theories and methods of studying human behaviour to the field of health-related behaviours. Initial successes have been achieved in such areas as promoting smoking cessation, adherence to prescribed medications, regular physical exercise and fitness, safe sex practices, stress management, and modification of CAD lifestyle risk factors. However, further theory-based research is needed to enhance our ability to understand, predict, and modify health-related behaviours. Among the most promising theoretical approaches is the transtheoretical model of change which attempts to integrate key constructs from several theoretical models in order to develop a more comprehensive understanding of health-related behaviours and enhance our ability to promote health-protective behaviour change. (See also 'The health belief model', 'Old age and health behaviour', 'Physical activity and health'.)

REFERENCES

Adler, N.E., Boyce, T., Chesney, M.A., Cohen, S., Folkman, S., Kahn, R.L. & Syme, S.L. (1994). Socioeconomic status and health: the challenge of the gradient. *American Psychologist*, **49**, 15–24.

Ajzen, I. & Fishbein, M. (1980). *Understanding attitudes and predicting behavior*. Englewood Cliff, N.J.: Prentice-Hall.

Antonovsky, A. (1990). Personality and health: testing the sense of coherence model. In H.S. Friedman (Ed.). *Personality and disease*; pp. 155–177. New York: Wiley.

Bandura, A. (1982). Self-efficacy mechanism in human agency. *American Psychologist*, **37**, 122–42.

Bandura, A. (1986). *Social foundations of thought and action*. Englewood Cliffs, N.J.: Prentice-Hall.

Carmody, T.P. (1990). Preventing relapse in the treatment of nicotine addiction: Current issues and future directions. *Journal of Psychoactive Drugs*, **22**, 211–38.

Carmody, T.P., Brischetto, C.S., Matarazzo, J.D., O'Donnell, R.P.& Connor, W.E. (1985). Co-occurrent use of cigarettes, alcohol, and coffee in healthy community-living men and women. *Health Psychology*, **4**, 323–35.

Denollet, J. (1993). Biobehavioral research on coronary heart disease: where is the person? *Journal of Behavioral Medicine*, **16**, 115–41.

Eysenck, H.J. (1970). *The structure of human personality*. 3rd edn. London: Methuen.

Eysenck, H.J. (1988). Behaviour therapy as an aid in the prevention of cancer and coronary heart disease. *Scandinavian Journal of Behavior Therapy*, **17**, 171–87.

Friedman, H.S. (Ed.). (1992). *Hostility, coping, and health*. Washington, D.C.: American Psychological Association.

Funk, S.C. (1992). Hardiness: a review of theory and research. *Health Psychology*, **11**, 335–45.

Glanz, S.A. (1993). *Tobacco industry response to passive smoking*. Paper presented at a meeting of the Tobacco-related Disease Research Program, San Francisco.

Herman, C.P. & Polivy, J. (1980). Restrained eating. In A.J. Stunkard (Ed.). *Obesity*, pp. 208–225. Philadelphia: Saunders.

Istvan, J. & Matarazzo, J.D. (1984). Tobacco, alcohol, and caffeine use: a review of their interrelationships. *Psychological Bulletin*, **95**, 301–26.

Janis, I.L. & Mann, L. (1968). A conflict-theory approach to attitude change and decision making. In A. Greenwald, T. Brook, & T. Ostrom (Eds.). *Psychological foundations of attitudes*, pp. 327–360. New York: Academic Press.

Kaplan, R.M. & Toshima, M.T. (1990). Social relationships in chronic illness and disability. In I.G. Sarason, B.R. Sarason, & G.R. Pierce (Eds.). *Social support: An interactional perspective*. New York: Wiley.

Kirscht, J.P. (1988). The health belief model and predictions of health actions. In D. Gochman (Ed.). *Health behavior*, pp. 27–41. New York: Plenum Press.

Kobasa, S.C. (1979). Stressful life events, personality, and health: an inquiry into hardiness. *Journal of Personality and Social Psychology*, **37**, 1–11.

Lazarus, R.S. & Folkman, S. (1984). *Stress, appraisal, and coping*. New York: Springer.

Leventhal, H. & Cameron, L. (1987). Behavioral theories and the problem of compliance. *Patient Education and Counseling*, **10**, 117–38.

Lowe, M.R. (1993). The effects of dieting on eating behavior: a three-factor model. *Psychological Bulletin*, **114**, 100–21.

Marlatt, G.A. & Gordon, J.R. (1985). *Relapse Prevention*. New York: Guilford Press.

Matthews, K.A. (1982). Psychological perspectives on the Type A behavior pattern. *Psychological Bulletin*, **91**, 293–323.

Mills, C.J. & Noyes, H.L. (1984). Patterns and correlates of initial and subsequent drug use among adolescents. *Journal of Consulting and Clinical Psychology*, **52**, 231–43.

Niaura, R.S., Rohsenow, D.J., Binkoff, J.A., Monti, P.M., Pedraza, M. & Abrams, D.B. (1988). Relevance of cue reactivity to understanding alcohol and smoking relapse. *Journal of Abnormal Psychology*, **97**, 133–52.

Prentice-Dunn, S. & Rogers, R.W. (1986). Protection motivation theory and preventive health: Beyond the health belief model. *Health Education Research*, **1**, 153–61.

Prochaska, J.O. & DiClemente, C.C. (1984). *The transtheoretical approach: crossing traditional boundaries of change*. Homewood, IL: J. Irwin.

Prochaska, J.O., Velicer, W.F., DiClemente, C.C. & Fava, J. (1988). Measuring processes of change: applications to the cessation of smoking. *Journal of Consulting and Clinical Psychology*, **56**, 520–8.

Prochaska, J.O., Velicer, W.F., Rossi, J.S., Goldstein, M.G., Marcus, G.H., Rakowski, W., Fiore, C., Harlow, L.L., Redding, C.H., Rosenbloom, D. &

Rossi, S.R. (1994). Stages of change and decisional balance for 12 problem behaviors. *Health Psychology*, **13**, 39–46.

Rozin, H.P. (1984). The acquisition of food habits and preferences. In J.D. Matarazzo, S.M. Weiss, J.A. Herd, N.E. Miller & S.M. Weiss (Eds.). *Behavioral health: A handbook of health enhancement and disease prevention*, pp. 590–607. New York: Wiley.

Scheier, M.F. & Carver, C.S. (1987). Dispositional optimism and physical well-being: the influence of generalized outcome expectancies on health. *Journal of Personality*, **55**, 169–210.

Scherwitz, L. & Rugulies, R. (1992). Lifestyle and hostility. In H.S. Friedman (Ed.). *Hostility, coping, and health*, pp. 77–98. Washington, DC: American Psychological Association.

Selye, H. (1980). The stress concept today. In I.L. Kutash, L.B. Schlesinger *et al.* (Eds.). *Handbook on stress and anxiety*, pp. 127–129. San Francisco: Jossey-Bass.

Skinner, B.F. (1953). *Science and human behavior*. New York: Macmillan.

Smith, T.W. & Christensen, A.J. (1992). In H.S. Friedman (Ed.). *Hostility, coping, and health*, pp. 33–48. Washington, DC: American Psychological Association.

Steptoe, A. & Wardle, J. (1992). Cognitive predictors of health behaviour in contrasting regions of Europe. *British Journal of Clinical Psychology*, **31**, 485–502.

Strickland, B.R. (1989). Internal-external control expectancies: from contingency to creativity. *American Psychologist*, **44**, 1–12.

Sugarman, J.R., Warren, C.W., Oge, L. & Helgerson, S.D. (1992). Using the Behavioral Risk Factor Surveillance System to monitor year 2000 objectives among American Indians. *Public Health Reports*, **107**, 449–56.

Sutton, S.R. (1982). Fear arousing communications: a critical examination of theory and research. In J.R. Eiser (Ed.). *Social psychology and behavioral medicine*, pp. 303–338. New York: Wiley.

US Public Health Services (1988). *The surgeon general's report on nutrition and health*. Washington, DC: US Department of Health and Human Services.

US Public Health Services (1990). *The health consequences of smoking: a report of the surgeon general*, CDC Report No 89–8411. Rockville, MD: US Department of Health and Human Services.

Velicer, W.F., DiClemente, C.C., Prochaska, J.O. & Brandenburg, N. (1985). Decisional balance measure for assessing and predicting smoking status. *Journal of Personality and Social Psychology*, **48**, 1279–89.

Walker, S.N., Sechrist, K.R. & Pender, N.J. (1987). The Health-Promoting Lifestyle Profile: development and psychometric characteristics. *Nursing Research*, **36**, 76–81.

Weinstein, N.D. (1993). Testing four competing theories of health-protective behavior. *Health Psychology*, **12**, 324–33.

Zuckerman, M., Buschbaum, M. & Murphy, D. (1980). Sensation-seeking and its biological correlates. *Psychological Bulletin*, **88**, 187–214.

Hospitalization in adults

MARIE JOHNSTON

Department of Psychology, University of St Andrews, Fife, Scotland, UK

INTRODUCTION

Hospitalization occurs when symptoms of illness can no longer be tolerated in the individual's domestic environment, when technical investigations need to be performed, or when treatments requiring specific equipment or 24-hour patient monitoring are to be undertaken. One might therefore expect that, at least for a substantial minority, hospitalization would be viewed as a source of relief or reassurance, or would hold out the possibility of offering a better understanding of symptoms or even resolution of symptoms. However, in the psychological literature, it is primarily conceptualized as a source of stress. Positive evaluations of hospitalization are largely restricted to literatures dealing with carer burden, e.g. for patients with Alzheimer's disease. On the other hand, discharge from hospital is seen as a stressful time and Ley (1988) has reported high levels of depression in patients in the period following discharge.

The Hospital Stress Rating Scale (Volicer & Bohannon, 1975) describes 49 events associated with being in hospital which may be stressful. The most stressful, thinking you might lose your sight, relates to the threat of illness as does the fourth, knowing you have a serious illness. Major sources of stress in hospital are the investi-gations and treatments, which may involve pain and uncertainty of outcome, e.g. knowing you have to have an operation (18) and other studies have found that anticipating painful treatments and proced-ures is a source of apprehension or distress for the great majority of patients. Other items relate to being away from family and home, e.g. missing your spouse (12) or being hospitalized far away from home (17), or to being in a new environment (Lucente & Fleck, 1972) which lacks privacy (see Architecture and health, Part 2, this Section), is shared by other people who are ill and receiving treat-ment, e.g. unfamiliarity of surroundings. Dependency on hospital staff and the possibility of poor communications in hospital can also be a source of stress as indicated by items such as not having your questions answered by the staff (13) or not being told what your dia-gnosis is (6).

Overall, surgical patients show higher levels of stress than med-ical patients. They score higher on unfamiliarity of surroundings, loss of independence and threat of severe illness, but lower on lack of information and financial problems.

Hospitalization obviously affects other people in the patient's social network, in addition to the patient. However, the effects on them have not been studied.

[121]

EVIDENCE OF STRESS

Emotional State

Many studies use scales that have been developed specifically to measure patients' anxiety about hospitalization but others use scales that have been used to measure mood or distress in other situations and populations. These latter scales have usually been extensively developed and validated and allow comparison of hospitalized patients with normal mood levels, with people undergoing other kinds of threat or with patients having mood disorders. An important consideration is whether the scale confuses symptoms of the patient's illness or of the effects of treatment with somatic mood effects; for example, patients may report feeling lethargic because of thyroid disorder or the after-effects of anaesthesia rather than as a feature of depressed mood. Some scales have been developed to either separate or omit such somatic items.

Numerous studies show evidence of high levels of psychological distress in hospitalized patients when compared with normal populations, including high rates of clinical emotional disorder. For example, surgical patients assessed on the day prior to surgery, show levels of anxiety that, on average, fall between normal levels and levels reported by psychiatric patients with diagnosed anxiety disorder, but are similar to those found in students prior to examinations. Anxiety levels continue to be high after surgery (Johnston, 1980), suggesting that the anxiety is caused not only by the threat of surgery but also by the ongoing discomforts and uncertainties.

Cognitions

When the concerns of hospital patients have been examined, it is clear that they have significant worries which are unrelated to the hospital environment, often concerning the welfare of their family at home in the patient's absence, or even ongoing everyday worries irrelevant to health and hospital (Johnston, 1988). Hospital worries may address both their medical condition and its treatment. While research has tended to focus on worries about treatment procedures, patients are more likely to be concerned about treatment outcomes, or even, the outcome of the disease whether or not treatment is possible. To some extent, these worries are inevitable because of the unpredictable nature of these outcomes, but this is exacerbated by the lack of information available to patients. Studies of psychological preparation for medical procedures demonstrate that provision of information or enhancing the patient's ability to tolerate the uncertainties can reduce the stressfulness of the experience.

Physiological

Physiological stress responses can be induced both by psychological stressors and by the physical procedures associated with medical treatment. For example, one study found raised levels of cortisol in patients on the evening before surgery, but could not identify whether these effects were due to the physical manipulations associated with shaving and enema or to the psychological implications of these procedures. A study by Corenblum and Taylor (1981) used blocking agents to demonstrate that prolactin increases due to the physical trauma were mediated by different physiological mechanisms from prolactin increases due to apprehension about surgery.

These physiological effects may interact with physiological disease and recovery processes, and might be part of the explanation of the poorer recovery of anxious surgical patients and the enhanced recovery of patients receiving psychological preparation.

INDIVIDUAL DIFFERENCES

People who are anxious by disposition are more likely to be highly anxious in the hospital situation than people low in trait anxiety. Hospital would appear to provide the threatening situations which elicit this underlying personality. People with high levels of anxiety may also use different coping strategies in dealing with the situation.

Coping strategies can be divided into problem-focused and emotion-focused strategies, the former attempting to reduce the impact of stress by removing the source, while the latter aims to minimize the emotional impact without necessarily dealing with the source. It has been suggested that some patients having surgery may try to deal with the threats by using an avoidant strategy which includes minimizing the dangers and directing one's attention to other matters, and such patients would tend to have low scores on tests of anxiety. Initially, it was proposed by Janis (1958) that such a strategy would result in poor outcomes for the patient as they would fail to do the necessary cognitive preparation, or 'work of worrying', and as a result would find the postoperative period unexpectedly harsh. Janis proposed that patients with low and high anxiety scores would do badly postoperatively and that a moderate level of anxiety was necessary to achieve optimal preparation. However, empirical studies have not found support for this hypothesis and instead patients having low levels of preoperative anxiety or those using avoidant coping strategies have done well postoperatively; it would appear that avoidant coping is adaptive for stressors of relatively short duration (Suls & Fletcher, 1985).

Factors which influence responses to hospitalization may be different in children (q.v.) or in elderly people (q.v.). Those with particular clinical conditions may also have different issues to contend with. For example, hospital staff on a surgical ward may have difficulty in ascertaining the level of support necessary for a disabled patient or the supervision and support required by a psychiatric patient. There is some evidence that patients whose condition results in some way from their own behaviour may receive different treatment and, for example, patients with AIDS may be treated less favourably (see 'Attitudes of health-care professionals'; Part 2, Section 3).

PSYCHOLOGICAL PREPARATION

While little work has been done to prepare adult patients for hospitalization *per se*, there is now very strong evidence that psychological preparation for surgery can result in better outcomes (Johnston & Vogele, 1993). A variety of methods have been used including:

- behavioural instruction: teaching techniques such as breathing and relaxation;
- procedural information: giving patients information about the procedures they will undergo;
- sensory information: giving patients information about the sensations they will experience;
- cognitive coping: teaching methods of reinterpreting apparent threats in a more positive light, using distraction, etc.

All of these methods have been shown to be effective. They have been found to improve a wide variety of important outcomes, including:

- anxiety
- pain
- pain medication
- behavioural recovery
- physiological indices
- length of stay.

Thus benefits are not confined to benefits in psychological functioning, but include outcomes of physiological significance and outcomes that affect health care costs.

Surgical patients have also been found to benefit by spending the preoperative period with patients who have already had the operation they are about to undergo (Kulik & Mahler, 1987). This study suggests that there is considerable potential for improving patient care by organizational as well as direct patient care interventions.

Interventions have also been designed for patients undergoing non-surgical procedures. Such procedures differ from the typical surgical procedure in that the patient is conscious and may be required to co-operate to ensure an efficient and effective procedure, e.g. in endoscopy. Sensory information and cognitive coping procedure have been found to be effective (Kendall & Epps, 1990).

There has been some concern that psychological preparation might be damaging for patients using avoidant coping strategies as the preparation might disrupt the patient's coping. While there is some evidence to support this view, a study by Shipley *et al.* (1978) suggests that the problem can be overcome by giving adequate preparation. Patients awaiting a stressful medical procedure saw a preparatory videotape either once or three times. Those with an avoidant coping style showed higher levels of anxiety during the endoscopy compared with a control group who saw an irrelevant control video, but only when they had seen the video once; they showed neither detrimental nor beneficial effects when they had seen it three times. Patients with attention coping styles showed benefit whether the video was shown one or three times. Thus the more thorough preparation resulted in benefits without the damaging side-effects for the avoidant copers.

COMMUNICATION BETWEEN PATIENTS AND STAFF

Patients in hospital depend on staff for their care and treatment, for information about their treatment and progress, and even for meeting their basic needs when the patient is severely disabled or restricted even temporarily as in the case of surgical patients. While patients may be diffident about asking for information, and the ethos of the hospital may imply that the 'good patient' takes a more passive role, studies have consistently shown that patients are dissatisfied with the amount of information they receive (Ley, 1988). Doctors and nurses have been wary of giving information which might be misinterpreted or which might alarm the patient, but even in serious illness such as cancer, over 90% of patients want to know about their diagnosis and treatment (Reynolds *et al.*, 1981), and in patients with motor neurone disease (q.v.), a disease which is progressively disabling and eventually terminal, incurable and lacking palliative treatments, the majority of patients have reported positive aspects of being given the diagnosis. By contrast, patients resent finding out important information by indirect means such as overhearing professional conversations.

Health-care professionals may lack the skills to identify patients concerns or to communicate effectively (Ley, 1988). Nurses underestimate patients' pain, and are poor at identifying which patients are worried about particular matters. Courses to develop communication skills are now an integral part of the training of doctors and nurses in many colleges.

Professionals may also fail to communicate effectively because communicating bad news or talking to very ill patients is particularly stressful (Parkes, 1985) and doctors and nurses are observed to have high levels of stress and may even demonstrate burnout (see Part 2, Section 3). (See also 'Coping with chronic illness', 'Attributions and health', 'Effects of hospitalization on children'.)

REFERENCES

Corenblum, B. & Taylor, P.J. (1981). Mechanisms of control of prolactin release in response to apprehension stress and anaesthesia. *Fertility and Sterility*, 365, 712–15.

Janis, I. (1958). *Psychological stress*. New York: Wiley.

Johnston, M. (1980). Anxiety in surgical patients. *Psychological Medicine*, 10, 145–52.

Johnston, M. (1988). Impending surgery. In S. Fisher & J. Reason (Eds.). *Handbook of life stress, cognition and health*. London: Wiley.

Johnston, M. & Vogele, C. (1993). Benefits of psychological preparation for surgery: a meta-analysis. *Annals of Behavioral Medicine*, 15, 245–56.

Kendall, P.C. & Epps, J. (1990). Medical treatments. In M. Johnston & L. Wallace (Eds.). *Stress and medical procedures*. Oxford: Oxford University Press.

Kulik, J.A. & Mahler, H.I.M. (1987). Effects of preoperative room-mate assignment on preoperative anxiety and recovery from coronary by-pass surgery. *Health Psychology*, 6, 525–43.

Ley, P. (1988). *Communicating with patients*. London: Croom Helm.

Lucente, F.E. & Fleck, S. (1972). A study of hospitalisation anxiety in 408 medical and surgical patients. *Psychosomatic Medicine*, 34, 304–12.

Parkes, K.R. (1985). Stressful episodes reported by first year student nurses: a descriptive account. *Social Science Medicine*, 20, 945–53.

Reynolds, P.M., Sanson-Fisher, R., Poole, A. & Harker, J. (1981). Cancer and communication: information giving in an oncology clinic. *British Medical Journal*, 282, 1449–51.

Shipley, R.H., Butt, J.H., Horwitz, B. & Farbry, J.E. (1978). Preparation for a stressful medical procedure: effect of amount of stimulus pre-exposure and coping style. *Journal of Consulting and Clinical Psychology*, 46, 499–507.

Suls, J. & Fletcher, B. (1985). The relative efficacy of avoidant and nonavoidant coping strategies: a meta-analysis. *Health Psychology*, 4, 249–88.

Volicer, B.J. & Bohannon, M.W. (1975). A hospital stress rating scale. *Nursing Research*, 24, 352–9.

Hospitalization in children

LOTHAR R. SCHMIDT

University of Trier, Department of Psychology,
Germany

INTRODUCTION

Due to the sheer number of children in hospitals today, the effects of hospitalization on these patients is without doubt an important one. In many countries, roughly half of the children are hospitalized at least once during childhood (disregarding the stay for their own birth). Many children have to go to hospitals repeatedly, and may receive complicated sequences of treatments because of severe illnesses. According to several authors, the prevalence of chronic illness conditions among children under 18 years of age has a range from 10% to 30% (Johnson, 1994; Newacheck & Taylor, 1992; Seiffge-Krenke *et al.*, 1996; Pless *et al.*, 1989).

In spite of marked changes in the hospital situation, the hospitalization of children is still a very emotional topic (even for professionals) which may lead to misinterpretations of the results and intentions of researchers (Eiser, 1988; Saile, Burgmeier & Schmidt, 1989).

Most of the studies which are quoted as main references for the severe, negative influences of hospital stays are rather old (Eiser, 1985). It seems rather useless to compare the results of studies which are more than 25 years old with more recent ones. The situation of children in the hospital has changed dramatically, mainly for the better. Thus, for example, the deprivation of children in hospitals, which was a frequent claim in the older literature, has now often been superseded by overstimulation.

There have been many initiatives from parents and professionals, resulting in very liberal visiting hours, permission to room-in, shorter hospital stays and the adequate preparation of the children. In addition, the hospitals frequently offer play groups, allow the children to bring in their own toys or games, and provide facilities like TV, walkmans etc. The professionals, especially the nurses, are better prepared with regard to the main needs of children in hospitals. In order to normalize the structure of the wards, many changes took place in the architecture, e.g. more openness of the rooms or more play rooms.

Saile (1987) explored 80 mothers one week after discharge of their children (mean age 3 years) from a German children's hospital. The psychological state and the behaviour of the children were rated by the mothers. There were only a few changes observed by the mothers, which were mainly modest.

Altogether, in Germany as in many other countries, the complaints of the 1950s and 1960s about inhumane conditions for children in hospital are just no longer true for most children's hospitals and wards. However, there are exceptions with regard to some special clinics or wards and with respect to certain children, especially boys, who are sometimes placed on an adult ward (e.g. for tonsillectomy).

FACTORS INFLUENCING THE EFFECTS OF HOSPITALIZATION

There are many different events and influences which make the hospital a potentially stressful place (Eiser, 1985; Rudolph, Denning & Weisz, 1995; Schmidt, 1992; Saile & Schmidt, 1990; Smorti & Tani, 1990) for example:

- separation from the mother, the father and the siblings
- fantasies and unrealistic anxieties about darkness, monsters, murders and wild animals (Smorti & Tani, 1990), which are not specifically related to hospitals but initiated by the strange situation;
- deprivation of social contacts (which does not seem to pose a major problem today, since other children and visitors can come to the bed without restrictions);
- social demands and threats;
- pain and other complications of the illness or surgery;
- stressful medical procedures, especially extremely *painful* procedures such as burn wound debridement or bone-marrow aspirations (Pruitt & Elliott, 1990);
- fears of disablement and death.

Children's concepts of hospitals and illness should be carefully assessed; in particular, magical thinking has to be regarded. Feelings of guilt, the belief in punishment from higher forces, etc. are frequent in young children and not unusual in older children and even adults.

On the other hand, the hospital may become a potentially compensatory and positive place, may even provide a 'kick' by

- enabling the child to become a 'hero' afterwards;
- offering opportunities for social experiences with other children and adults;
- offering intellectual stimulation, especially for underserved children.

In the above study (Saile, 1987), most of the few, yet strong changes in children's psychological states after hospitalization were in a positive direction (e.g. more vivacious, quicker, more active, more cheerful).

In a review, Saile and Schmidt (1990) provided a comprehensive framework of factors influencing hospitalization in childhood, which include:

- contextual factors, e.g. type of hospital and ward, special facilities for rooming-in, professional structure, architecture
- amount and kind of former experiences with hospitals and medical procedures including vicarious experiences, information and attitudes about hospitals

- variables of the children, e.g. age, sociodemographic situation, development, personality structure
- variables of the parents, e.g. rooming-in, educational practice and attitudes, personality structure, own experiences within the medical field.

Only few of these factors can, and will, be discussed here briefly.

There are many different types of hospitals and wards, like specialized hospitals for children, special wards for children in general hospitals or hospitals mainly for adults yet which also treat children, university clinics (often more geared towards medical research, further removed from the community and thus affording fewer visits, etc.) vs the regular type of hospital in the community or close to it, and finally, intensive care units for premature children or for older children with severe illnesses.

Deprivation is no longer a general problem for children in a hospital, rather, the overstimulation through noise and social contacts is. However, in special conditions, isolation might be required in the sequence of several treatments. Thus, deprivation and, in particular, the lack of direct communication may still be harmful.

Disregarded in this context are hospitals for psychiatric diseases as well as seizures or long-time visible handicaps (Merkens et al., 1989) since these patients need special care and show special problems which cannot be analyzed here. Also disregarded are the special psychological problems of children who are abused or mistreated by their parents.

Crucial to the effects of hospital stays are the reasons (causes) for the hospital admission, e.g. psychiatric disorders, conduct disorders, psychosomatic disorders, neurology (infections or chronic diseases), intensive care (premature birth, impairment, injuries), disabilities, infectious diseases, chronic diseases (cancer, dialysis, heart diseases, diabetes), elective surgery, major surgery and injuries (burns, ill treatment). Some of the conditions are remedied with one single stay in hospital, many of them, however, require multiple stays.

Usually, multiple hospital stays and the stressfulness of the treatment are related. The psychologically positive pole is one stay for an elective procedure without a major disease for children who are not younger than 4 years of age. In this case, usually no major psychological complications should be expected. On the other hand, if the children are very young, or if the procedures are very unpleasant and repeatedly applied, the staff should be alert in order to prevent as much disturbance as possible. If the probability of complications is low, the child and the parents should find a calm, confident, determined staff to serve as a model for them.

Previous hospital experiences with former hospitalizations may have negative effects (Melamed, 1984). Therefore, it is extremely important to try to finish each hospital stay, especially the first one, with an emotionally positive result for the child and the family.

It seems quite clear that the hospital situation actualizes patterns of interaction between mother and child that are not specific to the hospitalization *per se*. In other words, some interactional problems are brought to the hospital rather than being created through the hospitalization. Some of the illnesses which are the reason for the hospitalization may even stem from conflict patterns in the family.

The role of the *mother* is underscored in almost any publication and is usually regarded as a positive influence without further reflection. This was the main reason to fight for the rooming-in option. However, empirical studies show that the main effects of

rooming-in are often not impressive (Saile, 1987; Gutezeit, Daudert & Pehrs, 1991).

Saile (1987) analysed the emotional reactions of children between the age of 1.6 and 4.6 years with and without rooming-in. The children were hospitalized for elective surgery and had no major diseases. The positive effects of rooming-in could only be found for children of less than 3 years of age. In this hospital, however, the climate was very positive and many mothers also cared for children other than their own.

Gutezeit et al. (1991), measuring state anxiety in preschool children with and without rooming-in, who underwent strabotomy, were surprised about the small effects of rooming-in. They conclude that 'personality traits of the mother and the kind of attitude towards physicians and strabotomy neutralize the effect of rooming-in.' (p. 264) Therefore, they call for a preparation programme, especially for insecure mothers.

Glazebrook, et al. (1994) analysed implications for maternal presence in the anaesthetic room of children who were admitted for minor surgery

'More distress was shown by younger children and those scoring highly on temperament traits of intensity of response and withdrawal from new situations. There was also evidence that maternal presence in the anaesthetic room was associated with less distress . . . and children accompanied by mothers had significantly better behavioural adjustment at one week post-operation.' quotation (p. 55)

For children with chronic illnesses, the steady care of the mother seems extremely important. However, for mothers these tasks are often unresolvable (especially when there are other siblings to care for, or conflicting goals and attitudes in the family) and may lead to the state of 'miscarried helping' (Anderson & Coyne, 1993).

The Miscarried Helping Theory addresses the reality that parents with chronically ill children are faced with two sometimes conflicting sets of tasks: first, taking responsibility for implementing a regimen at home and warding off the immediate threat of medical crises; and second, establishing a context in which the child takes developmentally appropriate strides in assuming self-responsibility. In meeting the first set of tasks, particularly when driven by a sense of urgency and impending disaster or not adequately informed about their limits of influence over the disease, the child may be seen as an object or obstacle. The parent may resort to coercive or hostile-critical responses that achieve immediate compliance but make it more difficult to achieve compliance in the long run or to develop the child's self-responsibility. (Anderson & Coyne, 1993, p. 88).

PSYCHOLOGICAL PREPARATION

The psychological preparation of children and family members, especially mothers, has different perspectives depending on the contextual factors and the illness of the child. Essentially, one has to differentiate between (i) the general preparation for hospitalization, (ii) the preparation for specific medical procedures, and (iii) the preparation with regard to severe and chronic illnesses in general and to specific treatments for chronic illness (i.e. chemotherapy or bone marrow transplantation).

The general preparation for hospitalization can be accomplished by hospital tours with children in the kindergarten or in school. A quite popular and economic procedure is the showing of modelling films or videos.

However, instead of using one available video, each hospital should provide videos tailored to their own clinic, in order to create as much familiarity as possible with the personal and physical surroundings. In addition, it might be helpful to present different videos with problems which are related to the problems of the given child (surgery, chemotherapy, etc.).

A main area of psychological research and practice is the preparation for distinct medical procedures, e.g., blood tests, punctures, cardiac catheterization or different kinds of surgery (Rudolph *et al.*, 1995; Saile, Burgmeier & Schmidt, 1988). The preparation techniques and methods in these studies are modelling, cognitive behavioural interventions, treatment packages, supportive care, expressive techniques, providing information and relaxation techniques.

In a meta-analysis of controlled intervention studies, the effect of preparation methods was assessed quantitatively by Saile *et al.* (1988). The analysis was limited to 75 studies of children under 13 years of age who showed no other impairments. In almost all the cases, the children were prepared for an actual event. Only five studies prepared chronically ill children for highly aversive diagnostic and therapeutic measures.

In 125 controlled comparisons, the mean treatment effect was .44. This effect is statistically highly significant. However, in overlapping normal distribution curves it leads only to a 17 rank improvement. Thus, the individual or clinical importance of this main effect seems to be rather modest. The preparation did not have very marked differential effects. The most frequently used method of preparation, (modelling films) had below-average effects. A more recent meta-analysis led to comparable results (Saile & Krause, 1994).

However, in the present literature, the children who can be regarded most at risk often are not reached, since the preparation is most usually practised with older children for minor to moderate, one-time procedures.

Severe problems arise with chronic disease and especially with dying children. In these cases, the hospital is only *one* condition, working in combination to the existential threats, the complex sequences of procedures, and the resulting handicaps. There are special programmes which deal with the psychosocial aspects of children with chronic disease.

The effects of long term stays should be analyzed and discussed carefully. As Newacheck and Taylor (1992) have shown, the burden is uneven. About 5% of all chronically ill children have severe handicaps and multiple hospital stays. They and their parents are especially in need for help.

According to Pless *et al.* (1989, p. 753)

> . . . the prognosis for the social circumstances of the chronically
> physically ill child was remarkably good . . . The findings on mental
> state are confusing however. Between 15 and 26 years, those
> chronically physically ill in childhood reported more emotional problems
> than the other cohort members.

In order to provide optimal psychological preparation, psychologists should be consistently represented on the wards. They should find out which children are in need of psychological preparation in which situations. In addition, they could work with groups of children and take care that children do not induce anxiety by telling horrifying stories. Instead, they should try to find mastery models for the forthcoming treatments of a given child.

RESEARCH

Most studies on the effects of hospital stays in children do not employ a rigorous methodology. Very often, the data consist only of straight observations during the hospital stay or the answers of mothers to a simple questionnaire. Drawings of the children during their stay in the hospital often look very interesting, but it is almost always very hard to accomplish a valid interpretation of them.

In many studies, the different types of diseases, procedures, etc. are not regarded in a systematic way. Thus, very heterogenous samples of children might be confounded in the same study or by comparing studies which do not rely on the same hospital populations. As Standen (1990, p. 242) claims,

> Often research concentrates on particular age groups and so we still do
> not know enough about changes associated with all ages.

An exact documentation of procedures and experiences of children is needed, in order to change whatever is not necessary or helpful to them. During the hospital stay, emotions like anxiety should be measured as well as aggression and attachment towards the parents and siblings at home. In intensive care units and during the process of chronic illness in children, attachment and transference processes have to be carefully analysed.

CONCLUSIONS

Altogether, the situation of hospitalized children should neither be exaggerated nor undervalued. For most children, the problems are manageable indeed and do not have a long-lasting, negative impact. As mentioned above, psychologists should be present on the ward in order to prevent severe negative effects. They can also correct some of the problems of mothers who are overly anxious, emotionally unstable, or aggressive.

In spite of a lot of progress in the care for hospitalized children, whenever possible, ambulant care should have the first priority. Unnecessary hospital stays should be avoided for routine procedures as well as for chronic illnesses. Nevertheless, as Standen (1990) claims, there are many aspects to be regarded if young surgical patients are cared for at home. Especially with regard to chronic illness, frequent hospitalization might lead to a further fixation on medical care and the organic illness conditions. However, it seems important to keep as much relative health as possible in any illness condition (American Academy of Pediatrics, 1993).

In this respect, the behaviour of many children in hospitals might serve as a model for adults (patients and professionals) in hospitals and with diseases and disabilities. Even in dialysis, children often react quite naturally in comparison to adults. They do not care too much about the apparatus and the blood flow, but seem primarily interested in playing, doing their schoolwork, etc. In general, children try to change their surroundings in order to make a 'normal' life possible. The optimism and positive attitude in children can be exaggerated and, in severe illness conditions, can lead to severe consequences.

The different processes of coping have to be reflected upon (Rudolph *et al.*, 1995). Children, with their limited capacity to anticipate consequences, show more defensive and functional optimism. They do not only trust in the physicians and nurses, but especially in their parents. Sometimes, this trustful attitude changes drastically if chronically ill children find out that even their parents are not able to save their life or to provide them with a decent life.

Eiser (1988, p. 137) emphasizes in a very emotional comment on preparation procedures,

> *the continuing need to develop, improve, and make available preparation techniques for all hospitalized children.*

This is definitely not my position and one not inferred from the literature. For the many children who have no problems in the hospital, too much care might be harmful. On the other hand, any child in need of psychological assistance should find it.

One could argue that some children cannot articulate their psychological needs. This is a major problem, especially with very young or very shy children. On the other hand, nobody knows if a routine preparation procedure for these children is adequate. Even protagonists of behavioural medicine like Melamed (1984) found the same preparation procedures to have marked differential effects for different children.

Arguments with a naive, humanistic touch have a great chance of being accepted with regard to the situation of children in hospitals, because here, professional and personal attitudes are confounded in many of us. Such arguments may make mothers and professionals on the wards unnecessarily tense in the interaction with the child. It seems to be the main duty of psychologists to strengthen professional positions, which are in accordance with psychological experiences and with the results of psychological studies. (See also 'Hospitalization in adults' 'Children's perceptions of illness and death'.)

REFERENCES

American Academy of Pediatrics (1993). Child life programs. *Pediatrics*, **91**, 671–3.

Anderson, B.J. & Coyne, J.C. (1993). Family context and compliance behavior in chronically ill children. In N.A. Krasnegor, L. Epstein, S.B. Johnson & S.J. Yaffe (Eds.). *Developmental aspects of health compliance behavior*, pp. 77–89. Hillsdale, N.J.: Erlbaum.

Eiser, C. (1985). *The psychology of childhood illness.* New York: Springer.

Eiser, C. (1988). Do children benefit from psychological preparation for hospitalization? *Psychology and Health*, **2**, 133–8.

Glazebrook, C.P., Lim, E., Sheard, C.E. & Standen, P.J. (1994). Child temperament and reaction to induction of anaesthesia: implications for maternal presence in the anaesthetic room. *Psychology and Health*, **10**, 55–67.

Gutezeit, G., Daudert, E. & Pehrs, C. (1991). Children during hospitalization with regard to rooming-in and the state-anxiety of their mothers. In G. Biondi (Ed.). *Psychology in hospital*, pp. 259–265. Rome: Nuova Editrice Spada.

Johnson, S.B. (1994). Chronic illness in children. In G.N. Penny, P. Bennett & M. Herbert (Eds.). *Health psychology: a lifespan perspective*, pp. 31–50. Chur: Harwood.

Melamed, B.G. (1984). Health intervention: collaboration for health and science. In B.L. Hammonds & C.J. Scheirer (Eds.). *Psychology and health*, pp. 45–119. Washington, DC: APA.

Merkens, M.J., Perrin, E.C., Perrin, J.M. & Gerrity, P.S. (1989). The awareness of primary physicians of the psychosocial adjustment of children with a chronic illness. *Developmental and Behavioral Pediatrics*, **10**, 1–6.

Newacheck, P.W. & Taylor, W.R. (1992). Childhood chronic illness: Prevalence, severity, and impact. *American Journal of Public Health*, **82**, 364–71.

Pless, I.B., Cripps, H.A., Davies, J.M.C & Wadsworth, M.E.J. (1989). Chronic physical illness in childhood psychological and social effects in adolescence and adult life. *Developmental Medicine and Child Neurology*, **31**, 746–55.

Pruitt, S.D. & Elliott, C.H. (1990). Paediatric procedures. In M. Johnston & L. Wallace (Eds.). *Stress and medical procedures*, pp. 157–174. Oxford: Oxford University Press.

Rudolph, K.D., Denning, M.D. & Weisz, J.R. (1995). Determinants and consequences of children's coping in the medical setting: conceptualization, review and critique. *Psychological Bulletin*, **118**, 328–57.

Saile, H. (1987). *Entwicklungspsychologische Beiträge zur psychischen Belastung von Kindern durch einen Krankenhausaufenthalt. Eine Untersuchung zum Einfluß von Rooming-in und Temperament.* Frankfurt: Lang.

Saile, H. & Krause, S. (1994). Psychologische Vorbereitung von Kinder auf medizinische Maßnahmen: Replikation einer Metaanalyse. *Zeitschrift für Gesundheitspsychologie*, **2**, 176–93.

Saile, H. & Schmidt, L.R. (1990). Krankenhausaufenthalte bei Kindern. In I. Seiffge-Krenke (Ed.). *Krankheitsverarbeitung bei Kindern und Jugendlichen (= Jahrbuch der Medizinischen Psychologie.* Vol. 4), pp. 225–242. Berlin: Springer.

Saile, H., Burgmeier, R. & Schmidt, L.R. (1988). A meta-analysis of studies on psychological preparation of children facing medical procedures. *Psychology and Health*, **2**, 107–32.

Saile, H., Burgmeier, R. & Schmidt, L.R. (1989). Under which conditions do children benefit from psychological preparation for medical procedures? Comment on Eiser's critique. *Psychology and Health*, **3**, 143–44.

Schmidt, H-L. (1992). *Kinder erleben das Krankenhaus. Deprivation und Trennungstraumata im Lichte neuerer psychologischer Forschung.* Eichstätt: Kaufmann.

Seiffge-Krenke, I. Boeger, A., Schmidt, C., Kollmar, F., Floß, A. & Roth, M. (1996). *Chronisch kranke Jugendliche und ihre Familien.* Stuttgart: Kohlhammer.

Smorti, A. & Tani, F. (1990). Ängste von Kindern auf einer offenen pädiatrischen Station und die Einstellung ihrer Eltern zum Krankenhausaufenthalt. In I. Seiffge-Krenke (Ed.). *Krankheitsverarbeitung bei Kindern und Jugendlichen (= Jahrbuch der Medizinischen Psychologie.* Vol. 4), pp. 243–260. Berlin: Springer.

Standen, P. (1990). Psychological issues in child health. In P. Bennett, J. Weinman & P. Spurgeon (Eds.). *Current developments in health psychology*, pp. 229–245. Chur: Harwood.

Hospitalization in the elderly

SHULI REICH

Elderly Care Unit, St Thomas' Hospital, London,
UK

The disadvantages and debilitating effects of long-term hospitalization and institutional care have been well documented. In comparison, the potentially harmful impact of short-term hospitalization for the acutely medically ill elderly is a relatively neglected field. The present review focuses on this group of patients.

Elderly patients in acute geriatric and general medical wards may vary substantially in terms of their physical ability. The majority of patients who are admitted to these wards, particularly to geriatric wards that offer an age-related service (i.e. admitting all acutely ill patients over 75 years), make a complete recovery from their acute illness after only a few days in hospital. A sizeable proportion of patients (20–50%) however, may be chronically disabled and have a worse prognosis with higher rates of morbidity and mortality. The disability experienced by these patients generally results from a combination of the impairments associated with ageing and those associated with chronic diseases, most commonly chronic obstructive airways disease, degenerative arthritis, diabetes, heart failure, dementia and stroke. The impact of chronic disability in these patients is often compounded by their social isolation. For example, in an inner city, deprived catchment area, roughly half of all patients live alone with few, if any, social contacts outside statutory services. Almost all patients are admitted acutely on the day of referral following a GP visit or from the Accident and Emergency department and approximately 10% of these patients will be readmitted within a one-month period. The majority of patients live at home and the median age in a typical service is about 80 years.

The purpose of this chapter is to review the characteristics of the acute hospital setting and the attitudes and management styles of its staff in the context of the above group of patients in order to identify the potential risks and hazards of short periods of hospitalization.

Consider the following scenario: an elderly widow with chronic osteoarthritis and moderate chronic obstructive airways disease is admitted to hospital from her home with a chest infection. Prior to her recent illness, she was able to walk with a stick slowly and with difficulty around her flat and had been managing independently with the assistance of a weekly home help to do her shopping and cleaning. After a few days on the ward, she appears to have recovered from the chest infection but has failed to regain her former level of mobility. She has great difficulty in trying to stand, requiring the assistance of two members of staff, and hyperventilates in anticipation of any physical exertion. When questioned about her discharge, she reiterates the newly adopted views of her daughter and son-in-law that she could not possibly cope if she were to return home saying, 'Look my dear, I have lived through two World Wars and now I want to be looked after'! Although this may be an infrequent example of hospital-induced dependency, it provides an extreme illustration of a common dilemma that confronts the multidisciplinary team. Apparent changes in attitude of patients, who are potentially able to mobilize and return home but appear to be 'unmotivated to do so', are not rare occurrences.

ANTECEDENT STRESSORS

Although there may be several factors associated with the hospital environment that may have triggered this change of attitude, there may have also have been a series of events that predated the admission to hospital and which predisposed the elderly patient to a dependent style of thinking. Elderly people in the community are required to adapt to a series of stressful life events such as a death of spouse or friends, retirement, reduced finances, and moving away of family and friends. In addition, a sizeable number of patients admitted to acute geriatric or medical units are likely to be at least mildly physically disabled and have had to already adapt to more than one chronic illness. Although the ability to cope with stress and illness is not compromised by age *per se*, effective coping is more likely in the presence of a strong social network of family and friends (Kiyak & Borson, 1992).

When physical, social and emotional resources for coping are reduced, elderly people are rendered more vulnerable to depression and further medical problems and are less capable of adapting to new circumstances (Engel & Schmale, 1967; Locker 1991). Lack of social support is known to reduce the perceived quality of life in the community after an acute myocardial infarction. The presence of moderate dementia with its associated cognitive impairment is also known to reduce the range of adaptive coping responses to further stressors. Instead of a problem-orientated or information-seeking strategy to reduce and adapt to stress, more primitive coping strategies such as denial or ignoring the problem are employed (Kiyak & Borson, 1992). In these circumstances, patients may have been determined to be independent and maintain their own lifestyle while at home, but feel helpless and incapacitated in the face of further stresses that are incurred by an emergency admission to hospital.

HOSPITAL PROCEDURES

Hospitalization is a frightening experience for patients of all ages and leads to feelings of isolation, disorientation and anxiety. Fear of the disease and of its impact on the person's life is compounded by the strange, impersonal and institutional environment of a hospital with its lack of privacy and new procedures. Despite the modernization of acute hospital wards so as to accommodate small informal bays of four to six beds, little attention has been devoted to creating an environment that will stimulate and promote independence in patients. The design of seating arrangements could also be improved and more opportunities made available for patients, particularly those who have difficulty in walking to engage in conversation or meaningful activities. Some consideration has been given to reducing the stressful impact of medical procedures. A range of approaches including training in coping strategies and preparation before surgery have led to a reduction in the length of stay and the consumption of postoperative analgesics in young adults (Newman, 1984). Middle-aged and elderly patients were found to benefit from an intervention that provided information about how they would feel and what they should do after cataract surgery (Hill, 1982). Although there was no effect on measures of anxiety, depression or length of hospital stay, patients in the intervention group were quicker to venture out of their homes after surgery than patients who received interventions based on the provision of factual information about medical procedures and the nature of cataracts.

In practice, however, systematic preparation of the elderly undergoing surgery or even less invasive procedures is rarely adopted. In certain cases, the lack of preparation may be unavoidable. The delay between requesting a surgical opinion for say, below knee amputation, and the date of operation is usually minimal so as to reduce medical risks such as septicaemia and other complications. However, in most cases there is adequate time for preparation and greater efforts could be made to inform, offer coping strategies and to discuss patients' fears about the forthcoming procedure. In a community-based study, patients with chronic obstructive airways disease were targeted with short community-based interventions of combined cognitive and behavioural strategies for managing shortness of breath and exercise programmes. Significant improvements were obtained on measures of physical functioning, respiratory symptoms and emotional distress immediately after the intervention and at one year follow-up (Fishman & Petty, 1981).

Some have drawn attention to the medical and psychological complications of even several days bedrest after surgery. The combined effects of bedrest on muscle strength and respiratory function in an environment with strange sounds and smells can produce a cascade of symptoms leading to disorientation, weakness, delirium, fear and dependency (Inouye et al., 1993; Creditor, 1993). Such patients may feel that they have no control over the lives, and will never regain their former level of physical functioning.

A further obstacle to the successful recovery and discharge home of the elderly patient may be his/her belief about particular disease processes. The elderly and their carers often incorrectly attribute curable diseases to the mechanisms of normal ageing and delay in seeking medical advice. Deterioration of vision, hearing, strength and continence are endured with little recourse to help in the belief that they are inevitable and irreversible. Carers of elderly patients living in the community with a mild degree of dementia often do not consider their relatives to be demented or even to be suffering from a disease. Instead, they attribute the loss of memory and periods of confusion to aspects of the normal ageing process (Pollitt et al., 1989).

AGEISM AND ILLNESS BELIEFS
Why should elderly people and their families have such unrealistic and negative beliefs about the consequences of ageing? The elderly, particularly in western society are subject to, and may share, the extensive negative stereotyping in terms of beliefs, attitudes and behaviours directed towards them. Common stereotypes include notions that all elderly are demented, incompetent and unable to make decisions or care for themselves. This ageist view is not only held by the lay public, but is also commonly consciously or unconsciously adopted by health professionals. This view may be expressed in terms of a distorted and overly pessimistic perception of the physical status, capabilities and prospects of elderly inpatients (Hopper et al., 1993; Reich et al., 1993). The behavioural consequences of these beliefs may be paternalistic or custodial decision-making on behalf of the elderly by hospital staff and patients relatives (Norman, 1980). Staff may act in a protective manner and even infantilize their patients, such that they deprive them of information, choices and rights that are critical to a sense of well-being and independence. Even the assistance with tasks that patients are capable of performing for themselves may undermine their sense of control and task performance. Minor risks such as falls may be considered unacceptable by staff and relatives who may react by setting excessive limits on the patient. Unnecessary care and 'protection' in hospital and in the community may be advocated. In extreme cases, the patient's wishes may be ignored and involuntary relocation to institutionalized care in residential and nursing homes may be recommended. Elderly patients who do not actively participate in, or agree with, this discharge decision are known to be at increased risk of disorientation, apathy, morbidity and mortality in residential and nursing homes.

MULTIDISCIPLINARY TEAMS
Discharge to the patient's own home in line with their wishes may also represent a major stressor to elderly people after even a brief hospital stay. Specialized discharge teams have been developed to continue the work of the ward rehabilitation team in the home and to ease the psychological transition of returning home after a debilitating illness. This approach has led to a significant reduction in the incidence of readmissions in elderly patients (Martin, Oyewole & Moloney, in press). Specialized geriatric inpatient management in the form of a stroke rehabilitation unit has also been effective in reducing the length of stay of frail elderly stroke patients compared to management on general medical wards (Kalra, Dale & Crome, 1993). Whether the different groups of health professionals varied in their attitudes and expectations, as well in their knowledge of the elderly and in their use of multidisciplinary teams, remains to be determined. However, although geriatricians and their teams of staff may incorporate a holistic approach to the care and management of the elderly as part of their philosophy, the psychological sequelae of illness and hospitalization are rarely tackled in a systematic or explicit manner. Furthermore, the cohesive operation of the multidisciplinary team, whether based on geriatric wards or associated with medical firms, may be hindered by varying goals, attitudes, beliefs, decision-making practices and inadequate communication between different team members. Different approaches to the assessment and management of risks may lead to conflicts regarding inpatient goals and discharge plans. The presence of new physical disability in the frail elderly patient may cause anxiety and reduce the threshold of certain staff members for the acceptability of risks in hospital and in the community. The resultant discharge planning may then be focused on risk prevention and restrictions on the patient's freedom rather than on maximizing the quality of life of patients in their own homes.

THE MEDICAL CONSULTATION

Ageist beliefs and paternalistic attitudes towards the elderly, by general practitioners and hospital physicians, may also adversely affect the medical consultation process. The most common style of communication that is used by GPs with outpatients of all ages is one where the doctor is considered to be the expert, and the patient is required to co-operate. The consultation is characterized by paternalistic behaviour by the GPs who employ closed questions and rarely engage in participative discussions with their patients. Patients of low social status, such as the elderly or low social classes, are less likely to insist on more equal participation in the consultation or to make additional requests for information or clarification. Similarly, in a set of medical outpatient consultations, physicians were less responsive to topics raised by the elderly than by younger patients (Greene et al., 1987). Although the communication style of hospital physicians has not been examined in the context of elderly acute inpatients, it is likely that these encounters would not differ markedly from those in outpatient settings. Although consultations which are brief, diagnosis centred and authoritative may appear cost effective in the short term, they are associated with reduced satisfaction and compliance after discharge (Tuckett et al., 1985). The elderly, in particular, may feel disenfranchised, not listened to, and out of control of the workings of their own bodies. These feelings, when they occur repeatedly, are not likely to be conducive to patients taking responsibility for their own health such as quitting smoking or taking more exercise. In the hospital setting, the effects of these repeated encounters is to generate feelings of depersonalization, disempowerment and anxiety (Morgan, 1991).

SENSE OF CONTROL AND INDEPENDENCE

Feelings of lack of control of one's health, actions and environment and the relinquishing of powers to significant others such as doctors are often associated with adverse outcomes. A belief system of externalized control, referred to as external locus of control, has been found to be inversely correlated with physical recovery from stroke, and adjustment to a low constraint retirement home (Partridge & Johnston, 1989; Wolk, 1976). Others have argued that elderly inpatients with an external locus of control may be less distressed and feel less constrained in an acute hospital setting than patients who strongly believe in their ability to affect their own health outcomes (Cicirelli, 1980). Although repeated hospitalizations might be expected to decrease the belief of patients that they are in control of their health outcomes, the number of reported previous hospitalizations has, so far, been found to be unrelated to the perceived control by elderly patients (Hunter et al., 1980; Brown & Granick, 1983). In a more recent study, dependent attitudes of 33 acute geriatric inpatients were found to be positively correlated with duration of previous inpatient hospitalization (Eddington et al., 1990). Dependent attitudes were also negatively correlated with patients' ratings of their own well-being but were not related to the actual physical status of patients as rated by themselves or by nursing staff. The lack of consistency between the results of the different studies may be due to differing cohorts and characteristics of elderly patients sampled, as well as to the different scales and measures employed. Even if a clear relationship between external locus of control and the number of inpatient hospitalisations had been obtained, it would not be possible to conclude that the hospitalizations had actually influenced the patients' attitudes and beliefs. Other environmental factors associated with the acute hospital admission may also play a key role.

Specific manipulations that were designed to increase the perception of control in groups of elderly patients have been more useful in this regard. Interventions such as involvement and participation of patients in decisions to relocate to nursing homes have been found to have short- and long-term benefits for perceptions of control and physical health (Rodin, 1986). However, Rodin emphasizes that the effective improvements in patients beliefs in their own ability to control events may only become apparent when the environmental situation provides the opportunity for the increased sense of independence to be utilized. If patients are thwarted or sabotaged in their attempts to participate and influence the routine and interactions of staff, the beneficial effects of a positive intervention may be undermined. Most of these intervention studies have been conducted in the community or in preparation for residential/nursing homes. Little is known about the impact of these interventions in an acute hospital setting in preparation for patients being discharged to their own homes. Explicit discussion with patients regarding their fears and concerns in returning home and engaging their participation in the discharge decision-making process may be helpful in easing the transition.

In summary, brief periods of hospitalization may act as a trigger for the emergence of harmful and maladaptive coping strategies. A significant proportion of elderly patients that are admitted to acute geriatric and general medical wards have pre-existing chronic disability and are often already compromised in terms of their physical and psychological health. They are likely to be particularly vulnerable to the adverse effects of hospitalization and may be at risk of becoming more physically and psychologically dependent as inpatients and after discharge. Since the medical requirement for acute hospital admission in this group is usually essential, it may be advantageous to give more consideration to the level of choice, participation in decision-making, information and training in coping strategies for patients during their stay.

REFERENCES

Brown, B.R. & Granick, S. (1983). Cognitive and psychosocial differences between internal and external locus of control aged persons. Experimental Aging Research, 9, 107–10.

Cicirelli, V.G. (1980). Relationship of family background variables to locus of control in the elderly. Journal of Gerontology, 35, 108–14.

Creditor, M.C. (1993). Hazards of hospitalization of the elderly. Annals Internal Medicine, 118, 219–23.

Eddington, C., Piper, J., Bhavna, T., Hodkinson, H.M. & Salmon, P. (1990). Relationships between happiness, behavioural status and dependency on others in elderly patients. British Journal Clinical Psychology, 291, 43–50.

Engel, G.E. & Schmale, A.H. (1967). Psychoanalytic theory of somatic disorder: conversion, specificity and the disease onset situation. Journal of the American Psychoanalytic Association, 15, 344–365.

Fishman, D.B. & Petty, T.L. (1981). Physical, symptomatic and psychological improvement in patients receiving comprehensive care for chronic airway obstruction. *Journal of Chronic Disease*, 24, 775–85.

Greene, M.G., Hoffman, S., Charon, R. & Adelman, R. (1987). Psychosocial concerns in the medical encounter: a comparison of interactions of doctors with their old and young patients. *The Gerontologist*, 27, 164–8.

Hill, B.J. (1982). Sensory information, behavioural instructions and coping with sensory alteration surgery. *Nursing Research*, 31, 17–21.

Hopper, A., Boland, M., Benson, P., Richardson, P. & Reich, S. (1993). Effect of attitudes on clinical decisions. Paper presented at the 15th Congress of the International Association of Gerontology, Budapest.

Hunter, K.I., Linn, M.W., Harris, R. & Pratt, T. (1980). Discriminators of internal and external locus of control orientation in the elderly. *Research on Aging*, 2, 49–60.

Inouye, S.K., Viscoli, C.M., Horwitz, R.I., Hurst, L.D. & Tinetti, M.E. (1993). A predictive model for delirium in hospitalized elderly medical patients. *Annals Internal Medicine*, 119 474–81.

Kalra, L. Dale, P. & Crome, P. (1993). Improving Stroke Rehabilitation: a controlled study. *Stroke*, 24 1462–7.

Kiyak, H.A. & Borson, S. (1992) Coping with chronic illness and disability. In M.G. Ory, R.P. Abeles & P.D. Lipman (Eds.). *Aging, health and behaviour*. Sage Publications.

Locker, D, (1991). Living with chronic illness. In G. Scambler (Ed.). *Sociology as applied to medicine*. 3rd ed. Ballière Tindall.

Martin, F.C., Oyewole, A. & Moloney, A. (in press). A randomised controlled trial of high support hospital discharge team for elderly people. *Age and Ageing*.

Morgan, M, (1991). Hospitals and patients. In G. Scambler (Ed.). *Sociology as applied to medicine*. 3rd ed. Ballière Tindall.

Newman, S. (1984). Anxiety, hospitalization and surgery. In R. Fitzpatrick, J. Hinton, S. Newman, G. Scambler & J. Thomson (Eds.). *The experience of illness*. London: Tavistock Publications.

Norman, A. (1980). Rights and Risk. Centre for Policy on Ageing.

Partridge, C. & Johnston, M. (1989). Perceived control of recovery from physical disability: measurement and prediction.

British Journal of Clinical Psychology, 28, 53–9.

Pollitt, P.A. O'Connor, D.W. & Anderson, I. (1989). Mild dementia: perceptions and problems. *Ageing and Society*; 9 261–77.

Reich, S., Bracewell, C., Foster, C. & Hopper, A. (1993). Effect of medical education on clinical decisions. Paper presented at the 15th Congress of the International Association of Gerontology, Budapest.

Rodin, J. (1986). Health, control and aging. In M.M. Baltes & P.B. Baltes (Eds.). *Aging and the psychology of control*. Hillsdale. NJ: Lawrence Erlbaum.

Tuckett, D., Boulton, M., Olson, C. & Williams, A. (1985). *Meetings between experts: an approach to sharing ideas in medical consultations*. London: Tavistock Publications.

Wolk, S. (1976). Situational constraint as a moderator of the locus of control-adjustment relationship. *Journal Consulting and Clinical, Psychology*, 44 420–27.

Lay beliefs about health and illness

HOWARD LEVENTHAL

and

YAEL BENYAMINI

Institute for Health and Department of Psychology, Rutgers, The State University of New Jersey, New Brunswick, USA

An examination of the behavioural-health literature could lead an aspiring investigator to believe that two factors are sufficient to understand and predict the performance of actions to prevent, control and/or cure a health threat: intention (Fishbein & Ajzen, 1974), and self-efficacy, i.e. the belief that one is capable of performing the action (Bandura, 1976). With time for reflection, this investigator might wonder why so little attention has been given to motivation, i.e. that is to the factors affecting the selection of one among many possible actions, and the factors affecting the urge or need to act rather than to do nothing at all. It is indeed surprising that motivation is ignored given that its absence is so readily noticed by non-psychologists, e.g. when a TV interviewer asked a high school student about the value of training to say 'No' to drugs, the student replied, 'It is okay to know what to do but you have to want to do it'. There seem to be three reasons for the lack of concern with the two facets of motivation: (i) Many studies are conducted with the frame-

work of social learning theory which emphasizes the acquisition of behaviours that are specified *a priori*, e.g. quitting smoking; (ii) Investigators appear to accept the assertions of medical and public health authorities as to which actions are healthy and which are risky, further circumventing the need to examine choice; and (iii) Intentions and self-efficacy are easy to assess, good predictors of behaviour, and likely to produce publishable findings. Prediction, however, is not equivalent to explanation (Pedhazur, 1982).

COMMON-SENSE MODELS OF ILLNESS: THE SUBSTANCE AND IMPACT OF LAY BELIEFS

Studies of lay beliefs seek to describe the processes involved in the motivation of health and illness behaviours, i.e. to understand the factors underlying the selection, initiation, and long-term performance of healthy and risky behaviours. To facilitate this work, investigators have formulated a general systems model in which health

[131]

beliefs, i.e. the representation of health threats, along with coping procedures and rules for appraising outcomes, are conceptualized as major components in the system generating the individual's efforts at self and environmental regulation (Leventhal, Meyer & Nerenz, 1980; Meyer, Leventhal & Gutmann, 1985; Skelton & Croyle, 1991).

Attributes of illness representations

The representation of an illness, or the common-sense beliefs about it, defines the primary motivational variables in the system. Representations are identified by five sets of attributes: identity, i.e. the label and symptoms that define the threat (Lau, Bernard & Hartman, 1989); causes, i.e. its external (infectious agent; injury) or internal (genetic disposition) determinants (Baumann et al., 1989); time-line, i.e. its duration and rate of development; consequences, its somatic, social, and economic impact (Croyle & Jemmott, 1991); and its controllability, i.e. beliefs that it can be prevented, controlled, and/or cured (Lau & Hartmann, 1983).

The attributes of the representation have powerful effects upon the selection and maintenance of behaviours. For example, the label and symptoms, which are the abstract and concrete facets of the identity, are tightly joined to one another, symptoms typically functioning as direct indicators of the status of the underlying disease. As a consequence, the waxing and waning of symptoms can have a direct effect on motivation to seek medical care and use medications as prescribed. Thus, instances abound where treatment is stopped as soon as symptoms have disappeared and/or treatment terminated when it does not ameliorate symptoms. Unfortunately, symptomatic treatment can create problems. For example, for many infectious conditions treatment must continue post-symptom disappearance to ensure the elimination of disease agents. Hypertension provides yet another example, as the symptoms lay persons identify as signs of hypertension are unrelated to tonic levels of this condition (Baumann & Leventhal, 1985). While symptoms may be invalid guides to coping for many infectious diseases and hypertension, they may prove useful as guides to self-care for diseases such as asthma and arthritis if patients are appropriately trained to identify valid indicators and ignore others (Gonder-Frederick & Cox, 1991). We have described the bond between label and symptoms as an example of symmetry. Thus, if a person has symptoms s/he will seek a (diagnostic) label, and if labelled (diagnosed) s/he will seek symptoms (see Baumann et al., 1989; Croyle & Jemmott, 1991).

The second factor that has been shown to vary across persons and to affect adherence to treatment is time-line, or the perceived duration of an illness or health threat. For example, 40% of patients initiating treatment for hypertension for the very first time believe that it is an acute disease: 58% of these individuals drop out of treatment within 6 to 9 months in comparison to 17% who believe the disease is chronic (Meyer, Leventhal & Gutmann, 1985). The picture is different for cancer patients. While 40% of women in chemotherapy treatment for metastatic breast disease likened their illness to an acute, curable condition (measles), virtually none of these patients quits treatment; the proportion believing the disease is acute declined to 20% 6 months later (Leventhal et al., 1986). Time-line had no effect on adherence as the consequences of quitting, a rapid, painful death, and social pressures to remain in treatment, over-rode personal beliefs.

The effects of symptoms and time-line on adherence will vary, however, for different illnesses. For example, Klohn and Rogers (1991) found that young women at risk for osteoporosis, due to low consumption of calcium and inadequate weight-bearing exercise, expressed stronger intentions to adopt preventative behaviours when informed that the disease was likely to occur in the near, rather than remote, future and was disfiguring. The visibility and proximity of its consequences enhanced the apparent severity of the disease and stimulated intentions to take protective action.

Schemata and dimensions of difference

Studies of beliefs about specific illnesses and studies comparing beliefs for different illnesses, suggest the presence of schemata or prototypes of illness experience. In a series of elegant studies, Bishop and colleagues (summarized in Bishop, 1991) have shown that symptoms do indeed fall into sets, the more integrated sets are more quickly and more likely to be labelled, and the items within the more integrated sets are more easily recalled. Comparisons among illnesses, rather than the structure of a specific illness schema have generated a number of dimensions of difference which provide a somewhat different view of the beliefs domain (Lau et al., 1989). For example, Bishop's (1991) subjects generated two such dimensions, one of contagiousness and another of seriousness or life threateningness. Our studies of hypertensives (Meyer et al., 1985) and cancer patients (Leventhal et al., 1986) suggest the presence of three disease prototypes: acute, cyclic and chronic. The dimensions and clusters arising from comparative judgments appear to be important determinants of action.

PROCEDURES AND THE PROCESS OF COMMON SENSE CONSTRUCTIONS

In addition to the representation, a second component, variously labelled as action plans and/or coping procedures, is critical for adaptive behaviour. Both health promotive and health damaging behaviors depend upon the combined presence and action of factors from each of these two sets of factors, i.e. the representation which sets the target for coping, and the set of procedures from which a specific response is selected to reach the target.

Types of procedures

Information acquisition and self-treatments, two diverse categories, stand out for the frequency with which they serve both to define and to control illness. Waiting and watching, a relatively passive, information acquisition procedure is often reported at the onset of slowly developing episodes (Prohaska et al., 1987). Active procedures, e.g. reading about a disease or symptom, seeking out and talking to peers about similar health problems (Carver, Scheier & Weintraub, 1989), and seeking professional help (Cameron, Leventhal & Leventhal, 1993), will supplant passive ones when a symptom crosses a threshold of severity or duration. Active social comparison for symptom interpretation is extremely common among older adults (Cameron, Leventhal & Leventhal, 1993), and typically involving a family member (Glasser, Prohaska & Roska, 1992). The most likely direction for such communication appears to be from husband to wife (Stoller, 1993b).

Social comparisons, however, can occur rather automatically and with relatively little thought raising questions as to their active versus passive nature. For example, Jemmott, Ditto and Croyle

(1986) created a laboratory situation in which they tested individuals for a fictitious pancreatic disorder, TAA enzyme deficiency. The test, conducted on the participants' saliva, was arranged to yield positive findings for subjects under two conditions: one where the subject was told that he was the only person of the five present with a positive test, the other where he was told that he was one of four with a positive test. Subjects, ratings of the seriousness of the disorder, a judgement of its consequences, were affected by the social context; they judged the deficiency to be more severe when they were the only person with a positive test rather than one of four. Thus, a rapid and very likely 'thoughtless' scan of the social environment had an impressive impact on judging the consequences of an illness threat as more or less serious.

Procedures exist which may bias the information acquisition process and the evaluation of the information once it is received. Down-playing or 'normalizing' symptoms, suggesting that subjects have difficulty accepting that they are at risk, is widely reported. Normalizing is more common among elderly persons, particularly those who are healthy and less symptomatic than those with multiple chronic conditions (Stoller, 1993a); the latter individuals see health threats in almost any new symptom. Jemmott et al. (1986) also report clear evidence of minimization; in comparison to their not-at-risk peers, those given positive feedback judged the enzyme test to be less valid, and did that more so if they were the only person given a positive result.

Self-treatments, ranging from use of over-the-counter medication, to exercise and dietary programmes, are among the more active procedures that are used both to prevent disease and to control the symptoms of ongoing illness. For example, an individual suffering from burning, abdominal chest pain may take an antacid both to control and define the meaning of the pain: if the antacid relieves the pain, the pain is interpreted as gastric rather than cardiac. Stoller (1994) has reviewed the self-treatment procedures used by older adults and the conditions affecting their use.

Reciprocal shaping

The psychological literature typically describes coping procedures, particularly those focused on problem rather than emotion control, in terms of outcome expectations and self-efficacy. The systems formulation suggests, however, that the selection and performance of specific coping procedures also reflects the reciprocal, or integral relationship among representations and procedures. Integrality (Garner, 1962) implies that representations and procedures form natural gestalts, i.e. units in which the representations shape coping procedures and procedures shape representations.

The integrality concept suggests that representations motivate not only by generating a generalized need or urge to act (or to avoid action), but by generating specific questions and expectations regarding the utility of available coping procedures. For example, a person who believes that hypertension is symptomatic is more likely to use an electronic blood pressure machine while at a shopping mall if he feels his heart beating and has a headache than if he is asymptomatic and feels well. As there is no motivation to test when asymptomatic, and as untreated, tonic blood pressure will be elevated both when symptomatic and asymptomatic, symptom-based readings provide a biased view of the validity of symptoms as indicators of elevated blood pressure.

Similarly, both the label, hypertension, and the symptoms, convey the idea that elevated blood pressure is caused by stress (Blumhagen, 1980). Integral to this belief is the implication that opposite procedures, e.g. relaxing, ignoring and/or reinterpreting life stressors, are appropriate treatments. And, if relaxation reduces headache symptoms, it will reinforce the causal belief. The interactions among representations and procedures will generate changes in both during the course of an illness episode, the changes reflecting the reciprocal relationships among these active components, and the institutional and social context in which these transactions take place. Thus, while one will expect to identify commonalities in illness models across persons, the process should also generate a substantial degree of specificity by disease, culture and the individual.

Working cognition

We have used the phrase 'working cognition' to identify the cognition and procedures involved in the elaboration and evaluation of illness representations: they are the product and the source of representations and procedures and reflect the integral nature of the two. Working cognitions are *hypothesis or question* based: Is the burning I feel gastric or cardiac? Is my headache due to stress or is it more serious? These hypothesis-based questions link specific procedures and representations (if it is gastric, take an anti-acid, if a headache, take an aspirin) and they define outcome expectations and criteria for appraisals (if the pain goes away it is gastric / a stress headache). These questions and their associated procedures reflect basic assumptions about the organization of illness and they play a critical role in defining illness labels, beliefs about susceptibility to control, and the evaluation of the efficacy of one's resources for prevention, cure and control. They reflect both the substance of specific illness schemata (symptoms/labels; time-lines, etc.) and the dimensions generated by comparisons among these schemata.

It is clear that it will be possible to identify broad themes underlying working cognition. For example, Bishop's (1991) subjects are averse to contact with individuals suffering from contagious diseases but not averse to contact with individual's suffering from life-threatening diseases: a disease combining the two would arouse both avoidance and fear. Other dimensions can be seen in anthropologists' reports of health beliefs and practices in cultures other than our own; while they are present in our western culture, their familiarity reduces their visibility. For example, procedures may be motivated by questions concerning their geographical and/or mechanical relationship to symptoms and disease. This can be seen in direct manipulation of the location or organ system from which the symptom is believed to emerge. Weller et al. (1993) describe the Latino folk illness empacho, a disorder characterized by vomiting, stomach pain, and swollen stomach, that is believed to be caused by an intestinal obstruction due to overeating, or consuming poorly prepared food. Procedures for treating empacho include abdominal massages, rolling an egg on the stomach, ingesting teas, oils and purgatives, all of which are designed to dislodge the obstruction. Molera caida, or fallen fontanelle, an illness caused by dehydration (Kaye, 1993), is treated by physical manipulations designed to return the fontanelle to its normal position, e.g. holding the infant by the heels, sucking on the fontanelle or pressing on the soft palate.

Abstracting principles such as these from descriptive data will provide a compendium of the factors that people use to elaborate and verify their representations of biological reality. Understanding these 'working cognition' will prove critical for the development of theory, and for the practical issues of developing disease representations and treatment procedures that are shared by patient and practitioner.

THE SOCIAL CONTEXT AND THE DEVELOPMENT AND CHANGE OF ILLNESS REPRESENTATIONS

The social context, from informal social relationships to family, formal institutions, culture and language, impacts beliefs and procedures for managing health threats. These factors work together and independently in generating representations, coping procedures and rules for outcome appraisals.

Immediate social context

The family provides the earliest context for the acquisition of explicit memories and implicit skills for the exploration, labelling and management of symptoms. Parental expressions of concern from asking the toddler 'Where does it hurt?' to experiencing and observing various family nostrums for the treatment of symptoms in specific organ systems, creates an interpersonal context for developing cognitive representations of illness episodes. These interchanges can teach a child that illness is acute and self-limiting, something to be or not to be anxious about, and curable or not curable with nostrums ranging from chicken soup to aspirin.

Encounters with the medical care system are a second, major source for the development of illness representations. From the initial greeting 'How do you feel today?' to the review of systems (the head to toe symptom inquiry) which is conducted in the search for new problems and possible consequences of existent disease, the doctor–patient interchange encourages symptomatic representations of disease. This does not, however, insure shared perspectives. Practitioners and patients may arrive at quite different representations of the cause, course and appropriate treatment of a disorder from what is presumed to be the 'same' data base. Such outcomes are readily apparent when the patient's representation and criteria for treatment evaluation incorporate symptoms that are medically 'irrelevant', i.e. unrelated to the status of the underlying disease process. These encounters, along with information from friends and family, can reinforce the symptomatic identity of a problem and the use of common-sense treatments. As tincture of time cures most conditions, the common-sense approach is usually harmless. There are, however, conditions under which common-sense procedures such as sharing medications, may involve definite risk, e.g. drug interactions, etc. (Stoller, 1994).

Culture

One can detect the influences of cultural belief systems and language for virtually every attribute of illness representations. For example, the label for high blood pressure, i.e. hypertension, suggests that physical and mental hyper-activity and tension are both signs and causes of elevated blood pressure (Blumhagen, 1980) and very likely

encourages a variety of common-sense stress reduction methods for treatment. Religious and spiritual beliefs that are culture-wide can have a direct influence on causal representations, e.g. disease attributed to immoral behaviours, or an indirect effect, e.g. creating a background of mystical beliefs which set the stage for beliefs in 'possession' as causes of disease and atonement and good works as procedures for cure.

The relationship between culture and disease representations is, however, reciprocal. Both the biology of disease and beliefs about disease have shaped the medical care system and the system in turn has shaped and maintained these beliefs. For example, infectious illness and representations of these illness as symptomatic, communicable, time limited and curable, created a fee for service care system that treats disease and ignores prevention. Once in place, this service framework encourages and sustains the readiness to represent and manage chronic conditions as one manages acute, infectious conditions. The shaping of the health care system by infectious disease and health beliefs was a process that took place over decades and centuries; the effect became salient with the shift from acute to life threatening chronic conditions resulting from the increasing large number of elderly in the population (Knowles, 1977).

CONCLUDING COMMENT

The research examining the effects of lay beliefs on health behaviour and health disease management, has been largely descriptive in nature. Thus, it has focused upon the identification of the content of representations, types of procedures and the rules defining their inter-relationships. While the information generated by these studies has increased our understanding of behaviour to prevent and control illness and has improved our understanding of motivational processes, the systems framework has yet to demonstrate its utility as a platform for developing behavioural interventions. Recent studies on the development of interventions for self-management of arthritis suggest that long-term self-management depends upon three steps: accepting arthritis as a chronic (lifelong) condition; separating the underlying disease from its somatic manifestations (stiffness, pain); and learning to cope with, and regulate, these manifestations. These conditions lead to minimal disruption of an active life style (Pimm, Byron, Curson & Weinman, 1994).

Promising developments such as these suggest that common-sense models can deepen our understanding as to how the framing of a health threat can lead to the development of valid outcome expectations and an increased sense of efficacy at self-management. As our knowledge expands, we should have a better understanding of the motivational processes driving the behavioural system, an important step towards improving our skills as educators and health facilitators. (See also 'Attributions and health', 'Coping with chronic illness', 'Cultural and ethnic factors in health', 'Perceived control and health behaviour', 'Risk perception and health behaviour', 'Self-efficacy and health behaviour', 'Theory of planned behaviour', 'Trans-theoretical model of behaviour change'.)

ACKNOWLEDGEMENT

Preparation was supported by Grant AG 03501 and AG 12072 from the National Institute on Aging.

REFERENCES

Bandura, A. (1977). Self efficacy: toward a unifying theory of behavioural change. *Psychological Review*, **84**, 191–215.

Baumann, L.J. & Leventhal, H. (1985). 'I can tell when my blood pressure is up, can't I?' *Health Psychology*, **4**, 203–18.

Baumann, L.J., Cameron, L.D., Zimmerman, R. & Leventhal, H. (1989). Illness representations and matching labels with symptoms. *Health Psychology*, **8**, 449–69.

Bishop, G.D. (1991). Understanding the understanding of illness: lay disease representations. In J.A. Skelton & R.T. Croyle (Eds). *Mental representation in health and illness*, pp 32–59. New York: Springer-Verlag.

Blumhagen, D. (1980). Hyper-tension: a folk illness with a medical name. *Culture, Medicine, and Psychiatry*, **4**, 197–227.

Cameron, L., Leventhal, E.A. & Leventhal, H. (1993). Symptom representations and affect as determinants of care seeking in a community dwelling adult sample population. *Health Psychology*, **12**, 171–9.

Carver, C.S., Scheier, M.F. & Weintraub, J.K. (1989). Assessing coping strategies: a theoretically based approach. *Journal of Personality and Social Psychology*, **26**, 267–83.

Croyle, R.T. & Jemmott, J.B. III (1991). Psychological reactions to risk factor testing. In J.A. Skelton & R.T. Croyle, (Eds.) *Mental representation in health and illness* pp 85–107. New York: Springer-Verlag.

Ditto, P.H. & Jemmott, J.B., III (1989). From rarity to evaluative extremity: effects of prevalence information on evaluations of positive and negative characteristics. *Journal of Personality and Social Psychology*, **57**, 16–26.

Fishbein, M. & Ajzen, I. (1974). Attitudes towards objects as predictors of single and multiple behavioral criteria. *Psychological Review*, **81**, 59–74.

Garner, W.R. (1962). *Uncertainty and structure as psychological concepts*. New York: Wiley.

Glasser, M., Prohaska, T. & Roska, J. (1992). The role of the family in medical careseeking decisions of older adults. *Family and Community Health*, **15**, 59–70.

Gonder-Frederick, L.A. & Cox, D.J. (1991). Symptom perception, symptom beliefs, and blood glucose discrimination in the self-treatment of insulin-dependent diabetes. In J.A. Skelton & R.T. Croyle, (Eds.). *Mental representation in health and illness*, pp. 220–46. New York: Springer-Verlag.

Jemmott, J.B., III, Ditto, P.H. & Croyle, R.T. (1986). Judging health status: effects of perceived prevalence and personal relevance. *Journal of Personality and Social Psychology*, **50**, 899–905.

Kay, M. (1993). Fallen Fontanelle: culture-bound or cross-cultural?, *Medical Anthropology*, **15**, 137–56.

Kleinman, A. (1980). *Patients and healers in the context of culture*. Berkeley: University of California Press.

Klohn, L.S. & Rogers, R.W. (1991). Dimensions of the severity of a health threat: the persuasive effects of visibility, time of onset, and rate of onset on young women's intentions to prevent osteoporosis. *Health Psychology*, **10**, 323–9.

Knowles, J.H. (1977). *Doing better and feeling worse: health in the United States*. New York: W.W. Norton.

Koss-Chioino, J. & Canive, J. (1993). The intersection of popular and clinical diagnostic labeling: the case of embrujado, *Medical Anthropology*, **15**, 171–88.

Lau, R.R. & Hartmann, K.A. (1983). Common sense representations of common illnesses. *Health Psychology*, **2**, 167–85.

Lau, R.R., Bernard, T.M. & Hartman, K.A. (1989). Further explorations of common-sense representations of common illnesses. *Health Psychology*, **8**, 195–219.

Leventhal, H. (1970). Findings and theory in the study of fear communications. *Advances in Experimental Social Psychology*, **5**, 119–86.

Leventhal, H., Meyer, D. & Nerenz, D. (1980). The common sense representation of illness danger. In S. Rachman (Ed.). *Contributions to medical psychology*, **Vol. II**, pp. 7–30. New York: Pergamon Press.

Leventhal, H., Easterling, D.V., Coons, H., Luchterhand, C. & Love, R.R. (1986). Adaptation to chemotherapy treatments. In B. Andersen (Ed.). *Women with Cancer*, pp. 172–203. New York: Springer-Verlag.

Meyer, D., Leventhal, H. & Gutmann, M. (1985). Common-sense models of illness: the example of hypertension. *Health Psychology*, **4**, 115–35.

Pedhazur, E.J. (1982). *Multiple regression in behavioral research: explanation and prediction*. New York: Holt Rinehart and Winston.

Pimm, T.J., Byron, M.A., Curson, B.A. & Weinman, J. (1994). Personal illness models and the self management of arthritis. Paper presented at British Society of Health Psychology.

Prohaska, T.R., Keller, M.L., Leventhal, E.A. & Leventhal, H. (1987). Impact of symptoms and aging attribution on emotions and coping. *Health Psychology*, **6**, 495–514.

Skelton, J.A. & Croyle, R.T. (1991). *Mental representation in health and illness*. New York: Springer-Verlag.

Stoller, E. (1993a). Interpretations of symptoms by older people: a health diary study of illness behavior. *Journal of Aging and Health*, **5**, 58–81.

Stoller, E. (1993b). Gender and the organization of lay health care: a socialist-feminist perspective. *Journal of Aging Studies*. **7**, 151–70.

Stoller, E. (1994). The dynamics and process of self-care in old age. National Invitational Conference on Research Issues Related to Self-Care and Aging. Washington, DC.

Weller, S., Pachter, L., Trotter, R. & Baer, R. (1993), Empacho in four Latino groups: a study of intra- and inter-cultural variation in beliefs. *Medical Anthropology*, **15**, 109–36.

Life events and health

TIRRIL HARRIS

Department of Social Policy and Social Science,
Royal Holloway and Bedford New College,
University of London,
UK

INTRODUCTION

The notion of life events adversely affecting health is deeply embedded in popular consciousness. However, among theorists there have been interesting variations. Some early thinkers pursued general theories involving homeostasis, viewing disease in terms of 'illness as a whole'. The best known were Cannon's (1932) fight–flight reaction and Selye's (1956) general adaptation syndrome. These detailed a number of biological reponses to environmental demands, presenting them as an orchestrated pattern, almost regardless of the specific nature of these demands. These generalized patterns included responses which were easy to measure in early psychological laboratories, such as heart rate or sweating, and this may partly have accounted for the interest shown in this model of illness. Others pursued theories involving more specificity, believing that particular disorders arise from specific circumstances. During the 1950s this was accepted by followers of Franz Alexander and the School of Psychosomatic Medicine. Another example was Flanders Dunbar's influential set of ideas that specific personality types were more vulnerable to certain illnesses (Dunbar, 1954). But these views were often seen as linked with the notion that symptoms 'communicate symbolically', and thus with some type of psychodynamic approach, so acquiring all the suspicion attending psychoanalysis. The experimental work of Graham and colleagues concerning attitude specificity (Graham, Stern & Winokur 1958), which built many controls into research, producing the predicted specific physical changes after hypnotic induction of specific attitudes, avoided this psychoanalytic aura, but much of the other evidence in the specificity tradition then was fragmentary. Moreover, the specificity considered nearly always involved the person's underlying attitude rather than the specific way the environment impinged in the form of a life event. However, more recent research has suggested the value of examining the latter in relation to particular health outcomes and this chapter aims to convey this perspective.

LIFE EVENTS, DIFFICULTIES AND MEANING

Conceptual level of stress analysis

One important difference between various perspectives on stress involves what may be called their conceptual level. Five such levels can be distinguished:

(i) Microunit: incidents such as insults, which in aggregate amount to an experience at the next level, such as an estrangement.

(ii) Unit: the basic life event of most research instruments, an estrangement, house-move, job-change, or death.

(iii) Specific qualities of units: what type of event? a loss, humiliation, danger, frustration, challenge, or intrusion? Would it induce guilt or fatigue in most people?

(iv) General qualities of units: less specific characteristics such as positive/negative, severely vs mildly unpleasant.

(v) Person's summary score (not all instruments): where scores for individuals characterize their total experience, say of severely unpleasant events, during a given period.

Level (i), the incident level, is usually identified with the Hassles and Uplifts scale (Kanner *et al.*, 1981). While the distinction between hassles and uplifts suggests the positive/negative distinction at level (iv), many studies looking at health outcomes with this instrument ignore the effects at level (ii) and it thus becomes difficult to interpret how much stress a person is under at level (v). In other words, by concentrating attention on altercations with parking attendants and troubles getting computers to function, this instrument is in danger of missing the impact of more serious experiences such as children leaving home. Most instruments, however, do operate from level (ii), although the location of inclusion thresholds varies between them. The earliest measure, the Schedule of Recent Experiences (SRE: Holmes & Rahe, 1967) sees life events as anything involving significant change/readjustment, but leaves the estimate of this significance to the respondent: The respondent indicates whether a 'serious illness' or 'loss of someone close' has occurred. However, there is a potential bias, as the more anxious respondents will define as 'serious' illnesses which more sanguine personalities will consider only minor (say a bout of bronchitis), and respondents who have become depressed may look back and redefine their neighbour who has moved to Australia as 'very close', while those who have not suffered depressive onset may continue to feel friendly but not romanticize the degree of closeness of the relationship before the move (Brown, Harris & Hepworth, 1974).

The SRE then moves straight up to level (v). Each event on the checklist has been allotted a 'typical life-change unit score' from 0 (no change/distress likely) to 100 (maximum change/distress). Scores for each experience are then summed to give each individual a total score, and this, rather than the occurrence of more specific experiences, is the most frequently used measure employed in analyses of the SRE's impact on health outcomes. Another major disadvantage of this approach is its failure to deal with the meaning of events for individuals: a planned first pregnancy in a secure marital and financial situation has a different significance from an unplanned pregnancy for a single parent where there are already three children, cramped housing and a shortage of money; but both would get the same 'pregnancy' score on the checklist system.

Approaches to stress measurement such as the Life Experiences Survey (Sarason, Jonson & Siegel, 1978) or the Life Events Inventory (Tennant & Andrews, 1976) which do consider level (iv) can, of course, take account of the difference in the 'undesirability' between two such pregnancies. But they usually leave it entirely to the respondent to define 'undesirable', and here again there are dangers of bias in that sick and well subgroups may well vary systematically in their self-defined threshold for this. One approach, the Life Events and Difficulties Schedule or LEDS (Brown & Harris, 1978) attempts to capture such variations in the 'context' of the pregnancy without specifically taking account of the actual emotional appraisal of the individual concerned. For this contextual method of rating a judgement is made by the investigator about the likely meaning of each event for the person concerned, on the basis of what most people would feel in such a situation given biography, prior plans and current circumstances, but ignoring what he/she reports as the actual response. Based on a semistructured face-to-face interview, obtaining a full coherent account of any relevant incident, the interviewer uses a set of previously developed rules embodied in training manuals to decide which of 68 different types of possible event or ongoing difficulty can be included as having occurred during a defined period (level (ii)). The verbal interview and the detailed manuals give the LEDS three other advantages:

(a) an ability denied to simple questionnaires to deal more precisely with the relative timing of stressor and onset/ exacerbation of disorder by allowing cross-questioning and backtracking during the interview, relating symptoms to each other, and to events such as National Holidays (as well, of course, as to the stressful events under study).

(b) a wealth of narrative material which supplements specific probes designed to make distinctions at level (iii) as well as level (iv), and thus allows analysis by specific subtypes of unpleasant event. This permits exploration within the debate outlined earlier between general and specific theories of the impact of stress on health.

(c) a check on various types of investigator bias, along with control over respondent biases, through manuals with extensive lists of precedents and consensus meetings with other research workers, who are unaware of the subject's symptoms and reactions. This also ensures high rates of inter-rater reliability (Tennant *et al.*, 1979; Parry, Shapiro & Davies, 1981).

Because of these advantages the remainder of this chapter will concentrate on findings using the LEDS approach.

Vulnerability to the impact of life events and difficulties
Reference to the multifactorial nature of illness aetiology has become like grace before meals, often repeated but rarely followed through. Research still tends to focus on one factor while paying lip

service to the others. It will be argued here that the impact of life events on health can only be understood in the light of knowledge about what makes some people more likely than others to become ill after particular types of life event. In other words, without an understanding of vulnerability, understanding of the relationship between stress and health will remain limited.

Early work with the LEDS in Camberwell, London in the late 1960s focused on depressive disorder. Parallel findings in patient and random community female samples identified severe events and major difficulties as factors provoking onset of depression. These provoking agents constitute only a small minority of all stressors recorded by the LEDS instrument and largely involved interpersonal crises, such as discoveries of partners' infidelities, children's stealing or estrangements from former good friends or family, but depression was also linked with more material stressors such as threats of eviction or unemployment. It was noteworthy that events such as house moves, not rated severe because they involved only hassle and were only mildly unpleasant, were not associated with depression. Nor were events which were severe in the short but not the long term, such as a child with a threatened diagnosis of meningitis which turned later out to be migraine. Although extremely distressing during the first few days, such 'non-severe' events were, by definition, largely resolved by the end of two weeks.

A thorough exploration of the background and social network variables suggested that four 'vulnerability factors' might be at work. Two of them involved lack of supportive relationships, the first with a partner currently, the second, loss of mother by death or long-term separation before age 11, in the past. The other two, lack of employment and household containing three or more children, were closely linked with current roles, suggesting that women trapped at home were more vulnerable. Speculation on the common theme uniting these four factors suggested they were all likely to be associated with an intrapsychic state such as poor self-esteem or low mastery which would itself cause minor feelings of depression (likely in anyone experiencing such events) to generalize into the full-blown clinical state (for detailed discussion see Brown & Harris, 1978).

Later prospective work in North London confirmed these speculations. Self-esteem was deliberately measured at first interview, and at follow-up those who had shown negative self-evaluation were nearly three times more likely than the rest to become clinically depressed after a provoking agent (Brown *et al.*, 1986). At the same time, the specific nature of the unpleasant provoking events was examined more minutely (a task at level (iii)): they largely involved experiences of loss if that is defined broadly to include losses of cherished ideas as well as of persons or objects. Severe events not involving loss were only half as likely to be followed by depression (Brown, Bifulco & Harris, 1987). Further refinement revealed that it was really losses involving humiliation, entrapment or death that played the key role, others were only a quarter as likely to produce depression (Brown, Harris & Hepworth, 1995).

This brief account of the historical development of the LEDS perspective on depression shows how increasing refinement from the side of vulnerability – the move from gross demographic factors such as lack of employment or supportive partner to the allied low self-esteem – can lead to increasing specificity in the nature of the life events seen as critical: from 'severe' in level (iv), to 'loss' in level (iii), and then to humiliation, a subtype of loss even more likely to resonate with negative self-evaluation than other losses, such as adult children emigrating to gain promotion, or markedly reduced family income after partner's job loss.

Specificity of life-event stress resonates with specificity of vulnerability to produce specific illnesses

The LEDS has now been used to investigate a range of disorders, both psychiatric and somatic, and while there is no space here to go into details it may be of use to highlight particular causal chains which seem to have been identified.

(a) Humiliation/entrapment, low self-esteem and depression (see above).

(b) Danger, vigilance and anxiety disorder (Finlay Jones, Chapter 3 in Brown & Harris, 1989).

(c) Intrusiveness, sensitivity to criticism and schizophrenia (Awaiting further confirmation Brown & Harris, 1989, chapter 16, p.451).

(d) Goal-frustration, striving stubbornness and peptic ulcer disease (Craig, Chapter 9 in Brown & Harris, 1989).

(e) Goal-frustration/work difficulties, irrascibility/type-A, and myocardial-infarction (Neilson et al., in Brown & Harris, 1989, Chapter 12).

(f) Challenge, dedication and secondary amenorrhoea (Harris in Brown & Harris, 1989, Chapter 10).

(g) Conflict over speaking out, punctiliousness and functional dysphonia (Andrews & House in Brown & Harris, 1989, Chapter 13).

(h) Severe events (perhaps loss) and functional illness: abdominal pain, menorrhagia and somatization (Brown & Harris, 1989, Chapter 16).

A number of LEDS studies suggest that the old distinction between functional and organic disorder still has some value. In one early study with patients undergoing appendectomy, pathologist's reports on the appendices were only consulted after the life events had been rated (Creed in Brown & Harris, 1989 Chapter 8). This lends all the greater credibility to his finding that the same type of severe events associated with depressive onset were more than twice as common in the nine months before appendectomy for those without appendicitis as for both those with acute inflammation, and those in a community comparison group. The author suggested that pain in the absence of inflammation may form part of a cluster of psychiatric symptoms in response to a more severely threatening event, as may increases in gut motility (also invoked to account for functional abdominal pain). Further research with a range of gastrointestinal disorders confirmed this perspective (Craig, op. cit.). Again, those without signs of tissue damage showed a raised proportion with at least one of the severe events associated with depression, while those with other 'organic' conditions resembled the community comparison group. A similar patterning was found for functional menorrhagia, although here the high number with depression meant that a large number of these severe events were humiliations and losses (Harris, op. cit.). One study of somatization took particular care to distinguish somatizers with functional somatic symptoms from other mixed physical/psychiatric cases (Craig et al., 1993). Its findings not only confirmed the picture of preceding severe depresso-

genic-type events but also highlighted another parallel with depression: a high rate of neglect by parent figures in childhood. However, as children, somatizers, in addition, more often than pure psychiatric cases had experience of either their own or their parents' physical illness. The authors suggest that these produced the somatizers' particular form of coping with the loss of hope consequent upon the provoking event, namely presenting with a physical symptom, which might have become their habitual way to elicit care and support.

Severe events have also been implicated in the development of such 'organic' conditions as multiple sclerosis (Grant in Brown & Harris, 1989, Chapter 11), relapse in breast cancer (Ramirez et al., 1989), stroke (House et al. 1990), and diabetes mellitus (Robinson & Fuller, 1985).

These findings also suggest that depression may mediate between the occurrence of severe events and the onset of somatic illness, but that this could operate in at least two different ways. First, even though there is no organic tissue damage, it may render people more likely to interpret themselves as ill along the following lines:

Events and difficulties → Psychiatric → Increased sensitivity
caseness — to physical abnormality/pain without gross organic damage

Secondly the results on multiple sclerosis and breast cancer suggest the possibility of a chain of the following kind:

Provoking agent → Depression of → Disorders consequent
at least — on decreased borderline-case — immunological level — competence

Both of these pathways might be seen as characterized by a measure of disengagement from usual functioning. In other instances, anxiety, anger, and tension may operate as mediating factors, and these might be considered disorders of overengagement, such as ulcers, heart disease and even secondary amenorrhoea.

These diagrams highlight the need to specify the intervening physiological mechanisms serving to relate the emotional meaning of the stress experienced to the biochemistry of the disease. Henry and Stephens (1977) have counterposed the pituitary-adreno-cortical (PAC) and the sympatho-adreno medullary (SAM) systems, relating the former to conservation-withdrawal (like 'disengagement') and the latter to the fight–flight complex of reactions to stress (more like 'overengagement'). Calloway and others (1984) reported higher levels of urinary-free cortisol in those of their depressed patients who had undergone a severe event before illness onset. Changes in corticosteroid levels may have 'extensive and complex effects upon the immune system' (Stein, Keller & Schleifer, 1981), suggesting that studies of physical illness resulting from disorders of immune function should pursue hypotheses involving humiliation, loss, low self-esteem, and depressive response.

In summary, the specificity perspective on life events and health promises to encourage a multifactorial approach, in which data on life events, meaning and psychosocial vulnerability should be collected alongside detailed physiological data. (See also 'Noise effects on health', 'Perceived control and health behaviour', 'Stress and disease'.)

ACKNOWLEDGEMENTS

The life-events research described was originally conceived by Professor George Brown, and largely supported by the Medical Research Council. I am indebted to all the colleagues who have been members of the research team over the last 20 years who participated in the data collection, to Laurie Letchford and Sheila Williams for work with the computer and to all those who have taken the trouble to respond to our questions by telling of such painful and private experiences.

REFERENCES

Alexander, F. (1950). *Psychosomatic Medicine*. New York: Norton.

Brown, G.W. & Harris, T. (1978). *Social origins of depression: a study of psychiatric disorder in women*, New York: London and Free Press. Tavistock Press.

Brown, G.W. & Harris, T.O. (1989). *Life events and illness*. New York: Guilford & London: Unwin Hyman.

Brown, G.W., Andrews, B., Harris, T.O., Adler, Z. & Bridge, L. (1986). Social support, self-esteem and depression. *Psychological Medicine*, 16, 813–31.

Brown, G.W., Bifulco, A. & Harris, T. (1987). Life events, vulnerability and onset of depression: some refinements. *British Journal of Psychiatry*, 150, 30–42.

Brown, G.W., Harris, T.O. Hepworth, C. (1995). Loss and depression: a patient and non-patient comparison. *Psychological Medicine* (25, 7–21).

Calloway, S.P., Dolan, R.J., Fonagy, P., De Souza, F.V.A. & Wakeling, A. (1984). Endocrine changes and clinical profiles in depression: 1. The dexamethasone suppression test. *Psychological Medicine*, 14, 749–58.

Cannon, W.B. (1932). *The wisdom of the body*. 2nd edn. New York: Norton.

Craig, T.K.J, Boardman, A.P., Mills, K., Daly-Jones, O. & Drake, H. (1993). The South London Somatisation Study I: longitudinal course and influence of early life experiences. *British Journal of Psychiatry*, 163, 579–88.

Dunbar, H.F. (1954). *Emotions and bodily changes: a survey of literature on psychosomatic interrelationships*. New York: Columbia University Press.

Graham, D.T., Stern, J.A. & Winokur, G. (1958). Experimental investigation of the specificity of attitude hypothesis in psychosomatic disease. *psychosomatic Medicine*, 20, 446–57.

Holmes, T.H & Rahe, R.H. (1967). The Social Readjustment Rating Scale. *Journal of Psychosomatic Research*, 11, 213–18.

Henry, J.P. & Stephens, P.M. (1977). *Stress, health and the social environment. A sociobiological approach to medicine*, New York: Springer Verlag.

House, A., Dennis, M., Mogridge, L., Hawton, K. & Warlow, C. (1990). Life events and difficulties preceding stroke. *Journal of Neurology, Neurosurgery and Psychiatry*.

Kanner, A.D., Coyne, J.C., Schaefer, C. & Lazarus, R.S. (1981). Comparison of two methods of stress measurement: daily hassles and uplifts versus major life events. *Journal of Behavioral Medicine*, 4, 1–39.

Parry, G., Shapiro, D.A. & Davies, L. (1981). Reliability of life event ratings: an independent replication. *British Journal of Clinical Psychology*, 20, 133–4.

Ramirez, A., Craig, T.K.J., Watson, J.P., Fentiman, I.S., North W.R.S. & Rubens, R. (1989). Stress and the relapse of breast cancer. *British Medical Journal*, 298, 291–3.

Robinson, N. & Fuller, J.H. (1985). The role of life events and difficulties in the onset of diabetes mellitus. *Journal of Psychosomatic Research*, 29, 583–91.

Sarason, I., Jonson, J.H. & Siegel, J.M. (1978). Assessing the impact of life changes: development of the life experiences survey. *Journal of Consulting and Clinical Psychology*, 46, 932–46.

Selye, H. (1956). *The stress of life*. New York: McGraw-Hill.

Stein, M., Keller, S. & Schleifer, S. (1981) The hypothalamus and the immune response. In H. Weiner, M.A. Hofer & A.J. Stunkard (Eds.). *Brain, behaviour, and bodily disease*, New York: Raven Press.

Tennant, C. & Andrews, G. (1976). A scale to measure the stress of life events. *Australian & New Zealand Journal of Psychiatry*, 10, 27–32.

Tennant, C., Smith, A., Bebbington, P. & Hurry, J. (1979). The contextual threat of life events: the concept and its reliability. *Psychological Medicine*, 9, 525–8.

Noise: effects on health

STAFFAN HYGGE

Royal Institute of Technology, Kungl Tekniska Högskolan-Centre for Built Environment, Gävle, Sweden

NOISE: NATURE AND MEASUREMENT

Noise is commonly defined as unwanted sound or sound with an adverse effect. What is sweet music for one person may be noise to someone else, or even to the person himself if it interferes with other activities. Thus, noise is a psychological construct influenced both by physical and psychosocial properties.

Sound is created by the rapidly changing pressure of air molecules at the eardrum. A single tone, such as that from a tuning fork, can be depicted as a fixed wavelength sinusoidal pressure distribution across time. The number of pressure cycles per second, measured in Hertz (Hz), is the basis for the sensation of pitch. A healthy young ear is sensitive to sounds between approximately 20 Hz and up to 20 kHz. Infrasound is defined as the frequency range below 20 Hz and ultrasound as the range above 20 kHz. The amplitude of the sine wave (measured as root mean square, RMS), is perceived as loudness. To accommodate the wide dynamic power range of the human ear and in accordance with the Weber–Fechner law stating a logarithmic relationship between stimulus strength and response for hearing, a logarithmic magnitude scale for sounds has been introduced. Its unit is the decibel (dB), which is defined as:

$$\text{Sound pressure level (SPL) in dB} = Lp = 20 \times {}^{10}\log \frac{p}{p_0}$$

$$= 10 \times {}^{10}\log \frac{p^2}{p_0^2}$$

where p is the sound pressure being measured (in Pa) and p_0 is the reference level 20 μPa, which is about the minimum pressure detectable by a healthy human ear.

Since SPLs in dB are logarithms of ratios between pressures, they can not be added to yield a sum. SPLs in dB must first be converted to intensities expressed as squared sound pressures. The squares must then be summed up to a total intensity and converted back to dB units, as in the following example where three independent sources of 65, 69 and 68 dB re 20 μPa are added:

$$\text{Sum of squared pressures re 20 μPa} = 10^{\frac{65}{10}} + 10^{\frac{69}{10}} + 10^{\frac{68}{10}} =$$

$$= (3.16 + 7.94 + 6.31) \times 10^6 = 1.74 \times 10^7$$

$$L_{p_{tot}} = 10 \times {}^{10}\log(1.74 \times 10^7) = 72.4 \text{ dB re 20 μPa}$$

Adding two independent sound sources of the same SPL dB level will yield a sum that is ≃ 3 dB higher than one of them alone. However, the subjective effects of a change in 3 dB amounts to a just perceptible change. A change of around 10 dB is needed to experience the sound as twice as loud.

The hearing threshold for pure tones is lowest in the frequency range 500–4000 Hz, which also is the range where human speech has its maximum energy content. In order to compensate for the ear's frequency sensitivity, and to make units that are comparable across the audible frequency range, standardized weighting curves or filters have been defined for sound level meters (see Fig. 1.)

For calibration and reference purposes, the filters A, B, C, and D have a compensation value of zero (re SPL in dB) at 1000 Hz. The A-filter is intended to mirror hearing thresholds, the C-filter is supposed to mirror the ears's sensitivity to high intensities, and the B-filter to intermediate intensities. The main difference between the A, B, and C-filters is in how great the compensation is of low frequencies. Although the dBA-filter was designed for hearing thresholds of pure tones, it is the most commonly used filter across all intensities. Experience has shown it to have a very high overall correlation with, e.g. hearing loss and loudness ratings. However, when the low frequency components of a sound dominate, such as in HVAC-noise, dBA underestimates perceived noise.

Several indices have been suggested to represent fluctuating sound across time. A simple one is that of maximum level, L_{max}, which can be combined with a number index for how many times a certain L_{max}-level has been exceeded. Such measures have been employed for aircraft noise and for finding the best correlation with sleep quality. The Lp-measure, as in L_1 and L_{50}, states the percentage of time a certain value (in dB, dBA, etc.) is exceeded. The equivalent continuous sound pressure level, L_{eq}, is the constant level across the time period that represent the total energy of the variable sound. The L_{eq} levels are commonly used for codes and regulations and can be weighted to dBA, dBB etc. The L_{eq}-measure is strongly influenced by high peak values, but is very insensitive to increases in background sound levels.

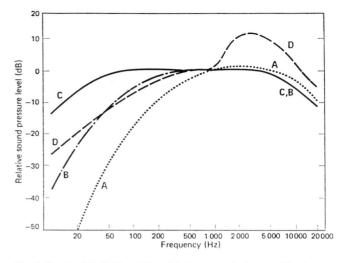

Fig. 1. Standard A, B, C, and D-weighting networks for sound level meters.

In addition to the filters and indices listed here, an array of others have been proposed (Kryter, 1985). These include attempts to incorporate masking, critical bands, rise-time, predictability, fluctuations and designing ratio-scales for the measurement of annoyance and perceived loudness.

AUDITORY HEALTH EFFECTS

Hearing impairment

Prolonged exposure to intense sounds result in noise-induced hearing loss. Three types of noise-induced hearing losses can be distinguished: (i) temporary threshold shifts (TTS), (ii) permanent threshold shifts (PTS), and (iii) acoustic trauma. TTS show an increase with SPL-levels and exposure time, starting somewhere around 70 dB for noise bands around 4 kHz and around 75 dB for bands around 250 Hz when the noise is presented for several hours. TTS is reversible but requires silent recovery periods. PTS is the effect of prolonged exposure to high intensity sounds with insufficient silent recovery periods in between. The effect to the inner ear is irreversible destruction of hair cells. To reduce the risk of PTS, most Western countries have restricted sound exposure in the work environment to 85 or 90 dBA for 8 hours a day, five working days a week for several years when no hearing protection is worn. However, that is not a decision purely guided by the concern to avoid hearing loss, since it has been estimated that around 10% of those so exposed to 85 dBA will accrue a hearing loss. The figure is estimated to drop to 4% if the levels are reduced to 80 dBA. Thus, converging evidence suggests exposure levels of around 75 dBA will be safe from the point of hearing impairment, temporary or permanent.

Noise-induced acoustic trauma involves very short exposure to very intense sounds, such as riveting, gunfire, explosives, toy pistols, clicking toys. These impulse sounds are treacherous because of their short duration, which falls short of the integration time of the brain, but not of the inner ear. Thus, their perceived loudness is much lower than the damage caused to the hair cells in the inner ear.

Degree of hearing impairment is assessed by audiometry, which normally consists of measuring hearing thresholds for pure tones in the frequency range 500–8000 Hz. The resulting audiograms are evaluated against standardized age-corrected audiograms for unimpaired hearing. Hearing impairment caused by broadband noise often starts in the frequency range 3000–6000 Hz, with a downward spread to 500–1000 Hz as the impairment grows worse. A slight impairment in the 3000–6000 Hz range does not much affect speech comprehension in an otherwise silent environment. However, when the frequency range from 2000 Hz and downwards is affected, speech comprehension is markedly affected.

Hearing impaired persons need up to a 10 dB better signal-to-noise ratio than normal hearing persons to understand speech.

During the last decades the importance of noisy leisure activities, rather than industrial work noise, have become more important as contributors to hearing impairment. In particular, chainsaws, lawn-mowers, snow mobiles, water scooters, loud concert and disco music, guns and rifles, explosives and certain toys with loud click sounds may cause hearing impairment by itself or by blocking recovery from TTS accrued at work.

NON-AUDITORY HEALTH EFFECTS

The World Health Organization defines health as *the state of complete physical, mental and social well-being, and not merely an absence of disease and infirmity.* Therefore, the health effects of noise should include a broader array of adverse effects than damage to organs and tissue.

Stress reactions and cardiovascular disorders

Noise has often been implicated as a contributing cause to the development of stress reactions and cardiovascular disorders. Correlational studies report higher systolic or diastolic blood pressure (BP) or elevated stress hormone levels in hearing impaired or noise exposed industrial workers (Evans & Cohen, 1987). Children and adults chronically exposed to aircraft noise have been found to have higher BPs and elevated levels of stress hormones compared to controls matched on sociodemographic characteristics (Cohen et al., 1986). Correlational and cross-sectional studies suffer from methodological flaws, primarily from possible selection bias and inability to rule out other possible causes for the stress reactions and cardiovascular disorders, such as a hazardous chemical environment and other stress inducing work related factors. Experimental studies, which for practical and ethical reasons must be restricted to acute rather than chronic noise effects, show noise effects on several non-specific physiological measures associated with stress reaction, including BP, heart-rate, stress hormone output and vasoconstriction. These reactions habituate to a large extent and thus its not clear how they can build up to a chronic effect (Evans & Cohen, 1987). However, stress reactions to chronic noise exposure have been shown in experimental study by Peterson et al. (1981). Rhesus monkeys were exposed to loud noise for 9 months. BPs increased by one third and high BP-levels were maintained for a one-month follow-up period after noise cessation.

It is probably fair to conclude that chronic exposure to high intensity noise increases the risk of cardiovascular problems. Because of this, and of fairly well controlled studies where noise has also been shown to increase secretion of stress hormones, it can be claimed that noise plays a role in a general stress response. Since detailed dose – response relationships are not fully specified, this conclusion must be restricted to high-intensity noise at this point.

With regard to other medical symptoms reportedly linked to noise, e.g. ulcers, miscarriage, weight at birth, consumption of medication, visits to doctors, infectious diseases, the evidence is still too meagre to be conclusive (Cohen et al., 1986).

Mental health

Since noise effects annoyance and prolonged annoyance may be conducive to mental illness, it has been argued that noise impairs mental health. Studies on mental health or mental-hospital admissions around Heathrow airport in London, Schiphol in Amsterdam, and the different airports in Los Angeles, give correlational support for such claims. However, in most of these cases, critics have shown that more stringent and proper controls for sociodemographic variables has strongly diminished the correlations between noise levels and various dependent measures. Thus, the results are conflicting and there is not a solid empirical basis for arguing strong effects of noise on mental health (Stansfeld et al., 1993).

Sleep

Sleep and sleep quality are among the most noise sensitive human activities. From laboratory studies is has been concluded that 20–35% of normal and self-reported noise sensitive persons have problems falling asleep, change sleep stage or are awakened by a number of peaks as low as 50 dBA L (Öhrström, 1993). There seems to be some agreement that peak-levels below 40 dBA, or equivalent noise levels below 35 dBA, do not have much effect on sleep.

Drowsy or sleeping people have difficulties in actively identifying and recognizing sounds, and consequently they have a problem in adapting or habituating to sounds. Children change sleep-stages less often than adults because of noise and are less easily awakened than adults, but the opposite is true for the elderly.

Effects of sleep deprivation on task performance the next day vary with the difficulty of the task, but no conclusive dose response relationships can be stated at this time.

Performance and cognition

In laboratory studies fairly high noise levels (80–90 dB in intermittent bursts) have been shown to affect attention, signal-detection, vigilance, short-term memory, etc. However, there are some noteworthy exceptions to this rule (cf. reviews by Broadbent, 1983; Jones, 1990; Smith, 1993). Exceptions involve speech-like noise, verbal material, and aftereffects to controllable and non-controllable noise.

In experiments on speech-like noise and short-term memory serial recall, a set of 7 – 9 digits or letters are presented visually at a fixed rate. A rehearsal period follows from the presentation of the last item to a prompt to reproduce the series in correct order. Speech in the rehearsal period, even devoid of semantic content such as a foreign tongue, or vocals in a song, interfere with recall, but broadband noise does not (see overviews by Jones & Macken, 1993; Jones & Morris, 1992). The effect is stable across sound levels ranging down to around 50 dBA, and has been shown to extend to a range of non-speech sounds. However, the serial nature of the memory task seems to be crucial. The effects or irrelevant speech on more cognitive tasks such as proof-reading and understanding is not as marked and less consistent.

Classroom experiments of recall one week after a learning task (Hygge, 1996) have shown impairment from aircraft and road traffic noise of 66 dBA *L* during a 15 min noise exposure. No impairment was shown from train noise and verbal noise of the same level, nor did any of the noise sources affect long-term recognition. A replication of the aircraft and road traffic noise at 55 dBA *L*, again showed impairment from aircraft noise, but no impairment from road traffic noise.

Vulnerability to noise of the language, reading and understanding processes, particularly in children, fits with findings from cross-sectional studies of school achievement and cognitive performance in noisy and less noisy areas (Evans & Lepore, 1993).

In a study of children around the new and old airports in Munich, cross-sectional analyses at the old airport before the close down showed that the chronically aircraft exposed children, compared to their matched control group, had higher levels of stress hormones, higher blood pressure while resting and at work, an indication of perceptual adaptation to noise (not only aircraft noise) and impaired motivation, long-term memory, reading and word-skills. (Evans, Hygge & Bullinger, 1995).

A longitudinal analysis of long-term memory, reading and word-skills at the old airport of the aircraft noise exposed children showed improvement in relation to the matched controls after the airport was closed. Parallel impairments in the very same cognitive functions have been shown at the new airport when it was opened (Hygge, Evans & Bullinger, 1996).

In a well-known series of experiments, Glass and Singer (1972) reported performance after-effects on the number of times their subjects attempted to solve insoluble geometric puzzles and proof-reading errors. The noise they used was a mixture of office-machines and foreign languages presented in aperiodic bursts in intensity ranges from 60 to 108 dBA depending on experiment. Their main findings were that the noise had deleterious effects on postnoise behaviour when the noise was uncontrollable or unpredictable by the subjects. The introduction of perceived control by making the noise predictable or controllable eliminated the adverse noise effect even when compared to a silent control group. These adverse effects of uncontrollable and unpredictable noise have been replicated in several studies for various types of noise, as well as for other stressors than noise (Cohen, 1980). Thus, research on the aftereffects of noise points to psychological coping mechanisms that may be basic and central to others stressors as well.

Social behaviour

In the laboratory, noise has consistently interacted with anger in provoking aggression as measured by the delivery of electric shocks to a confederate of the experimenter. That is, the presence of noise at the time of aggression is not by itself sufficient for increased aggression, but when the subject is made angry the presence of noise adds to the aggression shown. For helping behaviour, a mixture of experimental studies in the field and the lab show less helping when exposed to noise. However, the noise effect on helping is not as consistent and marked as that on aggression (Cohen & Spacapan, 1984).

THEORETICAL ACCOUNTS OF THE NOISE EFFECTS

There really are no theories regarding the noise-induced physical damage of hair cells in the inner ear. However, the empirical findings that physical energy of a certain intensity, frequency composition, duration, onset-time, etc causes a certain amount of impairment has been well documented.

Stress theories of noise effects have two prospects. One prospect explores the physiological effects, the other the psychological outcomes. The physiological theories have pointed to the roles played by epinephrine and norepinephrine secretion in the activation of the sympathetic–adrenal medullary system, and to hormone output from the pituitary – adrenocortical axis (Evans & Cohen, 1987). Psychological stress theories such as Lazarus (1966) view the person's psychological appraisal of a stimulus as threatening as a first stage, followed by a stage where the individual evaluates their resources to cope with the threat. If they perceive that they can cope, no stress response occurs, but they may later reappraise their coping ability. If they do not perceive that they can cope or are uncertain, stress is experienced.

Psychological theories of the performance effects of noise have relied primarily on two constructs: arousal and informational load. Arousal refers to nonspecific brain activity signifying different levels of general alertness. The Yerkes–Dodson law (Kahneman, 1973) of arousal and performance assumes an inverted U-relationship between performance and arousal. Too high or too low arousal, with reference to the optimum level, impairs performance. The exact optimal level depends on the difficulty of the task and individual skill on the task. Easterbrook (1959) forwarded the idea that over-arousal narrows the attention to focal parts of the task. If the focal cues are the relevant cues for successful performance, as in easy tasks, performance is improved. If the task is difficult and the relevant cues are not focal, performance is impaired. In practice, arousal theory and the inverted U-hypothesis suffer from several shortcomings (Hockey & Hamilton, 1983), including the multidimensionality of the construct and the problem of finding data-independent locations of the optimum level. On the other hand, it may be a convenient theoretical vehicle to accommodate combined and interactive effects of many different stressors, noise just being one.

Another line of theorizing (Smith & Jones, 1992) has emphasized dominant strategy selection, and reduced efficiency in the control processes while working in noise.

An information overload model, such as presented by Cohen *et al.* (1986), puts an emphasis on shrinking cognitive capacity as a result of attention allocation during noise and stress exposure, and the individual's adaptation to demands on information processing. One implication of this theory is that cumulative cognitive fatigue effects should show up as residuals also after the cessation of the noise, as in after-effects of non-controllable noise. Another important implication of the model is that both noise itself as a stressor, plus individual efforts to cope with the noise, can create adverse effects. (See also 'Life events and health', 'Perceived control and health behaviour', 'Stress and disease'.)

FURTHER READING

For more detailed accounts of noise, noise measurement, the effects on people, and and theories see relevant sections and references in Cohen *et al.* (1986), Jones and Chapman (1984), Kryter (1985), Smith & Jones (1992), and Tempest (1985).

REFERENCES

Broadbent, D.E. (1983). Recent advances in understanding performance in noise. In G. Rossi (Ed.). *Proceedings of the 4th International Congress on noise as a public health problem, Vol. 2*, pp. 719–738. Milan: Centro Ricerche e Studi Amplifon.

Cohen, S. (1980). After effects of stress on human performance and social behavior: review of research and theory. *Psychological Bulletin, 88*, 82–108.

Cohen, S. & Spacapan, S. (1984). The social psychology of noise. In D.M. Jones & A.J. Chapman (Eds.). *Noise and society.* London: Wiley.

Cohen, S., Evans, G.W., Stokols, D. & Krantz, D.S. (1986). *Behavior, health, and environmental stress.* New York: Plenum Press.

Easterbrook, J.A. (1959). The effect of emotion on cue utilization and the organization of behavior. *Psychological Bulletin, 66*, 183–201.

Evans, G.E. & Cohen, S. (1987). Environmental stress. In D. Stokols & I. Altman (Eds.). *Handbook of environmental psychology*, pp. 571–610. New York: Wiley.

Evans, G.W. & Lepore, S.J. (1993). Nonauditory effects of noise on children. A critical review. *Children's Environments, 10*, 31–51.

Evans, G.W., Hygge, S. & Bullinger M. (1995). Chronic noise and psychological stress. *Psychological Science, 6*, 333–8.

Glass, D.C. & Singer, J.E. (1972). *Urban stress: Experiments on noise and social stressors.* New York: Academic Press.

Hockey, R. & Hamilton, P. (1983). The cognitive patterning of stress states. In R. Hockey (Ed) *Stress and fatigue in human performance*, pp. 331–362. New York: Wiley.

Hygge, S. (1996). The effects of combined noise sources on long-term memory in children aged 12–14 years. In A. Schick & M. Klatte (Eds.), *Contributions to psychological acoustics. Result of the seventh Oldenburg symposium on psychological acoustics.* Oldenburg, Germany: Bibliotheks- und Informationssystem der Universität Oldenburg.

Hygge, S., Evans, G.W. & Bullinger, M. (1993). The Munich airport noise study: psychological, cognitive, and quality of life effects on children. In M. Vallet (Ed.). *Noise as a public health problem. Proceedings of the 6th International Congress. Vol. 3*, pp. 301–308. Arcueil, France: Inrets.

Hygge, S., Evans, G.W., & Bullinger, M. (1996). The Munich airport noise study: Cognitive effects on children from before to after the change over of airports. Invited paper to Inter Noise 96, Liverpool 30 July – 2 August 1996.

Jones, D.M. (1990). Progress and prospects in the study of performance in noise. In B. Berglund & T. Lindvall (Eds.). *Noise as a public health problem. Vol 4: New advances in noise research, Part 1*, pp. 383–400. Stockholm: Swedish Council for Building Research.

Jones, D.M. & Chapman, A.J. (Eds.). (1984). *Noise and society.* London: Wiley.

Jones, D.M. & Macken, W.J. (1993). Irrelevant tones produce an irrelevant speech effect: Implications for coding in phonological memory. *Journal of Experimental Psychology: Learning, Memory and Cognition, 19*, 369–81.

Jones, D.M. & Morris, N. (1992). Irrelevant speech and cognition. In A.P. Smith & D.M. Jones (Eds.). – *Handbook of human performance: vol. 1. The physical environment*, pp. 29–54. London: Academic Press.

Kahneman, D. (1973). *Attention and effort.* Englewood Cliffs, NJ: Prentice Hall.

Kryter, K. (1985). *The effects of noise on man.* 2nd edn. New York: Academic Press.

Lazarus, R.S. (1966). *Psychological stress and coping processes.* New York: McGraw-Hill.

Öhrström, E. (1993). Research on noise and sleep since 1988: Present state. In M. Vallet (Ed.). *Noise as a public health problem. Proceedings of the 6th International Congress. vol. 3* pp. 331–338. Arcueil, France: Inrets.

Peterson, E.A., Augenstein, J.S., Tanis, D.C. & Augenstein, D.G. (1981). Noise raises blood pressure without impairing auditory sensitivity. *Science, 211*, 1450–2.

Stansfeld, S., Gallacher, J., Babisch, W. & Elwood, P. (1993). Road traffic noise, noise sensitivity and psychiatric disorder: preliminary prospective findings from the Caerphilly study. In M. Vallet (Ed.). *Noise as a public health problem. Proceedings of the 6th International Congress. vol. 3* pp. 268–273. Arcueil, France: Inrets.

Smith, A.P. (1993). Recent advances in the study of noise and human performance. In M. Vallet (Ed.). *Noise as a public health problem. Proceedings of the 6th International Congress. vol. 3* pp. 293–300. Arcueil, France: Inrets.

Smith, A.P. & Jones, D.M. (1992). Noise and performance. In A.P. Smith & D.M. Jones, (Eds.). *Handbook of human performance: vol. 1. The physical environment*, pp. 1–28. London: Academic Press.

Tempest, W. (Ed.). (1985). *The noise handbook.* London: Academic Press.

Old age and health behaviour

SIOBHAN HART

Essex Rivers Health Care Trust, Essex County Hospital, Colchester, UK

Old age is a rather vague and arbitrarily defined portion of the lifespan. Nevertheless, there can be no doubt that the number of elderly people in our society has grown at a remarkable rate and will continue to do so for the foreseeable future. This is particularly true of those aged 80 years or more who constitute the fastest growing cohort in British society. Such demographic changes have profound implications for the allocation of health-care resources, since the impact of acute illness is often more severe in older people, and

[143]

recovery more protracted than in younger adults and, more importantly, because of the high prevalence of chronic diseases, some of which are also major causes of death. The majority of individuals aged 65 years or more suffer from at least one chronic condition and many suffer from two or more simultaneously. Lifestyle and behavioural factors are important in many of the major causes of morbidity and/or mortality that affect elderly people. These may increase the likelihood of acquiring the condition (e.g. vascular disorders and lung cancer) or be critical determinants of whether a condition is detected sufficiently early to allow for effective treatment (e.g. breast cancer). Strict behavioural management can also play an important role in limiting the extent of morbidity produced by chronic disorders (e.g. diabetes). However, negative stereotypes regarding elderly people which are widely held amongst health-care professionals, and often by elderly people themselves, have proved significant barriers to the provision of optimal treatment for elderly people when ill. These have also thwarted the promotion and/or adoption of healthier lifestyles and behavioural practices aimed at prevention of illness, let alone realization of more positive ideals such as those embodied in the World Health Organization's definition of health as 'a state of complete physical, mental and social well-being and not simply the absence of disease and infirmity'. It is widely held that old age is a time of inevitable decline exacerbated by a lifetime of poor health practices, that elderly people are generally unable and/or unwilling to modify their lifestyles and behaviours, that their compliance with therapeutic interventions is poor and that in any case the benefits to be derived from lifestyle and behavioural change at this stage of the life-cycle is minimal. This chapter aims to confront such nihilism and replace it with a more optimistic, though nevertheless realistic, appraisal of the health-related behaviours of elderly people that is based on empirical data, and to consider also the behaviour of health-care personnel as it pertains to elderly people.

Metrics such as hospital bed occupancy and the number of prescriptions dispensed per individual all support the view that elderly people are disproportionate consumers of health-care resources (see Hart, 1990). More contentious issues concern the efficacy and/or appropriateness of this resource expenditure. Although some data have suggested that elderly people overutilize health-care resources by presenting with non-serious complaints, many studies have painted a rather different picture. Indeed, Brody and Kleban (1981) concluded that 'Large numbers of uncomfortable and distressing symptoms are borne in silence', all too often being '. . . accepted helplessly and hopelessly as part of "normal aging" or as a form of distress about which "nothing can be done" . . .' In Stoller, Forster & Portugal's (1993) study of illness behaviour in a sample of older people living in community settings, it emerged that the most common response to symptoms was self-management without recourse to formal health-care services. Use of over-the-counter medications was a frequently employed strategy, although a decision to take no action was also a common initial response to many symptoms. It is clearly important to improve understanding by elderly people of the significance of symptoms and to promote greater awareness of the treatment options available to them so that needless suffering is prevented.

In the event that elderly people do seek help from formal service agencies, the attitudes and behaviours of health professionals become important determinants of whether elderly people receive the best treatment available or become the victims of unjustified nihilism. For example, although hypertension is well recognized as a major cause of morbidity and mortality amongst elderly people, there has been a persistent reluctance to treat this condition in older patients because physicians often fear that efforts to reduce blood pressure in elderly patients might do more harm than good. However, recent data (Beard *et al.*, 1992) indicate that hypertension can be actively treated in elderly people and that such treatment is associated with significant reductions in the incidence of fatal and non-fatal strokes. Similarly Derby (1991) has drawn attention to ageism in cancer care, arguing that elderly people are disadvantaged by a paucity of information that would allow for the design of optimal treatment regimens. Fentiman *et al.* (1990) have urged that fitness for general anaesthesia, rather than chronological age, should determine whether elderly patients with cancer are considered for surgical intervention.

One aspect of health-care resource utilization by elderly people that has drawn considerable comment is the extent to which they comply with prescribed treatment regimens. A particular, though by no means exclusive, focus of concern has been the consumption of prescribed drugs. Of course, non-compliance is not a phenomenon that is unique to elderly people. Indeed, a number of comparative studies have shown that the compliance of elderly people can be greater than that of younger contemporaries (see Hart, 1990). However, for a variety of reasons, the consequences of non-compliance by elderly individuals may be particularly serious and hence noteworthy. Age-related changes in pharmacokinetics and pharmacodynamics may render them particularly sensitive to the effects of certain compounds including undesired side-effects. Polypharmacy, which is common because of multiple pathologies, allows opportunities for drug interactions and exacerbates the likelihood of dosing errors. This problem may be further compounded by self-medication with non-prescription preparations of which prescribing physicians may be unaware. Reductions in sensory acuity and manual dexterity can also impede compliance. Atkin *et al.* (1994) found that, when admitted to an acute geriatric hospital service, some 41% of elderly people were unable to execute one or more of the motor acts necessary to allow them access to the medicines they had been prescribed. Considerable attention has been directed towards the important influence of cognitive factors in determining compliance. Not surprisingly levels of compliance are poorer when individuals have little knowledge about the nature of their condition(s), the purpose(s) of their medication(s) and/or are unable to remember their dosing regimen. What needs to be challenged is the stereotypical assumption that this is the natural state of affairs for elderly people. While there are indeed age-related declines in cognitive functioning, the magnitude of these is comparatively small for most individuals. Only a minority of elderly people suffer from dementia. Morrow, Leirer & Sheikh (1988) concluded that non-adherence is primarily caused by 'poor communication' between health professionals and their elderly clients. Clearly, the onus is on health professionals to prescribe the simplest possible treatment regimens that are commensurate with the goals of therapy and to make every effort to maximize their clients' levels of understanding.

The importance of treatment aimed at limiting the morbidity and mortality of established conditions in elderly people should not eclipse more ambitious goals such as early detection of disease at pre-symptomatic levels or control of risk factors so as to diminish the likelihood of conditions developing.

A number of studies have sought to determine what factors influence the decision by elderly people to take part in screening programmes or carry out self-examinations to detect pathology at an early stage. Grady's (1988) investigation of breast self-examination indicated that older women responded readily to an intervention designed to increase the frequency of this behaviour. Indeed, their long-term compliance exceeded that of many of the younger subjects in this comparative study. These results favour optimism regarding the possibility of involving older people in active self-monitoring so as to promote early detection of treatable disease. However, Grady's results also pointed to deficiencies in the current theoretical frameworks attempting to predict health-related behaviour. Somewhat surprisingly, they suggested that it was individuals with an external locus of control who were most compliant, that is those who downgraded personal responsibility for health in favour of fate, luck and chance and/or control by powerful others. However, other studies have reported that an internal locus of control is a better predictor of breast self-examination. Grady, like many others, also found that the Health Belief Model was inadequate for predicting the behaviour of elderly individuals. If nothing else, the contradictory results of investigations into breast self-examination attest to the heterogeneity of elderly women, something that can all too easily be obscured by the application of a group label such as 'the elderly'.

The under-representation of elderly people in cancer screening activities cannot entirely be attributed to their own beliefs, intentions and behaviours. Screening programmes are often not directed at individuals over 65, despite the increased prevalence of cancers in this age-group. Furthermore, physicians' expressed attitudes to cancer screening in older people may be at variance with their behaviour. Black, Sefcik & Kapoor (1990) reported that physicians who gave assent to recommendations that elderly people be screened for cancer often did not put this into practice.

Since the 1989 revision of their NHS contracts, general practitioners in the UK have been obliged to offer all patients over 75 years an annual health check and home visit. It is too early to evaluate the full impact of these procedures but preliminary data suggest that, although elderly people welcome the provision of annual check-ups, many physicians are sceptical about their worth. Criticisms have included low rates of detection, the induction of unnecessary anxiety in those assessed or paradoxically an inappropriate sense of reassurance. It has rightly been asserted that screening programmes are of little use unless appropriate resources are available to deal with positive outcomes. The focus of screening programmes might also be questioned. Indeed, it has been argued that they perpetrate an undesirable 'problem focus' and that there should be a shift away from medically orientated attempts to identify specific diseases in favour of a broader focus on functional capacity and quality of life (Perkins, 1991).

In recent years, considerable effort has been expended in promoting healthier lifestyles in middle-aged and younger individuals. There is empirical evidence that many elderly people too engage in a wide variety of behaviours (not necessarily related to formal health-care systems) to protect and promote their health (Amir,

1987; Jensen, Counte & Glandon, 1992) and indeed may do so more diligently than younger contemporaries (Leventhal & Prohaska, 1986). These activities include regular exercise, dietary control, maintaining social support networks, adopting psychological strategies to reduce stress as well as more general safety practices such as wearing seat belts in cars and checking electrical appliances in the home. Among the factors which might contribute to an age-related trend towards increased self-care are a growing sense of vulnerability to the debilitating effects of illness and a selective survivor effect, whereby those who have regularly carried out health-protective behaviours come to represent an increasing proportion of the cohort. Engagement in health-protective behaviours is associated with lower levels of morbidity and mortality (Amir, 1987) and, of course, there are abundant data pointing to the adverse consequences of unhealthy lifestyles.

Despite its obvious importance, there are relatively few empirical studies of the benefits to be derived from adopting healthier lifestyles *de novo* in later life. However, the evidence available points to efficacy. The positive effects of stopping smoking are comparable in younger and older individuals with coronary artery disease or after myocardial infarction in terms of minimizing morbidity and preventing further deterioration. Ceasing to smoke in later life can increase bone mineral density although its beneficial effects on respiratory function, for men at least, may be age related. Physical exercise in old age increases physical strength, decreases falls and associated injuries, enhances cardiovascular status and improves cognitive functioning in the virtual absence of serious cardiovascular or musculoskeletal complications (Elward & Larson, 1992). Of course, all benefits derived from participation in exercise programmes cannot be attributed to the physiological effects of exercise *per se*. Factors such as the physical setting and social context in which exercise occurs are also important.

The health of an individual at any age is the outcome of a complex interplay between biological, psychological and social factors. In old age, the boundaries between these spheres are even less well defined and their interactions more powerful. Consequently, when caring for elderly individuals, health professionals must adopt a holistic approach, giving due recognition to the importance of broader contextual issues, including gender and cultural heritage, which might exacerbate the power differential entailed in any clinical encounter. They must also take account of the impact upon an individual's life of socioeconomic factors, especially how the occurrence of multifaceted changes are psychologically construed and evaluated in relation to the perceived availability of coping resources. Empowering elderly individuals with the knowledge necessary to allow them to make informed choices, and to assume an appropriate level of responsibility for their own health outcomes, is a desirable goal provided that any associated tendency to attribute ill health to personal negligence is tempered by a historical perspective. While long-standing negative health practices have contributed to the ill health of many elderly people, it is only relatively recently that the dangers associated with practices such as smoking have come to be fully recognized. Furthermore, many older people confront, often simultaneously or in rapid succession, life events which, directly or indirectly, have adverse health consequences. These include retirement, bereavement, diminished social status and financial resources, disease and injury, relocation, pain and reduced mobility. Often individuals have little personal control over the occurrence of such events, but their effects may be exacerbated by behavioural responses. One maladaptive response is increased consumption of alcohol. A sizeable proportion of elderly people with alcohol-related problems only commence alcohol abuse in old age.

We are a long way from understanding the determinants of health behaviour in elderly people. All that is certain is the complexity of the causal web. Studies such as those of Jensen *et al.* (1992) highlight the fact that, even with quite sophisticated modelling, only a small proportion of the total variance can be accounted for. A key issue is the meaning of health for elderly people. Most research indicates that elderly people are often surprisingly optimistic when assessing their own health status, perhaps because they are making comparative judgements with their peers and/or their own ageist expectations of inevitable decline. Self-assessed health is the strongest single predictor of life satisfaction in elderly people. The health of elderly people is an issue that goes beyond increasing longevity. It is about successful ageing, that is sustaining independence, avoiding unnecessary disability, optimizing functional capacities and quality of life. Health behaviour in old age has a critical part to play in achieving this goal and efforts must be made to ensure that it is not thwarted by ageist nihilism. (See also 'The health belief model', 'Health-related behaviours: common factors'.)

REFERENCES

Amir, D. (1987). Preventive behaviour and health status among the elderly. *Psychology and Health*, 1, 353–77.

Atkin, P.A., Finnegan, T.P., Ogle, S.J. & Shenfield, G.M. (1994). Functional ability of patients to manage medication packaging: a survey of geriatric inpatients. *Age and Ageing*, 23, 113–16.

Beard, K., Bulpitt, C., Mascie-Taylor, H., O'Malley, K., Sever, P. & Webb, S. (1992). Management of elderly patients with sustained hypertension. *British Medical Journal*, 304, 412–16.

Black, J.S., Sefcik, T. & Kapoor, W. (1990). Health promotion and disease prevention in the elderly. Comparison of house staff and attending physician attitudes and practices. *Archives of Internal Medicine*, 150, 389–93.

Brody, E.M. & Kleban, M.H. (1981). Physical and mental health symptoms of older people: who do they tell?. *Journal of the American Geriatrics Society*, 29, 442–9.

Derby, S.E. (1991). Ageism in cancer care of the elderly. *Oncological Nursing Forum*, 18, 921–6.

Elward, K. & Larson, E.B. (1992). Benefits of exercise for older adults. A review of existing evidence and current recommendations for the general population. *Clinical Geriatric Medicine*, 8, 35–50.

Fentiman, I.S., Tirelli, U., Monfardini, S., Schneider, M., Festen, J., Cognetti, F. & Aapro, M.S. (1990). Cancer in the elderly: why so badly treated? *Lancet*, 335, 1020–2.

Grady, K.E. (1988). Older women and the practice of breast self-examination. *Psychology of Women Quarterly*, 12, 473–87.

Hart, S. (1990). Psychology and the health of elderly people. In P. Bennett, J. Weinman & P. Spurgeon (Eds.). *Current Developments in Health Psychology*, pp. 247–275. London: Harwood Academic Publishers.

Jensen, J., Counte, M.A. & Glandon, G.L. (1992). Elderly health beliefs, attitudes, and maintenance. *Preventive Medicine*, 21, 483–97.

Leventhal, E.A. & Prohaska, T.R. (1986). Age, symptom interpretation and health behaviour. *Journal of the American Geriatrics Society*, 34, 185–91.

Morrow, D., Leirer, V. & Sheikh, J. (1988). Adherence and medication instructions. Review and recommendations. *Journal of the American Geriatrics Society*, 36, 1147–60.

Perkins, E.R. (1991). Screening elderly people: a review of the literature in the light of the new general practitioner contract. *British Journal of General Practitioners*, 41, 382–5.

Stoller, E.P., Forster, L.E. & Portugal, S. (1993). Self-care responses to symptoms by older people. A health diary study of illness behavior. *Medical Care*, 31, 24–42.

Pain: a multidimensional perspective

DENNIS C. TURK

Department of Anesthesiology, University of Washington, USA

Pain has been the focus of philosophical speculation as well as scientific attention since earliest recorded times, dating back at least 4000 years to discussion of treatment in the Ebers Papyrus. Yet, despite its lengthy history; advances in knowledge of sensory physiology, anatomy, and biochemistry, and the development of potent analgesic medications and other innovative medical and surgical interventions that have evolved over time, pain relief remains elusive. At the present time, pain continues to remain one of the most challenging problems for the sufferer, health-care providers, and for society.

Although pain is an almost universal experience, there is little consensus how to define it. One factor that has contributed to the debate about what pain is relates to the fact that pain is a subjective experience, unlike blood pressure, there is currently no objective way to determine the extent of pain that an individual has or should have. Thus the only way to know how much pain one has is to ask the individual or make inferences from his or her voluntary (e.g. facial expression, ambulation) or involuntary (e.g. autonomic activity) behaviour.

A difficulty with understanding and treating pain is that it is a symptom associated with many diseases and syndromes and may result from diverse sources of pathology. Another factor that has contributed to confusion concerns differential characteristics of pain (e.g. sensory characteristics, duration).

These different ways of classifying subtypes of pain are important because they illustrate the differential contributions of affective, cognitive, behavioural, as well as sensory factors. Pain induced in the laboratory is not likely to generate the same level of emotional arousal as is experienced by a patients with cancer. Patients with acute pain such as postsurgical pain can expect elimination of pain in a reasonably short timeframe whereas, in the case of patients with chronic back pain, time course is indefinite, if not forever. The impact of interpretations of the meaning of the pain, expectancies for the future will influence behavioural responses and in some instances has been shown to influence physiology associated with the transduction of sensory information that is interpreted as pain (e.g. Flor, Turk & Birbaumer, 1985) as well as biochemical neurotransmitters associated with modulation of pain (e.g. Bandura et al., 1987).

UNDERSTANDING PERSISTENT PAIN: ALTERNATIVE CONCEPTUALIZATIONS

In order to understand the basis for the current treatment of pain, it is useful to consider the most common currently held conceptualizations. These can be loosely grouped as dualistic sensory–psychogenic, motivational, operant conditioning, gate control, and multidimensional models.

The dualistic model

The traditional biomedical (sensory) conceptualization of pain dates back several hundred years and is based on a simple linear view that assumes a close correspondence between a biological state and symptom perception. From this perspective, the extent of pain severity is presumed to be directly proportionate to the amount of tissue damage. Thus, the greater the physical pathology, the greater should be the patient's report of pain.

There are several perplexing features of persistent pain complaints that do not fit within the biomedical model. A particular conundrum is that fact that pain may be reported even in the absence of identified physical pathology. For example, in up to 80% of the cases, the cause of back pain is unknown (Deyo, 1986) and, in the case of the majority of persistent headaches, there is no identifiable physical pathology. Moreover, the clinical significance of identifiable structural abnormalities has also been challenged. For example, several investigators have found that spinal radiographic abnormalities based on plain CAT scans (Wiesel et al., 1984) and Magnetic Resonance Imaging (MRI; Boden et al., 1990) believed to be associated with pain can be identified in a significant number of asymptomatic individuals.

As is frequently the case in medicine, when physical explanations prove inadequate to explain symptoms, psychological alternatives are entertained. If the pain reported is disproportionate to objectively determined physical pathology, or if the complaint is recalcitrant to 'appropriate' treatment, then it is assumed that psychological factors must be involved. Several variants of psychogenic aetiological models have been proposed. For example, a model of a 'pain-prone' personality (Engel, 1959) suggests that persistent pain complaints occur in individuals who are predisposed to experience pain because of family history or specific, long-standing personality characteristics. The American Psychiatric Association (1987) has created a psychiatric diagnosis, Somatoform Pain Disorder, that is based on the absence of specific physical pathology or other psychiatric disorders in the presence of reports of pain.

These psychogenic views are posed as alternatives to purely physiological models. If the patient's report of pain occurs in the absence of or is 'disproportionate' to objective physical pathology, ipso facto, the pain reports have a psychological basis.

Motivational view

A variation of the dichotomous somatogenic – psychogenic views is a conceptualization that is ascribed to by many third-party payers. They suggest that, if there is insufficient physical pathology to justify the report of pain, the complaint is invalid, the result of symptom exaggeration or outright malingering. The assumption is that reports of pain without objective physical evidence are motivated by financial gain. It has been suggested by Koplow (1990) that it is fear of malingering that drives the entire American Social Security Disability System.

Operant conditioning model

A conceptualization based on operant conditioning (Fordyce, 1976) has been proposed as an alternative to the more traditional causal biomedical and psychogenic views of pain describe above. The operant conditioning model stands in marked contrast to the biomedical model of pain described above. This model proposes that, when an individual is exposed to a stimulus that causes tissue damage, the immediate response is withdrawal and attempts to escape from noxious sensations. This may be accomplished by avoidance of activity believed to cause or exacerbate pain, help seeking to reduce symptoms, and so forth. These behaviours are observable and, consequently, subject to the principles of operant conditioning. The operant conditioning model focuses on overt manifestations of pain and suffering—'pain behaviours'—such as limping, moaning and avoiding activity and not the physical basis of pain. Emphasis is placed on the communicative function of these behaviours.

According to the operant conditioning model, positive reinforcement such as attention and by avoidance of undesirable or feared activities may serve to maintain the pain behaviours even in the absence of noxious sensory input. In this way, respondent behaviours that occur following an acute injury may be maintained by reinforcement after any tissue damage has resolved.

A particularly important feature of conditioning models of pain is pain avoidance. Fordyce, Shelton, and Dundore (1982) hypothesized that avoidance behaviour does not necessarily require intermittent sensory stimulation from the site of bodily damage, environmental reinforcement, or successful avoidance of aversive social activity to account for the maintenance of protective movements. They suggested that protective behaviours could be maintained by anticipation of aversive consequences based on prior learning since non-occurrence of pain is a powerful reinforcer. Fordyce et al. confirmed their hypotheses in a case study.

The operant principle of stimulus generalization is also important as patients may come to avoid more and more activities that they

[147]

believe are similar to those that previously produced pain. Reduction of activity leads to greater physical deconditioning, more activities eliciting pain and consequently even greater disability. Moreover, it is quite probable that the deconditioning resulting from reinforced inactivity can result directly in increased noxious sensory input. Muscles that were involved in the original injury generally heal rapidly but due to under-use of these muscle, they become weakened and subject to noxious stimulation when called into action.

Several studies have provided evidence that supports the underlying assumptions of the operant model (for review, see Keefe & Williams, 1989). The operant model has, however, received some criticism (e.g. Schmidt, Gierlings & Peters, 1989).

SEARCH FOR ALTERNATIVE CONCEPTUALIZATIONS OF CHRONIC PAIN
The inadequacies of the biomedical, psychogenic, operant, and motivational views have instigated attempts to reformulated thinking about the complex and subjective phenomenon – pain. It is important to make a distinction between nociception and pain.

Nociception is the activation of sensory transduction in nerves that convey information about tissue damage. This information is capable of being perceived as painful. Pain, because it involves conscious awareness, selective abstraction, appraisal, ascribed meaning, and learning is best viewed as a perceptual not purely sensory process. From this description, it should be apparent that there is no isomorphic association between nociception and pain. Rather, the extent of pain and suffering is associated with an interpretive process.

Focus on chronic pain
The greatest amount of work on the role of psychological factors has been directed toward patients with chronic pain. Thus, it is worth considering the large and growing category of pain.

For the individual experiencing chronic pain, there is a continuing quest for relief that often remains elusive and leads to feelings of demoralization, helplessness, hopelessness, and outright depression. The health-care provider shares these feelings of frustration as his or her patients' reports of pain continue despite the health-care provider's best efforts and, at times, in the absence of pathology, that is sufficient to account for the pain reported. On a societal level, pain creates a major burden in lost productivity and disability benefits. Third-party payers are confronted with escalating medical costs, disability payments, and frustration when patients remain disabled despite extensive treatment and rehabilitation efforts. In short, pain is a major health problem in society that affects millions of people and costs billions of dollars in health care and lost productivity, in addiction to the incalculable human suffering.

In short, chronic pain is a demoralizing situation that confronts the individual, not only with the stress created by pain but with a cascade of ongoing stressors that compromise all aspects of the life of the sufferer. Living with chronic pain requires considerable emotional resilience and tends to deplete one's emotional reserve, and taxes not only the individual but also the capacity of significant others who provide support.

A multidimensional model of chronic pain
The variability of patient responses to nociceptive stimuli and treatment is somewhat more understandable when we consider that pain is a personal experience influenced by attention, meaning of the situation, and prior learning history, as well as physical pathology. Biomedical factors, in the majority of cases, appear to instigate the initial report of pain. Overtime, however, psychosocial and behaviour factors may serve to maintain and exacerbate levels of pain, influence adjustment and disability. Following from this view, pain that persists over time should not be viewed as either solely physical or psychological, but rather the experience of pain is maintained by an interdependent set of biomedical, psychosocial, and behavioural factors. The range of interacting factors that affect an individual with chronic pain suggest that the phenomenon is quite complex and requires a broader perspective than those discussed above.

Gate control model
Melzack and his colleagues (Melzack & Casey, 1968; Melzack & Wall, 1965) proposed the gate control theory of pain emphasizing the modulation of pain by peripheral as well as by central nervous system processes. This model provides a physiological basis for the role of psychological factors in chronic pain. Melzack and Casey (1968) differentiate three systems related to the processing of nociceptive stimulation: motivational – affective, cognitive – evaluative, and sensory – discriminative, all thought to contribute to the subjective experience of pain.

Although the physiological details of the gate control model have been challenged (e.g. Nathan, 1976), it has had a substantial impact on basic research and in generating a wide range of treatment modalities. The gate control model was developed as a static, cross-sectional model, consequently it has not incorporated the role of reinforcement and learning factors that are especially salient if one takes a more dynamic, longitudinal view of pain.

Cognitive – behavioural perspective
Although both the operant and gate control models depart significantly from the sensory – physiological models, each has a somewhat limited view and is inadequate in explaining the experience of chronic pain. The operant model fails to consider the role of the patient's appraisal of pain. The gate control model fails to take into consideration the interactions of environmental influences, physical factors, and pain perceptions and responses over time.

From the cognitive – behavioural perspective, people with chronic pain are viewed as active processors of information. They have negative expectations about their own ability and responsibility to exert any control over their pain. Moreover, they often view themselves as helpless. Such negative, maladaptive appraisals about their condition, situation, and their personal efficacy in controlling their pain and problems associated with pain serve to reinforce their experience of demoralization, inactivity, and the over-reaction to nociceptive stimulation. Such cognitive appraisals are posed as having an effect on behaviour, leading to reduced effort, reduced perseverance in the face of difficulty and activity, and increased psychological distress (Bandura, 1977).

The cognitive – behavioural perspective suggests that behaviour, emotions, and in some cases physiology are influenced by interpretations of events, rather than solely by physiological factors and characteristics of events *per se*. According to this model, it is patients' perspectives, based on their idiosyncratic attitudes, beliefs, and unique schema, that filter and interact reciprocally with emotional factors, sensory phenomenon, and behavioural responses.

[148]

Moreover, patients' behaviours elicit responses from significant others that can reinforce both adaptive and maladaptive modes of thinking, feeling, and behaving.

For chronic pain sufferers, certain ways of thinking and coping are believed to influence the perception of nociception, the distress associated with it, or factors that may increase nociception directly. As an illustration, pain that is interpreted as signifying on-going tissue damage or life-threatening illness is likely to produce considerably more suffering and behavioural dysfunction than pain which is viewed as being the result of a minor injury, although the amount of nociceptive input in the two cases may be equivalent. Flor *et al.* (1985) found that, when discussing pain or stress, back pain patients had significantly elevated muscle tension in their back, but not in their forehead or forearm. However, when these back pain patients were resting and not discussing pain or stress, their back muscle tension level was no higher than the non-back pain, pain patients or healthy individuals. Conversely, neither non-back pain, pain patients nor healthy individuals showed elevations in the EMG tension activity of specific back muscles when discussing severe stresses.

The studies reviewed in the preceding paragraph focused on the effects of thoughts on the autonomic nervous system. Cognitive factors have also been shown to have influence biochemical factors associated with pain. For example, Bandura *et al.* (1987) have demonstrated that the efficacy of cognitive coping strategies in studies of laboratory-induced pain can be attenuated by injection of a chemical agent (naloxone) that is known to block receptors for endogenous opiates (enkephalins and endorphins).

O'Leary *et al*, (1988) provided cognitive – behavioural stress management treatment to rheumatoid arthritis (RA) patients. RA is a disease that may result from impaired functioning of the suppressor T-cell system. Degree of self-efficacy (expectations about the ability to control pain and disability) enhancement was correlated with treatment effectiveness. Those with higher self-efficacy and greater self-efficacy enhancement displayed greater numbers of suppressor T-cells and reduced joint impairment. Thus, it appears that psychological factors can directly influence the musculoskeletal system, and neurotransmitter receptor access as well as the production of hormones believed to be associated with pain.

Chronic pain sufferers can develop ways of thinking and coping that in the short term seem adaptive, but in the long term serve to maintain the chronic pain condition and result in greater disability. As noted, because the fear of pain is aversive, the anticipation of pain is a strong motivator for avoidance of situations or behaviours that are expected to produce nociception. Moreover, the belief that pain signals harm further reinforces avoidance of activities believed to cause pain and increase physical damage. Through the process of stimulus or situational generalization, more and more activities are avoided in order to prevent exacerbation of pain. The undesirable results of this avoidance is greater physical deconditioning and increased disability.

Inactivity may also lead to preoccupation with the body and pain and these cognitive – attentional changes increase the likelihood of amplifying and distorting pain symptoms and perceiving oneself as being disabled. At the same time, the pain sufferer limits opportunities to identify activities that build flexibility, endurance, and strength without the risk of pain or injury. Moreover, distorted movements and postures used to avoid pain can cause further pain

unrelated to the initial injury. For example, when an individual limps, he or she protects muscles on one side of the back but may stress the muscles on the other side of the back, and this protective action (e.g. limping) may produce a new painful condition. Thus, avoidance of activity, although it is a seemingly rational way to manage a pain problem, can actually play a large role in increasing and facilitating nociception, the chronic pain condition, and disability, when maintained for extended periods.

Chronic pain sufferers often develop negative expectations about their own ability to exert any control over their pain. These negative expectations lead to feelings of frustration and demoralization when 'uncontrollable' pain interferes with participation in recreational, occupational, and social activities. Pain sufferers frequently terminate efforts to develop new strategies to manage pain and, instead, turn to passive coping strategies such as inactivity, self-medication, or alcohol to reduce emotional distress and pain. They also absolve themselves of personal responsibility for managing their pain and instead rely on family and health care providers. These strategies may have detrimental consequences.

Recent studies have supported the cognitive – behavioural model and demonstrated the important role of cognitive distortions, coping strategies, and self-efficacy in the experience of pain (Turk & Rudy, 1992). For example, Reesor and Craig (1988) showed that the primary difference between chronic low back pain patients who were referred because of the presence of many 'medically incongruent' signs (not consistent with physical pathology identified) and those who did not display these signs was maladaptive thoughts.

The cognitive activity of chronic pain patients may contribute to the exacerbation, attenuation, or maintenance of pain, pain behaviour affective distress, and dysfunctional adjustment to chronic pain (Turk & Rudy, in press, 1992). If psychological factors can influence pain in a maladaptive manner, they can also have a positive effect. Individuals who feel that they have a number of successful methods for coping with pain may suffer less than those who feel helpless and hopeless. Some of the psychological interventions commonly used in the treatment of chronic pain have been shown to be effective in helping people with persistent pain either to eliminate their pain or, if pain cannot be eliminated, to reduce their pain, distress, and suffering. These studies have demonstrated that how patients think about their pain may be important mediating mechanisms associated with improvement (Tota-Faucette *et al.*, 1993). Moreover, it has been demonstrated that patients' interpretations of their ability to control pain may be more closely associated with improvement than either the extent of physical pathology or changes in actual behaviour (Jensen, Turner & Romano, 1994).

From the cognitive – behavioural perspective, chronic pain is viewed not as the result of passive transmission of nervous impulses but as a dynamic interpretive process. Chronic pain sufferers tend to develop maladaptive psychological and behavioural responses to their plight. Assessment of the patient with persistent pain requires a comprehensive strategy that looks at psychological (e.g. current mood, beliefs, appraisals, expectancies), sociocultural, and behavioural factors along with pathophysiology (Turk & Rudy, 1994).

Summary and concluding comments

In summary, the unidimensional models of pain that focus on only one aspect of pain, whether it be sensory, affective, or behavioural, seem inadequate to explain such a complex phenomenon. More recent attempts to integrate the range of medical – physical, psychosocial, and behavioural within a broad multidimensional framework have been proposed, and a body of research appears to support the appropriateness of this conceptual model, at least in chronic pain. The application of the comprehensive model has received much less attention in other areas, despite the research demonstrating the moderating and modulating influences of cognitive, affective, and operant conditioning factors. Research is needed to extend the multidimensional model to these areas as to examine treatments that target not only the sensory component of the pain experience.

Patients all come to treatment with diverse sets of attitudes, beliefs and expectancies. What the research reviewed suggests is the importance of addressing these subjective factors, as they are likely to influence how patients present themselves and respond to treatments offered. Viewing all patients with the same medical diagnosis as similar is likely to prove unsatisfactory. It would seem prudent to (a) attempt to identify pain patients' idiosyncratic beliefs, (b) identify the environmental contingencies of reinforcement, (c) address those beliefs and environmental relationships that are maladaptive, and (c) to match treatment interventions both to physical characteristics of the diagnosis but also to relevant psychosocial and behavioural ones (Turk, 1990). (See also 'Coping with chronic pain'.)

REFERENCES

American Psychiatric Association (1987). *Diagnostic and statistical manual*, 3rd edn. Washington, DC: American Psychiatric Association.

Bandura, A. (1977). Self-efficacy: toward a unifying theory of behavior change. *Psychological Review*, **84**, 191–215.

Bandura, A., O'Leary, A., Taylor, C.B., Gauthier, J. & Gossard, D. (1987). Perceived self-efficacy and pain control: opioid and nonopioid mechanisms. *Journal of Personality and Social Psychology*, **53**, 563–71.

Boden, S.D., Davis, D.O., Dina, T.S., Patronas, N.J. & Wiesel, S.W. (1990). Abnormal magnetic-resonance scans of the lumbar spine in asymptomatic subjects. *Journal of Bone and Joint Surgery*, **72-A**, 403–8.

Deyo, R.A. (1986). The early diagnostic evaluation of patients with low back pain. *Journal of General Internal Medicine*, **1**, 328–38.

Engel, G.L. (1959). 'Psychogenic' pain and the pain-prone patient. *American Journal of Medicine*, **26**, 899–918.

Flor, H., Turk, D.C. & Birbaumer, N. (1985). Assessment of stress-related psychophysiological responses in chronic pain patients. *Journal of Consulting and Clinical Psychology*, **35**, 354–64.

Fordyce, W.E. (1976). *Behavioral methods for chronic pain and illness*. St Louis: C.V. Mosby.

Fordyce, W.E., Shelton, J. & Dundore, D. (1982). The modification of avoidance learning pain behaviors. *Journal of Behavioral Medicine*, **4**, 405–14.

Jensen, M.P., Turner, J.A. & Romano, J.M. (1994). Correlates of improvement in multidisciplinary treatment of chronic pain. *Journal of Consulting and Clinical Psychology*, **62**, 172–9.

Keefe, F.J. & Williams, D.A. (1989). New directions in pain assessment and treatment. *Clinical Psychology Review*, **9**, 549–68.

Koplow, D.A. (1990). Legal issues. Paper presented at the annual scientific session of the American Academy of Disability Evaluating Physicians, Las Vegas, Nevada.

Melzack, R. & Casey, K.L. (1968). Sensory, motivational and central control determinants of pain: a new conceptual model. In D. Kenshalo (Ed.). *The skin senses*, pp. 423–443. Springfield, IL: Thomas.

Melzack, R. & Wall, P.D. (1965). Pain mechanisms: a new theory. *Science*, **50**, 971–9.

Nathan, P.W. (1976). The gate control theory of pain: a critical review. *Brain*, **99**, 123–58.

O'Leary, A., Shoor, S., Lorig, K. & Holman, H.R. (1988). A cognitive-behavioral treatment for rheumatoid arthritis. *Health Psychology*, **7**, 527–44.

Reesor, K.A. & Craig, K. (1988). Medically incongruent chronic pain: physical limitations, suffering and ineffective coping. *Pain*, **32**, 35–45.

Schmidt, A.J.M., Gierlings, R.E.H. & Peters, M.L. (1989). Environment and interoceptive influences on chronic low back pain behavior. *Pain*, **38**, 137–43.

Tota-Faucette, M.E., Gil, K.M., Williams, D.A., Keefe F.J. & Goli, V. (1993). Predictors of response to pain management treatment. The role of family environment and changes in cognitive processes. *Clinical Journal of Pain*, **9**, 115–23.

Turk, D.C. (1990). Customizing treatment for chronic pain patients: who, what and why? *Clinical Journal of Pain*, **6**, 255–70.

Turk, D.C. & Rudy, T.E. (1992). Cognitive factors and persistent pain: a glimpse into Pandora's box. *Cognitive Therapy and Research*, **16**, 99–122.

Turk, D.C. & Rudy, T.E. (1994). An integrated approach to pain treatment: beyond the scalpel and syringe. In C.D. Tollison (Ed.). *Handbook of chronic pain management*. pp. 136–154. 2nd edn. Baltimore, MD: Williams & Wilkins.

Wiesel, S.W., Tsourmas, N., Feffer, H. *et al.* (1984). A study of computer-assisted tomography. 1. The incidence of positive CAT scans in an asymptomatic group of patients. *Spine*, **9**, 549–51.

Perceived control and health behaviour

KENNETH A. WALLSTON

School of Nursing, Vanderbilt University,
Nashville, Tennessee, USA

Health behaviours are those activities engaged in by people who are basically healthy that have an impact upon their health status (Kasl & Cobb, 1966). Included in this classification are such activities as: seeking information about health-related matters; going to the doctor, clinic, or dentist for check-ups, prophylaxis, or immunizations; engaging in exercise and good nutritional practices; wearing seat belts; practising 'safe sex'; periodic self-examinations of breasts or testes; and moderate use of alcohol. Also under the rubric of health behaviours are those activities that place one's health at risk, such as: smoking cigarettes; misusing drugs; drinking to excess; and sharing needles. Kasl and Cobb (1966) distinguish health behaviours from illness behaviours (e.g. seeking a diagnosis) and sick-role behaviours (e.g. adhering to a medical regimen once diagnosed).

By definition, then, both 'positive' and 'negative' health behaviours affect health status. Psychologists study behaviour. Health psychologists, therefore, are particularly interested in isolating the factors which might affect health behaviours, not only so they might better understand the processes involved, but also so that they might change the behaviours in order to optimize health status.

Among the many factors that have been associated with whether or not a person engages in some form of health behaviour is the person's perception of control. Perception of control means the subjective determination of the ability to determine or influence something. In this context, the 'something' refers either to the behaviour itself or to the consequences of the behaviour. Take, for example, the health behaviour of going to the doctor for an annual physical examination. Perceived control, in this example, can refer to the person's belief that he or she can choose whether or not to go to the doctor, when to go to the doctor, and, even, which doctor to go to, or it can refer to the person's belief that he or she can improve or maintain his or her health status by going to the doctor for a check-up. In either case, from a theoretical standpoint, the more a person perceives control in this situation (either over the behaviour or its consequences), the more likely the person is to engage in the behaviour in question all other things being equal.

Most of the research that has been done examining the linkage between perceived control and health behaviour has been based on some form of social learning theory. Two of the major social learning theorists, Julian Rotter and Albert Bandura, have each contributed key psychological constructs to the literature relevant to perceived control. These two constructs, locus of control and self-efficacy, have dominated the research literature.

Rotter's social learning theory (Rotter, 1954; 1982; Rotter, Chance, & Phares, 1972) states that, in any given situation, the likelihood that a person will engage in a particular behaviour (or set of behaviours) is a function of two things: the person's expectancy that the behaviour will lead to a particular outcome (or reinforcement) in that situation, and the value of the reinforcement to the person in that situation. Expectancies, however, are not always strictly situation-specific. Through a variety of learning experiences, individuals develop generalized expectancies that cut across situations.

Locus of control (Rotter, 1966) is one such generalized expectancy in Rotter's social learning theory. It refers to the person's belief as to whether control over valued reinforcements is internal or external to the person. (Locus is the Latin word for 'place'.) A person with an internal locus of control orientation believes that reinforcements are a consequence of either some action (or set of actions) in which the person engages, or of some relatively enduring characteristic (or set of characteristics) of the actor. Typically, an internal locus of control orientation is equated with a perception of control over reinforcements. A person with an external locus of control orientation believes that reinforcements are the result of forces outside of the person, either the situation itself or the action(s) of other people. Also included under 'external' locus of control is the belief that reinforcements are only determined by fate, luck or chance. An external belief orientation is typically equated with a perception of lack of control over reinforcements.

Rotter (1966) conceived of locus of control as a unidimensional construct with internality at one end of a continuum and externality at the other. Rotter developed the I–E Scale (Rotter, 1966) to assess individual differences along this continuum. Because generalized expectancies, such as locus of control, are learned through experiences in a variety of situations, they are thought to be stable over time, at least in adults. Thus, a generalized locus of control belief orientation is often conceived of as a personality-like construct (Phares, 1976) and is mostly utilized in research as an independent or predictor variable. Scores on the I–E Scale are either treated as a continuous variable and are correlated with other continuous measures (such as the frequency of behaviours), or, more typically, persons at one end of the I–E continuum are classified as 'internals' and those at the other end are classified as 'externals'.

The early research linking internal-external expectancies and health-related behaviours was reviewed by Strickland (1978) and B.S. Wallston and K.A. Wallston (1978). As an example of this early research, MacDonald (1970) showed that, among single female college students nearly twice the percentage of 'internals' (62%) reported practising contraception than did 'externals' (37%). Similarly, Dabbs and Kirscht (1971) found that college students they termed 'internal' were more likely to be inoculated against influenza than those they termed 'external'.

The unidimensionality of the locus of control construct has not stood up either empirically or theoretically. Levenson (1973, 1981) posited that internality and externality were orthogonal to one another (i.e. statistically independent; uncorrelated) rather than being opposite ends of a continuum. Furthermore, Levenson felt that externality was itself multidimensional. She developed the I, P and C Scales as separate indicators of: (i) a generalized internal locus of control orientation; (ii) the belief that 'powerful other people' controlled important reinforcements; or (iii) chance externality. Because the I Scale was only slightly correlated with the P and/or C Scales, this multidimensionality allowed a person to be simultaneously internally and externally orientated. Long *et al.* (1988) administered the I, P and C Scales to a group of college students along with an assessment of lifestyles in four domains: work, social, health, and leisure. High and low groups were formed for each locus of control dimension by taking the top and bottom 20% of the distribution. The high internals, low powerful others and low chance groups obtained significantly higher work and health scores than did their counterparts.

Responding to Rotter's (1975) suggestion that measures of expectancy that were specific to a given domain (such as health) might account for more variance in domain-specific criterion measures, the Wallstons and their associates developed a series of health-related locus of control scales in an attempt to explain individual differences in health behaviours and health status. Following Rotter, the first such measure, the HLC Scale (Wallston *et al.*, 1976) was unidimensional. It was soon followed, however, by Forms A and B of the Multidimensional Health Locus of Control (MHLC) scales (Wallston, Wallston & DeVellis, 1978) which, like Levenson's I, P and C Scales, contained separate assessments of internality (IHLC), powerful others (PHLC) and chance (CHLC) externality. Lau and Ware (1981) developed similar scales. Health locus of control beliefs are not conceived of as being as stable as more generalized locus of control beliefs; because they can be modified by significant health-related experiences, they are less reflective of personality than are more generalized belief orientations.

In Rotter's social learning theory expectancies (such as locus of control beliefs) were not the sole determinants of 'behaviour potential'. Given equal theoretical weight (although largely ignored in the early research literature) was the construct of 'reinforcement value' (i.e. how important a particular reinforcement is to the individual in a particular situation). The Wallstons made a strong theoretical case for examining interactions of health locus of control beliefs and health value in predicting health behaviours (Wallston & Wallston, 1984; Wallston, 1991). Only for persons who valued health should perceptions of control over health be deterministic of behaviour.

Early research with the health locus of control scales, especially studies accounting for variations in health value (for reviews see Lau, 1988; Wallston & Wallston, 1981, 1982), consistently supported the theoretical proposition that, among persons for whom health was valued, high scores on IHLC (or 'selfcare' in Lau & Ware's terminology) or low scores on CHLC were correlated with various indices of health behaviours. For example, Lau (1988) administered the Lau and Ware Health Locus of Control Scale along with a measure of health values to entering freshmen students at Carnegie Mellon University. The women in the sample were asked how frequently they practised breast self-examination (BSE) both at baseline and again at the end of their junior year. For the women who did not value health highly, self-control beliefs were

uncorrelated with BSE practice, but, for those who did value health, there was a significant positive correlation between self-control beliefs and BSE. Scores on the PHLC scale (or 'provider control' in Lau & Ware's parlance) have been less reliably predictive of preventive health behaviours, although, theoretically, such beliefs should be more predictive of illness and sick-role behaviours than of health behaviours. In all of these studies, however, the amount of variance in health behaviours explained by the health locus of control scores has been typically very small, seldom exceeding 10% (Wallston, 1992), thus calling into question the clinical significance of this statistical association.

The construct of self-efficacy (Bandura, 1977, 1991; O'Leary, 1985; Schwarzer, 1992) has proven to be a much more potent predictor of health behaviours than has locus of control. Self-efficacy refers to a person's subjective estimation that he or she is capable of engaging in a particular action (or set of actions) in a particular situation (Bandura, 1977). It is similar to, but different from locus of control, because the latter refers to control over an outcome and self-efficacy refers to control over a behaviour (K. A. Wallston *et al.*, 1987). As borne out by numerous studies (see chapter on 'Coping with chronic illness' in this Handbook for a review), a person who is self-efficacious in regard to a particular behaviour is likely to engage in that behaviour. Self-efficacy, as originally conceived of by Bandura, is highly behaviour – and situation-specific. According to this viewpoint, perceiving control over the behaviour in a certain situation does not necessarily generalize to other behaviours or other situations.

Wallston (1992) modified Rotter's social learning theory, substituting self-efficacy for locus of control as the major generalized expectancy construct. Generalized self-efficacy (which is, perhaps, more appropriately referred to as 'mastery' or 'competence') is the belief that one is capable of doing whatever the situation requires in order to obtain valued reinforcements. This is a more global conceptualization of self-efficacy than Bandura originally had in mind, but measures based on this construct can be quite predictive of health behaviour. For example, Pender *et al.*, (1990) studied a sample of 589 employees enrolled in six employer-sponsored health promotion programmes and found that perceived personal competence was the single most robust predictor of their measure of health-promoting lifestyles.

In Wallston's (1992) modification of Rotter's theory, locus of control is considered a moderator variable (Baron & Kenny, 1986). Assuming health is a valued reinforcer, internality and self-efficacy interact to predict health behaviour. A person who is motivated by health but who does not believe that his or her health status is controlled by his or her health behaviour will not likely engage in health behaviour *even if he or she is capable of doing so*. In the case of both an internal locus and high health value, however, health behaviour is largely, but not entirely, influenced by one's perceptions of control over that behaviour (i.e. by self-efficacy beliefs). Ajzen's (1988) Theory of Planned Behaviour similarly incorporates behavioural control as a major determinant of intentions and behaviour, particularly in instances where the behaviour is not under the volitional control of the actor. In tests of the Theory of Planned Behaviour, perceived behavioral control is operationalized similar to measures of self-efficacy. Protection Motivation Theory (Rogers, 1975) was revised in 1983 by Maddux and Rogers to incorporate self-efficacy in the prediction of intentions and behaviour, and the Health Belief Model, which has a 30-year history of being applied to the prediction of health behaviours, was revised in 1988 to emphasize the critical role of self-efficacy (see Rosenstock, Strecher & Becker, 1988) despite the fact that a lack of *self-efficacy* could have always been construed as a 'barrier' to engaging in 'positive' health behaviours. Finally, Schwarzer's recent attempt at combining the best elements from the Health Belief Model, Protection Motivation Theory, and the Theory of Planned Behavior, which he termed the Health Action Process Approach (see Schwarzer, 1992), specifies self-efficacy as both a mediator of intentions and as a direct predictor of action during the volitional process phase of his model.

The antithesis of perceiving control is to feel helpless. Learned helplessness theory (Abramson, Seligman & Teasdale, 1978) states that, when a person comes to believe that his or her outcomes are not contingent on his or her behaviour, there are significant motivational, emotional and behavioural consequences. Feeling helpless is similar to feeling incompetent, non-self-efficacious, and to having a chance locus of control orientation. People who feel helpless either do not engage in 'positive' health behaviours or abandon those behaviours before they can have a 'positive' effect on health status. Because of the link with helplessness and depression (Seligman, 1975) and depression with 'negative' health behaviours such as substance abuse and attempted suicides (Attkisson & Zich, 1990; Wells *et al.*, 1989), there is even some reason to believe that the lack of perceived control can be life-threatening. Psychologists, however, can often successfully treat depression using such techniques as cognitive–behaviour therapy (Beck, 1973; Dryden & Golden, 1987; Kendall & Hollon, 1979). (See also 'Attributions and health', 'Lay beliefs about health and illness', 'The health belief model', 'Self-efficacy and health behaviour', 'Stress and disease', 'theory of Planned behaviour 'Behaviour change: transtheoretical model of', 'Life events and health', 'Noise effects on health'.)

REFERENCES

Abramson, L.Y., Seligman, M.E.P. & Teasdale, J.D. (1978). Learned helplessness in humans: critique and reformulation. *Journal of Abnormal Psychology*, 87, 49–74.

Ajzen, I. (1988). *Attitudes, personality, and behaviour.* Milton Keynes: Open University Press.

Attkisson, C.C. & Zich, J.M. (Eds.). (1990). *Depression in primary care: screening and detection.* London: Routledge.

Bandura, A. (1977). Self-efficacy: toward a unifying theory of behavior change. *Psychological Review*, 84, 191–215.

Bandura, A. (1991). Self-efficacy mechanism in physiological activation and health-promoting behavior. In J. Madden (Ed.). *Neurobiology of learning, emotion and affect*, pp. 229–270. New York: Raven Press.

Baron, R.M. & Kenny, D.A. (1986). The moderator–mediator variable distinction in social psychological research: conceptual, strategic, and statistical considerations. *Journal of Personality and Social Psychology*, 51, 1173–82.

Beck, A.T. (1973). *The diagnosis and management of depression.* Philadelphia: The University of Pennsylvania Press.

Dabbs, J.M. & Kirscht, J.P. (1971). Internal control and the taking of influenza shots. *Psychological Reports*, 28, 959–62.

Dryden, W., & Golden, W.L. (Eds.). (1987). *Cognitive-behavioural approaches to psychotherapy.* Washington, DC: Hemisphere.

Kasl, S.A. & Cobb, S. (1966). Health behavior, illness behavior, and sick role behavior: I. Health and illness behavior. *Archives of Environmental Health*, 12, 246–66.

Kendall, P.C. & Hollon, S.D. (1979). *Cognitive behavioral interventions: theory, research, and practice.* New York: Academic Press.

Lau, R.R. (1988). Beliefs about control and health behavior. In D.S. Gochman (Ed.). *Health behavior: emerging research perspectives* (pp. 43–63). New York: Plenum Press.

Lau, R.R. & Ware, J.E. (1981). Refinements in the measurement of health-specific locus of control beliefs. *Medical Care*, 19, 1147–58.

Levenson, H. (1973). Multidimensional locus of control in psychiatric patients. *Journal of Consulting and Clinical Psychology*, 41, 397–404.

Levenson, H. (1981). Differentiating among internality, powerful others, and chance. In H. Lefcourt (Ed.). *Research with the locus of control construct (Vol. 1).* New York: Academic Press.

Long, J.D., Williams, R.L., Gaynor, P. & Clark, D. (1988). Relationship of locus of control to lifestyle habits. *Journal of Clinical Psychology*, 44, 209–14.

MacDonald, A.P.Jr. (1970). Internal–external locus of control and the practice of birth control. *Psychological Reports*, 27, 206.

O'Leary, A. (1985). Self-efficacy and health. *Behavior Research Therapy*, 23, 437–51.

Pender, N.J., Walker, S.N., Sechrist, K.R. & Frank-Stromberg, M. (1990). Predicting health-promoting lifestyles in the workplace. *Nursing Research*, 39, 326–32.

Phares, E.J. (1976). *Locus of control in personality.* Morristown, NJ: General Learning Press.

Rogers, R.W. (1975). A protection motivation theory of fear appeals and attitude change. *Journal of Personality*, 91, 93–114.

Rosenstock, I.M., Strecher, V.J. & Becker, M.H. (1988). Social learning theory and the health belief model. *Health Education Quarterly*, 15, 175–83.

Rotter, J.B. (1954). *Social learning and clinical psychology.* Englewood Cliffs, NJ: Prentice-Hall.

Rotter, J.B. (1966). Generalized expectancies for internal versus external control of reinforcement. *Psychological Monographs*, 80 (whole No. 609, 1).

Rotter, J.B. (1975). Some problems and misconceptions related to the construct of internal vs. external control of reinforcement. *Journal of Consulting and Clinical Psychology*, 43, 56–67.

Rotter, J.B. (1982). *The development and applications of social learning theory: selected papers.* Brattleboro, VT: Praeger.

Rotter, J.B., Chance, J. & Phares, E.J. (1972). *Applications of a social learning theory of personality.* New York: Holt, Rhinehart & Winston.

Schwarzer, R. (1992). *Self-efficacy: thought control of action.* Washington, DC: Hemisphere.

Seligman, M.E.P. (1975). *Helplessness.* San Francisco, CA: Freeman.

Strickland, B.R. (1978). Internal–external expectancies and health related behaviors. *Journal of Consulting and Clinical Psychology*, 46, 1192–211.

Wallston, K.A. (1991). The importance of placing measures of health locus of control beliefs in a theoretical context. *Health Education Research, Theory and Practice*, 6, 251–2.

Wallston, K.A. (1992). Hocus-pocus, the focus isn't strictly on locus: Rotter's social learning theory modified for health. *Cognitive Therapy and Research*, 16, 183–99.

Wallston, B.S. & Wallston, K.A. (1978). Locus of control and health: a review of the literature. *Health Education Monographs*, 6, 107–17.

Wallston, B.S. & Wallston, K.A. (1981). Health locus of control. In H. Lefcourt (Ed.). *Research with the locus of control construct (Vol. 1).* New York: Academic Press.

Wallston, K.A. & Wallston, B.S. (1982). Who

is responsible for your health? The construct of health locus of control. In G. Sanders & J. Suls (Eds.). *Social psychology of health and illness*, pp. 65–95. Hillsdale, NJ: Erlbaum.

Wallston, B.S. & Wallston, K.A. (1984). Social psychological models of health behavior: an examination and integration. In A. Baum, S. Taylor & J.E. Singer (Eds.). *Handbook of psychology and health, Volume 4: Social aspects of health*, pp. 23–53 Hillsdale, NJ: Erlbaum.

Wallston, B.S., Wallston, K.A., Kaplan, G.D. & Maides, S.A. (1976). Development and validation of the health locus of control (HLC) scale. *Journal of Consulting and Clinical Psychology*, **44**, 580–5.

Wallston, K.A., Wallston, B.S. & DeVellis, R. (1978). Development of the multidimensional health locus of control (MHLC) scale. *Health Education Monographs*, **6**, 101–5.

Wallston, K.A., Wallston, B.S., Smith, S. & Dobbins, C. (1987). Perceived control and health. *Current Psychological Research and Reviews*, **6**, 5–25.

Wells, K.B., Stewart, A., Hays, R.D. Burnam, M.A., Rogers, W., Daniels, M., Berry, S., Greenfield, S. & Ware, J. (1989). The functioning and well-being of depressed patients: results from the Medical Outcomes Study. *Journal of the American Medical Association*, **262**, 914–9.

Physical activity and health

NEVILLE OWEN

School of Human Movement, Deakin University, Victoria, Australia

PHILIP VITA

University of Sydney, Australia

INTRODUCTION

The habit of regular physical activity is associated with a number of health benefits, particularly in relation to the prevention of cardiovascular disease. Psychological research has made some useful contributions to the understanding of physical activity as a pattern of behaviour, and has generated practical guidelines for how to encourage people to be more active. In this chapter, we present a selective commentary on research which examines the determinants of people's participation in physical activity, using examples likely to be of interest to medical practitioners, psychologists and allied health practitioners. These determinants include social and biological characteristics; past and present activity patterns; psychological characteristics; knowledge, attitudes and beliefs; and, environmental characteristics. We also describe a theoretical model of the stages that are involved in taking up and maintaining physical activity habits, and present some brief, practical exercise-counselling guidelines which may be used by health practitioners to help patients become more active.

The past 20 years have seen a marked increase in the contribution of psychological research, which aims to understand participation in physical activity. This trend has been driven by the accumulating body of evidence that regular physical activity results in a number of health benefits, particularly reduced risk of cardiovascular disease; there is now good evidence that regularly taking part in moderate-level physical activities (for example, recreational walking or cycling) can have significant health-protective benefits (Blair *et al*, 1992).

There has been considerable interest in understanding and promoting higher levels of involvement in physical activity in industrialised countries, particularly in North America and Australia. Research on physical activity has been directed towards a number of different levels of analysis within the overall discipline of psychology, ranging from psychophysiology through to population studies and social marketing (Dishman, 1988; Lee & Owen, 1986).

The behavioural epidemiology of physical activity and inactivity

At its most basic level, the epidemiological study of physical activity is concerned with the identification of those patterns of activity and inactivity which may be causally linked to disease. One step removed from this relationship between behaviour and disease is the epidemiological study of physical activity as a behaviour in itself, the study of who is active, who is inactive, why they are inactive, and how we might help them become more active. The focus is on the distribution and determinants of physical activity and inactivity and not on the disease outcomes which may be influenced by these behaviours (Owen & Bauman, 1992). Soundly based psychological perspectives on the determinants of physical activity as a lifestyle behaviour can be used not only to guide initiatives which health practitioners might take to help individual patients to be more physically active, but also to influence the development of large-scale interventions and public policy (Booth *et al.* 1993; Owen & Lee, 1989).

Stephens (1987) concluded that, in the mid-1980s, there was probably a lower proportion of inactive persons in the North American population, compared to a decade earlier, largely due to an increase in activity by women and older people. This finding is consistent with more recent Australian surveys (Bauman, Owen & Rushworth, 1990; Owen & Bauman, 1992). These Australian surveys indicate that, despite a slight increase in those people reporting that they took part in vigorous physical activities, and a significant decline in the proportion who reported being totally sedentary (33% to 25%), only between 10% and 20% of the Australian population engaged in regular vigorous physical activity. While these apparent trends may seem to be encouraging for those involved in physical activity promotion they do not diminish the need to understand the determinants of participation, so that the characteristics of inactive groups may be identified, and appropriate services and public policies may be developed.

THE DETERMINANTS OF PHYSICAL ACTIVITY

Research has identified a number of characteristics related to physical activity involvement, although much of it has been concerned with participants in quite formal exercise programmes. Here, we present a selective commentary of some of the relevant studies. We use the term 'determinant', as it is often used elsewhere in the literature, to denote a reliable association or predictive relationship, not necessarily causation (Owen & Bauman, 1992).

Demographic and biological characteristics

Some personal characteristics have consistently been found in studies of supervised activities and in general population studies. These findings indicate that women tend to be less vigorously active than are men, the better educated are more likely to exercise, and that activity decreases with advancing age (Bauman & Owen, 1992), although women are more likely than are men to adopt and maintain moderate activity routines such as walking (Sallis, *et al*, 1986). Such variations in exercise habits as a function of sociodemiographic characteristics provide useful background against which psychological factors may be interpreted.

Past and present activity patterns

In supervised programmes where activity can be directly observed, past participation in the programme is the most reliable correlate of current participation (Oldridge, 1984). The rate of participation typically drops sharply within the initial three to six months, and then declines very gradually (Oldridge, 1984). Individuals who are still active after six months are likely to remain active a year later for both supervised and free-living activity (Sallis et al., 1986). North American population studies have found that about two-thirds of adults with a history of participation in two or more sports in their youth were physically active. Moreover, they were almost three times more likely to be performing vigorous activities than people who had not participated in sports in their youth. While exercise or sport experience in youth may be an influence on exercise behaviour in adults, its influence may be overriden by other personal and environmental factors (Dishman, 1988).

Psychological characteristics

Self-motivation is a generalized tendency to persist in the absence of extrinsic reinforcement and to be largely independent of situational influence (Dishman, 1988). It is likely to be socially learned through the observation of others and through the influences of opportunities and reinforcement, and also to be dependent upon the individual's ability at self-reinforcement. Successful endurance athletes have consistently scored high on self-motivation, and self-motivation has discriminated between adherents and dropouts across a variety of settings, including athletic conditioning, adult fitness, cardiac rehabilitation and corporate fitness programmes. An interaction between self-motivation and biological traits in influencing exercise adherence has been found in several studies. Compared to drop-outs, adherers tend to be leaner, lighter and more self-motivated. Dishman (1990) has suggested that the lack of specificity for self-motivation in predicting drop-out from physical activity supports the idea that psychological traits probably interact with aspects of the physical activity setting to determine behaviour.

Programmes with strong social support, or reinforcement in settings requiring low-frequency, low-intensity activity, may negate differences in self-motivation. A role for personal motivational traits as determinants of physical activity is supported by early findings that those who exhibit Type. A behaviour were early dropouts from cardiac rehabilitation (see Dishman, 1988). Perceived self-efficacy, or confidence in one's ability to exercise, has predicted future activity (Sallis *et al.*, 1986). Self-efficacy has been found to differentiate between employees who intended to exercise and those who had maintained regular vigorous exercise (Marcus & Owen, 1992). Self-perceived mood disturbance has been found to relate to early dropout from adult fitness and cardiac rehabilitation programmes (see Dishman, 1988).

Knowledge, attitudes and beliefs

Knowledge of health and exercise has been associated with regular activity of moderate intensity in a population-based study, but did not predict participation in vigorous activity (Sallis *et al.*, 1986). There is evidence that those who strongly value exercise, who believe they have control over the outcome in their lives, and who expect personal health benefits from exercise are more likely to engage in physical activity (Dishman, 1988). However, it is difficult to determine the role of these factors from studies of those who enter supervised programmes, because they all may have quite positive attitudes and beliefs about exercise, high self-perceptions of exercise ability, and feelings of responsibility for maintaining their own health.

Environmental characteristics

Environmental factors may contribute to, or hinder, the adoption of physical activity both in community and clinical programmes. However, due to the fact that environmental barriers have usually been assessed by self-reported perceptions of participants and non-participants, the objectivity, validity, and reliability of these barriers are difficult to verify scientifically. Consequently, the degree to which the true origin of the determinant resides in the person or the environment has not been determined. The findings of several independent researchers show a similar pattern of answers.

The most common reason identified for either not adopting exercise, or for dropping out of programmes is lack of time (Owen & Bauman, 1992). Both perceived convenience of the exercise setting and actual geographical proximity to home or place of employment are consistent predictors of entry and continued participation in programmes (Dishman, 1988). Reasons people give for not maintaining exercise may be biased by social demand characteristics and by the relative salience of social and environmental cues (Lee & Owen, 1986). Dishman (1988, 1990) has argued that investigating the effects of the physical and social environment on activity habits may not contribute significantly to the understanding of exercise patterns, since considerations such as time, money, and convenience are not relevant to those who have not made the decision to exercise, while active people are already attuned to the environmental barriers.

Stages in the adoption and maintenance of exercise habits

The Prochaska and DiClemente transtheoretical model of behaviour change (see Marcus & Owen, 1992, for an application of this model to physical activity), identifies a precontemplation stage, in which change is not being considered; a contemplation stage, in which change is being considered; a preparation stage; an action stage;

maintenance of change; and, relapse (in which a person may return to one of the earlier stages). This model has been used to identify correlates of different stages in a population study of the adoption of physical activity (Booth *et al.*, 1993). The transtheoretical model is a promising conceptual development, with practical applications to the development of interventions for a number of the behaviours central to heart-disease prevention, and particularly to exercise promotion (see Donovan & Owen, 1994).

People probably progress through these stages at varying rates and they may leave and re-enter the behaviour–change continuum at varying points. As a consequence, taking up and maintaining physical activity may be better seen as a cyclical rather than as a linear sequence. It seems that many are unable to effect lasting changes with their first attempt. It is also likely that individuals revert to preintervention behaviour before they embark on subsequent attempts to move through the stages to successful maintenance.

Recent exercise programme results indicate that 50% of programme volunteers have experienced previous failures (Dishman, 1988). Given that various stages appear to be involved in the acquisition of physical activity habits, it follows that characteristics associated with the adoption of exercise may not be the same as those that relate to the successful maintenance of behaviour change (Lee & Owen, 1986). Separate processes probably are operating during the adoption phase and maintenance phase of physical activity. Marcus & Owen (1992) examined the relationship of self-efficacy and aspects of a decisional-balance model with different stages of exercise adoption and maintenance. Self-efficacy, or confidence, reliably differentiated between the different stages. Furthermore, the pattern of results indicated a significant trend of increased self-efficacy as subjects classified themselves through the behaviour–change sequence from precontemplation to maintenance. These results serve to support the notion that different psychological processes may be involved in the different stages of the adoption and maintenance of exercise habits.

APPROACHES TO EXERCISE COUNSELLING AND BEHAVIOURAL CHANGE

There are some patient counselling and more general behaviour–change principles (see Meichenbaum & Turk, 1987; Owen & Lee, 1989; Russell, 1986) which, if kept in mind, can be helpful in guiding exercise counselling. Often, patients or clients fail to make changes or to maintain them because of forces in their own lives or work settings, or because the advice they have received, or the goals they have set, are not realistic.

Help patients to set realistic physical activity goals
First steps towards a change in any health-related behaviour must be achievable. Some small amounts of regular exercise or some modest amounts of weight loss are better than none, and simple increases in incidental exercise such as walking up stairs each day can be beneficial. Help patients to choose long-term goals for exercise, but also help them to find things to do that will allow them to succeed initially.

Be specific in the advice you give
The more specific a message or advice can be about the type, the duration, the intensity and the context of physical activity, the greater its likelihood of success. Patients are more likely to respond to options for specific actions than to exhortations to do something in general.

Provide choice and variety
If people feel they have chosen a course of action for themselves, they are more likely to persist with it than if they feel it has been forced upon them. It is important there be an appropriate range of physical activity options made clear to patients, but that they not be presented with a confusing array of ideas and choices.

Encourage patient initiatives and independence
Conveying the most appropriate knowledge and fostering the skills, which patients might need to develop in order to take initiatives to change, will increase their chances of continuing with those changes. People should not become dependent on a very specific programme, or on only one type of exercise; they should be helped to learn about a variety of physical activity options, and to do things for themselves.

Help the patient to focus on the intrinsic value of exercise
Physical activities which are interesting because they provide enjoyment, skill development, competition, feedback on ability, and variety, or which offer opportunities for socializing, are more likely to encourage people to take up exercise and to maintain it than are dull and routine activities.

Be aware of patient's stage of readiness to exercise
Changes in behaviour often proceed through developing relevant awareness and knowledge, then motivation to change, adoption of new behaviour, and maintenance of change. Different approaches are needed to influence the different stages of change.

Consider the appropriateness and the convenience of exercise settings that are available to patients
The less travelling time, expenditure, and disruption of other activities required, the more likely that a person will enter a programme or continue with an activity. Settings for physical activity need to be readily available and pleasant. Help patients to identify what will be most appropriate and convenient for them.

CONCLUSIONS

In this overview chapter, it has only been possible to comment briefly and to give a few examples from the extensive body of psychological research on the determinants of exercise participation. The brief set of practical guidelines on ways to involve patients in healthier levels of physical activity indicate approaches which are likely to be helpful, and to show where there is more information relevant to physical activity counselling and behavioural change. Helping patients (and whole communities) to become more physically active is integral to clinical and population approaches to disease prevention and health promotion, and also to some important areas of disease treatment. Health researchers and practitioners need to be aware of the potential benefits to patients and communities of being more physically active, and should strive to maintain a well-informed perspective on this important health-related behaviour. (See also 'The health belief model', 'Health-related behaviours: common factors'.)

REFERENCES

Bauman, A., Owen, N. & Rushworth, R.L. (1990). Recent trends and socio-demographic determinants of exercise participation in Australia. *Community Health Studies*, **14**, 19–26.

Blair, S.N., Kohl, H.W., Gordon, N.F. & Paffenbarger, R.S. (1992). How much physical activity is good for health? *Annual Review of Public Health*, **12**, 99–126.

Booth, M., Macaskill, P., Owen, N., Oldenburg, B., Marcus, B. & Bauman, A. (1993). The descriptive epidemiology of stages of change in physical activity. *Health Education Quarterly*, **20**, 431–40.

Dishman, R.K. (1988). *Exercise adherence: its impact on public health.* Champaign, IL.: Human Kinetics Books (2nd ed. 1994).

Dishman, R.K. (1990). Determinants of participation in physical activity. In C. Bouchard, R. Shephard, T. Stephens, J.R. Sutton, & McPherson (Eds.). *Exercise, fitness, and health.* Champaign, IL: Human Kinetics Books.

Donovan, R.J. & Owen, N. (1994). Social marketing and mass interventions. In R.K. Dishman (Ed.). *Exercise adherence: its impact on public health* (2nd edn.). Champaign, Illinois: Human Kinetics.

Lee, C. & Owen, N. (1986). Exercise persistence: contributions of psychological theory to the promotion of regular physical activity. *Australian Psychologist*, **21**, 427–66.

Marcus, B.H. & Owen, N. (1992). Motivational readiness, self-efficacy and decision-making for exercise. *Journal of Applied Social Psychology*, **22**, 3–16.

Meichenbaum, D. & Turk D.C. (1987). *Facilitating treatment adherence: a practitioner's guidebook.* New York: Plenum Press.

Oldridge, N.B. (1984). Adherence to adult exercise fitness programs, In J.D. Matarazzo, S.M. Weiss, J.A. Herd, N.E. Miller & S.M. Weiss (Eds.). *Behavioural health: a handbook of health enhancement and disease prevention*, pp. 467–487. New York: Wiley.

Owen, N. & Lee, C. (1989). Development of behaviorally-based policy guidelines for the promotion of exercise. *Journal of Public Health Policy*, **10**, 43–61.

Owen, N. & Bauman, A. (1992). The descriptive epidemiology of physical inactivity in adult Australians. *International Journal of Epidemiology*, **21**, 305–10.

Russell, M.L. (1986). *Behavioural counselling in medicine.* New York: Oxford University Press.

Sallis, J.F., Haskell, W.L. Fortmann, S.P., Vranizan, K., Taylor, C.B. & Solomon, D.S. (1986). Predictors of adoption and maintenance of physical activity in a community sample. *Preventive Medicine*, **15**, 331–41.

Stephens, T. (1987). Secular trends in adult physical activity: exercise boom or bust? *Research Quarterly for Exercise and Sport*, **58**, 94–105.

Risk perception and health behaviour

BARUCH FISCHHOFF

Department of Engineering and Public Policy,
Department of Social and Decision Sciences,
Carnegie Mellon University, Pittsburgh, USA

INTRODUCTION

Health depends, in part, on deliberate decisions. Some of these decisions are private, such as whether to wear bicycle helmets and seatbelts, read and follow safety warnings, buy and use condoms, and fry or broil food. Other decisions involve societal issues, such as whether to protest the siting of hazardous waste incinerators and half-way houses, vote for fluoridation and 'green' candidates, and support sex education in the schools.

In some cases, single choices can have a large effect on health risks (e.g. buying a car with airbags, taking a dangerous job, getting pregnant). In other cases, the effects of individual choices are small, but can accumulate over multiple decisions (e.g. repeatedly ordering broccoli, wearing a seatbelt, or using the escort service in parking garages). In still other cases, choices intended to affect health risks do nothing at all or the opposite of what is expected (e.g. responding to baseless cancer scares, subscribing to quack treatments).

In order to make health decisions wisely, individuals need to understand the risks and benefits associated with alternative courses of action. They also need to understand the limits to their own knowledge and to the advice proffered by various experts. This chapter reviews the research base for systematically describing people's degree of understanding about health risk issues, as well as

for designing and evaluating messages to improve that understanding.

There are several issues that deserve full accounts of their own, including the roles of emotion, individual differences (personality), culture, and social processes in decisions about risk, which are not addressed in this chapter.

QUANTITATIVE ASSESSMENT

Estimating the size of risks

A common presenting symptom in experts' complaints about lay decision-making is that 'they do not realize how small (or large) the risk is'. Where that is the case, the mission of health communication is conceptually simple (if technically challenging): transmit credible risk estimates (Kahneman, Slovic, & Tversky, 1982; Weinstein, 1987). Research suggests that lay estimates of risk are, indeed, subject to biases. Rather less evidence clearly implicates these biases in inappropriate risk decisions.

In one early study (Lichtenstein *et al.*, 1978), subjects judged the annual number of deaths in the US from each of 30 causes (e.g. botulism, tornados, motor vehicle accidents), using one of two response modes. One task presented pairs of causes; subjects chose the more frequent, then estimated the ratio of frequencies. In the second task, subjects directly estimated the deaths tolls, after being told the answer for one cause (an anchor), in order to give an order-of-magnitude feeling for what numbers were appropriate. The study reached several seemingly robust conclusions.

(a) Estimates of relative frequency were quite consistent across response mode. Thus, subjects seemed to have a moderately well-articulated internal risk scale, which they could express even in unfamiliar response modes.

(b) Direct estimates were influenced by the anchor given. Subjects told that 50 000 people die annually from car accidents produced estimates which were two to five times higher than those produced by subjects told that 1000 die from electrocution. Thus, people seem to have less of a feel for absolute frequency, rendering them sensitive to the implicit cues in how questions are posed.

(c) Subjects' mean estimates showed less dispersion than did the statistical estimates. The overall trend was to overestimate small frequencies and underestimate large ones. However, the anchoring bias suggests that this pattern might have changed with different procedures, making the compression of lay estimates the more fundamental result.

(d) Some causes of death consistently received higher estimates than others of equal frequency. They tended to be causes that are disproportionately visible (e.g. homicide vs. asthma), suggesting a tendency to estimate frequency by the ease with which events are remembered or imagined, while failing to realize what a fallible index such availability is (Kahneman et al., 1982).

(e) In a subsequent study, subjects assessed the probability of having chosen the more frequent of the paired causes of death. They tended to be overconfident (e.g. choosing correctly only 75% of the time when they were 90% confident of having done so). This result is a special case of a general tendency to be inadequately sensitive to the extent of one's knowledge, which can produce both over and underconfidence (Yates, 1989).

One recurrent obstacle to assessing or improving lay people's estimates of risk is reliance on verbal expressions of quantitative risks such as 'very likely' or 'rare'. Such terms can mean different things to different people and even to the same person in different contexts (e.g. likely to be fatal vs. likely to rain) (Wallsten et al., 1986) sometimes even within communities of experts. The patterns in the 'causes of death' study could only be observed because it elicited quantitative estimates.

Evaluating the accuracy of lay estimates required credible statistical estimates, against which they can be compared. Performance might be different (poorer?) for risks whose magnitude is less certain than those in public health statistics. Furthermore, laypeople may (legitimately?) not see population risks as personally relevant.

One partial way to avoid these problems is asking subjects whether they are more or less at risk than others in (more or less) similar circumstances (Weinstein, 1987). People typically see themselves as facing less risk than average others (which could be true for only half a population). Several processes could account for such a

bias toward optimism, including both cognitive ones (e.g. the greater availability of the precautions that one takes) and motivational ones (e.g. wishful thinking). Such a bias could prompt unwanted risk-taking (e.g. because warnings seem more applicable to other people). Adults and adolescents have been found to respond similarly, despite the common belief that teens take risks, in part, because of a unique perception of invulnerability (Quadrel et al., 1993).

These studies measure health risk perceptions under the assumption that people define 'risk' as 'probability of death'. However, in scientific practice, 'risk' means different things for different analysts. For some, it is expected loss of life of expectancy; for others, it is expected probability of premature fatality (with the former definition placing a premium on deaths among the young). Some disagreements regarding the magnitude of risks reflect differing definitions of risk (National Research Council, 1989).

Investigators have examined the correlations between quantitative judgments of 'risk' and various subjective features (e.g. voluntariness of exposure, scientific uncertainty, controllability). Looking at the correlations among features (Slovic, 1987), they have found a remarkably robust picture, typically revealing two or three dimensions of risk, which are relatively similar across elicitation method, subject population (e.g. experts vs. laypeople), and risk domain. Core concepts in defining these dimensions include how well a risk seems to be understood and how much of a feeling of dread it evokes. The locations of individual hazards in this 'risk space' do vary with individual and group, in ways related to preferred risk management policies (e.g. how tightly a technology should be regulated). Relatively little is known about the role of these dimensions in individual risk decisions.

QUALITATIVE ASSESSMENT

Event definitions

Scientific estimates of the magnitude of a risk require detailed specification of the conditions under which it is to be observed. When investigators ask about the size of risks without providing these needed details, they make it very hard to provide sensible answers. In order to respond correctly, subjects must first guess the question, and then know the answer to it. Consider, for example, a survey asking, 'How likely do you think it is that a person will get the AIDS virus from sharing plates, forks, or glasses with someone who has AIDS?'. For responses to be meaningful, all subjects must spontaneously assign the same value to missing details such as what kind of sharing is intended (e.g. eating from the same bowl, using utensils that have been through a dishwasher) and how frequently it occurs. Then investigators must guess what subjects decided.

Aside from their methodological importance, the details that subjects infer can be substantively interesting. Quadrel (1990) asked adolescents to think aloud as they estimated the probability of several deliberately ambiguous events (e.g. getting into an accident after drinking and driving, getting AIDS through sex). Her subjects wanted to know the 'dose' involved with most risks (e.g. how much drinking, how much driving), when that was not provided. However, those subjects seldom asked about the amount of sex, either in a question about the risks of pregnancy or another question about the risks of HIV transmission. They seemed to believe that an individual either is or is not sensitive to the risk, regardless of the amount of the exposure. Indeed several reviews (e.g. Morrison, 1985) have concluded that between one-third and one-half of sexually active adolescents explain not using contraceptives with variants of, 'I thought I (or my partner) couldn't get pregnant'. Adults may not be that much better in estimating the rate at which risk accumulates through repeated exposure. One corollary of this bias is not realizing the extent to which seemingly small differences in single-exposure risks (e.g. contraceptive failure rates) can lead to large differences in cumulative risk.

Mental models of risk processes

These intuitive theories of how risks accumulate were a byproduct of research intended to improve the elicitation and communication of quantitative probabilities. Often, however, people are not poised to decide anything. Hence, they need no estimates. Rather, they just want to know what the risk is and how it works. The term 'mental model' is often applied to intuitive theories that are elaborated well enough to generate predictions in diverse circumstances. They have a long history in psychology (Gentner & Stevens, 1983).

If these mental models contain critical bugs, then they can lead to erroneous conclusions, even among people who are otherwise well informed. For example, not knowing that repeated sex increases the associated risks could undermine much other knowledge. Another study (Morgan et al., 1992) found that many people know that radon is a colourless, odourless, radioactive gas. Unfortunately, they also associate radioactivity with permanent contamination. However, this widely publicized property of high-level radioactive waste is not shared by radon. Not realizing that the relevant radon byproducts have short half-lives, homeowners might not even bother to test (believing that there was nothing that they could do, should a problem be detected). Leventhal and his colleagues (e.g. Leventhal & Cameron, 1987) have demonstrated how misunderstanding the physiology and phenomenology of maladies like hypertension can reduce compliance with treatment regimes.

In principle, the best way to detect such misconceptions would be to capture people's entire mental model on a topic. Doing so would also identify those accurate beliefs upon which education could build. One wants neither to induce nor to dispel misconceptions, either through leading questions or subtle hints. The interview should neither preclude the expression of unanticipated beliefs nor inadvertently steer subjects around topics. Morgan et al. (1992) describe one possible method.

CREATING COMMUNICATIONS

Selecting information

The first step in designing communications is to select the information that they should contain (Fischhoff, 1992). In many existing communications, this choice seems arbitrary, reflecting some expert or communicator's notion of 'what people ought to know'. Poorly chosen information can both waste recipients' time and be seen as wasting it. Recipients will be judged unduly harshly if they are uninterested in information that, to them, seems irrelevant.

One possible strategy for selecting information is to bridge the gap between mental models of a hazard held by laypeople and by experts. That could mean adding missing concepts, correcting mis-

takes, strengthening correct beliefs, and de-emphasizing peripheral ones.

A second possible strategy is to concentrate on critical 'bugs' in recipients' beliefs, cases where people confidently hold incorrect beliefs that could lead to inappropriate actions (or, where they lack enough confidence in correct beliefs to act on them).

A third possibility is providing those pieces of information having the largest possible impact on pending decisions. That requires formal modeling in order to determine the sensitivity of decisions to different information. For example, Merz (1991) applied value-of-information analysis to deciding whether to undergo carotid endarterectomy, a procedure which involves scraping out an artery leading to the head. He found that knowing about a few, but only a few, of the many possible side-effects would change the preferred decision for a significant portion of patients.

The choice among these approaches to selecting information would depend on, among other things, how much time is available for communication, how well the decisions are formulated, and what scientific risk information exists.

Formatting information

Once information has been selected, it must be presented in a comprehensible way. That means taking into account the terms that recipients use for understanding individual concepts and the mental models they use for integrating those concepts. It also means respecting the results of research into text comprehension, such as: (a) comprehension improves when text has a clear structure, (b) critical information is more likely to be remembered when it appears at the highest level of a clear hierarchy, and (c) readers benefit from 'adjunct aids', such as highlighting, advanced organizers (showing what to expect), and summaries (Kintsch, 1986).

Evaluating communications

Misdirected communications can prompt wrong decisions, create confusion, provoke conflict, and cause undue alarm or complacency. Indeed, poor communications can have greater public health impact than the risks that they attempt to describe. It may be no more acceptable to release an untested communication than an untested drug. Because communicators' intuitions about recipients' risk perceptions cannot be trusted, there is no substitute for empirical validation.

CONCLUSION

Communicating risks can be as complicated as assessing them. Research in this area is fortunate in being able to draw on well-developed literatures in such areas as cognitive, health, and social psychology, survey research, psycholinguistics, psychophysics, and behavioural decision theory. It is unfortunate in having to deal with unfamiliar topics, surrounded by unusual kinds of uncertainty, without stable vocabularies, and raising difficult threatening tradeoffs.

Health risk decisions are not just about cognitive processes. Emotions play a role, as do social processes. None the less, it is important to get the cognitive part right, lest people's ability to think through decisions be underestimated, underserved, and undermined. (See also 'The health belief model', 'Lay beliefs about health and illness', 'Medical decision-making'.)

REFERENCES

Fischhoff, B. (1992). Giving advice: decision theory perspectives on sexual assault. *American Psychologist*, **47**, 577–88.

Gentner, D. & Stevens, A.L. (Eds.). (1983). *Mental models*. Hillsdale, NJ: Erlbaum.

Kahneman, D., Slovic, P. & Tversky, A. (Eds.). (1982). *Judgement under uncertainty: heuristics and biases*. New York: Cambridge University Press.

Kintsch, W. (1986). Learning from text. *Cognition and Instruction*, **3**, 87–108.

Leventhal, H. & Cameron, L. (1987). Behavioral theories and the problem of compliance. *Patient Education and Counseling*, **10**, 117–38.

Lichtenstein, S., Slovic, P., Fischhoff, B., Layman, M. & Combs, B. (1978). Judged frequency of lethal events. *Journal*
of Experimental Psychology: Human Learning and Memory*, **4**, 551–78.

Merz, J.F. (1991). Toward a standard of disclosure for medical informed consent: development and demonstration of a decision–analytic methodology. PhD dissertation. Carnegie Mellon University.

Morgan, M.G., Fischhoff, B., Bostrom, A., Lave, L. & Atman, C.J. (1992). Communicating risk to the public. *Environmental Science and Technology*, **26**, 2048–56.

Morrison, D.M. (1985). Adolescent contraceptive behavior: a review. *Psychological Bulletin*, **98**, 538–68.

National Research Council (1989). *Improving risk communication*. Washington DC.

Quadrel, M.J. (1990). Elicitation of adolescents' risk perceptions: qualitative
and quantitative dimensions. PhD dissertation. Carnegie Mellon University.

Quadrel, M.J., Fischhoff, B. & Davis, W. (1993). Adolescent (in)vulnerability. *American Psychologist*, **48**, 102–16.

Slovic, P. (1987). Perceptions of risk. *Science*, **236**, 280–5.

Wallsten, T.S., Budescu, D.V., Rapoport, A., Zwick, R. & Forsyth, B. (1986). Measuring the vague meanings of probability terms. *Journal of Experimental Psychology*, **115**, 348–65.

Weinstein, N. (1987). *Taking care: understanding and encouraging self-protective behavior*. New York: Cambridge University Press.

Yates, J.F. (1989). *Judgment and decision making*. Englewood Cliffs, NJ: Prentice Hall.

Self-efficacy and health behaviour

ALBERT BANDURA

Department of Psychology, Stanford University, California, USA

People have always striven to exercise control over events that affect their lives and well-being. By exerting influence in spheres over which they command some control, they are better able to realize desired futures and to forestall undesired ones. People's level of motivation, affective states and behaviour are based more on what they believe than what is objectively the case. Hence, it is people's beliefs in their causative capabilities that is the major focus of interest.

Perceived self-efficacy refers to people's beliefs in their capabilities to organize and execute the courses of action required to deal with prospective situations. Such beliefs influence what courses of action people choose to pursue, how much effort they put forth in given endeavours, how long they will persevere in the face of obstacles and failure experiences, their resilience to adversity, whether their thought patterns are self-hindering or self-aiding, how much stress and depression they experience in coping with taxing environmental demands, and the level of accomplishments they realize (Bandura, 1992*a*, 1997).

Perceived self-efficacy operates as an important determinant of health promotive behaviour (Bandura, 1992*b*; Schwarzer, 1992). There are two levels at which a sense of personal efficacy plays an influential role in human health. At the more basic level, people's beliefs in their capability to cope with the stressors in their lives activate biological systems that mediate health and disease. The second level is concerned with the exercise of direct control over the modifiable behavioural aspects of health and the rate of ageing.

BIOLOGICAL EFFECTS OF EFFICACY BELIEFS IN COPING WITH STRESSORS

Many of the biological effects of beliefs of personal efficacy arise in the context of coping with stressors. Stress has been implicated as an important contributor to many physical dysfunctions (Krantz, Grunberg & Baum, 1985; O'Leary, 1990). Controllability is a key organizing principle regarding the nature of stress effects. It is not stressful life conditions *per se*, but the perceived inability to manage them that produces the detrimental biological effects (Bandura, 1992*b*; Maier, Laudenslager & Ryan, 1985; Shavit & Martin, 1987).

In social cognitive theory, stress reactions arise from perceived inefficacy to exercise control over aversive threats and taxing environmental demands (Bandura, 1986). If people believe they can deal effectively with potential environmental stressors, they are not perturbed by them. But, if they believe they cannot control aversive events, they distress themselves and impair their level of functioning. The causal impact of beliefs of controlling efficacy on biological stress reactions is clearly verified in experimental studies in which people are exposed to stressors under perceived inefficacy and after their beliefs of coping efficacy are raised to high levels through guided mastery experiences (Bandura, 1992*b*). Exposure to stressors without perceived efficacy to control them activates autonomic, catecholamine and endogenous opioid systems. After people's perceived coping efficacy is strengthened, they manage the same stressors without experiencing any distress, autonomic agitation or activation of stress-related hormones.

The types of biochemical reactions that accompany a weak sense of coping efficacy are involved in the regulation of the immune system. Hence, exposure to uncontrollable stressors tends to impair the function of the immune system in ways that can increase susceptibility to illness (Kiecolt-Glaser & Glaser, 1987; Maier *et al.* 1985; Shavit & Martin, 1987). Epidemiological and correlational studies indicate that lack of behavioural or perceived control over perturbing conditions increases susceptibility to bacterial and viral infections, contributes to the development of physical disorders and accelerates the rate of progression of disease (Schneiderman, McCabe & Baum, 1992).

Most human stress is activated in the course of learning how to exercise control over environmental demands and developing and expanding competencies. Stress activated in the process of acquiring coping efficacy may have very different physiological effects from stress experienced in aversive situations with no prospect of ever achieving any self-protective efficacy. Indeed, stress aroused while gaining coping mastery over threatening situations can enhance different components of the immune system (Bandura, 1992b). Providing people with the means for managing acute and chronic stressors increases immunological functioning. There are substantial evolutionary benefits to experiencing enhanced immunocompetence during development of coping capabilities vital for effective adaptation. It would not be evolutionarily advantageous if acute stressors invariably impaired immune function, because of their prevalence in everyday life. If this were the case, people would be bedridden most of the time with infections or they would quickly perish.

The field of health functioning has been heavily preoccupied with the physiologically debilitating effects of stressors. Self-efficacy theory also acknowledges the physiologically strengthening effects of mastery over stressors. A growing number of studies are providing empirical support for physiological toughening by successful coping (Dienstbier, 1989). The psychosocial modulation of health functioning is concerned with the determinants and mechanisms governing the physiologically toughening effects of coping with stressors as well as their debilitating effects.

SELF-EFFICACY IN HEALTH PROMOTIVE BEHAVIOUR

Lifestyle habits can enhance or impair health. This enables people to exert some behavioural control over their vitality and quality of health. Efficacy beliefs affect every phase of personal change: whether people even consider changing their health habits; whether they enlist the motivation and perseverance needed to succeed should they choose to do so; and how well they maintain the habit changes they have achieved (Bandura, 1992b). People's beliefs that they can motivate themselves and regulate their own behaviour play a crucial role in whether they even consider changing detrimental health habits. They see little point to even trying if they believe they do not have what it takes to succeed. If they make an attempt, they give up easily in the absence of quick results or setbacks.

Effective self-regulation of health behaviour is not achieved through an act of will. It requires development of self-regulatory skills. To build people's sense of efficacy, they must develop skills on how to influence their own motivation and behaviour. In such programmes, they learn how to monitor the behaviour they seek to change, how to set attainable subgoals to motivate and direct their efforts, and how to enlist incentives and social supports to sustain the effort needed to succeed (Bandura, 1986). Once equipped with skills and belief in their capabilities, people are better able to adopt behaviours that promote health, and to eliminate those that impair it.

Habit changes are of little consequence unless they endure. Maintenance of habit change relies heavily on self-regulatory capabilities and the functional value of the behaviour. Development of self-regulatory capabilities requires instilling a resilient sense of efficacy as well as imparting skills. Experiences in exercising control over troublesome situations serve as efficacy builders. This is an important aspect of self-management because, if people are not fully convinced of their personal efficacy, they rapidly abandon the skills they have been taught when they fail to get quick results or suffer reverses. Studies of health habits, that are amenable to change but difficult to maintain, show that a low sense of efficacy increases vulnerability to relapse (Bandura, 1992b; Marlatt, Baer & Quigley, 1995).

Health-care expenditures are soaring at a rapid rate. With people living longer and the need for health care services rising with age, societies are confronted with major challenges on how to keep people healthy throughout their lifespan, otherwise they will be swamped with burgeoning health costs. This requires intensifying health promotion efforts and restructuring health delivery systems to make them more productive. Efficacy-based models have been devised combining knowledge of self-regulation of health habits with computer-assisted implementation that provides effective health-promoting services in ways that are individualized, intensive and highly convenient (Bandura, 1992c). Self-management programmes based on the self-efficacy model improve the quality of health in cost-effective ways.

Chronic disease has become the dominant form of illness and the major cause of disability. The treatment of chronic disease must focus on self-management of physical conditions over time rather than on cure. This requires, among other things, pain amelioration, enhancement and maintenance of functioning with growing physical disability and development of self-regulative compensatory skills. Holman and Lorig (1992) have devised a prototypical model for the self-management of different types of chronic diseases that improves psychophysical functioning and greatly reduces utilizations of medical services. The more the self-management programme enhances patients' sense of efficacy to exercise control over their health functioning, the greater the health benefits they achieve.

The diverse lines of evidence taken as a whole indicate that the self-efficacy mechanism plays an influential role in mediating the impact of psychosocial factors both on biological systems that interrelatedly alter physical functioning and on health habits that impair or enhance the quality of health. Knowledge concerning the determinants of efficacy beliefs and the processes through which they exert their effects provide explicit guidelines on how to structure operative models for health promotion.

IMPACT OF PROGNOSTIC JUDGEMENTS ON EFFICACY BELIEFS AND HEALTH OUTCOMES

Much of the work in the health field is concerned with diagnosing maladies, forecasting the likely course of different physical disorders and prescribing remedies. Medical prognostic judgements involve probabilistic inferences from knowledge of varying quality and inclusiveness about the multiple factors governing the course of a given disorder. One important issue regarding medical prognosis concerns the range of determinants included in a prognostic model. Because psychosocial factors account for some of the variability in the course of health functioning, inclusion of self-efficacy determinants in prognostic models enhances their predictive power (Bandura, 1992c).

Prognostic judgements are not simply inert forecasts of a natural course of a disease. Prognostic expectations can affect patients' beliefs in their physical efficacy. Therefore, diagnosticians not only foretell but may partly influence the course of recovery from disease.

Prognostic expectations are conveyed to patients by attitude, word and the type and level of care provided them. People are more likely to be treated in enabling ways under positive than under negative expectations. Differential care that promotes in patients different levels of personal efficacy and skill in managing health-related behaviour can exert stronger impact on the trajectories of health functioning than simply conveying prognostic information. Prognostic judgements have a self-confirming potential. Expectations can alter patients' sense of efficacy and behaviour in ways that confirm the original expectations. The self-efficacy mechanism operates as one important mediator of self-confirming effects. (See also 'The health belief model', 'Perceived control and health behaviour'.)

REFERENCES

Bandura, A. (1986). *Social foundations of thought and action: a social cognitive theory.* Englewood Cliffs, NJ: Prentice-Hall.

Bandura, A. (1992a). Exercise of personal agency through the self-efficacy mechanism. In R. Schwarzer (Ed.). *Self-efficacy: thought control of action*, pp. 3–38. Washington, DC: Hemisphere.

Bandura, A. (1992b). Self-efficacy mechanism in psychobiologic functioning. In R. Schwarzer (Ed.). *Self-efficacy: thought control of action*, pp. 355–394. Washington, DC: Hemisphere.

Bandura, A. (1992c). Psychological aspects of prognostic judgments. In R.W. Evans, D.S. Baskin & F.M. Yatsu (Eds.). *Prognosis of neurological disorders*, pp. 13–28. New York: Oxford University Press.

Bandura, A. (1997). *Self-efficacy: the exercise of control.* New York: Freeman.

Dienstbier, R.A. (1989). Arousal and physiological toughness: Implications for mental and physical health. *Psychological Review*, 96, 84–100.

Holman, H. & Lorig, K. (1992). Perceived self-efficacy in self-management of chronic disease. In R. Schwarzer (Ed.). *Self-efficacy: thought control of action*, pp. 305–323. Washington, DC: Hemisphere.

Kiecolt-Glaser, J.K. & Glaser, R. (1987). Behavioral influences on immune function: evidence for the interplay between stress and health. In T. Field, P.M. McCabe & N. Schneiderman (Eds.). *Stress and coping across development*, Vol. 2, pp. 189–206. Hillsdale, NJ: Erlbaum.

Krantz, D.S., Grunberg, N.E. & Baum, A. (1985). Health psychology. *Annual Reviews in Psychology*, 36, 349–83.

Maier, S.F., Laudenslager, M.L. & Ryan, S.M. (1985). Stressor controllability, immune function, and endogenous opiates. In F.R. Brush & J.B. Overmier (Eds.). *Affect, conditioning, and cognition: essays on the determinants of behavior*, pp. 183–201. Hillsdale, NJ: Erlbaum.

Marlatt, G.A., Baer, J.S. & Quigley, L.A. (1995). Self-efficacy and addictive behavior. In A. Bandura (Ed.). *Self-efficacy in changing societies*, pp. 289–315. New York: Cambridge University Press.

O'Leary, A. (1990). Stress, emotion, and human immune function. *Psychological Bulletin*, 108, 363–82.

Schneiderman, N., McCabe, P.M. & Baum, A. (Eds.). (1992). *Stress and disease processes: perspectives in behavioral medicine.* Hillsdale, NJ: Erlbaum.

Schwarzer, R. (1992). Self-efficacy in the adoption and maintenance of health behaviors: theoretical approaches and a new model. In R. Schwarzer (Ed.). *Self-efficacy: thought control of action*, pp. 217–243. Washington, DC: Hemisphere.

Shavit, Y. & Martin, F.C. (1987). Opiates, stress, and immunity: animal studies. *Annals of Behavioral Medicine*, 9, 11–20.

Sexual behaviour

ALAN J. RILEY

Human Sexuality Unit, St George's Hospital Medical School, London, UK

Sexual behaviour can be defined broadly as behaviour aimed at inducing sexual arousal or enhancing sexual arousal progressively through the phases of the sexual response leading to resolution of the increasing sexual tension associated with sexual arousal. Thus an individual may indulge in a particular sexual behaviour to resolve his or her spontaneous sexual arousal. This could be considered an homeostatic process maintaining the body in a state of non-sexual arousal. On the other hand, an individual may indulge in a particular sexual behaviour to induce his or her sexual arousal *de novo*. An extension of self-orientated sexual behaviour to interpersonal beha-

viour is obviously necessary. Hence an individual may indulge in a behaviour that is aimed at inducing or increasing sexual arousal in another individual. This normally has a self rewarding motive in that its purpose frequently, though not exclusively, is to induce reciprocal sexual behaviour.

It is axiomatic that sexual behaviour is a prerequisite for sexual reproduction, but sexual behaviour serves other important roles. It is important for bonding relationships, and the pleasure and release of tension usually associated with either auto-sexual or interpersonal sexual behaviour is important for self-esteem and mental health.

The separation of these roles for sexual behaviour from the procreative role is not restricted to humans; many animals indulge in homosexual activities and masturbation even when a receptive female is available.

Sexual behaviour may be classified as proceptive where an individual seeks out sexual arousal or receptive where the individual accepts sexual behaviour directed at him or her by another individual. Human sexual behaviour is diverse and a product of many variables including personality, biological drive, hormonal status, learning, social conditioning and environmental and cultural circumstances. The person's internal perception of being male or female, so-called gender identity, also influences the pattern of sexual behaviour. There is evidence that factors, especially hormonal stimulation, occurring during foetal development can influence patterns of sexual behaviour in later life.

INDUCERS OF SEXUAL BEHAVIOUR

As with any behaviour, sexual behaviour has a drive or appetitive component. The most important change that has occurred during evolution is the increased influence of higher brain centres on sexual behaviour and the dissociation of behaviour patterns from direct hormonal control linked to optimizing reproduction. This is not to say that hormones do not play a role in human sexual behaviour; they do, but not to the same extent as in lower animals. For example, many female mammals will only indulge in copulatory behaviour during oestrus, the fertile phase of their ovarian cycle. In contrast, women may indulge in sexual behaviour throughout their menstrual cycles, and several studies have shown women to have highest levels of sexual activity during the pre- and postmenstrual phase stages of the menstrual cycle when fertility is lowest.

Complex central neural mechanisms control sexual behaviour. These mechanisms provide both stimulatory and inhibitory influences on sexual behaviour. The medial preoptic area of the hypothalamus appears to be important for stimulation of sexual behaviour, and has been described as the sex drive centre. However, other areas of the brain are also important in the generation of sexual drive, including the medial amygdala. Other areas of the brain are thought to have an inhibiting role on sexual behaviour. The paragigantocellular region of the brainstem reticular formation appears to be especially important in this respect.

Processes occurring in the brain can generate sexual drive, which may then induce sexual behaviour. Sexual drive is that process that induces perceptual changes that increase the chances of sexual behaviour. The sudden experience of sexual thoughts or fantasies, or the occurrence of spontaneous sexual arousal in the absence of sexual stimulation are prime examples of centrally generated sexual drive. However, sexual thoughts and fantasies can also be contrived consciously and may lead to sexual arousal. In addition, sexual drive can be triggered by stimuli received by the special senses. For example, it is not abnormal for men and women to become sexually aroused in response to such voyeuristic experiences as seeing sexually stimulating images or hearing sexually stimulating noises. Interpreting such images or noises as being sexually stimulating must depend on previous association between the generalized stimulus and sexual arousal. For example, a child with no experience of sexual intercourse would not become sexually aroused while watching (for example, on video) human sexual intercourse. Children can, however, become sexually aroused spontaneously or in response to genital stimulation.

Not all behaviour that appears sexual in nature is sexually driven. It is not unknown for a person to masturbate to relieve pain (endorphines are released during the sexual response) or to relieve non-sexual tension, and people indulge in sexual activity for material gain (e.g. prostitution). Hence sexual behaviour has a motivational element which works at two levels. First, we can be motivated to indulge in sexual behaviour without any prior sexual arousal or drive, and secondly the progression of sexual drive to sexual behaviour requires motivation to allow this to happen or indeed motivation not to let it happen. Such control of sexual behaviour requires there to be cognitive processing of the awareness of sexual arousal. If our aspiration is for sexual behaviour to progress, then being aware of early sexual arousal acts to reinforce the arousal process. On the contrary, if the aspiration is not to behave sexually, then awareness of early sexual arousal initiates inhibitory signals which turn off sexual arousal. This cognitive feedback is processed by the cerebral cortex and is effected through the limbic system. Disturbances in this cognitive feedback process can cause or contribute to sexual difficulties.

From a clinical perspective, it is often useful to distinguish between sexual drive and sexual desire although, at the present time, such distinction is rarely made in the literature where sexual drive, desire, interest, libido and appetite are all used synonymously. Sexual drive can be considered as a omnipotent inducer of sexual activity which can initiate all types of sexual behaviour, for example, masturbation, fantasy, interpersonal sexual activity. Sexual desire is a focused sexual drive. Thus a person may present with lack of desire for sexual activity with their partner and yet have strong sexual drive manifested by frequent masturbation or sexual activity with another partner. Many factors may be involved in the focusing of sexual drive into different sexual behaviours. Obviously, the non-availability of a willing partner normally precludes interpersonal sexual behaviour and in this situation sexual drive may proceed to masturbation unless there are particular cultural or religious reasons not to masturbate. Thus culture and religion can have strong influences on the pattern of sexual behaviour. These influences are learnt through the process of socialization which occurs during childhood and continues throughout adulthood.

Operant conditioning plays an important role in the development and continuation of human sexual behaviour. Orgasm may be seen as a reward or reinforcer. Hence a behaviour that induces it will be repeated and may replace other sexual behaviours that do not provide orgasmic release. However, although orgasm may be a primary reinforcer, other positive results of a particular sexual behaviour can also have a reinforcing role, even if orgasm does not occur. These may include social reinforces in the form of praise from the sexual partner or the conditioned reinforcer of feeling at one with one's partner during sexual activity. On the other hand, a behaviour that results in pain or punishment leads to avoidance of that particular behaviour. For example, the experience of pain during sexual intercourse, perhaps caused by lack of genital lubrication, may lead to infrequent sexual intercourse and eventual loss of sexual desire. However, recent research has shown that punishments are less effective than rewards in shaping behaviour. Thus a parent may reprimand a child caught masturbating but the child will continue to masturbate in a place where he is unlikely to be observed by the parent. Unfortunately, in this case, future masturbation may be associated with guilt which can have a negative influence on the child's developing sexuality and which may cause sexual difficulties in later life.

To some extent, sexual behaviour in humans is scripted in much the same way as is the precopulatory and copulatory behaviour of animals. Just as acting on the theatre stage usually follows a prewritten script, patterns of sexual behaviour follow scripts based on prior learning. Scripts tell us what to do, when and with whom to do it; in many ways they lay down an etiquette of sexual behaviour. For example, in a given culture, an accepted progression of heterosexual behaviour during courtship might be holding hands, kissing, touching body parts through clothes, touching breasts under clothes, manual genital stimulation, oro-genital stimulation and finally sexual intercourse. As there are cultural differences in patterns of acceptable sexual behaviour, sexual behaviour scripting is culturally determined.

NORMAL AND ABNORMAL SEXUAL BEHAVIOUR

Cross-cultural studies provide evidence of the vast variations in human sexual behaviour. The diversity of accepted sexual behaviour patterns between different cultures makes it impossible to define a repertoire of normal sexual behaviour. Although it may be easier to define abnormal sexual behaviour, even in this respect there are some surprising cultural differences. In western cultures, any sexual behaviour that causes unwanted physical or psychological trauma is considered abnormal. The number of people practising sadomasochistic behaviour associated with sexual activity is probably greater than is generally realized.

AUTOSEXUAL BEHAVIOUR

The most important conscious elements of autosexual behaviour are masturbation and sexual fantasies, while sexual daydreams are unconscious components of sexual behaviour. Masturbation is the stimulation of the genitalia with the purpose of inducing or enhancing sexual arousal and excitement. The practice is not restricted to humans; it occurs among many other species of mammals. Of all sexual activities, masturbation in the human has been the most widely discussed and condemned and yet most extensively practised. Because it has been so violently condemned and erroneously considered to cause adverse physical and psychological effects, many people, especially women, have high levels of guilt association with masturbation. Masturbation should be considered a normal activity and one which helps people realize their full sexual potential.

Masturbation usually begins in infancy. At about 15 to 19 months of age, both boy and girl infants explore their genitals and start to self-stimulate them experiencing the pleasure so induced. This behaviour is probably induced initially by the infant's natural instinct to explore his/her body and maintained by the pleasure derived from it. It is normal for children to continue touching their genitals, and the frequency and intensity of the practice increases during adolescence. With the increase in gonadal hormones that occurs during puberty, genital self-stimulation becomes sexually driven. Sexual fantasies may be used to enhance arousal during masturbation. Sexual fantasies are consciously orchestrated sexual thoughts, the content of which is always fantastic or unreal. In con-

trast, sexual daydreams, which also start to be experienced during adolescence, are sexual thoughts that occur spontaneously and whose content may be either fantastic or realistic. In a minority of people, orgasm can be induced solely by fantasy without any genital manipulation.

It is common for the adolescent to become interested in sexual and erotic imagery. They may use erotica such as sexy magazines or videos to enhance their sexual arousal whilst masturbating. This can be seen as the first step in their autosexual behaviour becoming interpersonal; they may use models in the pictures as imaginary partners for their sexual activity.

INTERPERSONAL SEXUAL BEHAVIOUR

Interpersonal sexual behaviour involves activities undertaken to attract and maintain a partner and, having achieved this, to induce sexual arousal in both partners so that sexual intercourse becomes possible. The process of maintaining a partner usually involves the development of 'love' and being 'in love'. The latter is a desire to maintain closeness to the partner and when this is achieved without conflict intimacy follows naturally. Important attributes of this state is the ability to be loved whilst loving one's partner, and a desire to encourage growth and happiness of the loved one. Sexual activity between the couple acts both to reinforce this state of love, the need each partner has of the other, and to act as a catalyst for further development of the relationship.

How individuals interact sexually depends to a great extent on their perception of the behavioural and attitudinal expectations for their gender. Traditionally, women have been passive and sexually non-demanding, whereas men are sexually active and assertive. There is now a trend towards women becoming more sexually assertive and, interestingly, this is having a positive effect on male sexual functioning.

Normal elements of interpersonal sexual behaviour include looking and listening to each other, touching, kissing and caressing, especially the erotic zones of the body. The behaviour progresses to manual and oral stimulation of the female breasts and nipples of both sexes, mutual stimulation of the genitalia (known inappropriately as mutual masturbation), and oro-genital contact. Oro-genital contact is known as fellatio or cunnilingus when the object is the penis or vulva, respectively. Although in heterosexual relationships the biological conclusion of interpersonal sexual behaviour is sexual intercourse, this is by no means a necessity nor is it desirable for every sexual advance to lead to sexual intercourse. Sexual relationships are known to flourish without penetrative sexual activity. It is not abnormal for people to fantasize during interpersonal sexual activities.

An important aspect of interpersonal sexual behaviour is sexual satisfaction. This has physiological and psychological components. Physiologically, sexual satisfaction depends essentially on the sensual aspects of the sexual interaction and relief of sexual tension that occurs with orgasm. In contrast, the psychological component of sexual satisfaction relies heavily on emotional interaction. There is a gender difference in importance of these two components; men place greater emphasis on the physiological component whilst, for women, the psychological component is more important. For women, sexual satisfaction relies very much on the qualities of the relationship in which the sexual behaviour occurs.

[164]

SEXUAL ORIENTATION

Whilst heterosexuality is essential for procreation, homosexuality can not nowadays be considered psychopathological. About 5% of adult men and women are exclusively homosexual throughout their lives, and probably about twice this number are predominantly homosexual for at least part of their lives. Over the years many theories have been postulated to explain the aetiology of homosexuality. Initially, these were based on psychological factors especially that homosexuality is a learned or conditioned condition. More recent focus has been on biological factors, particularly prenatal exposure to an abnormal hormonal milieu and altered brain structure. It is interesting that genetic studies reveal a higher incidence of homosexual concordance among monozygotic twins than among dizygotic twins, and that homosexual men have more brothers who are also homosexual than do heterosexual men. These observation may suggest a genetic predisposition. However, available data do not point to any single factor as the cause.

FURTHER READING

Bancroft, J. (1989). *Human sexuality and its problems.* 2nd edn. Edinburgh: Churchill Livingstone.

Cole, M. (1988). Normal and dysfunctional sexual behaviour: frequencies and incidences. In Cole, M. & Dryden, W. (Eds.). *Sex therapy in Britain.* Milton Keynes: Open University Press.

Marmor, J. (Ed.) *Homosexual behavior.* New York: Basic Books.

Sleep, circadian rhythms and health

MICHAEL HERBERT

Department of Behavioural Medicine
International Medical College, Kuala Lumpur,
Petaling Jaya,
Selangor, Malaysia

The emergence of Health Psychology as a discipline has done much to reorientate doctors towards behavioural aspects of the medical profession. Even so, it will be readily apparent to most practitioners that there is a reciprocity between human behaviour and biological functioning. This can be seen clearly in the study of sleep and in the various biological rhythms, which underlie our daily activities. Our lifestyles and psychological state exert influences on how well we sleep and conversely, the quality of our sleep can affect how well we function during the day. The same reciprocity exists between behaviour and the rhythmic fluctuations in our physiological and hormonal states. This chapter examines some of these relationships.

SLEEP

All animals, including humans, experience a state of periodic, voluntary loss of consciousness which is termed 'sleep'. On average, most people spend about 8 hours per day in this state so that, by the time we have reached age 60, most of us have spent approximately 20 years in relative oblivion. For this reason alone, sleep would seem to be important, although explanations as to why we do it remain in dispute (Shapiro & Flanigan, 1993). Sleep certainly does appear to be central to medical practice, since complaints about inadequate, unrefreshing or disturbed sleep are a frequent cause of people seeking help. The size of the problem is reflected in the fact that, according to one estimate, about one in ten nights' sleep in the United Kingdom is induced pharmacologically. The present discussion will focus on normal sleep and on some common problems people have with it.

Normal sleep

Psychophysiological studies of sleep are usually approached by recording the EEG from electrodes placed over the frontal and occipital cortex, from others placed alongside the eyes and yet others placed below the chin. The sleep of a healthy, young adult (18–25 years) displays a characteristic profile. Following conventional scales of sleep depth, determined by the frequency and amplitude of the EEG, there is a rapid 'descent' from the alpha pattern (12–14 Hz, low voltage) which is characteristic of relaxed wakefulness, to 'delta' activity (2–4 Hz, high voltage) normally associated with profound loss of consciousness. Approximately once every 90 minutes there is a remarkable change in the EEG which then displays evidence of strong activation, placing this kind of sleep close to wakefulness in physiological terms. This state is accompanied by bursts of rapid, jerky eye movements, increased brain temperature and blood flow, secretion of catecholamines, marked lability of blood pressure, heart rate, respiration rate, twitching of the extremities (fingers and toes) and a general loss of muscle tonus apart from in those needed to maintain life. This kind of sleep is the now well-known Rapid Eye Movement (REM) phase of sleep with which dreaming is associated. REM episodes become longer and more physiologically intense as the night progresses, and dreams correspondingly become more vivid.

Young adults spend around 25% of their sleep in REM and another quarter in delta-wave sleep, also known as slow wave sleep (SWS) or sometimes as 'deep' sleep. The remaining 50% is spent in a stage intermediate between these two. There are needs for REM and SWS demonstrated by the fact that deprivation of either one of them by deliberate, laboratory experimentation or by pharmacological and environmental demands, results in a 'rebound' phenomenon, whereby an attempt is made to regain the lost sleep when allowed to sleep naturally.

Psychosocial influences on sleep

Insomnia, defined as the chronic inability to obtain adequate sleep, is a major reason for people seeking medical help. Problems with insomnia fall into three major kinds. Since intense mental activity such as studying hard can delay the onset of sleep quite considerably in otherwise healthy people, it will be of little surprise that psychological factors which raise cortical arousal also have a similar effect. Sleep onset insomnia is often associated with elevated cortical activation linked with prolonged worry or anxiety and may require treatment by cognitive or other kinds of psychotherapeutic interventions.

Early morning awakening is a second kind of insomnia. There are few problems in falling asleep but thereafter there is an inability to maintain sleep beyond a few hours. When persistent, this is frequently a sign of severe clinical depression which may need appropriate referral.

Many people, especially in industrialized countries, are required to work at unusual hours of the day and night. Shift workers who regularly alternate their hours during which sleep can be taken frequently experience sleep maintenance insomnia. For such people, sleep is spasmodic. There are generally few difficulties in falling asleep initially, but the sleep which follows is, after a few hours, fragmented with frequent wakenings often for prolonged periods. The major reason lies in the conflict between the need to lower arousal levels to permit sleep and the biological rhythms underlying our daily functioning which are gearing us for normal waking activity. The problem may be exacerbated by increased noise and light levels during daytime hours.

Sleep complaints are particularly obvious among the elderly who wake more often and for longer periods during the night. This inability to maintain sleep may be a function of the reduced need for SWS which occurs in the elderly. There is a gradual reduction in the daily requirement for SWS from the 25% obtained by young people to around 2% in people between 60 and 70 years. A useful way to envisage the problems faced by the elderly is to regard the daily need for SWS as a 'weight' which 'pulls' people into sleep and keeps them asleep. Any reduction in this need makes falling and staying asleep harder. The ageing process seems to have this effect, which can be made worse by taking naps during the day. Daytime naps, which are hard to resist especially after retirement, may 'use up' much of the already diminished SWS need, thereby magnifying nocturnal sleep difficulties.

Many other factors can influence the sleep profile. These include medical illnesses particularly those which are painful, new sleeping environments, and noisy or hot bedrooms. It is therefore not surprising that complaints about sleep in hospital are frequent and are usually dealt with by the routine prescription of hypnotics. The trouble is that hypnotics can result in reduced REM sleep, leading to the rebound phenomenon after discharge home. The heightened physiological activation which normally accompanies REM is even more intense during such a rebound and may be potentially serious for people with cardiovascular problems.

Sleep Deprivation

For whatever reason, if people have insufficient sleep, they are in danger of experiencing the consequences of sleep loss. In cases of prolonged total sleep deprivation, hallucinations can occur, although there appear to be no serious long-term physiological complications. Shorter periods of total sleep loss are associated with lowered arousal levels during the following day which are manifested in periods of inability to maintain concentration interspersed between normal periods of normal functioning. The inability to sustain concentration is more evident during the morning hours than the late afternoon, probably because of increasing arousal levels as the day progresses. Sleep loss may also be accompanied by an increase in 'microsleeps' which are very brief periods when individuals seem incapable of registering input or focusing attention. Naturally, undertaking hazardous activities such as driving vehicles while in this state can be dangerous.

Most people do not regularly experience total sleep loss. More often we undergo partial sleep loss. For the average person who sleeps around 8 hours per night, cognitive functioning does not seem to be impaired until less than 2 hours' sleep have been achieved on any one night. However, if the sleeper is going to undergo a prolonged period of reduced sleep, then the evidence suggests that there is a minimum need for at least 6 hours per night.

Need for Sleep

Most laypeople assume that individuals need 8 hours sleep per night, and will often complain if this perceived need goes unmet. While it is true that the average need lies around 7.5 to 8 hours per day, there is variation around this mean. Some people need as much as 10 or 11 hours per day, while others need only around 3 hours or so. Inappropriate expectations may lead the naturally short sleeper to seek and become dependent on hypnotics. The naturally long sleeper on a ration of eight hours may end up in a chronically sleep-deprived state.

Sleep Hygiene

Some suggestions based on psychological grounds have been put forward to help people with sleep problems. Clearly, anxiety states precluding sleep onset can be dealt with by appropriate psychological therapy. For those who have difficulty falling asleep and for those who have difficulty in maintaining sleep, a useful suggestion is to avoid lying in bed for hours in a state of full alertness. An explanation based on Classical Conditioning would maintain that this simply serves to associate wakefulness with cues from the bedroom environment. It may be helpful if the sleeper were to move from the bedroom and carry out such things as household chores before trying again to sleep. For similar reasons, it has even been suggested that changing the bedroom decorations may function to break the association between environmental cues and wakefulness.

Relaxation by non-stimulating reading material or regular bedtime routines can also aid the rapid onset of sleep. In like fashion, maintaining regular hours of going to bed and arising have been shown to result in the most beneficial sleep resulting in maximum efficiency and subjective alertness the next day. The reasons for that will become apparent in the next section.

CIRCADIAN RHYTHMS

Underlying practically all human functioning are rhythmic fluctuations in biological variables (Waterhouse, 1993). In addition to circadian (24–hour) rhythms, there are supradian rhythms (longer than 24 hours) evident in the menstrual cycle, and infradian cycles (less than 24 hours) manifested in periodic fluctuations every 90 minutes. The 24–hour rhythms are clearly seen in body temperature, but are also evident in hormonal secretions such as in Growth Hormone.

These periodic fluctuations are also reflected in psychological functioning. Humans are at their least efficient maintaining concentration, and correspondingly more likely to make errors, in the early hours of the morning when arousal levels, as reflected in body temperature, are at their nadir. Maximum alertness tends to be in the late afternoon or early evening. However, there are suggestions that divisions of people into Morning and Evening types may have some validity.

In a now famous series of studies, Aschoff and his coworkers investigated a number of factors which exert influences on how the temporal regularity of our functioning is organized. By putting volunteers into environments from which all cues about time of day were excluded, they were able to demonstrate that the delicate balance of these rhythms are synchronised by various physical and social cues (Zeitgebers) such as sleep onset, light and social hints about real clock time. In the absence of such cues, humans start to 'free-run', whereby the normal temporal relationship between the various parameters becomes disjointed. Interestingly, Aschoff noted that in humans who had been free-running for some time, there were periods when the various bodily cycles naturally reunited. It was during these times that the volunteers reported that they felt well.

Perhaps one of the major negative influences on the temporal harmony of our various circadian rhythms is a behavioural one. People frequently are employed on some kind of shift work. According to one estimate, about 20% of the workforce is employed at unusual hours of the day. Shift work comes in many permutations of rotating and alternating patterns of working weeks or days. Only rarely does a worker sustain a regular sleep-wake pattern which does allow eventual adaptation to the new routine. The usual effect of shift work is to disrupt the temporal harmony of the various endogenous bodily rhythms, which then have corresponding adverse effects on sleep and health.

Shift workers have been reported to suffer from more gastrointestinal disorders than expected although this conclusion is complicated by the fact that people who cannot tolerate unusual working hours may self-select out of jobs which require disjointed working routines. Stomach disorders may be exacerbated because gastric juices are secreted at the wrong time and because only poor quality food is generally available during the night. Reports suggest that approximately 25% of shift workers have no breakfast and 11% have no lunch. Although the majority of shift work is probably done by men, women are obviously not immune from its adverse consequences. Female cabin crew on aircraft experience constant desynchrony of biological rhythms due to time zone changes and are therefore more prone to menstrual cycle irregularity.

Social problems also face shift workers. Because society is normally geared towards the light – dark cycle, there are potential difficulties in fulfilling parental and marital roles. The afternoon shift (from 2–10pm) tends to disrupt the parental role. The shift worker gets up late and so does not see the children in the morning before school. On arriving home at night, the children are usually in bed. There is no evening relaxation, play or mealtime discussions. The only available time is at weekends and this can be a cause of frustration and resentment within the family

The marital role tends to be most disrupted by having to work night shifts. Sexual relationships are obviously endangered by the husband and wife sleeping at different times and this may be reflected in the higher divorce rate amongst shift workers. However, this may be a chicken and egg situation because those choosing to do shift work maybe those who have pre-existing marital conflicts.

Human beings are biological, psychological and social creatures. A disruption in any one of these aspects of our functioning has repercussions in the others. It is therefore necessary for medical practitioners to take full account of all the influences being exerted on individuals in order to provide effective and efficient health care.

REFERENCES AND ADDITIONAL READING

Broughton, R.J. & Ogilvie, R.D. (Eds). (1992). *Sleep, arousal and performance.* Boston: Birkhauser.

Guilleminault, C. (1987). *Sleep and its disorders in children.* New York: Raven Press.

Horne, J. *Why we sleep.* (1989). Oxford: Oxford University Press.

Shapiro C.M. & Flanigan M.J. (1993). Function of sleep. *British Medical Journal* **306**, 383–5.

Waterhouse, J. (1993). Circadian rhythms. *British Medical Journal* **306**, 448–51.

The reader is also referred to a series of articles which appeared in the *British Medical Journal* in April–May 1993, Volume 306 under the general series title of 'ABC of sleep disorders'.

Social support and health

THOMAS ASHBY WILLS

Ferkauf Graduate School of Psychology and
Department of Epidemiology and Social Medicine,
Albert Einstein College of Medicine, Bronx, New
York, USA

This chapter considers evidence on social support as a protective factor. Epidemiological research indicates two conclusions in this area: (a) social support is related to a lower level of mortality among the general population, and (b) social support is related to better recovery from illness in clinical samples. Protective effects of social support have been replicated over studies and national populations and the effect of social support is comparable across causes of mortality, hence seems to function as a general resistance resource. The mechanism of these effects is still a topic of active investigation. The following sections discuss methods, findings, and theories in this area.

METHODS

In epidemiological studies, social support has been defined and measured in two different ways. One approach is to determine the number of social relationships in which the subject is a participant. This approach, derived from research on the structure of social networks, establishes variables such as whether the subject is married; has relatives in the vicinity; knows and visits neighbours; has friends with whom he/she regularly communicates; has children; is a member of a community organization (e.g. sports team, school board); or is a member of a church or other religious organization. The sum of these items provides a total score for social integration because it indexes the number of established social relationships in which the subject participates (e.g., Berkman & Syme, 1979). In this approach, information on the quality of the relationships is not acquired because the goal is to determine the total number of social connections and, by inference, the person's level of integration in the community.

A second approach administers scales determining the extent to which the subject perceives various supportive functions to be available from his/her social relationships. The supportive functions include emotional support, the availability of persons in whom one can confide and share feelings and problems; instrumental support, the availability of useful goods and services from other persons (e.g. money, transportation, assistance with house work or child care); informational support, the availability of useful information, advice, and guidance; and social companionship, the availability of persons with whom the subject can pursue recreational and cultural activities. The goal of these measures is to establish the extent to which a subject knows persons who would provide these kinds of resources if a need existed. A score for functional support provides an index of the perceived quality of the supportive function(s) available (e.g. Blazer, 1982). Emotional support has proved to be the function most broadly useful for coping with a range of life stressors, but independent effects for functions of instrumental and informational support have been demonstrated for contexts such as adolescent adjustment, postpartum depression, and problems of the elderly (Krause, 1987; Wills, 1991).

Epidemiological research methods have focused on prediction of mortality. In the typical prospective design, a representative sample of community residents or hospital patients is assessed at study outset with measures of social integration and/or functional support, together with measures of current health status and measures of other possible confounders such as socioeconomic status. The sample is followed over a reasonable time period (5–10 years in several studies) and morbidity or mortality status is determined for all traceable participants (> 95% of the initial sample in most studies). The relative risk of mortality over the follow-up interval is determined for subjects with high vs. low social integration or functional support, with statistical adjustment for factors such as age, gender, and socioeconomic status.

In this true prospective design, results are amenable to causal inferences about the effect of social support on health because the predictor measures are obtained prior in time to the disease outcome, and analyses can rule out confounding variables as explanations for the observed effect. It is particularly important to rule out the possibility that persons who are ill at study outset have lower levels of social support because of physical or emotional restriction; this process could also generate findings of an inverse relationship between initial social support (lower among diseased persons) and subsequent mortality (higher among diseased persons). This question can be resolved in analyses by controlling statistically for initial health status. This interpretation and other confounders have been ruled out in several prospective studies (see House, Landis & Umberson, 1988).

Two different models of action for social support have been tested. One model suggests support would be beneficial for persons irrespective of current stress level. The alternative model posits that social support will have the greatest effect for persons currently experiencing a high level of life stressors. This is termed the stress-buffering model because adequate support serves as a 'buffer' that protects a person from the otherwise adverse impact of stressful occurrences. Research designs comparing these models obtain a measure of life stress together with a measure of social support, and test whether support is differentially effective for persons with high vs. low stress. Research on physical and psychological morbidity has generally indicated stress-buffering effects for functional support measures (Cohen & Wills, 1985; Wills, 1991).

SOCIAL SUPPORT AND MORTALITY IN GENERAL POPULATIONS

Prospective studies with general-population samples have shown that persons with a higher level of social integration have a reduced risk of mortality, and the effect of social support is independent of factors such as gender and ethnicity. For example, Berkman and Syme (1979) studied a sample of 4725 community residents in the Western US, obtaining a score for social integration based on marital status, contacts with friends and relatives, church membership, and informal group membership. Over a 9-year follow-up, the relative risk of mortality for subjects with low vs. high social integration was 2.3 for men and 2.8 for women. This finding was replicated in a study of 2754 community residents in the Midwestern US, followed over a 9–12 year period (House, Robbins & Metzner, 1982), for whom relative risks were 2.0–4.0. House et al. (1982) measured initial health status through a direct medical examination that included electrocardiogram (ECG), blood pressure, and forced expiratory volume (FEV). The inverse relation between social support and mortality was shown not to be confounded with baseline health status, replicating a similar finding from Berkman and Syme (1979). The higher mortality for those with low social integration was comparably distributed across all causes (including cardiovascular disease, cancer, and infectious disease) and was not concentrated in any one disease category.

A prospective study with a sample of 331 persons > 65 years of age obtained measures of initial health status and a functional support measure indexing the availability of persons who were perceived as confidants, understood and cared about the respondent, and would help if the respondent were ill (Blazer, 1982). Relative risk of mortality over a 30-month follow-up period for persons with low vs. high support was 3.9, and this effect was shown to be independent of gender, ethnicity, economic resources, and baseline health status. Thus the protective effect of social support is not restricted to younger populations, and is not attributable simply to augmentation of economic resources.

In a prospective study of mortality in Gothenburg, Sweden by Rosengren et al. (1993) a sample of 756 men (all 50 years of age at baseline) completed a direct examination by a physician together with a measure of emotional support and a measure of stressful life events during the previous year. At a 7-year follow-up, results indicated social support was inversely related to mortality, with an effect size comparable to that for cigarette smoking, self-perceived health status, and life stress. Though the number of deaths in this study was relatively small (41 in total), a significant stress × support interaction suggested a stress-buffering process. Among men with low emotional support the relative risk for mortality attributable to life stress was 15.1 (95% confidence interval (CI) 3.5–64.9); among men with high support the relative risk was 1.2 (95% CI 0.4–3.8).

Effects of social support have been demonstrated across different national populations. An inverse relation between social integration and all-causes mortality has been demonstrated in predominantly rural areas in eastern Finland and the southeastern US, and in urban areas in Sweden and the western US (House et al., 1988). Similar findings have occurred in studies of Japanese-American immigrants, Israeli nationals, and other ethnic groups (Cohen & Syme, 1985), so the effect of social support on health has considerable generality.

Studies disagree on whether increased mortality occurs only among the very isolated, but several large prospective studies have shown a continuous gradient in mortality across levels of support (House et al., 1988); a conservative interpretation of the evidence assumes a dose–response relationship.

SOCIAL SUPPORT, MORBIDITY, AND RECOVERY FROM ILLNESS

Several studies have shown social support related to lower rates for a particular type of morbidity: pregnancy or delivery complications. Following from Sosa's original study in Guatemala, experimental studies have shown the presence of a supportive companion during labour related to lower rates of delivery complications. For example, a randomized trial by Kennell et al. (1991) assigned a sample of 616 women to a supported group or two comparison groups. Results indicated the supported group had shorter duration of labour, fewer cesarean sections for delivery, and fewer neonatal problems. An observational study by Collins et al. (1993) with a sample of 129 low-income women followed for six months showed that women with better quality support had better labour progress and their infants had higher Apgar scores; women with larger social networks had babies with higher birth weight.

Social support has been shown to be related to lower rates of mortality after onset of clinical illness in several studies. For example, Williams et al. (1992) studied an inception cohort of 1368 patients (82% male) with CAD. Patients were recruited through an angiography unit and enrolled in the study if found to have significant CAD (≥ 75% stenosis of at least one major artery). At study outset, patients completed a social support measure that included marital status and availability of a confidant. A medical risk score was composed from ten physical variables measured at intake, and empirically was a strong predictor of survival. Results from an average 9-year follow-up indicated that patients with low support, defined as unmarried and without a confidant, had a significantly lower survival rate (50%) compared with those having high support (82%). This effect of social support was found to be independent of medical risk and of economic resources.

Related findings have occurred in other studies of chronic illness. For example, Littlefield et al. (1990) studied a sample of 158 adults with IDDM. Patients completed a functional support measure together with measures of depression and of illness-related disability. Analyses indicated a buffering effect for social support: The relationship between disability and depression was reduced among patients with high support. A study of 194 elderly persons with myocardial infarction, followed for 6 months after the illness, showed that those with greater emotional support had a significantly lower rate of mortality (Berkman, Leo-Summers & Horwitz, 1992). Findings from other contexts on the relation of social support to compliance with medical regimens and adjustment to illness are discussed in other sources (Berkman, Vaccarino & Seeman, 1993; Cohen & Syme, 1985).

A randomized trial by Spiegel et al. (1989) was conducted with 86 patients who had metastatic breast cancer. Patients were assigned to participate in a 1-year support-group experience with other women who had breast cancer, or were assigned to a usual-care condition. Results indicated that women who participated in the support group had a significantly longer survival time. This provocative study has suggested an important new topic for research on social support effects among persons with advanced illness.

THEORIES OF EFFECT

While the relation between social support and health status has been consistently replicated, there is less direct evidence on mechanisms of this effect. Several different mechanisms have been suggested and are coherent with existing biological and psychological knowledge (see Cohen, 1988). It is possible that social support may act to avert the onset of disease, to reduce severity of disease, or to enhance recovery from illness; and effects may occur through physiological or behavioral mechanisms. The testing of these mechanisms is currently a topic of active investigation (Uchino, Cacioppo & Kiecolt-Glaser, 1996). Following is a conceptualization of generic mechanisms, which are not mutually exclusive and may be complementary.

Effect on Neuroendocrine Responses

The presence of persons perceived as supportive may have an effect for reducing sympathetic-nervous-system arousal through the hypothalamic–pituitary – adrenocortical (HPA) axis. The calming effect of a supportive companion may reduce anxiety and muscular tension in a fairly rapid manner. A linkage of catecholamines to risk for CAD and pregnancy complications also has a plausible biological basis.

Effect on Self-esteem

The perception by a patient that there are people who care about him/her and can be confided in about problems is related to increased self-esteem. This mechanism was suggested by Krause (1987) to account for the relation between support and reduced depression in the elderly. This type of emotional support may come from health professionals, from friends and family, or from other sources such as counsellors and ministers. The perception that a person is integrated in the larger community and accepted in a number of social roles may also have an impact on self-esteem, hence may be involved in the observed relation of social integration measures to health outcomes.

Effect on Depression

A number of studies have shown social support related to reduced levels of depression (Cohen & Wills, 1985). The role of social support for decreasing depression is thought to occur because the perception that support is available decreases the perceived severity of stressors, thus decreasing anxiety, and increases person's ability to cope with stressful situations (Wills & Cleary, 1996). Depressive affect states may relate to health outcomes through reducing immune-system function, increasing disability, or decreasing motivation to comply with medical regimens (Cohen, 1988; Uchino et al., 1996). Social integration may provide useful information about prevention and treatment resources in the community, and also provide advice and feedback about coping efforts (Wills, 1991).

Effect on Substance Use

Persons with high social integration and good emotional support show lower rates of smoking and alcohol abuse. Though epidemiological studies have found an effect of social support on mortality independent of health behaviours, they have also shown an inverse correlation between support and substance use, so this may represent part of the mechanism through which social support relates to health outcomes.

CONCLUSIONS

The research discussed in this chapter indicates that social support is a significant protective factor, related to lower rates of mortality and better recovery from illness. These findings have been demonstrated in a variety of national populations and in several types of medical patient groups. While a number of research questions are still being addressed, these findings have a plausible theoretical basis in both physiological and behavioural mechanisms. Interventions to enhance social support may have beneficial effects for patients with early illness or patients with advanced disease. (See also 'Family influences and health', 'Socioeconomic Status and health'.)

REFERENCES

Berkman, L.F., Leo-Summers, L. & Horwitz, R.I. (1992). Emotional support and survival after myocardial infarction: a prospective, population-based study of the elderly. *Annals of Internal Medicine*, **117**, 1003–9.

Berkman, L. & Syme, S.L. (1979). Social networks, host resistance, and mortality: a nine-year follow-up study of Alameda County residents. *American Journal of Epidemiology*, **109**, 186–204.

Berkman, L.F., Vaccarino, V. & Seeman, T. (1993). Gender differences in cardiovascular morbidity and mortality: the contribution of social networks and social support. *Annals of Behavioral Medicine*, **15**, 112–18.

Blazer, D.G. (1982). Social support and mortality in an elderly community population. *American Journal of Epidemiology*, **115**, 684–94.

Cohen, S. (1988). Psychosocial models of the role of social support in the etiology of physical disease. *Health Psychology*, **7**, 269–97.

Cohen, S. & Syme, S.L. (Eds.). (1985). *Social support and health*. Orlando, FL: Academic Press.

Cohen, S. & Wills, T.A. (1985). Stress, social support, and the buffering hypothesis. *Psychological Bulletin*, **98**, 310–57.

Collins, N.L., Dunkel-Schetter, C., Loebel, M. & Scrimshaw, S.C.M. (1993). Social support in pregnancy: correlates of birth outcomes and postpartum depression. *Journal of Personality and Social Psychology*, **65**, 1243–58.

House, J.S., Landis, K.R. & Umberson, D. (1988). Social relationships and health. *Science*, **241**, 540–5.

House, J.S., Robbins, C. & Metzner, H.L. (1982). The association of social relationships and activities with mortality. *American Journal of Epidemiology*, **116**, 123–40.

Kennell, J., Klaus, M., McGrath, S., Robertson, S. & Hinkley, C. (1991). Continuous emotional support during labor in a US hospital: a randomized controlled trial. *Journal of the American Medical Association*, **265**, 2197–201.

Krause, N. (1987). Life stress, social support, and self-esteem in elderly populations. *Psychology and Aging*, **2**, 349–56.

Littlefield, C.H., Rodin, G.M., Murray, M.A. & Craven, J.L. (1990). Influence of functional impairment and social support on depressive symptoms in persons with diabetes. *Health Psychology*, **9**, 737–49.

Rosengren, A., Orth-Gomer, K., Wedel, H. & Wilhelmsen, L. (1993). Stressful life events, social support, and mortality in men born in 1933. *British Medical Journal*, **307**, 1102–5.

Spiegel, D., Bloom, J., Kraemer, H. & Gottheil, E. (1989). Effect of psychosocial treatment on survival of patients with metastatic breast cancer. *Lancet*, ii, 888–91.

Uchino, B.N., Cacioppo, J.T. & Kiecolt-Glaser, J.K. (1996). The relationship between social support and physiological processes: a review with emphasis on underlying mechanisms and implications for health. *Psychological Bulletin*, **119**, 488–531.

Williams, R.B., Barefoot, J.C., Califf, R.M., Haney, T.L., Saunders, W.B., Pryor, D.B., Hlatky, M.A., Siegler, I.C. & Mark, D.B. (1992). Prognostic importance of social resources among patients with CAD. *Journal of the American Medical Association*, **267**, 520–4.

Wills, T.A. (1991). Social support and interpersonal relationships. In M.S. Clark (Ed.). *Review of personality and social psychology*, Vol. 12, pp. 265–289. Newbury Park, CA: Sage.

Wills, T.A. & Cleary, S.D. (1996). How are social support effects mediated: a test for parental support and adolescent substance use. *Journal of Personality and Social Psychology*, **71**, 937–52.

Socioeconomic status and health

DOUGLAS CARROLL
School of Sport and Exercise Sciences, University of Birmingham, UK

GEORGE DAVEY SMITH
Department of Social Medicine, University of Bristol, UK

PAUL BENNETT
Gwent Psychology Services, and Department of Psychology, University of Bristol, UK

In the fifteenth century, the city of Florence operated a *Monte delli doti*, a fund into which the relatively affluent fathers of female offspring could deposit dowry investments. Morrison, Kirshner and Molha (1977) compared the size of these investments with the subsequent ages at death of the women concerned. A gradient of decreasing mortality was seen from those accompanied by a dowry of 49 florins or less to those with dowries greater than 100 florins (Fig. 1). Early in the nineteenth century, the city of Glasgow established a number of splendid urban burial grounds to commemorate its worthy decedents. Davey Smith *et al.*, (1992a) recently measured the heights of the obelisks that commonly serve as monumental markers in these 'cities of the dead', on the reasonable presumption that, since form is standard, height would have determined cost and, accordingly, reflect the socioeconomic status of the decedents. Height of obelisk was then compared with age at death of the first generation of families commemorated; a reliable positive association emerged for both the men and women (Fig. 2).

Contemporary data confirm that health continues to vary markedly with socioeconomic status. Whether indexed by occupation-based classifications systems, such as the Registrar General's social class scheme (Townsend & Davidson, 1982), or by arguably more direct asset-based measures, such as income (Berkman & Breslow, 1983), housing tenure and car ownership (Whitehead, 1988), those in more favourable social and material circumstances enjoy substantially lower rates of premature mortality than those in less favourable circumstances. For example, analysis of the multiple risk factor intervention trial (MRFIT) screening sample of over 300 000 middle-aged American men (Davey Smith *et al.*, 1992b) reveals a continuous association between 12-year mortality and median income of area of residence at time of entry to the study (Fig. 3).

The relationship between socioeconomic status and mortality holds not only for all-cause mortality, but also for most of the major cause of death groupings. Various indices of morbidity display similar patterns of stratification (Blaxter, 1989; Marmot *et al.*, 1991), and health variations with socioeconomic locus appear to typify women much as they do men (Arber, 1989), as well as appearing to be characteristic of all western countries studied in this context.

The size and persistence of such health differentials, together with their robustness to the use of different measures of socioeconomic status and mortality, defy their dismissal as artefact. The available evidence also renders unlikely explanations in terms of health-related social selection, i.e. that those in poor health tend to move down the social scale, whereas those in good health move up (see, Blane, Davey Smith & Bartley, 1993; Carroll, Bennett & Davey Smith, 1993). There is, for example, a clear mismatch between the years during which social mobility is most common and those during which impaired health is prevalent, i.e. the years between labour market entry and early middle age are characterized by low mortality and morbidity, yet it is in these early years of working life that social mobility is most likely. More concrete evidence emerges from the Longitudinal Study (Goldblatt, 1988, 1989). Mortality differentials among those not changing social class group were similar to overall mortality differentials. Were social selection at work, we would have expected the differentials to be concentrated among those changing social class.

Evidence also suggests that the differential propensity of different social groups to engage in unhealthy behaviours, such as smoking, excessive alcohol consumption, and poor diet, affords only a partial explanation of health variations. Let us consider the case of smoking. Cigarette smoking clearly contributes to ill-health, and there is a differential prevalence of smoking among different social groups. However, inequalities in health remain even when differential smoking rates are taken into account. In the 10-year follow-up of the Whitehall I study, mortality was three times greater for men in the lowest, relative to those in the highest civil service employment grades. Importantly, the mortality differentials by employment grade and car ownership for those men who had never been smokers were much the same as those which characterized the whole sample

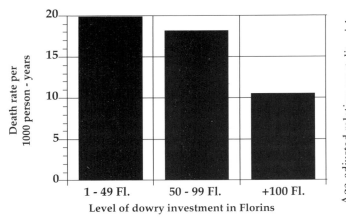

Fig. 1. Deaths per 1000 person–years for females receiving different levels of dowry investment as young girls (adapted from Morrison, Kirshner, and Molho, 1977).

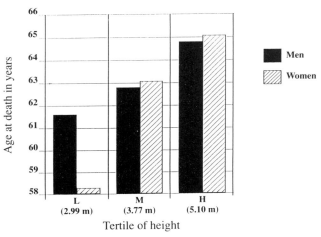

Fig. 2. Age of death according to height of obelisks (adapted from Davey Smith, Carroll, Rankin & Rowan, 1992).

Regression coefficient per metre of height = 1.42* for men *p <.005
2.19* for women

Regression coefficient per metre of height = 1.93* for men
adjusted for year of death 2.92* for women

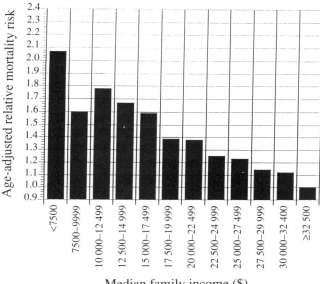

Fig. 3. Relative all-cause mortality risk by level of median family income for zipcode of residence for white men screened for MRFIT (adapted from Davey Smith, Neaton, Stamler & Wentworth, 1992).

(Davey Smith & Shipley, 1991). In addition, Davey Smith, Shipley & Rose (1990) reported large occupationally related mortality differentials for causes of death not regarded as smoking related. The socioeconomic gradient in coronary heart disease has received particular attention in this context. In the Whitehall I study (Marmot, Shipley & Rose, 1984), occupational status-related differentials in death rates from ischaemic heart disease persisted when variations in smoking, obesity, plasma cholesterol, and blood pressure were taken into account. Corroborative evidence emerges from a recent 17-year prospective study of coronary heart disease in Danish men (Hein, Suadicani & Gyntelberg, 1992). Adjusting for age, blood pressure, body mass index and alcohol consumption, men in the lowest social class registered an incidence 3.6 times that of men in the highest social class. Further more, while smoking, as has been observed consistently, was strongly associated with overall

ischaemic heart disease risk, additionally adjusting the incidence data for smoking habits left the relative risk with social class essentially unchanged at 3.5.

If socioeconomic health gradients are not, for the most part, attributable to variations in unhealthy behaviour, the major influences must reside in the broader social and material fabric of people's lives. While the persistent ecologies of those in different social loci vary in a number of ways, variations in exposure to physical pathogens undoubtedly play a part. For example, the health damaging effects of exposure to physicochemical hazards, primarily a feature of working class occupations, have long been recognized (Hunter, 1955). Low quality, damp accommodation has been found to be associated with poor health, particularly with higher prevalence rates for respiratory disease (Martin, Platt & Hunt, 1987; Platt, et al., 1989). The strikingly higher rates of mortality suffered by the inhabitants of Glasgow relative to those of Edinburgh are paralleled by, among other things, stark differences in winter air pollution levels. Concentrations of smoke and sulphur dioxide recorded in 1972–3 were almost twice as high in Glasgow (Watt & Ecob, 1992). While the material correlates of morbidity and mortality have received substantially less attention in recent years than the behavioural correlates, the available evidence suggests that material influences are likely to be substantial.

This could be taken as testimony that psychological factors are little involved in socioeconomic health variations. However, at least two considerations argue otherwise. First of all, the available data indicate that socioeconomic health gradients persist into the materially better-off social strata, i.e. health stratification is not simply a matter of the most immiserated in society suffering exceedingly poor health. It was, after all, the prosperous in fifteen century Florence who attracted dowry investment, and the relatively affluent of Glasgow who were interred in its 'cities of the dead'. Contemporary confirmation emerges from ecological research comparing mortality

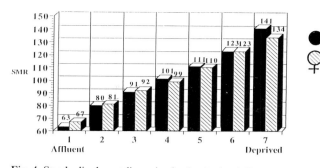

Fig. 4. Standardized mortality ratios for deprivation/affluence categories (ages 0–64). Deprivation scores based on: overcrowding, low social class, male unemployment, no car (adapted from Carstairs & Morris, 1991).

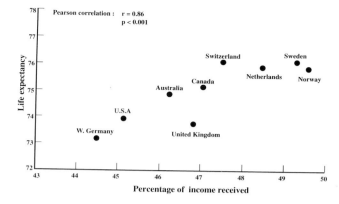

Fig. 5. Relationship between life expectancy at birth and percentage of post tax and benefit income received by the least well-off 70% of families. (adapted from Wilkinson, 1990, 1992).

rates in different Scottish postal code areas classified according to a composite measure of deprivation/affluence based on social class, male unemployment, household overcrowding, and access to a car (Carstairs & Morris, 1991). Their analysis reveals a continuous gradient of increasing mortality from the most affluent to the most deprived (Fig. 4).

Secondly, recent comparisons of life expectancy across different western countries appear to add further weight to the view that non-material factors may be involved. Wilkinson (1990, 1992) reported that life expectancy variations among such countries are only modestly predicted by Gross National Product. However, income distribution, defined as the percentage of total post-tax income and benefit received by the least well-off 70% of 'families' is substantially predictive (Fig. 5). It is interesting to note that this analysis did not include Japan. The Japanese now have the longest life expectancy in the world (Marmot & Davey Smith, 1989) and also the most equitable distribution of income of any OECD country (Wilkinson, 1992). What these analysis appear to indicate is that, for the majority of people in western countries, health hinges on relative as well as absolute living standards, implying that psychological processes may be at work. As Wilkinson (1990) concluded,

'It looks as if what matters about our physical circumstances is not what they are in themselves, but where they stand in the scale of things in our society. The implication is that our environment and standard of living no longer impact on our health primarily through direct physical causes, regardless of our attitudes and perceptions, but have come to do so mainly through social and cognitively mediated processes.' (p.405).

Given the difficulties which attend life expectancy as a measure, that it is substantially influenced by infant mortality rates, Wilkinson's conclusion may be somewhat overstated. Nevertheless, his analysis and the continuous character of socioeconomic health

gradients invite a search for mediating processes of a psychological nature.

What might these psychological mediators be? We have, as yet, only preliminary indications, largely derived from observational epidemiological studies; with such methodologies it is notoriously easy to produce spurious associations due to confounding (Davey Smith & Phillips, 1990). Nevertheless, recent reviews (Alder et al., 1994; Carroll, Bennett & Davey Smith, 1993; Williams, 1990) have identified psychological stress, personal control, social support, and hostility as possible candidates, and evidence also points to inequalities in the distribution of these psychological factors among different occupational groups (Barefoot et al., 1991; Marmot et al., 1991).

Deciphering key psychological variables and the primacy of their influence in this context is unlikely to be an easy task, given the interactions and overlaps which undoubtedly exist Nevertheless, it is a task worth undertaking, given the magnitude and persistence of socioeconomic health variations, and at least preliminary evidence implicating psychological factors. At the same time, though, it is important to appreciate that gross social and material division almost certainly remain the basic source of such health inequalities (Williams, 1990). Accordingly, the most compelling intervention strategies in this regard are unlikely to be psychological. Rather they will be those which directly counter socioeconomic inequalities (Carroll, Davey Smith & Bennett, 1996). (See also Family influences on health', 'Social Support and health.') As inequalities in income have increased in societies such as the UK and USA in recent years (see, e.g. Millar, 1993), so, too, have health inequalities (McCarron, Davey Smith & Wormsley, 1994; Pappas, Queen, Hadden & Fisher, 1993; Phillimore, Beattie & Townsend, 1994).

REFERENCES

Adler, N.E., Boyce, T., Chesney, M.A., Cohen, S., Folkman, S., Kahn, R.L. & Syme, S.L. (1994). Socioeconomic status and health: the challenge of the gradient. *American Psychologist*, **49**, 15–24.

Arber, S. (1989). Gender and class inequalities in health: understanding the differentials. In J. Fox (Ed.). *Health inequalities in*

European countries. Aldershot: Gower Publishing Co.

Barefoot, J.C., Peterson, B.L., Dahlstrom, W.G., Siegler, I.C., Anderson, N.B., & Williams, R.B. (1991). Hostility patterns and health implications: Correlates of Cook-Medley hostility scale scores in a national survey. *Health Psychology*, **10**, 18–24.

Berkman, L.F. & Breslow, L. (1983). *Health and ways of living: the Alameda Country Study*. Oxford: Oxford University Press.

Blane, D., Davey Smith, G. & Bartley, M. (1993). Social selection: what does it contribute to social class differences in health? *Sociology of Health and Illness*, **15**, 1–15.

Blaxter, M. (1989). A comparison of measures of inequality in morbidity. In J. Fox (Ed.) *Health inequalities in European countries*. Aldershot: Gower Publishing Co.

Carroll, D., Bennett, P & Davey Smith, G. (1993). Socio-economic health inequalities: their origins and implications. *Psychology and Health*, 8, 295–316.

Carroll, D., Davey Smith, G. & Bennett, P. (1996). Some observations on health and socio-economic status. *Journal of Health Psychology*, 1, 23–39.

Carstairs, V. & Morris, R. (1991). *Deprivation and health in Scotland*. Aberdeen: Aberdeen University Press.

Davey Smith, G., Carroll, D., Rankin, S. & Rowan, D. (1992a). Socioeconomic differentials in mortality: evidence from Glasgow graveyards. *British Medical Journal*, 305, 1554–7.

Davey Smith, G., Neaton, J.D., Stamler, J. & Wentworth, D. (1992b). Income differentials in mortality risk among 305,099 white men. Paper presented at the British Sociological Association/European Society of Medical Sociology Joint Conference. Edinburgh, Scotland.

Davey Smith. G. & Phillips, A.N. (1990). Declaring independence: why we should be cautious. *Journal of Epidemiology and Community Health*, 44, 257–8.

Davey Smith, G. & Shipley, M.J. (1991). Confounding of occupation and smoking: Its magnitude and consequences. *Social Science and Medicine*, 11, 1297–300.

Davey Smith, G & Shipley, M.J. & Rose, G. (1990). The magnitude and causes of socio-economic differentials in mortality: further evidence from the Whitehall study.

Journal of Epidemiology and Community Health, 44, 265–70.

Goldblatt, P. (1988). Changes in social class between 1971 and 1981: could these affect mortality differentials among men of working age? *Population Trends*, 51, 9–17.

Goldblatt, P. (1989). Mortality by social class, 1971–85. *Population Trends*, 56, 6–15.

Hein, H.O., Suadicani, P. & Gyntelberg, F. (1992). Ischaemic heart disease incidence by social class and form of smoking: the Copenhagen male study – 17 years' follow-up. *Journal of Internal Medicine*, 231, 477–83.

Hunter, D. (1955). *The diseases of occupations*. London: Hodder and Stoughton.

McCarron, P., Davey Smith, G. & Wormsley, J. (1994). Deprivation and mortality in Glasgow: changes from 1980 to 1992. *British Medical Journal*, 309, 1481–2.

Marmot, M.G. & Davey Smith, G. (1989). Why are the Japanese living longer? *British Medical Journal*, 299, 1547–51.

Marmot, M.G., Shipley, M.J. & Rose, G. (1984). Inequalities in health–specific explanations of a general pattern? *Lancet*, i, 1003–6.

Marmot, M.G., Davey Smith, G., Stansfeld, D., Patel, C., North, F., Head, J., White, I., Brunner, E. & Feeney, A. (1991). Health inequalities among British civil servants: the Whitehall 11 study. *Lancet*, 337, 1387–92.

Martin, C.J., Platt, S.D. & Hunt, S. (1987). Housing conditions and health. *British Medical Journal*, 294, 1125–7.

Millar, J. (1993). The continuing trend in rising poverty. In A. Sinfield (Ed.). *Poverty, inequality, and justice*, Edinburgh: University of Edinburgh.

Morrison, A.S., Kirshner, J. & Molha, A. (1977). Life cycle events in 15th century Florence: records of the Monte Delle Doti. *American Journal of Epidemiology*, 106, 487–92.

Pappas, G., Queen, S., Hadden, W. & Fisher, G. (1993). The increasing disparity in mortality between socioeconomic groups in the United States, 1960 and 1986. *The New England Journal of Medicine*, 329, 103–9.

Phillimore, P., Beattie, A. & Townsend, P. (1994). Widening inequalities of health in northern England, 1981–1991. *British Medical Journal*, 308, 1125–8.

Platt, S.D., Martin, C.J., Hunt, S. & Lewis, C.W. (1989). Damp housing, mould growth and symptomatic health state. *British Medical Journal*, 298, 1673–8.

Townsend, P. & Davidson, N. (1982). *The Black Report* Harmondsworth: Penguin.

Watt, G.C.M. & Ecob, R. (1992). Mortality in Glasgow and Edinburgh: a paradigm of inequality in health. *Journal of Epidemiology and Community Health*, 46, 498–505.

Whitehead, M. (1988). *The health divide*. Harmondsworth: Penguin.

Wilkinson, R.G. (1990). Income distribution and mortality: a 'natural' experiment. *Sociology of Health and Illness*, 12, 391–412.

Wilkinson, R.G. (1992). Income distribution and life expectancy. *British Medical Journal*, 304, 165–8.

Williams, D.R. (1990). Socioeconomic differentials in health: a review and redirection. *Social Psychology Quarterly*, 53, 81–99.

Stress and disease

ANDREW STEPTOE

Department of Psychology, St George's Hospital Medical School, University of London, UK

The notion that psychological stress influences vulnerability to disease is one of the major themes in health psychology, and has spawned a tradition of animal and human research dating back more than 50 years. Nevertheless, the relevance of stress to the development of disease has remained on the margins of biomedical science. In part, this is the result of lack of awareness among some clinicians of the advances that have been made in systematic studies of stress and health. However, scepticism concerning the role of stress has also arisen because of the grandiose claims made by some investigators; too often stress has been put forward as a cause when the pathophysiology of a condition is not understood, only to be discarded after the discovery of precise aetiological factors.

DEFINITION OF STRESS

The definition of stress remains controversial, and it is probably unwise to employ the word as more than a general term embracing a range of phenomena (Weiner, 1992). Hans Selye's original definition of stress as the 'nonspecific response of the body to any demand' has not proved helpful, first because stress responses are not non-specific but patterned according to the situations encountered and the coping behaviours deployed, and secondly because it begs the question of what conditions provoke this response pattern. Most research in the health field is based on a transactional model, in which stress responses are said to arise when demands exceed the personal and social resources that the individual is able to mobilize. The transactional approach acknowledges that almost any event, however unpleasant or distressing, may produce different responses in two people, or even in the same person on different occasions. The stress response itself is multidimensional, involving adjustments at the cognitive level (such as impairments in decision-making), affective changes and reductions in emotional well-being, a wide range of behavioural responses, and physiological adjustments in the autonomic, neuroendocrine and immune systems.

METHODOLOGICAL AND RESEARCH DESIGN ISSUES

A major difficulty that has beset investigators of stress and disease is the design of studies. Early research on stress relied on cross-sectional comparisons between patients suffering from particular diseases and healthy controls, and this remains a common procedure. The basic difficulty in such studies lies in teasing out cause/effect relationships. The observation that stress levels are elevated in patients with a particular illness does not mean that stress responses predated illness onset and contributed to it. People's lives and psychological characteristics may change with disease, and retrospective biases occur as patients search for meaning in their experiences. More compelling evidence is provided by prospective designs, in which stress parameters are assessed in initially disease-free individuals who are then followed up to discover who becomes ill. These studies are, however, difficult to conduct for many medical conditions, since the precise timing of disease onset can be uncertain, and there are many co-factors that contribute to risk and have to be measured.

A second important methodological issue is the role of negative affectivity. Negative affectivity refers to undifferentiated dysphoria and the disposition to experience aversive emotional states, and has been indexed by a variety of mood and personality measures related to anxiety, depression and neuroticism. It has been argued that negative affectivity increases vulnerability to stressors, thereby increasing health risk. Friedman and Booth-Kewley (1987), for example, have argued that a 'disease-prone personality' increases susceptibility to a range of disorders, and can be variously measured by anxiety, depression, hostility and anger scales. On the other hand, several lines of evidence suggest that associations between negative affect and disease may be in part spurious. High negative affect predicts somatic complaints and subjective symptoms independently of underlying disease severity (Watson & Pennebaker, 1989). Negative affect can also influence perceptions of stress, the recall of negative life events, ratings of social supports, and decisions to seek medical care. Studies of stress and disease that rely on subjective reports of illness without taking account of negative affectivity therefore run the risk of identifying erroneous associations. This problem highlights the need to assess objective behavioural and physiological markers of disease and disease risk whenever possible.

One of the major changes to have taken place in stress research over recent decades has been the shift from considering certain physical illnesses as being caused exclusively by psychological factors (as in the psychosomatic tradition), to viewing stress-related processes as contributors to multifactorial disease risk. Stress factors may be relevant to a variable extent in a wide range of medical conditions, contributing to early aetiology in some cases, the rate of progression of established illness in other cases, and even to the precipitation of acute clinical events (such as myocardial infarction) in individuals with advanced disease.

A greater understanding of the role of stress in disease may stem from considering the range of studies that are employed (for illustrations of these findings, see Steptoe & Wardle, 1994). They include the following.

Animal studies

Studies of animals provide the best controlled evidence for stress being relevant to disease, since they involve random assignment, exposure to precisely defined conditions, and strict regulation of factors such as diet and exercise that may contribute to disease risk. Important findings from animal studies include the development of gastric lesions in rats subject to uncontrollable as opposed to controllable shock, the influence of aversive stimulation on immune competence and on the rate of development of malignant tumours, the effects of social conflict on the induction of hypertension in mice, and the role of social stress in coronary atherosclerosis in monkeys. There are many species differences and methodological complications in studies of stress and disease in animals. Such studies are best interpreted as showing that stress processes can influence disease development, rather than that these factors are necessarily important in the clinical context.

Studies of pathophysiology

Pathophysiological studies are relevant to understanding the role of stress in that they may identify the metabolic and regulatory processes that are disturbed by stimulation from the central nervous system. If no plausible biological mechanism is delineated, then arguments about the role of stress must remain speculative. Examples of important pathophysiological findings include the presence of sympathetic nervous system activity in early hypertension, the influence of parasympathetic activity and immune dysfunctions in bronchial asthma, the role of sympathetic activation in cardiac arrhythmia and catecholamine release in thrombus formation in patients with coronary artery disease, and the relevance of electromyographic disturbances in different groups of patients suffering from chronic pain.

Mental stress testing

Mental stress testing involves the monitoring of autonomic, neuroendocrine and immune responses during acute exposure to demanding tasks or emotionally charged situations. It is widely used in the investigation of stress in relation to cardiovascular disorders, headache, rheumatoid arthritis and other conditions. The aim of mental stress testing is to understand how pathophysiological

[175]

mechanisms may be disturbed by behavioural demands. These methods are used particularly commonly in studies of hypertension and coronary heart disease, but the relevance of acute physiological stress responses to disease processes is fiercely debated (Turner, 1994). Mental stress testing provides a laboratory model for studying stress and disease, and has limitations similar to those of other laboratory models.

Field studies

Field studies of stress and disease involve the measurement of physiological parameters associated with health risk in groups of people exposed to threatening or demanding situations. The aim is to determine whether disturbances in function that are of clinical significance occur in real-life conditions, and not just in the rarefied atmosphere of the laboratory or clinic. Examples include studies of impaired immune function in people looking after relatives with Alzheimer's disease, monitoring of blood pressure from people working in jobs characterized by high demands and low control, and measurement of neuroendocrine function in individuals living in crowded or noisy conditions.

Clinical and epidemiological studies

Studies of people suffering from clinical disorders remain a strong theme in stress research. A variety of strategies are used, from investigations of personality and behaviour patterns to life events and social networks. On the larger scale, psychosocial epidemiological methods are now being employed to evaluate the contribution of stress-related processes, using large cohort designs, prospective methods, stratified population sampling and careful evaluation of co-factors to study experiences such as unemployment, social isolation and work patterns. On the grander scale still, stress has been proposed as being relevant to major sociocultural influences on health such as socioeconomic status and migration. It can be argued that, without evidence at these levels of study, no amount of experimental or pathophysiological data can prove the role of stress-related processes in health risk. On the other hand, clinical and epidemiological studies are rarely conclusive because of the impossibility of random assignment of people to different experiences, and the difficulties of measuring and controlling for every possible confounding factor. Ultimately, the hypothesis that psychological stress is linked with disease depends on a comprehensive evaluation of evidence from all levels of study, and on the combined weight of corroborative findings from several research strategies.

DEMANDS, RESOURCES AND PREDISPOSITIONS

Greater understanding of the contribution of stress processes to health risk can be gained through characterizing the major elements (see Goldberger & Breznitz, 1993).

Psychosocial demands

Psychosocial demands (or stressors) are quantified with a variety of methods including the assessment of major life events, everyday minor events and hassles, and perceived stress. Long-term demands are particularly relevant since they may stimulate chronic physiological adjustments and behaviour change. Generalizing across a wide range of studies, the experiences that are associated with the most damaging stress responses are typically severely threatening situations that are unpredictable, uncontrollable, and make complex demands on the individual.

Psychosocial resources

The resources that are relevant to stress responses include social support, and certain personality characteristics and behaviour patterns that influence susceptibility to stressors. Among the factors that may be protective are optimism, defined by Scheier and Carver (1992) as a bias towards positive outcome expectancies, and a constellation of characteristics that make up the 'hardy' personality formulated by Suzanne Ouellette. There is evidence that these factors do reduce likelihood of ill-health in people exposed to high stressor levels, although the research has been criticized on methodological grounds. Other personal dispositions, such as high levels of neuroticism and tendencies to repress or inhibit emotional expression, may increase susceptibility. These social and psychological factors are mediated through psychological coping responses, defined here as behavioural and cognitive processes mobilized by the individual in an effort to manage the situation and its emotional consequences. There is considerable interest in defining what forms of coping are adaptive for health in particular situations.

Disease vulnerability

Models linking stress processes with disease must account for why not all people exposed to the same adverse life experience become ill, and why different people develop different types of disorder. One explanation for these individual differences relates to biological and genetic predispositions. The extent to which stress processes contribute to risk depends on constitutional vulnerability, with factors such as genetic make-up, pre-existing pathology, nutritional status and physical fitness being relevant. Stress processes do not act in isolation, but interact with risk factors identified in conventional biomedical research.

PATHWAYS TO DISEASE

The mechanisms through which stress responses impinge on disease processes can be specified. Apart from the influence of stress on subjective symptomatology and illness behaviour, there are two major pathways, involving behaviour changes and psychophysiological responses (Adler & Matthews, 1994).

Behavioural pathways

Activities such as cigarette smoking, dietary choice, certain sexual practices and alcohol consumption affect disease risk. One way stress transactions may influence health is through altering the frequency or pattern of health behaviours. Associations between adverse life events and alcohol consumption or relapse following smoking cessation have been described, while demanding working conditions have been related to sedentary lifestyles and high dietary fat intake. Adherence to advice concerning health screening and medical treatment may also be adversely affected by stress processes (Anderson, Kiecolt-Glaser & Glaser, 1994). The social supports mobilized in efforts to cope with upsetting situations can increase exposure to pathogens. Thus the influence of stress on disease may be mediated in part through changes at the overt behavioural level.

Psychophysiological pathways

A second set of mechanisms linking stress with illness involves the autonomic, neuroendocrine and immune responses that are stimulated during stress transactions. The central components of the psychophysiological stress response are activation of the pituitary–adrenocortical axis leading to release of corticosteroids, and the sympathoadrenal pathway, stimulation of which activates the sympathetic nervous system and release of catecholamines from the adrenal medulla (Stanford & Salmon, 1993). A variety of cardiovascular, metabolic, gastrointestinal and immune responses are elicited, and their pattern is influenced by the precise nature of the demands and resources mobilized.

Within the psychophysiological framework, there are a number of distinct mechanisms that may be relevant. The first involves psychophysiological hyper-reactivity, or exaggerated stress responsivity. Vulnerable individuals may show exaggerated responsivity in certain physiological parameters, such as blood pressure or catecholamine release; if these responses are repeated or sustained over lengthy periods, they may lead directly to functional and structural pathology. This process underlies much research on stress and illness, but the best evidence for its action is in the field of cardiovascular disease risk (Steptoe & Tavazzi, 1996). A related process through which psychophysiological responses influence disease is by affecting the progression or stability of existing conditions. This process may operate in many disorders. Disturbances in mood and perceived stress may, for example, provoke physiological responses that trigger painful episodes in patients prone to headache, lead to disturbances in insulin regulation in diabetes mellitus, or even trigger episodes of cardiac arrhythmia and coronary ischaemia in patients with coronary artery disease.

A third possibility is that health is compromised not by the direct influence of physiological responses, but by reducing the organism's vulnerability and resistance to pathogens. Emotionally induced immunosuppression may increase the likelihood of infections becoming established and provoke inflammatory episodes in auto-immune disorders (Cohen & Williamson, 1991). The influence of stress processes on host vulnerability may also underlie connections between stress and cancer (Anderson et al., 1994). It is important to recognize that stress does not play a causal but a facilitating role under these circumstances. Whether or not the person succumbs to disease will depend on the stress-induced vulnerability coinciding with exposure to infection and the presence of pathogens. (See also 'Life events and health', 'Noise effects on health', 'Perceived control and health behaviour', 'Type A behaviour, hostility and coronary artery disease'.)

REFERENCES

Adler, N. & Matthews, K.A. (1994). Health Psychology: why do some people get sick and some stay well? *Annual Review of Psychology*, **45**, 229–59.

Anderson, B.L., Kiecolt-Glaser, J.K & Glaser, R. (1994). A biobehavioral model of cancer stress and disease course. *American Psychologist*, **49**, 389–404.

Cohen, S. & Williamson, G.M. (1991). Stress and infectious disease in humans. *Psychological Bulletin*, **109**, 3–24.

Friedman, H.S. & Booth-Kewley, S. (1987). The 'disease-prone' personality: a meta-analytic view of the construct. *American Psychologist*, **42**, 539–55.

Goldberger, L. & Breznitz, S. (Eds.). (1993). *Handbook of stress* (2nd edn.). New York: Free Press.

Scheier, M.F. & Carver, C.S. (1992). Effects of optimism on psychological and physical well-being: theoretical overview and empirical update. *Cognitive Therapy and Research*, **16**, 201–28.

Stanford, S.C. & Salmon, P. (Eds.). (1993). *Stress: from synapse to syndrome*. London: Academic Press.

Steptoe, A. & Wardle, J. (Eds.). (1994). *Psychosocial processes and health: a reader*. Cambridge: Cambridge University Press.

Steptoe, A. & Tavazzi, L. (1996). The mind and the heart. In D.G. Julian, A.J. Camm, K. Fox, R. Hall & P.A. Poole-Wilson (Eds.) *Diseases of the heart*. Second edition. London: WH Saunders.

Turner, J.R. (1994). *Cardiovascular reactivity and stress*. New York: Plenum.

Watson, D. & Pennebaker, J.W. (1989). Health complaints, stress, and distress: explaining the central role of negative affectivity. *Psychological Review*, **96**, 234–54.

Weiner, H. (1992). *Perturbing the organism: the biology of stressful experience*. Chicago: Chicago University Press.

Theory of planned behaviour

STEPHEN SUTTON

Department of Epidemiology and Public Health,
University College London, UK

The Theory of Planned Behaviour (Ajzen, 1988, 1991) is an extension of the Theory of Reasoned Action (Ajzen & Fishbein, 1980). Both models are widely used in research on health behaviours. Since the Theory of Reasoned Action is a special case of the Theory of Planned Behaviour and continues to be used in its own right (e.g. Terry, Gallois & McCamish, 1993), it will be described first. Then Ajzen's extension to the model will be discussed.

THE THEORY OF REASONED ACTION

The Theory of Reasoned Action specifies the causal relationships between beliefs, attitudes, intentions and behaviour. The model assumes that most behaviours of social relevance (which would include most health-related behaviours) are under volitional control, and that a person's intention to perform a behaviour is both the immediate determinant and the single best predictor of that behaviour. Intention, in turn, is held to be a function of two basic determinants, one personal and the other reflecting social influence. The personal factor is the individual's positive or negative evaluation of performing the behaviour. This is referred to as attitude toward the behaviour (AB). The second determinant represents the perceived expectations of important others with regard to his/her performing the behaviour in question, and is called the subjective norm (SN). Generally speaking, people will have strong intentions to perform a given action if they evaluate it positively, and if they believe that important others think they should perform it. These two components, attitude toward the behaviour and subjective norm, are assumed to combine additively to determine behavioural intention (BI):

$$BI = w_1(AB) + w_2(SN)$$

where w_1 and w_2 are weights representing the relative importance of the personal–attitudinal and the social–normative components. The relative importance of the two factors will vary across behaviours and situations. In some cases, the attitudinal component will be more important; in other cases, normative considerations will predominate.

The theory also specifies the determinants of AB and SN. Attitude toward the behaviour is held to reflect the person's salient beliefs concerning the possible personal consequences of the action. Generally speaking, a person who believes that performing a given behaviour will lead to mostly positive outcomes will hold a favourable attitude toward the behaviour, and conversely, a person who believes that the action will result in mostly negative personal outcomes will hold an unfavourable attitude. Subjective norm is also a function of beliefs, namely the person's beliefs that specific individuals or groups think he or she should perform the behaviour. Generally speaking, a person who believes that most significant referents think he/she should perform the behaviour will perceive social pressure to do so. In short, a person's behavioural intentions, and hence behaviour, depend ultimately on their beliefs concerning (a) the possible consequences for them of performing the behaviour and (b) the expectations of important others. It follows that, in order to change behaviour, it is necessary to change these underlying beliefs.

Fishbein and Ajzen argue that variables other than BI, AB, SN and their component beliefs, that is variables 'external' to the model, can influence intentions, and hence behaviour, only by influencing AB, SN or the relative importance of these two components. For example, the intention to perform a given action may be related to age or neuroticism. However, according to Fishbein and Ajzen, the effects of these variables on intentions would be entirely mediated by their effects on AB and SN. Thus, the Theory of Reasoned Action specifies the proximal and sufficient determinants of intentions and behaviour.

According to Fishbein and Ajzen, a measure of intention will not always be an accurate predictor of behaviour. There are at least two factors that influence the strength of the observed relationship between intention and behaviour. The first is the degree of 'correspondence' between the measures. In order to predict behaviour accurately, it is essential that the two concepts are measured at the same level of specificity or generality. For example, to predict whether or not a person will smoke cigarettes at the departmental

Christmas party, the measure of intention should be phrased specifically in terms of 'smoking cigarettes at the departmental Christmas party'. The second factor that influences the strength of the intention–behaviour relationship is the stability of intentions. Clearly, if a person's intention changes in the interval between the measurement of intentions and behaviour, this will reduce the accuracy of prediction. This is likely to be a problem in most applications of the model to health behaviours. The longer the time interval, the greater the probability that events will occur that produce changes in intention, and therefore the lower the observed relationship between intention and behaviour.

THE THEORY OF PLANNED BEHAVIOUR

Many health behaviours cannot simply be performed at will; they require skills, opportunities, resources, or cooperation for their successful execution. The Theory of Planned Behaviour was an attempt to extend the Theory of Reasoned Action so that it could be applied to behaviours that are not entirely under volitional control, for example giving up smoking or using a condom. To accommodate such behaviours, Ajzen added a variable called perceived behavioural control to the model. This refers to the perceived ease or difficulty of performing the behaviour and it is assumed to reflect past experience as well as anticipated obstacles. It is similar to Bandura's (1982) concept of self-efficacy. According to Ajzen, perceived behavioural control is a function of control beliefs in just the same way as subjective norm is a function of normative beliefs. It is assumed to have a direct influence on intention: the more control a person believes themselves to have over the behaviour in question, the stronger will be their intention to perform the behaviour. Perceived behavioural control may also have a direct influence on behaviour, for two reasons. First, holding intention constant, an individual with higher perceived behavioural control is likely to try harder and to persevere for longer than an individual who has lower perceived control. Second, people may be able to anticipate real barriers to executing the behaviour successfully; thus, perceived behavioural control can often be used as a proxy for a measure of actual control. Figure 1 summarizes the Theory of Planned Behaviour in the form of a causal model.

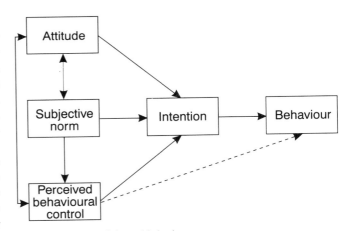

Fig. 1. The theory of planned behaviour.

OPERATIONALIZING THE THEORIES

The components of the theories are typically operationalized using questionnaire ratings in semantic differential format. Table 1 gives examples for a (fictitious) study of the decision to stop smoking in the New Year, based on the recommendations made by Ajzen and Fishbein (1980, Appendix A, pp. 261–263). The table includes only the global or direct measures of the components. The reader should consult Ajzen and Fishbein (1980) and recent applications of the models for examples of the way that beliefs are operationalized. In the table, the number of indicators per construct varies. This reflects standard practice. For example, it is quite common to use several indicators of AB but only one indicator of BI and one indicator of SN. However, to minimize random measurement error (maximize reliability), it is preferable to use multiple indicators of each construct. Even with multiple indicators, the main components of the theories can be measured using a fairly short questionnaire. However, if indirect measures are used (e.g. measures of behavioural beliefs and outcome evaluations with respect to a set of outcomes), questionnaires can become prohibitively long for many practical situations.

HOW WELL DO THE THEORIES PERFORM?

A meta-analysis of 87 studies that applied the Theory of Reasoned Action to diverse topics (not specifically health-related) found a mean correlation (weighted by sample size) of 0.53 for the intention-behaviour relationship and a mean multiple correlation of 0.66 for predicting intention from attitude and subjective norm (Sheppard, Hartwick & Warshaw, 1988). An analysis of 23 independent samples in which smoking intentions were predicted from attitude and subjective norm found multiple correlations ranging from 0.43 to 0.83 with an overall (unweighted) mean correlation of 0.63 (Sutton, 1989). Thus, the Theory of Reasoned Action typically explains around 25% of the variance in behaviour (from intention alone) and somewhat less than 50% of the variance in intentions. These effects are sufficiently large to be useful for practical predictive purposes, though from a theoretical perspective they suggest that the theory does not provide an adequate explanation of intention and behaviour. The Theory of Planned Behaviour would be expected to do better because of the inclusion of an additional explanatory variable. Ajzen (1991) summarized the results from a number of studies that used the extended model. In nearly every case, perceived behavioural control added significantly to the prediction of intention and behaviour.

CRITICISMS OF THE THEORIES

The Theories of Reasoned Action and Planned Behaviour have attracted a large amount of critical comment. Some of the main criticisms are outlined below:

(i) It has been argued that a distinction should be made between behavioural intentions, which refer to a person's plans about his/her own future behaviour, and behavioural expectations or self-predictions, which refer to the person's perceived likelihood of performing a given behaviour (Warshaw & Davis, 1985). For example, a non-smoking adolescent may think it likely that he/she will be a smoker in five years' time without having a definite plan to take up smoking. Although intention can be seen as having a causal effect on behaviour, a behavioural self-prediction may, or may not, influence behaviour directly.

Table 1. *Recommended operationalizations of the components of the theory of reasoned action/planned behaviour for the decision to 'stop smoking in the New Year'*

Behavioural intention (BI)
I intend to stop smoking in the New Year.

    likely —:—:—:—:—:—:— unlikely

Attitude toward the behaviour (AB)
My stopping smoking in the New Year would be

harmful	—:—:—:—:—:—:—	beneficial
good	—:—:—:—:—:—:—	bad
rewarding	—:—:—:—:—:—:—	punishing
undesirable	—:—:—:—:—:—:—	desirable

Subjective norm (SN)
Most people who are important to me think

    I should —:—:—:—:—:—:— I should not

stop smoking in the New Year.

Perceived behavioural control (PBC)
How much control do you feel you have over your smoking?

    very little —:—:—:—:—:—:— a lot

How easy or difficult would you find it to stop smoking in the New Year?

    very easy —:—:—:—:—:—:— very difficult

(ii) The theories say little about how an intention is translated into action. In Schwarzer's (1992) terms, the model focuses on the motivational phase of decision-making and neglects the action phase.

(iii) In the subjective expected utility (SEU) model from which the theories are derived, the subjective normative aspects of a behaviour are treated in the same way as other perceived rewards and costs; they are not accorded any special status. For example, gaining the approval of one's spouse is treated as just another potential benefit of quitting smoking. A number of problems stem from splitting off the normative aspects from the rest (Miniard & Cohen, 1981; Sutton, 1989).

(iv) The theories have been criticized as being unrealistically complex (e.g. Eiser & van der Pligt, 1988). In some applications, subjects may be asked to rate as many as 50 possible outcomes of a behaviour. Critics argue that, when people make decisions, they typically consider only a small number (say < 10) aspects of the problem and they use simplifying heuristics or rules of thumb rather than engage in a complex integration of multiple outcomes. However, in any application, the measuring instrument needs to be comprehensive enough to cover all the outcomes that might be important to the subjects who are taking part. Using a large number of outcomes is simply a device to ensure that this happens; it does not imply that a particular respondent will consider all or even most of these outcomes when making a decision. Nevertheless, the theories may not provide a valid description of the process by which people make decisions, and most 'tests' of the model do not actually test the expectancy-value assumption (the multiplicative combination of beliefs and evaluations) that underlies the model.

(v) The theories have also been criticized for being too simple and too parsimonious. Many other variables (perceived behavioural control among them) have been proposed as additional explanatory factors. When studying repeated health behaviours, one potentially important variable for understanding current intention and future behaviour is the person's current or past behaviour (Bentler & Speckart, 1979; Sutton, 1994). Indeed, it is often the case that the best predictor of future behaviour is an earlier measure of the same behaviour. Furthermore, past behaviour frequently bypasses intention and has an independent predictive effect on future behaviour.

CONCLUSIONS

The Theories of Reasoned Action and Planned Behaviour postulate a small number of proximal and sufficient determinants of intentions and behaviour. The measures are fairly well standardized and can easily be adapted to a new health behaviour. Since behavioural intention is central to the theories, they will nearly always provide useful predictive power. Detailed examination of the beliefs that are assumed to underlie intentions may help to guide interventions. The theories seem best suited for studying one-off or occasional behaviours such as having a tetanus booster rather than frequently repeated behaviours like wearing a seat belt or going jogging. Most applications of the theories have been correlational, and there have been few experimental tests of the theories (for an exception, see Fishbein, Ajzen & McArdle, 1980). Although the theories are useful for prediction, they may not provide an accurate description of how people make health-related decisions.

REFERENCES

Ajzen, I. (1988). *Attitudes, personality, and behavior*. Milton Keynes: Open University Press.

Ajzen, I. (1991). The theory of planned behavior. *Organizational Behavior and Human Decision Processes*, 50, 179–211.

Ajzen, I. & Fishbein, M. (1980). *Understanding attitudes and predicting social behavior*. Englewood Cliffs, NJ: Prentice-Hall.

Bandura, A. (1982). Self-efficacy mechanism in human agency. *American Psychologist*, 37, 122–47.

Bentler, P.M. & Speckart, G. (1979). Models of attitude–behavior relations. *Psychological Review*, 86, 452–64.

Eiser, J.R. & van der Pligt, J. (1988). *Attitudes and decisions*. London: Routledge.

Fishbein M., Ajzen, I. & McArdle, J. (1980). Changing the behavior of alcoholics: effects of persuasive communications. In I. Ajzen & M. Fishbein (Eds.). *Understanding attitudes and predicting social behavior*, pp. 217–242. Englewood Cliffs, NJ: Prentice-Hall.

Miniard, P. & Cohen, J.B. (1981). An examination of the Fishbein–Ajzen behavioral intentions–model's concepts and measures. *Journal of Experimental Social Psychology*, 17, 309–39.

Schwarzer, R. (1992). Self-efficacy in the adoption and maintenance of health behaviors: theoretical approaches and a new model. In R. Schwarzer (Ed.). *Self-efficacy: thought control of action*, pp. 217–243. Washington: Hemisphere.

Sheppard, B.H., Hartwick, J. & Warshaw, P.R. (1988). The theory of reasoned action: a meta-analysis of past research with recommendations for modifications and future research. *Journal of Consumer Research*, 15, 325–43.

Sutton, S.R. (1989). Smoking attitudes and behavior: applications of Fishbein and Ajzen's theory of reasoned action to predicting and understanding smoking decisions. In T. Ney & A. Gale (Eds.). *Smoking and human behavior*, pp. 289–312. Chichester: John Wiley & Sons.

Sutton, S.R. (1994). The past predicts the future: interpreting behaviour–behaviour relationships in social psychological models of health behaviour. In D.R. Rutter & L. Quine (Eds.). *Social psychology and health: European perspectives*, pp. 71–88. Aldershot: Avebury.

Terry, D.J., Gallois, C. & McCamish, M. (Eds.). (1993). *The theory of reasoned action: its application to AIDS-preventive behaviour*. Oxford: Pergamon Press.

Warshaw, P.R. & Davis, F.D. (1985). Disentangling behavioral intention and behavioral expectation. *Journal of Experimental Social Psychology*, 21, 213–28.

Transtheoretical model of behaviour change

STEPHEN SUTTON

Health Behaviour Unit, Department of Epidemiology and Public Health, University College London,

The transtheoretical or stages of change model (Prochaska & DiClemente, 1986; Prochaska, DiClemente & Norcross 1992) claims to offer a general, comprehensive, and theoretically coherent account of behaviour change. Most applications of the model have been to smoking cessation but it has also been applied to other problem behaviours such as cocaine use, condom use, and weight control (Prochaska, 1994).

The transtheoretical model comprises a number of components or dimensions. This chapter gives an overview of the model in terms of its two main components: the stages of change and the processes of change. The implications for intervention are discussed and an overall assessment of the usefulness of the model is made.

THE STAGES OF CHANGE

The latest version of the model postulates five stages: precontemplation (not seriously thinking about changing); contemplation (seriously thinking about changing); preparation (ready to change); action (attempting to change); and maintenance (change achieved). The model holds that individuals move through these stages from precontemplation to action or maintenance but will typically relapse

Table 1. *Categorical definition of stages (from DiClemente* et al., *1991)*

Precontemplation (PC)
Currently smoking and not seriously considering quitting within the next 6 months.

Contemplation (C)
Currently smoking and seriously considering quitting within the next 6 months but either (1) not planning to quit within the next 30 days or (2) has not made at least one 24-hour quit attempt in the past year, or both.

Preparation (PA)
Currently smoking, seriously considering quitting within the next 6 months, planning to quit within the next 30 days, and has made at least one 24-hour quit attempt in the past year.

Action (A)
Currently not smoking; quit in last 6 months.

Maintenance (M)
Currently not smoking; quit > 6 months ago.

back to precontemplation and cycle through the stages several times before achieving termination of the problem.

The most commonly used method of assessing stages of change is the staging algorithm approach in which each subject is assigned to one of a set of mutually exclusive and exhaustive categories on the basis of their responses to a small number of questionnaire items. Table 1 gives an example. Note that current smokers are classified on the basis of both their intentions and their recent behaviour (quit attempts) whereas ex-smokers are classified using a simple behavioural criterion (how long they have been abstinent). A serious inconsistency in this scheme is that smokers can only be in the preparation stage if they have made a recent quit attempt. It follows that first-time quitters can never have been in the preparation stage at any time in their smoking history. The time periods referred to (6 months, 30 days) are to some extent arbitrary and, in interpreting data on the prevalence of different stages, it should be borne in mind that changing the time frame may well lead to a change in prevalence. For example, if preparation were defined in terms of planning to quit in the next 7 days (rather than the next 30 days), one would expect the prevalence of smokers in the preparation stage to be lower.

Movement through the stages

The concept of stage implies ordering or sequence. Several studies have assessed subjects (smokers and ex-smokers) on two or more occasions enabling movement between stages to be examined. Prochaska *et al.* (1991) reported data on a sample of 544 self-changers who provided information about stage of change every six months for two years. Only 16% of subjects, showed a stable progression over the two years from one stage to the next in the sequence (e.g. precontemplation to contemplation) without suffering any reverses (e.g. PC–PC–PC–C–C). There were apparently no subjects who showed a stable progression through three or more stages (e.g. PC–PC–C–C–A); two was the maximum. Of subjects, 12% moved backwards one or two stages (e.g. C–C–C–PC–PC). Of subjects, 36% showed a flat profile, that is they stayed in the same stage across the five waves of measurement (e.g. PC–PC–PC–PC–PC).

This study in effect took five 'snapshots' over a two-year period. It is quite possible that many subjects moved through other stages in the six-month periods between measurements. The study did not attempt to find out what went on between follow-ups; only the subject's current stage was recorded. With this caveat, the findings as reported show clearly that forward progressive movement through the stages is far from being the modal pattern of change among volunteer self-changers.

It is possible that in treatment settings movement between stages will be more systematic and more consistent with the sequence postulated by the model. Relevant data have been reported by DiClemente *et al.* (1991). Smokers participating in a self-help cessation programme were divided into precontemplators, contemplators, and those who were prepared for action. Stage of change at baseline predicted the probability of attempting to quit as well as smoking status at 1 and 6 months (i.e. movement to the action stage). This is consistent with the stages of change model but it is also consistent with continuum models that hold that the probability of making an attempt to quit depends on current intentions and past behaviour (prior quit attempts) (Sutton, Marsh & Matheson, 1987). Indeed, rather than being viewed as discrete stages, precontemplation, contemplation, and preparation can be regarded simply as a convenient way of summarizing where people lie on a continuum of intention or readiness to change.

Stage models can vary in terms of the sequences and transitions they allow. At one extreme, a stage model may postulate an invariant sequence: everyone will move through the same sequence of stages. A less extreme, and more realistic, version of the model would state that if someone moves at all, they can move forwards to the next stage or backwards to the preceding stage but that forward movement is more likely. An even less strict version would allow people to skip stages, both forwards and backwards, but would still hold that the most likely transition (apart from staying put) will be to the next stage in the putative sequence. Less strict still is the 'lifetime model' which postulates only that to enter a particular stage in the sequence you must have been in the preceding stage at some earlier time in your life. At the other extreme from the invariant stage model, the notion of a sequence of stages can be abandoned completely. In this approach, stages of change are replaced by states of change. Unlike stages, states carry no implication of ordering or sequence; a person can in principle move from one state to any other state (Sutton, 1996).

THE PROCESSES OF CHANGE

The second core dimension of the model is the processes of change. These are covert or overt activities that people engage in to help them progress towards recovery. They are assumed to be common to self-change and to change that occurs within a formal treatment programme. Examples are consciousness raising (increasing information about self and problem), self-reevaluation (assessing how one feels and thinks about oneself with respect to a problem), counterconditioning (substituting alternatives for problem behaviours), and reinforcement management (rewarding oneself or being rewarded by others for making changes). In the transtheoretical model, the processes of change are integrated with the stages of change in the sense that different processes are assumed to be emphasized in different stages.

Table 2. *Processes of change listed under the stages in which they are emphasized most and least.*

Precontemplation	→	Contemplation	→	Action	→	Maintenance
Eight processes used the least		Consciousness raising				
			Self-reevaluation[a]			
			Self-liberation			
			Helping relationship			
			Reinforcement management			
				Counter-conditioning[a]		
				Stimulus control[a]		

[a]Processes emphasized in two stages are shown overlapping both stages. From Prochaska J.O. & DiClemente, C.C. (1983). Stages and processes of self-change of smoking: toward an integrative model of change, *Journal of Consulting and Clinical Psychology*, **51**, p. 394. Copyright 1983 by the American Psychological Association. Adapted by permission.

A 40-item questionnaire designed to assess the ten basic processes of change in smoking cessation was described by Prochaska *et al.* (1988). The respondent is asked to rate the frequency of use of each process in the last month on a five-point scale from 1 = never to 5 = repeatedly.

The coverage of processes is inadequate. There are many things that smokers may do prior to making a quit attempt (e.g. setting a target date, cutting down, and switching to a low tar brand) which are not included in the list of processes. A further limitation of the model is that it focuses only on positive processes. Processes that may hinder movement toward smoking cessation (e.g. procrastination, avoidance, wishful thinking) are not represented in the questionnaire.

A key hypothesis in the stages of change model is that different processes will be used in different stages. In a cross-sectional study of smokers and ex-smokers, Prochaska and DiClemente (1983) found significant differences in the processes used across stages; these are summarized in Table 2. Not surprisingly, precontemplators reported using eight of the ten processes less frequently than the other groups. Again, not surprisingly, behavioural processes tended to be used more frequently in the action and maintenance stages (i.e. by those who had stopped smoking). Some processes seemed to be emphasized in two consecutive stages. For example, counterconditioning and stimulus control (removing reminders of smoking) were used more than average in both action and maintenance. Prochaska and DiClemente interpret this as indicating that these processes bridge the two stages and as supporting the idea that engaging in these processes will help to shift the individual from action to maintenance.

Prochaska *et al.* (1985) reported the results of discriminant function analyses predicting movement between stages over a six-month period in a large sample of smokers and exsmokers. All but one of the ten processes (environmental reevaluation) occurred in one or more of the six discriminant functions (prediction equations) that emerged from the analysis. However, more frequent use of a process was sometimes predictive of progression to a more advanced stage and sometimes predictive of no movement or regression to an earlier stage; positive and negative predictive relationships occurred with about equal frequency. For example, one discriminant function dis-

tinguished contemplators who became precontemplators from those who became recent quitters. The latter group was relatively high in self-reevaluation but relatively low in consciousness raising. A second discriminant function distinguished contemplators who became recent quitters from those who stayed in the contemplation stage. Those who took action were those who had been low in self-reevaluation and low in social liberation.

It is difficult to draw any clear recommendations for treatment or self-change from these results. The findings also show some important discrepancies with those of Prochaska and DiClemente (1983). For example, in that study, consciousness raising was emphasized in the contemplation stage. But in the Prochaska *et al.* (1985) paper, more frequent use of consciousness raising appeared to have an adverse effect.

STAGE-MATCHED INTERVENTIONS

One attraction of a stage model is that it suggests the possibility of stage-matched interventions in which subjects in different stages of change receive different versions of an intervention package rather than the same standard package. Prochaska and colleagues (Prochaska *et al.*, 1993; Velicer *et al.*, 1993) developed stage-based self-help smoking cessation manuals and tested them in a randomized controlled study against the best available manuals. Participants in the 'individualized manual' condition were sent the manual matched to their individual stage of change and manuals for all the subsequent stages. Using a criterion of prolonged abstinence, there was no significant advantage for the individualized manuals. Abstinence rates were around 3% at 12 months and 7% and 5% at 18 months in the stage-matched and standardized conditions, respectively. Other conditions involving repeated contact with participants roughly doubled these success rates.

Several other controlled studies of stage-matched intervention programmes for smokers, problem drinkers and drug users are in progress, but the results are not yet available.

CONCLUSIONS

The transtheoretical model has intuitive appeal and heuristic value. With few exceptions (Davidson, 1992; Sutton, 1996), commentators have been unanimous in their praise and enthusiasm for the model. However, the empirical evidence, particularly from longitudinal studies, does not strongly support the model. For example, using particular processes in particular stages does not consistently predict movement to subsequent stages. Many of the findings that are interpreted as supporting the model are also consistent with other widely used models (e.g. the Theory of Reasoned Action) that do not postulate a sequence of discrete stages. A major problem is that the model is not specified clearly enough. The assumptions about causal pathways are not made explicit. For example, what is the presumed causal relationship between the processes of change and the pros and cons for changing? Stage definitions and measures vary widely between studies. Nevertheless, the model is useful in a number of ways. For example, stage of change can be used as an outcome variable in treatment and intervention studies. Any forward progression can be regarded as a success. The transtheoretical model can be thought of as a prescriptive model, a model of ideal change (Sutton, 1996). As such, it provides a useful framework which may contribute to the development of more effective interventions.

REFERENCES

Davidson, R. (1992). Prochaska and DiClemente's model of change: a case study?, *British Journal of Addiction*, **87**, 821–2.

DiClemente, C.C., Prochaska, J.O., Fairhurst, S.K., Velicer, W.F., Velasquez, M.M. & Rossi, J.R. (1991). The process of smoking cessation: an analysis of precontemplation, contemplation, and preparation stages of change. *Journal of Consulting and Clinical Psychology*, **59**, 295–304.

Prochaska, J.O. (1994). Strong and weak principles for progressing from precontemplation to action on the basis of twelve problem behaviors. *Health Psychology*, **13**, 47–51.

Prochaska, J.O. & DiClemente, C.C. (1983). Stages and processes of self-change of smoking: toward an integrative model of change. *Journal of Consulting and Clinical Psychology*, **51**, 390–5.

Prochaska, J.O. & DiClemente, C.C. (1986). Toward a comprehensive model of change.

In W.R. Miller & N. Heather (Eds.). *Treating addictive behaviors: processes of change*, pp.3–27. New York: Plenum.

Prochaska, J.O., DiClemente, C.C., Velicer, W., Ginpil, S. & Norcross, J.C. (1985). Predicting change in smoking status for self-changers. *Addictive Behaviors*, **10**, 395–406.

Prochaska, J.O., Velicer, W., DiClemente, C.C. & Fava, J. (1988). Measuring processes of change: applications to the cessation of smoking. *Journal of Consulting and Clinical Psychology*, **56**, 520–8.

Prochaska, J.O., Velicer, W., Guadagnoli, E., Rossi, J.S. & DiClemente, C.C. (1991). Patterns of change: dynamic typology applied to smoking cessation. *Multivariate Behavioral Research*, **26**, 83–107.

Prochaska, J.O., DiClemente, C.C. & Norcross, J.C. (1992). In search of how people change: applications to addictive behaviors. *American Psychologist*, **7**, 1102–14.

Prochaska, J.O., DiClemente, C.C., Velicer, W. & Rossi, J.S. (1993). Standardized, individualized, interactive, and personalized self-help programs for smoking cessation. *Health Psychology*, **12**, 399–405.

Sutton, S.R. (1996). Can 'stages of change' provide guidance in the treatment of addictions? A critical examination of Prochaska and DiClemente's model. In G. Edwards & C. Dare (Eds.). *Psychotherapy, psychological treatments, and the addictions*, pp.189–205, Cambridge: Cambridge University Press.

Sutton, S.R., Marsh, A. & Matheson, J. (1987). Explaining smokers' decisions to stop: test of an expectancy-value approach. *Social Behaviour*, **2**, 35–49.

Velicer, W., Prochaska, J.O., Bellis, J.M., DiClemente, C.C., Rossi, J.S., Fava, J.L. & Steiger, J.H. (1993). An expert system intervention for smoking cessation. *Addictive Behaviors*, **18**, 269–90.

Type A behaviour, hostility and coronary artery disease

WILLEM J. KOP
and
DAVID S. KRANTZ

The Department of Medical and Clinical Psychology, Uniformed Services University of the Health Sciences, Bethesda, USA

ORIGINS AND EARLY RESEARCH

In the late 1950s, cardiologists Friedman and Rosenman initiated systematic research on a behaviour pattern that appeared to be related to increased risk of myocardial infarction. This behaviour was labelled the Type A Behaviour Pattern (TABP) and was defined as:

> ... *an action-emotion complex that can be observed in any person who is aggressively involved in a chronic, incessant struggle to achieve more and more in less and less time, and if required to do so, against the opposing efforts of other things or persons*, ...

(Friedman & Rosenman, 1959). In other words, Type A behaviour is characterized by: an excessive competitive drive, impatience, hostility, and vigorous speech characteristics. The complement of TABP was called Type B behaviour and was described as the relative absence of Type A characteristics. A Structured Interview (SI) was developed to assess Type A behaviour. In the SI, the subject is interrupted and challenged by the interviewer to evoke behavioural responses such as vigorous speech and competition of control over

the interview. Apart from the behavioural observations, the SI also allows for a content analysis of the answers. Since the clinical assessment of subjects' behaviours is an essential part of this technique, special training is required to administer and score the SI. As an alternative assessment procedure, several self-administered questionnaires have been developed (e.g. the Jenkins Activity Survey (JAS: Jenkins, Zyzanski & Rosenman, 1971), and the Bortner Type A scale (Bortner, 1969)). Because Type A questionnaires rely solely on self-report, only modest correlations are observed between the SI and self-report questionnaires.

The early reports of Friedman, Rosenman and co-workers have resulted in numerous epidemiological and experimental investigations on the relationship between TABP and manifestations of coronary artery disease. In the 1960s and 1970s, most epidemiological studies supported the association between TABP and risk of future coronary artery disease (CAD) in men and women. The magnitude of these associations was comparable to that of traditional risk factors for CAD and also independent of these factors, such as hypertension, and elevated cholesterol levels. One major study in this area was the Western Collaborative Group Study (WCGS) in which 3200 males were followed up for 8.5 years (Rosenman *et al.*, 1975). It was observed that individuals with Type A behaviour were more than twice as likely to suffer coronary disease than their Type B counterparts. Another important study was the Framingham Heart Study (Haynes, Feinleib & Kannel, 1980). Type A behaviour was found to be predictive of CAD in white-collar professioned men and in women working outside the home. These findings led a review committee of the National Heart Lung and Blood Institute to construe that Type A behaviour was a risk factor for CAD in middle-aged US citizens (1981). Later studies, however, have failed to show an association between TABP and clinical coronary disease (for review, see Matthews & Haynes, 1986).

EQUIVOCAL RESULTS OBTAINED IN TYPE A BEHAVIOUR RESEARCH

The Multiple Risk Factor Intervention Trial (MRFIT) and a subsequent longer follow-up analysis of the WCGS revealed the most compelling evidence against the association between TABP and subsequent manifestations of CAD. In the MRFIT study (Shekelle *et al.*, 1985), both the SI and the JAS were administered in high risk men, and neither was associated with future cardiac disease. Ragland and Brand (1988) reported on the recurrence of myocardial infarction in men who participated in the WCGS and who survived their first myocardial infarction. Unexpectedly, Type A behaviour was found to be protective in this sample. Thus, the predictive value of Type A behaviour in populations with elevated risk of coronary disease remains controversial. Furthermore, since 1979, virtually no positive reports have been published that support the relationship between questionnaire-assessed Type A behaviour and CAD.

Is this to say that Type A behaviour is no longer an important construct for cardiovascular health? The answer to this question is 'no' for several reasons. First, one must consider methodological issues in the interpretation of the studies with negative findings. Studies that revealed negative findings regarding TABP and prediction of future cardiac disease investigated 'high-risk' populations. Because Type A behaviour may be related to the presence and persistence of several coronary risk factors and adverse health behaviour (e.g. smoking, unhealthy diet, etc.), this may attenuate the observed association between TABP and cardiac disease in high risk populations. In addition, several negative studies included patients who participated in treatment trials (either drugs or behaviour modification), which may have biased recruitment and reduced the magnitude of the associations observed between TABP and cardiac disease. Moreover, TABP may be associated with specific non-survival of first cardiac events. That is, Type A persons who suffer their first myocardial infarction may be less likely to survive this incident than Type Bs. If this is correct, then study samples that are limited to survivors of myocardial infarction do not include the high risk Type A individuals.

HOSTILITY AS TOXIC COMPONENT OF TYPE A BEHAVIOUR

Research findings have accumulated that underline the importance of hostility as a risk factor for CAD (e.g. Helmer, Ragland & Syme, 1991). Like Type A behaviour, hostility is defined as a psychological *trait*. Hostility is characterized by a negative attitudinal set, a cynical view of the world, an antagonistic style, and the presence of negative expectations as to the intentions of other people (Siegman & Smith, 1994). The attitudinal trait of hostility is distinct from anger, which is an emotional *state* and often leads to aggressive behaviour. Type A behaviour and hostility relate to anger in the sense that thus affected individuals experience an elevated number of episodes of anger. Therefore, Type A behaviour hostility, and anger share common characteristics, but they also are independent to a considerable degree.

Hostility is most commonly assessed with the Cook–Medley Hostility Inventory (a self-report questionnaire; Cook & Medley, 1954), or alternatively with the Structured Interview initially developed to assess Type A behaviour. The Cook–Medley scale is a 50-item questionnaire derived from the Minnesota Multiphasic Personality Inventory. Many studies show that the two measures of hostility share some common variance, but classifications of individuals may vary considerably. This is, again, likely caused by the fact that the SI classification is dependent on behavioural observations such as speech characteristics, whereas the Cook–Medley depends on self-reports of a cynical or a hostile demeanor. Several papers report on subfactors that may comprise the Cook-Medley questionnaire, of which 'cynicism', 'aggressive responding', and 'hostile affect' appear to have the strongest relationships with CAD. Also, other questionnaires are available to assess hostility (e.g. the Buss–Durkee Hostility Scale). In sum, hostility is considered to be a psychological trait that can be assessed by either the Cook–Medley questionnaire or Structured Interview.

It is conceivable that the consequences of a chronic hostile attitude are not limited to physiological changes that make individuals more prone to develop coronary disease. Hostility also appears to have psychological repercussions. Glass (1977) proposed a psychological model in which Type A individuals were hypothesized to experience a state of frustration and exhaustion, a 'prodromal depression', preceding myocardial infarction. The basic assertion was that Type A individuals exert intense efforts to control stressful events. These active coping attempts eventually extinguish and lead to frustration and psychic exhaustion. This notion provides a model accounting for why Type A behaviour and hostility may interact with constructs such as Depression and Vital Exhaustion, which also are factors that may affect the progression of coronary artery disease (Carney *et al.*, 1988; Kop *et al.*, 1994). It may be that there is more to the coronary prone hostile personality than a simple antagonistic and offensive basic attitude; other psychological factors such as insecurity and a lack of reliable emotional bonds may drive this overt behavioural style (Siegman & Smith, 1994).

TYPE A BEHAVIOUR AND HOSTILITY AS RELATED TO CORONARY DISEASE

Measures of hostility derived from the Structured Interview have been shown to be predictive of severity of coronary artery disease in samples where global Type A behaviour was not similarly predictive (Dembroski *et al.*, 1989). On the other hand, the Cook–Medley questionnaire does not unequivocally predict severity of CAD (see Siegman & Smith, 1994). One study (Siegman, Dembroski of Ringel, 1987) suggests the particular importance of the behavioural manifestation of hostility in the relationship with CAD severity.

Several longitudinal studies have addressed the predictive value of hostility in the development of clinical manifestations of CAD. SI-assessed hostility predicts cardiac events in initially healthy subjects and in patients at high risk of coronary disease who were participants in the Recurrent Coronary Prevention Project (RCPP; Friedman *et al.*, 1986) and the MRFIT (Dembroski *et al.*, 1989). On the other hand, the Cook–Medley questionnaire has yielded mixed results in follow-up studies of healthy individuals. This may partially be due to particular circumstances in which subjects completed the inventories (often as part of a job or university selection procedure), and the use of very long follow-up durations (often more than 20 years).

Apparently, the behavioural component of hostility, which is more likely to be detected by the SI, is an essential feature in the elevated risk of cardiac end-points (Helmer *et al.* in Siegman & Smith, 1994). It is noteworthy that both cross-sectional studies and longitudinal studies support the notion that the relationship between hostility and coronary artery disease is most evident among individuals younger than 60 years of age. This may be due to the fact that younger hostile persons encounter provocative situations more often.

PSYCHOBIOLOGICAL MECHANISMS

Psychological stressors result in elevations in heart rate, blood pressure, increases in blood-lipids and catecholamines, and also in platelet activity and blood clotting factors. The predominant mechanism suggested to explain associations between hostility and coronary disease proposes an increased physiological response to environmental stressors among hostile individuals (Williams *et al.*, 1991; Krantz *et al.*, 1988).

High blood pressure may promote damage to the coronary vessel wall, especially at sites where turbulence in coronary blood flow exists (e.g. branching points). In the setting of this mild coronary injury, deposition of lipids may occur which further enhances vascular damage. The progression of coronary atherosclerosis is determined by an intermittent process of blood clot formation and degradation that may finally develop into coronary obstruction and, consequently, clinical manifestations of coronary disease. This suggests that psychological stress may affect different biological processes at different disease stages.

In a series of animal studies by Kaplan, Manuck, and colleagues, it was found that high dominant male monkeys (macaques) in socially unstable circumstances showed more coronary atherosclerosis at necropsy (Kaplan *et al.*, 1982). In other studies, this research group established that individual differences in the consequences of aggressive behaviour can be explained in part by the psychosocial context in which these behaviours are displayed.

As for Type A behaviour and hostility in humans, several reports support the contention that psychobiological over-reactivity is characteristic of hostile individuals, particularly when these individuals are exposed to situations that elicit hostile behaviour. Thus, prolonged exposure to elevated responses to stress in blood pressure, heart rate, catecholamines and blood clotting factors may account for the elevated risk of disease progression in hostile individuals.

MODIFICATION OF HOSTILITY

Several studies have reported positive effects of behaviour modification in patients with cardiovascular disease. The majority of these studies have been directed at reducing Type A behaviour. Because hostility appears to be a significant feature of Type A, these studies are applicable to strategies aiming at modifying hostility. Hostile persons are more likely to encounter stressful situations, which increases the prevalence of angry experiences. In addition, hostile persons do typically not have the advantage of stress-decreasing resources such as social support, which is partly due to the antagonistic behaviour that hostility portrays. Thus, hostile persons may be more prone to develop coronary disease both because of an overall increased reactivity and because of a more frequent exposure to conditions in which anger occurs. In general, intervention studies indicate that control over angry emotional experiences can be enhanced by 'behavioural' approaches (e.g. addressing issues such as patience when driving, taking sufficient time for the daily meals), whereas the hostile attitude might be altered using 'cognitive' strategies (i.e. managing unreasonable expectations and ideas).

In general, hostility intervention groups are conducted in a group setting consisting of ± 10 participants. First, an attempt is made to gain insight into the triggers of angry incidents. Usually, participants are asked to self-monitor their behaviour to determine the circumstances in which irritation occurs. Secondly, new strategies to cope with aggravating situations are introduced, such as learning to voluntarily insert a delay between the provoking incident and the reaction to it. At later stages of the intervention, a more cognitive approach is followed, where unrealistic beliefs and expectations are addressed. This may eventually result in opportunities to address provoking situations in a 'problem solving' way.

The efficacy of these interventions is supported in a number of studies. For example, in the RCPP, the number of reappearing myocardial infarctions was significantly lower in patients who received Type A intervention (7.2% versus 13.2%, during 3 years of follow-up; Friedman *et al.*, 1986). A substantial decrease in Type A behaviour occurred far more often in a Type A treatment group than in a control group. Moreover, patients who were successful in considerably decreasing their Type A behaviour, suffered a re-infarction four times less than those who failed to do so.

These results indicate that psychological interventions are capable of reducing antagonistic behaviour patterns, thereby leading to a reduction of cardiovascular risk. Further studies are needed to investigate the biological concomitants of hostility. For example, it has been suggested that a relative depletion of the neurotransmitter serotonin is characteristic of hostile individuals. On the other hand, this deficiency has been purported for numerous psychological abnormalities, of which depression is the most well established. It may be, however, that a combined behavioural and pharmacological approach proves to be successful in ameliorating hostility. Interventions that address hostility may enhance both the length and the quality of life in patients at risk of coronary disease. (See also 'Stress and disease'.)

ACKNOWLEDGEMENTS

Preparation of this paper was supported by USUHS Protocol R07233, and a grant from the NIH (HL47337). The opinions and assertions expressed herein are those of the authors and should not be construed as reflecting those of the USUHS or of the Department of Defense.

REFERENCES

Bortner, R. (1969) A short rating scale as a potential measure of pattern A behavior. *Journal of Chronic Diseases*, **22**, 87–91.

Buss, A.H. & Durkee, A. (1989). An inventory for assessing different kinds of hostility. *Journal of Counseling Psychology*, **21**, 343–9.

Carney, R., Rich, M., Freedland, K., Saini, J., te Velde, A., Simeone, C. & Clark, K. (1988). Major depressive disorder predicts cardiac events in patients with coronary heart disease. *Psychosomatic Medicine*, **50**, 627–33.

Cook, W.W. & Medley, D.M. (1954) Proposed hostility and pharisaic-virtue scales for the MMPI. *Journal of Applied Psychology*, **38**, 414–18.

Dembroski, T., MacDougall, J., Costa, P. & Grandits, G. (1989) Components of hostility as predictors of sudden death and myocardial infarction in the Multiple Risk Factor Intervention Trial. *Psychosomatic Medicine*, **51**, 514–22.

Engebertson, T.O. & Matthews, K.A. (1992) Dimensions of hostility in men, women, and boys: Relationships to personality and cardiovascular response to stress. *Psychosomatic Medicine*, **54**, 311–23.

Friedman, M. & Rosenman, R. (1959) Associations of specific overt behavior pattern with blood and cardiovascular findings: blood cholesterol level, blood clotting time, incidence of arcis senilis and clinical coronary artery disease. *Journal of the American Medical Association*, **169**, 1286–96.

Friedman, M., Thoresen, C.M., Gill, J.J. *et al.* (1986) Alteration of Type A behavior and its effect on cardiac reoccurrence in post myocardial infarction patients: summary results of the recurrent coronary prevention project. *American Heart Journal*, **112**, 653–65.

Glass, D.C. (1977). *Behavior pattern, stress and coronary disease*. Hillsdale: Lawrence Erlbaum.

Haynes, S.G., Feinleib, M. & Kannel, W.B. (1980). The relationship of psychosocial factors to coronary heart disease in the Framingham study, III; eight year incidence of coronary heart disease. *American Journal of Epidemiology*, **3**, 37–58.

Helmer, D.C., Ragland, D.R. & Syme, S.L. (1991). Hostility and coronary artery disease. *American Journal of Epidemiology*, **133**, 112–22.

Jenkins, C.D., Zyzanski, S.J. & Rosenman, R.H. (1971). Progress towards validation of a computer-scored test for the Type A coronary-prone behavior pattern. *Psychosomatic Medicine*, **33**, 193–202.

Kaplan, J.R., Manuck, S.B., Clarkson, T.B., Lusso, F.M. & Taub, D.R. (1982). Social status, environment and atherosclerosis in cynomolgus macaques. *Arteriosclerosis*, **2**, 359–68.

Kop, W.J., Appels, A.P.W.M., Mendes de Leon, C.F., de Swart, H.B. & Bär, F.W. (1994). Vital exhaustion predicts new cardiac events after successful coronary angioplasty. *Psychosomatic Medicine*, **56**, 281–7.

Krantz, D.S., Contrada, R.J., Hill, D.R. & Friedler, E. (1988). Environmental stress and biobehavioral antecedents of coronary heart disease. *Journal of Counseling and Clinical Psychology*, **56**, 333–41.

Matthews, K.A. & Haynes, S.G. (1986). Type A behavior pattern and coronary disease risk; update and critical evaluation. *American Journal of Epidemiology*, **123**, 923–60.

Ragland, D.R. & Brand, R.J. (1988). Type A behavior and mortality from coronary heart disease. *New England Journal of Medicine*, **318**, 65–9.

Review Panel. (1981) Coronary-prone behavior and coronary heart disease; a critical review. *Circulation*, **63**, 1199–215.

Rosenman, R.H., Brand, R.J., Jenkins, C.D., Friedman, M., Straus, R. & Wurm, M. (1975). Coronary heart disease in the Western Collaborative Group Study; follow-up experience after 8½ years. *Journal of the American Medical Association*, **233**, 872–7.

Shekelle, R.B., Hulley, S.B., Neaton, J., Billings, J., Borhani, N., Gerace, T., Jacobs, D., Lasser, N., Mittlemark, M. & Stamler, J. (1985). The MRFIT behavioral pattern study II; type A behavior pattern and risk of coronary death in MRFIT. *American Journal of Epidemiology*, **112**, 559–70.

Siegman, A.W., Dembroski, T.M. & Ringel, N. (1987) Components of hostility and the severity of coronary artery disease. *Psychosomatic Medicine*, **49**, 127–35.

Siegman, A.W. & Smith, T.W. (1994) *Anger, hostility and the heart*. Hillsdale NJ: Lawrence Erlbaum.

Smith, T.W. (1992). Hostility and health; current status of a psychosomatic hypothesis. *Health Psychology*, **11**, 139–50.

Williams, R.B., Suarez, E.C., Kuhn, C.M., Zimmerman, E.A. & Schanberg, S.M. (1991) Biobehavioral basis of coronary prone behavior in middle aged men; part 1, evidence for chronic SNS activation in Type As. *Psychosomatic Medicine*, **53**, 517–27.

Unemployment and health

STANISLAV V. KASL

Department of Epidemiology,
Yale University School of Medicine,
Connecticut, USA

INTRODUCTION

By far the most dominant methodological issue in unemployment research centres on the distinction between causation and selection. Does the observation of poorer physical and/or mental health reflect the impact of unemployment or does it, instead, denote the influence of prior characteristics of the individuals who later become unemployed. The latter alternative, biased selection into exposure status, could reflect either: (a) the direct influence of health status, i.e. persons with poorer health are more likely to become unemployed, or (b) indirect influence of characteristics, such as disadvantaged social status and unstable occupational career, which lead both to greater likelihood of unemployment and of poorer health status. The interpretive dilemma, causation vs. selection, also applies to studies in which the independent (exposure) variable is either length of unemployment or the contrast between re-employed vs. continued unemployment. The poorer health of those with prolonged unemployment could again be either because this reflects a higher dose of the exposure variable, or because those with prior poorer health have a lower chance of being re-employed.

Since studies of the impact of unemployment on health are based on a variety of observational (non-experimental) designs, the absence of experimental control (i.e. random assignment) to exposure status, employed vs. unemployed, precludes a definitive answer to the causation vs. selection dilemma. The strong observational designs have included: (a) studies of factory closures in which all employees lose their jobs and are then followed for health status changes (Morris & Cook, 1991); (b) longitudinal follow-up studies of employed and unemployed individuals on whom baseline health status data allow for statistical adjustments of possible selection biases (e.g. Morris, Cook & Shaper, 1994); and (c) follow-up studies of unemployed individuals in which the benefits of re-employment can be examined and adjusted for selection biases. Weak designs have included: (a) longitudinal follow-ups of employed and unemployed persons on whom baseline data are too limited (e.g. age and education only) to adequately control for selection factors; and (b) cross-sectional comparisons in which selection factors cannot be easily separated from causation. Retrospective accounts of reasons for job loss (i.e. whether or not it is health-related) allow for some control of selection biases, but their adequacy is difficult to assess.

It is necessary to mention one additional approach which has a long history in unemployment research (see Kasl, 1982); analysis of aggregate ('ecologic' or 'macroeconomic') data in which annual fluctuations in some economic indicator, often the nationwide percentage of the labour force that is unemployed, are related to annual changes in some outcome, such as total mortality, cause-specific mortality, alcohol consumption, and acts of domestic violence (e.g. Brenner, 1987). These business cycle analyses are currently seen as highly problematic and controversial, often involving data analyses which are difficult to follow and understand (Dooley & Catalano, 1988). Consequently, many authors feel that they do not have sufficient grounds either to dismiss the methodology, or to trust it and accept the findings.

It is also important to realize that the experience of job loss and unemployment is likely to be multifaceted and thus the results can be complex, especially when one is also trying to study intervening processes and moderating influences. For example, Jahoda (1979) suggests that a job, aside from meeting economic needs, has additional 'latent functions': (a) imposes time structure on the day; (b) implies regularly shared experiences and contacts with others; (c) links an individual to goals and purposes which transcend his/her own; (d) defines aspects of personal status and identity; (e) enforces activity. At minimum, we should try to distinguish the effects of economic hardships in unemployment from the noneconomic effects of being without a job. We must also remember that, for some individuals, job loss may represent the termination of exposures, such as work stress or specific work hazards, which themselves may have been adverse influences on health while employed.

IMPACT ON MORTALITY AND MORBIDITY

There are about five to six epidemiologic studies which have examined the relationship between unemployment and mortality during the last decade. Studies using data for Great Britain, Sweden, Finland, Denmark, and Italy are in agreement in demonstrating an excess mortality associated with unemployment. The excess may be as high as 50%–100%, but is reduced to about 20%–30% by adjustments for confounders which reflect pre-existing characteristics. When those who became unemployed for health reasons are excluded, aspects of social class are stronger confounders than baseline health (usually assessed with limited data) and lifestyle habits. Men and women appear to show comparable impact, as do wives of unemployed men. Younger persons seem to be at risk for greater impact, while occupational groupings do not suggest much variation in impact. Cause-specific analyses suggest that suicides, accidents, violent deaths and alcohol-related deaths tend to be especially elevated, but do not explain all of the excess mortality.

It is noteworthy that the one study which used US data but otherwise similar methodology (Sorlie & Rogot, 1990), failed to detect any impact of unemployment on mortality. This discrepancy with the European data is not easily explained, particularly since it is believed that the 'social net' protecting the unemployed is stronger in these European countries than in the US.

Overall, the conclusion that unemployment increases the risk of total mortality is prudent but not unassailable. Selection factors are clearly present as contributory influences, and fully controlling for them has not yet been possible.

Studies of unemployment and morbidity introduce potentially a new concern not applicable to mortality studies: the procedure for measuring health status outcomes. There are at least two concerns: (i) The influence of psychological distress on some measures could be substantial: that is, measured physical symptoms and complaints could be due to the distress rather than some underlying physical condition, or psychological distress could lower the threshold for reporting existing physical symptoms. (ii) Measures based on seeking and/or receiving care could indicate differences in illness behaviour rather than underlying illness. In addition, it may be occasionally simply too difficult to determine what is being measured. Thus in a nicely designed prospective study of closure of a sardine factory in Norway (Westin, 1990), the rates of disability pension observed over a 10-year follow-up period were higher, compared to rates at a nearby 'sister factory' which didn't close. While these pensions are 'granted for medical conditions only', it is still difficult to know what exactly is being assessed and what health status differences would have been observed with other types of measurements.

There is reasonable agreement from several longitudinal studies that the job loss experience has a negative impact on health, though the precise nature of this impact is difficult to pinpoint. For example, in a Canadian study of GE factory closure (Grayson, 1989), former employees reported on a survey a high number of ailments. However, the elevated rates were for such a wide range of conditions that the authors suggested that the results indicate higher levels of stress which produce 'a series of symptoms that people mistake for illness itself'. A British study of factory closure examined the impact on general practice consultation rates (Beale & Nethercott, 1988). Comparisons of rates were made both before vs. after factory closure as well as changes over time among cases vs.

controls. The factory closure was clearly associated with increased rates of consultation, referrals, and visits to the hospital. More refined analyses revealed that illnesses which were indicative of relatively 'chronic' conditions (i.e. those with previous high rates of consulting) were the ones which showed the increase. Thus it is not clear if these conditions were exacerbated by the factory closure, or if there was simply an increased rate of consulting, without any underlying clinical changes.

A number of other reports, based both on longitudinal and cross-sectional data, offer confirmatory evidence regarding an adverse impact of unemployment on morbidity. The range of outcome variables is quite wide: hospital admissions, medical consultations, use of prescribed drugs, reports of chronic conditions, disability days, activity limitations, and somatic symptoms. The difficulty is that these studies typically show a selected impact rather than a uniform one across all indices examined, and little consistency emerges when one tries to identify those variables which are particularly sensitive to the experience across studies. And, at present, it is not possible to offer any convincing explanations of the variability in results, such as that it is due to the differential cost sensitivity of the indirect health status indicators across different study samples.

IMPACT ON BIOLOGICAL AND BEHAVIOURAL RISK FACTORS

The biological variables which have been examined in relation to unemployment include: (a) indicators of 'stress' reactivity, such as serum cortisol, which do not have a well-documented relationship to specific diseases; (b) a very diverse set of indicators of immune functioning which are linked to possible disease outcomes theoretically rather than empirically; and (c) risk factors for specific diseases, typically cardiovascular disease, where the presumption is that a chronic impact on these due to unemployment translates into higher risk for clinical disease.

Studies using neuroendocrine variables or indicators of immune functioning find broad support for the conclusion that these biological parameters are sensitive to some aspect of the unemployment experience. Specifically, the findings strongly suggest the presence of anticipation effects (i.e. before job loss has taken place) and short-term elevations, but generally do not demonstrate the continuation of elevated levels with continuation of unemployment. It appears that these biological parameters are better suited for describing or detecting acute phases of reactivity rather than chronic effects suggestive of increased risk of future disease.

Investigations of cardiovascular risk factors in relation to unemployment reveal that the threat of unemployment (i.e. holding a job with an insecure future) may be associated with higher levels of risk factors, particularly total serum cholesterol and low density lipoproteins. Otherwise, the results suggest a pattern somewhat similar to the neuroendocrine findings. For example, analyses of blood pressure and serum cholesterol change from a Michigan study of plant closure (Kasl & Cobb, 1980) revealed a substantial sensitivity of these variables to the experience of anticipating the closing of the plant, losing the job, and going through a period of unemployment, and finding a new job. However, these were acute effects reflecting specific transitions. Men who continued to be unemployed did not stay at higher levels, but declined even in the absence of finding a new job. Two years after the event, the men had

'normal' blood pressure levels and somewhat below normal cholesterol levels.

There are also studies of very young adults and they suggest the possibility that cardiovascular risk factors may not be sensitive to unemployment in this age group. It is not clear, however, if this is an age effect *per se*, or if the unemployment experience so close to the end of formal schooling is different from unemployment later in the life cycle.

There are several reports which are concerned with the impact of unemployment on health habits and behavioural risk factors. The typical variables examined include cigarette smoking, alcohol consumption, body weight, and physical exercise. Cigarette smoking tends to be relatively stable, while body weight shows an impact in some studies (i.e. an increase) but not in others. Alcohol consumption has been of greatest interest, but the picture is distinctly a mixed one (e.g. Hammarstrom, 1994). On balance, the majority of studies fails to show an increase, though one well-designed longitudinal study showed an increase in the diagnosis of clinically significant alcohol abuse attributable to being laid off (Catalano *et al.*, 1993). That same study also showed that employed persons working in communities with high unemployment rates were at a reduced risk of becoming alcohol abusers. It is worth noting that the examined health habits are also likely to represent selection factors; that is, there is evidence that higher levels of smoking and heavy drinking will predict a greater likelihood of subsequent unemployment.

IMPACT ON MENTAL HEALTH AND WELL-BEING

There is little doubt that unemployment has a negative impact on mental health and well-being. (This statement does not preclude or pre-empt a second conclusion, namely that selection dynamics are likely to play a role as well.) However, moving beyond this broad generalization, in order to formulate additional more specific conclusions, becomes difficult because the evidence is less consistent and/or less complete.

Longitudinal studies strongly support the expectation that unemployment will have an adverse impact on subclinical symptomatology or symptoms of poor mental health (e.g. Warr, Jackson & Banks, 1988); it is unlikely that the impact is also on overt diagnosable clinical disorder. Longitudinal studies also generally (but not always) demonstrate that becoming re-employed is associated with a reduction in symptomatology (e.g. Kessler, Turner & House, 1988; Warr *et al.*, 1988). In general, it would appear that depressive symptoms are the most sensitive indicators of impact of unemployment. However, because symptom checklists tend to be well intercorrelated, often similar findings are obtained with other scales such as anxiety or somatization (psychophysiological symptoms). Other impact has been described, such as lower self-confidence and higher externality (one's life is beyond one's control); self-esteem may be impacted only on items which reflect self-criticism (Warr *et al.*, 1988).

The considerable literature on the psychological impact of unemployment permits the following additional conclusions:

1. Findings on young adults generally show a similar negative impact but also point to the considerable importance of the nature of the first (or early job): symptoms of distress were

highest among dissatisfied workers, lowest among satisfied workers, with the unemployed at intermediate levels.

2. Evidence for possible gender differences in impact is inconclusive, but there is some suggestion that women may be less likely to benefit (i.e. reduction of symptoms) from the unemployment-to-re-employment transition than men. Among wives of husbands who have been laid off, symptoms do go up, but with some delay. Not surprisingly, we have no studies of impact of wives' layoff on husbands.

3. Evidence for rural – urban differences is limited but fairly suggestive: the impact on symptoms of distress may be weaker in the rural setting, but rural workers are more likely to miss aspects of work and work-linked activities (Kasl & Cobb, 1982).

4. The magnitude, duration, and time course of impact are not easily linked to duration of unemployment in the many studies, suggesting that adaptive processes may attenuate or alter the impact.

5. Financial difficulties and additional life events are two likely mediators of impact of unemployment on mental health.

6. Buffers which moderate the impact include high levels of social support, participation in social – leisure activities, absence of psychiatric history, and high sense of mastery and self-esteem. High work commitment aggravates the negative impact of becoming unemployed, but among those going from unemployment or re-employment, high work commitment enhances the degree of recovery.

ACKNOWLEDGEMENT

This review was facilitated by a grant from the American Industrial Health Council.

REFERENCES

Beale, N. & Nethercott S. (1988). The nature of unemployment morbidity. 2. Description. *Journal of the Royal College of General Practitioners*, **38**, 200–2.

Brenner, M.H. (1987). Economic change, alcohol consumption, and heart disease mortality in nine industrialized countries. *Social Science and Medicine*, **25**, 119–32.

Catalano, R., Dooley, D., Wilson, G. & Hough, R. (1993). Job loss and alcohol abuse: a test using data from the Epidemiologic Catchment Area Project. *Journal of Health Social Behavior*, **34**, 215–25.

Dooley, D. & Catalano, R. (1988). Recent research on psychological effects of unemployment. *Journal of Social Issues*, **44**, 1–12.

Grayson, J.P. (1989). Reported illness after CGE closure. *Canadian Journal of Public Health*, **80**, 16–19.

Hammarstrom, A. (1994). Health consequences of youth unemployment-review from a gender perspective. *Social Science and Medicine*, **38**, 699–709.

Jahoda, M. (1979). The impact of unemployment in the 1930s and the 1970s. *Bulletin of the British Psychological Society*, **32**, 309–14.

Kasl, S.V. (1982). Strategies of research on economic instability and health. *Psychological Medicine*, **12**, 637–49.

Kasl, S.V. & Cobb, S. (1980). The experience of losing a job. Some effects on cardiovascular functioning. *Psychotherapy and Psychosomatics*, **34**, 88–109.

Kasl, S.V. & Cobb, S. (1982). Variability of stress effects among men experiencing job loss. In L. Goldberger & S. Breznitz (Eds.). *Handbook of stress*, pp. 445–465. New York: The Free Press.

Kessler, R.C., Turner, J.B. & House, J.S. (1988). Effects of unemployment on health in a community survey: main, modifying, and mediating effects. *Journal of Social Issues*, **44**, 69–85.

Morris, J.K. & Cook, D.G. (1991). A critical review of the effect of factory closures on health. *British Journal of Industrial Medicine*, **48**, 1–8.

Morris, J.K., Cook, D.G. & Shaper, A.G. (1994). Loss of employment and mortality. *British Medical Journal*, **308**, 1135–9.

Sorlie, P.D. & Rogot, E. (1990). Mortality by employment status in the National Longitudinal Mortality Study. *American Journal of Epidemiology*, **132**, 983–92.

Warr, P., Jackson, P. & Banks, M. (1988). Unemployment and mental health: some British studies. *Journal of Social Issues*, **44**, 47–68.

Westin, S. (1990). The structure of a factory closure: individual responses to job-loss and unemployment in a 10-year controlled follow-up study. *Social Science and Medicine*, **31**, 1301–11.

Weight control

VIVIEN J. LEWIS

Psychology Service, Shelton Hospital, Bicton Heath, Shrewsbury, Shropshire, UK

PSYCHOLOGICAL CONSEQUENCES OF OVERWEIGHT

One of the strongest and most frequent of the concerns about health among the general public in western societies over recent years has been to eat and drink in a way that seeks to attain or maintain a slim body shape. Such uses of foods and beverages are popularly known as 'dieting'. Whether slimming or weight loss is desired because of health considerations or sociocultural ideals, it provides one of the most powerful motivations for dietary change in people not suffering from specific health disorders such as renal disorders, diabetes and coronary heart disease.

More than 50% of women and an increasing number of men in

the UK diet in an attempt to lose weight (and maintain that loss) at least once in their lives, but very few achieve and maintain their desired body weight. Nevertheless, the consequences of excess body weight for morbidity are well documented. Epidemiological evidence and indications from clinical science point to excessive fat deposition in the abdominal region as a sign of risks to the cardiovascular system, as well as for diabetes and certain cancers (Garrow, 1988). However, the psychological effects of overweight or, indeed, perceived overweight, as well as repeated fluctuations in body weight, are far more complex.

Arising from the seminal work of Herman and his colleagues in the early 1970s, a growing body of research has confirmed an association between dieting and a tangle of worries about eating and body weight such that, if restricted food intake breaks down into a 'binge', variations in body weight ensue. 'Dietary restraint' is unlikely to be a unitary personal trait, but rather a 'dieter' may select cyclically, occasionally or persistently from the variety of eating habits, beliefs, values and emotions perceived as options within the informal institution of 'dieting' (Booth, Lewis & Blair, 1990). Anecdotal clinical experiences of associations between both actual and perceived overweight and depressive episodes, if not actual depression *per se*, have been confirmed by recent research. Emotional eating has been found to be positively correlated with Body Mass Index (Wardle, 1987) and also to interfere with attempts to reduce body weight (Blair, Lewis & Booth, 1990).

The distinction between actual and perceived overweight is not an arbitrary one. For a substantial number of individuals in the general population as well as those presenting at the health professional's clinic stating that they wish to lose weight, current body weight falls within the desired range for their age and height, and they have no weight-associated health disorder. Indeed, a significant proportion of women are dissatisfied with what is, in fact, a healthy weight, and aspire to body weights as much as 9% lower than those which are recommended in published tables of 'ideal weights' (Lewis, 1991). Thus individuals become dissatisfied with their physical appearance, prompting dieting behaviour which is generally ineffective and may develop into a long-term preoccupation. Dysfunctional behaviour, thoughts and emotions regarding body shape and weight control therefore occur widely among those who feel fat as well as those who are actually obese. Some argue that dieting to control body weight may have a causal role in the onset of both anorexia nervosa and bulimia nervosa (Lewis & Blair, 1991).

Social messages and stereotypes portray individuals who are overweight, to a greater or lesser degree, with negative attributes such as being weak, out of control and undesirable (Wadden & Stunkard, 1985). Together with negative emotional consequences of overweight and repeated attempts to lose body weight, individuals experience a significant reduction in general self-esteem and low confidence in ability to control weight.

SOCIAL–PSYCHOLOGICAL INFLUENCES ON BODY WEIGHT CONTROL

In recent years there has been an increasing emphasis in western cultures on the positive attributes of slender and healthy bodies, in particular for women (Wooley & Wooley, 1984). This 'culture of slenderness' is increasingly well documented, and rooted in an his-

torical context where a woman's physical appearance has previously acted as an object representing a husband or father's status and is still ascribed social value through the 'public gaze' (see Lewis & Blair, 1993). Thus overweight is perceived as deviance from the currently prescribed sociocultural norm, with the negative attributions which have already been mentioned.

Within this context of prescribed slenderness and healthfulness, the pressures for women to attain and maintain a slim body shape and, increasingly, for men to attain healthy muscularity, conflict in relatively affluent societies with a comparative abundance of easy-to-prepare and densely calorific foods. Furthermore, for women, traditional roles of mothering and the purchase, preparation and provision of food create situations in which they feel required to cater for others, while at the same time denying themselves. More widely, contradictory pressures on women as 'passive–dependent' and 'assertive–independent' create scenarios wherein emotional eating, often in secret, is the sole source of emotional nurturance.

The concept of dieting, therefore, is often imbued into the young child at an early age. The child experiences peer pressure to conform to the 'ideal body shape' and may witness the mother restricting her food intake. Children themselves are often 'put on a diet' at an early age, and children as young as 11 years old report significant levels of body shape dissatisfaction (Salmons *et al.*, 1988). The context, therefore, for weight control is one in which some individuals inaccurately perceive themselves as overweight and others maintain a genuinely unhealthy degree of overweight.

PSYCHOLOGICAL INTERVENTIONS FOR WEIGHT CONTROL

An effective conception of weight control has to work within the facts of physics: except for transient water losses, weight loss requires a period of negative energy balance and the maintenance of that loss requires the avoidance subsequently of any running-average positive energy balance. For anybody, an appropriate level of exercise is worth attaining and maintaining. However, the greatest scope for achieving negative energy balance is a reduction in energy intake relative to that individual's own intake when gaining weight or maintaining overweight. In addition, there may be changes in lifestyle that are necessary over and above whatever can be done about energy expenditure. The thermodynamics of dieting therefore requires the learning of dietary habits and preferences likely to result in lower energy intake together with the monitoring of their impact on body weight over time in the particular individual. 'Success' is eating sufficiently less to move towards a healthy weight, however slowly. 'Failure' is either never eating that much less, stopping eating that much less too soon, eating that much less for too long, or alternating eating much less with eating much more.

The physics of weight control is straightforward, but the sociology, psychology and physiology of weight control and dietary behaviour generally are far more complex. Although often effective in the short term, all current interventions for weight control, including surgical, pharmacological and psychological have proved to be relatively ineffective in long-term maintenance of reduced body weight. Major reasons for this comparative lack of success may be failure to enable the individual overweight person to deal with emotional problems about body shape, an individual's low confidence in ability to control weight, and lack of attention to the complex array of associated psychological factors.

At this point in time, the psychological interventions which have offered the most promise for weight control, both in terms of loss of body weight and maintenance of that loss, have been the cognitive–behavioural therapies. Individuals' confidence that they can act in a desired way has been found to be predictive of success in changing behaviour relevant to health and, in the particular case of weight control, higher initial self-efficacy has been found to be positively related to weight loss (Edell *et al.*, 1987). Thus more successful interventions have aimed to empower individuals to determine their own balance of values between appearance and health and, where then appropriate, to choose sustainable habits of eating and exercise that can contribute substantially to negative energy balance and to avoid situations that undermine intentions to attain target weight (Lewis, Blair & Booth, 1992).

In the last two decades, a variety of behavioural, cognitive and cognitive–behavioural techniques have been applied to interventions for weight control. These have included, for example, systematic desensitization, aversive conditioning, modelling, behavioural rehearsal, assertion training and cognitive restructuring. The premise which underlies most of these interventions is that, for weight loss and the maintenance of that loss to occur, the eating habits of the individuals concerned need to be modified on a permanent basis. Although behavioural interventions have been shown to have some success in terms of initial weight loss in both adults and children, behaviour therapies in isolation have so far tended to be relatively ineffective in facilitating long-term weight loss. For example, Stalonas, Perri and Kerzner (1984) found that, 5 years after participating in a behavioural programme, clients reported being slightly heavier on average than they were before the programme.

Stunkard (1987) has proposed that the effectiveness of psychological therapies for weight control could be improved by the inclusion of contracts involving monetary or material penalties for non-attendance, poor weight loss or poor maintenance. However, incentives might be of benefit only while they are present such that subsequent maintenance of weight loss could be poor, unless permanently sustainable changes in intake behaviour, exercise or thermogenesis had been initiated. Indeed, largely extrinsic material and social motivations could reveal deficiencies in intrinsic motivation for effective and enduring weight-reducing and loss-maintaining behaviour.

Most of these approaches take the form of 'packages', comprising some of various behavioural and cognitive techniques such as self-monitoring of food intake, reinforcement and contingency management, avoiding discriminative stimuli for eating, changing responses to stressful situations, nutrition education, cognitive restructuring and physical activity (Stunkard, 1987). However, this necessarily makes it difficult to establish which techniques have been most effective in terms of promoting and maintaining weight loss (Bennett, 1987).

There are many problems attached to the evaluation of behavioural and cognitive interventions for weight control. For example, there is a considerable degree of variability in the amounts of weight lost between individuals in the same treatment programmes. This could reflect that different components of the treatment packages are differentially effective for different individuals. If so, then generalized packages cannot account for a necessary personalization of intervention strategies, and obesity in different individuals may be caused and maintained by different factors.

Losing weight produces little (if any) benefit unless that weight loss is maintained. Often, while treatment weight losses are fairly well maintained, target weights are not achieved since weight loss does not continue after treatment. Various factors may be involved in poor maintenance and continuation of weight loss, such as compensatory metabolic changes, the abandoning of techniques advocated during treatment, and the non-acquisition of skills required to cope with physical or psychological stressors inappropriately precipitating overeating episodes. If the latter is occurring, then dealing with stress by the use of alternative strategies which are more appropriate and incompatible with eating should promote self-control and prevent relapse.

The balance of evidence, to date, suggests that the most effective forms of cognitive-behavioural packages for weight control are those which do not necessarily focus on weight loss *per se*, but on encouraging self-efficacy in weight control and self-assertion in body image. The behavioural component of such packages informs both about the behaviour of dieting and also about dietary health-risk factors, including nutritional and dietary education as well as information about exercise, behavioural strategies and practical supports which have been found to be effective at facilitating permanent loss of body weight. The core cognitive elements adapt cognitive therapeutic approaches (Beck, 1976) to the moderation of dieting emotions, in particular, emotional overeating and binge-eating. In addition, cognitive strategies aim to increase personal effectiveness and might include assertion training, both with a generic orientation and also with a more specific focus on issues of food and body shape. Finally common reasons for dieting and attitudes to body shape and appearance are elucidated, with a view to enabling self-assertion against social pressures. Although the package is generalized, its effectiveness depends on the extent to which it can be personalized for each individual encountered (Lewis, Blair & Booth, 1992).

IMPLICATIONS FOR HEALTH CARE

Wooley and Wooley (1984) raised the question of whether obesity should be treated at all, and there are certainly a significant number of arguments that it should not. First, in many instances an individual's degree of overweight is not sufficient to provide a significant health risk, and it is rather the perception of overweight that is the central issue. Secondly, there is evidence that both anorexia nervosa and bulimia nervosa are associated with incidences of dieting, if not caused by dieting. Thirdly, the chances of attaining and maintaining a reduced body weight are still not clinically significant. Nevertheless, health professionals, self-help dieting groups and marketing strategists still promote weight control strategies and products without due consideration for their need and their potential effectiveness. In such cases, interventions might be better designed to aim for increased body shape satisfaction rather than body weight reduction.

However, there are a significant number of individuals for whom their excess body weight is a serious risk due to health concerns. It is encumbent then upon health professionals to reconceptualize 'treatment' for weight control. Interventions of choice at this time would be broadly based upon cognitive–behavioural strategies, but would aim to increase personalization of programmes of information and skill transfer. The health professional would no longer be an 'expert clinician' acting upon the 'patient', but rather an informed counsellor whom people actively desiring to change could use as they felt appropriate. The health professional would therefore not attempt to force clients to accommodate themselves to fixed treatment regimes, but would rather enable them to assimilate expert knowledge into their existing social milieu.

REFERENCES

Beck, A.T. (1976). *Cognitive therapy and the emotional disorders.* New York: International Universities Press.

Bennett, G.A. (1987). Behavior therapy in the treatment of obesity. In R. A. Boakes, D.A. Popplewell & M.J. Burton (Eds.). *Eating habits: food, physiology and learned behaviour,* pp. Chichester: Wiley.

Blair, A.J., Lewis, V.J. & Booth, D.A. (1990). Does emotional eating interfere with success in attempts at weight control? *Appetite,* 15, 151–7.

Booth, D.A., Lewis, V.J. & Blair, A.J. (1990). Dietary restraint and binge eating: pseudo-quantitative anthropology for a medicalised problem habit? *Appetite,* 14, 116–19.

Edell, B.H., Edington, S., Herd, B., O'Brien, R.M. & Witkin, G. (1987). Self-efficacy and self-motivation as predictors of weight loss. *Addictive Behaviours,* 12, 63–6.

Garrow, J.S. (1988). *Obesity and related diseases.* Edinburgh: Churchill Livingstone.

Lewis, V.J. (1991). Approaches to permanent weight control. *Appetite,* 17, 162.

Lewis, V.J. & Blair, A.J. (1991). The social context of eating disorders. In R. Cochrane & D. Carroll (Eds.). *psychology and social issues. A tutorial text,* pp. 22–30. London: Falmer Press.

Lewis, V.J. & Blair, A.J. (1993). Food and body image: dieting and distress. In C. Nivien & D. Carroll (Eds.). *The health psychology of women,* pp. 107–20. Switzerland: Harwood.

Lewis, V.J., Blair, A.J. & Booth, D.A. (1992). Outcome of group therapy for body-image emotionality and weight-control self-efficacy. *Behavioural Psychotherapy,* 20, 155–65.

Salmons, P.H., Lewis, V.J., Rogers, P., Gatherer, A.J. & Booth, D.A. (1988). Body shape dissatisfaction in schoolchildren. *British Journal of Psychiatry,* 153, 88–92.

Stalonas, P.M., Perri, M.G. & Kerzner, A.B. (1984). Do behavioral treatments of obesity last? A 5-year follow-up investigation. *Addictive Behaviors,* 9, 175–83.

Stunkard, A.J. (1987). Behaviour therapy for obesity. In A.E. Bender & L.J. Brookes (Eds.). Body weight control: the physiology, clinical treatment and prevention of obesity,) pp. Edinburgh: Churchill Livingstone.

Wadden, T.A. & Stunkard, A.J. (1985). Social and psychological consequences of obesity. *Annals of internal medicine,* 103, 1062–7.

Wardle, J. (1987). Eating style: a validation study of the Dutch eating behavior questionnaire in normal subjects and women with eating disorders. *Journal of psychosomatic Research,* 31, 161–9.

Wooley, S.C. & Wooley, O.W. (1984). Should obesity be treated at all? *Association of Research into Nervous and Mental Disease,* 62, 185–92.

SECTION 2: Psychological assessment and intervention

Behaviour therapy
Biofeedback
Cognitive behaviour therapy
Community-based
 interventions
Counselling
Disability assessment
Group therapy

Health education
Health status assessment
Hypnosis
Neuropsychological assessment
Neuropsychological rehabilitation
Pain management
Placebos
Psychodynamic psychotherapy

Reality orientation
 therapy
Relaxation training
Repertory grids
Self-management
Social skills training
Stress management
Work-site interventions

Behaviour therapy

GERALD C. DAVISON

Department of Psychology
University of Southern California, USA

Behaviour therapy, sometimes also called behaviour modification, developed initially during the 1950s through the work of people like B.F. Skinner (1953) and Joseph Wolpe (1958). The attempt was to create an approach to intervention that relied on experimentally tested principles of learning. In its earliest years the emphasis in behaviour therapy was on classical and operant conditioning, and throughout the 1960s and thereafter, a number of therapeutic techniques were developed that purportedly rested on these experimental foundations. The word 'purportedly' is used intentionally here because an ongoing scientific controversy has surrounded the extent to which behaviour therapy techniques truly derive their effectiveness from learning principles developed primarily from infrahuman experimentation. Suffice it to say that the most innovative techniques came from practising clinicians whose thinking was guided and enriched by their awareness of certain learning principles and by their creative attempts to apply them in the complex and often chaotic domain of clinical intervention. There is considerable evidence from numerous research settings worldwide that many of these techniques are helpful for dealing with a wide range of psychological disorders (see Davison & Neale, 1996).

An early behaviour therapy effort was by Andrew Salter (1949), whose book *Conditioned reflex therapy* represented an attempt to rationalize assertion training in Pavlovian conditioning terms. Salter was perhaps the first to argue that many anxious and depressed individuals could be helped by encouraging them to express openly to others both their likes and dislikes. He used Pavlovian theorizing to argue that much human psychological suffering arises from an excess of cortical inhibition, a state that could be reversed by an increase in emotional expressiveness. While the theorizing is doubtful, the approach in general is widely employed and even has links with humanistic emphases on meeting and expressing one's basic needs.

Also in the classical conditioning camp is Joseph Wolpe, whose book *Psychotherapy by reciprocal inhibition* has had an enormous impact on the thinking and practices of scientifically orientated clinicians. Trained in medicine and basing his work on Mary Cover Jones's (1924) classic case study with a fearful child, Wolpe conducted experiments with cats to show that graduated exposure to conditioned aversive stimuli (harmless situations that had been paired with painful electric shock) could markedly reduce, if not altogether eliminate, the acquired fear and avoidance. Extrapolating from this and related research on conditioned fear (e.g. Miller, 1948; Mowrer, 1939), Wolpe devised his technique of systematic desensitization, which entails training the patient in deep muscle relaxation, constructing with the patient a hierarchy of situations that elicit varying degrees of unwarranted and unwanted fear, and presenting each situation seriatim to the imagination of the person in a relaxed, non-anxious state. The idea is to countercondition the fear, that is, enable the patient to confront a fearsome event without experiencing the usual anxiety, thereby changing the response to the presumed conditioned stimulus from fear to neutrality or even positive interest. It would appear that the applicability of this technique is limited only by the ingenuity of the clinician in construing a patient's problems in terms that permit the construction of an anxiety hierarchy. Usually these imaginal exposures are supplemented, sometimes even replaced, by real-life exposures to what the person needlessly fears, cf. *in vivo* desensitization.

Another approach usually considered to derive its efficacy from classical conditioning is aversion therapy, which involves pairing an undesirably attractive event or stimulus with a negative emotional state such as fear or disgust. The effectiveness as well as the morality of aversive procedures have been a subject of heated debate over the past three decades, but many reports attest to its usefulness in dealing with problems such as excessive drinking of alcohol, smoking, overeating, and the paraphilias.

The general approach other than classical conditioning that historically lies at the core of behaviour therapy is operant conditioning, deriving from Skinner's work on the importance of contingencies in behaviour, that is, whether a given response is followed by a positive reinforcer like food or praise, or by a negative reinforcer like pain or disapproval. Withholding of a positive reinforcer can have punishing effects. Operant techniques attracted a great deal of favourable attention in the 1960s through the work of investigators like Azrin (e.g., Ayllon & Azrin, 1968) and others, who showed that reinforcement contingencies could favourably affect such problems as regressive crawling in children, poor academic performance, inappropriate social behaviour of various kinds, and non-compliance to therapeutic instructions. A notable achievement took the form of the token economy, a procedure whereby tokens are awarded for desirable behaviour and sometimes also taken away for undesirable behaviour, and later exchanged for goodies like candy or access to better dining facilities for hospitalized adult patients. In a functional sense, the token economy brings to the institutionalized setting the orderliness of a market economy, whereby particular behaviours are given a certain value within the parameters of a monetary system.

A major example of a token economy is provided by Paul and Lentz (1977), who studied three methods of rehabilitating severely impaired chronic mental patients. As compared to a milieu therapy, which essentially set expectations for the patients but without the highly structured contingencies of the token economy; and as compared to a routine hospital management group, which entailed continued usage of heavy doses of neuroleptic medication; the token economy achieved better success in reducing symptomatology and shaping useful self-care and social skills. It should be mentioned that there were cognitive elements as well within the token economy condition, an issue we turn to below.

While difficult to categorize as a behaviour therapy, modelling is widely used by behaviour therapists as an efficient way to teach complex patterns of behaviour. The early research programme of Albert Bandura (Bandura & Walters, 1963) documented the powerful effects of observing another person perform sometimes lengthy chains of behaviour. Evidence suggested that people can acquire behavioural patterns without reinforcement, but that their performance of what they have learned is indeed influenced by expected contingencies. A noteworthy application of modelling can be found in role-playing or behaviour rehearsal (Lazarus, 1971), whereby a therapist models effective behaviour and then encourages the patient to follow suit. Irrational fears can also be reduced by watching a fearless model interact with the frightening stimulus (Bandura & Menlove, 1968). The fact that something important is learned by watching another person suggests that cognitive processes are important.

The foregoing summarizes briefly the techniques and approaches usually associated with the phrases behaviour therapy or behaviour modification. But, since the late 1960s, there has been increasing recognition of the role of cognitive processes in therapeutic behaviour change, not only in the form of the cognitive therapies described in a separate entry but within those therapies judged to rely on classical and operant conditioning. For example, Wolpe's systematic desensitization has been conceptualized as a cognitive change technique or at least a procedure that relies on the patient's cognitive abilities (Davison & Wilson, 1973). After all, patients imagine what is troubling them, and these symbolic exposures lead to anxiety reduction in actual fearsome situations.

What then is behaviour therapy? Does it include explicit attention to cognition, or should it be restricted to conditioning principles? Indeed, what is to be included under the rubric of 'behaviour?' Only overt behaviour, as the Skinnerian legacy would have us concentrate on; or also on mediating behaviours in the tradition of Mowrer, Miller, and Wolpe? Answers depend on who is responding. To this writer and many others, behaviour therapy refers most generally and most usefully to a laboratory-based, empirical approach to therapeutic change. There need not be any prior allegiance to particular theories or principles of change. Behaviour therapists strive to use rigorous standards of proof rather than to rely on untested and sometimes even untestable concepts such as the Freudian unconscious. In sum, behaviour therapy/behaviour modification is an attempt to change abnormal behaviour, thoughts, and feelings by applying in the clinical context the epistemologies, methods, and discoveries made by non-applied behavioural scientists in their study of both normal and abnormal behaviour. Viewed this way, any consideration of behaviour therapy would be incomplete without the inclusion of cognitive concepts (See also 'Biofeedback', 'Cognitive behaviour therapy', 'Group therapy').

REFERENCES

Ayllon, T. & Azrin, N.H. (1968). *The token economy: a motivational system for therapy and rehabilitation.* New York: Appleton-Century-Crofts.

Bandura, A. & Menlove, F.L. (1968). Factors determining vicarious extinction of avoidance behavior through symbolic modelling. *Journal of Personality and Social Psychology*, 8, 99–108.

Bandura, A. & Walters, R.H. (1963). *Social learning and personality development.* New York: Holt, Rinehart & Winston.

Davison, G.C. & Neale, J.M. (1996). *Abnormal psychology.* Revised 6th edn. New York: Wiley.

Davison, G.C. & Wilson, G.T. (1973). Processes of fear-reduction in systematic desensitization: cognitive and social reinforcement factors in humans. *Behavior Therapy*, 4, 1–21.

Jones, M.C. (1924). A laboratory study of fear: the case of Peter. *Pedagogical Seminary*, 31, 308–15.

Lazarus, A.A. (1971). *Behavior therapy and beyond.* New York: McGraw-Hill.

Miller, N.E. (1948). Studies of fear as an acquirable drive: I. Fear as motivation and fear-reduction as reinforcement in the learning of new responses. *Journal of Experimental Psychology*, **38**, 89–101.

Mowrer, O.H. (1939). A stimulus–response analysis of anxiety and its role as a reinforcing agent. *Psychological Review*, **46**, 553–65.

Paul, G.L. & Lentz, R.J. (1977). *Psychosocial treatment of chronic mental patients: milieu versus social learning programs.* Cambridge, MA: Harvard University Press.

Salter, A. (1949). *Conditioned reflex therapy.* New York: Farrar, Straus.

Skinner, B.F. (1953). *Science and human behavior.* New York: Macmillan.

Wolpe, J. (1958). *Psychotherapy by reciprocal inhibition.* Stanford, CA: Stanford University Press.

Biofeedback

ROBERT J. GATCHEL

Department of Psychiatry
University of Texas Southwestern Medial Center
at Dallas, USA

Before Harry Houdini performed one of his famous escapes, a skeptical committee would search his clothes and body. When the members of the committee were satisfied that the great Houdini was concealing no keys, they would put chains, padlocks and handcuffs on him . . . Of course, not even Houdini could open a padlock without a key, and when he was safely behind a curtain he would cough one up. He could hold a key suspended in his throat and regurgitate it when he was unobserved . . . The trick behind many of Houdini's escapes was in some ways just as amazing as the escape in itself. Ordinarily when an object is stuck in a person's throat he will start to gag. He can't help it – it's an unlearned, automatic reflex. But Houdini had learned to control his gag reflex by practicing hours with a small piece of potato tied to a string.
(Lang, 1970, page 2).

Over the years, there have been other unusual instances of voluntary control of physiological functions noted in the scientific literature. For example, the early literature reported a case of a middle-aged male who had the ability to control the erection of hairs over the entire surface of his body (Lindsley & Sassaman, 1938). Numerous early instances of voluntary acceleration of heart rate were reported by Ogden and Shock (1939). Moreover, the Russian psychologist Luria (1958) described a mnemonist who had attained remarkable control of his heart rate and skin temperature. This individual could abruptly alter his heart by 40 heart beats per minute. He could also raise his skin temperature of one hand while simultaneously lowering the temperature of the other hand. McClure (1959) also noted the case of an individual who could voluntarily produce complete cardiac arrest for periods of several seconds at a time. Finally, it has also been well documented that many yogis can control various physiological responses at will (Bagchi & Wenger, 1957).

The above reported acts of bodily control have traditionally been viewed as rare feats that only certain extraordinarily gifted or unusual individuals could accomplish. However, starting in the 1950s, behavioural scientists started to develop techniques and demonstrate that the 'average person on the street' could learn a significant degree of control over physiological responding. The primary training method developed and utilized in this learning process has been labelled biofeedback. This initial research began to stimulate an interest, among both the scientific community and the general public, in the area of biofeedback, because of its many potentially important clinical and medical applications. For example, it would be therapeutically valuable if we could teach patients with hypertension how to lower their blood pressure, or teach patients with headaches how to control the vasodilation process involved in the pain process. Indeed, Birk (1973) was the individual who coined the term behavioural medicine to describe the application of a behavioural treatment technique (biofeedback) that could be applied to medicine or medical problems (e.g. headache pain).

WHAT IS BIOFEEDBACK?

The biofeedback technique is based on the fundamental learning principle that we learn to perform a specific response when we receive feedback or information about the consequences of the response we have just made and then make appropriate adjustments. That is to say, biofeedback can be viewed as any consequence of biological performance which is perceived by a behaving subject. Indeed, this is how we learn to perform the wide variety of motor skills and behaviours we use in everyday activities. Thus, for example, we learn how to drive a car by receiving continuous feedback about how much we need to turn the steering wheel in order to turn the car a certain distance, or how much pressure to apply to the accelerator in order to make the car move at a certain speed or slow down. If we are denied this feedback (as, for instance, by being blindfolded), we would never receive useful information about the consequences of our driving responses. Most likely, we would therefore never be able to learn the appropriate adjustments needed to perform a certain successful manoeuvre needed with a car. Thus, information feedback is very important. A review of numerous experimental studies has clearly demonstrated the important role of feedback in learning and performance of a wide variety of motor skills (Annent, 1969).

The availability of feedback is also important in learning how to control internal physiological responses. However, much of our biological behaviour is concerned with maintaining a constant internal 'homeostasis' and is not readily accessible to conscious awareness. Indeed, we do not consciously experience some interoceptive awareness of internal biological activity such as muscle tension or our pulse because there is normally adaptive advantage to not having to consciously attend or control these activities on a continuous basis. Moreover, interoceptors do not normally have the extensive afferent representation at the cortical level which is needed for a high degree of perceptual acuity or the fine discriminability characteristics of audition or vision.

Since we do not normally receive feedback of these internal events in day-to-day situations, we cannot be expected to control them. However, if an individual is provided biofeedback of, say, blood pressure via a visual display monitor, he or she can become more aware of the consequences of blood pressure changes and how adjustments can be made to modify and eventually control it. Receiving feedback thus removes one's 'blindfold', enabling one to voluntarily control a response. The recent development of sensitive physiological recording devices and digitalogic technology has made it possible to detect small changes in visceral events and provide subjects with immediate feedback of these biological events.

Today, biofeedback is broadly and loosely defined as a technique for transforming some aspect of physiological behaviour into electrical signals which are made accessible to exteroception or awareness (usually vision or audition). Sometimes, the feedback signal is combined with a tangible reward such as money or the opportunity to view attractive pictures in an attempt to motivate the individual and strengthen the effect of the targeted physiological response. In other instances, the clinician provides verbal praise for success in addition to feedback. These latter practices also are forms of biofeedback, since they too convey information to the learner about his or her biological performance. In most instances, however, response contingent lights or tones alone can be shown to augment voluntary control.

HISTORICAL DEVELOPMENT OF BIOFEEDBACK

Borrowing heavily from operant conditioning techniques, the early biofeedback investigators demonstrated some degree of operant or voluntary control in a wide variety of visceral, central nervous system, and somatomotor functions. Although the prevailing *zeitgeist* argued against the possibility of operant control of internal physiological events, as early as 1938 Skinner tried (and failed) to condition vasoconstriction through positive reinforcement. One of the first experiments successfully demonstrating that human subjects could learn to voluntarily control a visceral response was conducted by the Russian psychologist, Lisina (1958). She initially tried to train human subjects how to constrict or dilate blood vessels in their arms in order to avoid electric shock (avoidance of shock was used as a reinforcement). Her initial efforts to condition or produce these vascular changes were unsuccessful. However, control of constriction and dilation was obtained when subjects were permitted to watch their vascular changes displayed on a recording device; that is, they were given biofeedback.

Shearn (1962) was the first investigator to demonstrate the operant conditioning or control of heart rate. He trained subjects to control their heart rates by allowing them to listen to amplified feedback of their heart beats while learning how to avoid a mild electric shock by increasing their heart rate to a specified level during different parts of the experiment. Lang and colleagues were the first American investigators to provide a visual type of continuous feedback in training subjects how to stabilize their heart rates (Lang, Sroufe & Hastings, 1967). These investigators, who did not use shock avoidance, found that subjects learned to significantly decrease the amount of heart rate variability while performing a task, and this ability improved with practice. They found that the biofeedback task itself was intrinsically rewarding and that subjects learned a considerable degree of heart control without any special incentives.

At about this same time when various investigators were demonstrating this voluntary control of heart rate, Kamiya (1969) reported that human subjects could learn to control the appearance of alpha rhythm in brain-wave activity by providing them with biofeedback (subjects were given external feedback such as brief lights or tones when alpha rhythms were present). The maintenance of a high level of alpha was reported to be related to relaxation, pleasant effect, and a 'letting go' experience.

Of all the modalities, blood pressure control initially had, perhaps, the most potential for clinical significance. The first study of blood pressure control via biofeedback in humans was reported by Shapiro et al. (1969). They documented that normal subjects were able to decrease (and to a lesser extent increase) their systolic blood pressures as a consequence of being provided beat-to-beat feedback of Korotkoff sounds (and additional reinforcement for blocks of successful trials). The amount of change during the one session study was small, not exceeding an average of 5 mm Hg. However, this study provided impetus for subsequent investigations that attempted to increase the amount of change to clinically significant levels and to induce such changes in clinical hypertensives.

Since the time of these above discussed pioneering studies, there have been demonstrations of this learned control by human subjects of a wide range of 'involuntary responses': cardiac ventricular rate, systolic and diastolic blood pressure, peripheral vascular responses, electrodermal activity, gastric motility, skin temperature, penile tumescence, and various brain-wave rhythms. Gatchel and Price (1979) provided an early review of this research.

CLINICAL APPLICATIONS OF BIOFEEDBACK

Encouraged by these early successes which demonstrated voluntary control of normal physiological activity, medical and psychological clinicians soon began to question whether pathophysiological activity could also be controlled with the goal of restoring health or preventing illness. This stimulated a rapid growth of the biofeedback literature evaluating the clinical effectiveness of biofeedback. This research has been reviewed in a number of different sources (e.g. Hatch, Fisher & Rugh, 1987). There is also a journal (*Biofeedback and Self-Regulation*), as well as a professional society which specializes in biofeedback and self-regulation (Association for Applied Psychophysiology and Biofeedback) which celebrated its 25th year in 1994. There are also a number of useful practitioner guides that have been published (e.g. Basmajian, 1989; Schwartz, 1987).

To date, it has been amply demonstrated that some degree of self-control is possible over behaviours long assumed to be completely involuntary. It has also been shown that, with biofeedback, it

[198]

is possible to extend voluntary control to pathophysiological responding in order to modify this maladaptive behaviour in the direction of health. These are highly significant achievements. However, many important questions still remain as to how medically effective biofeedback will be. Unfortunately, research evaluating therapeutic effectiveness of biofeedback procedures has been plagued by a number of problems. To date, very few well-controlled clinical outcome studies have been conducted using large numbers of patients having well-confirmed medical diagnoses. Moreover, the few comparative outcome studies that have been performed compared the relative effectiveness of biofeedback to various other behavioural techniques (such as simple relaxation training). It would be extremely helpful to also compare biofeedback techniques with more traditional medical treatments, some of which have fairly well-established success rates. Combinations of medical and behavioural techniques should also be explored and evaluated. However, these studies will be most informative if investigators design them so that the unique contribution of each individual technique, as well as the combined effect, can be isolated and reliably measured.

Unfortunately, there have been claims for the therapeutic efficacy of biofeedback which have been grossly exaggerated and even wrong. Overall, it is justified to conclude that relevant and encouraging data do exist, but at the present time the value of clinical training and biofeedback still has to be questioned in some areas. Moreover, terms such as 'biofeedback therapists' and 'biofeedback clinic', which are now regularly encountered in many medical centres, are difficult to justify. They imply that a form of treatment exists which is more or less generally applicable to a variety of ills. Worse yet, they imply, at least in the minds of some, that biofeedback is a new alternative treatment modality. Currently, in the majority of areas in which it is applied, biofeedback should be viewed merely as an adjunctive treatment.

A LOOK TO THE FUTURE

In the future, the potential of biofeedback in the diagnosis, aetiology, prevention, and rehabilitation of various disorders should continue to be tested. Indeed, biofeedback is a good example of the new 'biobehavioural' model of health and disease. Health and illness are viewed as aspects of an individual's overall biobehavioural response to daily living. Thus, biofeedback as a form of behavioural medicine still has a great deal of potential application. Some of its most important contributions may also prove to be conceptual rather than technological or directly therapeutic. Moreover, as the author has emphasized earlier, in order for the field of biofeedback to continue to effectively develop and progress:

'. . . the clinician or researcher employing biofeedback needs knowledge in a number of different areas: the pathophysiology of the disorder being treated and the physiology of the response systems to be voluntarily regulated, the relation of such response systems to the etiology and symptoms of the particular disorder, the electrical functioning of the feedback device itself, the nature of the self-regulation process involved in biofeedback 'learning', and the knowledge and use of appropriate methodology. Without such expertise, it cannot be expected that useful and reliable biofeedback treatment procedures can be developed.' (Gatchel & Price, 1979, page 235).
(See also 'Behaviour therapy', 'Group therapy'.)

REFERENCES

Annent, J. (1969) *Feedback and human behavior.* Baltimore: Penguin Books.

Bagchi, B.K. & Wenger, M.A. (1957) Electro-physiological correlates of some yogi exercises. *Electroencephalography and Clinical Neurophysiology*, supplement 7, 132–49.

Basmajian, J.V. (Ed.). (1989) *Biofeedback: principles and practice for clinicians.* Baltimore: Williams & Wilkins.

Birk, L. (Ed.) (1973). *Biofeedback: behavioral medicine.* New York: Grune & Stratton.

Gatchel, R.J. & Price, K.P. (Eds.). (1979). *Clinical applications of biofeedback: appraisal and status.* Elmsford, New York: Pergamon.

Hatch, J.P., Fisher, J.G. & Rugh, J.D. (Eds.). (1987). *Biofeedback: studies in clinical efficacy.* New York: Plenum.

Kamiya, J. (1969). Operant control of the EEG alpha rhythm and some of its reported effects on consciousness. In C. Tart (Ed.). *Altered states of consciousness.* New York: Wiley.

Lang, P.J. (1970) Autonomic control or learning to play the internal organs. *Psychology Today.*

Lang, P.J., Sroufe, L.A. & Hastings, J.E. (1967). Effects of feedback and instructional set on the control of cardiac rate variability. *Journal of Experimental Psychology*, 75, 425–31.

Lindsley, D.B. & Sassaman, W.H. (1938). Autonomic activity and brain potentials associated with 'voluntary' control of pilomotors. *Journal of Neurophysiology*, 1, 342–9.

Lisina, M.I. (1958). The role of orientation in the transformation of involuntary reactions to voluntary ones. In L.G. Voronin, A.N. Leontiev, A.R. Luria, E.N. Sokolov & O.B. Vinobradova (Eds.). *Orienting reflex and exploratory behavior.* Washington: American Institue of Biological Sciences.

Luria, A.R. (1958). *The mind of a mnemonist,* trans. by L. Solotaroff. New York: Basic Books.

McClure, C.M. (1959). Cardiac arrest through volition. *California Medicine*, 90, 440–8.

Ogden, E. & Shock, N.W. (1939). Voluntary hypercirculation. *American Journal of the Medical Sciences*, 198, 329–42.

Schwartz, M.S. *Biofeedback: a practitioner's guide.* (1987). New York: Guilford Press.

Shapiro, D., Tursky, B., Gershon, E. & Stern, M. (1969) Effects of feedback and reinforcement on the control of human systolic blood pressure. *Science*, 163, 588–90.

Shearn, D.W. (1962). Operant conditioning of heart rate. *Science*, 137, 530–1.

Cognitive behaviour therapy

DONALD MEICHENBAUM

University of Waterloo, Ontario, Canada

INTRODUCTION

The practitioner of contemporary psychotherapies is confronted with a conundrum. More than 250 different forms of psychotherapy have been proposed, each with its own advocates and supposed claims of efficacy. How is one to make sense of this array of psychotherapeutic techniques, especially in an era of managed health care where the issues of 'accountability' and 'efficacy' are so prominent?

Cognitive behavioural therapies (CBT) are designed to penetrate this labyrinth of diversity by proposing a model of general psychopathology and a theory of behaviour change that integrates diverse psychotherapeutic procedures, that is sensitive to a biopsychosocial perspective of medical and psychiatric disorders, and that is tied to empirically demonstrated interventions. In the past, various schools of psychotherapy (e.g. psychodynamic, behavioural and humanistic) have been offered as competing approaches, with little proposed overlap. In recent years, there has been an effort to develop an 'integrative' approach of psychotherapeutic techniques that has a demonstrated empirical basis of efficacy. CBT has been at the forefront of this integrative movement. CBT has led the way in demonstrating the beneficial effects of psychotherapy in not only alleviating distress, but also in reducing the likelihood of subsequent relapse.

In this brief account the following will be attempted:

(a) to define CBT and describe its theoretical perspective;
(b) to put CBT in some historical perspective;
(c) to briefly review some illustrative findings;
(d) to describe some of the limitations of CBT;
(e) to indicate possible future directions, in terms of treating both medical and psychiatric clinical problems.

As a result, the reader should better appreciate the reasons for the enthusiasm that CBT has generated, and at the same time become a more 'critical consumer' of the CBT literature.

WHAT IS CBT?

While this appears to be a simple and straightforward question, the answer is somewhat complex. As Mahoney and Arnkoff (1978) observe, subsumed under the heading of CBT are a number of diverse therapeutic procedures including cognitive therapy, cognitive restructuring procedures, rational – emotive psychotherapy, problem-solving interventions, coping skills training such as stress inoculation training, panic control techniques, and self-instructional training. As will be seen, one should not impose a 'uniformity myth' on these diverse therapeutic procedures since they hold different theoretical perspectives and have differential outcomes.

Despite these differences, there are some common features to CBT approaches that can be highlighted. These features include the following.

1. At the theoretical level, CBT embraces a biopsychosocial perspective that highlights the reciprocal interdependence of feelings, thoughts, behaviour, resultant consequences, social context, and physiological processes, namely, a reciprocally deterministic approach as described by Bandura (1978). While some CBT theorists have highlighted cognitions as being central or primary in the psychotherapeutic process, proposing that cognitions, in the form of 'irrational beliefs' (Ellis, 1977) or cognitive distortions and errors (Beck, 1976), can cause emotional disturbance and maladaptive behaviour, more recent forms of CBT have taken issue with such a 'rationalist' and 'objectivist' position. As Neimeyer (1985) and Mahoney (1988) observe, rationalistic therapeutic approaches attempt to have clients monitor and correct 'disturbed' or 'irrational' beliefs and 'faulty logic'. The 'rationalist' approach attempts to help clients develop more accurate and objective views of 'reality' by such means as logical disputation, instruction, personal experiments, whereby the clients can collect empirical evidence in order to test their beliefs against external reality.

In contrast, the emergent forms of CBT have embraced a more constructivist perspective (Meichenbaum & Fitzpatrick, 1993). The constructivist perspective is based on the notion that individuals are 'architects' or 'constructors' of their environment and it highlights that how individuals behave may inadvertently, perhaps unwittingly, and even unknowingly, create reactions in others that confirm their beliefs about themselves and the world. The constructivist perspective highlights that individuals 'construct' their personal realities or 'narrative stories' and create their own representational models of the world. It is not, as if, there is one reality and our clients distort that reality, thus contributing to their problems. Rather, constructivists propose that there are multiple realities, and the task of therapy is to help clients become aware of how they create their realities and the consequences of such personal constructions. The shift from a 'rationalist – objective' perspective to a 'constructivist' perspective is not a mere shift in semantic emphasis, but a shift that has important implications for both assessment and treatment.

2. A second feature of CBT is that it tends to be short term (less than 20 sessions), although Linehan, Heard and Armstrong (1993) have used a one-year CBT intervention to reduce parasuicidal behaviour with borderline patients. No matter what the length of the CBT treatment the intervention tends to be highly collaborative, using Socratic questioning techniques and discovery-focused interventions. It also tends to be proactive in encouraging clients to perform 'personal experiments' or 'homework' between sessions. Another feature of all CBT interventions is the inclusion of relapse prevention (RP) procedures. While RP was initially emphasized by CB therapists Marlatt and Gordon (1985) in their work with clients who had problems with addiction, the concept of RP is relevant to

all forms of CB intervention. In RP, clients explore the nature of high-risk situations that are likely to contribute to lapses and that can escalate into becoming a full-blown relapse. In therapy, clients rehearse how to anticipate and handle such lapses.

3. CBT is particularly sensitive to the critically important role of relationship and emotional factors in the therapeutic process. In addition to collaboration such factors as warmth, empathy, emotional atunement, acceptance, providing hope, bolstering client efficacy, and nurturing a therapeutic alliance are each emphasized by CB therapists (See Meichenbaum, 1994; Meichenbaum & Turk, 1987, for a discussion of how these relationship factors are incorporated into CBT). As Safran and Segal (1990) observe, CBT recognizes the 'inseparability of therapy techniques, personal qualities of the therapist, and the therapeutic relationship (p.35)'.

CBT IN HISTORICAL PERSPECTIVE

In order to appreciate the diverse CBT approaches, it is helpful to consider briefly the historical cross-currents that have contributed to the CBT approach. As documented by Raimy (1975), a long tradition of semantic therapists have highlighted the role of cognitive factors in psychopathology and behaviour change. Illustrative of this tradition are Pierre Janet (1893) who believed that hysterics suffered from 'fixed ideas', while Paul Dubois (1904–1907) who argued that 'incorrect ideas' produced psychological distress, and George Kelly (1955) who discussed the role of 'personal constructs' as being critical to how individuals construe themselves and the world.

But these semantic therapists were predated by Greek, Roman, and Eastern philosophers and religious leaders (e.g. Epictetus, Gautama Buddha, Immanuel Kant, and others). Modern day cognitive therapists such as Aaron Beck, Albert Ellis and Arnold Lazarus, and other CB therapists owe their lineage to this semantic tradition.

Much more contemporary, CBT emerged out a growing dissatisfaction with both the theoretical and empirical bases of a strictly behavioural therapeutic approach (e.g. see Breger & McGaugh, 1965; Brewer, 1974; McKeachie, 1974). Each of these authors questioned the adequacy of 'learning theory' explanations of both psychopathology and behavioural change. It soon became apparent that, if behaviour therapy techniques were altered to become more sensitive and inclusive of the client's thoughts and feelings, then treatment efficacy would improve (Mahoney, 1974; Meichenbaum, 1977).

At the same time a 'cognitive revolution', as Dember (1974) characterized it, was taking place. Whether it was the adoption of an information processing perspective, the development of social learning theory, or the inclusion of a Vygotskian 'internalization' perspective (see Vygotsky, 1978), the irreversible tide toward CBT had been established. From its origins in the 1970s, CBT has emerged as one of the most endorsed therapeutic procedures (second next to eclectic) therapeutic approaches (Smith, 1982). Is such interest and enthusiasm warranted by the data? This question sets the stage for a brief consideration of the empirical status of CBT.

SOME ILLUSTRATIVE FINDINGS

Space does not permit a detailed meta-analysis of CBT procedures for diverse clinical populations. A number of comprehensive reviews exist (e.g. Barlow, 1992; Clark & Salkovskis, 1991; Haaga & Davison, 1993; Hollon, 1990; Hollon & Beck, 1993; Meichenbaum,

1993). Two clinical populations that have received most research attention are those patients suffering from anxiety and depressive disorders.

After reviewing the literature on anxiety disorder Magraf *et al.* (1993) concluded that 81–90% of panic disordered patients who received CBT were panic free at 1- to 2-year follow-ups, compared with 50–55% of pharmacologically treated anxious patients, and 25% of those receiving supportive therapy. Similar stability of treatment results is evident for patients with generalized anxiety disorders and social phobias (Hollon & Beck, 1993). An overwhelming majority (80%) of anxious patients are symptom free at 1–2 years, often with significant improvement on other dimensions. As Magraf *et al.* (1993) conclude:

We are no longer dealing with experimental treatments that still have to prove themselves. Instead, cognitive behavioral treatment rests on firm experimental evidence that justifies their application is everyday practice (p.6)

A similar favourable picture exists in the treatment area of unipolar depression. For example, in summarizing the CBT with depressives, Hollon, DeRubeis & Seligman (1992) concluded that,

Patients treated to remission with cognitive therapy had a relapse rate of 26% versus a relapse rate of 64% for those treated with pharmacotherapy (p.90)

Thase *et al.* (1991) reported that the results at a 1-year follow-up indicated that cognitive therapy of depressed clients reduced relapse rates to 30%, compared to 70% for pharmacologically treated patients. The combination of cognitive therapy and medication has been typically associated with only a modest advantage over either single modality (about only one-quarter of a standard deviation) (Hollon *et al.*, 1992). In short, there is an enduring effect for CBT on depressives with only about 20% of all treatment responders relapsing or seeking additional treatment within the first 12–24 months following treatment termination, compared to about 50% relapsing of responders to pharmacotherapy alone (Hollon & Beck, 1993).

While these initial results with anxious and depressed clients are encouraging, CBT is no panacea. As Chambless and Gillis (1992) caution, even more powerful CBT interventions are needed in order to yield long-term significant change with clients who have chronic disorders, who have accompanying personality disorders, who experience marital distress and interpersonal difficulties (also see Robins & Hayes, 1993).

CB therapists have recently extended their efforts to new and more challenging clinical populations including schizophrenic patients, patients with bipolar disorders, HIV patients with depression, patients with personality disorders, sexual offenders, drug addicts, alcoholics, eating disordered patients, distressed couples, and other clinical groups (for a description of this work, see Beck, 1993).

The relative effectiveness of CBT is not limited to psychiatric problems, but has been extended to physical disorders. As Turk and Salovey (1993) report:

The clinical effectiveness of cognitive-behavioral interventions have been demonstrated with a wide range of chronic illness and disabilities, including headaches, arthritis, temporomandibular disorders, low back pain, spinal cord injuries, atypical chest pains, functional somatic symptoms, and cancer. These approaches have been used with patients across the age span from adolescents to geriatric patients. (pp. 32–33)

In a recent study in which the author was a consultant nurses were trained to provide CBT to patients with various chronic medical conditions. Not only did the CBT improve the patients' levels of adjustment relative to control groups, but CBT also significantly reduced medical utilization costs, Roberts *et al.* (1994). In these days of concern about the monetary costs of medical treatments, these results have very significant implications for the future application of CBT.

One of the future directions of CBT will be to 'give CBT away', so nurses, probation officers, coaches, as well as computers, will be able to conduct CBT. Meichenbaum (1993), in a recent review of 20 years of stress inoculation training, has indicated the widespread potential application of CBT on both a prevention and a treatment basis (also see Hollon *et al* 1992). For example, Meichenbaum (1994) discusses how CBT can be applied to populations of individuals who have been exposed to traumatic stress disorders, the emerging disorder of the 1990's, given the widespread incidence of natural and manmade disasters. CBT is likely to lead the way in formulating treatment and prevention programmes. But such extension of CBT must be accompanied by a commitment to evaluative research.

In summary, the history of CBT has been marked by commitments to research on basic psychosocial processes, sound empirical evaluations, and theoretical development. The field of psychotherapy is 'maturing' as it searches for an integrative perspective and for effective empirically demonstrated procedures. CBT has played, and will continue to play, a pivotal role in these developments. (See also 'Coping with chronic illness', 'Behaviour therapy', 'Biofeedback', 'Group therapy'.)

REFERENCES

Bandura, A. (1978). The self-system in reciprocal determinism, *American Psychologist*, 33, 344–58.

Barlow, D.H. (1992). Cognitive–behavioral approaches to panic disorders and social phobia. *Bulletin of the Menninger Clinic*, 56, 14–28.

Beck, A. (1976). *Cognitive therapy and the emotional disorders*. New York: International Universities Press.

Beck, A.T. (1993). Cognitive therapy: past, present and future. *Journal of Consulting and Clinical Psychology*, 61, 194–9.

Breger, L. & McGaugh, J. (1965). Critique and reformulation of 'learning theory': approaches to psychotherapy and neurosis. *Psychological Bulletin*, 63, 338–58.

Brewer, W. (1974). There is no convincing evidence for operant or classical conditioning in adult humans. In W. Weiner & D. Palermo (Eds.) *Cognition and the symbolic processes*. New York: Halsted Press.

Chambless, D.L. & Gillis, M.M. (1992). Cognitive therapy of anxiety disorders. *Journal of Consulting and Clinical Psychology*, 61, 248–60.

Clark, D.M. & Salkovskis, P.M. (1991). *Cognitive therapy with panic and hypochondriasis*. New York: Pergamon Press.

Dember, W. (1974). Motivation and the cognitive revolution. *American Psychologist*, 29, 161–8.

Dubois, P. (1904/1907). *The psychic treatment of nervous disorders*. New York: Funk & Wagnell.

Ellis, A. (1977). *The basic clinical theory of rational–emotive therapy*. New York: Springer.

Haaga, D.A. & Davison, G.C. (1993). An appraisal of rational–motive therapy. *Journal of Consulting and Clinical Psychology*, 61, 215–21.

Hollon, S.D. (1990). Cognitive therapy and pharmacotherapy for depression. *Psychiatric Annals*, 20, 249–58.

Hollon, S.D. & Beck, A.T. (1993). Cognitive and cognitive–behavioral therapies. In S.L. Garfield & A.E. Bergin (Eds.). *Handbook of psychotherapy and behavior change: an empirical analysis* (4th edition). New York: Wiley.

Hollon, S.D., DeRubeis, R.J. & Seligman, M.E. (1992). Cognitive therapy and the prevention of depression. *Applied and Preventative Psychology*, 1, 89–95.

Janet, P. (1893). *Nerveuses et idée fixes* (2 vols.). Paris: Alcan.

Kelly, G. (1955). *The psychology of personal constructs* (2 vols.). New York: Brunner/Mazel.

Linehan, M.M., Heard, L. & Armstrong, H.E. (1993). Naturalistic follow-up of a cognitive behavioral treatment for chronically parasuicidal borderline patients. *Archives of General Psychiatry*, 50, 971–4.

Magraf, J., Barlow, D.H., Clark, D.M. & Telch, M.J. (1993). Psychological treatment of panic: Work in progress in outcome, active ingredients, and followup. *Behaviour Research and Therapy*, 31, 108–18.

Mahoney, M. (1988). Constructive metatheory: implications for psychotherapy. *International Journal of Personal Construct Psychotherapy*, 1, 299–315.

Mahoney, M. & Arnkoff, D. (1978). Cognitive and self-control therapies. In S. Garfield and A. Bergin (Eds.). *Handbook of psychotherapy and behavior change*. New York: Wiley.

Mahoney, M.J. (1974). *Cognition and behavior modification*. Cambridge, MA: Ballinger.

Marlatt, A. & Gordon, J. (1985). *Relapse prevention*. New York: Guilford.

McKeachie, W. (1974). The decline and fall of the laws of learning. *Educational Researcher*, 3, 7–11.

Meichenbaum, D. (1977). *Cognitive behavior modification: an integrative approach*. New York: Plenum.

Meichenbaum, D. (1993). Stress inoculation training: a twenty-year update. In R.L. Wolfolk & P.M. Lehrer (Eds.). *Principles and practice of stress management*. New York: Guilford.

Meichenbaum, D. (1994). *Clinical handbook/ treatment manual on PTSD*. Waterloo, ON: Institute Press.

Meichenbaum, D. & Turk, D. (1987). *Facilitating treatment adherence: a practitioner's guidebook*. New York: Plenum.

Meichenbaum, D. & Fitzpatrick, D. (1993). A constructivist narrative perspective of stress and coping: stress inoculation applications. In L. Goldberger & S. Breznitz (Eds.). *Handbook of stress*. New York: Free Press.

Neimeyer, R.A. (1985). Personal constructs in clinical practice. In P. Kendall (Ed.). *Advances in cognitive behavioral research and therapy*. New York: Academic Press.

Raimy, V. (1975). *Misunderstanding of the self: cognitive psychotherapy and the misconception hypothesis*. San Francisco: Jossey-Bass.

Roberts, J., Browne, G.B., Streiner, D., Gafni, A., Pallister, R., Hoxby, H., Jamieson, E. & Meichenbaum, D. (1994). Promoting adjustment and reducing health service utilization. Unpublished manuscript, McMaster University, Ontario.

Robins, C.J. & Hayes, A.M. (1993). An appraisal of cognitive therapy. *Journal of Consulting Clinical Psychology*, 61, 205–15.

Safran, J. & Segal, Z. (1990). *Interpersonal processes in cognitive therapy*. New York: Basic Books.

Smith, D. (1982). Trends in counseling and

psychology. *American Psychologist*, **37**, 802–9.

Thase, M.E., Eimons, A.D., Cahalone, J.F. & McGeary, J. (1991). Cognitive behavior therapy of endogenous depression. *Behavior therapy*, **22**, 457–67.

Turk, D.C. & Salovey, P. (1993). Chronic disease and illness behaviors: a cognitive-behavioral perspective. In P. Nicassio & T.W. Smith (Eds.). *Psychosocial management of chronic illness*. Washington, DC: American Psychological Association.

Vygotsky, L.S. (1978). *Mind in society: the development of higher psychological processes.* Cambridge, MA: Harvard University Press.

Community-based interventions

KENNETH HELLER

CHRISTIE M. KING

ANA M. ARROYO

and

DEBORAH E. POLK

Department of Psychology, Indiana University, Bloomington, USA

Psychologists who design community-based, health interventions base their work on the proposition that social and environmental processes impact upon health and well-being, and contribute to health decline, malnutrition, disease, and mortality. This assumption is based upon the now large body of research evidence linking poverty and social disorganization to despair and negative health practices which, in turn, have cumulative negative effects on health. Furthermore, rather than assuming that negative environmental conditions are fixed and immutable aspects of industrial society, community psychologists believe that with encouragement and education, citizens can become more active in modifying unhealthy lifestyles. The goals of community health interventions, then, are to help set in place social structures that support and reinforce individual and group efforts at improving the quality of life.

The emphasis on facilitative social structures is not intended to minimize the efforts that individuals can take to improve their own health. Indeed, much can be accomplished by encouraging patients to change unhealthful practices that contribute to increased risk for disease. For example, convincing patients to adopt a healthy diet, decrease smoking, drug and alcohol intake, and engage in moderate exercise have been prime ingredients in the reduction of cardiovascular risk that has taken place within the last two decades. However, there is a limit to what individuals can do on their own when confronted with adverse environmental conditions. The barriers to continued improvements in community health are not in the individual citizen's knowledge of proper health practices, but in political, social and economic factors that maintain risk-producing social conditions. Since there is now a substantial body of research indicating that rates of morbidity and mortality are linked to social conditions such as poverty, unstable living conditions, community disintegration, poor education, social isolation and lack of employment opportunities (Adler *et al.*, 1994; Williams *et al.*, 1992), the dilemma for modern community health practice is how to deal with these negative social conditions.

While the correction of adverse social conditions can be difficult to accomplish, we believe that health practitioners need not wait for some golden age of social enlightenment before acting to improve community health. There are many examples of local projects in which citizens have developed effective action plans in collaboration with health professionals. The key ingredients in these efforts involve a mobilized and informed community group in which social structures have been developed that encourage concerted action. The idea is to find ways to encourage the development of groups that can provide the structure for citizens to become proactive in health maintenance.

COMPONENTS OF SUCCESSFUL COMMUNITY-BASED HEALTH INTERVENTIONS

We now know what it takes to expedite the formation of successful community action groups. For example, research indicates that citizens are most likely to come together when they have an opportunity to share common experience, develop emotional closeness and recognize that they have a common identity or destiny (McMillan & Chavis, 1986). They are most likely to take concerted action when they have the necessary skills and resources (Heller, 1990) and belong to organizations that have a task focus, clear roles for participating members, and use democratic decision-making procedures (Wandersman & Florin, 1990). These key ingredients can be illustrated by several of the community health projects described below.

How can a health provider activate a citizen's constituency? Kelly (1988) describes the steps to be taken in the development of a viable community intervention. The process starts with 'reconnaissance', or finding out about the community and how it operates. Kelly believes that no matter what the presenting problem, community-based programmes will not succeed unless one understands and respects existing community traditions for responding to problems, develops a cadre of citizens willing to work on the project, and provides a social setting in which their talents can be engaged. In other words, community intervention is not a 'solo enterprise' in which a health professional can expect to achieve success by working alone without the involvement of influential community members. One needs to understand that preventative health activities are usually adopted through informal social influence. People discuss health behaviours with those whom they know, and choose advisers of equal or slightly higher status. Influential opinion leaders are not only those with the most credibility, but also those who understand and can show empathy with the individual's concerns and attempts to change.

The operation of these principles can be seen in a project aimed at the reduction of behaviour problems among low-income Mexican–American children in Houston (Johnson, 1988). To gain the co-operation of parents, the staff first conducted door-to-door surveys of families in the Houston barrios asking about their aspirations for their children. These ideas were brought to a group of representative families for discussion. The parents then were encouraged to form a Parents' Advisory Council which would become the setting to facilitate and sanction programme activity. Final programme goals and procedures were developed in collaboration with this Council, whose members also served as both advisers and project spokespersons throughout the course of the programme. For example, the citizen advisers noted that Mexican culture frowns on women participating in public programmes outside the home. This meant that the first contacts with potential participants had to be in their own homes, working with both mothers and fathers to demonstrate that the social development of children was a goal valued by the community. Without the parents' advice about how to proceed, this programme would probably have had few participants.

Sometimes, it is health professionals themselves who need to change in order for community programmes to be considered. This is because of the changes in attitudes and standard operating procedures that are sometimes required. One example can be seen in a medical centre in Israel as they considered modifying their treatment of women experiencing childbirth through caesarean section (Tadmor, 1988). Previous obstetric practice, which was initially designed to spare the mother unnecessary anxiety by withholding information about the procedure until the last minute, actually served to aggravate unrealistic fears and increase distorted perceptions. Also the lack of anticipatory guidance and support for the mother before the procedure was found to slow postoperative recovery and acceptance of the baby. Unfortunately, the well-meaning desire to save the mother unnecessary anxiety contributed to negative health outcomes. Thus, changes were needed in the attitudes of medical and nursing staff before any new programme could be implemented. These were accomplished through on-the-job training and staff workshops. Ultimately, the new programme that was adopted maximized information to new mothers preoperatively and facilitated their active involvement in the care of their infants. In addition, a postoperative, caesarean birth support group was developed in which mothers were encouraged to become active in helping one another in dealing with common problems encountered in caring for these infants. An important end product of these activities was the increased level of emotional attachment between mother and infant.

In this example, the training workshops for physicians and allied health professionals provided the social setting through which staff attitude change could be reinforced at a group level. At the same time, changing the role of mothers from passive recipients of staff ministration to active counsellors and teachers of other mothers increased the likelihood that they themselves would leave the hospital with new knowledge and coping skills that could be used in day-to-day infant care.

OVERCOMING IMPEDIMENTS TO COMMUNITY HEALTH PROGRAMMES: DISTRUST, LACK OF MOTIVATION AND SOCIAL AND CULTURAL BARRIERS

The model in clinical medicine of treating individuals in isolation from their social milieu has had limited effectiveness in dealing with the health problems of the vast majority of citizens (Ewart, 1991). This is because social factors play a large role in facilitating or inhibiting the adoption of effective health practices. Dealing with these social factors, then, becomes a key ingredient in community health programmes.

While the principles enunciated thus far seem simple enough, there are impediments that can undermine well-meaning, community-based health interventions. To begin with, those most at risk are usually those who are most reluctant to volunteer for community programmes. For example, Fink and Shapiro (1990) found that mortality rates from all causes were highest among women who refused to participate in a voluntary breast cancer screening programme conducted by their health insurance plan. Reaching these reluctant participants required personal contact and intensive outreach as demonstrated by Lacey et al., (1989). In their cancer screening project, public health outreach workers, culturally sensitive to the target population, visited places frequented by women (such as beauty shops, grocery stores, housing projects and currency exchanges) to bring word of the programme and allay fears that only surfaced after personal contact had been established.

Social and psychological motives that impact upon individual health practices can be quite diverse. For example, they can include concerns about personal appearance and the maintenance of esteem with one's peers, the desire to avoid social rejection, the need for material and financial security, as well as knowledge of effective health practices. Given that these factors can operate to either facilitate or impede programme adoption, the goal is to design interventions that ameliorate potential resistances to behaviour change that come from the social milieu.

Resistances can come from the immediate social environment (family and friends) or from broader economic and cultural forces. The importance of the family environment has been recognized by the growing practice of expanding clinical treatment regimens to include family members. Morisky et al., (1983) found that a hypertension programme that included a spouse or family member resulted in improved blood pressure control and reduced mortality compared with a treatment group that focused on the individual patient alone. However, more difficult to address are social factors that are maintained by broader socioeconomic or cultural forces. In the context of AIDS prevention, Mays and Cochran (1988) note the social pressures that make it difficult for low-income ethnic women to refuse unsafe sexual practices. Many of these women lack power in intimate relations because of economic dependance, or are culturally excluded from decisions about contraceptive use. Expecting them to say no to unsafe sex is not very realistic, without concomitant changes in cultural attitudes and standards of conduct that would reinforce their decision. It is also important to address the economic dependence of these women with school and job training programmes. For similar reasons, an important component in a health and wellness programme for pregnant teenagers emphasizes the mother remaining in school (Rhodes, 1993).

Problem-focused health training programmes usually are most effective when they expand their focus and deal with motivation and social pressure as well as teaching simple behavioural skills. For example, in order for behaviour change to occur, one has to believe that one is personally capable of performing the new behaviours, in addition to acquiring the skills to properly execute them. A major impediment in the adoption of diet and exercise programmes is the pessimistic belief of many obese individuals that they will be unable to follow the prescribed programme. Working to improve motivation and skills with individual patients is one possibility, but since the belief in personal efficacy and the acquisition of skills occurs in a social context, changing the social milieu is often more effective in producing the desired results. Thus, Botvin and Tortu's (1988) substance abuse prevention programme for adolescents focused not only on the negative health effects of smoking, but also included esteem-enhancing activities in a group context. By conducting the programme in schools with peer trainers presenting the programme, the emphasis was on producing changes in the peer culture itself. Indeed, evaluation indicated that the programme was more effective when it was peer led than when the teachers were adults.

Not all community interventions succeed and one has to be prepared that, despite one's best intentions, something can go wrong. However, examples of failed interventions are instructive because they often point to missing or overlooked programme elements. For example, Baumgarten et al., (1988) set up a mutual help network among the elderly residents of a government subsidized apartment building in Canada. Rather than improving morale and satisfaction, those receiving the intervention showed a decrease in satisfaction with the support they were receiving and a moderate increase in depression compared to control group residents of a similar building in the same neighborhood. While the reasons for the negative effects of the intervention are not clear, one possibility is the problems encountered in trying to bring together residents of ethnically diverse backgrounds. The basis of the intervention was the encouragement of increased interaction among residents, but they were of different religious and language backgrounds and had a prior history of intergroup tension. In retrospect, the authors believe that the residents may not have wanted increased interaction with other dissimilar residents, preferring instead to spend time alone or with close friends and family members. Obtaining prior data about the social life of the elderly residents and their feelings toward other residents might have produced a more needs-relevant intervention, and again points to the importance of understanding the groups with whom you work before assuming that you know how to intervene.

CONCLUSIONS

At the present time, there is an ongoing debate in medical education about the extent to which public health and prevention concepts should be taught in the medical school curriculum (Altman, 1990). Despite the value of community-based prevention programmes, the traditional focus in medicine has been on treatment not prevention. The reward structure in medicine favours those who specialize in treatment, especially in the treatment of uncommon disorders whose occurrence in the general population may be relatively infrequent. The general practitioner or public health physician receives much less admiration from medical colleagues and much less pay than the more exotic specialist. Engaging in prevention activities requires the acceptance of less tangible rewards for yet another reason. Primary prevention programmes often take years to show changes in community-wide rates of disease, so there is less immediate gratification than is experienced by the private practitioner who can usually provide quick symptomatic relief to patients who appear at the doctor's office. So, if the reward structure in medicine is so heavily tilted towards treatment, why should physicians in training want to learn how to engage in community-based prevention activities?

This is a hard question to answer because it involves value choices. Community interventionists recognize that social and economic inequities exist in society and hope that their efforts can play a small part in addressing these problems. They also recognize that health problems cannot be divorced from general social life, so we are not likely to make major inroads in improving public health simply by dealing with one individual patient at a time. A number of examples have been provided in this chapter to demonstrate that enhanced well-being and reduction in rates of disease are not likely to occur simply through the development of more sophisticated treatment strategies, but by major community-wide attitude and lifestyle changes. The challenge of community medicine, then, is to help build social structures and groups that discourage destructive lifestyles and behaviours, while empowering and reinforcing health-enhancing citizen activity.

REFERENCES

Adler, N.E., Boyce, T., Chesney, M.A., Cohen, S., Folkman, S., Kahn, R.L. & Syme, S.L. (1994). Socioeconomic status and health: The challenge of the gradient. *American Psychologist*, 49, 15–24.

Altman, L.K. (1990). A profession divided is finding it hard to teach prevention. *New York Times*, (Medical Science) August, 14, C3.

Baumgarten, M., Thomas, D., Poulin de Courval, L. & Infante-Rivard, C. (1988). Evaluation of a mutual help network for the elderly residents of planned housing. *Psychology and Aging*, 3, 393–8.

Botvin, G.J. & Tortu, S. (1988), Preventing adolescent substance abuse through life skills training. In R.H. Price, E.L. Cowen, R.P. Lorion & J. Ramos-McKay (Eds.). *14 ounces of prevention: a casebook for practitioners*, pp. 98–110. Washington, DC: American Psychological Association.

Ewart, C.K. (1991). Social action theory for a public health psychology. *American Psychologist*, 46, 931–46.

Fink, R. & Shapiro, S. (1990). Significance of increased efforts to gain participation in screening for breast cancer. *American Journal of Preventive Medicine*, 6, 34–41.

Heller, K. (1990). Social and community intervention. *Annual Review of Psychology*, 41, 141–68.

Johnson, D.L. (1988). Primary prevention of behavior problems in young children: The Houston Parent–Child Development Center. In R.H. Price, E.L. Cowen, R.P. Lorion & J. Ramos-McKay (Eds.). *14 ounces of prevention: a casebook for practitioners*, pp. 44–52. Washington, DC: American Psychological Association.

Kelly, J.G. (1988). *A guide to conducting prevention research in the community: first steps*. New York: The Haworth Press.

Lacey, L.P., Phillips, C.W., Ansell, D., Whitman, S., Ebie, N. & Chen, E. (1989). An urban community-based cancer prevention screening and health education intervention in Chicago. *Public Health Reports*, 104, 536–41.

Mays, V.M. & Cochran, S.D. (1988). Issues in the perception of AIDS risk and risk reduction activities by Black and Hispanic/Latina women. *American Psychologist*, **43**, 949–57.

McMillan, D.W. & Chavis, D.M. (1986). Sense of community: a definition and theory. *Journal of Community Psychology*, **14**, 6–23.

Morisky, D.E., Levine, D.M., Green, L.W., Shapiro, S., Russell, R.P. & Smith, C.R. (1983). Five-year blood pressure control and mortality following health education for hypertensive patients. *American Journal of Public Health*, **73**, 153–162.

Rhodes, J.E. (1993). Easing postpartum school transitions through parent mentoring programs. *Prevention in Human Services*, **10**, 169–78.

Tadmor, C.S. (1988) The perceived personal control preventive intervention for a Casearian birth population. In R.H. Price, E.L. Cowen, R.P. Lorion & J. Ramos-McKay (Eds.). *14 ounces of prevention: a casebook for practitioners*, pp.141–152. Washington, DC: American Psychological Association.

US Department of Health and Human Services (1986). *Integration of risk factor interventions: two reports to the Office of Disease Prevention and Health Promotion.* Washington, DC: ODPHP Health Information Center.

Wandersman, A. & Florin, P. (1990). Citizen participation. In J. Rappaport & E. Seidman (Eds.). *Handbook of community psychology*. New York: Plenum.

Williams, R.B., Barefoot, J.C., Califf, R.M., Haney, T.L. Saunders, W.B., Pryor, D.B., Hlatky, M.A., Siegler, I.C. & Mark, D.B. (1992). Prognostic importance of social and economic resources among medically treated patients with angiographically documented coronary artery disease. *Journal of the American Medical Association* **267**, 520–4.

Counselling

JOHN ALLEN
and
ROBERT BOR

Medical Counselling Unit, Psychology Department, City University, London, UK

INTRODUCTION

It has been estimated that as many as one-third of all patients who consult a doctor do so because they have a 'personal problem', or real physical symptoms, causing them distress and reflecting an underlying psycho-social problem (Pereira Gray, 1988). Often patients first present with such 'life-problems' or psychosomatic symptoms during a medical consultation lasting a matter of minutes. If the doctor has no psychological training, the 'life-problem', or psychosomatic symptoms may well be medicalized, i.e. treated solely or principally as an organic complaint. Treatment then tends to take the form of psychotropic drugs. The consequence may well be that the condition becomes chronic, or fails to improve, resulting in yet more frequent consultations and further prescriptions. Many observers have commented on the enormous amount of personal distress this scenario causes patients and the huge resulting costs to health-care providers.

Counselling, among other forms of psychological help, may well be beneficial for patients presenting with such problems. The counsellor working with people in medical settings can provide time in which patients may express feelings about loss of abilities, roles and self-esteem, and assist them in coming to terms and/or coping with these and other changes. In addition to the psychological benefits of counselling, there are at least some indications that the presence of a counsellor in the primary health-care team leads to: a reduction in patients' psychosomatic symptoms, a consequent reduction in drug prescription rates, and a reduction in the demand for the time of medical staff. Other claimed benefits include: a better shared understanding of the role of counselling in the work of the therapeutic team, fewer inappropriate referrals and investigations, and fewer hospital admissions. Moreover, it appears that the division of workload leads to increased satisfaction for GPs and greater mutual respect within the primary health-care team.

THE NATURE OF COUNSELLING

If counselling is to have these beneficial effects, it is imperative that the appropriate conditions should be provided for its effective practice. There needs to be a clear appreciation within each medical team of the nature of counselling and the ways in which it differs from other forms of helping. The definition of counselling has always been problematic but one which is espoused by the British Association for Counselling (BAC) states: 'people become engaged in counselling when a person, occupying regularly or temporarily the role of counsellor offers or agrees explicitly to offer time attention and respect to another person or persons temporarily in the role of client' (BAC, 1985). The Code for Counsellors published by the BAC also states:

> *the overall aim of counselling is to provide an opportunity for a client to work towards living in a more satisfying and resourceful way. . . . Counselling may be concerned with developmental issues, addressing and resolving specific problems, making decisions, coping with crisis, developing personal insight and knowledge, working through feelings of inner conflict or improving relationships with others. The counsellor's role is to facilitate the client's work in ways which respect the client's values, personal resources and capacity for self-determination. (BAC, 1992).*

One of the clear implications of the stress on self-determination is that in counselling, the patient or client, is involved in an active, and to a large extent autonomous, process of exploration, clarification and problem solving. (This autonomy is often explicitly recognized by the use of the preferred title of 'client' rather than patient in the counselling context.) The emphasis on enabling or facilitating the client's decision-making in 'client-centred' approaches to counselling can be sharply contrasted with the traditional 'doctor-centred', or biomedical model, of patient care. In counselling, the 'expert' role is abandoned in favour of a consultative style which values client responsibility and freedom. This may well involve the sharing of specialist knowledge, particularly about medical issues but the use of such information is seen ultimately as the client's responsibility.

THE IMPACT OF COUNSELLING ON MEDICAL PRACTICE

Interestingly in recent years the 'client-centred' approach in counselling has had a significant impact on medical practice especially among those practitioners who have become dissatisfied with the older 'doctor-centred' model of patient care. Both in general practice, and in postgraduate training, psychological and social approaches to the understanding of health and illness have led to alternative ways of working with patients. There has, for example, been increasing acceptance by medical practitioners that an understanding of the patient's view is vital to the process of consultation, and that medical treatment should be based on shared involvement in decision-making. To facilitate this in practice, many of the skills developed in the counselling context such as active listening, empathic responding and reflection have been adopted by medical practitioners. Davis and Fallowfield (1991) argue that the use of counselling skills within a 'patient-centred' approach to medical care results in many benefits for patients and health professionals. These include increased patient and professional satisfaction, greater diagnostic adequacy, and improved adherence to treatment. Where they occur, these benefits are thought to be largely due to improved communication between patients and health professionals. Certainly, poor communication between doctor and patient accounts for some of the reasons given by patients for unsatisfactory medical consultations (Ley, 1988) and is cited as central to the reasons why patients sue their professional carers (Beckman et al., 1994). It has been shown, for example, that doctors working in different settings received dissatisfaction ratings from patients ranging from 26% in general practice to 39% in psychiatry, possibly reflecting an unequal emphasis on communications skills across settings and varying constraints on time in consultations. Studies of patient satisfaction which address communication skills are not without methodological flaws (Fitzpatrick, 1984) but some important findings have emerged. For example, it is clear that simply improving doctors' communication skills through tutoring (e.g. Maguire, Fairburn & Fletcher, 1986) may not directly improve the patient's understanding of the diagnosis, enhance compliance with treatment, or help the family cope with illness in all cases. This is because patients: sometimes forget what they have been told; are influenced and constrained by complex processes when making decisions about treatment; and some families have rules which govern the dissemination of information which, among other outcomes, can lead to secrecy between its members. Current research and practice addresses how best to improve communication, taking into account inherent constraints in the medical consultation such as time, the complexity of information, high levels of anxiety and distress in patients, and ambiguity in the professional caring relationship.

COUNSELLING IN THE MEDICAL CONTEXT

The origins of professional counselling for medical problems lie in efforts to improve patients' knowledge in order to help them to make informed decisions about treatment and care (such as with counselling for treatment for infertility, HIV antibody test counselling and termination of pregnancy counselling among others). More recently, this has extended to psychological support counselling. Counselling in medical settings is frequently associated with the following issues or problems: post-traumatic stress, pain management, pre and postoperative stress, spinal injury, cancer, genetic counselling, multiple sclerosis, HIV disease, adjustment to coronary heart disease, substance misuse, renal disease, treatment non-compliance, infertility, anxiety, helping sick children and their families cope, among many others.

There is rapid growth in the area of counselling in primary health-care settings. Not only is this a context in which counsellors can work with patients at the first point of diagnosis, treatment and care, but it also provides an opportunity for focused health education and preventative counselling (McDaniel, Campbell & Seaburn, 1990). An increasing number of counsellors working in primary care settings provide brief, symptom-focused counselling sessions (Boot et al., 1994).

Many of the interactions between health-care professionals and patients may not involve counselling as defined above but they may involve the use of counselling skills. The distinction between the use of counselling skills and counselling as a discrete activity is an important one but one which is often not made explicit. Bond (1993) has pointed out that counselling skills may be seen as a group of interpersonal, or communication, skills which share the common purpose of assisting the self-expression and autonomy of the recipient. Thus the purpose or values they serve are similar, if not identical, to those of counselling; namely empowerment and the encouragement of self-determination.

Counselling skills can therefore, be regarded as providing ways of helping patients make informed choices from a range of health options. In this way counselling skills may be distinguished from the use of other communication skills such as those employed to advise, influence and persuade. Bond (1993) also points out that counselling and the use of counselling skills may be distinguished from each other, at least in part, by noting whether the contracting between the parties concerned is explicit or not. The BAC definition of counselling given earlier expressly addresses this issue by noting the need for a clear understanding of the roles of counsellor and client. Confusions of role have often arisen, particularly in health care and medical contexts because counselling has been practised by those who occupy dual roles such as counsellor and doctor, nurse or health visitor. Where dual relationships apply, it is especially important to make the boundaries between roles clear and appropriately manage overlap between professional roles. The pitfalls of dual relationships in the context of general practice have been insightfully examined by Kelleher (1989) and it seems that, in the context of health counselling, such problems can best be avoided by ensuring that where

[207]

Table 1.

Counselling skills – the provision of factual information and advice about medical conditions, assessment, laboratory tests, treatment, drug trials, disease prevention and health promotion
Counselling skills/Implications counselling – discussion with the patient and others which addresses the meaning of the information for the patient, personal relationships and taking into account the patient's unique circumstances
Support counselling – in which the emotional consequences of implications can be expressed and acknowledged in a caring environment, and
Therapeutic counselling – which focuses on healing, psychological adjustment, coping and problem resolution.
(Adapted from The King's Fund Report, 1991).

possible the role of counsellor is separate from the provision of other services.

It is possible to envisage the relationship between counselling skills as a continuum as described in Table 1 (although for a contrary view on the relationship between counselling and counselling skills see Pratt, 1990).

Here counselling skills and counselling are seen as overlapping activities which play more or less prominent roles in different kinds of health-related consultations.

EVALUATION OF COUNSELLING

In a climate in which competition for resources is acute, it is essential that the effectiveness of counselling be demonstrated in order to justify its continued support. There is now a well-recognized need to determine the efficacy of counselling in medical settings (King *et al.*, 1994). Some studies have attempted to do this by asking whether counselling is cost-effective. Maguire *et al.* (1982), for example, reported considerable savings to the NHS through the early recognition and treatment of psychiatric problems in counselled mastectomy patients, as compared with a control group. Other studies have examined changes in patients' use of medical services or reductions in the number of drugs prescribed following counselling. Whilst the results of these studies have generally been favourable, it is necessary to interpret these outcomes with caution. In many of these studies there have been serious methodological flaws such as: the absence of control groups; sample attenuation; non-independent evaluation; and lack of appropriate statistical comparison (Brown & Abel Smith, 1985).

Most evaluation studies have concentrated on psychological outcomes such as the alleviation of distress, psychological adjustment and the amelioration of psychiatric conditions. Here again methodological difficulties abound. As with the psychotherapies, efficacy depends on the goals of the counsellor, the conceptual framework used and the methodologies that are employed. The research literature contains many examples of evaluation studies where researchers have used outcome measures of doubtful validity and reliability, research designs have been oversimplified and data has been overinterpreted. Moreover, the situation is not eased by the determination among some researchers to apply almost identical criteria for conducting evaluation studies of counselling to those used in clinical drug trials (Andrews, 1993). However, some recent studies have addressed many of the flaws which bedevilled earlier attempts to

establish the psychological efficacy of counselling in the medical context. For example, Milne and Souter (1988) studied the effects of counselling on assessed levels of stress in a study, which used patients as their own controls by incorporating a waiting list before counselling began. Significant increases in the use of coping skills and decreases in the levels of strain were found. Moreover, these results were not the result of normal crisis resolution because those with the most chronic problems developed more adequate coping skills whilst showing increased stressor scores. Patients who improved showed significant reductions in treatment cost in terms of hospitalization, GP visits and drugs prescription rates.

Other studies have examined the efficacy of counselling as an adjunct to medical treatment of cardiovascular problems and cancer. Maes (1992) has pointed out that psychosocial interventions, including counselling, may affect cardiac rehabilitation in two ways. First, such interventions may facilitate psychosocial recovery and thus aid return to everyday activities. Secondly, they may play an important role in secondary prevention, by improving compliance with medical advice concerning medication and lifestyle changes. Many of the studies of counselling and cardiac rehabilitation have been reviewed by Maes (1992) and Davis and Fallowfield (1991), who conclude that there is now considerable evidence that counselling, and related forms of intervention, can have beneficial effects on reported stress levels, professional reintegration, necessary lifestyle changes, and even perhaps mordibity and mortality. Davis and Fallowfield (1991) also provide a review of studies in which counselling has been employed as an adjunct to physical treatment for many other medical conditions ranging from diabetes mellitus to spinal cord injury.

Although gross measures may indicate the effectiveness of counselling, we still know little about the psychological processes underlying such changes. We also need to know more about which kinds of counselling interventions are particularly beneficial for which patients and at what stage of their illness. This requires detailed consideration of patient characteristics, the nature and time course of the presenting problems, patients' previous coping strategies and the impact of family and other supports. Research into counsellor characteristics and their impact on counselling is also much needed.

TRAINING ISSUES

To date, there has been enormous variability in the experience and qualifications of those employed as counsellors in medical settings. The situation has been unsatisfactory partly because in the UK there are no statutory regulations governing the qualifications of counsellors. However, helpful recommendations have been drawn up by the BAC which also operates a voluntary counsellor accreditation procedure. The Counselling in Primary Health Care Trust has also been active in promoting courses at postgraduate level for counsellors working in general practice and other settings. Chartered counselling psychologists in the UK are governed by statutory regulations through a route to qualification regulated by the British Psychological Society. With more courses emerging in counselling and counselling psychology at masters and post-masters level, it can be hoped that the qualifications of those working as counsellors will improve and higher levels of professional practice will be provided.

REFERENCES

Andrews, G. (1993). The essential psychotherapies. *British Journal of Psychiatry*, **162**, 447–51.

Beckman, H., Markakis, K. Suchman, A. & Frankel, R. (1994) The doctor – patient relationship and malpractice. *Archives of Internal Medicine*, **154**, 1365–70.

Bond, T (1993). *Standards and ethics for counselling in action.* Sage.

Boot, D., Gillies, P., Fenelon, J., Reubin, R., Wilkins, M. & Grey, P. (1994). Evaluation of the shortterm impact of counselling in general practice. *Patient Education and Counselling*, **24**, 79–89.

Brown, P.T. & Abel Smith, A.E. (1985). Counselling in medical settings. *British Journal of Guidance and Counselling*, **13**, 75–88.

British Association for Counselling (1985). *Counselling definitions of terms in use with expansion and rationale.* Rugby: British Association for Counselling.

British Association of Counselling (1992). *Code for counsellors.* Rugby: British Association for Counselling.

Davis, H. & Fallowfield, L. (1991). *Counselling and communication in health care.* Chichester: John Wiley.

Fitzpatrick, R. (1984). Satisfaction with health care. In Fitzpatrick, R., Hinton, J., Newman, G., Scambler, G. & Thompson, J. (Eds.). *The experience of illness.* London: Tavistock.

Kelleher, D. (1989). The GP as counsellor: an examination of counselling in general practice. *Counselling Psychology Section Review*, **4**, 7–13.

King, M., Broster, G., Lloyd, M. & Horder, J. (1994) Controlled trials in the evaluation of counselling in general practice. *British Journal of General Practice*, **44**, 229–32.

King's Fund Report (1991). *Counselling for regulated infertility treatments.* London: The King's Fund.

Ley, P. (1988). *Communicating with patients: improving communication, satisfaction and compliance* London: Chapman & Hall.

McDaniel, S., Campbell, T. & Seaburn, D. (1990). *Family oriented primary care.* New York: Springer-Verlag.

Maes, S. (1992). Psychosocial aspects of cardiac rehabilitation in Europe. *British Journal of Clinical Psychology*, **31**, 473–83.

Maguire, P., Oentol, A., Allen, D., Tait, A., Brooke, M. & Sellwood, R. (1982). Cost of counselling women who undergo mastectomy. *British Medical Journal*, **284**, 1933–5.

Maguire, P., Fairburn, S. & Fletcher, C. (1986). Consultation skills of young doctors. *British Medical Journal*, **292**, 1573–8.

Milne, D. & Souter, K. (1988). A re-evaluation of the clinical psychologist in general practice. *Journal of the Royal College of General Practitioners*, **38**, 457–60.

Pereira Gray, D. (1988). Counselling in general practice. *Journal of the Royal College of General Practitioners*, **38**, 50–1.

Pratt, J.W. (1990). The meaning of counselling skills. *Counselling*, **1**, 21–2.

Disability assessment

RAY FITZPATRICK

Nuffield College,
Oxford, UK

THE CONCEPT OF DISABILITY

Much of the work of health care is concerned with addressing the consequences for patients of disease. A plethora of terms variously refer to such consequences in terms of 'functional status', 'dependency', 'disability' and 'handicap'. The World Health Organization (1980) has developed an important schema for delineating relationships between these concepts: the International Classification of Impairments, Disabilities and Handicaps (ICIDH). The ICIDH schema defines impairment as any loss or abnormality of psychological, physiological or anatomical structure or function. Impairment therefore refers to failure at the level of organs or systems of the body. Disability refers to any restriction or lack of ability to perform an activity in the manner considered normal for a human being. The emphasis is therefore on things that individuals cannot do. Handicap is any disadvantage for an individual, resulting from impairment or disability, that limits the fulfilment of a role for that individual. It refers to the social disadvantages that may follow from disease.

Although there may be a linear progression from disease through impairment, disability to handicap, this is not necessary. Individuals may, for example, experience considerable handicap because of an impairment without any significant level of disability. A facial dis-figurement may result in no disability for an individual, but, because of embarrassment or stigma, may result in considerable handicap. Relationships between impairment, disability and handicap are often quite weak. For example, in asthma, levels of pulmonary function may only modestly correlate with experience of handicap in daily life. A variety of social and psychological factors intervene to influence levels of disability and handicap arising from disease.

Recent independently measured estimates of the prevalence of disability in the USA and UK come to rather similar conclusions, with approximately 14% of adults being considered disabled due to ill-health. Arthritis, blindness, stroke, coronary heart disease and bronchitis are the disorders most commonly responsible for disability in these estimates.

Assessment has, to date, largely focused on disability, although measures are beginning to address handicap more systematically. The most fundamental question is to determine which problems of function are relevant to disability. It is common to distinguish between two levels of functioning: basic and instrumental activities of daily living (ADL). Basic ADL functions are those that are essential for self-care such as bathing, dressing and feeding. Instrumental ADL are those activities such as doing laundry, shopping, housekeeping, getting around by driving or public transport that are necessary for someone to maintain a level of independent living, especially in the absence of a carer. Problems with instrumental ADL (IADL) are far more common than for basic ADL so that the prevalence of disability is very much influenced by whether the broader range of IADLs are included in operational measures.

PURPOSES OF ASSESSMENT

Assessments of disability may serve a number of different purposes. It is essential to be quite clear about the purpose to which any particular measure is to be put. A particular measure of disability may, for example, be very useful as a population survey instrument for measuring the prevalence of disability in a population, but not perform well as a measure of outcome in clinical trials or evaluation studies.

Assessment of need

Earliest attempts to measure disability were intended to provide more standardized and objective assessments of the nature and severity of disability in patient groups in order to provide estimates of need for nursing or other forms of health professional care. Instruments such as the Index of ADL (Katz et al., 1963) were originally developed in a hospital context. As described below, the Index of ADL depends on trained assessors observing patients' performances over a range of functions. A related purpose of disability assessment is to determine eligibility for benefits.

More structured and explicit methods of assessing disability are considered important because of widespread evidence that health professionals underestimate the extent of disability in their patients. Thus in one study of a group of US doctors working in primary medical care, doctors were asked to assess disability in their patients and results compared to evidence obtained directly from patients (Calkins et al., 1991). Doctors failed to recognize or underestimated 66% of disability. Structured methods such as screening questionnaires may reduce such problems.

Increasingly, measures of disability are used to assess need on a population basis, whether to assist purchasers in determining their priorities or to help providers of care to identify patients in need of services. It is much less realistic to have trained observers make assessments of whole populations. So, recently much emphasis has been given to developing measures of disability that can be obtained from self-completed mailed questionnaires. The emphasis in instruments like the Lambeth Disability Screening Questionnaire (Charlton, Patrick & Peach, 1983) is upon measures that can screen for the presence of disability with some confidence rather than provide detailed or specific information about the nature of disabilities for any individual.

Prediction of problems

A related use of disability assessments is in the prediction of problems, either in terms of increased risk of deterioration in health or mortality, or in terms of demands placed upon health services. Thus a brief self-completed questionnaire assessing instrumental ADLs which was sent to elderly individuals living in the community proved to be a significant predictor of mortality independently of demographic and other social factors over a four-year period (Reuben et al., 1992). Amongst survivors, poor disability scores at baseline were also associated with poorer self-reported health at follow-up.

Measures of outcome

Disability measures may be used to assess the progress of patients over time, and by extension to assess outcomes of health care in quality assurance, evaluation studies or clinical trials. Thus, in a randomized controlled trial of oral gold over a 24-week period, patients with rheumatoid arthritis were shown to obtain significantly greater benefits from the active drug compared with the placebo in terms of a simple disability score from the Health Assessment Questionnaire as well as for other outcomes such as pain, stiffness and tender joints (Bombardier et al., 1986). The scope for therapeutic benefits from interventions is often so modest that disability assessments need to be sensitive to quite subtle changes. In general, information about outcomes obtained from disability measures provides evidence of the effects of interventions that most directly address patients' concerns.

MEASUREMENT REQUIREMENTS

The measurement properties required for disability assessments are the same as for all other health status and psychometric instruments. Assessments need to be reliable, valid, sensitive to change, acceptable, relevant and practical to use. However, a proliferation of disability instruments has occurred in which the majority of instruments have still not been evaluated against such criteria. Test–retest reliability is one important component of measures but, for observer-based measures of disability, inter-rater reliability is also of importance. There are no 'gold standard' criteria against which to measure validity. Instead, a battery of approaches should be used that includes the important stage of informal examination of whether the content of measures is appropriate to the intended use and encompasses all relevant dimensions. More formal assessment of validity involves construct validity by comparing results with other related measures or predictive validity in which scores are examined against subsequent health status or health-care use.

Sensitivity to change requires particular attention in disability assessment. It cannot be assumed that, because an instrument has been shown to be valid in terms of distinguishing degrees of severity of disability between patients that it will also be sensitive to important changes over time in disability within patients. One problem is that measures of disability may make only a small number of broad distinctions between levels of disability. For example, the standard American Rheumatism Association (ARA) functional classification distinguishes just four levels of disability ranging from 'complete functional capacity' to 'largely or wholly incapacitated'. There is a substantial amount of change that can occur to patients in degree of disability whilst remaining within a single grade of the ARA scale. Such broad categories can therefore understate the effects of health care interventions. Simple changes to instruments such as increasing the number of response categories may increase sensitivity to change without increasing respondents burden. Some evidence for increased sensitivity in measuring disability for patients with strokes is reported for the Barthel Index when functional items (feeding, dressing, etc) were coded on a range of five points from 'unable to do task' to 'fully independent' instead of the conventional three (Shah, Vanclay & Cooper, 1989).

Another problem that can limit disability measures sensitivity to change derives from so called 'ceiling' and 'floor' effects. Instruments may not leave scope for patients to express further improvement or deterioration beyond the items included in the instrument. Thus, for example, the Health Assessment Questionnaire (HAQ) was completed by patients with rheumatoid arthritis at the beginning and end of a five-year period. Patients with the poorest (highest disability) initial scores for HAQ generally rated their disability as worse five years later. However, they experienced very little deterioration in HAQ scores. By comparison, other groups with initially lower disability scores and who also at the end rated their disability as having declined less, nevertheless experienced larger deterioration according to HAQ scores. The most likely explanation for such patterns is that HAQ may not register severest degrees of decline in disability.

TYPES OF ASSESSMENTS

Direct clinical testing

Traditionally clinicians have used a number of physical tests to assess aspects of function and disability, for example, by timing patients required to walk particular distances or perform tasks such as buttoning and unbuttoning. One problem with such assessments is that they may be unrepresentative of the challenges faced by the patient in his or her usual environment. However, a more fundamental problem is that such tests are remarkably unreliable (Pincus, Brooks & Callahan, 1991). By standardizing the instructions to patients and methods of recording observations, it is possible to obtain very good inter-rater reliability (Pincus et al., 1991). Clinical tests such as walking time are inevitably limited in scope because of inherent difficulties of directly observing many IADLs such as shopping and use of transport.

Observer-based assessments

Far more widely used are a number of standardized assessments made directly of disability by trained observers. One of the first, and still commonly used, of such assessments is the Index of ADL developed by Katz and colleagues (1963). Individuals are rated by observers on a three-point scale of degree of independence for each of six activities: bathing, dressing, toileting, transfer (moving in and out of bed and chairs), continence and feeding. Evidence of reliability and validity is not as readily available as for many more recent methods of assessment. It concentrates only on more basic ADLs and uses rather broad categories so that it may not be appropriate as an outcome for the majority of interventions from which only modest benefits are expected.

A somewhat similar observer-based instrument that is widely used is the Barthel Index. The Barthel index exists in a variety of forms which differ in items and methods of scoring but all require observers' ratings of a number of basic ADLs. There appears to be somewhat more evidence available to support the Barthel Index (Wade & Collin, 1988). Like the Index of ADL it may not be sensitive to more modest benefits commonly considered in rehabilitation of physical disability. The Barthel Index focuses upon what individuals actually do rather than on what they can do (two quite distinct issues) and may be influenced by the context in which assessment is made.

Standardized interviews and questionnaires

Most recently disability has been assessed via instruments that can take the form of standardized interviews or, in many cases are usable as self-completed questionnaires. Probably the most widely used instrument to date is the Sickness Impact Profile (SIP) (Bergner et al., 1981) It comprises 136 statements with 'yes' or 'no' responses. Items contribute to one of 12 scales: walking, body care and movement, mobility, work, sleeping and rest, eating, housework, recreation, emotion, social interaction, alertness and communication. The first three scales can be combined to produce a 'physical scale' which most closely resembles a disability assessment. Scoring of items are weighted on the basis of extensive rating exercises of panels to assess severity. It has been shown to be reliable, valid and responsive for a quite wide range of chronic diseases. Because of its length it requires 20–30 minutes to complete and is therefore not appropriate for some settings. As with all instruments, use as a self-completed instrument may be limited for individuals with significant cognitive impairment.

It is increasingly becoming clear that, for some purposes such as screening or evaluation of outcomes, shorter questionnaires may perform almost or completely as well as longer formats (Katz et al., 1993). A questionnaire, the Lambeth Disability Questionnaire (Charlton et al., 1983), has been developed from the SIP to perform as a screening instrument for disability. It comprises just 22 items and requires only five minutes to complete. Some aspects of validity have been examined; it distinguishes between disabled and non-disabled individuals as determined by other measures (Charlton et al., 1983).

Another shorter form instrument designed for self-completion is the SF-36 which comprises 36 items and is rapidly becoming the most widely used of shorter health status questionnaires (Brazier et al., 1992). It contains two dimensions highly relevant to disability: physical functioning and role limitations due to physical problems. It has been quite widely applied and examined for measurement properties.

In addition to instruments such as SF-36, which may be used to assess disability across a wide range of diseases, a number of short disability assessments have been developed for use in specific disorders. Probably the most familiar and most widely used is the Health Assessment Questionnaire (HAQ) (Fries, Spitz & Young, 1982) for use in rheumatoid arthritis. It contains 20 items across eight areas of function: dressing and grooming, rising, eating, walking, hygiene, reach, grip and outside activity. It has been shown to fulfil a number of functions: screening, clinical assessment, outcome measure to a satisfactory standard. Evidence has been cited above of possible ceiling effects in the HAQ, which may be an important problem, given that disability in rheumatoid arthritis can deteriorate quite substantially beyond the scope of the scale (Gardiner et al., 1993).

It should be noted that many of the more recent instruments such as SIP and SF-36 contain items and dimensions which really address aspects of handicap as well as disability according to WHO criteria in examining issues such as occupational problems and social support. It may be argued that such instruments do not very clearly distinguish the two levels.

ISSUES FOR THE FUTURE

The majority of current forms of assessment involve the use of standardized instruments. However an important approach to rehabilitation is based on 'goal attainment scaling' in which patient and therapist jointly set priorities in terms of specific targets for particular functional problems. It is possible to adapt such individualized assessment of whether goals are achieved with more conventional standardized measurement systems. Tugwell and colleagues (1990) developed an instrument to assess disability in rheumatoid arthritis (the Patient Preference Disability Questionnaire) in which patients identify up to five functional problems of concern to them arising from their disease. Patients were then recruited to a placebo-controlled randomized trial of a particular drug, methotrexate. Patients completed the newly devised instrument as well as a number of standard disability and rheumatological measures before and after therapy. The individualized instrument produced greater differences between active drug and placebo than did many of the standard measures. There is a great deal more scope for making disability measures relate more closely to individual priorities, although work will also be needed to clarify the statistical analysis of such data.

The work of Tugwell and colleagues also illustrates quite clearly the need for more direct 'back to back' comparisons of the value of different disability measures in particular applications, especially with regard to sensitivity to change. A study has already been cited above (Katz et al., 1993) in which it was demonstrated that shorter disability measures were as sensitive as longer measures to changes in patients' disability. A study was designed to examine comparatively the sensitivity to change of the major functional measures in rheumatoid arthritis (Fitzpatrick et al., 1993). Patients completed at three-monthly intervals the Health Assessment Questionnaire, the Sickness Impact Profile and two other assessments commonly used to assess disability in RA. No single instrument proved consistently more sensitive to the changes that patients themselves reported in response to more global questions about the progress of their disease. It was possible to conclude that simpler and shorter instruments like the Health Assessment Questionnaire are as sensitive as more detailed instruments, whilst being more practical to complete and therefore more plausible as outcome measures in routine practice.

At present, there is a diverse range of assessments in this field and more important than further development of additional measures is the task of directly testing the value and relevance of existing measures.

REFERENCES

Bergner, M., Bobbitt, R., Carter, W. & Gilson, B. (1981). The Sickness Impact Profile: development and final revision of a health status measure. *Medical Care*, **19**, 787–805.

Bombardier, C., Ware, J., Russell, I., Larson, M., Chalmes, A., Read, J. & of the Auranofin cooperating Group. (1986). Auranofin therapy and quality of life in patients with rheumatoid arthritis: results of a multi-center trial. *American Journal of Medicine*, **81**; 565–78.

Brazier, J., Harper, R., Jones, N. et al. (1992). Validating the SF-36 health survey questionnaire: new outcome measure for primary care. *British Medical Journal*, **305**, 160–4.

Calkins, D., Rubenstein, L., Cleary, P. Davies, A., Jette, A., Fink, J., Kosecoff, R., Young R., Brook, R. & Delbanco, T. (1991). Failure of physicians to recognize disability in ambulatory patients. *Annals of Internal Medicine*, **114**, 451–3.

Charlton, J., Patrick, D. & Peach, H. (1983). Use of multivariate measures of disability in health surveys. Journal of Epidemiology and community Health 37, 296–304.

Fitzpatrick, R., Ziebland, S., Jenkinson, C.,

Mowat, A. & Mowat, A. (1993). A comparison of the sensitivity to change of several health status instruments in rheumatoid arthritis. *Journal of Rheumatology*, **20**, 429–36.

Fries, J., Spitz, P. & Young, D. (1982). The dimensions of health outcomes: the Health Assessment Questionnaire, disability and pain scales. *Journal of Rheumatology*, **9**, 789–93.

Gardiner, P., Sykes, H., Hassey, G. & Walker, D. (1993). An evaluation of the Health assessment Questionnaire in long term longitudinal follow-up of disability in rheumatoid arthritis. *British Journal of Rheumatology*, **32**, 724–8.

Katz, S., ford, A., Moskowitz, R., Jackson, D. & Jaffer, M. (1963). Studies of illness in the aged: the Index of ADL: a standardized measure of biological and psychosocial function. *Journal of the American Medical Association*, **85**, 914–19.

Katz, J. Larson, M., Phillips, C., Fossel, A. & Liang, M. (1993). Comparative measurement sensitivity of short and longer health status instruments. *Medical Care*, **30**, 917–25.

Pincus, T., Brooks, R. & Callahan, L. (1991). Reliability of grip strength, walking

time and button test performed according to a standard protocol. *Journal of Rheumatology*, **18**, 997–1000.

Reuben, D., Rubenstein, l., Hirsch, S. & Hays, R. (1992). Value of functional status as a predictor of mortality: results of a prospective study. *American Journal of Medicine*, **93**, 633–9.

Shah, S., Vanclay, F. & Cooper, B. (1989). Improving the sensitivity of the Barthel Index for stroke rehabilitation. *Journal of Clinical Epidemiology*, **42**, 703–9.

Tugwell, P., Bombardier, C., Buchana, W., Goldsmith, C., Grace, E. & Hanna, B. (1990). Methotrexate in rheumatoid arthritis: impact on quality of life assessed by traditional standards item and individualized patient preference health status questionnaires. *Archives of Internal Medicine*, **150**, 59–62.

Wade, D. & Collin, C. (1988) The Barthel ADL Index: a standard measure of physical disability? *International Disability Studies*, **10**, 64–7.

World Health Organization (1980). International Classification of Impairments, Disabilities and Handicaps. Geneva: World Health Organization.

Group therapy

PETER HAJEK

*Psychology Section, Department of Human Science
and Medical Ethics, St Bartholomew's and the
Royal London School of Medicine and Dentistry,
London, UK*

This chapter will (i) outline the main approaches to using groups to help people deal with psychological problems, (ii) examine briefly the relevant outcome research, and (iii) describe the main applications of group therapy, with particular focus on groups in medical setting.

MODELS OF GROUP THERAPY

There is an obvious intuitive and experiential validity in the notion that cohesive groups can provide considerable support and psychological help to their members. Throughout our lives the features of our membership in various groups such as the primary and secondary family, school class, work groups, and networks of friends are of great importance. Social interactions within such structures are one of the major sources of human happiness and fulfilment, as well as of human misery.

Various religious and secular groups have always helped to alleviate their members' psychological distress. However, the idea of creating groups for an explicitly therapeutic purpose is relatively new. The first account of such groups was published in 1907. Rather surprisingly, this pioneering report is from a general medical rather than a psychiatric setting. An American internist, Joseph Pratt, organized group meetings to provide support and encouragement to patients with tuberculosis, and to demonstrate the benefits of compliance with the therapeutic regimen of the day. In recent years, support groups for people with physical or externally based problems are becoming popular again. Throughout the intervening period, however, group therapy has been practised primarily in psychiatric and psychological settings, and the most influential approaches were informed predominantly by the work with neurotic populations.

Groups are a complex and multivariate tool and there exists a large number of styles of group work. Well over 100 'group therapies' have been described in the literature. Most of them, however, derive from four basic approaches, and could be in broad terms allocated to one of them, or to their combinations. These four major strands can be labelled analytical, interpersonal, experiential, and didactic. They correspond to the main work styles a group can adopt, i.e. to analyse motives for group members' behaviour; to provide an opportunity for social learning; to generate emotional experiences; and to impart information and teach new skills.

In practice, group therapists working with similar types of clients often converge on a similar integrated package of interventions and skills, spanning these different approaches. For an observer it would often be impossible to say to which particular 'school' the therapist subscribes. Throughout this chapter, this amalgam which characterizes the practice of many experienced group therapists is labelled 'mainstream practice'. Even the principal proponents of the four alternative forms of group treatment include at least some elements of the other approaches in their work.

The analytical approach

This has a historical primacy as the first to apply a theory of psychological functioning and disorders to group treatment. It remains influential in the UK, and has left clear marks on the eclectic mainstream practice of group therapy. In broad terms, the goal of treatment is to uncover and resolve hypothetical unconscious conflicts. This is expected to lead to the patient's recovery. The mainstream practice has adopted elements of two particular hallmarks of group analytical treatments, i.e. attention to hidden motivation behind group members' interactions, and attention to the relationship of group members to the group leader (transference).

The interpersonal approach

This emphasizes the opportunity for social learning which groups can provide. Its origin is in 'laboratory' groups initiated by Kurt Lewin in 1947 and intended as an *in vitro* social environment in which group members can learn about how groups function and how participants behave in them. Treatment applications of a combination of this and other approaches are associated primarily with the work of I. Yalom. The mainstream practice has adopted the concept of social feedback (i.e. allowing group members to learn how their behaviour affects others), and an empirically derived outline of typical developmental processes and stages in an unstructured group. 'Training groups' also provide a model for training group therapists in awareness of group processes.

The experiential approach

The experiential approach to groups is characterized by working primarily with the clients' current awareness of their experience. The most important sources for this approach were 'encounter groups' inspired by Carl Rogers and aimed primarily at experiences of closeness and acceptance. Jacob Moreno's psychodrama and more recent developments such as gestalt therapy by Fritz Perls represent other important influences. The contribution of this approach to mainstream practice is primarily in encouraging group therapists to use techniques aimed at stimulating desirable group experiences. (The label 'experiential' is used here for convenience. It often appears in various other contexts as well).

[213]

Didactic approaches

There are associated primarily with behavioural and cognitive treatments administered in groups, but are also widely practised in various health promotion/education contexts. The therapist usually has a set agenda for each session, group members are given concrete tasks, and group interaction and group processes are not the main focus of attention. Behaviour and cognitive therapists and health education workers usually lack a background in group dynamics, and tend automatically to adopt the simplest group model we are all familiar with, i.e. that of a classroom with a teacher and pupils. Behavioural approaches have developed in opposition to the older models, and there has been little cross-fertilization so far. This is unfortunate as there is some evidence that employing group processes can increase the efficacy of behavioural treatments.

Further details of different approaches to group treatment, and descriptions of group processes and of practical skills involved in running groups can be found in, e.g. Yalom, 1995; Hansen, Warner & Smith, 1980; Aveline & Dryden, 1988.

THERAPEUTIC FACTORS IN GROUP THERAPY

There are a number of hypothetical processes through which groups are supposed to exercise their therapeutic effects. Different applications of group treatment concentrate on different therapeutic factors. A description of group treatment in terms of therapeutic factors expected to foster specific treatment goals is a useful practical alternative to describing a groupwork style only in terms of the therapist's theoretical persuasion. This 'transtheoretical' approach to group treatment is also amenable to empirical research

Several categorizations of therapeutic factors have been proposed. Table 1 provides one of them, based on a list by Bloch and Crouch (1985) with the last item, Group Pressure, added by the

Table 1. *Therapeutic factors in group therapy*

1. *Acceptance* – the patient feels a sense of belonging and being valued (cohesiveness).
2. *Universality* – the patient discovers that he is not unique with his problems.
3. *Altruism* – the patient learns with satisfaction that he can be helpful to others in the group.
4. *Instillation of hope* – the patient gains a sense of optimism about his potential to benefit from treatment.
5. *Guidance* – the patient receives useful information in the form of advice, suggestions, explanation, and instruction.
6. *Vicarious learning* – the patient benefits (e.g. by learning about oneself) by observing the therapeutic experience of fellow group members.
7. *Self-understanding* – the patient learns something important about himself (insight).
8. *Learning from interpersonal action* – the patient learns from his attempts to relate constructively and adaptively within the group (interpersonal learning).
9. *Self-disclosure* – the patient reveals highly personal information to the group and thus 'gets it off his chest'.
10 *Catharsis* – the patient releases intense feelings which brings him a sense of relief.
11. *Group pressure* – the patient alters undesirable behaviours/attitudes to gain or to retain group approval.

present author. The pressure to conform to group norms has a somewhat ominous ring, and listing it as a potentially therapeutic force seems to go against the selfactualization philosophy endorsed in most writings on groups and therapy. However, where the goal of the group includes, e.g. modification of health behaviours, drug use, or antisocial behaviour, and where the group manages to establish norms conducive to desirable behaviour change, group pressure can be a major therapeutic influence. Different factors become prominent in different types of groups. For example, a group aimed at uncovering hidden motives behind self-defeating neurotic behaviours would focus on self-understanding more than on guidance; an Alcoholics Anonymous group would rely on instillation of hope more than on catharsis; and a support group for patients diagnosed with cancer would emphasize universality and altruism more than insight.

EFFICACY OF GROUP THERAPY

The main and obvious argument in favour of group treatments is that, assuming there is little difference in efficacy between individual and group approaches, treating people in groups is much more cost-effective. Running a group with ten patients for the same length of time per session as individual treatment would take, means that group therapy achieves the same effect as individual therapy ten times more cheaply; or to put the argument differently, for the same cost, group therapy helps ten times as many people as the individual approach.

A more involved issue concerns the specificity of any group treatment effects. Group treatment (like most psychological treatments) has been shown in many instances to be better than no treatment; and direct and meta-analytical comparisons have not found much difference between individual and group approaches (Smith, Glass & Miller, 1980, Rose & LeCroy, 1991). This, however, could be due to various non-specific factors. It is the basic assumption of all types of group therapy that the processes generated in group setting (which are not available in an individual setting) are conducive to patients' recovery. To demonstrate empirically this hypothetical active ingredient of group treatment is not easy. The broad question of specific efficacy of a treatment which can be applied in different forms with different conditions may appear too unfocused. However, to consider any treatment approach valid and deserving of further study, some proof is needed of the existence of the presumed effect in whatever form and context.

Research in efficacy of psychological treatments is generally difficult and plagued with methodological problems. Research into the efficacy of group treatments has the additional handicap of extra demands on sample size because the units of observation are groups rather than individual patients; and it is even more difficult to find a suitable control condition for group treatments than it is for individual treatments. Comparisons of groups treatment with no treatment or with individual treatments cannot demonstrate the specific effects of groups. More promising are mutual comparisons of group treatments which only differ in group-specific variables. One area uniquely suited to this type of research is that of smoking cessation groups. This is because there is an almost unlimited supply of patients, treatment is brief, and outcome (i.e. tobacco abstinence) is clearly defined and can be verified objectively. In this population, it has been shown that variations in group format and in group size affect outcome, and that an individual's chances of success are significantly determined by group membership, i.e. being a member of a 'good' group enhances an individual's member's chance of success. (Hajek *et al.*, 1985, Hajek 1994). At least in this particular area, groups have specific effects on therapeutic outcome.

The most recent review of studies of group therapy, including both outcome and process research, can be found in Bednar and Kaul (1994).

APPLICATIONS OF GROUP THERAPY

Table 2 lists some of the standard uses of group therapy. The remainder of this chapter concentrates on groups for physically ill people.

The physically ill people can derive a number of benefits from participating in a support group. For instance, in several studies, cancer patients allocated to groups were reported to be less depressed and fatigued with fewer maladaptive coping responses, higher self-esteem, and reporting more life satisfaction than controls (Davis & Fallowfield, 1991; Blanchard, 1994). Medical care traditionally focuses on medical illness, and patients' concerns tend to remain unexplored. Yet it is obvious that learning that one has a terminal or debilitating illness has a profound psychological impact, which deeply affects patient's psychological well-being, and can affect the course of the illness itself. It appears that group support can ameliorate some of these effects.

The goals of groups with the physically ill differ from the focus of traditional group therapy. Most 'medical' groups concentrate primarily on providing general support to group members, although some would also aim at influencing their health behaviours (e.g. cardiac rehabilitation groups). The group camaraderie and 'common bond in common disease' have already been described by Joseph Pratt. In the current revival of medical groups, the emphasis on sharing mutual concerns and feeling understood and accepted remains central. Other elements include relinquishing the unhealthy 'silent sufferer' role often adopted to protect others; the opportunity to learn from other group members ways of coping with illness; sharing relevant information and resources; maintaining social interest and involvement; etc. Groups are often also an ideal forum for health professionals to impart and discuss medical advice affecting patients' lifestyle. Groups with patients are usually dependent on health professionals in both their organization and content. Within the health service, group leaders come from diverse professional background, including, e.g. psychology, medicine, social work, psychiatry, nursing, and rehabilitation.

Examples of 'disease management' groups include groups for chronic pain sufferers (in addition to general support, cognitive–behavioural principles are usually included), patients with coronary

Table 2. *Common uses of group therapy*

1. *Groups for normals* – assisting personal development in individuals who are not experiencing specific problems. Examples: staff groups, sensitivity groups, parents groups, women groups, etc.
2. *Group counselling for externally based problems.* Examples: groups for rape victims, disaster victims, relatives of alcoholics, relatives of mentally or terminally ill, etc.
3. *Group support for physically ill patients.* Examples: Cardiac rehabilitation, pain management, groups for cancer patients, HIV positive patients, etc. (see text)
4. *Group treatment for antisocial and addictive behaviours.* Examples: Groups and therapeutic communities for delinquents, inmates, drug addicts, alcoholics, etc.
5. *Group therapy for people with neurotic problems and personality disorders.* Traditional area of group therapy, usually psychiatric outpatients
6. *Groups for people with severe mental disorders.* Psychiatric in-patients and out-patients (rehabilitation, occupational therapy, 'living skills', etc.)

artery disease (cardiac rehabilitation programmes are possibly the largest application of disease management groups, and typically include exercise, modification of type A behaviour, and health education in addition to group support), cancer patients, diabetics, patients with AIDS, etc. Even in didactically orientated groups, elements of group support tend to have bigger impact than other components (e.g. Rahe, Ward & Hayes, 1979).

An important branch of this work concerns groups with relatives of patients with chronic debilitating conditions. These groups often have a self-help format. If health professionals are involved at all, it may be only in the initiation stage, or possibly in an on-going consulting capacity. Support groups for patients' families have been described for parents of newborn children who died, family members of cancer patients, of patients with Alzheimer's disease, etc. Particulars of some of the developments in groups for physically ill and their families can be found in Roback (1984) and Davis & Fallowfield (1991).

Group counselling for patients with serious medical conditions and for their families is by no means commonplace. However, the merits of this approach are increasingly recognized and the number of such groups is steadily increasing. The idea of using group support to alleviate the psychological distress accompanying certain diseases and to improve disease management, has taken root, and is likely to continue to develop. (See also 'Coping with chronic illness', 'Behaviour therapy', 'Biofeedback', 'Cognitive behaviour therapy'.)

REFERENCES:
Aveline, M. & Dryden, W. (Eds.). (1988). *Group therapy in Britain.* Milton Keynes: Open University Press.
Bednar, R. & Kaul, T. (1994). Experiential group research. In A. Bergin, & S. Garfield, (Eds.). *Handbook of psychotherapy and behavior change.* New York: Wiley.
Blanchard, E. (1994). Behavioral medicine and health psychology. In A. Bergin & S.

Garfield (Eds.). *Handbook of psychotherapy and behavior change.* New York: Wiley.
Bloch, S. & Crouch, E. (1985). *Therapeutic factors in group psychotherapy.* Oxford: Oxford Medical Publications.
Davis, H. & Fallowfield, L. (Eds.). (1991). *Counselling and communication in health care.* Chichester: Wiley.

Hajek, P. (1994). Helping smokers to overcome tobacco withdrawal: background and practice of withdrawal-oriented therapy. In R. Richmond (Ed.). *Interventions for smokers: an international perspective.* Baltimore: Williams and Wilkins.
Hajek P., Belcher M. & Stapleton J. (1985). Enhancing the impact of groups: an evaluation of two group formats for

smokers. *British Journal of Clinical Psychology*, **24**, 289–94.

Hansen, J., Warner, R. & Smith, E. (1980). *Group counseling. Theory and process.* Chicago: Rand McNally.

Rahe, R., Ward, H. & Hayes, V. (1979). Brief group therapy in myocardial infarction rehabilitation: three-to four-year follow-up

of a controlled trial. *Psychosomatic Medicine*, **41**, 229–42.

Roback, H. (Ed.). (1984). *Helping patients and their families cope with medical problems.* San Francisco: Jossey-Bass.

Rose, S. & LeCroy, C. (1991). Group methods. In F. Kanfer, & A. Goldstein,

(Eds.). *Helping people change.* New York: Pergamon.

Smith, M., Glass, G. & Miller, T. (1980). *The benefits of psychotherapy.* Baltimore: Johns Hopkins University Press.

Yalom, I. (1995). *The theory and practice of group psychotherapy.* 4th ed. New York: Basic Books.

Health education

GERJO KOK

Department of Health Education, University of Limburg, Maastricht, The Netherlands

HEALTH EDUCATION, HEALTH PROMOTION AND PREVENTION

Health education is a planned activity, stimulating learning through communication, to promote healthy behaviour. The concept of health education needs to be distinguished from the concepts of prevention and health promotion. Three types of prevention are the goals of health promotion: (i) primary prevention, (ii) early detection and treatment, and (iii) patient care and support. Health education is one of the means to achieve these goals. Other health promotion instruments are resources and regulation. Health education is based on voluntary change, while regulation is based on forced compliance and will only be effective in combination with control and sanctions. Health promotion is the combination of goals and means. In general, interventions that are directed at several levels and that use more means, will be more effective (Milio, 1988; Simons-Morton *et al.*, 1988).

To provide an example of this last statement, let us look at the prevention of drunken driving. There is regulation: most countries have laws against driving under the influence of alcohol. Often there is control: drivers are stopped by the police and may be tested, although countries differ in their commitment to these control activities. There are resources: public transportation, especially in the weekends and during the night, cheap taxis for adolescents. There is education: about the rules and possible sanctions, about resources, and about drunken driving itself, i.e. the consequences of drunken driving, but also ways to prevent getting into that situation. The combination of control, resources and education is optimally effective; only control, only resources, or only education would probably not have much effect.

Health education as an intervention for patient care, and support is usually called patient education instead of health education. Sometimes patient education supports patients who recover, for instance, after surgery. Sometimes the focus is on chronic patients, such as patients with asthma or diabetes. Patient education also includes support for people who are dying, for instance in case of lung cancer or AIDS. Patient education is not only directed at the patient but also at their family and at health professionals. Health

workers such as physicians and nurses are the primary providers of patient education. Frequently, many different health workers are involved in the treatment of the same patient. Patient education by each of these professionals is not always attuned to the needs of the patient. This calls for the development of patient education programmes that co-ordinate the educational activities of the different health professionals involved, for example, by developing protocols for continuity of care (Mesters, Meertens & Mosterd, 1991).

THE PLANNING OF HEALTH EDUCATION

Health education is a planned activity. The best known and most often used planning model in health education and health promotion is Green's Precede/Proceed model (Green & Kreuter, 1991); see Fig. 1.

In short, Green starts with the social diagnosis: what is the quality of life of a certain group, community or country, and the epidemiological diagnosis: is health relevant for the quality of life and if it is, what are the most serious health problems? With the behavioural and environmental diagnosis, we analyse the determinants of health in terms of behaviour/lifestyle and environment. With the educational and organizational diagnosis we analyse the determinants of the relevant behaviours, in terms of predisposing, reinforcing and enabling factors, and select the variables that we might want to influence. With the administrative and policy diagnosis we analyse the possible usefulness of health education and other potential interventions: resources, regulations. Next, we turn to the implementation of health promotion interventions, including the health education intervention. We then evaluate the process, impact, and outcome of these interventions, resulting in feedback and improvement of the interventions.

Let us look at a planning example. In most western countries such as the Netherlands, the quality of life in general is high. People value health as one of the most important aspects of their quality of life. What are the most important health problems? In terms of mortality these are: cardiovascular disease (CVD) and cancer. What are the determinants of CVD and cancer? In terms of environment these are for instance: industrialization and unhealthy working

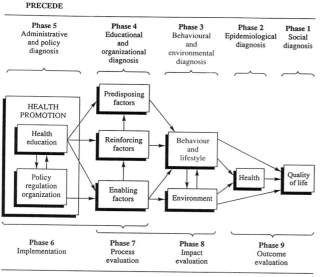

Phase 5
Administrative and policy diagnosis

Phase 4
Educational and organizational diagnosis

Phase 3
Behavioural and environmental diagnosis

Phase 2
Epidemiological diagnosis

Phase 1
Social diagnosis

Phase 6
Implementation

Phase 7
Process evaluation

Phase 8
Impact evaluation

Phase 9
Outcome evaluation

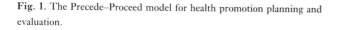
PROCEED

Fig. 1. The Precede–Proceed model for health promotion planning and evaluation.

environment. In terms of behaviour and lifestyle, for instance, smoking and unhealthy diet. Let us select smoking and, in particular, the prevention of the onset of smoking, as a relevant behaviour that we might want to influence. Why do adolescents start smoking? Not because they like it and not because they don't know about the dangers. They start smoking basically as a result of social pressure, mostly from peers, family or mass media. In terms of predisposing factors adolescents often don't know how to resist social pressure. In terms of reinforcing factors: belonging to a peer group is very important for adolescents. In terms of enabling factors: cigarettes are easy to get, and sanctions against smoking are weak. What can we do? In terms of health education, we want to improve adolescents' self-efficacy in resisting social pressure. There are a number of techniques that help adolescents to learn how to resist pressure to smoke (of which 'just say no' is the least effective!), for instance, through positive role modelling (see Evans *et al.*, 1978). In terms of resources and regulation we want to develop anti-smoking policies, for instance, at schools, or through community action against vendors that sell cigarettes to adolescents under legal age. The implementation of such a health promotion programme is organized in co-operation with schools, parents and students. Finally, the effectiveness of the programme is measured. In terms of process evaluation the central question is: was the programme implemented as planned and was the supposed self-efficacy improvement actually realized? In terms of impact evaluation: did fewer students in our programme group start smoking than in a comparison group? It may be clear that an improvement in terms of outcomes, reduction of CVD and cancer, and quality of life, cannot be expected for several years.

QUALITY OF THE PLANNING

The process of planning health education programmes is a cumulative and iterative process. On the one hand, we need answers on earlier planning questions to decide about later phases. On the other

hand, the process is not rigid but flexible and we go back and forth through the model. During the planning process we make use of existing knowledge that is systematized in theories, and that is available as empirical data. Why does it have to be so complex? Certainly not because health educators admire complicated models, but because careful planning is essential if we strive for effect. A very important study in this respect is a meta-analysis by Mullen, Green & Persinger (1985) on 70 studies about the effectiveness of patient education. They looked at studies that were methodologically sound and that included knowledge and compliance as effect variables. Several diseases and several types of interventions were represented.

We will focus here on one very interesting aspect of this study, namely the estimation of the quality of the educational interventions as a predictor of effectiveness. Mullen *et al.* estimated the quality of the interventions using six criteria that they derived from the literature and that can also be seen as guidelines for intervention development:

1. Consonance: the degree of fit between the programme and the programme objectives.
2. Relevance: the tailoring of the programme to knowledge, beliefs, circumstances, and prior experiences of the learner, as assessed by pretesting or other means.
3. Individualization: the provision of opportunities for learners to have personal questions answered or instructions paced according to their individual progress.
4. Feedback: information given to the learner regarding the extent to which learning is being accomplished (e.g. blood pressure reading).
5. Reinforcement: any component of the intervention that is designed to reward the behaviour (other than feedback) after the behaviour has been enacted (e.g. social support).
6. Facilitation: the provision of means for the learner to take action and/or means to reduce barriers to action (e.g. subsidies).

Mullen *et al.* show that the best predictor of success was the rating score for the quality of the educational intervention. The choice for a specific educational technique was not related to effectiveness, again demonstrating that there is no such thing as a 'magic bullet'. Thus, the effectiveness of a health education intervention is determined by the quality of the planning process.

In the six criteria that Mullen *et al.* used, we recognize different concepts from Green's planning model: the choice of relevant behavioural objectives, tailoring to determinants of behaviour, learning (health education), reinforcement and support, and facilitation (health promotion). There are also some concepts that have not been described in the Precede/Proceed model, but are selected from behavioural science theories. Before we continue to comment on the use of theories in health education, we will describe some common pitfalls in health education planning.

PLANNING PITFALLS

Since the quality of the planning process is the best predictor of success, planning mistakes are the best predictor of failure. A very common mistake is to jump from the health problem to some kind of intervention, without answering the intermediate planning questions. Furthermore, since evaluation is rare, the ineffectiveness of such interventions often remain hidden. Another popular mistake is the assumption that information about risks is enough to change people's behaviour: it is not (as all smoking health professionals illustrate). Recently, we have seen this mistake in the proposal to stop educating gay men about Aids 'because they all know the risks and obviously do not want to change their behaviour', without any recognition of the importance of skills that need to be learned to achieve such a change. In terms of determinants of behaviour, knowledge is hardly ever an important factor. People need a motive for behavioural change, but that is just the first step in the long road to consistent behaviour change.

At different moments in the planning process there are pitfalls (Kok & Bouter, 1990):

1. Problem: the pitfall of developing an intervention for a non-existing or quite irrelevant problem.
2. Behaviour: the pitfall of developing an intervention addressing behaviour that lacks a clear relationship with the problem, for instance, because that relationship is vague or the problem is mostly determined by environmental factors.
3. Determinants of behaviour: the pitfall of developing an intervention that is based on a misconceived idea about the determinants of the behaviour. Earlier we mentioned that the onset of smoking is not caused by risk knowledge but by insufficient skills to resist social pressure to smoke.
4. Intervention: the pitfall of developing an inadequate intervention. For instance, education while resources are still lacking, or insufficient tailoring to the target group.
5. Implementation: the pitfall of developing a potentially effective intervention with the wrong implementation. For instance, a school programme on Aids that is not used because teachers do not agree with the content.
6. Evaluation: the pitfall of unjustified satisfaction with the intervention and the failure to evaluate the process, the impact and the outcome thoroughly.

USING THEORIES IN HEALTH EDUCATION: DETERMINANTS

At different phases in the planning process we use theories. The first phases rely on epidemiological theories; the later phases, when we develop the educational intervention, rely on theories from the behavioural sciences, especially social psychology. In this and the next two paragraphs we will describe theories that can be applied in the three phases: determinants, intervention and implementation.

In the educational diagnoses we try to understand why people behave as they do. Current social psychological models indicate three types of determinants of behaviour (Ajzen, 1988; Bandura, 1986):

1. Attitude: beliefs about advantages and disadvantages of behaviour resulting in an attitude about the behaviour, also described as outcome expectations.
2. Social influence: beliefs about social norms, behaviour of others (modeling).
3. Self-efficacy: beliefs about perceived control, self-efficacy expectations.

Models about determinants of behaviour do not imply a one-directional influence; attitudes, social influence and self-efficacy can be antecedents as well as consequences of behaviour (Zimbardo & Leippe, 1991). In educational interventions we try to change determinants in order to change behaviour, but we also use techniques that influence behaviour rather directly, such as commitment procedures and systematic experiences with the behaviour followed by feedback and reinforcement. Positive experiences with behaviour, in turn, may change psychosocial determinants of behaviour, thus creating reciprocal determinism (Bandura, 1986).

USING THEORIES IN HEALTH EDUCATION: INTERVENTIONS

Current general social psychological models on behaviour change distinguish steps, phases or stages of change. Within those steps, a number of different specific theories can be applied. One general framework for theories on behaviour change is provided by McGuire's (1985) persuasion – communication model. He describes different steps that people take, from the initial response to the educational message to, hopefully, a continuous change of behaviour in the desired direction. Simplified, the first steps indicate successful communication, the following steps involve changes of determinants and behaviour, and the last step is concerned with maintenance of that behaviour change. Going through these steps, McGuire argues that the educational interventions should change with each step. The choices that have to be made about the message, the target group, the channel, and the source, will be different, or may even be conflicting, depending on the particular step that is addressed.

Prochaska & DiClemente's (1984) stages of change model distinguishes stages of change within the person: precontemplation, contemplation, preparing for action, action, and maintenance or relapse. Their model does not refer to the communication process, but the similarities between this model and McGuire's are evident. An important contribution of the stage model is the specific tailoring of educational efforts to groups of people in different stages. Interventions based on this model normally have completely different methods or strategies for each stage.

Within these general frameworks, a number of other theories can be applied (Zimbardo & Leippe, 1991; Glanz, Lewis & Rimer, 1996). To get people motivated for change, we apply theories on risk perception (Weinstein, 1987), for instance, to help people maintain their behavioural change, we apply relapse prevention theories (Marlatt & Gordon, 1985). Although these theories often cover only steps, or even only parts of steps, they can be helpful in developing interventions that focus on particular aspects of change. Using McGuire's framework, for instance, can be helpful in stimulating programme planners to recognize neglected variables and to recognize appropriate theories that can be applied.

Theories can suggest techniques, but the actual application of these techniques in the educational intervention requires practical experience, creativity and thorough pretesting (Bartholomew et al., 1991; Parcel et al., 1989; Schaalma & Kok, 1994).

USING THEORY IN HEALTH EDUCATION: IMPLEMENTATION

Development of an educational intervention includes making plans for programme implementation. The adoption of innovations is a systematic process, following the pattern of diffusion (Rogers, 1983). A number of characteristics of the intervention are related to faster adoption: compatibility, relative advantage, flexibility, observability, trialability, low risk, reversibility, low complexity.

Currently, diffusion researchers stress the importance of carefully developing the linkage between the change agent system and the target group system (Havelock *et al.*, 1973; Oldenburg *et al.*, 1996; Orlandi *et al.*, 1990). In the example of smoking prevention in schools, it is important to involve teachers and students in the development of the programme, as well as principals and parents (Parcel, B.G. Simons-Morton & Kolbe, 1988). In the example of co-operation among different health professionals to achieve continuity of care, it is important to involve all those groups in the development of the protocol.

EPILOGUE: PLANNED HEALTH EDUCATION

Health education is a planned activity, stimulating learning through communication, to promote healthy behaviour. Health education can contribute to prevention, in combination with other types of interventions, regulation and resources. Health education planning involves a series of phases where quality of life, health problems, health behaviour, determinants of behaviour and possible interventions are successively analysed, followed by the development and implementation of the intervention and evaluation of the process, impact and outcome. Careful planning is important, since quality of planning has been shown to determine effectiveness of the educational intervention. Unfortunately, we see a lot of planning mistakes in practice.

A wide range of theories from the behavioural sciences may contribute fruitfully to the analysis of determinants, and the development and implementation of health education interventions.

REFERENCES

Ajzen, I. (1988). *Attitudes, personality, and behavior.* Milton Keynes, UK: Open University Press.

Bandura, A. (1986). *Social foundations of thought and action.* Eaglewood Cliffs, NJ: Prentice-Hall.

Bartholomew, L.K., Parcel, G.S., Seilheimer, D.K., Czyzewski, D., Spinelli, S.H. & Congdon, B. (1991). Development of a health education program to promote the self-management of cystic fybrosis. *Health Education Quarterly*, 18, 429–34.

Evans, R.I., Rozelle, R.M., Mittelmark, M.G., Hansen, W.B., Bane, A.L. & Havis, J. (1978). Deterring the onset of smoking in children: knowledge of immediate psychological effects and coping with peer pressure, media pressure and parental modeling. *Journal of Applied Social Psychology*, 8, 126–35.

Glanz, K., Lewis, F.M. & Rimer, B. (1996). *Health behavior and health education.* 2nd edn. San Francisco: Jossey-Bass.

Green, L.W. & Kreuter, M.W. (1991). *Health promotion planning; an educational and environmental approach.* Mountain View, CA: Mayfield.

Havelock, R.G., Guskin, A., Frohman, M., Havelock, M., Hill, M. & Huber, J. (1973). *Planning for innovation through dissemination and utilization of knowledge.* Institute for Social Research, University of Michigan: Ann Arbor.

Kok, G. & Bouter, L.M. (1990). On the importance of planned health education.

The American Journal of Sports Medicine, 18, 600–5.

McGuire, W.J. (1985). Attitudes and attitude change. In G. Lindsay & E. Aronson (Eds.). *The handbook of social psychology,* vol. 2, pp. 233–346. New York: Random House.

Marlatt, G.A. & Gordon, J.R. (1985). *Relapse prevention; maintenance strategies in the treatment of addictive behaviors.* New York: Guilford.

Mesters, I., Meertens, R. & Mosterd, N. (1991). Multidisciplinary co-operation in primary care for asthmatic children. *Social Science and Medicine*, 32, 65–70.

Milio, N. (1988). Strategies for health promoting policy: a study of four national case studies. *Health Promotion International*, 3, 307–11.

Mullen, P.D., Green, L.W. & Persinger, G. (1985). Clinical trials for patient education for chronic conditions; a comparative meta-analysis of intervention types. *Preventive Medicine* 14: 753–81.

Oldenburg, B., Hardcastle, D.M. & Kok, G. (1996). Diffusion of innovations. In K. Glanz, F.M. Lewis & B.K. Rimer (Eds.). *Health behavior and health education: theory, research and practice,* 2nd edn., San Fransisco: Jossey-Bass.

Orlandi, M.A., Landers, C., Weston, R. & Haley, N. (1990). Diffusion of health promotion innovations. In Glanz, K., Lewis, F.M. & Rimer, B.K. (Eds.). *Health behavior and health education; theory, research and practice,* pp. 288–313. San Francisco, CA: Jossey Bass.

Parcel, G.S., Simons-Morton, B.G. & Kolbe, L.J. (1988). Health promotion: integrating organizational change and student learning strategies. *Health Education Quarterly*, 15, 435–50.

Parcel, G.S., Taylor, W.C., Brink, S.G., Gottlieb, N., Enquist, K., O'Hara, N.M. & Erikson, M.P. (1989). *Family and Community Health*, 12, 1–13.

Prochaska, J.O. & DiClemente, C.C. (1984). *The transtheoretical approach: crossing traditional boundaries of therapy.* Illinois: Dow Jones-Irwin Homewood.

Rogers, E.M. (1983). *Diffusion of innovations.* New York: The Free Press.

Schaalma, H.P. & Kok, G. (1994). Developing AIDS education; a systematic approach based on research, theories and co-operation. In D. Rutter (Ed.). *The social psychology of health and safety; European perspectives.* Alsershot, UK: Avebury.

Simons-Morton, D.G., Simons-Morton, B.G., Parcel, G.S. & Bunker, J.F. (1988). Influencing personal and environmental conditions for community health: a multilevel intervention model. *Family and Community Health*, 11, 25–35.

Weinstein, N.D. (1987). *Taking care; understanding and encouraging self-protective behavior.* Cambridge University Press.

Zimbardo, Ph.G. & Leippe, M.R. (1991). *The psychology of attitude change and social influence.* Philadelphia: Temple University Press.

Health status assessment

STEPHEN WRIGHT

Department of Medical Psychology, Leicester
General Hospital, UK

INTRODUCTION

The primary aim of this chapter will be to provide a framework to enable the reader to make sense of the extensive literature on health status assessment. With a few notable exceptions, published studies on this topic typically pay little attention to broader issues and assumptions around health and health status. A brief attempt will be made here to rectify this unfortunate omission. In this context, and with the purpose of informing decisions about choice of measure, a selection of published measurement instruments will be briefly reviewed and used to illustrate some general points. Discussion will be almost entirely restricted to self-completion questionnaire instruments.

The validity of very simple single-item measures of self-perceived health status also bears noting at the outset. The evidence supporting a strong association between self-assessed health and mortality has recently been comprehensively reviewed by Idler (1992). The six large-scale (minimum sample size = 1078) studies she discusses essentially tested the value of self-perceived health as a *predictor* of subsequent mortality, with follow-up periods ranging from 4–14 years. Self-assessed health contributed significantly to the prediction of mortality even after controlling for a wide array of 'objective' health indicators (e.g. sociodemographic and health practice variables). This provides powerful evidence in support of the criterion validity of self-assessed health status.

WHAT DO WE MEAN BY HEALTH STATUS?

There are two main alternatives here. The first approach involves health status being defined by the researcher in terms of the questions included and the response options provided in a health status assessment (HSA) instrument. Traditionally, the content of such instruments has been largely at the whim of scale developers, although psychometric considerations have been brought into play in the final stages of their evolution. Only rarely have the views of the potential pool of respondents and other relevant experts been sampled (to assess appropriateness, comprehensiveness and redundancy) in a structured way during scale development (see Sprangers *et al.*, 1993).

This approach is typified by multi-item HSA measures. Given the growing number of HSA instruments and the limited overlap between these in terms of content, it is worth drawing attention to the necessary trade-off between breath and depth in order to keep the resulting instrument within practical limits. If a scale is to cover a broad range of health attributes, it can only do so at a relatively shallow level. If the depth/detail of coverage is important, the scale will need to be limited in terms of the range of attributes covered. Fig. 1 illustrates this diagrammatically.

The breadth of researchers' conceptualization of health status has increased over the past decades. The traditional central component was function/dysfunction, i.e. what respondents could do (e.g. Karnofsky *et al.*, 1948). A subsequent addition was symptom status, i.e. physical sensation or a state of *being*. More recently, there has been some agreement that four components can be distinguished, namely (i) physical symptoms, (ii) psychological distress, (iii) social interaction and (iv) functional status (e.g. Aaronson, Bullinger & Ahmedzai, 1988). This broadening in views of health status is notable in two respects. First, it has encouraged the increasing use and acceptance of an alternative label for this area of research, namely 'health-related quality of life'. Secondly, it has led to a growing awareness of overlap between lay and academic concepts of health and health status. Reviewing research on lay representations, Wright (1990b) summarized this work in terms of three components:- health as *being*, health as *doing* and health as *having* (a resource/reserve of health). This analysis provides a useful means of distinguishing health and health status. Whilst the latter is viewed concretely as overall well-being at a particular point in time, with the focus on function and somatic sensation, the former is more abstract, referring to a potentiality, focusing particularly on reserves/resources.

The second alternative involves leaving the definition of 'health status' to the respondent. This approach is best exemplified in single-item self-ratings in which respondents are simply asked to rate their 'current state of health'. Two comments bear noting. First, there is evidence that conceptualizations of health vary as a function of age and sex (Wright, 1986/1990*a*), social class (D'Houtaud & Field, 1984) and culture (e.g. Currer & Stacey, 1986). Secondly, until very recently, there was very little 'qualitative' research into lay representations of health and health status. Taking both of these points into account leaves open two options. The first is to employ single-item self-ratings of health status in combination with assessments of the content of respondent representations (e.g. Wright 1990b). The second is to utilize a flexible approach to assessment, whereby the specification of item content is left to respondents (e.g. Ruta *et al.*, 1994).

It is also worth noting that existing HSA instruments focus almost exclusively on the effects of illness, i.e. employing a 'negative'/health-in-a-vacuum conceptualization of health and thus ignoring positive health states (see Wright, 1990a/b). This approach classifies respondents as either not–ill (i.e. 'healthy') or as in varying states of ill-health. Published scales have not been designed to show sensitivity to variations within the former group and are thus prone to 'ceiling' effects or a negative skewing in the distribution of scores when applied to non-ill individuals. However, available instruments

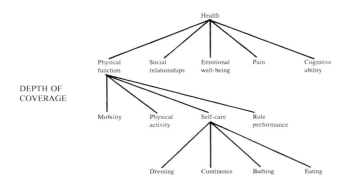

Fig. 1. Possible attributes for a health state classification system.

do show some variations in this regard with a recent comparison of the EuroQol and the SF-36 demonstrating that the latter shows a less skewed distribution of scores (Brazier, Jones & Kind, 1993).

WHAT IS THE PURPOSE OF MEASURING HEALTH STATUS?

Two broad purposes of measurement can be distinguished although, in practice, elements of both are usually involved in specific research studies. It is the balance between the two which varies. The first focuses on comparisons between two or more groups and is exemplified in the classical double-blind, randomized clinical trial (RCT). The primary function of such a trial is evaluative, i.e. assessing the efficacy of a new treatment. The most desirable characteristic of HSA instruments in this context is maximum sensitivity to real differences in health status between experimental/criterion groups. Single-item self-ratings may be a viable option here. Considering multi-item options, the most appropriate will depend on the comparison being made. Maximizing sensitivity may be best achieved by greater breadth or depth. Thus, a 'deeper/narrower' instrument may be most appropriate in the trial of a new drug which is claimed to decrease pain and swelling and increase function in affected joints in rheumatoid arthritis. However, a 'broader/shallower' instrument may be more appropriate where the hypothesis being tested is whether an experimental treatment improves health status overall (i.e. to ascertain whether its advantages outweigh its disadvantages).

A subdivision is often made here between assessment for the purposes of a comparison between alternative forms of treatment for the same medical condition (as above) and comparisons to inform decisions about resource allocation within health services. In a time of increasing demand and limited budgets within the public sector, moves to determine the most effective use of funds have been growing, largely at the initiative of health economists. Given the need to compare the respective health gains resulting from comparable interventions across medical conditions, this type of enterprise is best served by generic HSA instruments. The Quality Adjusted Life Year [QALY] index (Kind & Rosser, 1988) has been widely employed in this context.

The second purpose of assessment hinges on furthering process-orientated knowledge, fulfilling a primarily descriptive function. An essential feature of such studies is their relatively long-term pro-

spective/longitudinal design; whilst RCTs often involve follow-ups, these are usually relatively short-term. The most important attributes of HSA instruments here are that they can used repeatedly and provide assessments in sufficient depth/detail to allow the testing of process-orientated hypotheses. The former requires that measures are fairly brief and not too onerous to complete. The latter tends to encourage the use of 'deep/narrow', rather than 'broad/shallow', HSA instruments. Single-item self-ratings of health status are of limited value here.

HOW CAN HEALTH STATUS BE MEASURED?

Broad Scale Types and Format Options
Three broad types of HSA instrument may be distinguished. The first involves single-item self-ratings of overall health status, typically in response to the following question:- 'How would you rate your current state of health?'. Some researchers have added an explicit comparison, e.g ' . . . compared to other people of your age [and sex]'. In the absence of such *explicit* comparisons, it seems clear that implicit comparisons play an important part in self-ratings of health status. Wright (1987) reported health satisfaction self-ratings according to age to be an almost perfect inverse function of the discrepancy between perceived current and perceived best possible health status. Thus, the narrower the gap between the latter, the higher the satisfaction.

This underlines the importance of collecting two sets of additional data, as single-item data in isolation are of limited conceptual value (Wright, 1990b; pp. 100–1). First, other single-item health ratings to provide a framework within which to make better sense of current self-ratings. Examples include self/previous best, self/best possible, estimated age/sex average and self/health satisfaction. Secondly, quantitative (e.g. Wright 1990a) or qualitative data on respondents' conceptualizations of health.

Two response option alternatives have been employed in published studies. The more popular has been verbal ratings featuring 4- (VRS-4) or 5- (VRS-5) point scales, with the most popular of these being a VRS-4 offering the following options: 'Excellent', 'Good', 'Fair' or 'Poor' (see Idler, 1992). There is now widespread evidence of the reliability of VRS measures, whilst impressive evidence in support of their validity was mentioned in the introductory section (see above). The less widely used, so far, has been the visual analogue scale (VAS), typically utilizing an undivided 100 mm line, with the poles labelled 'Poor' and 'Perfect' (e.g. Wright, 1987). Provisional evidence of the reliability and validity of VAS health self-ratings in a 'healthy' sample has been provided by Wright (1986), whilst similar evidence in a sample of end-stage renal failure patients is reported by Wright et al. (1994).

The two remaining types of HSA instrument both comprise multi-item scales. The difference between the two hinges on whether or not health state valuations are included. Those multi-item instruments which include valuations are known as Index HSA scales, whilst those which do not are known as Profiles. In both cases, a range of items are included comprising symptoms and/or health problems, with ratings providing quantitative data on the extent of health difficulties experienced. HSA profiles, however, make no attempt to combine scores on separate subscales. In the case of index measures, the items/subscales are weighted according to relative importance, usually based on consensual data collected from a representative sample, so that the individual scores can be added together to give an overall total or index score. This total score typically ranges between 0 (= dead) and 1 (= perfectly healthy).

The valuations from which these weightings derive are typically obtained through a series of interviews which are used to collect data on how much worse or better respondents judge each health state to be compared to every other one. 'Health state' refers to each of the possible constellations of levels on the health attributes included in the index. A simple example would be the 32 possible combinations of positions on the disability (8 levels) and distress (4 levels) attributes of the QALY index (Kind & Rosser, 1988). Although valuations are usually based on consensual data (as above), there are available methods for individualizing these (e.g. the Patient Generated Index (PGI; Ruta et al., 1994) and the Leicester Uraemic Symptom Scale (Wright et al., 1994)).

Examples of HSA profiles include the Sickness Impact Profile [SIP] (Bergner et al. 1981), the Nottingham Health Profile [NHP] (Hunt, McEwan & McKenna, 1986), the SF-36 (Ware & Sherbourne, 1992), the Arthritis Impact Measurement Scales [AIMS] (Meenan, Gertman & Mason, 1980), the EORTC Quality of Life Questionnaire-Core [QLQ-C] (Aaronson et al., 1993). The first two are both generic instruments with well-established reliability and validity. The SIP is a 136-item scale comprising 12 categories of activity (ambulation, body care and movement, mobility, household management, recreation and pastime, social interaction, emotion, alertness, sleep and rest, eating, communication, work) and also divisible into two dimensions (physical, including categories 1 to 4 above; psychosocial, including categories 5 to 9 above). Scores on the SIP subscales indicate the extent of dysfunction in each of the activity categories. However, completion of the scale simply requires respondents ticking those (out of the total 136) statements which apply to them on a given day [and which they judge to relate to their state of health]. In essence, it offers respondents a yes/no response option and is therefore compromised in its sensitivity to change. The NHP has a similar format but is divided into six sections (sleep, energy, pain, social isolation, emotional reactions, physical mobility) with the resulting profile comprising scores on each of these dimensions. Two major criticisms of this instrument have been made. First, that its sensitivity is compromised (like the SIP) by its yes/no response format; this can also make it unacceptable to potential respondents. Secondly, that the sections may not be independent; for example, the pain and physical mobility category scores tend to be highly correlated.

The SF-36 is a further generic HSA profile and the product of extensive work over the past decade in the US Medical Outcomes Study. It was designed to bridge the gap between the 'lengthy health surveys used successfully in research projects and the relatively coarse single-item health measures used in national surveys and numerous clinical investigations' (Ware & Sherbourne, 1992; p.474). This instrument comprises 36 items forming 8 subscales (physical functioning, role limitations due to physical health problems, role limitations due to emotional problems, social functioning, bodily pain, general mental health, vitality, general health perceptions) and is constructed for self-completion and administration in person or by telephone by a trained interviewer. Three recent UK studies using large general population samples (range 1582–

9332) have documented its acceptability to respondents and provided further evidence in support of its internal consistency and validity (Brazier et al., 1992; Garratt et al., 1993; Jenkinson, Coulter & Wright, 1993). Brazier et al. (1993) also report that it compares favourably with the EuroQol in terms of showing a less skewed distribution of scores and Jenkinson et al. (1993) include normative data derived from a large sample of UK adults of working age.

The AIMS and QLQ-C are HSA profile instruments specific to arthritis and cancer respectively. The former assesses nine dimensions of health and functional ability including mobility, physical activity (walking, bending, lifting), activities of daily living, dexterity, household activities (management of money, medication, housekeeping), pain, social activity, depression and anxiety. Additional items cover general health and health perceptions. Factor analyses of the AIMS have identified three constituent factors, namely physical function, psychological function and pain.

The QLQ-C initially took the form of a 36-item scale, subsequently reduced to 30 items; a 33-item version is currently being field-tested. In order to provide an alternative to the stark choice between broad/generic and narrow/specific HSA instruments, the EORTC Quality of Life Study Group has pioneered a third option whereby assessment combines the two through the use of a core instrument (the QLQ-C), applicable to all diagnostic groups/treatment conditions, as well as modular scales which are diagnosis and/or treatment specific. The QLQ-C30 incorporates five functional scales (physical, role, cognitive, emotional, social) and seven symptom scales (fatigue, nausea and vomiting, pain, dyspnoea, sleep disturbance, appetite loss, constipation) as well as two general items assessing 'overall physical condition' and 'overall quality of life'. It is reported to be acceptable to respondents, taking on average 11–12 minutes to complete with little or no assistance (Aaronson et al., 1993). These authors report acceptable internal consistency and evidence of the instrument's validity.

Examples of HSA indexes include the QALY index (Kind & Rosser, 1988), the Quality of Well-Being Scale (Kaplan & Bush, 1982), the Index of Health-Related Quality of Life [IHQL] (Rosser et al., 1992) and the EuroQol (EuroQol Group, 1990). The QALY has been in use since the mid-1970s and has been one of the most widely employed HSA index instruments. It has a two-dimensional structure, featuring the attributes of disability and distress. By distinguishing eight levels of the former and four of the latter, it yields a total of [8 × 4 =] 32 possible health states; however, three of these are excluded for practical purposes since the authors judge distress to be a constant with the disability level 'unconscious'. Health state classification of study subjects is based on observation and/or interview by a trained rater. Valuations for each of the health states were obtained from interviews with a sample of 70 individuals, including groups of experienced doctors (n=10), experienced nurses (n=20), patients (n=20) and healthy volunteers (n=20). Out of the 29 possible health states, 3 received valuations worse than death (i.e. below zero).

More recently, a second generation British HSA index, the IHQL, has been developed by Rosser and her colleagues (Rosser et al., 1992). This has a three-dimensional structure, distinguishing physical (discomfort) and emotional (distress) components within the QALY distress dimension. The three dimensions are subdivided into a total of seven attributes as follows: Disability (dependence, dysfunction), Discomfort (pain/discomfort, symptoms), Distress (dysphoria, disharmony, fulfilment). These are further subdivided into 44 scales (e.g. mobility, cognitive function, sensory deficits) subsuming 107 descriptors (e.g. walk, memory loss, hearing). This yields in the order of 10^{52} possible health states. Three versions of the IHQL are available: a self-completion questionnaire, an observer-completion version for use in interviews and a relative-completion version to be completed on behalf of the patient by a relative or close friend. Given the vast number of theoretically possible health states, a complex multistage category-rating technique was employed to obtain valuations. Publication of psychometric evaluation data regarding this instrument is awaited with interest.

The EuroQol was developed with the aim of producing a standardized non-disease-specific instrument for describing health-related quality of life and to generate a single index value for each health state. The resulting instrument is designed for self-completion and capable of use in postal surveys. It consists of two sections. Part 1 requires respondents to select one option from two or three alternative statements addressing six dimensions (mobility, self-care, main activity, family/leisure activities, pain/discomfort, anxiety/depression). Taken together these define a total of 216 possible health states. Part 2 requires a 100-point visual analogue scale health status self-rating. Either part can be used to generate index scores. Valuations were obtained during piloting of the questionnaire. As with the IHQL, psychometric evaluation data are awaited. However, the instrument is more prone to 'ceiling' effects than its most comparable HSA cousin, the SF-36 (Brazier et al., 1993).

Comparison and evaluation

A wide variety of HSA instruments is now available, each of which may be positioned at a unique point in multidimensional space. The major dimensions include length, breadth of coverage, depth of coverage, applicable specificity, tendency to skewness in the distribution of scores, consistency and nature of response format and availability in other languages. In addition, for multi-item scales, there is an important choice between index and profile measures. Although the former typically involve considerably more work at the development stage, they are a conceptual requirement for certain research applications (e.g. resource allocation). It is increasingly evident that no individual measure can be expected to satisfy all requirements, so there can be no single 'gold standard' as far as HSA is concerned. The precise purpose of assessment continues to be the most important consideration when deciding on instrumentation.

The comparative psychometric properties of possible HSA options are a further important factor. It is increasingly accepted that sensitivity to change, in addition to adequate reliability and validity, is a desirable property of scales used to assess change over time. The most appropriate form of reliability index for HSA instruments is internal consistency, given the inappropriateness of test-retest reliability assessment as health status is expected to change over the sort of period of time needed to minimize the contamination of responses.

Available instruments continue to focus almost exclusively on health problems or difficulties and, as such, are more accurately labelled as measures of illness-related quality of life. Viewed from the perspective of current assessment practice, 'health status' represents the outcome of interactions between biopsychosocial health reserves/resources (see below) and biomedical disease.

HEALTH AS A STATE OR A TRAIT?

Current approaches to HSA are entirely founded on the view of health as a state, i.e. assessing (point-in-time) health status and changes over time. However, interest has been growing in the possibility that there may be consistencies within individuals in health status. This has led to the development of constructs such as 'hardiness' (Kobasa, 1979), 'sense of coherence' (Antonovsky, 1993) and 'dispositional optimism' (Scheier & Carver 1985), all of which may be summarized in terms of dispositional resilience. There is already considerable support for the hypothesis that this variable is an important influence on health status-related outcomes (e.g. Anson et al., 1993). This may provide an additional element, along with social support and psychoneuroimmunological function, in the explanatory construct of biopsychosocial health reserves or resources (health as having; see above) viewed as a health status-related predisposition. It is important to emphasize that 'state' and 'trait' approaches are not mutually exclusive, they are complementary. As in all such research, the real question is to determine the relative importance of state and trait components both in general and in particular contexts. However, it is worth noting that it was self-ratings of *health*, rather than health status, which were found to predict medium- and long-term mortality in the studies reviewed by Idler (1992).

ACKNOWLEDGEMENTS

Valuable comments on an earlier version of this chapter by Dr Neil Aaronson are gratefully acknowledged.

REFERENCES

Aaronson, N.K., Bullinger, M. & Ahmedzai, S. (1988). A modular approach to quality-of-life assessment. *Recent Results in Cancer Research*, 111, 231–49.

Aaronson, N.K., Ahmedzai, S., Berman, B., Bullinger, M., Cull, A., Duez, N.J., Filiberti, A., Flechtner, H., Fleishman, S.B., de Haes, J.C.J.M., Kaasa, S., Klee, M., Osoba, D., Razavi, D., Rofe, P.B., Schraub, S., Sneeuw, K., Sullivan, M., Takeda, F. EORTC QoL Study Group (1993). The EORTC QLQ-C30: A quality of life instrument for use in international clinical trials in oncology. *Journal of the National Cancer Institute*, 85, 365–76.

Anson, O., Paran, E., Neumann, L. & Chernichovsky, D. (1993). Gender differences in health perceptions and their predictors. *Social Science and Medicine*, 36, 419–27.

Antonovsky, A. (1993). The structure and properties of the Sense Of Coherence scale. *Social Science and Medicine*, 36, 725–33.

Bergner, M., Bobbitt, R.A., Carter, W.B. & Gilson, B.S. (1981). The Sickness Impact Profile: development and final revision of a health status measure. *Medical Care*, 19, 787–805.

Brazier, J.E., Harper, R., Jones, N.M.B., O'Cathain, A., Thomas, K.J., Usherwood, T. et al. (1992). Validating the SF-36 health survey questionnaire: new outcome measure for primary care. *British Medical Journal*, 305, 160–4.

Brazier, J.E., Jones, N. & Kind, P. (1993). Testing the validity of the EuroQol and the SF-36 health survey questionnaire. *Quality of Life Research*, 2, 169–80.

Currer, C. & Stacey, M. (1986). *Concepts of health, illness and disease*. Leamington Spa: Berg.

D'Houtaud, A. & Field, M.G. (1984). The image of health: variations in perception by social class in a French population. *Sociology of Health and Illness*, **65**, 40–59.

EuroQol Group (1990). EuroQol: a new facility for the measurement of health related quality of life. *Health Policy*, **16**, 199–208.

Garratt, A.M., Ruta, D.A., Abdalla, M.I., Buckingham, J.K. & Russell, I.T. (1993). The SF 36 health survey questionnaire; an outcome measure suitable for routine use within the NHS? *British Medical Journal*, **306**, 1440–4.

Hunt, S.M., McEwan, J. & McKenna, S.P. (1986). *Measuring health status*. London: Croom Helm.

Idler, E.L. (1992). Self-assessed health and mortality: a review of studies. In S. Maes, H. Leventhal & M. Johnston (Eds.). *International review of health psychology vol 1*. Chichester: J. Wiley.

Jenkinson, C., Coulter, A. & Wright, L. (1993). Short form 36 (SF36) health survey questionnaire: normative data for adults of working age. *British Medical Journal*, **306**, 1437–40.

Kaplan, R.M. & Bush, J.W. (1982). Health-related quality of life measurement for evaluation research and policy analysis. *Health Psychology*, **1**, 61–80.

Karnofsky, D.A., Abelmann, W.H., Craver, L.F. *et al.* (1948). The use of nitrogen mustards in the palliative treatment of carcinoma. *Cancer*, **1**, 634–56.

Kind, P. & Rosser, R. (1988). The quantification of health. *European Journal of Social Psychology*, **18**, 63–77.

Kobasa, S.O. (1979). Stressful life events, personality and health: an enquiry into hardiness. *Journal of Personality and Social Psychology*, **39**, 1–11.

Meenan, R.F., Gertman, P.M. & Mason, J.R. (1980). Measuring health status in arthritis: the Arthritis Impact Measurement Scales. *Arthritis and Rheumatism*, **23**, 146–52.

Rosser, R., Cottee, M., Rabin, R. & Selai, C. (1992). Index of health-related quality of life. In A. Hopkins (Ed.). *Measures of the quality of life and the uses to which such measures may be put*. London: Royal College of Physicians of London.

Ruta, D.A., Garratt, A.M., Leng, M., Russell, I.T. & MacDonald, L.M. (1994). A new approach to the measurement of quality of life: the Patient Generated Index. *Medical Care*, **32**, 1109–26.

Scheier, M.F. & Carver, C.S. (1985). Optimism, coping and health: assessment and implications of generalized outcome expectancies. *Health Psychology*, **4**, 219–47.

Sprangers, M.A.G., Cull, A., Bjordal, K., Groenvold, M. & Aaronson, N.K. (1993). The European Organisation for Research and Treatment of Cancer approach to quality of life assessment: guidelines for developing questionnaire modules. *Quality of Life Research*, **2**, 287–95.

Ware, J.E. & Sherbourne, C.D. (1992). The MOS 36-item short-form health survey (SF-36). I. Conceptual framework and item selection. *Medical Care*, **30**, 473–83.

Wright, S.J. (1986). Age, sex and health: a summary of findings from the York Health Evaluation Survey (Discussion paper 15, May 1986). York: University of York, Centre for Health Economics.

Wright, S.J. (1987). Self-ratings of health: the influence of age and smoking status and the role of different explanatory models. *Psychology and Health*, **1**, 379–97.

Wright, S.J. (1990a). Conceptions and dimensions of health. In R. Shute & G. Penny (Eds.). *Psychology and health promotion: proceedings of the Welsh branch of the British Psychological Society conference on 'psychology and health promotion'*, Gregynog Hall 1988. Cardiff: BPS Welsh Branch.

Wright, S.J. (1990b). Health status measurement: review and prospects. In P. Bennett, J. Weinman & P. Spurgeon (Eds.). *Current developments in health psychology*. London: Harwood.

Wright, S.J., Stein, A., Boyle, H., Moorhouse, J. & Walls, J. (1994). Health-related quality of life assessment in end-stage renal failure. *Quality of Life Research*, **3**, 63–4.

Hypnosis

MICHAEL HEAP
Centre for Psychotherapeutic Studies,
Department of Psychiatry,
University of Sheffield,
UK

THE NATURE OF HYPNOSIS

Hypnosis is a complex psychological phenomenon. It is an interaction between two people, one of whom is identified as the 'hypnotist', the other as the 'hypnotic subject' (or there may be a group of subjects). In practice it involves a variety of psychological processes and phenomena: selective attention, usually (though not necessarily) relaxation, imagery, expectation, role-playing, compliancy, and attribution. The salience of each of these ingredients varies according to the situation.

There are two further processes, related to the above and to each other, namely trance and suggestion. Trance is here defined as a waking state in which the subject's attention is detached from his or her immediate environment and is absorbed by inner experiences such as feelings, cognitions and imagery. As a rule, this experience is facilitated by eye closure.

It is useful to distinguish between 'inner experiences' which are consciously driven (that is, effortful, verbal, reality-based, etc.) and those which are less so (not goal-directed, not concerned with immediate realities, creative, involving spontaneous imagery, etc.), the latter type being more associated with therapeutic trance experience.

Further properties of trance, as defined above, have been determined by empirical research and include the following which, though not guaranteed, may be said to have an increased probability of occurrence due to trance:

(i) particularly in the case of the second type of trance experience, with regular practice, alleviation of the effects of stress (Benson, 1975);

(ii) alteration in the experience of the passage of time, usually leading to underestimation (von Kirchenheim & Persinger, 1991);

(iii) some amnesia for events which clearly registered because the subject responded overtly to them;

(iv) attenuation of the experience and increased tolerance of ongoing discomfort and pain;

(v) an enhanced predisposition to go to sleep (Anderson, Dalton & Basker, 1979).

This definition of trance includes everyday daydreaming or meditative states, and the aforementioned properties may be exploited formally or informally for beneficial purposes. Such is obviously the case with property (i); the regular practice of self-hypnosis is a common component of hypnotherapy. Properties (ii) and (iv) are useful in treatments for pain management, either where the pain results from some physical condition or where the patient is undergoing some uncomfortable medical intervention. The possibility of selective amnesia (property (iii)) is occasionally exploited in analytical applications of hypnosis (see later) where unconscious material may be elicited during hypnosis but may otherwise remain unconscious until such time as the patient is able to consciously assimilate it. Finally, the obvious application of property (v) is in the area of insomnia.

This brings us to another, rather more contentious property of trance, namely that it facilitates access to unconscious material: memories, feelings, fantasies, and so on which are normally below the level of conscious awareness but which may nevertheless exert an influence on the patient's behaviour, thoughts and feelings. Evidence for this tends to come from single case illustrations rather than from empirical research.

There is in fact a tradition in hypnotherapy of perceiving the unconscious in two ways, firstly in the psychoanalytic manner as a repository of anxiety – and guilt-provoking memories, impulses, conflicts and so on, and secondly as a store of untapped or underused strengths and resources which the patient may be assisted in bringing to bear on his or her problem. Recently the latter idea has been associated with the late American psychiatrist Milton Erickson who was influential in the field of hypnotherapy and, particularly since his death in 1980, has become a cult figure in a way not dissimilar to Mesmer in the eighteenth century. Other features of the Ericksonian approach are, as in this chapter, a broad definition of trance, and the use of story and metaphor as therapeutic communications by the hypnotist. The latter approach is now popular in the use of hypnosis with children.

Typically, in hetero-hypnosis, as distinct from self-hypnosis, subjects are encouraged by the hypnotist's communications to assume an inner focus of awareness, and to let immediate realities and concerns become part of the background of their experience. However, the hypnotist does not 'become part of the background'; subjects must attend to the hypnotist and allow him or her to guide and orchestrate the content of their subjective inner world. In this context the term 'suggestion' is used to denote the type of communication delivered by the hypnotist.

A suggestion is a communication conveyed verbally by the hypnotist which directs the subject's imagination in such a way as to elicit intended alterations in the way he or she is behaving, thinking or feeling.

The word 'intended' is meant to convey a key defining property which is that the alterations in behaviour, thinking and feeling approximate those which would occur were the imagined events to be taking place in reality. (The reader may also find that the term 'suggestion' is often used to denote the process of responding by the subject to the communication.)

A corollary of the above is that the subjective experience of responding to suggestion has an automatic or involuntary quality. For example, the hypnotist may ask the subject to concentrate on his or her arm; suggestions are then conveyed that the arm is becoming very light and beginning to rise in the air. Associated imagery may be provided – for instance a helium-filled balloon tugging at the wrist. The arm may indeed lift up, but the subjective impression must be that the arm is lifting unaided (or largely so) by conscious effort; the intended response is not that the subject compliantly lifts the arm to placate the hypnotist.

Suggestions which elicit changes in motor behaviour are described as 'ideomotor' and those directed at somatosensory experience (e.g. glove anaesthesia) as 'ideosensory'. Suggestions may also describe olfactory and gustatory experiences ('You are now smelling and tasting an orange'), visual and auditory experiences ('You can see your best friend in front of you'; 'You can hear a wasp buzzing round your head'), alterations in autonomic responding (e.g. handwarming and heart rate decrease) and complex changes such as amnesia, time distortion, and regression to an earlier developmental stage.

Suggestions may be intended either to take effect immediately or some time after the session of hypnosis. The latter type, termed 'posthypnotic suggestions' are widely used in hypnotherapy. Two examples which illustrate their characteristic form are 'Each and every time you put a cigarette to your lips, you will immediately experience this terrible taste in your mouth' and 'Between now and your next session you will have a dream at night which will help you understand your problem and how to overcome it'.

Trance and suggestion have a two-way relationship in that the one tends to facilitate the other. So, a suggestion such as arm levitation encourages the subject to focus awareness away from the external surroundings and to concentrate on a physical experience; hence suggestions in themselves tend to encourage the subject to have a trance experience as defined earlier. However, encouraging the subject to assume a trance state itself may increase his or her responsiveness to suggestion (Hilgard, 1965); clearly he or she is more likely to experience the intended changes if attention is focused away from events or concerns relating to the surrounding environment.

Accordingly, it is customary to precede hypnotic suggestions with a series of suggestions specifically aimed at encouraging the subject to assume a trance state. These suggestions are collectively termed the 'hypnotic induction' and usually involve methods of relaxation such as progressive muscular relaxation and appropriate guided imagery, although many therapists include a procedure such as arm levitation, which allows the patient to experience automatic responding. The later stages of this manoeuvre are termed 'deepening'.

Induction and deepening are probably not as essential to hypnotic responsiveness as was once thought, but they do have the useful therapeutic role of providing the patient with a relaxation routine (self-hypnosis) which he or she is encouraged to practice unaided between sessions with the purpose of gaining mastery over tense and anxious feelings.

THE CLINICAL APPLICATION OF HYPNOSIS

The above description of hypnosis in terms of trance and suggestion contains most of the ingredients we need in order to develop therapeutic strategies for a wide range of problems. A traditional hypnotherapeutic intervention consists of the following overlapping stages:

(i) a pre-hypnotic stage of rapport-building, information-gathering, allaying of misconceptions, and so on;

(ii) hypnotic induction and deepening which, as was stated earlier, usually consist of suggestions and imagery conducive to relaxation, an internal focus of attention, and perhaps the experience of automatic responding;

(iii) the treatment phase, which consists of various kinds of suggestions and imagery, either intended to promote the desired changes in experience and responding or to facilitate access to unconscious processes which may have a bearing on the patient's problem;

(iv) a consolidation phase incorporating post-hypnotic suggestions aimed at reinforcing the therapeutic strategies adopted; this stage often includes a series of positive suggestions of a general nature, intended to encourage a sense of self-confidence and optimism, and termed 'ego-strengthening';

(v) the alerting of the patient and the post-hypnosis phase of enquiry, clarification of the therapeutic work done, recapitulation of instructions for homework assignments, and so on.

We may also include as an additional stage the practice of self-hypnosis by the patient between appointments. The purpose of this for patients may simply be to learn to control and alleviate anxiety and tension but they may also be instructed to rehearse suggestions and imagery specific to their problem. For example, migraine sufferers may imagine hand-warming, or smokers or slimmers may repeat self-statements (affirmations) concerning the reasons for their not smoking or over-eating. The self-hypnosis routine may be practised with the aid of an audiotaped recording.

SPECIFIC CLINICAL APPLICATIONS OF HYPNOSIS

The above format lends itself well to the treatment of a wide range of medical and psychological disorders and there is virtually no problem for which one can confidently assert that hypnosis has no conceivable role. There exist, however, certain distinctions and constraints which regulate the useful application of hypnotherapeutic procedures.

12 Firstly, we may draw a distinction between hypnosis intended for direct symptom alleviation as opposed to hypnosis for uncovering and resolving memories, feelings, conflicts, and so on which may underlie the presenting problem. Examples of the former approach, which is often termed 'suggestive', are provided by the use of suggestion and posthypnotic suggestion, ego-strengthening, and self-hypnosis, for problems such as smoking, obesity, social anxiety, medical complaints which may be aggravated by psychological factors (e.g. irritable bowel syndrome, skin disorders and migraine) and painful conditions. We may include here the use of hypnosis to help patients undergo painful or stressful medical or surgical interventions (such as chemotherapy for cancer and, for the anxious patient, dental treatment and childbirth).

The second approach of hypnosis is termed 'hypnoanalysis' and is based on a rather simplistic dichotomy of the conscious and unconscious mind. This model has generated a variety of ingenious therapeutic manoeuvres. Examples are the uncovering of material by asking the patient to imagine a theatre stage or cinema screen as a metaphor for the unconscious mind, dream suggestion and interpretation, age regression, and the use of ideomotor finger signals to denote the responses 'Yes', 'No', 'Don't know', etc. to questions posed by the therapist concerning the possible unconscious origins of the patient's problem. Hypnoanalysis may be used for many of the above problems, but it tends to be favoured for those in which there is evidence of past trauma.

A second distinction is due to Wadden & Anderton (1982) in their influential review of outcome studies using the suggestive approach. They contrasted certain problems such as overeating, smoking and alcoholism with others such as warts, asthma, and clinical pain, referring to the former as 'self-initiated' and the latter as 'non-voluntary'. They concluded that the effects of suggestive hypnotherapy for the former were probably largely non-specific and placebo based. There was, however, good evidence for the specific effects of hypnosis in the treatment of 'non-voluntary' disorders.

We are probably justified in extending the category 'non-voluntary' to a wider range of problems which have a predominantly somatic component and for which we find good support in the research literature for the effectiveness of suggestive hypnotherapy (see Gibson & Heap, 1991). Amongst these are certain gastrointestinal disorders such as irritable bowel syndrome and peptic ulceration, and eczema. Relaxation and stress control are a substantial component of therapy, but suggestions also target the affected organ or body part. Examples are imagining the warm, healing rays of the sun on the skin in the case of eczema, and the release of colonic spasm and the smooth passage of stool in the case of irritable bowel syndrome. Whorwell (1991) who has, with his colleagues, undertaken a major study of hypnosis for irritable bowel syndrome, insists that in the treatment of this disorder, suggestions must focus on bowel activity itself (hence the term 'gut-directed hypnotherapy'); suggestions of general relaxation and ego-strengthening are insufficient. This claim raises the question of how specifically one can target an autonomic or physiological response by hypnotic suggestion.

Next, we may note that it is most appropriate to think of hypnosis not so much as a therapy itself but as a procedure (or a set of procedures) which may be used to augment a broader course of treatment. In fact, there is a spectrum of treatments ranging from those where the entire therapy consists of just one or a small number of sessions based on the format outlined earlier, to those where hypnotherapy constitutes a small component of a much more extensive treatment programme. Typifying the former is the single session treatment of warts (induction, deepening, posthypnotic suggestions of symptom removal, ego-strengthening and de-hypnotizing); similarly a single session treatment for smoking cessation.

At the other end of the spectrum we see the judicious use of manoeuvres such as age regression and dream suggestion in a course of long-term analytical psychotherapy (Karle, 1988) and the augmentation of a programme of cognitive therapy by hypnotic suggestions and imagery calculated to reinforce the restructuring of maladaptive beliefs and cognitions (Alladin & Heap, 1991; Ellis, 1993).

CONTRAINDICATIONS AND PRECAUTIONS

It is not easy to define succinctly those occasions when hypnosis should be proscribed. It is generally inadvisable to use it with psychotic patients, although its application here has occasionally been reported. Some caveats concerning hypnosis are applicable to psychological therapies generally, such as the importance of a thorough medical examination, the recognition and treatment of clinical depression, and the inclusion of the patient's spouse and family in treatment when they are implicated in the presenting problem. There is concern nowadays about the authenticity of traumatic memories elicited by the indiscreet use of regressive methods, particularly where sexual abuse is claimed. However, probably the most common consequence of misapplying hypnosis is simply timewasting if a preferred treatment exists, such as exposure in the case of a phobia or response prevention in the case of obsessive-compulsive disorder.

CONCLUSIONS

In practice hypnosis is a relatively benign procedure. Its clinical application continues to suffer through being uninformed by a rigorous body of academic knowledge and by the unwillingness or incapacity of many practitioners, and indeed authors, on the subject, to commit themselves to a proper scientific understanding. Nevertheless it provides techniques that are simple and of proven efficacy and it can be unreservedly recommended for inclusion in the clinical practitioner's range of therapeutic skills.

REFERENCES

Alladin, A. & Heap, M. (1991). Hypnosis and depression. In Heap & W. Dryden (Eds). *Hypnotherapy: a handbook*, pp. 49–67. Buckingham: Open University Press.

Anderson, J. A. D., Dalton, E. R. & Basker, M. A. (1979). Insomnia and hypnotherapy. *Journal of the Royal Society of Medicine*, 72, 734–9.

Benson, H. (1975). *The relaxation response*. New York: William Morrow & Co.

Ellis, A. (1993). Hypnosis and rational emotive therapy. In J. W. Rhue, S. J. Lynn & I

Kirsch (Eds.) *Handbook of Clinical Hypnosis*, pp. 173–86. Washington DC: American Psychological Association.

Gibson, H. B. & Heap, M. (1991). *Hypnosis in Therapy*. Hove: Lawrence Erlbaum Associates.

Hilgard, E. R. (1965). *Hypnotic Susceptibility*. New York: Harcourt, Brace & World

Karle, H. W. A. (1988) Hypnosis in analytic psychotherapy. In M. Heap (Ed.) *Hypnosis: current clinical, experimental and forensic practices*, pp. 208–20. London: Croom Helm.

Von Kirchenheim, C. & Persinger, M. A. (1991). Time distortion: a comparison of hypnotic induction and progressive relaxation procedures. *International Journal of Clinical and Experimental Hypnosis*, 39, 63–6.

Wadden, T. A. & Anderton, C. H. (1982). The clinical use of hypnosis *Psychological Bulletin*, 91, 215–43.

Whorwell, P. J. (1991). Use of hypnotherapy in gastrointestinal disease. *Bristish Journal of Hospital Medicine*, 45, 27–9.

Neuropsychological assessment

JANE POWELL

Department of Psychology, Goldsmith's College,
University of London, UK

Organic injury to the brain can have complex and interacting psychological effects, not only at the level of intellectual impairment but also at the levels of affective and behavioural disturbance. These sequelae may be directly or indirectly caused by the brain injury, and may vary in severity from those which are gross and obvious to those which are subtle and detectable only on detailed assessment. Nevertheless, even those which are subtle can have pervasive effects on a patient's social and occupational functioning, whilst those which are gross may arise from a variety of causes with different treatment implications. In either case neuropsychological assessment can be highly germane to clarification of the problem, to prediction of the functional consequences, and to the development of appropriate interventions or environmental adaptations.

To illustrate this, consider the case of a young man who has sustained a head injury in an assault. A year after the incident he has made a good physical recovery, but is very aggressive and has lost his job as a sales manager because of hostility towards colleagues and a general lack of organization in his work. These problems might, on the one hand, arise from organic damage to regions of the brain involved in the genesis or inhibition of aggression, or, on the other, be a psychological reaction to some more subtle cognitive deficit such as a generalized reduction in the efficiency with which information is processed or a mild but specific impairment of memory. In the former case, a pharmacological treatment to control the emotional reactions might be most appropriate, whilst in the latter it would be more relevant to address the underlying cognitive deficit directly and/or to help the patient adjust his lifestyle and outlook to his new limitations.

PURPOSES OF NEUROPSYCHOLOGICAL ASSESSMENT

The form taken by any neuropsychological assessment will depend critically on the question which is to be answered. Frequent issues for assessment include the following:

- description and measurement of organically based cognitive deficits
- differential diagnosis (e.g. to ascertain whether memory problems arise from organic injury or mood disturbance)
- prediction of the consequences of neurosurgical excision of brain tissue (e.g. the cost-benefits likely to accrue from a temporal lobectomy)
- monitoring improvement or deterioration associated with recovery from, or exacerbation of, a neurological condition
- evaluation of the neuropsychological effects, positive or adverse, of pharmacological and non-pharmacological treatments (e.g. to determine whether a psychological intervention has improved attention, or whether an anticonvulsant might impair learning)
- guiding rehabilitation strategies
- predicting or explaining deficits in social, educational, or occupational functioning
- medico-legal evaluations (e.g. contributing to determination of compensation awards, ascertaining fitness to plead, etc.).

DIMENSIONS AND LEVEL OF ASSESSMENT

The extensiveness of, and methods employed within, any individual assessment will be largely determined by the specific referral question, though a wide range of other factors will also be influential. These will include characteristics of the patient which affect either their ability or their willingness to carry out certain tests, as well as resource-based considerations such as the location in which the assessment is to take place or the amount of time which is available.

A key part of many neuropsychological assessments is likely to be concerned with the patient's intellectual functioning, usually tested via formal pen-and-paper or computerized test procedures. However, this is neither the only form of assessment used nor necessarily the most important. If the presenting problem is one of behavioural or emotional disturbance, assessment may concentrate on the systematic collection of information either from the patient or from others concerning factors which may trigger the reactions. Thus, although neuropsychological assessment is often perceived as a special form of cognitive assessment, it is very often much broader than this. In practice, a referral to a neuropsychologist will often result in a multidimensional assessment in which the problem is analysed from a number of perspectives rather than from just one. In some cases there may in fact be no formal cognitive testing, with brain-behaviour relationships imputed from other sources of information.

In general, it may be useful to categorize aspects of neuropsychological assessment into those which are primarily descriptive and those which are explanatory. The former represents an attempt to identify the type and severity of any problems, whilst the latter entails more theoretically driven procedures designed to illuminate the causes or consequences of an observed deficit. These two aspects will be differentially important depending on the nature of the initial question. So, if the purpose of the assessment is to quantify the extent of any memory deficits (e.g. for the purposes of monitoring change over time, or for medico-legal purposes), then a standardized measurement of different aspects of the patient's memory relative to their general intellectual level may suffice. By contrast, if the purpose of the assessment is to determine why the patient has difficulty in remembering information in daily life and to make therapeutic recommendations, then more detailed probing of potential causes for the memory problem become relevant. For instance, it may be that the memory deficit is secondary to poor concentration or impaired perception, or that it is related to the form in which the information is presented (e.g. verbally vs. visually). If an understanding of why the patient has particular problems can be generated, then specific treatment implications should follow.

Descriptive assessments will also vary in terms of their breadth, and this again is likely to reflect the referral question. In one case the requirement may be to determine whether a brain injury has resulted in any impairment, whilst in another the emphasis may be particularly on a certain aspect of the patient's functioning. The basis for focusing on one aspect more than on others may consist in observations which have already been made (e.g. that the patient appears forgetful) or on the basis of what is known about the aetiology or location of the brain injury (e.g. that there is a focal lesion to a part of the brain which is implicated in memory functions). The prediction of neuropsychological sequelae which are likely to arise from damage to specified areas of the brain has become an increasingly sophisticated exercise over the last decade or so with the emergence of complex information-processing models of cognitive function, a framework which is considered briefly below.

COGNITIVE NEUROPSYCHOLOGY

This framework guides much of contemporary neuropsychological assessment, and derives from an integration of theory and research bearing on the elements of information-processing involved in normal cognition ('cognitive psychology') with that relating organic brain injury to alterations in psychological function defined more broadly to incorporate not only cognition but also mood and behaviour ('neuro-psychology').

To illustrate the clinical utility of this approach, consider acquired deficits of spelling which can follow brain injury. Anatomically, impairments of spelling and writing seem predominantly to be associated with lesions of the left posterior region of the brain (see, e.g. McCarthy & Warrington, 1990, for an overview). Although this by no means implies either that all patients with left posterior lesions will have such deficits, or that the presence of such a deficit definitively indicates left posterior damage, nevertheless the observed association is important in guiding the form of the clinical assessment. Thus, if a patient is known to have sustained an injury to the left parietal or occipital lobe, the neuropsychologist is able to make an informed decision to include within the assessment tests which will be specifically sensitive to spelling or writing difficulties.

At this point, analysis of the information-processing operations entailed in spelling allows the neuropsychologist to identify the presence of specific deficits. These can vary in their impact, from those which give rise to extensive and very obvious difficulties for the person to those which produce much more subtle effects that may be less obvious at first glance but which may nevertheless have the effect of slowing the patient down or causing him to underperform in certain situations. For instance, Ellis and Young (1988) have proposed that one route to writing down a single word which is spoken out loud entails the sequential occurrence of the following operations:

- auditory analysis (extraction of individual speech sounds from the speech wave)
- representation of word as a series of individual distinctive speech sounds (phoneme level)
- mapping of sounds on to spellings (phoneme–grapheme conversion)
- representation of letters involved in the spelling (grapheme level)
- representation of the particular form in which the letters are to be written, e.g. in upper vs. lower case (allograph level)
- generation of motor programme for writing the letters (graphic motor patterns)
- writing (activation of the motor programme)

This sequence has been derived from a combination of theoretical analysis, experimentation with healthy individuals, and evidence from brain-injured patients that some of these processes can be disrupted independently of others. Other aspects of the model are yet to be confirmed, and it is in a continuing process of development.

Using the above framework, the clinical neuropsychologist may test whether the patient's difficulty in writing to dictation reflects difficulty at the level of acoustic analysis, at the level of phoneme–grapheme conversion, or at one of the other stages. The implications are quite different: if the patient has specific difficulty at the level of acoustic analysis, then in parallel with the above problem he may have considerable difficulty in understanding other people's speech but be unimpaired in copying written words or in writing down his own thoughts. By contrast, if the deficit arises at the level of phoneme–grapheme conversion, he is not likely to have a problem in comprehending normal speech but may experience some difficulty in keeping written notes, etc. It may be that a deficit of the latter type actually has very little practical impact, in that alternative routes to spelling (e.g. from vocabulary) may be undamaged; on the other hand, if these alternative routes are not spontaneously used by the patient, then the assessment may have the practical benefit of focusing rehabilitation on training and practice in use of these or other functional mechanisms.

APPROACHES TO ASSESSMENT OF COGNITIVE FUNCTIONS

Test of cognitive abilities can be functionally grouped in various ways. In a recent overview, Benton (1994) has categorized tests of differentiable neuropsychological impairments under the following headings:

- verbal capacities and aphasia (*includes expression, comprehension, fluency*)
- visuoperceptual capacities (*e.g. object recognition, visual discrimination, processing of spatial relationships*)
- audition (*e.g. recognition and identification of sounds; auditory localization; phoneme / word discrimination*)
- somesthesis (*e.g. identification of objects through touch; perception of sensory stimulation on the skin*)
- motor skills and praxis (*e.g. fine motor co-ordination and manual dexterity; manipulation of objects; ability to execute purposeful motor acts on verbal command or by imitation*)
- learning, memory and orientation
- executive functions and abstract reasoning (*the higher level cognitive capacities such as concept formation, judgement, mental flexibility, creativity, decision-making, insight, and planning*)

Other, more general, dimensions of neuropsychological assessment frequently include overall 'intelligence', effectively a composite index of the effectiveness of an individual's functioning across all of the above domains, and 'intellectual efficiency' which may be manifest (for instance) in the speed with which simple information is processed, or in the ability to maintain vigilance or concentration over an extended period.

These functions are inevitably inter-related, in that deficits in some areas are likely to have adverse effects on functioning in others: for example, an impairment of verbal comprehension will impede verbal learning and memory, and will be associated with a deterioration on many reasoning tasks. Likewise, attentional deficits will limit the extent to which new information is taken in and is retrievable from memory.

Some neuropsychologists in some settings routinely adopt the approach of conducting a comprehensive descriptive assessment, systematically testing all of the main areas of cognitive function using a standardized battery of tests such as the Halstead–Reitan or Luria Nebraska. A brief description and consideration of these batteries, can be found in Kolb and Whishaw's (1989) valuable reference text. In Britain the more common clinical practice is to employ a combination of smaller sets of standardized tests pertaining to restricted domains of cognitive function and to supplement these with other tests which are of particular relevance to the individual patient.

The best-known and most widely used instrument is almost certainly the Wechsler Adult Intelligence Scale – Revised (WAIS-R; Wechsler, 1981), which comprises 11 sub-tests together yielding 'intelligence quotients' (IQ scores). Separate IQ scores can be computed for the tests strongly influenced by verbal reasoning abilities, and for those which are less obviously language-based (Performance tests). This battery, or a shortened version of it, is often used to yield an anchor point against which to evaluate a patient's other test scores: so, if a patient of superior intelligence scores only in the average range on tests of memory, this is more likely to represent a deterioration than similar memory test scores in a patient of average IQ. This example highlights the importance of considering the overall profile of a patient's performance on tests rather than considering individual results in isolation. The same philosophy also holds at the finer levels of description highlighted within the cognitive neuropsychological approach: thus, the interpretation of a spelling deficit will vary depending on whether it is associated with concomitant abnormalities of comprehension, perception, etc.

[229]

Within each area, there may exist any number of tests to probe the patterning of a patient's deficits and residual abilities (see, e.g. Lezak 1995, for a wide-ranging inventory and discussion of specific neuropsychological instruments). Of the tests used, many have been standardized so that a patient's performance can be evaluated by comparison with normative data, but there is, in addition, a significant role for more informal, unstandardized tests which may be sensitive to idiosyncratic or qualitative aspects of a patient's functioning. These may be generated *ad hoc* during the assessment, as the neuropsychologist formulates hypotheses about the patient's underlying impairments and tests them out in an individualized way.

For instance, if a patient performs poorly on a test of mental arithmetic, he might have a problem either with generating strategic aspects of the computation or with remembering details of the question. The neuropsychologist might decide to pit these explanations against each other, either by presenting the question in a written format (thereby reducing the memory load but keeping the complexity of the calculation constant), or by presenting a strategically 'easier' problem containing approximately the same number of to-be-remembered facts. Although these variations on the basic theme are not standardized, they permit an individualized analysis of the stage at which an observed deficit arises.

INTEGRATION WITH OTHER NEUROLOGICAL INDICES

Neuropsychological assessment has a distinctive role within the multiplicity of tests the patient may undergo following brain injury, and one which is an important complement to other types of information. Physiological, biochemical, and neuroimaging techniques are able to identify, often with great precision, the locus or biological mechanism giving rise to a brain lesion, and this information is likely to be critical in informing medical treatment and often in making a general prognosis. Neuropsychology contributes a detailed analysis of the individual patient against a background understanding of brain–behaviour relationships, and thereby allows the consequences of the lesion for the patient's current and future functioning to be determined. An integration of the physiological and the neuropsychological information is therefore critical, both at the level of development of theory, and at the level of understanding, predicting, and treating the consequences of a neurological event for an individual patient.

REFERENCES

Benton, A.L. (1994). Neuropsychological assessment. *Annual Review of Psychology*, 45, 1–23.

Ellis, A.W. & Young, A.W. (1988). *Human cognitive neuropsychology*. Hove, UK: Lawrence Erlbaum Associates.

Kolb, B. & Whishaw, I.Q. (1989). *Fundamentals of human neuropsychology*, 3rd ed. San Francisco: Freeman.

Lezak, M.D. (1995). *Neuropsychological assessment*, 3rd ed. Oxford: Oxford University Press.

McCarthy, R.A. & Warrington, E.K. (1990). *Cognitive neuropsychology: an introduction*. London: Academic Press.

Wechsler, D. (1981). *WAIS-R manual*. New York: The Psychological Corporation.

Neuropsychological rehabilitation

BARBARA A. WILSON
MRC Applied Psychology Unit, Cambridge

INTRODUCTION

Neuropsychological rehabilitation is concerned with the assessment, treatment and recovery of brain-injured people, and aims to reduce the impact of disability and handicapping conditions and, indirectly, improve the quality of life of patients.

For the most part, neuropsychological rehabilitation concentrates on cognitive deficits following brain injury, although physical, social, emotional and behavioural disorders are also addressed. It can therefore be distinguished from cognitive rehabilitation in that it encompasses a wider range of deficits.

Modern rehabilitation of brain-injured people probably began in Germany during World War I as a result of improvements in survival rates of head injured soldiers (Goldstein, 1942). Goldstein stressed the importance of cognitive and personality deficits following brain injury, and described principles that are almost identical to those used in current neuropsychological rehabilitation.

A further impetus to neuropsychological rehabilitation came during World War II, with developments in Germany, the UK, the Soviet Union and the USA (Boake, 1989; Prigatano, 1986). An important paper by Zangwill (1947) discussed principles of re-education and referred to three main approaches. These were: compensation, substitution, and direct retraining.

At the same time, Luria and his colleagues were treating head-injured soldiers in the Soviet Union, and describing their activities (Luria, 1979). These early papers by Zangwill and Luria still provide a rich source of ideas for contemporary neuropsychologists interested in rehabilitation.

CURRENT APPROACHES TO NEUROPSYCHOLOGICAL REHABILITATION

These can be classified in a number of ways and, in order to make certain comparisons that have fuelled recent debates, the following have been selected: (a) theory driven, (b) patient driven, (c) holistic, (d) impairment specific, and (e) (following on from Zangwill) those focusing on compensation, substitution and direct retraining.

Theory driven and patient driven approaches

Neuropsychological rehabilitation involves patients, their families and therapists, and is influenced by many disciplines including neurology, geriatric medicine, physical medicine, clinical psychology, occupational therapy, social work, psychotherapy, physiology, and education. However, the major theoretical influences have come from cognitive neuropsychology and behavioural psychology, the latter also being heavily influenced by learning theory.

In recent years there has been a lively debate among cognitive neuropsychologists concerning the relevance of theory to therapy. On the one hand, there are the views of those, such as Coltheart, Bates, and Castles (1991) who argue that theories from cognitive neuropsychology can, and should, guide practice; and on the other hand there are those, such as Baddeley (1993) who remain unconvinced that theoretical approaches have played a major role in this area. Baddeley (1993) suggests that cognitive neuropsychology has learned a great deal from the study of brain-injured patients over the past 20 years, while it remains unclear as to how much patients have benefited from the theoretical input of cognitive neuropsychology. Wilson and Patterson (1990) made a similar argument, claiming that recent interest by neuropsychologists in treatment has been almost entirely for the benefit of the scientist rather than the patient.

The major argument in favour of theory-driven approaches suggests that, in order to treat a deficit, it is necessary to fully understand the nature of that deficit, and to do this adequately one needs a model of how function is normally achieved. Coltheart *et al.* (1991), using the example of anomia, sum up the position in the following manner:

> One needs to have in mind a model of how naming is normally achieved before one can begin to seek to understand impairments of naming consequent upon brain damage: and one needs this understanding before one determines what kinds of treatment could be appropriate. (pp. 216–217)

The opposing point of view suggests that, while treatment models are extremely useful for identifying the nature of the deficit, and for explaining observed phenomena, they provide little or no information as to how to treat the deficit. The models may tell us what is wrong, but they do not appear to be able to tell us what actions we might take in order to overcome, modify, or compensate for what is wrong. It would seem therefore that theoretical models from cognitive neuropsychology, while being of considerable indirect influence on therapy by increasing the sophistication of assessment and promoting understanding of the nature of particular deficits, cannot as yet inform therapists how, precisely, to treat neuropsychological deficits.

Behavioural psychology continues to exert considerable influence on the rehabilitation of brain damaged patients. There are examples in abundance of the application of behavioural principles to the treatment of neurologically impaired patients (see, for example, Wilson, 1991). While it can be argued that behavioural psychology's influence has been more in the domain of therapeutic techniques and strategies than in theoretical input, it has neverthe-

less brought considerable success to the field of rehabilitation. When faced with a choice between strict adherence to theory or adapting behavioural models to solve problems, behavioural psychologists typically opt for the latter. In other words, the approach is patient rather than theory driven. Treatment programmes are typically designed for individual patients, following a set of principles, while the influence of theory remains in the background. This is not an argument for doing away with theory. Without its indirect influence therapists might lead themselves into time-wasting cul-de-sacs. Until such time as there should be a theory of rehabilitation, however, therapists must continue developing treatment programmes that are patient driven while at the same time welcoming the support of a theoretical framework within which to work. In other words, theory's influence tends to be, apart from its direct help in providing specific diagnoses, of a more general kind as far as treatment is concerned.

This is not to say that there are not times when theory makes a direct impact upon treatment. Nor do I wish to preclude future developments of theoretical models that might indeed exert direct influence upon treatment. For example, a recent series of experiments, which has combined theoretical influences from cognitive neuropsychology and behavioural psychology for the benefit of brain-injured patients with severe memory impairments, involves an errorless learning approach (Wilson *et al.*, 1994). Influenced by studies of implicit memory from cognitive neuropsychology and errorless discrimination learning from behavioural psychology, Wilson *et al.* demonstrated that people with severe memory disorders learn better when trial-and-error learning is prevented. The explanation seems to be that errors are likely to be reinforced by people with poor episodic memory because of their reliance upon implicit memory, which is poor at error elimination.

Holistic approaches and remediation of specific impairments

Although cognitive problems are among the most handicapping for brain injured people, they are not generally seen in isolation. Emotional and behavioural problems are common, and may indeed worsen over time. Depression, anxiety, irritability and aggression may all occur. Social isolation is often reported by brain injured people and their families. Different personality characteristics and premorbid lifestyles may exacerbate or diminish the relevance of current problems for everyday functioning, and may influence the effectiveness of rehabilitation.

Such a multitude of sequelae following brain injury has led to the development of holistic approaches whereby rehabilitation programmes attempt to deal with the 'whole person'. The original holistic neuropsychological rehabilitation regime for brain-injured people appears to be that of Ben Yishay and his colleagues in Israel in 1974 (Prigatano, 1986), with a few others following Ben Yishay's model elsewhere in the USA and in Europe.

Major themes of these programmes include the development of increased awareness, acceptance and understanding, cognitive retraining, development of compensatory skills, and vocational counselling. Evidence is provided of increased self-esteem among patients, reduction in anxiety and depression, and greater social interaction.

Holistic units such as those above are rare, particularly outside the USA. Many brain-injured people are seen by individual therapists or psychologists on an outpatient basis. Remediation of cognitive deficits can, nevertheless, be effective when efforts are focused upon specific impairments as is reflected in articles written over the past four years in the *Journal of Neuropsychological Rehabilitation*. Some rehabilitation units that do not run on holistic lines have adopted more pragmatic policies and attempt to deal with impairments in everyday functioning as directly as possible, while others attempt to treat a basic underlying deficit. At this stage in the development of neuropsychological rehabilitation, there are no hard and fast rules as to the best ways of treating patients, and judged by research and treatment reports in journals, any one of the above approaches can justifiably claim certain levels of success.

Compensation, substitution and direct retraining

As mentioned earlier, Zangwill (1947) was the first to categorize approaches to rehabilitation in this manner while, later, others have developed, modified and extended this basic classification. Zangwill worked mostly with aphasic patients although, in addition to language deficits, he also addressed problems involving attention and initiative. He was concerned with the extent to which brain-injured people might be expected to compensate for their disabilities, and the extent to which the human brain is capable of re-education. These questions are, of course, as pertinent today as they were so years ago.

By 'compensation' Zangwill meant reorganization of psychological function in order to minimize or circumvent a particular disability. He believed that compensation, for the most part, took place spontaneously without explicit intention by the patient, although in some cases compensation could occur through the patient's own efforts or as a result of instruction and guidance from a psychologist.

'Substitution', in Zangwill's interpretation, meant building up new methods of response to replace the response damaged irreparably by a cerebral lesion. He recognized this was a form of compensation, but one taken further and requiring specific reeducation. Lip reading for deaf people, and Braille for blind people would be examples of substitution.

Zangwill's third approach, and the one he regarded as training at its highest level, was 'direct retraining', that is retraining the damaged function. His arguments in favour of this approach were, however, rather tentative, and he admitted that he had no strong evidence in its support.

Variations on these approaches have been propounded by a number of neuropsychologists including Luria *et al.* (1969) and Wilson and Patterson (1990). Luria *et al.* (1969), for example, discuss 'functional adaptation' whereby patients are encouraged or taught to use an intact skill to compensate for a damaged one. This appears to be one of the most successful procedures in rehabilitation, with its underlying principle of finding alternative solutions to help patients compensate for neuropsychological impairments. In short, the principle argues that, 'If you cannot achieve your goal in one way, find an alternative way to achieve the goal'. Such a principle encompasses Zangwill's earlier approaches of compensation and substitution.

In addition to the above approaches to rehabilitation, Wilson and Patterson (1990) regard environmental control as a further strategy to use with severely intellectually handicapped patients. This approach attempts to bypass or avoid problems through changing, restructuring or reorganizing the environment. The origin of this approach can be found within the discipline of behaviour modification, and has been used to decrease undesirable behaviour in people with mental handicaps.

Teaching people to use their residual skills more efficiently is yet another approach described by Wilson and Patterson (1990) and is possibly one of the most widely used in memory rehabilitation where direct retraining is probably impossible. Through using rehearsal and study methods, and mnemonics (Wilson, 1995), amnesic patients can be helped to capitalize on their residual albeit damaged skills.

The approaches described above are not mutually exclusive and can be used in combination. For example, a memory impaired person may be helped by (a) reorganizing the environment to reduce the load on memory; (b) being taught the appropriate use of compensatory memory strategies, thereby using functional adaptation; and (c) being encouraged to learn new information through the use of study and rehearsal techniques, that is being helped to adapt residual skills more efficiently.

THE APPLICATION OF NEW TECHNOLOGY TO NEUROPSYCHOLOGICAL REHABILITATION

In the early part of the 1980s there was considerable excitement concerning the use of computers, which were expected to revolutionize cognitive rehabilitation. It was thought they would assist neuropsychologists with assessment, monitoring treatment effectiveness, and retraining. Numerous software programmes appeared, despite the fact that they were not subjected to controlled investigation at that time. Robertson (1990) published a review of computerized rehabilitation and focused on programmes for language, memory, attention, visuoperceptual and visuospatial disorders. His concern was with adults with non-progressive, acquired brain damage, so he excluded computer programmes used for assessment, recreation, teaching aids, or prosthetic devices. He found no evidence that computerized memory, visuoperceptual or visuospatial training produced significant changes in cognitive functioning. Language training programmes fared a little better, although there was no published evidence for general effectiveness of computerized language training. Only in attention training were there some positive results, although even here the evidence was contradictory. Since Robertson's (1990) review further studies of computerized attentional training programmes appear to support the tentative evidence available in the 1980s.

Already useful as prosthetic devices for people with language or physical impairments, computers are likely to play more important roles in other areas of cognitive disability. For example, they could be used as aids in activities of daily living by providing series of cues to guide patients through the steps needed to perform practical tasks such as cooking, janitorial activities or money management. Glisky (1995) points out that computers have great power for storing and producing on demand all kinds of information relevant to an individual's functioning in everyday life.

Another area of current interest is in the use of computers as memory aids. Much of the work in memory rehabilitation involves teaching people to compensate for their impairments by employing aids such as diaries, tape recorders and electronic organizers. Work in this area of rehabilitation is difficult, however, because remembering to use an aid is in itself a memory task that brain injured people may forget to employ. Additionally, memory impaired people will probably experience great difficulty in learning to programme an electronic or computerized aid or they may use them in unsystematic and inefficient ways. Kapur (1995) discusses a number of external memory aids and suggests ways of teaching their use. Wilson (1995) reports on one particular computerized memory aid, NeuroPage, developed by a neuropsychologist, Neil Hersh, and Larry Treadgold, the engineer father of a head injured son. Neuro-Page is a simple and portable paging system with a screen that can be attached to a waist belt. The system uses an arrangement of microcomputers linked to a conventional computer memory and, by telephone, to a paging company. The scheduling of reminders or cues for each individual is entered into a computer and from then on no further human interfacing is required. On the appropriate date and time, the reminder is transmitted to the individual, and all that person has to learn is to press one fairly large and obvious button on receipt of the signal. Preliminary reports from California and from Cambridge in England look promising and suggest that brain-injured people have been enabled to achieve greater independence in such tasks as household chores, taking medication, attending college classes and feeding pets. NeuroPage may well prove to be of considerable benefit to other brain-injured people, such as those with attention or planning disorders, and to people with psychiatric conditions such as schizophrenia, and to normal elderly people with age-related memory decline.

CONCLUSIONS

Neuropsychological rehabilitation has reached an exciting stage of development with a worldwide growing interest in the subject as reflected in numerous conferences, debates, books and papers in journals relevant to the field. This interest has been stimulated by scientific research, on the one hand, and by improved and more sophisticated clinical practice, on the other. A wide range of methodologies is available to practitioners of neuropsychological rehabilitation, including those from cognitive neuropsychology, learning theory, developmental psychology, linguistics and, more recently, connectionist modelling. It is to be hoped that, as a result of combined efforts in the areas of theoretical debate, scientific research, and good clinical practice, a substantial and all embracing theory of neuropsychological rehabilitation will eventually emerge to inform psychologists and therapists working in the field.

REFERENCES

Baddeley, A.D. (1993). A theory of rehabilitation without a model of learning is a vehicle without an engine: a comment on Caramazza and Hillis. *Neuropsychological Rehabilitation*, 3, 235–44.

Boake, C. (1989). A history of cognitive rehabilitation of head-injured patients, 1915 to 1980. *Journal of Head Trauma Rehabilitation*, 4, 1–8.

Coltheart, M., Bates, A. & Castles, A. (1991). Cognitive neuropsychology and rehabilitation. In M.P. de Partz & M. Leclercq (Eds.). *La rééducation neuropsychologique de l'adulte*. Paris: Publications de la Société de Neuropsychologie de Langue Française.

Glisky, E. (1995). Computers in memory rehabilitation. In A.D. Baddeley, B.A. Wilson & F. Watts (Eds.). *Handbook of memory disorders*. Chichester: Wiley.

Goldstein, K. (1942). *Aftereffects of brain injury in war*. New York: Grune and Stratton.

Kapur, N. (1995). Memory aids in rehabilitation of memory disordered patients. In A.D. Baddeley, B.A. Wilson & F. Watts (Eds.). *Handbook of memory disorders*. Chichester: Wiley.

Luria, A.R. (1979). In M. Cole & S. Cole (Eds.). *The making of mind: a personal account of Soviet psychology*. Cambridge, Mass: Harvard University Press.

Luria, A.R., Naydin, V.L., Tsvetkova, L.S. & Vinarskaya, E.N. (1969). Restoration of higher cortical function following local brain damage. In P.J. Vinken & G.W. Bruyn (Eds.). *Handbook of clinical neurology*, vol. 3. Amsterdam: North Holland.

Prigatano, G.P. (1986). Personality and psychosocial consequences of brain injury. In G.P. Prigatano, D.J. Fordyce, H.K. Zeiner, J.R. Roueche, M. Pepping & B. Case Wood (Eds.). *Neuropsychological rehabilitation after brain injury*, pp. 29–50. Baltimore and London: The Johns Hopkins University Press.

Robertson, I. (1990). Does computerized cognitive rehabilitation work? A review. *Aphasiology*, 4, 381–405.

Wilson, B.A. (1991). Behaviour therapy in the treatment of neurologically impaired adults. In P.R. Martin (Ed.). *Handbook of behavior therapy and psychological science: An integrative approach*, pp. 227–252. New York: Pergamon Press.

Wilson, B.A. (1995). Management and remediation of memory problems in brain damaged adults. In A.D. Baddeley, F. Watts & B.A. Wilson (Eds.). *Handbook of memory disorders*. Chichester: Wiley.

Wilson, B.A. & Patterson, K.E. (1990). Rehabilitation and cognitive neuropsychology: does cognitive psychology apply? *Journal of Applied Cognitive Psychology*, 4, 247–60.

Wilson, B.A., Baddeley, A.D., Evans, J.J. & Shiel, A. (1994). Errorless learning in the rehabilitation of memory impaired people. *Neuropsychological Rehabilitation*, 4, 307–326.

Zangwill, O.L (1947). Psychological aspects of rehabilitation in cases of brain injury. *British Journal of Psychology*, 37, 60–9.

Pain management

STEPHEN MORLEY

*Division of Psychiatry and Behavioural Science in
Relation to Medicine, School of Medicine,
University of Leeds, UK.*

PSYCHOLOGICAL ANALYSIS OF PAIN AS A CONSTRUCT

In order to understand psychological approaches to pain management, it is necessary to examine the contemporary psychological analysis of pain. This analysis conceives of pain as a meta construct, that is a set of interrelated components none of which uniquely defines pain. Moreover, each component is itself a complex construct and the subject of scientific and clinical investigation. The various components interact in with a degree of reciprocal determination and will be present in varying degrees in pain patients. The experimental analysis of these components has developed considerably in recent years but many problems remain. As a result of this, psychological treatments are only partly based on a fully rational analysis of the problem.

Biological

The main elements in this are the neurobiological processes underlying nocioception, transmission and modification of nocioceptive inputs, the central representation of pain and physiological responses to painful stimuli, e.g. increased muscle tension and sympathetically mediated responses. Although many biological pain processes are not directly addressed by psychological treatments, it is clear that psychological management must be sensitive to variation in biological causes of pain. Some psychological methods have been applied to modify the putative physiological basis of pains (biofeedback) and to alter the reactive component (relaxation).

Subjective experience of pain

This concerns the perceived quality of the pain. Current thinking conceptualizes the subjective experience as comprising of three interrelated domains, sensory quality (reflected by descriptors such as 'throbbing' and 'shooting'), intensity ('mild', 'strong'), and affective ('unpleasant', 'agonising'). In developing treatments for this component psychology has construed the problem as one involving selective attention mechanisms. Treatments have been developed to train patients to switch the focus of their attention and to generate new contents for attention

Cognitive

The phrase 'cognitive' is used very broadly to refer to a wide range of psychological phenomena, including a person's attitudes and beliefs about pain as well as more fundamental appraisal mechanisms which incorporate attention, perception and memory processes. It also refers to the mental activity in which people engage while experiencing pain. Current research indicates that certain types of activity, such as thinking about possible catastrophic outcomes (catastrophizing), may intensify the experience of pain and distress.

Pain behaviour

This is a complex construct and refers to a wide range of directly observable behaviours: para-vocalizations and facial expressions induced by changes in pain intensity, verbal complaints and expressions of pain, postural changes, general activity level, medication consumption and a range of other placatory behaviour. Psychological theorizing has applied the concepts of Pavlovian (respondent) and Operant conditioning in the analysis of these aspects of pain. It should be noted that pain behaviour is essentially observable by a third party, and it is therefore subject to modification by social reinforcement contingencies. This process has been invoked to explain variation in pain behaviour between individuals and conversely applied as a therapeutic tactic. The major behavioural treatment is concerned with analysis of the contingent relationship between pain and behaviour and the subsequent modification of the contingencies (Fordyce, 1976).

Emotional

In addition to the immediate affective quality of pain, pain frequently induces strong, negative, emotional states. Common ones are anxiety, depression, anger and frustration. Cognitive behavioural therapies developed within a psychiatric context (Hawton *et al.*, 1989) have been adapted for use with pain patients.

Social context

Finally, we must consider the social context in which pain occurs. Factors known to influence several aspects of pain include the age and gender of the person, family characteristics, culture and the behaviour of professionals and carers (Moore, 1990). In addition to these feature there are influences due to work and employment status and in some cases the legal status of the person, i.e. whether compensation claims are pending (Mendelson, 1994).

Implications

This brief résumé indicates the breadth of factors considered by psychological approaches to pain management. Clearly, not all treatments embrace all the factors and one major challenge facing psychology is to specify the interrelations between the several constructs which comprise the concept of pain. The preceding analysis implies that assessment and measurement in relation to management should incorporate multiple measures. Furthermore, we can expect that measures are not necessarily concordant (highly correlated); neither will they display synchrony when they change, as each is likely to be controlled by different psychological processes. These characteristics mean that we are faced with complex data sets which require detailed consideration to interpret their meaning.

PSYCHOLOGICAL TREATMENTS IN THE MANAGEMENT OF PAIN

Psychological approaches to pain management are multimodal, presenting the patient with a series of interventions throughout treatment. Evaluating the impact of treatment has been generally focused on the problem of chronic pain but the methods can be applied to acute pain, e.g. preparation for childbirth and surgery, with success. There are also many laboratory studies on acute experimental pain. Meta-analytic reviews of the psychological management of pain (Malone & Strube, 1988) and of multidisciplinary approaches incorporating substantial psychological components (Flor, Fydrich & Turk, 1992), testify to the effectiveness of psychological approaches to pain management. A current focus of research is to determine the contributions and mechanisms of effect of specific treatments (see below).

Philosophy and stages of therapy

Although current treatments are derived from concepts in behavioural and cognitive behavioural psychology, they also overlap with approaches derived from the general psychotherapy literature. Psychological management is characterized by several features which are common to treatment programmes despite variations in their content. Psychological treatments require the active engagement of the patient, who becomes involved in planning and executing their treatment, rather than being a passive recipient of a treatment delivered by a professional. The patient is explicitly assigned some personal responsibility for their treatment. Patients are provided with educational material about pain mechanisms in general and about their particular pain. This aspect of management provides the therapist with information about the patient's understanding/misunderstanding of their pain and is part of the assessment process which seeks to determine the attitudes, beliefs and cognitive state of the patient. Conversely, the educational aspect provides patients with alternative ways of construing their experience. Specific emphasis is placed on the covariation between psychological states and the experience of pain. For example, patients are frequently required to keep pain diaries to help them discover the reciprocal influences between events, their mood, behaviour and pain. Psychological management also requires patients to set specific goals for treatment and specify ways in which they may be achieved. In the case of chronic pain, goal setting often requires the patient to shift from unrealistic outcome expectations of no-pain to expectations that they will be able to manage their pain, so that its impact on their life is reduced. The aim of management is to elaborate the patient's view of pain and in doing so help them generate a range of treatment options which they will be able to apply outwith the clinic. Psychological management therefore explicitly considers how treatments may be generalized and maintained out of the clinic and over a prolonged period of time. Research on this aspect of treatment has, however, not kept pace with practice (Turk & Rudy,

1991). These features closely mirror the phases which have been identified in general psychological treatments: (i) remoralization, the provision of hope and motivation to learn new ways of managing their problems; (ii) remediation, the acquisition of new ways of coping and behaving; and (iii) rehabilitation, the extension of treatment gains into daily living and plans for the future (Howard, Orlinsky & Lueger, 1994).

SPECIFIC TREATMENTS

Education

Education is always part of multidisciplinary pain treatment programmes. Descriptions of programmes indicate that the educational process is largely active and requires patients to reflect on their own understanding of pain. Once elicited this is compared with contemporary accounts of a pain, largely an elaboration of the Gate Control Theory (see Turk's chapter in this Handbook). Patients are encouraged to think about the implications of the different models of pain, and this process is frequently reinforced by the establishment of self-monitoring, diary-keeping exercises (Hanson & Gerber, 1990). The educational component of treatment is an integral part of contemporary psychological management (Turk & Meichenbaum, 1994) and serves to engage the patient as an active collaborator in the process of treatment. The impact of the educational component does not appear to have been evaluated as a separate entity and this is understandable as it is specifically integrated into other active treatment components.

Psychobiological treatments

There are two broad classes of treatments, biofeedback and relaxation, which are aimed at modifying a biological aspect of pain. In biofeedback physiological signals (e.g. EMG, skin temperature) are processed and displayed as auditory or visual information to the patient. The patient is instructed to attempt to change a feature of the display in a direction corresponding to the required change in physiological functioning. For example, the pitch of an auditory signal might correlate with EMG activity, so that reduction in EMG will be reflected by a lowering of pitch. Biofeedback has been extensively investigated as a standalone treatment over 25 years (Jessup & Gallegos, 1994: Malone & Strube, 1988). There is substantial evidence that it can be effective in the treatment of a variety of painful disorders, e.g. headache. Recent reconsideration of biofeedback as a treatment has been stimulated by experimental analysis of chronic pain problems which has identified specific peripheral dysfunctions hypothesized to be responsible for nociceptive input. For example, Flor and Birbaumer (1993), treated patients with low back pain and temporomandibular pain with EMG biofeedback derived from the appropriate paraspinal or facial muscles. The data indicated that biofeedback training was more effective than a relatively brief cognitive-behavioural programme and standard, conservative, medical treatment.

As described, biofeedback targets physiological dysfunction hypothesized to be related to nociception. It may also be used nonspecifically to help induce a general state of relaxation. Relaxation is widely used component of psychological treatment packages. The primary purpose of relaxation is to reduce the psychophysiological arousal frequently associated with pain. It is also frequently taught as a coping resource which patients can use at times of heightened pain and distress. Biofeedback procedures are not generally necessary as there is a range of relaxation procedures (active progressive relaxation, autogenic training, varieties of breathing exercises) which are relatively easily applied within a clinical setting.

Attention and distraction

Methods designed to modify attentional focus are a frequently incorporated into cognitive-behavioural pain management programmes and presented as part of a relaxation strategy. The rationale for this approach is a widely held view that the content of conscious awareness is determined by a limited capacity channel with attentional mechanisms controlling which aspects of a person's external and internal environment enter into consciousness (Cioffi, 1991). Pain may be considered as a stimulus which vies for finite attentional resources. The purpose of treatment is therefore to teach patients to switch attention to other sources of stimulation or to change the interpretation placed on the current focus of awareness. For example, a patient may be taught to construct a vivid mental image which includes features from a number of sensory dimensions, e.g. cutting a lemon and squeezing a drop of the juice onto the tongue. The elaborated sensory features of this image compete with the painful stimulus and reduce its impact. Alternatively, the patient may be encouraged to alter the focus of their attention to the pain without switching attention directly away from the pain. In this instance, the subject may be asked to focus on the sensory quality of the pain and transform it to a less threatening quality. For example, a young man with a severe 'shooting' pain was able to reinterpret the sensory quality into an image which included him shooting at goal in a soccer match. As a result of this transformation, the impact of the pain was greatly reduced although its shooting quality remained.

Fernandez (1986) suggested a naturalistic classification of attentional manipulation strategies which reflects this basic distinction. While these procedures are undoubtedly popular, empirical evidence for their effectiveness is mixed and experimental investigation of the mode of action is difficult (Eccleston, 1995). On balance, it would appear that attention switching/distraction strategies do have a role to play in the management of pain although it is probable that they are most effective at low to medium levels of pain intensity (Jensen & Karoly, 1991). Hypnotic methods may also be employed to modify the subjective experience of pain (Spanos, Carmanico & Ellis, 1994).

Cognitive–behavioural strategies

Cognitive–behavioural interventions are predicated on the hypothesis that it is a person's interpretation of events rather than the events themselves which determines the subjective experience and behavioural response to the event. In the context of pain the critical determinants of a person's emotional and behavioural adaptation to the pain are their thoughts, (appraisals, expectations, and beliefs about the origin and consequences of the pain), rather than the nociceptive and biological events *per se*. Cognitive–behavioural methods seek to modify a person's thinking about pain, and in doing so to change their pattern of adaptation to it. The central technique of cognitive–behavioural strategies is the identification of the

sequence of thoughts and actions exhibited during painful episodes. A common content of patient's mental activity is 'catastrophization', the expectation of worst-state outcomes (see Lestor & Keefe, this volume). These and other dysfunctional methods of thinking about pain can be modified by a set of techniques which include cognitive challenges to the belief, provision of alternative ways of construing events (reattribution) and self-instructional behavioural experimentation with alternative more adaptive coping responses. Treatment is delivered through guided rehearsal under the supervision of a therapist with subsequent monitoring and modification as the patient introduces the methods into their daily life (Hanson & Gerber, 1990; Turk & Meichenbaum, 1994; Turner & Jensen, 1993).

Behavioural

Behavioural approaches to pain are directed at modifying pain behaviour rather than the subjective experience of pain. Pain behaviour includes maladaptive postural changes, excessive resting and dysfunctional rest–activity cycles. The application of principles of operant behaviour modification have been paramount in the development of behavioural treatments (Fordyce, 1976; Keefe & Lefebvre, 1994). Frequent targets for intervention are patients' activity levels (physical fitness), medication intake and social interactions with family members. Behavioural assessment identifies the events which precede (discriminative stimuli) the target pain behaviour and the consequences of the behaviour (the reinforcers). Treatment consists of manipulating the contingencies between these events in order to decrease non-functional responses and increase positive adaptive ways of behaving. Features of behavioural treatments include graded programmes to increase exercise and alter the contingent relationship between exercise and pain, modification of social reinforcement given by solicitous spouses and family members, and modifying the contingencies between pain and medication intake. Behavioural treatments have been frequently delivered as in-patient programmes as this allows the treatment environment to be carefully controlled. Staff are trained not to reinforce maladaptive pain behaviour and to interact in a consistently therapeutic manner. A behavioural approach to pain also implies that it is necessary for family members to change their behaviour towards the patient The typical pattern of behaviour between spouses is described as 'solicitous'; the patient's partner is unduly attentive and responsive to signs of pain thereby positively reinforcing patterns of rest and non-participation in family and household activity. Family members are therefore, frequently involved in treatment programmes (e.g. Turner et al., 1990). Finally, behavioural approaches may be implemented through carefully designed self-control methods in which the patient is taught how to modify and change their own contingencies and reinforcers (Hanson & Gerber, 1990).

Social and family

As noted above, operant behavioural techniques explicitly target patterns of spouse and family interaction. Psychodynamic and systems theory approaches to understanding the social context of pain have also been incorporated into management programmes but there is a lack of empirical analysis in this field (Rowat, Jeans & LeFort, 1994).

CONCLUSIONS

Generally speaking, psychological management of pain has drawn from a range of theoretical ideas in psychology and developed a correspondingly catholic approach to treatment. The main features of this have been noted. In addition to the range of treatments, psychology has developed a distinctive approach to delivering the treatment which encourages the active participation of the patient in deciding the goals of therapy and monitoring its progress. Current research is attempting to unravel the mechanisms of effect and relative importance of the various treatment methods. (See also 'Coping with chronic pain', 'Placebos', 'Relaxation training'.)

REFERENCES

Cioffi, D. (1991). Beyond attentional strategies: a cognitive–perceptual model of somatic interpretation. *Psychological Bulletin*, **109**, 25–41.

Eccleston, C. (1995). Chronic pain and distraction: an experimental investigation into the role of sustained and shifting attention in the processing of chronic persistent pain. *Behaviour Research and Therapy*, 33, 391–406.

Fernandez, E. (1986). A classification of cognitive coping strategies for pain. *Pain*, **26**, 141–51.

Flor, H. & Birbaumer, N. (1993). Comparison of the efficacy of electromyographic biofeedback, cognitive-behavioral therapy, and conservative medical interventions in the treatment of chronic musculoskeletal pain. *Journal of Consulting and Clinical Psychology*, **61**, 653–8.

Flor, H., Fydrich, T. & Turk, D.C. (1992). Efficacy of multidisciplinary pain treatment centers: a meta-analytic review. *Pain*, 49, 211–30.

Fordyce, W.E. (1976). *Behavioral methods for chronic pain and illness.* St Louis: CV Mosby.

Hanson, R.W. & Gerber, K.E. (1990). *Coping with chronic pain: a guide to patient self-management.* New York: Guilford Press.

Hawton, K., Salkovskis, P.M., Kirk, J. & Clark, D.M. (1989). *Cognitive behaviour therapy for psychiatric problems: a practical guide.* Oxford: Oxford University Press.

Howard, K.I., Orlinsky, D.E. & Lueger, R.J. (1994). Clinically relevant outcome research in individual psychotherapy: new models guide the researcher and clinician, *British Journal of Psychiatry*, 165, 4–8.

Jensen, M.P. & Karoly, P. (1991). Control beliefs, coping efforts, and adjustment in chronic pain. *Journal of Consulting and Clinical Psychology*, 59, 431–8.

Jessup, B.A. & Gallegos, X. (1994). Relaxation and biofeedback. In P.D. Wall & R. Melzack (Eds.). *Textbook of pain, 3rd edn.*, Edinburgh: Churchill Livingstone.

Keefe, F.J. & Lefebvre, J.C. (1994) Behavior therapy. In P.D. Wall & R. Melzack (Eds.). *Textbook of pain, 3rd edn.*, Edinburgh: Churchill Livingstone.

Malone, M.D. & Strube, M.J. (1988). Meta-analysis of non-medical treatments for chronic pain, *Pain*, 34, 231–44.

Mendelson, G. (1994). Chronic pain and compensation issues. In P.D. Wall & R. Melzack, (Eds.). *Textbook of pain 3rd edn.*, Edinburgh: Churchill Livingstone.

Moore, R. (1990). Ethnographic assessment of pain coping perceptions. *Psychosomatic Medicine*, 52, 171–81.

Rowat, K.M., Jeans, M.E. & LeFort, S.M. (1994). A collaborative model of health care: patient, family and health professionals. In P.D. Wall & R. Melzack (Eds.). *Textbook of pain*, 3rd edn . Edinburgh: Churchill Livingstone.

Spanos, N.P., Carmanico, S.J. and Ellis, J.A. (1994). Hypnotic analgesia. In P.D. Wall & R. Melzack (Eds.). *Textbook of pain (3rd edn)*. Edinburgh: Churchill Livingstone.

Turk, D.C. & Rudy, T.E. (1991). Neglected topics in the treatment of chronic pain patients–relapse, noncompliance, and adherence enhancement. *pain*, 44, 5–28.

Turk, D.C. & Meichenbaum, D. (1994). A cognitive–behavioural approach to pain management. In P.D. Wall & R. Melzack (Eds.). *Textbook of pain (3rd edition)*, Edinburgh: Churchill Livingstone.

Turner, J.A. & Jensen, M.P. (1993). Efficacy of cognitive therapy for chronic low back pain. *Pain*, 52, 169–77.

Turner, J.A., Clancy, S., McQuade, K.J. & Cardenas, D.D. (1990). Effectiveness of behavioral therapy for chronic low back pain: a component analysis. *Journal of Consulting and Clinical Psychology*, 58, 537–79.

Placebos

PHILIP HUGHES RICHARDSON

Division of Psychiatry and Psychology,

UMDS (London University),

Guy's Hospital,

London, UK

Psychological factors have been widely implicated in patients' responses to medical treatments. Research on placebos and placebo effects provides one important means to examine such factors. Despite the frequent use of placebos in treatment evaluation research, however, there has been limited agreement as to what, in fact, constitutes a placebo. The definition both of placebo and placebo effect has been widely debated and the viability of the placebo concept has itself been challenged (Richardson, 1989). The earlier and, some would say confusing, terminology of 'specific' and 'non-specific' factors is rapidly giving ground to Grünbaum's more recently proposed conceptual framework. This distinguishes 'characteristic' features of a treatment, which are specified by a theory of therapy to be remedial for a particular disorder, from 'incidental' treatment ingredients, which are not so specified. Placebo effects are therefore described as those effects on a target disorder which are brought about by incidental treatment ingredients, whether or not the treatment itself is a non-placebo or a placebo (i.e. none of its characteristic ingredients is, in fact, remedial for the disorder) (Grünbaum, 1981).

Placebo therapy has been delivered in many shapes and sizes, extending far beyond the traditional stereotype of the sugar pill. Most conventional treatments (injections, surgery etc) can, and have, been delivered in bogus form. Treatments based on modern technology (ultrasound, transcutaneous nerve stimulation, etc) are particularly amenable to administration in a theoretically inactive way, and completely bogus treatments (e.g. subconscious reconditioning therapy) have been developed to capitalize on the inherently high credibility of modern science (Richardson, 1994). Anonymous surveys indicate that placebo use is far from rare in everyday hospital practice, though the reasons commonly given to justify their use (e.g. fobbing off the demanding patient, 'proving' that the symptom thereby reduced was psychogenic in origin) betray a poor knowledge of relevant empirical research findings and limited levels of psychological sophistication among users.

Early research findings concerning the effects of placebos typically reported symptom relief in placebo-treated patients on the basis of improvements from pre- to post-treatment assessment. In many cases the placebo was administered as the only control condition in the evaluation of some putatively nonplacebo treatment. Instances of spontaneous symptom fluctuation could thus be erroneously attributed to the placebo as could the effects of other methodological artefacts (e.g. reactivity of measurement, statistical regression). Recent studies, incorporating a no-treatment control condition, provide more compelling evidence that symptom relief which can be observed to follow placebo administration can, in fact, be attributed to the placebo itself, and hence be considered a true placebo effect.

Placebo-induced symptom relief has been reported in an impressively wide range of illnesses, including allergies, angina pectoris, asthma, cancer, cerebral infarction, depression, diabetes, enuresis, epilepsy, insomnia, Meunière's disease, migraine, multiple sclerosis, neurosis, ocular pathology, Parkinsonism, prostatic hyperplasia, schizophrenia, skin diseases, ulcers and warts (see White, Tursky & Schwartz, 1985). The number of patients appearing to benefit from placebos varies from study to study, with response rates ranging from 0% to 100% for the same condition (Ross & Olson, 1982). Pain, which is the commonest symptom leading to medical consultation, has been the commonest outcome measure in studies of the placebo effect. Laboratory studies of experimentally induced pain generally yield low response rates; typically 16% of subjects showing a 50% reduction on whichever pain measure is employed. Response rates are higher for clinical pain, and an average response rate of 35% has been reported by a number of reviewers. Studies where the primary focus of interest is the placebo effect itself have often yielded much higher response rates still, as have those in which the primary symptom being treated is itself psychological (e.g. anxiety, depression). As well as accounts of symptom reduction reported by patients and doctors, there have been a number of studies demonstrating placebo effects on objective measures of various bodily processes. These include GSR, blood pressure, lung func-

tion, postoperative swelling, and gastric motility (Richardson, 1989, 1994). For example, Hashish, Feinman & Harvey reported significantly greater reductions in post-operative swelling in dental patients who had received placebo ultrasound than in those who were simply monitored over the same period of time without treatment (Hashish et al., 1988). Reported adverse effects of placebo administration have included dependence, symptom worsening (the 'nocebo' effect) and a variety of side-effects, both subjective (e.g. headache, concentration difficulties, nausea) and 'objective' (e.g. skin rashes, sweating, vomiting). Placebo and drug effects have proved hard to differentiate. Several studies have reported parallel time effect curves, dose–response relationships and similar performance on other parameters by both placebos and the drugs with which they have been compared (Ross & Olson, 1982).

Two broad kinds of strategy can be discerned in studies designed to further our understanding of placebo effects: first exploratory studies seeking to identify which variables are significantly associated with an increased or reduced likelihood of occurrence of a placebo response; and secondly theory-driven research aimed at testing hypotheses about presumed mechanisms of the effect. Exploratory studies have focused either on patient variables, treatment characteristics, or aspects of the therapist and therapist–patient interaction.

Individual differences among placebo responders have long been a focus of research interest. Investigations of sociodemographic characteristics including age, gender, educational level, SES, and ethnicity have generally yielded mixed and inconclusive findings (Shapiro & Morris, 1978; Richardson, 1994). More recent studies of individual differences have broadened in scope to include measures of intelligence and personality. Locus of control, field dependence, emotional dependence, extraversion, introversion, neuroticism, suggestibility, autonomic awareness, acquiescence, tolerance of ambiguity, affiliation, autonomy and impulsivity have all featured as potential predictors of the placebo response (Richardson, 1994). Once again, however, a repeated pattern of conflicting and equivocal findings (e.g. both extraversion and introversion have emerged as predictors of placebo responsiveness) renders the likelihood of identifying the characteristics of the archetypal placebo responder increasingly remote. Two further considerations are relevant here. First, studies that have sought to demonstrate the cross-situational consistency of placebo responsiveness have generally failed to do so (Shapiro & Morris, 1978). Secondly, conditioning studies have demonstrated that previous non-responders can be turned into responders (see below). These findings appear to converge in suggesting that placebo responsiveness may not be an enduring trait. Patient-centred research on the placebo effect may yield more fruitful results if (variable) psychological processes replace (fixed) psychological characteristics as the focus of attention.

Effects of the physical characteristics of placebos on the size and nature of the patient's response have also been investigated. The size and colour of pills and capsules have been repeatedly manipulated, but with little reliable impact. Grosser variations in the form of treatment delivery may be more influential, in that more serious or 'major' procedures appear to have stronger effects. For example, injections would appear to have a greater placebogenic impact than pills and early studies of placebo surgery reported unusually high positive response rates. For example, in the work of Cobb et al.,

85% of patients with angina made improvements on a range of measures, including ECG and exercise tolerance test performance, following placebo surgery in which they received only an operation scar (Cobb *et al.*, 1959; Dimond, Kittle & Cockett, 1960). Treatment procedures making use of sophisticated technical equipment may also have enhanced placebo power. For example, Langley and colleagues obtained a higher than usual 55% response rate to placebo transcutaneous nerve stimulation when the equipment was dressed up with additional technological trappings (oscilloscope, flashing lights, dials; Langley *et al.*, 1984). The reasons why certain treatments provoke stronger placebo responses than others remain unclear, though there is some evidence that technically sophisticated treatments have greater inherent credibility for the patient, and the capacity to generate stronger expectations of successful outcome (Petrie & Hazleman, 1985). Classical conditioning accounts of the placebo effect, on the other hand, propose that treatment characteristics which have been previously associated with the therapeutic action of powerful nonplacebos will be those which also promote stronger conditioned placebo responses (see below).

Although certain treatments may have inherent qualities which enhance the placebo effect, it would seem likely that the manner of treatment administration and associated qualities of the therapist might also moderate such processes. The potential importance of the impact of the therapist's expectations on the patient's response to treatment has long been recognized in the treatment evaluation literature, where the need for double-blind procedures in both treatment administration and patient assessment has been considered as virtually axiomatic. In fact, therapist variables have been extensively explored in the placebo literature and the majority of studies point towards their importance. Therapists with greater interest in their patients, greater confidence in their treatments, and of greater status, all appear to promote greater placebo responses on the part of their patients (Shapiro & Morris, 1978). The relevant therapist behaviours and the precise nature of their impact on the patient have as yet been poorly explored. Research in the allied field of doctor–patient communication has demonstrated the influence of certain therapist behaviours on patient satisfaction and adherence to medical advice, which may also be relevant to the outcome of placebo treatment. For example Horwitz *et al.* have shown that the risk of death during the year following myocardial infarction was substantially greater in patients who took less than 75% of their prescribed medication, regardless of whether the medication was a beta blocker or a placebo (Horwitz *et al.*, 1990). The mechanisms of this effect are unclear, however, and there has yet been little cross-fertilization between research on therapist influences on the placebo effect and the cognate and better developed fields of psychotherapy process research and studies of doctor–patient communication.

It might be thought that the rather piecemeal nature of the studies reported thus far derives from the lack of any integrating theoretical framework within which the mechanisms of the placebo effect may be understood. In fact, hypotheses concerning the mode of action of placebos are numerous and have been couched in terms of: operant conditioning, classical conditioning, guilt reduction, transference, suggestion, persuasion, role demands, hope, faith, labelling, selective symptom monitoring, misattribution, cognitive dissonance reduction, control theory, anxiety reduction, expectancy effects, endorphin release, as well as in terms of various artefacts of study design and/or measurement (Richardson, 1994). Sadly, however, the investigations that have been driven by such theories are small in number and, in many cases non-existent.

The possibility that most reported placebo effects are simple artefacts of study design or measurement has surfaced in two major forms: first in the idea that real symptom change occurs but is falsely attributed to placebo administration; and secondly, that no change has occurred but measurement errors create the spurious impression of change. The first category includes instances of spontaneous patient improvement during the period of placebo treatment, change induced by the repeated measurement of symptoms, and statistical regression to the mean. That these phenomena occur is undisputed. They undoubtedly must temper our interpretation of all apparent placebo effects inferred from pre- to post-treatment change in placebo-treated cases. They have little or no relevance, however, to our understanding of placebo effects obtained in studies that have properly incorporated a no-treatment or waiting-list control condition.

The second category of potential artefact, data distortion through measurement error on the part of the investigator or patient, is perhaps more compelling, particularly in view of the extensive evidence for the power of experimenter biases and of therapist expectancy effects on patient outcome. Observer bias in the measurement of symptoms can be reduced in controlled studies by the use of assessors who are blind to the patient's treatment group allocation. It is harder however to blind the patient to the fact of having received treatment. Over-reporting of symptoms prior to treatment (e.g. to 'earn' treatment) and under-reporting of symptoms after treatment (e.g. to please the doctor) will create the impression of a positive treatment effect. Patients in the waiting list control condition who may have over-reported on the first pretreatment assessment have no reason to alter their report at the second assessment, if they are still awaiting treatment. This source of potential bias is therefore not eliminated by the inclusion of the usual no-treatment control group. Despite its potential role in accounting for some instances of the placebo effect, the likelihood that this kind of misreporting can account for all placebo effects is reduced by the frequent observation of objectively measured change in various bodily processes, including those of which the patient would normally have no awareness (e.g. blood pressure, lung function).

The psychological accounts of placebogenesis that have received greatest research attention would appear to be the anxiety-reduction, cognitive dissonance, expectancy and classical conditioning accounts.

Since much placebo research has focused on pain and its reduction, and since anxiety is believed to increase the experience of pain, it is not surprising that the reduction of anxiety has been proposed to account for a variety of placebo phenomena (Evans, 1974). For example, the reduced placebo response rates in experimental, as opposed to clinical, pain, have been accounted for by the fact that healthy experimental volunteers will be less anxious initially than patients who may be ill or injured; unlike the patient group they are less likely to experience anxiety reduction when offered (placebo) treatment, whereas the relief at being offered treatment may itself alleviate to some extent the symptoms of the patient group. Likewise the commonly observed pain relief associated with the

[239]

ingestion of a painkiller, yet which occurs well before any possible pharmacological effect could have occurred, might be explained by the immediate relief of anxiety which accompanies the knowledge of having received treatment. Experimental support for this interpretation of placebo effects is sparse. Evans *et al.* found that patients who experienced anxiety reduction after placebo administration later showed greater pain tolerance than a group for whom placebo administration led to higher anxiety. Other investigators, however, have found no association between changes in state anxiety and placebo-induced symptom change (Richardson, 1994), and the role of anxiety reduction in placebo-induced symptom change therefore remains unclear.

Cognitive dissonance theory proposes that the holding of two or more psychologically inconsistent beliefs creates a state of tension which will motivate the individual to reduce the inconsistency. The knowledge of having received treatment is inconsistent with the perception of no symptom change, and the resultant dissonance may motivate the patient to alter his/her experience of the symptom, to reduce the inconsistency. Laboratory studies have shown dissonance arousal to be a powerful force capable of producing physiological as well as psychological change (Zimbardo, 1969). There have been numerous demonstrations of the relevance of dissonance theory to clinical phenomena in general, and its relevance to the placebo effect has been most clearly established in a small series of experiments reported by Totman (Totman, 1987). Using various conventional dissonance-inducing experimental paradigms he was able to show that patients in whom greatest dissonance was aroused at the time of placebo administration were those who showed greatest subsequent symptom relief. His interpretation of these findings has not gone unquestioned however, and alternative anxiety-reduction accounts of his findings have been proposed (Richardson, 1994).

Expectancy-based accounts of placebo effects are ubiquitously encountered in the placebo literature. Patient expectations have been shown to be related to the outcome both of psychotherapy and of drug therapy and there is some evidence to suggest that expectancy manipulations may influence responses to a placebo. For example, Cami and colleagues showed that an expectancy manipulation influenced heart rate responses to a cannabis placebo (Cami *et al.*, 1991). A number of investigators have also found that therapeutic instructions may influence analgesic response both to a placebo and to standard painkillers (see Richardson, 1994). In contrast, however, a recent review of the research literature on cognitive coping strategies, concluded that verbal expectancy manipulations

alone were no more effective in reducing pain than no treatment (Richardson, 1994). This suggests that other aspects of treatment administration may interact with expectancy if the latter indeed plays some role in determining outcome. In addition, in comparative studies testing alternative mechanisms of the placebo effect, expectancy accounts have tended to fare worse (Richardson, 1994). Moreover, despite their commonsense appeal, expectancy-based accounts of the placebo effect are likely to have limited explanatory force in the absence of some further specification both as to how particular expectancies are formed and as to the precise mechanism(s) by which a particular expectancy translates itself into a particular form of symptom relief.

Classical conditioning accounts of placebo phenomena are based on the view that many of the standard accompaniments of effective nonplacebo treatments (e.g. doctors, syringes, stethoscopes) can become conditioned stimuli by virtue of their repeated association with symptom relief. Thus the habitually shorter latency of conditioned as opposed to unconditioned responses would also account for the phenomenon of unusually early pain relief as a placebo response to a painkiller (see above). Likewise the absence of the customary medical CSs in the laboratory would account for the lower rate of positive placebo responses in experimental than clinical pain. Classical conditioning of drug responses has been demonstrated in both animals and humans and a recent series of studies by Voudouris *et al.* has established the relevance of conditioning phenomena to our understanding of placebo effects in humans (Voudouris, Peck & Coleman, 1989, 1990). In these studies of experimentally induced pain, the pairing of reduced shock intensity with the application of a placebo 'analgesic' cream led to significantly lower pain ratings to a given level of nociceptive stimulation than when no prior conditioning trial had been run. Voudouris *et al.* also found that a verbal expectancy manipulation yielded less powerful placebo-induced pain relief than the conditioning procedure. Conditioning accounts of the placebo effect therefore appear promising but have yet to be tested directly on clinical populations.

It remains to be established which of the above theories of the placebo effect can best account for the psychological processes which commonly mediate patients' responses to their medical treatments. It seems unlikely that any single approach will successfully account for all placebo phenomena with respect to all symptoms and all response modalities. Only further empirical research will clarify these issues. (See also 'Coping with chronic pain', 'Pain management'.)

REFERENCES

Cami, J., Guerra, D., Ugena, B., Segura, J. & de la Torre, R. (1991). Effect of subject expectancy on the THC intoxication and disposition from smoked hashish cigarettes. *Pharmacology, Biochemistry and Behavior*, 40, 115–19.

Cobb, L.A., Thomas, G.I., Dillard, D.H. *et al.* (1959). An evaluation of internal-mammary-artery ligation by a double blind technique. *New England Journal of Medicine*, 260, 1115–18.

Dimond, E.G., Kittle, C.F. & Cockett, J.E.

(1960). Comparison of internal mammary-artery ligation and sham operation for angina pectoris. *American Journal of Cardiology*, 4, 483–6.

Evans, F.J. (1974). The placebo response in pain reduction. *Advances in Neurology*, 4, 289–96.

Grünbaum, A. (1981). The placebo concept. *Behaviour Research and Therapy*, 19, 157–67.

Hashish, I., Feinman, C. & Harvey, W. (1988). Reduction of postoperative pain

and swelling by ultrasound: a placebo effect. *Pain*, 83, 303–11.

Horwitz, R.I., Viscoli, C.M., Bermkan, L., Donaldson, R.M., Horwitz, S.M., Murray, C.J., Ransohoff, D.F. & Sindelair, J. (1990). Treatment adherence and risk of death after a myocardial infarction. *Lancet*, 336, 542–5.

Langley, G.B., Sheppeard, H., Johnson, M. & Wigley, R.D. (1984). The analgesic effects of transcutaneous electrical nerve stimulation and placebo in chronic pain patients. *Rheumatology International*, **2**, 1–5.

Petrie, J. & Hazleman, B. (1985). Credibility of placebo transcutaneous nerve stimulation and acupuncture. *Clinical and Experimental Rheumatology*, **3**, 151–3.

Richardson, P.H. (1989). Placebos: their effectiveness and modes of action. In A. Broome (Ed.). *Health psychology: processes and applications*, pp. 35–56. London: Chapman and Hall.

Richardson, P.H. (1994). Placebo effects in pain management. *Pain Reviews*, **1**, 15–32.

Ross, M. & Olson, J.M. (1982). Placebo effects in medical research and practice. In J.R. Eiser (Ed.). *Social psychology and Behavioural Medicine*, pp. 441–58. Chichester: John Wiley.

Shapiro, A.K. & Morris, L.A. (1978). The placebo effect in medical and psychological therapies. In A.E. Bergin & S. Garfield (Eds.). *Handbook of psychotherapy and behavioral change*. 2nd edn. pp. 369–410, New York: John Wiley.

Totman, R. (1987). *The Social Causes of Illness*, 2nd edn. Chapter 2, London: Souvenir Press.

Voudouris, N.J., Peck, C.L. & Coleman, G. (1989). Conditioned response of the placebo phenomena: further support. *Pain*, **38**, 109–16.

Voudouris, N.J., Peck, C.L. & Coleman, G. (1990). The role of conditioning and verbal expectancy in the placebo response. *Pain*, **43**, 121–8.

White, L., Tursky, B. & Schwartz, G.E. (1985). *Placebo: theory, research and mechanisms*, New York, London: Guilford Press.

Zimbardo, P.G. (1969). *The cognitive control of motivation*. Illinois: Scott, Foresman.

Psychodynamic psychotherapy

CHRIS EVANS

Psychotherapy Section, Department of General Psychiatry,
St, George's Hospital Medical School,
London, UK

INTRODUCTION

Psychodynamic psychotherapy attempts to remove unconscious conflicts or replace them with consciously acknowledged problems. The tools are models of the nature of the unconscious and of the leakage from unconscious to conscious which have their roots in the work of Sigmund Freud. As well as being a method of treatment, psychodynamic psychotherapy also raises strong questions about epistemology: the origins of knowledge and understanding. Because its roots lie in Freud's medical background and in the treatment of psychosomatic problems (hysterical symptoms), it has much to offer health psychology. There are a number of studies using conventional research methodology which provide strong support for psychodynamic methods with a range of conditions including somatic problems (e.g. Guthrie, 1991; Guthrie *et al.*, 1993; Milton, 1992). There are also excellent introductions to theories (Parry, 1983; Storr, 1979; Brown & Pedder, 1979; Symington, 1986; Malan, 1979; Greenberg & Mitchell, 1983; Sandler, Dare & Holder, 1973 in roughly increasing rigour). This chapter will not summarize those gallons in a pint pot but will identify the roots of psychodynamic psychotherapy in psychoanalysis and their implications for physical and mental health. This will reveal an epistemological challenge which questions the sufficiency and completeness of traditional research methods in health psychology.

THE PROBLEM (*REDUCTIO AD ABSURDUM*)

Like any epistemological challenge, this benefits from consideration in its most extreme form:

Why should someone with recurrent, crippling pain resembling angina but not associated with any other evidence of coronary disease, lie on another person's couch for fifty minutes a day at prearranged times five times a week over a period of five or more years? Why should that person attempt to say whatever comes into his or her mind? Why should the other attempt to maintain an 'evenly suspended attention' to this material, making comments at a frequency and in a manner that would be regarded as socially unacceptable in most other settings? Why should that person call comments 'interpretations' when both use the same language? Why would either believe that this might ultimately relieve the first person of the pain or its impact on his or her life?

This *reduction ad absurdum* describes, in bare outline, a pure form of psychoanalysis. By contrast, most psychodynamic psychotherapies involve less frequent meetings over shorter periods, rarely use the couch, and often involve the therapist in more overt engagement with the patient. Of course, all psychotherapies and counselling have a human relationship in common and much of their value is consequent upon this. However, this chapter is about differences between psychodynamic and other therapies, and putting these differences in their most extreme form is pertinent, not only because Sigmund Freud's theory of psychoanalysis continues to underpin all psychodynamic psychotherapies, but because it helps us decide what methods of enquiry will be congruent with the theory.

The use of the couch, the contrast between the ascetic abstention from conventional interaction coupled with the fascinatingly self-absorbed spending of such a high proportion of one's waking life concentrating on oneself and involving another in that concentration; these all arose from some basic postulates about the way people might show symptoms of apparently organic pathology (hysteria) and about the way we all think, feel and behave. In this chapter I suggest why we might still use these methods in the twenty-first century.

DEFINITIONS

The logic of the unconscious

Psychodynamic psychotherapies are distinguished from other therapies by their emphasis on unconscious determination: symptoms, like all thought, feeling and behaviour are believed to be non-random and to have determinants that are beyond conscious awareness. This unconscious is not the unconscious of associations set up in simple learning paradigms nor is it that of appraisal processes in cognitive theory, though it has elements in common with these. Two things are held in common with simple learning theories: (i) determination involves storage of earlier experiences; and (ii) the process itself is not subjectively appreciable although its results may be. The first of these is uncontroversial at first sight, but the second merits expansion as 'insight' in psychodynamic psychotherapies is often misunderstood. In strictly behavioural therapy the process by which behaviour has been acquired is considered only spuriously accessible to consciousness: conscious appreciation of the process may be reassuring but this is not the same as changing behaviour. For example, as a behaviourist, I may feel less stupid for appreciating that a conditioning process led me to grope for the light switch in its old position, but I believe that this appreciation contributes little or nothing to my becoming adept at hitting the switch in its new position. Similarly, as an analytic patient I may consider that my crippling responses to authority replicate an early relationship with parents but this appreciation will not necessarily change my responses: analytic change is thought to come about mainly by 'working through' those responses in relation to the analyst.[1] In this model, I might come to avoid my pathological responses without much conscious appreciation of how they arose, just as I will adapt to the new position of the light switch.

The parallels with the cognitive therapies are different. In marked contrast to the unconscious processes of simple learning theories and strict behavioural therapies, the unconsciousness of the psychodynamic and cognitive psychotherapies is complex both in algorithmic sophistication and in an element of recursion:[2] the processes postulated can involve internal representations of the self that is constituted by those processes.

So, although the psychodynamic unconscious has parallels with that of learning and cognitive psychologies, it differs from both in that it is not considered to obey the rules we use in formal logic and intuitive conscious thought. The critical difference is that the logic of the unconscious involves selective reversals, e.g. the internal representation of pain may involve the representation of its opposite,

pleasure. This may sound so absurd that it is hard to recognize that selective ignoring of differences is the fundamental characteristic of all thought: to recognize that two people are both human is to attend selectively to their similarities and temporarily ignore their differences. What makes this so formidable in the psychodynamic unconscious is that, because the process is 'unconscious', we do not recognize that this is what we have done when we substitute pain for pleasure or vice versa.

The other crucial idea about the psychodynamic unconscious is precisely that it is dynamic: an active process of repression keeps some contents unconscious because they are dangerous to acknowledge. The process of psychoanalysis is that of coming to be aware of these censorings so that conscious choices can be made. Simplifying, not perhaps unrealistically, the wish to have sexual intercourse with someone other than your partner, a wish perhaps thwarted by chronic chest pain, may come to be recognized and choices made about fidelity with consequent relief from the chest pain. (Note that this process may take time, as the licentious wish may actually have come to be gratified, perversely, as pain and pleasure become exchangeable once forced into the unconscious.)

The historical and ahistorical nature of the dynamic unconscious

The psychoanalytic model of development has been found disturbing in two different ways. The first is that the historical information used may be that of (infantile) fantasy, e.g. it may involve a fantasy of having been rejected rather than a reality (or it may involve both a reality and a fantasy). The second is that it tends to involve a much greater degree of sexuality than is generally considered to be present in the minds of young children.

Transfer from unconscious to conscious by repetition

The dimension of time provides the most clinically important of the ways in which it is possible for us to become conscious of our unconscious: this is the process of repetition, that we are 'doomed to repeat that which we cannot remember', the general clinical aspect of this is that symptoms often replay, in coded fashion, that which is unconscious, like the chest pain in our example. The specific clinical application is 'transference': the reenactment of the unconscious processes in the relationship between patient and analyst. For example, the patient may become worried that his relationship with the analyst is a form of disloyalty to his sexual partner, or, more likely, there may be subtle aspects of the relationship that suggest this, or unconscious reversal may exchange analyst for patient and the patient may experience the analyst as a disloyal lover for seeing other patients or for having a home life of his or her own.

Other leakages from unconscious to conscious

The earliest of these was hypnosis: the extraordinary extent to which consciousness can be suspended in hypnosis was one of the influences that led to the 'talking cure'. This was rapidly abandoned in favour of the 'royal road to the unconscious' dreams, or, in good clinical practice, the unravelling of the coded leakage from the unconscious through the patient's 'free associations' to recalled dreams. This, in turn, led to the general use of 'free association': the attempt to describe exactly what goes on in one's mind (and body) without censorship (matched by the 'evenly suspended attention' of

---

[1] This chapter is based on the individual analytic situation. The group analytic situation, in which 'working through' may relate more to a fellow patient, is not considered as it can be markedly more confusing to explain. I believe it to obey similar principles, the confusing aspects being simple functions of numerical and combinatorial complexity.

[2] A recursive process can invoke itself and can have great utility in computing. For example, consider finding the factorial of a number (four factorial, written as '4!' is 4*3*2*1 = 24, five factorial, 5! = 5*4*3*2*1 = 120). It can be seen that 4! = 4*3! = 4*3*2*1 . . . A recursive algorithm for this is 'If the number to act on is one, the answer is one, otherwise: find the factorial of one less than the number you're currently trying to act on and multiply it by the number your currently working on.'

the analyst with its own peculiar form of non-censorship). Finally, there are 'Freudian slips' and other hints that creep into language through metaphor and humour. Although Freudian slips are a small part of the clinical route to the unconscious, the general attention to language (non-verbal as well as verbal) in free association forms the matrix linking patient and analyst in a process of discovery.

Separation of subject and object

Partly because of Freud's roots in a very deterministic nineteenth-century science of hydraulics and separation of subject and researcher, it is only comparatively recently (around the late 1940s) that analysts first stated overtly that the unconscious of the analyst, reacting moment to moment in the session, might itself be informative and communicative rather than a technical error to be expunged by a second training analysis. Thus was the positive analysis of 'countertransference' introduced and the full complexity of the bilateral process of analysis acknowledged increasingly clearly.

UNCONSCIOUS DETERMINISM AND NON-DETERMINABILITY

One issue, much disputed among psychodynamic workers, is that these unconscious processes may be expected in the light of 'Chaos theory' (see e.g. Ruelle, 1991), to be likely to be highly idiosyncratic to individuals. Specifically, although general theory can be stated in a simple way, as above, it postulates an iterative[3] development of the unconscious, with both reality and fantasy constantly being incorporated in interaction with other people's unconsciousnesses (expressed in their behaviours). It is iterative in that the cumulative state of assimilated material affects the way new material is added. Not only is the process assumed to be iterative but also it is assumed to be non-linear (often described, even by Freud himself, as simply illogical). The maths of 'Chaos theory' suggests that iterative non-linear processes will, almost always, show extreme sensitivity to initial conditions so that the prediction of later states is nearly impossible on the basis of finite knowledge about earlier states. This sensitive dependence is such that the interaction between any one person (patient) and any other person (therapist) will be complex, so complex indeed that neither person could be replaced with another without the overall picture changing radically, perhaps unrecognizably. I will argue below that, if this bit of the theory is accepted, then testability will not be easily achieved.

Summary

The unconsciousness postulated in psychodynamic psychotherapy is not accessible to deliberate introspection nor does it obey an immediately obvious and coherent set of logical rules. However, it is believed to be profoundly influenced by biological, including sexual, drives from an early age. The psychodynamic psychotherapies all use these basic ideas, in very different guises and proportions, to find a story through which symptoms can either be understood or changed, or both understood and changed. Some of the biggest controversies in the theory turn on the degree to which 'biological' here may imply genetic determination, and on whether or not there is a 'biological' drive to interpersonal relatedness ('attachment') and, if so, what form or forms it takes.

THE PROBLEM AGAIN, BACKGROUND AND EXPANSION

These ideas were not new in 1895 when Freud started his codification of them and of their implications for treatment. He drew, with acknowledgement, on evidence in the works of poets, novelists and playwrights from Sophocles to Freud's contemporaries. He also drew, again with acknowledgement, upon Charcot's work on hysteria and on hypnotism. What makes Freud's work stand apart from that of his predecessors was that his was the most radical codification and that it was the first to be carried out with a determination to give the ideas and the practice the respectability of a 'science', of a 'psychology' whilst also locating them firmly within some of the traditions of nineteenth- (and twentieth-) century medicine. Most of the problems that have dogged psychoanalysis and all the psychodynamic psychotherapies since 1895 relate to the merits of this claim to scientific status and the ambivalent relationship with medicine and psychiatry.

The aspiration to scientific status is always problematical in the social and human sciences as many of the traditional qualities of scientific work: objectivity, replicability, open peer review, prediction, testability of predictions and strong (mathematical) internal coherence, rest upon the separation of the subject (scientist) and object (field of enquiry). The scientist may be composed of molecules, including molecules of hydrogen, but that is not considered to influence the behaviour of the hydrogen molecules he or she investigates. It is not so clear that our thoughts and the behaviours we investigate can remain so independent of our investigations. In fact, many of us believe that the processes described by Freud are unlikely to be applicable to us in the way they were to his own mind and that of his colleagues, acquaintances and patients, precisely because they have become the currency of our thought. If this is the case, and if much of the psychodynamic unconscious is unconscious because, for social and personal reasons, it must not reach consciousness, then the task of finding it will require recursively more effort now that our consciousness is imbued with this possibility.

Separation of subject and object breaks down at the extremes of modern theoretical physics but that does not invalidate its status as science. Equally, and very pertinently for our purposes, Gödel has shown (see, e.g. Nagel & Newman, 1958) that a number theory cannot be complete and at the same time entirely logically consistent, yet mathematicians have not abandoned number theory nor maths in general. More prosaically, much of psychology copes with this discomforting similarity of subject and experimenter and clear experimental technique including random allocation, 'blinding' of subjects and experimenters, together with good use of psychometrics and statistics, gives leverage on many psychological problems. All of that approach rests on two main assumptions: (i) that the measured processes are likely to be similar in all subjects under investigation; and (ii) that the topics to be investigated are not so private or intimate that their exploration and disclosure in the publication for peer review will necessitate deliberate falsification of potentially crucial foci of the processes under study.

Unfortunately, neither interchangeability nor easy disclosure is true in psychotherapy. Most people who seek psychodynamic

---

[3] An iterative process is one that repeats, e.g. finding a square root by repeated approximations above and below until sufficient precision is achieved.

psychotherapy are as interested in their uniqueness as individuals at least as much as in their commonalities with others. Equally, most would not wish their communications to be published in full, with full identificatory detail of their early lives, current partnerships and family dynamics, etc. Furthermore, no ethics committee will ever sanction such disclosure nor the even more alluring possibility of cloning people of identical upbringings to put them through essentially the same processes or different ones, allocated at random, so as to test the predictions implicit or explicit in the presentation of the first case report.

So the 'why?' in our *reductio ad absurdum* cannot be answered by the received processes of nomothetic science: there are no data that assert clearly that we can calculate a confidence interval for the likely success for 50 people going for 50 such analyses for cardiac pain on no known organic cause (this is actually no different from any other psychotherapy or medical therapy for this condition known to this author). Further, in contrast to behavioural or cognitive theories, psychodynamic theories suggest that we may be missing the point trying to acquire such estimates, unless our understanding of the unconscious and of psychotherapy develops far beyond its present state and reduces the supposition of individual idiosyncrasy both in the patient's and in the therapist's contributions to the therapy.

DISCUSSION

I believe these arguments leave psychodynamic psychotherapy incompatible with Popperian 'science'. However, perhaps most 'science' fails, at least in current forms, to satisfy Popperian criteria. It is also arguable that Popper's notion of falsifiability is itself profoundly problematical, not to say unfalsifiable. Extrapolation of Gödel's theorem suggests that no 'science' along Popperian lines can exist without extra-scientific underpinnings. Nevertheless, when this author wishes to consider the 'scientific' quality of behavioural and cognitive therapies, the Popperian criterion seems excellent as it is congruent with the theories of behavioural and cognitive theory. However, some problems of patients and speculations about the

nature of 'mind' and 'humanity' seem to go beyond those theories. Then there is a misfit between traditional experimental methods and the psychodynamic theory that helps understand these problems. In this dilemma one can take a Kuhnian position and argue either that psychodynamic psychotherapies (or all psychology) are currently only 'prescientific', i.e. that there is no received paradigm by which views are exchanged and evaluated. More anarchically, one can take the strong hermeneutic or social constructionist positions: that science is no more than understandings, and that the understandings of psychoanalysis have a respectability as great as the published data of a synchrotron experiment: both are received as part of a general discourse of interested people. A final position is (neo)Platonism: the belief that there are verities that transcend determinism and transcend constructionism, verities knowable only by their reflections in maths and other beauties (see e.g. Penrose, 1989).

Mathematics, epistemology and the general field of the social sciences have all, in parallel with psychoanalytic or psychodynamic theory, developed radically in the twentieth century. This has made possible a new rigour in the discussion of psychoanalytic theory and is probably about to lead to a new willingness to consider fully the problems of confidentiality and the nature of case material in psychodynamic therapies. This full consideration will neither dismiss the ethical and human problems nor rely uncritically on carefully massaged case reports. It will allow intelligent and conscientious use of video and audiotaped material for text and discourse analysis, just as it may already be supporting a new attention to surface and deep phenomenology in clinical psychology and psychiatry. Finally, this new sophistication in discussing psychoanalytic theory should link with the pure and applied mathematics of non-linear dynamic systems ('Chaos') and its recent extensions into control theories for non-linear dynamic systems and into the understanding of complex systems. Although these liaisons will strike terror into many on both sides as each misrepresents the other, I believe they will offer more hybrid vigour than ever came out of the attempted marriages of conventional positivist empiricism and psychoanalysis.

REFERENCES

Brown, D. & Pedder, J. (1979). *Introduction to psychotherapy. An outline of psychodynamic principles and practice.* London: Tavistock Publications.

Greenberg, J.R. & Mitchell, S.A. (1983). *Object relations in psychoanalytic theory.* Cambridge, Massachusetts: Harvard University Press.

Guthrie, E. (1991). Brief psychotherapy with patients with refractory irritable bowel syndrome. *British Journal of Psychotherapy,* 8, 175–88.

Guthrie, E., Creed, F., Dawson, D. & Tomenson, B. (1993) A randomized controlled trial of psychotherapy in patients with refractory irritable bowel syndrome. *British Journal of Psychiatry,* 163, 315–21.

Malan (1979). *Individual psychotherapy and the science of psychodynamics.* London: Butterworths.

Milton, J. (1992). Presenting the case for NHS psychotherapy services: a working bibliography. *Psychoanalytic psychotherapy,* 6, 151–67.

Nagel, E. & Newman, J.R. (1958). *Gödel's proof.* London: Routledge and Kegan Paul.

Parry, R. (1983). *Basic psychotherapy.* 2nd edn. Edinburgh: Churchill Livingstone.

Penrose, R. (1989). *The emperor's new mind.* London: Vintage.

Ruelle, D. (1991). *Chance and chaos.* Harmondsworth: Penguin Books.

Sandler, J., Dare, C. & Holder, A. (1973). *The patient and the analyst. The basis of the psychoanalytic process.* London: Maresfield.

Storr, A. (1979). *The art of psychotherapy.* London: Martin Secker & Warburg Ltd. and William Heinemann Medical Books Ltd.

Symington, N. (1986). *The analytic experience.* London: Free Association Books.

Reality orientation therapy

JANE VOLANS

Department of Clinical Psychology,
Oxleas NHS Trust, Bostall House, Goldie Leigh
Hospital, Lodge Hill, London, UK

INTRODUCTION AND BACKGROUND

Reality orientation is undoubtedly the best researched and evaluated of all psychological interventions used to date with dementia sufferers. Its importance must be judged not just in terms of its effectiveness as a therapy, but also in terms of its overall impact on policy and practice.

In spite of intensive and relatively well-funded research into physical treatments, it is now generally accepted that only tiny improvements can be effected in this way, and that it is the practical and psychosocial aspects of care that most require attention. Unfortunately, although clinical psychologists have played a major part in the development of psychosocial interventions in other client groups for several decades, few psychologists interested themselves in the older client group until the late 1960s, and those who did, tended to concentrate on the development of psychological testing batteries.

The first attempts at psychological interventions with older adults in a variety of forms of inpatient care were reported in the main in American journals. These tended to be vague about the interventions themselves, and the diagnoses of the patients involved. The development of the reality orientation (RO) approach had, in fact, begun in about 1959, initially in the Veterans Hospital in Topeka Ohio, and subsequently in Tuscaloosa, but the first reports did not appear for another six years or so. The approach comprised a set of strategies initially intended to ameliorate the general sensory and social deprivation that characterized the 'care' of long-stay psychiatric patients at that time. Subsequently it was also implemented with the more recently admitted dementia sufferers Folsom (1968). Even in the earlier publications, the approach was described in terms which were specific enough to allow some replication in other centres. Training courses for health professionals were set up at Tuscaloosa, which attracted therapists from both sides of the Atlantic. The charisma and enthusiasm of the Tuscaloosa group, together with the attraction of adopting an approach that was relatively tried and tested, as compared with what had gone before, ensured that RO was widely disseminated, well in advance of more formal evaluations.

WHAT IS RO?

There are three main forms of Reality Orientation. The best known and most extensively researched of these is 'Classroom RO'. Small groups of dementia sufferers assemble for half an hour or so with one or more group leaders. The main aim of the group is to provide information that will enhance orientation in time, place and person, and if possible to more general world or national news, in a form that will hold the attention of group members. The group is held near to a 'Reality Orientation Board' (a wall – mounted display focusing on day, date, and approximate time of day, possibly also including information about location, and a simple statement about weather conditions).

Generally the group will meet in a quiet place, away from interruptions, and the timing and location of the group will be kept constant. Other materials will be brought into the session as appropriate. These may include calendars, advent calendars, seasonal fruit or vegetables or other cues to season (fallen leaves, spring flowers, icicles), pictures from newspapers or magazines, or pieces of sporting equipment (e.g. tennis racquets during Wimbledon). Group members are encouraged to handle materials, to comment on them, and to use them as cues when posed questions. All group members will be given a chance to participate. All contributions are valued, but when possible mistakes are gently and tactfully corrected. The group leader conveys information, and encourages active rehearsal by questioning, seeking fact, subjective evaluation or more personal connections with the topic.

Although there have been no systematic attempts at task analysis, which might tease out the most essential elements of the RO package, the *Training manual*, produced by the American Hospitals' Association listed the key elements as early as 1976. These comprised: a calm environment, a set routine, simple direct responses to patients' questions, distinct and direct speech, reminders of time place and person, correction of 'rambling', full explanation of new procedures, allowing ample time for response, clear verbal and behavioural guidance, showing patients that they were expected to understand and comply, showing patients that they were expected to care for themselves as much as they were able, treating patients as respected dignified adults, showing interest and sincerity, showing kindness and politeness in a matter of fact way, and consistency in all the above.

These have been amplified more recently (Holden & Woods 1982, 1988). Both books contain detailed advice on the running of RO sessions, and useful summaries of the principles involved in making the sessions attractive to group members. They stress the need for creating a special atmosphere, for varying materials, and for making the sessions stimulating. Therapists are advised to use praise as much as possible, to maintain courtesy and take an interest in the individual group members, and to minimize signs of authority (e.g. uniforms) as much as possible. They also advise placing clients in groups which are relatively homogeneous with respect to severity of deficit, and mobilizing knowledge from long-term memory stores to promote confidence by ensuring some success.

In spite of the clarity of this advice, and the emphasis placed on maintaining the well-being of the group members the authors became aware during the mid-1980s of misuses of RO, and in the second edition of the book (Holden & Woods, 1988) they cite examples of studies in which the approach has been applied in a mechanical and over structured fashion. They advise that group leaders keep in mind the principles of RO, rather than adhere rigidly to a set of methods.

Twenty-four hour RO is even more difficult to implement. All staff who have a significant amount of contact with the patients or residents have to be trained in the approach. The main principles are:

(a) that a patient should never be misinformed;

(b) that a patient's mistakes and misperceptions should be tactfully corrected. (Holden & Woods (1988) counsel discretion in the use of tactful correction though, pointing out that, since the most important goal is to prevent the rehearsal in incorrect ideas, distraction may often be more successful than outright contradiction.)

(c) that attempts should be made during all interactions to convey information that will help to maintain their orientation.

Individual RO consists of individually tailored programmes, with specific, and individually relevant targets. Formulations of the problem behaviours or self-care deficits will generally include aspects of disorientation which maintain the problem, and interventions will include the use of rehearsal of key material, or environmental changes aimed at reducing disorientation, as appropriate. For example, Hanley (1986) describes a ward-orientation programme designed to help an 86 year-old lady regain continence by ensuring that she was enabled to learn to find her own way to the toilet.

DOES RO WORK?

Early reports about the efficacy of the whole RO package (Folsom, 1968) were enthusiastic, but largely uncontrolled. The earlier controlled studies focused largely on classroom RO. There have been several comprehensive reviews of this extensive literature, but different reviewers reach different conclusions in spite of the fact that they all cover the same core of studies. Powell-Proctor and Miller (1982) and Burton (1982) remain unconvinced that the techniques as they stand are clinically useful, while Holden and Woods (1982, 1988) and Hanley (1984) are cautiously optimistic. Overall, it seems that the more tightly controlled the study, the less generalized the effects appear to be, especially if the groups include only dementia sufferers. For example, when Woods (1979) compared the effects of RO with non-specific group discussion, across matched groups using a range of outcome measures, it turned out that the RO group did better than the controls on cognitive testing after treatment, but that there were no significant differences on behaviour rating scale scores. Holden and Sinebruchow (1979) were able to demonstrate some gains in social behaviour, which were attributable to RO, in a subsequent study, but not all of the patients who participated were dementia sufferers.

In contrast, 24-hour RO has been less extensively studied. Implementing the extensive changes in ward practices, and instituting training programmes for all ward staff for the purposes of an outcome study is seldom attempted. In the few studies that have been reported, it has turned out that, in spite of careful preparation and training, ensuring that the approach is actually being used consistently has been a major obstacle in demonstrating its effectiveness (Hanley, 1984).

Perhaps the most promising findings have been those reported for individual reality orientation programmes (Hanley, 1986). How much these owe to the RO approach *per se*, and to what extent they constitute clinical psychology in action, is open to debate. It is, however, possible that the fact that these studies could be performed at all, given the extent to which they were incorporated into the overall ward programme owes much to the enthusiasm generated by the RO movement.

CHALLENGES TO RO

Powell-Proctor and Miller (1982) are particularly outspoken in their criticisms of RO. In general, they doubt the wisdom of 'taking a popular technique off the shelf and applying it without further thought'. Some of their particular criticisms have been addressed in subsequent studies, but some issues remain unresolved.

(a) 'RO is vague and woolly and could mean anything in practice . . . such a claim would not be entirely without foundation'. This statement predates the publication of the handbooks (Holden & Woods 1982, 1988) which provide more detailed descriptions of good RO practice, but it is probably fair to say that the earlier lack of definition has increased the difficulty of evaluating some of the original outcome studies. Indeed, Holden and Woods themselves (1982, 1988) draw attention to indications that some of the earlier studies differed widely in terms of how well the techniques were implemented. Accounts of individual RO are, by contrast, highly specific, but these could also be cited as examples of how a very wide range of approaches has come to be labelled as RO.

(b) 'The general rationale behind RO is less than satisfactory' Miller and Powell-Proctor take issue both with the extent to which RO is supposed to attain all embracing goals, and with the salience of the competencies actually addressed by RO programmes.

In their view, it might be more pertinent to the well-being of long-stay, institutionalized patients to concentrate on everyday living skills, such as dressing and toiletting. While there is much to be said for this point of view, little attention has been given to assessing more directly which inputs might contribute most to the well-being of the dementia sufferers in practice. Even though their views can not always be sought in conventional ways, the question needs to be addressed further.

The other weakness in the rationale behind RO that Miller and Powell-Proctor comment upon, is the failure to take full account of factors known to enhance learning. This is probably symptomatic of a more general problem with the whole RO approach: in short we can only speculate about how it works. Holden and Woods (1982, 1988) make a number of creative suggestions about the probable processes involved, but are ready to admit that these are post hoc and essentially unresearched. In this regard, RO is very much out of step with the other psychological therapies described in this book, for which the theory practice links are much clearer.

(c) 'Whether it (RO) is better than alternative forms of intervention has yet to be securely established, but the pointers that do exist are not favourable'. The two forms of intervention that have been increasingly used with the client group are reminiscence therapy (Coleman, 1986 *a*, *b*) and validation therapy (Feil, 1982). Neither approach has a well-developed outcome literature, and subsequent research which attempts to compare the efficacy of these two approaches with RO has done little to clarify the issue (although it has raised some interesting questions).

Baines, Saxby & Ehlert (1987) describe a crossover trial of RO versus reminiscence therapy, in which the two therapies seemed to interact, the group which received RO followed by Reminiscence showing greater improvement than the group that received Reminiscence first, on both behavioural and cognitive measures. Baines *et al.* generate a reasonably plausible explanation for this finding, suggesting that skills learned during the RO phase may have helped patients to make use of the subsequent reminiscence sessions. The practical implication of this finding would seem to be that as the two therapies seem to be complementary, there is little point in forcing a decision between them.

Scanland and Emershaw (1993), on the other hand, reported no significant improvements over a four-month period for either RO or Validation Therapy, each held five times weekly. However, there was no matched no-treatment control group, or any attempt at time series analysis, so it is impossible to tell whether the apparent lack of change resulted from an underlying deterioration in the sample, which the two therapy approaches were powerful enough to offset.

DOES RO CHANGE THE AGENTS OF CHANGE?

Although formal training in 24 hour RO did not have the desired effect on staff behaviour, there is some evidence that the process of engaging in RO groups has a positive effect on staff attitudes. For example, Baines *et al.* (1987) reported that both RO and reminiscence groups helped staff to develop their knowledge of individual residents. Job satisfaction was also found to increase. Salmon (1993), on the other hand, points out that positive attitudes do not necessarily predict higher levels of positive interaction. He is, however, encouraged by the finding that it is during the RO sessions themselves that positive interactions between nurses and patients are most likely to occur, and concludes that, given the very low levels of interaction at other times, this is an important function of RO programmes, irrespective of their specific therapeutic value.

It is also worth noting that the advent of RO seemed to coincide with the end of the almost complete therapeutic nihilism that pervaded care policy for dementia sufferers. If the RO movement has played a part in this, then all of the efforts put into it will have been worthwhile, even if the case for its efficacy remains unproven.

CURRENT DEVELOPMENTS

At present, interest seems to have shifted away from the RO approach itself and there have been relatively few recent publications. However, at the same time there are signs of a growing interest in developing approaches to care which address more directly the well being of the Dementia sufferers (e.g Kitwood & Bredin, 1992), and in investigating different models of providing help for carers (Morris *et al.* 1992). It is to be hoped that this diversification of approach, and the more systematic groundwork involved, will lead to a gradual and secure extension of the therapeutic repertoire of those engaged with the care of dementia sufferers.

REFERENCES

American Hospitals Association (1976). *This way to reality – a guide to developing a reality orientation program.* Chicago, Illinois.

Baines, S., Saxby, P. & Ehlert, K. (1987). Reality orientation and reminiscence therapy: a controlled cross-over study of elderly confused people. *British Journal of Psychiatry*, **151**, 222–31.

Burton, M. (1982). Reality orientation for the elderly: a critique. *Journal of Advanced Nursing*, 7, 427–33.

Coleman, P.G. (1986a). Issues in the therapeutic use of reminiscence. In Hanley and M. Gilhooly (Eds) *Psychological therapies for the elderly.* London: Croom Helm.

Coleman, P.G. (1986 *b*). *The ageing process and the role of reminiscence.* Chichester: John Wiley.

Feil, N. (1982). *Validation: the Feil Method.* Cleveland Ohio: Edward Feil Productions.

Folsom J.C. (1968). Reality orientation for the elderly patient. *Journal of Geriatric Psychiatry*, 1, 291–307.

Hanley, I. (1984). Theoretical and practical considerations in reality orientation therapy. In I. Hanley & J. Hodge. (Eds). *Psychological approaches to the care of the elderly.* London: Croom Helm.

Hanley, I. (1986). Reality orientation in the care of elderly patients with dementia – three case studies. In I. Hanley R M. Gilhooly (Eds) *Psychological therapies for the elderly.* London: Croom Helm.

Holden, U & Sinebruchow, A. (1979). Validation of reality orientation therapy for use with the elderly. Unpublished manuscripts.

Holden, U. & Woods, R. (1982). *Reality orientation: psychological approaches to the 'confused' elderly.* London: Churchill Livingstone.

Holden, U. & Woods, R. (1988). *Reality orientation: psychological approaches to the 'confused' elderly.*–London: Churchill Livingstone.

Kitwood T. & Bredin K. (1992). *A guide to the care of those with failing mental powers.*– Bradford: Gale Centre Publications.

Morris, R., Woods, R., Davies K., Berry, J. & Morris, L. (1992). The use of a coping strategy focussed support group for carers of dementia sufferers. *Counselling Psychology Quarterly*, 5, 337–48.

Powell-Proctor, L. & Miller, E. (1982). Reality orientation: a critical appraisal. *British Journal of Psychiatry*, **140**, 457–63.

Salmon, P. (1993). Interactions of nurses with elderly patients: relationship to nurses' attitudes and to formal activity periods. *Journal of Advanced Nursing*, 18, 14–19.

Scanland, S. & Emershaw, L. (1993). Reality orientation and validation therapy: dementia, depression and functional status. *Journal of Gerontological Nursing*, 19, 7–11.

Woods, R. (1979). Reality Orientation and staff attention: a controlled study. *British Journal of Psychiatry*, **134**. 502–7.

Reality orientation therapy

Relaxation training

MICHAEL H. BRUCH

University College London Medical School,
Department of Psychiatry & Behavioural
Sciences, London, UK

INTRODUCTION

Procedures to relax body and mind have been known for thousands of years. In some cultures relaxation methods have even become an integral part of philosophical, religious value systems. In view of this, it is perhaps surprising that relaxation techniques have gained clinical interest only fairly recently. Early pioneers include J.H. Schultz (autogenic training; e.g. Schultz & Luthe, 1959) and Edmund Jacobsen (progressive muscle relaxation; Jacobson, 1929). Davidson and Schwartz (1976) found it surprising that the subject had been absent from psychological examination for so long despite obvious links between psychological and physiological arousal and emotional disorders. In their work they quote eminent scientists such as William James and Sigmund Freud. With respect to the latter '. . . he remained imperceptive to the possible significance of relaxation in psychotherapy. Although the cultivation of a low arousal state as a precondition for the spontaneous emergence of imagery (i.e. free association) was an important component of psychoanalytic therapy . . .' (p.399).

Furthermore, perhaps as a result of its varied nature and ideographic meaning for different individuals, there were no generally agreed definitions of the concept. Jacobson attempted to define relaxation by describing its effects as follows . . . 'respiration loses the slight irregularities, the pulse rate may decline to normal, the knee jerk diminishes or disappears along with the pharyngeal and flexion reflexes and nervous start, the esophagus . . . relaxes in all its parts, while mental and emotional activity dwindle or disappear for brief periods' (cf. Davidson & Schwartz, 1976; p.400).

In modern clinical psychotherapy and behavioural medicine the focus for relaxation is on emotional and health problems, which are perceived to be associated with increased levels of tension. In such clinical contexts, therapists make frequent use of stress reduction or relaxation techniques. The aim for the patient is to learn to control and modify somatic and cognitive responses in such a way that they become incompatible with subjective anxiety, pain or tension. Typical targets are reduction of muscular tension muscular, vasodilatation to reduce blood pressure, reduction of hyperventilation, reduction of tachycardia and reduction of gastrointestinal responses.

METHODS

To this day a vast array of methods and respective variations as well as combinations thereof has been reported. Lehrer and Woolfolk (1993) have recently published the second edition of their now classic handbook of stress management. They present and discuss at length the most commonly applied methods which have received research evaluation. These include progressive relaxation, autogenic training, breathing, meditational techniques (as developed from Hindu philosophy (i.e. Yoga) and Zen Buddhism, hypnosis, biofeedback, cognitive approaches, music therapy, aerobic exercises and pharmacological methods. Brief descriptions of the most important approaches are given below. As the present context does not allow a detailed introduction of these methods and their variations, the interested reader may be referred to the above-mentioned text.

Progressive relaxation

This technique was originally developed by Edmund Jacobson (1929). He regarded it as a therapeutic method to achieve muscular quiescence to effect cognitive and somatic relaxation. The patient is trained to recognize and to control decreasingly intense levels of muscular tension. As Woolfolk and Lehrer (1984) point out: 'The primary aim is to make the individual able to recognize and eliminate even the most minute levels of tension, to remain as tension free as possible at all times, and to eliminate unnecessary tension continuously during everyday activities.' (p.5). The method was originally designed as an independent psychotherapy to achieve deep relaxation. The emphasis was for the patient to discover minute changes in tension for himself. The therapist would not make suggestions regarding the expected effects but encourage proprioceptive experience to facilitate learning.

In later use the method was abbreviated for flexible and integrated use with other therapeutic approaches. According to Woolfolk and Lehrer (1984) this was also accompanied by a shift from awareness training to maximum relaxation effect. Such applications are more directive and suggestive with the aim of achieving deep relaxation as quickly as possible. Typical examples can be found within the fields of behavioural and cognitive therapies as described by Hawton and co-workers (1989). These deal mainly with anxiety states and phobic disorders. Such approach was first pioneered by Wolpe (1958) and labelled *systematic desensitization*. Here, relaxation is used as a stimulus for counter conditioning. A more recent development is applied relaxation, a comprehensive step-by-step guide building on progressive relaxation but also utilizing additional methods (Öst, 1987).

Autogenic training

This method was originally developed by Schultz in the early part of this century (English version by Schultz & Luthe, 1959) on the basis of his experience with hypnosis. Autogenic training (AT) can be described as a form of autosuggestion to influence physiological processes. Similar as in biofeedback facilitation of self-regulation processes is intended. The goal is to reduce excessive autonomic arousal and the patient is asked to concentrate on his bodily sensations in a passive, accepting style. As Linden (1993) has noted, it is especially the principle of passive concentration that distinguishes AT from progressive muscle relaxation and biofeedback, where emphasis is on active concentration. The method is supported by an impressive body of research (Linden, 1990) and, although slightly out of fashion in the past, there appears to be growing interest currently.

Meditational techniques

Meditational procedures can be found in many cultures, including western societies. Traditionally meditation was associated with philosophical and religious contexts. As discussed with Patel (1993) it was only recently that such methods were considered to be useful for the reduction of stress induced tension and anxiety. She describes the nature of meditation as follows: '. . . meditation practice involves taking a comfortable position . . . it then involves being in a quiet environment, regulating the breath, adopting a physically relaxed and mentally passive attitude, and dwelling single-mindedly upon an object . . . the ultimate idea is to learn the discipline of concentrating on one thing and only one thing at a time, to the exclusion of everything else . . . giving voluntary concentration to a subject not only enables a person to see and think about that subject with greater clarity, but also brings into consciousness all the different ideas and memories associated with the subject. A practical result is an increased ability to find a solution to any problem' (p.127) Thus it seems evident that meditation is attempting to address somatic as well as cognitive systems.

Biofeedback

Biofeedback is a fairly recent method which came into clinical use in the late 1960s. Biofeedback may be defined as any technique which increases the ability of a person to control voluntary physiological activities by providing information about those activities. Biofeedback is information about the state of biological processes. The concept was originally introduced by Neal Miller (1978) who stimulated an enormous interest, which has led to very productive research and development activities.

Biofeedback is the most technical of the major established relaxation methods as it requires sophisticated electronic equipment. The main intention is to teach the individual self-control over processes which are normally subject to autonomic functioning. Or, as Woolfolk and Lehrer (1993) put it . . . 'biofeedback is a method for representing somatic activity as information available to cognition' (p.7). The procedure is highly specific and focuses on one autonomic response system at a time. Rimm and Masters (1979) have compiled a comprehensive list of clinical applications which can involve heart rate, blood pressure, skin temperature, skin conductivity, EEG, EMG and other responses. According to Stoyva and Budzyenski (1993) also pioneers in the field, 'the object of such training is to achieve control over biological systems that previously have been operating in a maladaptive fashion and have been beyond conscious control . . . biofeedback training essentially involves three stages. The first stage is acquiring awareness of the maladaptive response . . . next, guided by the biofeedback signal, he or she learns to control the response. Finally, the client learns to transfer the control into everyday life.' (p.263). Although it is not entirely clear how feedback control is mediated and, despite mixed results, the method has been firmly established in the behavioural treatment of anxiety and stress disorders.

Cognitive techniques

The relationship between maladaptive thinking and anxiety/stress is well documented (e.g. Beck, Emery & Greenberg, 1985) and has inspired the development of cognitive behaviour therapy. It is assumed that negative, irrational thought patterns distort perception and evaluation of threatening stimuli and thus prevent adaptive and coping oriented behaviours. Cognitive approaches to effect relaxation would thus seek to modify negative and dysfunctional thought patterns which are seen to promote tension and anxiety in the first place. The causal role of cognitive appraisal in the genesis of pathological emotionality is emphasized. Typical treatments involve identification and reinterpretation of internal events such as thoughts, images, bodily sensations. Cognitive techniques are employed to raise awareness for negative thoughts, cognitive distortions, and dysfunctional schemas which may serve as an underlying condition.

Finally, Woolfolk and Lehrer (1993) list a number of additional relaxation techniques which are increasingly used by clinicians of various persuasions but have not yet been subject to scientific enquiry. These include Alexander technique which focuses on posture and movement of the body; Tai-Chi an ancient Chinese technique which focuses on '. . . balance, muscular relaxation, deep breathing, and mental concentration during a complex series of slow, dance-like movements' (p.4); also, the Japanese method of Akaido, which is based on Zen Buddhism, is becoming increasingly popular in the west.

THEORETICAL ISSUES

A decade ago, Schwartz (1984) pointed out that, despite recent rigorous development in clinical psychology and behavioural medicine, there were few attempts to develop general theories of relaxation. In a recent review, Lehrer and Woolfolk (1993) have merely identified three general frameworks, the relaxation response theory by Benson (1975), the multiprocess theory by Davidson and Schwartz (1976), and a hierarchical cognitive–behavioural model by Smith (1988).

The relaxation response theory postulates that all applied relaxation techniques produce a similar relaxation response which leads to reduction of sympathetic arousal. The antithesis to this is the multiprocess model which suggest specific effects of the various techniques. Smith's model proposes a hierarchical order of specific behaviours and cognitions, arranged according to level of difficulty, to achieve complete relaxation. Clearly, the model intends to accommodate the complexity of factors involved with relaxation but has yet to receive empirical support.

Lehrer and Woolfolk have reached the conclusion that, to date, most evidence supports the multiprocess theory which postulates specificity of treatment to match individual response patterns. Perhaps one should favour a compromise position as clinical evidence points to some generalized relaxation effect with most established techniques. At present a unifying framework is still missing as existing theories can only partially explain the effects of various techniques as well as respective interactions with individual responding and presenting problems.

Another concern is the gap between theoretical understanding and clinical application. For example, when the theorist–researcher attempts to clarify the efficacy of different techniques, the clinician may simply use intuition regarding selection or combination of several methods. Typically, clinicians tend to apply their favourite method and use it to maximum effect. It is not always clear to what extent non-specific aspects, such as the therapeutic relations, come into play, especially when similar results are achieved across different patients and disorders.

CLINICAL APPLICATION

Relaxation techniques have been applied as an independent therapeutic approach to relieve problems related to chronically elevated level of arousal. Examples include insomnia, nervousness, headaches, hypertension etc. The goal is to achieve a reduction of a chronically high level of arousal by sustained practice, initially under supervision of a therapist.

Also relaxation may be designed as an integral part of a comprehensive treatment programme. Stress inoculation training (Meichenbaum, 1993) or anxiety management training (Suinn, 1990) may serve as the typical examples. In this way relaxation training is employed as more active and flexible tool. Typically one starts with deep relaxation and once the patient is able to relax, a shortened and individualized version is directly applied to stress or anxiety inducing situations. This approach is designed to facilitate coping behaviours and prevent avoidances.

Another well-documented and successful relaxation programme in the Cognitive–Behavioural framework is the above mentioned applied relaxation (Öst, 1987). Such programmes typically last between 8 and 12 sessions and consists of the following steps: training in recognizing early signs of anxiety, progressive relaxation, tension release training, cue-controlled relaxation, differential relaxation, rapid relaxation, application training and maintenance. The main objectives are to provide a rationale and motivate the patient to enable short, effective techniques which can be applied in realistic anxiety situations as opposed to the consulting room. Emphasis is on intensive training and self-control.

Furthermore, the question arises as to whether relaxation techniques should be differentially applied, depending on the nature of problems as well as individual response mechanisms.

In clinical work it is useful to seek guidance by the tripartite response system analysis as originally put forward by Peter Lang (1969) who has proposed three loosely coupled systems: verbal–cognitive, autonomic–physiological, and behavioural–motoric components which are highly interactive. This conceptualization allows to examine the nature of subjective anxiety or stress. For example, one may be able to identify a dominant response mode which has causal impact on the other systems. In other cases there may be an enhancing interaction between cognitive and autonomic variables as is typical for the anticipatory anxiety syndrome.

Such investigations are expected to provide vital clues for relaxation procedures. For example, an anxiety response which is predominantly cognitively represented would obviously require a different therapeutic focus (eg cognitive restructuring) compared to a strong autonomic reaction (e.g. biofeedback).

All this would suggest that particular techniques may be espe-cially suitable for certain individuals. Woolfolk and Lehrer (1993) have extensively reviewed this issue by comparing techniques across problems as well as within problems with different individuals. They conclude the following: 'We find that each of the various techniques has specific effects, in addition to a global, undifferentiated relaxation effect. There are few kinds of problems for which one technique is clearly superior to another, but, for the most part, the effects of the various techniques are similar. Combinations of techniques often produce better results than single techniques do. Also, there is some evidence that particular individuals may be differentially motivated by and attracted to specific techniques.' (p. 11). However, most studies need cautious evaluation as techniques may have lost their clinical significance through abbreviation and standardization procedures, or non-clinical samples were used.

Lehrer and Woolfolk (1993) also emphasize the importance of motivation and compliance, especially in consideration of the enormous drop out rate. It seems important that clients understand the rationale of relaxation principles and are prepared to practise on a daily basis. Clients show individual preferences and some data suggest that compliance is best with meditation followed by progressive relaxation, autogenic training, and biofeedback. Subjects who feel more in control of themselves tend to do better with all techniques except for biofeedback.

CONCLUSIONS

In reviewing various relaxation approaches one can confirm the prevailing clinical view that the various techniques work differently with different individuals in different problem situations. In more detail, it appears that best results are obtained when modalities of individual responses are matched with corresponding treatments.

On the other hand, Lehrer and Woolfolk (1993) conclude from their review that most methods are likely to achieve also some general relaxation effect. Also, combinations of techniques tend to be more effective than singular treatments. Most experts in the field have developed such treatment packages to enhance relaxation effects (examples were given above). Clinicians tend to use relaxation techniques and combinations on a trial and error basis, which makes it difficult to assess the outcome of specific techniques in applied settings. Some clinicians have claimed synergistic effects when using a variety of modalities.

To facilitate relaxation it seems thus crucial to conduct a comprehensive cognitive–behavioural assessment of relevant target complaints to identify individual response modalities. Further, non-specific factors such as motivation, the therapeutic relationship, level of self-regulation ability, and expectations according to personal preferences need to be assessed. Linden (1993) has suggested that it may be useful to present model options and their rationale to the patient in order to encourage a choice. It is assumed what is understood well, credible, and self-chosen may work best for the individual patient. The ultimate goal is to generalize relaxation skills so it can be applied actively to all relevant settings reported by the sufferer.

Finally, relaxation techniques have been demonstrated to be highly successful in the fields of emotional disorders and behavioural medicine. With emotional disorders, the emphasis appears to be more 'cognitive' as one intends to adjust the perception and evaluation of stress and tension, whereas in behavioural medicine techniques tend to focus predominantly on the modification of somatic states, like pain, hypertension, or other physical conditions. (See also 'Coping with chronic illness', 'Coping with chronic pain', 'Pain management'.)

REFERENCES

Beck, A.T., Emery, G., & Greenberg, R.L. (1985). *Anxiety disorders and phobias.* New York: Basic Books.

Benson, H. (1975). *The relaxation response.* New York: Morrow.

Davidson, R.J. & Schwartz, G.E. (1976). Psychobiology of relaxation and related stress: a multiprocess theory. In D. Mostofsky (Ed.). *Behaviour modification and control of physiological activity.* Englewood Cliffs: Prentice-Hall.

Hawton, K., Salkovskis, P.M., Kirk, J. & Clark, D.M. (1989). *Cognitive behaviour therapy for psychiatric problems.* Oxford: Oxford Medical Publications.

Jacobson, E. (1929). *Progressive relaxation.* Chicago: University of Chicago Press.

Lang, P.J. (1969). The mechanics of desensitisation and the laboratory study of human fear. In C.M. Franks (Ed.). *Behaviour therapy: appraisal and status.* New York: McGraw-Hill.

Lehrer, P.M. & Woolfolk, R.L. (1993). *Principles and practice of stress management.* 2nd edn. New York: Guilford Press.

Linden, W. (1990). *Autogenic training: a clinical guide.* New York: Guilford Press.

Linden, W. (1993). The autogenic training method of J.H. Schultz. In P.M. Lehrer &

R.L. Woolfolk (Eds.). *Principles and practice of stress management.* 2nd ed. New York: Guilford Press.

Meichenbaum, D (1993). Stress inoculation training: a 20 year update. In R.L. Woolfolk & P.M. Lehrer (Eds.). *Principles and practice of stress management.* New York: Guilford Press.

Miller, N.E. (1978). Biofeedback and visceral learning. *Annual Review of Psychology,* **29**, 373–404.

Öst, L.G. (1987). Applied relaxation: description of a coping technique and review of controled studies. *Behaviour Research and Therapy,* **25**, 397–410.

Patel, C. (1993). Yoga-based therapy. In R.L. Woolfolk & P.M. Lehrer (Eds.). *Principles and practice of stress management.* New York: Guilford Press.

Rimm, D.C. & Masters, J.C. (1979). *Behaviour therapy.* 2nd ed. New York: Academic Press.

Smith, J.C. (1988). Steps toward a cognitive-behavioural model of relaxation. *Biofeedback and Self-Regulation,* **13**, 307–29.

Schultz, J.H. & Luthe, W. (1959). *Autogenic training: a psychophysiological approach to psychotherapy.* New York: Grune and Stratton.

Schwartz, G.E. (1984). Foreword. In R.L. Woolfolk & P.M. Lehrer (Eds.). *Principles and practice of stress management.* New York: Guilford Press.

Stoyva, J.M. & Budzyenski, T.H. (1993). Biofeedback methods in the treatment of anxiety and stress disorders. In P.M. Lehrer & R.L. Woolfolk (Eds.). *Principles and practice of stress management.* 2nd edn. New York: Guilford Press.

Suinn, R.M. (1990). Anxiety management training. New York: Plenum.

Wolpe, J. (1958). *Psychotherapy by reciprocal inhibition.* Stanford: Stanford University Press.

Woolfolk, R.L. & Lehrer, P.M. (1984). *Principles and practice of stress management.* New York: Guilford Press.

Woolfolk, R.L. & Lehrer, P.M. (1993). The context of stress management. In P.M. Lehrer & R.L. Woolfolk (Eds.). *Principles and practice of stress management.* 2nd edn. New York: Guilford Press.

Repertory grids

PEGGY DALTON

20 Cleveland Avenue, London, UK

ASPECTS OF THE THEORY BEHIND THE TECHNIQUE

In his *Psychology of Personal Constructs* (1955/1991), George Kelly put forward his theory of personality, based on his fundamental belief that the way we are is governed by the ways in which we have come to anticipate events. He described how we try to make sense of things by a process of comparison and contrast. We construe one person, perhaps, as like someone familiar to us in being 'kind', while a third is 'harsh' in the way he treats us. One situation we have experienced has been 'enjoyable', another 'uncomfortable' and we may anticipate that a third, new situation will be like the second because we have been told that it too will be crowded, noisy and hot. Such bipolar discriminations Kelly

refers to as constructs. It should be stressed that constructs are not simply verbalized thoughts; we construe through visual perception, hearing, touch, smell and our kinaesthetic sense. Many of our constructs are at a low level of awareness and may be experienced as 'gut reaction'.

Such constructions are seen as linked together to form networks of meaning, as where the person construed as 'kind' rather than 'harsh' may also seem 'warm' rather than 'cold', 'humorous', rather than 'dour' and so on. Some constructs will be at a higher level of meaning than others. 'Fulfilled' versus 'unfulfilled', for example, clearly has a wealth of possible meaning, while 'has warm clothes' versus 'has no clothes' may be seen as just one aspect of fulfilment. Some constructs may be of great significance to the person while

Rating scale 1 ← 4 → 7		elements	Father (1)	Mother (2)	Jane (sister) (3)	Me Now (4)	Kevin (admired) (5)	Tony (friend) (6)	George (disliked) (7)	As I'd like to be (8)	Alan (boss) (9)	Denis (colleague) (10)	Moira (friend) (11)	Chris (ex-friend) (12)	Grandmother (13)	Grandfather (14)
look after money	couldn't care less	1	3	5	4	3	4	7	2	4	1	2	4	1	7	2
strong/independent	passive/dependent	2	1	2	2	7	2	1	1	3	4	2	2	5	4	2
a certain 'looseness'	uptight	3	6	7	4	7	2	5	3	2	5	1	7	2	5	5
never gives way	will give way	4	1	1	5	7	1	4	1	4	6	4	4	1	4	2
make people depend on them	encourages responsibility	5	2	1	5	2	6	7	4	5	4	6	5	7	3	6
at ease with self	constantly stressed	6	5	7	4	7	2	1	4	4	2	4	2	7	2	4
gets on with people	a pain	7	5	5	2	7	2	2	5	2	3	4	1	3	4	2
aloof	warm	8	2	7	6	1	6	4	2	5	2	5	5	1	7	7
charismatic	boring	9	5	3	4	7	3	2	4	3	3	5	2	1	4	4
depressive	faces things	10	7	2	6	1	4	4	3	4	4	6	7	1	5	5
macho	effiminate	11	1	5	4	6	1	3	2	3	6	4	4	6	4	4
mature/adult	never grew up	12	3	6	3	7	2	2	2	2	4	2	2	5	5	3
goes out to life	stays inside	13	4	2	2	6	2	1	2	2	5	5	1	7	2	2

Fig. 1. A client's rated grid.

others are less important. The former are described as core constructs the latter as peripheral.

All these constructs, whether easily verbalized or experienced as feelings, abstract or more concrete, core or peripheral are linked together to form a construct system. And, it is through this system that a person develops theories about things in order to know how to approach the world. Experience of events and people will modify these theories and elaborate them as we grow older. Our sense of ourselves will change as we become involved in more aspects of life. Learning something new will initiate new ideas. New relationships will evoke new feelings. Validation or invalidation from others will contribute to the overall picture of ourselves at any point in time.

So brief a description of the nature of a construct and the formation of a construct system is only one aspect of Kelly's rich and complex theory as it is expounded in his original two volumes (1955). A fuller understanding of his ideas is essential to the responsible use of repertory grids in psychological intervention. Fransella and Bannister (1977) and Beail (1985) discuss the various forms and purposes of the technique within the context of the theory as a whole.

THE NATURE OF GRID TECHNIQUE

'The purpose of grids' say Fransella and Bannister (1977 p.3), 'is to inform us about the way in which our system is evolving and its limitations and possibilities. The results of the grid have often been looked on as a map of the construct system of an individual, a sort of idiographic cartography'. They describe the process as 'a particular form of structured interview'. Through it we can put ourselves in another's shoes and see things from his or her point of view. It should be stressed that any one grid will only present a sample of the person's construing. In setting it up, it will be important to focus our

enquiry on the area of particular concern, whether it be someone's relationships with others, their anticipations of certain events or their views of themselves and others with regard to a specific problem which is troubling them.

GRID ADMINISTRATION

The setting up of a grid generally proceeds in five stages: the choosing of elements (i.e. whatever is to represent the focus of enquiry), the elicitation of constructs, completion by the client, analysis of the data, interpretation.

Choosing the elements

The elements in a grid used in psychological intervention are, more often than not, significant people in clients' lives, although they may also be difficult situations which they encounter or, perhaps, various roles which they see themselves as called upon to play. If the first, a client might be asked to choose people who are important to them, such as parents and other family members and close friends. In order to obtain a spread of people, they may also be given titles, such as 'a person in authority', 'someone you dislike', 'someone you admire' and so on and asked to supply the names. 'Self' elements are also included (see examples in Fig. 1).

Eliciting the constructs

The usual method for eliciting constructs from the chosen elements is by asking the client to consider three of them in relation to one another in terms of some important way in which two of them are alike and thereby different from the third. The response might be that two of them are 'charismatic', while the third is 'boring'. Then other triads of elements are presented and the client asked the same question. Where this process seems too complicated, as for young

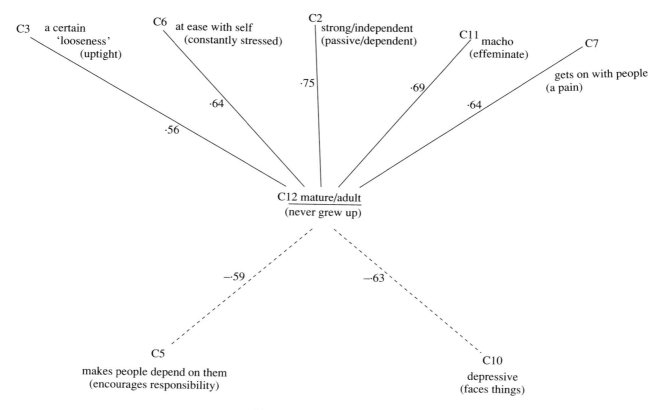

Fig. 2. First cluster of constructs.

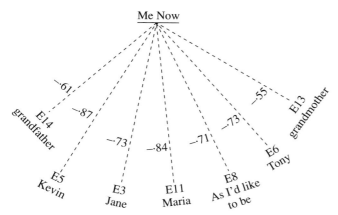

Fig. 3. First cluster of elements

people perhaps, the client might be asked just to compare two people or even say what is important about one and to give the contrast to what they describe. This goes on until the therapist feels that a representative sample of constructs has been produced (see Fig. 1). Techniques for exploring constructs further through 'laddering' and 'pyramiding' are described in Dalton and Dunnett (1992, pp. 124–128).

Grid completion

The elements in a grid are most often rated on a given scale or rank ordered. In Fig. 1 the client has used a seven-point scale, rating each construct in turn across the elements.

Analysis of grid data

The first level of grid analysis is direct scanning of the raw data. From Fig. 1 we can see at once that this client is not at all happy with himself. Looking down the two columns for 'Me Now' and 'As I'd Like to be' we see wide differences in many of the ratings: he sees himself as 'a pain', for example, but would like to be able to get on with people. He feels that he 'never grew up' but wishes he were 'mature/adult'. We would have been aware during the elicitation of the constructs of his concern with dependency (2, 5 and less directly, 12), and relating to people (7, 8, and 9) and he places Me Now very negatively on the scale for all these constructs. His admired person (Kevin) is, of course, rated similarly to As I'd like to be. The ways in which he rates the different constructs, too, have meaning. For 'strong/independent' vs 'passive/dependent', for example, he uses the positive pole for almost everyone except himself, whereas 'makes people dependent on them' vs 'encourages responsibility' is rated across the whole range of the scale, presenting a less crude discrimination.

For ease of comparison between the rating or ranking of constructs and elements Thomas and Shaw (1976) developed a procedure called focusing, which involves reordering the rows and columns to put like with like. Kelly maintained that the degree of similarity between constructs or elements could be given mathematical expression and a number of computer programs have been devised based on correlations between the rows and columns. Beail (1985) provides a comprehensive survey of programs using both factor analysis and cluster analysis. Probably still the most widely used example of the former is Slater's Ingrid (1964), which analyses the data into principal components, showing the relationships between constructs, elements and constructs with elements. A more recent package, Flexigrid 5.2 (Tschudi, 1992) contains programs for three different methods of analysis: Principal Component Analysis, a computer version of Focus or hierarchical clustering, and GAB (Grid Analysis for Beginners), the simplest form of clustering in use.

Interpretation for therapist and client

Some indication has been given of how the raw data might be explored and more often than not the client will be aware of the kinds of patterns emerging at this level. Graphic presentations from computer programs will, however, provide further indications of the ways in which the client is construing those aspects of his or her world which are focused on through the elements.

The first cluster of constructs from the client's grid (Fig. 2) shows that for him being mature and adult implies being strong and independent, at ease with self, macho, having a certain 'looseness', getting on with people and (since they are negatively correlated) the contrast poles of construct 10, 'faces things' and construct 5, 'encourages responsibility', none of which he regards as applying to himself as he is now. The first element cluster (Fig. 3) shows vividly his low sense of self, with very high negative correlations between Me Now, As I'd Like to be, his admired person, Kevin, and a number of friends and liked relatives. Sheehan (1985) found such self-construing to be typical of depressed clients.

Aspects of construing, such as cognitive complexity, can also be explored. 'The more loosely knit the constructs (the lower the correlations), the more complex is the person's system' (Fransella & Bannister, 1977). Conversely, a grid showing most of the constructs highly correlated with one another would suggest that the person construes things tightly, making black-and-white predictions with

little room for maneouvre. This has obvious implications for therapy and potential for change. Fransella and Bannister also discuss such features as extremity of rating and integration of the self and others within grids. (For many examples of grid interpretation see Beail, 1985).

REPERTORY GRID TECHNIQUE IN CLINICAL PRACTICE AND RESEARCH

Grid technique has been applied in a wide range of contexts, but the use for which it was originally conceived by Kelly, clinical practice, has been the area of richest development. Ryle (1985), devised the Dyad Grid for use with couples, where each partner rates the other and also how he or she believes himself or herself as being construed within the relationship. Proctor (1985) used grids with whole families. Grids have been specially designed for exploring particular problems. Brumfitt (1985) used them with aphasic people and Sheehan (1985) with people suffering from depression. Button's (1993) Self-Grid was designed originally for his clients with eating disorders. With elements such as Me at normal weight, Me at thinnest as well as the more usual Me Now and Ideal Self the client focuses on aspects of self-perception related to the presenting problem.

Since any grid aims at clarifying how the client views things at a given time, the technique clearly lends itself to tracing changes in construing over time and is therefore a useful tool for measuring therapeutic outcome. Winter (1985) sees repertory grid technique as an appropriate instrument for evaluating psychological intervention as it combines objectivity of scoring and sensitivity to psychological change. Not only are there a number of methods available for individual grid analysis but also for comparing pairs and groups of grids (eg contained in FLEXIGRID 5.2 (1992)). Research into outcome for populations of clients, therefore, may be facilitated.

REFERENCES

Beail, N. (Ed.). (1985). *Repertory grid technique and personal constructs*. London and Sydney: Croom Helm.

Brumfitt, S. (1985). The use of repertory grids with aphasic people. In N. Beail (Ed.). *Repertory grid technique and personal constructs*. London and Sydney: Croom Helm.

Button, E. (1993). *Eating disorders: personal construct therapy and change*. Chichester, New York, Brisbane, Toronto, Singapore: John Wiley.

Dalton, P. & Dunnett, G. (1992). *A psychology for living*. Chichester, New York, Brisbane, Sydney: John Wiley.

Fransella, F. & Bannister, D. (1977). *A*

manual for repertory grid technique. London, New York, San Fransisco: Academic Press.

Kelly, G.A. (1955/1991) *The psychology of personal constructs*. New York: Norton. (Re-printed by Routledge, London.)

Proctor, H. (1985). Repertory grids in family therapy and research. In N. Beail (Ed.). *Repertory grid technique and personal constructs*. London and Sydney: Croom Helm.

Ryle, A. (1985). The dyad grid and psychotherapy research. In N. Beail (Ed.). *Repertory grid technique and personal constructs*. London and Sydney: Croom Helm.

Sheehan, M.J. (1985). The process of change in the self-construing of a depressed

patient – Clare. In N. Beail (Ed.). *Repertory grid technque and personal constructs*. London and Sydney: Croom Helm.

Slater, P. (1964). *The principal components of a repertory grid*. London: Vincent Andrew.

Thomas, L.F. & Shaw, M.L.G. (1976). *Focus manual*. Brunel University: Centre for the Study of Human Learning.

Tschudi, F. (1992). *Flexigrid 5.2: Programmes for analyses of repertory grids*. Oslo: Tschudi System Sales.

Winter, D.A. (1985). Repertory grid technique in the evaluation of therapeutic outcome. In N. Beail (Ed.). *Repertory grid technique and personal constructs*. London and Sydney: Croom Helm.

Self-management

THOMAS L. CREER
and
KENNETH A. HOLROYD
Ohio University, Athens, USA

Self-regulatory, self-control, or self-management capabilities represent a distinctive human attribute. We not only react to external events, but are self-reactors with the capacity for self-evaluation and self-directed action. Self-regulatory capabilities permit us to exercise some control over our motivation and action (Bandura, 1986). In focusing on different problems, investigators have employed different operational and context-specific definitions of self-regulation, self-control, or self-management, and categorized regulatory processes, outcomes, and postulated mediators in various ways (Karoly, 1993). Despite the lack of consensus on a common paradigm for self-regulatory, self-control, or self-management research (the terms are used interchangeably by most investigators) a common definition has evolved:

> *Self-management refers to those processes, internal or transactional, that enable individuals to guide goal-directed activities over time and across settings. Self-management entails modulation of thought, affect, behavior, or attention through use of specific mechanisms and skills. (Adapted from Karoly, 1993).*

When self-management activities have the goal of preventing or controlling physical disorders, they often require that the patient collaborate with physicians or other health care personnel. Self-management activities also are determined by the nature of the physical disorder or disorders that are the focus of attention.

PROCESSES AND SKILLS OF SELF-MANAGEMENT

The process of self-management has been described by others (e.g. Ford, 1987; Karoly, 1993). Despite different terminology, there is considerable commonalty among descriptions; apparent differences often result from the different ways particular processes are partitioned into categories, not from real differences in conceptualization. Processes salient in the self-management of health problems include: (i) goal selection; (ii) information collection; (iii) information processing and evaluation; (iv) decision-making; (v) action; and (vi) self-reaction. These processes, as well as the skills required to execute given processes successfully, serve as the framework for the discussion that follows.

Goal selection

Goal selection occurs only after systematic preparation. In particular, two preparatory functions are necessary. Individuals must acquire knowledge of the health problem or condition that is to be prevented or managed and how risk factors or the disorder itself can be managed. Patient education provides the basis for self-management actions later performed by patients. After individuals have been provided with relevant health information and taught the skills they can perform to help prevent or control a disorder, specific individual goals must be identified that, if achieved, are likely to enhance the health and well-being of the individual. Typically these goals are established collaboratively through consultation with physicians or other health care professionals. There are three positive consequences of goal selection (Ford, 1987; Karoly, 1993): (i) it establishes preferences about what is a desirable outcome; (ii) it enhances the commitment of individuals to perform goal-relevant self-management skills; and (iii) it establishes expectancies on the part of individuals that trigger their effort and performance. Ideally, individuals begin to believe that in performing certain self-management activities, they can become partners with their physicians in managing their health, rather than passive recipients of health care interventions.

Successful collaboration between physicians and patients in goal selection guides individuals in organizing and applying self-management skills to achieve selected goals. Goal selection is the only activity where there is true collaboration between patients and their physicians. After goals have been established, it typically becomes the responsibility of individual patients to perform whatever self-management skills are necessary to attain the goals; physicians and other medical personnel are limited to tracking the individual's behaviour. This point has, at times, been misunderstood by physicians who seemingly assume there is active patient/physician collaboration throughout all phases of self-management. This confusion can be illustrated by an example regarding asthma, a disorder where there has been a concerted effort to develop and evaluate self-management programmes. A group of experts on asthma was convened to develop a consensus regarding diagnostic and treatment strategies. The resulting report is invaluable in that it established and clarified standards and procedures for the management of asthma (National Heart, Lung & Blood Institute, 1992). However, the report also highlights an existing misunderstanding in that it appears to assume self-management is characterized by an ongoing collaboration between physicians and their patients. There is no recognition in the report that the execution of the majority of self-management activities is the responsibility of patients only; thus, effective techniques will need to be developed to facilitate patients independent performance of complex self-management activities.

Information collection

Self-monitoring, or the self-observation and self-recording of data, is the basis of information collection. In pursuing the goals they have

[255]

helped establish, individuals must attend to, and record, information that bears upon their pursuit of these goals. Self-monitoring provides the foundation for self-management. Indeed, there are indications that self-monitoring is essential to the successful self-management of problems ranging from asthma (Creer & Bender, 1993) to weight (Baker & Kirschenbaum, 1993).

Several suggestions can be offered to improve the monitoring of health-related behaviours (Creer & Bender, 1993). First, individuals should attend only to phenomena that have been operationally defined as target behaviours or responses. Wherever possible, an objective measure, such as blood pressure in the case of hypertension or blood glucose in the case of diabetes, should be included. Secondly, in documenting information, it is imperative that individuals record data on a regular basis and, whenever possible, observe and record data only during specified windows of time.

Despite the above suggestions, self-monitoring is still a tedious and arduous task for many people. Kirschenbaum and Tomarken (1982), in fact, suggest that 'obsessive–compulsive self-regulation' was an apt term for describing the degree of persistent self-monitoring that is required by many self-management programmes. The extensive data collection demanded by many self-management programmes is problematic for many patients, particularly when they are asked to monitor numerous categories of information or to self-monitor constantly. In an attempt to better understand the self-management process, investigators have been tempted to ask patients to collect ever more detailed and varied information. For example, the numerous suggestions offered in the report by the NIH expert panel on asthma (National Heart, Lung & Blood Institute, 1992) make sense when considered individually; when combined, however, they are likely to overwhelm the average patient. At the same time self-monitoring becomes more involved, we, none the less, retain the hope that self-management training will not force patients to centre their lives around their disorder. The minimal essential elements of self-monitoring necessary for effective self-management need to be identified. Investigators also must remain aware that excessively complex self-monitoring requirements can produce unwanted side-effects.

Information processing and evaluation

Individuals must learn to process and evaluate the information they collect about themselves and their condition. Five distinct steps are involved:

First, individuals must be able to ferret out any significant changes that occur in the information they observe, record, and process about themselves. This may not be difficult when signs of a condition are gathered with an objective measure, e.g. a blood pressure monitor. The task becomes complex, however, when individuals are asked to monitor information about the subjective symptoms of a condition. This private information is available only to individuals, although they may be asked to reconcile the symptoms they experience against objective signs of the condition.

Secondly, standards must be established to permit individuals to evaluate the data patients process about themselves and their condition. Public standards exist for evaluating the severity of many disorders including hypertension, diabetes, asthma, and AIDS. However, there are no public standards for evaluating the severity of other disorders, including most recurrent and chronic pain dis-

orders. Attempts have been made to develop self-report and rating scales that can be used reliably to assess the severity of these disorders. However, as information about the severity of pain and other symptoms is only available to the individual, the assessment of these variables may be idiosyncratic to a given individual. Idiosyncratic criteria and standards used by one individual to evaluate symptoms may be invaluable in evaluating changes in his or her condition; however, these standards are likely to vary across individuals and thus be of limited help in assessing the performance of a group of individuals.

Thirdly, individuals must learn to evaluate and make judgements about the data they process. Making judgements may not be difficult with objective data; individuals can usually match any deviations from an objective standard if changes have occurred that may require some type of action on their part. Matching-to-standard becomes a more difficult task in the case of subjective symptoms. Individuals must acquire and refine their skills at matching their reactions to what, at the outset of their performance of self-management skills, were often ambiguous and fuzzy standards.

Fourthly, individuals must evaluate any changes that occur in terms of the antecedent conditions that may have led to the change, the behaviours they might perform to alter the changes, if necessary, and the potential consequences of their action. An analysis of the antecedents, behaviours performed, and consequences of that action often provides information necessary for making decisions about possible courses of action.

Finally, contextual factors must be considered in processing and evaluating information about a given health-related condition. There is a multidirectional interaction between the context and elements of self-management. In addition, contextual variables, including setting events, establishing stimuli, and establishing operations, may influence the course of self-management of a chronic health-related condition (Creer & Bender, 1993).

Decision-making

This is a critical function in self-management in that after patients collect, process, and evaluate data on themselves and their condition, they are asked to make appropriate decisions based upon the information. Despite an increasing amount of data available regarding medical decision-making, there is a paucity of information as to how individual patients make decisions. Yet, decision-making is at the core of successful self-management of any condition. One study compared decision-making by medical personnel and patients (Creer, 1990). The medical personnel included 30 medical students, 30 allergists who treated asthma, and seven physicians who were regarded by their peers as experts on asthma. All subjects described how they would approach treating asthma problems described in a series of vignettes. The patients included 84 asthmatic children and their parents who had been taught to use self-management skills to control asthma. They described how they managed actual asthma attacks experienced by the children. Results indicated that the physicians regarded as experts and the children and their parents who effectively applied self-management skills both utilized 12 effective judgement rules or decision-making strategies. These included: (a) considering each attack as a separate incident; (b) generating a number of testable treatment alternatives; (c) using a personal data base in selecting the most efficacious treatment strategy;

(d) adjusting stepwise treatment to fit changes in severity of attacks; (e) eschewing preconceived notions about attack management; (f) thinking in terms of probabilities regarding potential outcomes; and (g) avoiding an over-reliance on memory regarding asthma and its treatment. In short, patients and families who performed self-management skills and expert physicians used similar advanced cognitive strategies, coupled with remarkable flexibility, both in making decisions and in processing and evaluating information to generate hypotheses about the management of asthma.

Action

Action entails the performance of self-management skills to help control a physical disorder or health-related condition. Self-instruction underlies whatever action is taken by individuals; it includes the prompting, directing, and maintaining of the performance of self-management skills. How successful individual patients will be is, to a major extent, a function of the instruction they provide to themselves to initiate and maintain whatever action is required to achieve the goal they are pursuing. It is also dependent on contextual variables that may facilitate or impinge upon the performance of self-management skills.

Self-instruction is significant to self-management in two other ways (Creer & Bender, 1993). First, establishing control over a disorder or condition requires that individuals perform, often in a stepwise fashion, the strategies they have worked out beforehand with their physicians. Individuals must use self-management skills to attain the goals they and their physicians jointly selected prior to the acquisition and performance of these skills. Secondly, self-instruction can prompt other strategies for managing or coping with a disorder. These may include those summarized by Karoly (1993), including attentional resource allocation, effort mobilization, planning and problem-solving, verbal self-cueing, facilitative cognitive sets or expectations, stimulus control, and mental thought or cognitive control. Other strategies might include relaxation, self-desensitization, skill rehearsal, modelling, linking or unlinking of behavioural chains, and self-reinforcement (Creer & Bender, 1993).

Self-reaction

Self-reaction refers to the attention individuals direct toward evaluating their performance (Bandura, 1986). On the basis of their evaluation, individuals can establish realistic expectations about their performance, as well as evaluate whether they need more training and expertise. Individuals should also develop realistic expectations about the limits of self-management in attaining the goals they have helped select. They should realize that they are unlikely to be able to apply self-management skills to control every aspect of either their behaviour or their condition that they may wish to manage.

Self-efficacy influences the performance of self-management skills. Self-efficacy is the belief of individuals that they can adequately perform specific skills in a given situation (e.g. Bandura, 1977). Knowing self-management skills is not enough to ensure that these skills will be used appropriately; individuals must also believe they are capable of performing these skills to reach whatever goal they have helped set for themselves. Self-referent thought is credited as mediating the relation between selective goals and action. As noted by Karoly (1993), a belief in domain-specific efficacy, in contrast to beliefs individuals have regarding the consequences of their performance, 'is the self-referent, generative capability that stands out as a singularly powerful self-motivating force' (p. 37). Self-efficacy arises, in part, from performance accomplishments and guides and regulates future action. Self-efficacy has been shown to be a significant component of a number of self-management programmes including those designed for smoking cessation, chronic pain management, and asthma management.

DISCUSSION

Self-management procedures are being applied to an increasing number of health-related conditions (Holroyd & Creer, 1986). The potential for self-management is indicated by the report of a blue ribbon panel that included a prominent former Surgeon General of the United States, C. Everett Koop, that emphasized health-care costs in the United States could be sharply reduced by decreasing the need and demand for medical services (Fries et al., 1993). The key to their analysis, and to the large reductions in health-care costs they projected, was the contention that individuals could assume greater responsibility for their health through self-management.

Despite initial successes with self-management techniques, and the promise that the widespread application of these procedures could effectively reduce the demand for medical services and promote healthy lifestyles, the systematic application of self-management is in its infancy. The current state of affairs is not evident in a lack of enthusiasm regarding the application of self-management techniques; the techniques are being introduced with a widening pool of physical disorders. Rather, it is evident when we consider what is known about the processes of self-management. Knowledge regarding the stages of goal selection is well documented; numerous health education programmes have been developed and a significant number evaluated in controlled studies. Information also is available regarding physicians' selection of goals. In a systems approach, data is available concerning the input represented by patient education and goal selection. At the other end of the continuum, controlled evaluations of self-management programmes provide evidence of changes in outcome, indicating something has occurred between the input and output in the self-management activities of individuals. The question remains, however, exactly what self-management processes were involved in producing the observed outcomes? Processes thought to play a role in self-management were outlined in this discussion. However, these are suggested mechanisms that are only vaguely supported by the data. Research is needed to determine the exact role and function of each process in self-management. Once the processes have been identified, the next question is, how do the processes fit together into a stream of events from goal selection to self-reaction? This will prove a far more complex question to answer. As Karoly (1993, p. 26) noted:

An unfortunate consequence of the artificial (but artful) parsing of a complex, contextually embedded stream of events is the tendency for mechanisms to be analyzed singly (overlooking possible compound effects), by way of unique paradigmatic renderings, in relation to only a subset of potential outcomes, and with regard to but a portion of the complete regulatory cycle.

If the self-management process can be understood, there remains the additional query, how can this knowledge of self-management processes best be utilized to enhance the effectiveness of specific self-management programmes? Our limited understanding of the self-management process should not, at this point, deter clinicians and researchers from continuing to develop new self-management programmes or from improving existing programmes. These efforts are fully justified by the positive outcomes produced by such programmes. However, as our understanding of the process of self-management increases, this understanding should shape the development of future self-management programmes and allow us to increase the effectiveness of existing programmes.

REFERENCES

Baker, R.C. & Kirschenbaum, D.S. (1993). Self-monitoring may be necessary for successful weight control. *Behavior Therapy*, **24**, 377–94.

Bandura, A. (1977). Self-efficacy: toward a unifying theory of behavioral change. *Psychological Review*, **84**, 191–215.

Bandura, A. (1986). *Social foundations of thought and action: a social cognitive theory.* Englewood Cliffs, NJ: Prentice-Hall.

Creer, T.L. (1990). Strategies for judgment and decision-making in the management of childhood asthma. *Pediatric Asthma, Allergy, and Immunology*, **4**, 253–64.

Creer, T.L. & Bender, B.G. (1993). Asthma. In R.J. Gatchel & E.B. Blanchard (Eds.). *Psychophysiological disorders.* Washington, DC: American Psychological Association.

Ford, D.H. (1987). *Humans as self-constructing living systems: a developmental perspective on behavior and personality.* Hillsdale, NJ: Erlbaum.

Fries, J.F., Koop, C.E., Beadle, C.E., Cooper, P.P., England, M.J., Greaves, R.F., Sokolov, J.J., Wright, D. & the Health Project Consortium (1993). Reducing health care costs by reducing the need and demand for medical services. *New England Journal of Medicine*, **329**, 321–5.

Holroyd, K.A. & Creer, T.L. (1986). *Self-management of chronic disease: handbook of clinical interventions and research.* Orlando, FL: Academic Press.

Karoly, P. (1993). Mechanisms of self-regulation: a systems view. *Annual Review of Psychology*, **44**, 23–52.

Kirchenbaum, D.S. & Tomarken, A.J. (1982). On facing the generalization problem: the study of self-regulatory failure. In P.C. Kendall (Ed.). *Advances in cognitive-behavioral research and therapy*, vol. 1. New York: Academic Press.

National Heart, Lung & Blood Institute (1992). International consensus report on diagnosis and treatment of asthma. Washington, DC: US Department of Health and Human Services.

Social skills training (SST)

MICHAEL ARGYLE

Department of Experimental Psychology,
University of Oxford, UK

THE MEANING AND MEASUREMENT OF SOCIAL SKILLS

Social skills are patterns of social behaviour that make people more socially competent, that is, able to produce the desired effects on others. In everyday skills these effects are related to personal motivations, e.g. to be popular, to stay married, or to control children. In work situations there are task goals, e.g. to sell things, for subordinates to work better, pupils to learn more or for patients to recover, or to cope effectively with members of another culture.

Research has shown that the possession of social skills produces important benefits. They result in having more friends and staying married, and thus having more social support, which in turn leads to happiness and better physical and mental health. Social skills at work lead to greater work effectiveness, which is good both for the individual and for the organization. The lack of social skills is a common source of unhappiness and of failure at work.

There is a genetic component to social skills, and they are partly acquired in childhood. However, later learning experiences are also important, and social skills can be acquired by training; we shall describe how.

In order to plan the training, or study the success of training, of individuals or groups, it is necessary to assess their social competence and the nature of any social skill deficits. Several methods are commonly used. Interviews can find which social situations the client finds difficult, and what he or she thinks is going wrong. Questionnaires can do this more systematically; many have been constructed but none has been generally accepted (Spitzberg & Cupach, 1989), though the short self-report scale by Sarason works quite well, and we have used a list of situations, which the client rates for difficulty. Role-playing of some simple situations, with stooges, can give a clear idea of any weaknesses. Ratings by family, friends, hospital staff or colleagues are widely used, especially for work skills. Objective measures of work success, e.g. at selling or interviewing, have the greatest validity, but each individual may have a different work setting, not comparable with those of others.

THE EXTENT OF SOCIAL DIFFICULTIES AND THE NEED FOR SST

Everyday skills

Children may be aggressive bullies, may be rejected for other reasons, or may be simply neglected by other children. They may be disruptive in school. These kinds of behaviour, and the rejection they produce, may lead to mental disturbance later. Adolescents and young people may be lonely, shy, or have difficulties with the opposite sex. About 40% of students say that they are 'shy', 55% say that they are often lonely. Social behaviour problems are very widespread in this group, and can cause great unhappiness, but often pass with time and experience. Adults may have no friends, or may have marital difficulties (a third of marriages break up), or can't cope with their children. Old people may be lonely, may be quarrelsome and have difficulty keeping up relationships with kin.

Social skills at work

Most jobs involve dealing with other people, and for teachers, managers, salespersons and others this is the main job. Socially unskilled managers and supervisors produce high levels of discontent and consequent absenteeism, labour turnover and lack of motivation among their subordinates. Some salespersons sell four times as much as others in the same shop. Those who go to work abroad as salespersons, or for organizations like the Peace Corps, have a failure rate of up to 60% in some parts of the Middle or Far East, i.e. they come home before their one-or two-year term is completed. Lack of social skills is one of the main reasons for people losing their jobs. Many jobs require special skills; often the only training is experience on the job; evidently this often fails (Argyle, 1989). Some jobs require the social skills to deal with very difficult situations, as with social workers.

Mental patients

All kinds of mental patients have social behaviour problems. Schizophrenics and other psychotics have severe difficulties in this sphere; others find them very difficult to deal with and avoid them if they can. Many neurotics have social difficulties too; we found that about 25% of a sample of outpatients were seriously socially inadequate in a number of ways, corresponding to the components of social skill to be described below, such as lack of rewardingness, poor non-verbal communication and conversational skills (Trower, Bryant & Argyle, 1978).

THE MAIN COMPONENTS OF SOCIAL SKILLS

Social skills are rather like manual motor skills in that the performer uses a sequence of skilled moves to influence something else. In this case he or she uses verbal and non-verbal signals to influence other people. These skills can be divided into a number of components, each of which can go wrong and may need training (Argyle, 1994).

Rewardingness

This may consist of verbal moves such as praise, sympathy or encouragement, non-verbal ones such as smiles or head-nods, help of various kinds, presents, meals, advice, or doing enjoyable things together. Rewardingness leads to being liked, it is important in marriage and is often used in marital therapy, and is part of the skills of leadership, looking after subordinates.

Assertiveness

This is the capacity to influence or control others, but without damaging the relationship. It is quite different from both passive and from aggressive behaviour. Assertion is achieved partly by the use of verbal persuasion, giving the other reasons for doing what is wanted. It also uses certain non-verbal signals, a subtle combination of friendly signals and dominant ones, like a loud but friendly voice. However, to avoid damaging the relationship, it is necessary to be concerned with the other's interests and point of view (Galassi, Galassi & Vedder, 1981).

Non-verbal communication (NVC)

NVC plays several key parts in social performance. It is one of the main channels for expressing emotions and attitudes to others. Socially skilled individuals are found to use a common pattern of NVC, a high level of smiling, gaze, loud and expressive voice, other-directed gestures. In work situations it is necessary to control NVC, to produce the desired effects on others, rather than showing accurately what is being felt. NVC is also important in accompanying speech, adding to meaning by gestures and tone of voice, in synchronizing utterances, and providing feedback from listeners (Argyle, 1988).

Verbal communication

This lies at the heart of most social behaviour. Each utterance needs to be constructed and delivered so that it can be understood by, and has the desired impact on, the recipients. Utterances must be placed in sequence to construct a meaningful conversation; utterances and sequences take special forms for different situations, e.g. doctor–patient, teacher–pupil, selling, chat between friends. Speakers usually 'accommodate' to each other by moving towards one another's speech style for instance in accent or loudness, which leads to acceptance by the other. 'Politeness' avoids damaging another's self-esteem. or constraining their behaviour, for example, by indirect requests, and it too has positive results (Ellis & Beattie, 1986).

Empathy, co-operation and concern for other

These are found in socially effective individuals, and are lacking in the socially inadequate. Empathy is the capacity to see another's point of view, to share their emotions, and display this concern. Co-operative individuals take account of the other's goals, and co-ordinate behaviour so that both sets of goals can be reached, as in bargaining, when an 'integrative solution' is sought. Concern for others is essential in close relationships, and is found in marriage and close friendships.

Social intelligence

Social skill requires understanding and knowledge of social situations and relationships, and of the rules of each. Some SST clients for example do not know the purpose of a party or interview, or the rules governing these situations (Argyle, Furnham & Graham, 1981). They need the ability to decide which is the best way to handle difficult social situations. Some aspects of social skill are at this level of knowledge, awareness and planning, but others are at a lower, automatic level, such as most NVC.

Self-presentation

This is the sending of information about the self, particularly occupation and group membership, by means of clothes, accent, or general manner, mainly by NV cues. It is important for doctors, news readers, and others to look the part, or they are not taken seriously. Common errors are bogus claims, working too hard at presenting the self, or sending insufficient information. Self-disclosure usually takes place gradually, and is reciprocated.

SOCIAL BEHAVIOUR PROBLEMS IN MENTAL PATIENTS

Serious social difficulties are found in patients, including people with quite mild degrees of anxiety or depression (Hollin & Trower, 1986).

Neurotics

A great variety of problems are found here. A quarter or more of neurotics are found to be seriously inadequate in their social performance, some because they have social anxiety or phobia, and avoid situations. Social anxiety may be shown in trembling, blushing, nervous gestures, or gaze aversion. Some neurotics talk too much, very fast, with speech errors; others are unable to sustain a conversation at all. They are often very egocentric, think about their own concerns, and their own social performance. They are unassertive and found unrewarding, they often have difficulty making friends or keeping relationships.

Depression

The depressed mood is seen in facial expression, drooping posture, downward-directed gaze, crying, and low-pitched voice with falling pitch. Depressives speak little, with long pauses, often about their problems, which they see as hopeless, and for which they blame themselves. They have low self-esteem and think that others reject them more than they actually do. They, too, are unrewarding, and as a result are avoided, as well as being egocentric and socially ineffective.

Schizophrenia

This includes a variety of patients, but their social performance is often defective in a number of ways. Their NVC is disturbed, blank facial expression, need for a lot of personal space, self-touching gestures, flat and monotonous voice, untidy appearance. Some do not speak at all, the conversation of others is rambling and irrelevant. They cannot co-ordinate their behaviour with that of others or form social relationships.

Anti-social personalities (psychopaths)

These individuals appear to be socially competent, but have a total lack of empathy, or concern for others, and are unable to see anyone else's point of view. They are unable to form close or lasting relationships, and get into trouble because of their dishonesty, drunkenness and lack of restraint in aggressive and sexual behaviour.

METHODS OF SOCIAL SKILLS TRAINING

The 'classical' method: role-playing

Most varieties of SST are forms of role-playing, in which trainees try out the skill away from the real situation and are given some kind of coaching. The classical method has the following three phases:

Instruction and modelling

The trainer describes a particular aspect of the skill and either demonstrates how to do it, or shows a videotape of it being done.

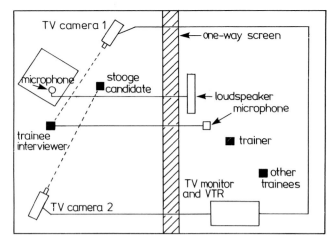

Fig. 1. A social skills training laboratory.

Role-playing

A problem situation is described; one or more stooges (or confederates) are produced, and the trainee role-plays for 7 – 8 minutes; the performance is usually videotaped.

Feedback

The trainer gives careful and constructive comments and suggestions, plays back the videotape, and other trainees join in the discussion. Trainees have to learn some new vocabulary, to refer to the different moves made, for example by teachers or sales staff, and the elements of NVC and conversation.

It is common to work with a group of about six, who can act as role-partners for each other; the whole session might last 1½ hours or more, and there would be 6–10 sessions, covering a carefully planned series of topics, based on the needs of the trainees. Most trainers use videotape, and there is evidence that this produces better results than verbal comments alone. The laboratory set-up is shown in Fig. 1. It includes a one-way screen, video cameras, mixer and monitors, and an ear microphone for the trainer to speak to a trainee during the role-playing, if needed.

A central problem with this method is how to enable trainees to generalize the new skills to their real-life situations. One solution is the use of 'homework', i.e. trainees are asked to try out each new skill several times between weekly sessions. If trainees are in an institution, training can be continued by the staff between formal training sessions.

Examples of this kind of training are microteaching for teachers, interviewer training, assertiveness training, and SST for neurotic outpatients (L'Abate & Milan, 1985).

However, role-playing is not very satisfactory if it is impossible to reproduce the trainees' problem situations in the laboratory or clinic, such as dealing with a drunken mob for the police, or with angry trade unionists for management. An alternative in these cases is training on the job, to which we turn later.

Other laboratory methods

Some of the components of social skill listed above can be trained by role-playing, e.g. assertiveness and rewardingness, but other components need slightly different treatment. Non-verbal communication can be trained by means of a mirror (for the face) and a tape-recorder (for the voice), and the modelling of photographs or tape-recordings. Verbal communication and conversation may need some detailed instruction on the construction of utterances or sequences of utterances, especially for some professional social skills. Self-presentation can be improved simply by advice about clothes and other aspects of appearance, or by speech training. Empathy and attention to others are difficult to train. Various exercises are used, e.g. carrying out simple interviews to find out another's opinions, thus focusing attention on the other. Social intelligence can be trained by presenting verbal descriptions of social problem situations, and asking trainees to think of ways of dealing with them (Shure, 1981).

Learning on the job

This has not always been successful in the past, and people often fail to learn the right skills after years of experience. However, on-the-spot coaching can be successful; it is necessary to have a coach or mentor who is an expert in the skill, who accompanies the trainee, and can give instant feedback. This method is widely used for teacher training, and in some areas for police training, given by 'tutor constables'.

Educational methods.

Lectures, discussion, reading and films can make an important contribution to SST. These have been found to have little effect when used alone, since social skills, like motor ones, need practice as well as instruction. However, these methods are useful where knowledge

or understanding are needed, as in cross-cultural training, and also for situations and relationships and their rules (Argyle, 1994).

HOW SUCCESSFUL IS SST?

Many experimental follow-up studies have been carried out, making comparisons with other forms of training, or with no training (Spence & Shepherd 1983).

Everyday skills

SST is very successful with adolescents and young adults, especially for assertiveness, loneliness, and heterosexual skills. Marital therapy is successful for older adults.

Work skills

Most firms use some kind of SST for supervisors and managers. This is effective in terms of the productivity and job satisfaction of subordinates (Burke & Day, 1986). Microteaching is useful in saving classroom training time, and in eliminating errors (Brown & Shaw, 1986). Much is known about the effective skills of doctors, and it seems likely that similar training for them is equally effective (Pendleton *et al.*, 1984).

Mental patients

SST is the most effective treatment for neurotics who are socially unskilled. For other patients it is certainly better than no treatment, and is often found to be as good as other treatments, for depression and a variety of other conditions (see Williams, 1986; and other chapters in Hollin & Trower, 1986). However, it is usually used in combination with other methods, such as drugs or cognitive therapy.

REFERENCES

Argyle, M. (1988). *Bodily communication.* 2nd edn. London: Methuen.

Argyle, M. (1989). *The social psychology of work.* 2nd edn. Harmondsworth: Penguin Books.

Argyle, M. (1994). *The psychology of interpersonal behaviour.* 5th edn. London: Penguin Books.

Argyle, M., Furnham, A. & Graham, J.A. (1981). *Social situations.* Cambridge: Cambridge University Press.

Brown, G. & Shaw, M. (1986). Social skills training in education. In C.R. Hollin & P. Trower (Eds.). *Handbook of social skills training,* vol 2, pp. 59–78, Oxford: Pergamon.

Burke, M.J. & Day, R.R. (1986). A cumulative study of the effectiveness of managerial

training. *Journal of Applied Psychology,* **71,** 232–45.

Ellis, A. & Beattie, G. (1986). *The psychology of language and communication.* London: Weidenfeld and Nicholson.

Galassi, J.P., Galassi, M.D. & Vedder, M.J. (1981). Perspectives on assertion as a social skills model. In J.D. Wine & M.D. Smye (Eds.). *Social competence.* New York: Guilford.

Hollin, C.R. & Trower, P. (Eds.). (1986). *Handbook of social skills training.* Oxford: Pergamon.

L'Abate, L. & Milan, M.A. (1985). *Handbook of social skills training and research.* New York: Wiley.

Pendleton, D., Schofield, T., Tate, P. & Havelock, P. (1984). *The consultation: an*

approach to learning and teaching. Oxford: Oxford University Press.

Shure, M. (1981). A social skills approach to child-rearing. In M. Argyle (Ed.). *Social skills and health.* London: Methuen.

Spence, S. & Shepherd, G. (Ed.). (1983). *Developments in social skills training.* London: Academic Press.

Spitzberg, B.H. & Cupach, W.R. (1989). *Handbook of interpersonal competence research.* New York: Springer.

Trower, P., Bryant, B. & Argyle, M. (1978). *Social skills and mental health.* London: Methuen.

Williams, J.M.G. (1986). Social skills training and depression. In C.R. Hollin & P. Trower (Eds.). *Handbook of social skills training.* Oxford: Pergamon.

Stress management

ANDREW STEPTOE

Department of Psychology, St George's Hospital
Medical School, University of London, UK

Stress management is the term used to describe a broad range of psychological procedures designed to modify stress responses and ameliorate the impact of potentially stressful experiences. Stress management was originally introduced in clinical settings to assist patients with acute and chronic illness adapt to their circumstances, and to promote effective coping with stressful medical procedures. However, the growth of this area has been rapid, and in the present day a wide variety of populations are considered to benefit from stress management, including occupational groups (notably healthcare workers, emergency services personnel, transport workers, students and teachers), and people in disadvantaged personal circumstances such as family caregivers for chronically sick relatives, single parents, the unemployed and victims of assault and abuse. Several of the major stress management procedures are described elsewhere in the *Handbook* including relaxation training, biofeedback and cognitive behaviour therapy (see also Lehrer & Woolfolk, 1993). This contribution will focus on the background to stress management, its basic elements and outcomes.

ORIGINS AND BACKGROUND TO STRESS MANAGEMENT

Stress management as it is currently practised can be seen to have emerged through the convergence of several psychological treatment approaches and perspectives.

Biofeedback and relaxation

Biofeedback and relaxation training methods such as progressive muscle relaxation and autogenic training were first introduced to counter stress-induced physiological activation in the early days of behavioural medicine. These techniques were applied to conditions such a tension and migraine headache, hypertension, Raynaud's disease and epilepsy, on the assumption that clinical status would be improved by direct modification of the underlying physiological dysfunction (Surwit *et al.*, 1982). However, two limitations emerged in clinical evaluations of these methods. The first was that training in quiet, calm clinical settings was found not necessarily to generalize to everyday situations, making it important to modify techniques so that skills could be acquired not in isolation, but in the context of coping with stressful situations. Secondly, discrepancies were apparent between therapeutic effects and putative psychophysiological mechanisms (Steptoe, 1989). The belief that biofeedback involves direct learning and control over autonomic responses proved difficult to confirm. Similarly, although relaxation training is associated with a diminution of muscle tension and with reduced activation of neuroendocrine parameters such as cortisol, it is not

clear that these physiological responses are responsible for clinical effects. It has consequently been proposed that biofeedback and relaxation may confer benefits through cognitive processes, such as providing clients with a greater sense of control, rather than through purely physiological mechanisms. Relaxation training and its variants have become an important element in stress management.

Behaviour therapy

Stress management owes a considerable debt to the methods of behaviour therapy developed in the 1950s and 1960s for the management of phobias, obsessive – compulsive disorders and other anxiety-related problems. Systematic desensitization, exposure techniques, modelling, role play and social skills training were originally formulated for assisting people with debilitating mental and behavioural disorders, but have since been adapted and integrated into stress management. Behaviour therapy itself has evolved in the hands of many clinicians into cognitive behavioural psychotherapy, as a distinction between pure behavioural methods and therapies involving the modification of attitudes and cognitions has become blurred.

A particularly important technique of behaviour therapy that has formed one of the backbones of stress management is systematic desensitization. Originally, systematic desensitization involved teaching patients with problems such as phobias to relax, then presenting them with anxiety-provoking stimuli (either *in vivo* or in imagination) at progressively more intense levels. This was adapted by Meichenbaum (1985) and colleagues into stress inoculation, in which people are exposed to stressful situations in a step-by-step fashion, and develop a repertoire of coping skills to help them manage these problems. Participants are encouraged to articulate thoughts related to preparing, confronting and coping with the situation and the feelings it engenders through a series of 'self-statements'. Similar methods were developed by Novaco (1973) for anger management.

Occupational psychology

The third strand in the development of stress management derives from study of the work environment and the problems of job satisfaction, absenteeism, poor productivity and employee health. Lennart Levi from Sweden was particularly influential in arguing that the adverse effects of work are not simply due to individual weaknesses and vulnerabilities, but that the organization of jobs and the psychosocial work environment are partly responsible. An important development in this context was the formulation of the demand-control model of work-related strain by Karasek & Theorell

(1990). They have suggested that job strain and risks to health arise not merely through high levels of demand, but when high demands are coupled with low personal control over how the job is carried out, and limited opportunities to develop skills. The implication has been that re-designing the way the workplace is organized in terms of control over decisions and allocation of responsibilities may be beneficial to emotional and physical well-being. It illustrates the point that stress management is not only a matter for the individual, but that environmental restructuring may be relevant.

ELEMENTS OF STRESS MANAGEMENT

A great variety of stress management approaches have been developed for different problems, making it difficult to generalize about techniques. For example, a stress management programme for helping patients with arthritis pain might include training in distraction methods, problem-solving to identify the triggers for pain and how to avoid them, exercise regimens, and education in appropriate use of medical services. Methods for the treatment of hypertension have been concentrated almost exclusively on relaxation training, while a programme for stress management to help health professionals cope with work might involve cognitive reappraisal of threatening situations, time management and mobilization of social support. Still other factors come into prominence with stress management for alcohol dependency, bereavement, or the victims of natural disasters. Stress management is not a standard procedure, but requires careful consideration of the circumstances surrounding the particular problem. Nevertheless, there are a number of elements that are fundamental and can be defined in general terms.

Environmental change

Stress responses arise through an imbalance between the demands and expectations on an individual, and abilities effectively to mobilize personal and social coping resources. It follows that one element of stress management is the exploration of environmental contingencies and methods of changing these. If particular situations tend to elicit stress responses, it may be possible to prevent them from developing, or to withdraw before severe stress responses arise. For example, particular social interactions with family members or work colleagues may elicit feelings such as anger, or may be associated with headache and other symptoms. Identification of these circumstances may make it possible to modify the chain of events at an early stage to prevent it from spiralling to damaging levels, or to suggest ways of appraising matters differently so that they are no longer perceived as stressful. In work settings, the modification of hierarchical management structures, the timing and flow of tasks, and control over how they are to be carried out, may prove beneficial (Murphy et al., 1995). These strategies are designed to alter the situations that give rise to stress responses, thereby blunting the magnitude of reactions.

Enhancement of coping resources

The other side of the equation is to enhance the coping skills and resources that are available to the person. Many stress management programmes help people to acquire a range of coping skills, and provide practice in their deployment. A number of methods of coping may be relevant, from relaxation and other calming responses to problem-solving, effective use of social support and assertive skills. The coping resources required during stress management may be quite specific to the particular problem, for instance, training in the regulation of breathing patterns to prevent hyperventilation, or practice in muscle contraction exercises to prevent stiffness during invasive medical examinations, or may be quite general. An important principle in stress management is that coping methods are applied flexibly. The best methods of dealing with one problem may be less relevant to others, so clients are encouraged to experiment with different approaches.

Enhancement of resistance

A third general element of stress management is that it is associated with efforts to maintain a healthy lifestyle. People who fail to manage stress effectively are often found to engage in unhealthy behaviours such as excessive alcohol consumption, cigarette smoking and unnecessary risk taking. The modification of these behaviours may be important to the success of stress management. Regular exercise has been proposed as a stress buffer, while adequate sleep and rest time and healthy diets may increase the individual's resistance to health risks.

The different elements outlined here cannot, of course, be strictly partitioned, and many stress management programmes use a variety of techniques to achieve their aims. An example is the Type A behaviour modification programme devised by Friedman and colleagues for the Recurrent Coronary Prevention Project (Friedman et al., 1986). This programme was developed to help Type A cardiac patients recognize the undesirable elements of the behaviour pattern, the beliefs and attitudes underlying its maintenance, and to provide training in alternative ways of responding. The programme involved relaxation training, the recognition of exaggerated arousal reactions, instruction in self-monitoring and self-observation methods, restructuring of the environment to eliminate excessive daily activities and demands, plus the use of cognitive methods, role play and self-management to identify and modify assumptions and beliefs about the world, substitute affection for irritability, and assertiveness for aggression, to establish new goals and extend social contacts. This package supplemented information about heart disease, and advice concerning exercise, diet, smoking and appropriate use of health care. Clearly, such an approach is very complex, and the factors that are most important in reducing cardiovascular risk are difficult to identify.

OUTCOMES OF STRESS MANAGEMENT

Stress management is applied to different problems for different purposes, so it is not possible to draw general conclusions about efficacy. None the less, a broad distinction between two types of outcome can be drawn.

Many stress management programmes are intended to help clients cope emotionally with particular distressing circumstances, in the hope that reducing emotional distress will promote psychological well-being and quality of life. This is the first important goal in work settings and for many clinical groups. However, a second possibility is that stress management not only influences emotional adaptation, but physiological processes that are relevant to health risk and illness outcome. The hope in some applications of stress management is that patients will both feel better and enjoy enhanced heath. For example, the stress management programme for Type A behaviour described earlier has been shown to reduce the risk of recurrent myocardial infarction (Friedman et al, 1986). Stress management programmes offered to men at the time of testing for HIV infection have been found to enhance immune defences as well as reducing the distress caused by positive tests (Antoni et al., 1991). Methods of preparing people psychologically for surgery may lead to reduced distress in hospital and to more rapid physical recovery (Johnston & Vögele, 1993). There is also evidence that supportive stress management groups for patients with primary breast cancer may be associated with prolongation of life (Spiegel et al., 1989).

The mechanisms underlying these responses have yet to be precisely defined. It is probable that psychophysiological processes (alterations in neuroendocrine activation and in autonomic tone) are involved, together with changes in health behaviours such as adherence to medical treatment, exercise, and nutrition. The fact that stress management may affect health directly holds out exciting prospects for advances in health care. Nevertheless, it should not diminish the importance of the primary aim of programmes, which is to improve emotional adjustment. Enhanced quality of life is of great value in itself, and remains the main justification for wider use of stress management techniques in health settings. (See also 'Relaxation training'; 'Cognitive behaviour therapy').

REFERENCES

Antoni, M.H., Baggett, L, Ironson, G., August, S., LaPerriere, A., Klimas, N., Schneiderman, N. & Fletcher, M.A. (1991). Cognitive–behavioral stress management intervention buffers distress responses and immunologic changes following notification of HIV-1 seropositivity. Journal of Consulting and Clinical Psychology, 59, 906–15.

Friedman, M., Thoresen, C.E., Gill, J.J., Ulmer, D., Powell, L.H., Price, V.A., Brown, B., Thompson, L., Rabin, D.D., Breall, W.S., Bourg, E., Levy, R. & Dixon, T. (1986). Alteration of type A behavior and its effect on cardiac recurrences in post myocardial infarction patients: summary results of the recurrent

coronary prevention project. American Heart Journal, 112, 653–65.

Johnston, M. & Vögele, C. (1993). Benefits of psychological preparation for surgery: a meta-analysis. Annals of Behavioral Medicine, 15, 245–56.

Karasek, R. & Theorell, T. (1990). Healthy work. New York: Basic Books.

Lehrer, P.M. & Woolfolk, R.L. (Eds.). (1993). Principles and practice of stress management, 2nd edn. New York: Guilford Press.

Meichenbaum, D. (1985). Stress inoculation training. New York: Pergamon Press.

Murphy, L.R., Hurrell, J.J., Sauter, S.L. & Keita, G.P. (Eds.) (1995). Job stress interventions. Washington, DC: American Psychological Association.

Novaco, R.W. (1973). Anger control: the development and evaluation of an experimental treatment. Lexington, MA: Lexington Books.

Spiegel, D., Bloom, J.R., Kraemer, H.C. & Gottheil, E. (1989). Effect of psychosocial treatment on survival of patients with metastatic breast cancer. Lancet, II, 888–91.

Steptoe, A. (1989). Psychophysiological interventions in behavioural medicine. In G. Turpin (Ed.). Handbook of clinical psychophysiology. Chichester: John Wiley.

Surwit, R.S., Williams, R.B., Steptoe, A. & Biersner, R. (Eds.). (1982). Behavioral treatment of disease. New York: Plenum Press.

Worksite interventions

JAMES R. TERBORG
University of Oregon, Eugene, Oregon, USA and Oregon Research Institute, Eugene, Oregon, USA

RUSSELL E. GLASGOW
Oregon Research Institute, Eugene, Oregon, USA

Health promotion programmes at the worksite have become increasingly popular in North America over the past 15 years (US Department of Health and Human Services, 1993). A casual reading of the research literature suggests the frequency of worksite interventions has also increased in Japan, Australia and Europe. Worksite Health Promotion (WHP) interventions are thought to be cost-effective for promoting health and reducing medical demand (Fries et al., 1993; Pelletier, 1993). This chapter summarizes research on WHP interventions. We conclude that worksite interventions hold substantial promise, but, because of variability in outcomes, both across studies and across worksites within a given study, current results are not widely generalizable.

WHAT IS WORKSITE HEALTH PROMOTION?

No single definition exists on what constitutes a WHP intervention. Does the distribution of weight loss pamphlets at work qualify as a worksite intervention? Does implementation of a smoking policy qualify? There is agreement, however, that a worksite intervention should include: (i) the periodic or continuing delivery of educational or behaviour change materials and activities that are designed to maintain or improve employee fitness, health and well-being; and (ii) changes in organizational practices and policies conducive to health promotion (Fielding, 1991; Glasgow & Terborg, 1988). Legislatively mandated programmes and activities in employee health and safety are generally excluded. Most worksite interventions focus on educational and skill building materials and activities. Interventions targeting changes in organizational practices and policies are less common. Few interventions emphasize both. WHP programmes vary along several dimensions, including facilities, budget, eligibility, scope, and target outcomes.

The US Public Health Service conducted a national survey of worksite health promotion activities in 1985 and again in 1992 (US Department of Health and Human Services). A total of 1507 worksites in the private sector with 50 or more employees were surveyed in 1992, and baseline data from the 1985 survey were used to estimate change. There was an increase in worksite health promotion activities, with 81% reporting health promotion information or activities in 1992 compared to 66% in 1985. Notable increases were found in programmes on nutrition, weight control, physical fitness, high blood pressure and stress management. Physical fitness and smoking control were the most prevalent activities (41% and 40% respectively) in 1992 and programmes on sexually transmitted diseases and prenatal education were the least prevalent (10% and 9%, respectively). Number of employees at the worksite was positively related to prevalence of health promotion activities. Unionized worksites and worksites in the services industry and in the transportation/communications/utilities industry were also more likely to offer health promotion activities. Formal evaluations of programme effects are rarely conducted, with less than 7% of worksites collecting data on such outcomes as health-care costs, health status, health behaviours, productivity or absenteeism.

WHY TARGET THE WORKSITE FOR HEALTH PROMOTION INTERVENTIONS?

The worksite provides an excellent setting for health promotion. Worksite interventions have potential to: reach people with health risks who might not otherwise participate; provide long-term social and environmental support for the adoption and maintenance of healthy behaviours; reduce company and employee health-care expenditures through provision of convenient and free, or low cost, preventative and early detection interventions; improve labour-management relations; improve productivity; reduce absenteeism due to illness and injury; and reduce voluntary turnover and insurance costs. Although the potential for benefits is high, there is substantial variability in results across worksites with health promotion programmes.

There is widespread belief that companies adopt health promotion programmes to reduce health-care costs and to improve employee productivity. But, research suggests the primary reasons companies adopt and maintain programmes have little to do with the economic 'bottom line'. Key reasons include: a strong personal commitment to healthy lifestyles by senior management; as a response to employee requests; as part of moving to new facilities; the desire to project a favourable corporate image; a belief that health promotion is an important benefit that improves employee recruitment; and as a means for improving employee morale and job satisfaction (Fielding, 1990; Wolfe, Slack & Rose-Hearn, 1993).

The relative importance of 'softer' human relations and morale outcomes over 'harder' outcomes such as cost savings and improved productivity is noteworthy for two reasons. First, optimistic claims for cost savings and productivity improvements made by some of the strongest proponents of worksite health promotion programmes

(see Fries et al., 1993; Pelletier, 1993) may not be particularly relevant to the adoption and maintenance of such programmes. Secondly, a de-emphasis on economics might be desirable for the long-term future of worksite programmes because there remain unanswered questions about positive and negative results of WHP interventions including their long-term cost-effectiveness (Kaman, 1995; Shephard, 1992; Warner et al., 1988).

WHP INTERVENTIONS: THEORY AND INTERVENTION DESIGN

The conceptual and theoretical underpinnings used to design WHP interventions are either eclectic or haphazard, depending on your point of view. Most studies have been loosely informed by social learning theory or the health-belief model and focus on a combination of educational, motivational, and skills training approaches. More sophisticated designs have adopted techniques of social marketing (e.g. audience segmentation). Few studies have focused on the public health model by attempting to encourage and evaluate the extent of participation by all employees (Glasgow, McCaul & Fisher, 1993). One of the few systematic applications of theory has been the Working Well Trial (Abrams et al., 1994), which applied a mix of social cognitive theory with systems/levels analysis. We are not aware of any attempts to examine competing theories in the same study.

Research studies typically report behavioural prevention strategies with an individual-focus, single risk-factor intervention targeted at primary prevention. Few studies have systematically varied environmental prevention strategies and policy changes (e.g. smoking bans; replacing high fat foods in cafeterias and vending machines; risk-rated insurance) or examined the interactive effects of behavioural and environmental prevention strategies. Such research should be encouraged.

An increasing number of studies report applying organizational change procedures following the action – research model, but these studies resemble consulting more than research. Exceptions to this minimal use of organizational change in worksite interventions are the Working Well Trial (Abrams et al., 1994) and the Take Heart Project (Glasgow et al., 1994). These investigations, which use the worksite as the unit of analysis, include the creation of employee committees to help direct the intervention strategy and to enhance employee involvement and ownership. Systematic collection of key organizational variables (e.g. industry, structure, technology, employee norms, financial performance) allows for an evaluation of factors related to the adoption, implementation and maintenance of worksite interventions.

WHP INTERVENTION: EVALUATION RESULTS

Fries et al. (1993) and Pelletier (1993) enthusiastically concluded that a growing number of studies provide evidence that at least some types of WHP interventions appear to be effective. Unfortunately, because many of these 'first generation' studies suffer from significant methodological and practical weaknesses (Glasgow et al., 1994; Jeffery et al., 1993; Warner et al., 1988), a more cautious evaluation is recommended.

Many WHP interventions report results only for employees who voluntarily participate in and complete treatment. These studies have limited internal and external validity because of biases

[265]

introduced through self-selection. Jeffery *et al.* (1993) report, for example, that recruitment of employees to worksite smoking programmes can range from 0% to 88% and that dropout rates from worksite weight loss programmes can range from 0.5% to 80%. Rarely is the effect of intervention assessed in terms of change in the entire worksite population.

A second limitation is the failure to analyse data at the worksite level of analysis. Consider the often cited work by Erfurt and associates (Erfurt, Foote & Heirich, 1991). This study examined four different worksite interventions in four manufacturing plants. Plants were randomly assigned to receive one of the following: health screen only; health screen plus health education; health screen, health education and follow-up counselling; and all of the above plus social organization of health promotion within the plant. Data were collected from volunteers in 1985 and again in 1988 on blood pressure, body weight and smoking. A one-way analysis of variance was conducted to identify mean differences among changes in employee risk factors across the four plants. Results of these analyses showed significant differences across the four plants/programmes. The authors concluded that, 'Worksite wellness programs that provide regular follow-up monitoring and counseling for employees with CVD risks seem to show better results in achieving and sustaining risk reductions than do programs that provide only one-shot health screening or health screening plus health education . . .' (p. 447). This design, however, does not allow one to draw definite conclusions regarding the effect of WHP interventions because, from a methodological perspective, the sample size in each intervention is not the number of employee participants in each plant, but the number of plants in the intervention. In this design, only one plant was assigned to each intervention. Analysing data at the employee level of analysis generally overstates true intervention effects because such designs ignore potential intra-class (e.g. within worksite) correlation. These designs also say little about generalizability across different worksites. As noted below, substantial differences have been found across different worksites receiving the same intervention (Jeffery *et al.*, 1993).

Another problem with some studies is reliance on relatively intensive, highly structured and expensive interventions delivered by highly trained research staff, such as the programme at the Adolph Coors Company (Henritze & Brammell, 1989). This intervention would be difficult to replicate and fund.

Finally, there are problems differentiating WHP effects from other variables, such as secular trends, changes in state or local health policies and regulations, and changes in medical insurance. The dramatic results reported by the City of Birmingham in Alabama, for example, are impossible to interpret with regard to the effect of the WHP intervention (Harvey *et al.* 1993).

Fortunately, several research projects recently have been designed that address many, if not all, of the methodological and practical problems noted above. Unfortunately, these larger and more methodologically sophisticated 'second generation' studies tend to report smaller effect sizes or failure to detect significant differences on one or more key risk factors (Fisher, Glasgow & Terborg, 1990; Jeffery *et al.*, 1993).

The most rigorous methodological design published at the time of this review is the Healthy Worker Project at the University of Minnesota (Jeffery *et al.*, 1993). This design randomly assigned 32 worksites to intervention or no intervention for two years. The worksite intervention targeted cigarette smoking and obesity and utilized state-of-the-art behaviour change programmes and cash incentives. Pilot work with 435 employees in one worksite established the short-term efficacy of the intervention. The main study examines intervention effectiveness across worksites.

Results using worksite as the unit of analysis were modest compared to 'first generation' studies using employee level analyses. No statistically reliable differences ($p < .05$) were observed between intervention and control worksites for weight loss, using both cohort and cross-sectional employee samples, and for smoking, using the cross-sectional sample. Furthermore, the statistically significant decrease in smoking found in intervention worksites with the cohort sample became non-significant when analyses were restricted only to employees who agreed to biochemical validation of smoking status. Jeffery *et al.* (1993) also report large variability across worksites in both baseline and change data, for both cohort and cross-sectional analyses.

The most definitive data on worksite health promotion interventions will be available in 1994 or 1995 from the National Cancer Institute sponsored collaborative Working Well Trial (Abrams *et al.*, 1994), which targets smoking, diet and medical screens for cancer. This study involves four research centres geographically dispersed across the United States and 114 worksites. Special features of this trial include using the worksite as the unit of randomization and analysis, a theory-driven conceptual model that targets both individual and organizational levels of change, and emphasis on both education and behaviour change programmes as well as on organizational practices and policies. Data also are forthcoming from the first phase of the Take Heart Project, sponsored by the National Heart, Lung and Blood Institute (Glasgow *et al.*, 1994) involving 38 worksites. Target outcomes are smoking, dietary fat, total blood cholesterol, organizational policies and practices, and long-term programme maintenance and effectiveness.

Analyses from first generation studies (e.g. Erfurt *et al.*, 1992), demonstrate that WHP interventions can facilitate behaviour change. Although reassuring, these reports say little about the generalizability and long-term effectiveness of worksite interventions across different worksites. The Healthy Worker Project suggests that WHP interventions may not be as effective as previously thought (Fries *et al.*, 1993; Pelletier, 1993).

ORGANIZATION ENVIRONMENT AND POLICY APPROACHES TO WHP

Organizational policies and characteristics of the worksite environment are powerful levers for health promotion; however, few studies have targeted environmental and policy change. The results are mixed and many, if not all, of the methodological shortcomings discussed earlier apply to environment and policy research.

The implementation of restrictive smoking policies at work is, by far, the most commonly studied policy intervention. Cross-sectional surveys suggest a weak association between smoking cessation and employment in a worksite that bans smoking (Brenner & Mielck, 1992). Longitudinal data collected before, and after, implementation of restrictive worksite smoking policies suggest that such policies may be effective in reducing tobacco use at work, but they have inconsistent effects on smoking prevalence (Gottlieb *et al.*, 1990). It is often recommended that smoking cessation programmes be offered at work when restrictive smoking policies are introduced, but no conclusive evidence supports this otherwise reasonable recommendation. The primary health benefit of restrictive worksite smoking policies appears to be a reduction in employee exposure to environmental tobacco smoke, which is a sufficient health reason for implementing such policies.

Growing interest is directed toward worksite policies regarding employee health benefits as a way to promote health and reduce health-care costs and utilization. Several companies have experimented with providing differential benefits, or benefit-related incentives, to employees based on their health status and health care cost experience. Although a strong financial argument can be made for using health benefits as an incentive for health promotion at the worksite, the data are limited and ethical challenges continually arise (Kaman, in press).

Almost no worksite policy research has been directed in areas other than restrictive smoking policies and changes in health benefits design. This is unfortunate because many worksite opportunities exist to promote low fat and high fibre diets (e.g. catering policies, healthful food in vending machines and cafeterias), exercise (e.g. attractive stairwells to promote walking instead of using the elevator, convenient bicycle storage), maintenance of proper body weight (e.g. scales in restrooms), and other healthful outcomes (Glanz, 1993). In fact, building such activities into the normal work day may have a greater long-term public health impact than more formal WHP interventions that target high-risk employees.

ECONOMIC IMPACT OF WHP INTERVENTIONS

Fries *et al.* (1993) and Pelletier (1993) conclude that WHP interventions show positive health benefits and favourable cost-effectiveness/cost–benefit outcomes. They blame academic conservatism for holding health promotion research and policy to a more stringent standard of proof than other widely accepted medical procedures. Pelletier (1993) states there is less information on the cost-effectiveness or cost-benefits of surgery than on WHP interventions, yet surgical procedures are widely used while WHP interventions meet resistance. These authors recommend widespread implementation of WHP interventions as a means to reduce health care costs by reducing the need and demand for medical services. They also point to additional savings at work resulting from reduced accidents and absenteeism and improved productivity.

A detailed review of the economic consequences of WHP interventions can be found in Kaman (1995), which supports the beneficial effects of WHP interventions but also suggests a more conservative interpretation than that provided by Fries *et al.* (1993) and Pelletier (1993).

Most research on cost-effectiveness or cost–benefits is hampered by the use of correlational or quasi-experimental designs and the inaccessibility of data necessary for accurate estimates of dollar costs and dollar benefits. Data suggest that employees with numerous health risks (e.g. high blood pressure, sedentary lifestyle, smoke cigarettes, overweight) have higher health-care utilization and costs than employees with few or no health risks. However, many factors impact utilization and cost, and little is known about the independent and synergistic effects of WHP interventions. Similarly, employee health risks have been positively associated with absentee-

ism from work and negatively associated with job productivity. But again, many factors impact absenteeism and productivity and the measurement of these outcomes often lacks acceptable reliability and validity.

Kaman (1995) concludes that a growing number of studies report favourable economic results. It is difficult to evaluate and compare these studies, however, because no widely accepted approach currently exits for estimating costs and benefits. Different authors use different assumptions in their estimates of WHP intervention costs and dollar benefits, and small changes in assumptions can have substantial effects. Furthermore, even though computer simulations of WHP interventions suggest that such programmes may be cost-beneficial, economic benefits primarily come from avoiding the opportunity costs of lost productivity rather than from real dollar decreases in health-care costs. Simulations also show that programme effects vary widely across different organizations and from year to year in the same organization (Kaman, 1995).

To our knowledge, no WHP intervention has established that reductions in health-care costs, health-care utilization or absenteeism, and increases in productivity, are causally dependent, either directly or indirectly, on improvements in health risk status brought about by WHP interventions. Until such research is forthcoming, a conservative interpretation of the economic benefits of WHPs is recommended. At the same time, however, data suggest few if any adverse effects on organizational effectiveness and continue to support the worksite as being a critical element in health policy directed at reducing the need and demand for medical services through health promotion and disease prevention.

CONCLUSIONS AND RECOMMENDATIONS

Research supports the worksite as a good setting for health promotion interventions. Numerous anecdotal reports, case studies, correlational designs and quasi-experimental designs have demonstrated that education and behaviour change programmes offered at work can be associated with healthful changes in employee behaviours, and with reductions in risk factors for heart disease and cancer. Data also suggest that WHP interventions can yield favourable cost-effectiveness and cost–benefit ratios. Relatively little work has focused on policy and environment changes at the worksite.

Programme evaluations generally suffer from serious methodological weakness. Rigorous evaluation designs using the worksite as the unit of analysis show considerable variability in outcomes across worksites and are less likely to report positive effects than less sophisticated designs. Estimates of cost-effectiveness and cost–benefits must be interpreted with considerable caution as this complex topic has yet to be addressed in a comprehensive way. Linkages among WHP interventions, employee behaviour, employee health and employee productivity are not well understood and require consideration of multiple levels of analysis, including individual, work group, organization and society.

In addition to research needs identified throughout the review, the following topics need attention: (i) what are the relative advantages and disadvantages of multiple risk factor vs. single risk factor WHP interventions; (ii) are programmes that emphasize widespread employee participation more efficacious than programmes that only target high-risk employees; (iii) how do continuous low cost/low intensity programmes compare to high-intensity programmes offered once or twice a year; (iv) what is the effectiveness of worksite interventions in small and moderate-sized worksites, which often lack resources; (v) what are the independent and synergistic effects of behaviour change programmes and environmental/policy changes; (vi) why are outcomes highly variable across worksites; and (vii) what must be done to produce consistent long-term results from WHP interventions?

As the focus of health-care reform moves towards health promotion and disease prevention, the worksite becomes an increasingly attractive setting. Research has shown the potential of WHP interventions. The task ahead is to understand how WHPs function so they can be reliably implemented and transferred across different worksites.

REFERENCES

Abrams, D.B., Boutwell, W.B., Grizzle, J., Heimendinger, J., Sorensen, G., & Varnes, J. (1994). Cancer control at the workplace: The Working Well Trial. *Preventive Medicine*, **23**, 15–27.

Brenner, H. & Mielck, A. (1992). Smoking prohibition in the workplace and smoking cessation in the Federal Republic of Germany. *Preventive Medicine*, **21**, 252–61.

Erfurt, J.C., Foote, A. & Heirich, M.A. (1991). Worksite wellness programs: incremental comparison of screening and referral alone, health education, follow-up counseling, and plant organization. *American Journal of Health Promotion*, **5**, 438–48.

Fielding, J.E. (1990). Worksite health promotion programs in the United States: Progress, lessons and challenges. *Health Promotion International*, **5**, 4–13.

Fielding, J.E. (1991). Health promotion at the worksite. In G.M. Green & F. Baker (Eds.). *Work, health and productivity*, pp. 256–276. New York: Oxford University Press.

Fisher, K.J., Glasgow, R.E. & Terborg, J.R. (1990). Worksite smoking cessation: a meta-analysis of controlled studies. *Journal of Occupational Medicine*, **32**, 429–39.

Fries, J.F., Koop, C.E., Beadle, C.E., Cooper. P.R., England, M.J., Greaves, R.F., Sokolov, J.J., Wright, D. & Health Project Consortium. (1993). Reducing health care costs by reducing the need and demand for medical services. *The New England Journal of Medicine*, **329**, 321–5.

Glanz, K. (1993). Environmental and policy approaches to cardiovascular disease prevention through nutrition. Paper presented at the workshop on Environmental and Policy Approaches to Cardiovascular Disease Prevention, Centers for Disease Control, Atlanta, Georgia, September 8–10, 1993.

Glasgow, R.E. & Terborg, J.R. (1988) Occupational health promotion programs to reduce cardiovascular risk. *Journal of Consulting and Clinical Psychology*, **56**, 365–3.

Glasgow, R.E., McCaul, K.D. & Fisher, K.J. (1993) Participation in worksite health promotion: A critique of the literature and recommendations for future practice. *Health Education Quarterly*, **20**, 391–408.

Glasgow, R.E., Terborg, J.R., Hollis, J.F., Severson, H.H., Fisher, K.J., Boles, S.M., Pettigrew, E.L., Foster, L.S., Strycker, L.A. & Bischoff, S. (1994) Modifying dietary and tobacco use patterns in the worksite: the Take Heart Project. *Health Education Quarterly*, **21**, 69–82.

Gottlieb, N.H., Eriksen, M.P., Lovato, C.Y., Weinstein, R.P. & Green, L.W. (1990). Impact of a restrictive work site smoking policy on smoking behaviour, attitudes, and norms. *Journal of Occupational Medicine*, **32**, 16–23.

Harvey, M.R., Whitmer, R.W., Hilyer, J.C. & Brown, K.C. (1993). The impact of a comprehensive medical benefits cost management program for the city of Birmingham: results at five years. *American Journal of Health Promotion*, **7**, 296–303.

Henritze, J. & Brammell, H.L. (1989). Phase II cardiac wellness at the Adolph Coors Company. *American Journal of Health Promotion*, **4**, 25–31.

Jeffery, R.W., Forster, S.A., French, S.H., Kelder, H.A., Lando, H.A., McGovern, D.R., Jacobs, D.R. & Baxter, J.E. (1993). The healthy worker project: a worksite intervention for weight control and smoking cessation. *American Journal of Public Health*, **83**, 395–401.

Kaman, R. (Ed.). (1995) *Worksite health promotion economics*. Champaign, IL: Human Kinetics Publishers.

Pelletier, K.R. (1993). A review and analysis of the health and cost-effective outcome studies of comprehensive health promotion and disease prevention programs at the worksite: 1991–1993 update. *American Journal of Health Promotion*, **8**, 50–62.

Shephard, R.J. (1992). A critical analysis of work-site fitness programs and their postulated economic benefits. *Medicine and Science in Sports and Exercise*, **24**, 354–70.

US Department of Health and Human Services (1992). 1992 national survey of worksite health promotion activities: summary. *American Journal of Health Promotion*, **7**, 452–64.

Warner, K.E., Wickizer, T.M., Wolfe, R.A., Schildroth, J.E. & Samuelson, M.H. (1988). Economic implications of workplace health promotion programs: review of the literature. *Journal of Occupational Medicine*, **30**, 106–12.

Wolfe, R., Slack, T. & Rose-Hearn, T. (1993). Factors influencing the adoption and maintenance of Canadian, facility-based worksite health promotion programs. *American Journal of Health Promotion*, **7**, 189–98.

Working Well Research Group. (in press) Cancer control at the workplace: the Working Well Trial. *International Journal of Preventive Medicine*.

SECTION 3: Health-care practice

Attitudes of health professionals
Breaking bad news
Burnout in health professionals
Compliance among health professionals
Compliance among patients
Doctor–patient communication
Health-care work environments
Medical accidents: adverse events in medical treatment

Medical decision-making
Nurse–patient communication: nursing assessment and intervention for effective pain control
Patient satisfaction
Psychological problems: detection
Psychological support for health professionals

Quality of life assessment
Recall by patients
Shiftwork and health
Stress in health professionals
Teaching communication skills
Training and the process of professional development
Training educators
Written communication

Attitudes of health professionals

HANNAH M. McGEE

*Department of Psychology, Royal College of
Surgeons of Ireland, Dublin, Ireland*

INTRODUCTION

Research on attitudes of health professionals has been a relatively marginal activity until recently. This has been because of what Marteau and Johnston (1990) describe as the implicit model of health professional attitudes and beliefs, i.e. that they are knowledge-based and invariant. Health professionals have been seen as having an 'empirically derived set of shared beliefs'. However, a developing literature demonstrates wide variability in health professional attitudes. The importance of this variability is illustrated here in a range of studies which depict the presentation of treatment options for health care users, the professional choices made about access to services and the overall outcome of health care for patients and professionals.

Many of the studies to date have been atheoretical, focusing instead on a description of attitudes themselves or on their associates. Attitudes of health professionals are often inferred rather than being directly assessed. For instance, previous experience is often assessed in relation to current behaviour with attitudes then inferred, as in current patterns of hospital referral for childhood gastroenteritis and the prior training experiences of general practitioners (McGee & Fitzgerald, 1991). Divergent current behaviour, e.g. higher levels of referral to cardiac surgery for male than female patients (King, Clark & Hich, 1992) are also documented and attitudinal influences inferred (in this case a range of attitudes including those relating to the severity of symptoms as presented by men and women). Some cognitive and social psychological constructs have been incorporated in research studies of health professional attitudes, and these are illustrated alongside methodological strategies in the next sections.

ATTITUDES OF HEALTH PROFESSIONALS TO VARYING CHARACTERISTICS OF HEALTH-CARE USERS

Health professionals attribute a range of treatment-relevant characteristics to service users based on information available to them. Thus patients who are reported to practice lifestyle habits associated with the disorder which has been diagnosed, e.g. smoking with lung cancer, are expected to be less concerned about their health and less adherent to medical recommendations (Marteau & Riordan, 1992). Recall of details regarding individuals is greater when it fits with the expected stereotypes of health professionals. For instance, when specific characteristics (e.g. 'promiscuous') were paired with particular background details (e.g. 'homosexual'), they were recalled more readily by counsellors (Casas, Brady & Ponterotto, 1983). Professional attributions may differ depending on the gender of patients. Cardiac staff have been shown to attribute psychological

difficulties following coronary artery bypass surgery to 'emotional problems' in women and to 'organic problems' in men (King *et al.*, 1992). Attitudes also vary in relation to the particular type of health professional involved and in relation to the type of health problem under consideration. In general, health professionals are less willing to be associated with more chronic disorders and with those individuals having a poorer prognosis. Margolies *et al.* (1983) demonstrated that medical students want more professional distance from psychiatric than from cancer patients and from cancer than myocardial infarction patients. Similarly, they want more distance from male than female patients and from those with a poor rather than good prognosis. With regard to differences associated with the type of health professional training undertaken, occupational therapists and physiotherapists have been found to rate the likely benefit of health care to disabled individuals as being higher than do nurses (Johnston *et al.*, 1987).

PROFESSIONAL CHOICES ABOUT ACCESS TO HEALTH SERVICES

It is difficult to directly document how professional attitudes *per se* influence choices about treatment for particular patients. A well-known experimental study by McNeil and colleagues (1982) demonstrated that the format in which information is presented can influence health-care choices for patients, students and physicians. The research task involved choosing between surgical and medical management of cancer given various facts about short- and long-term risks and framing the information in either a positive (survival statistics) or a negative (mortality statistics) manner. For all groups, information presented in a positive framework led to higher levels of adoption of the treatment alternative than did the same statistics presented negatively (i.e. as mortality data). Service availability may be influenced by implicit beliefs about appropriate behaviour by different groups, e.g. women and men in the hospital setting. In the postoperative management of a range of elective procedures, nurses have been shown to offer pain medication less often to men than to women undergoing comparable procedures and also to refuse requests for pain relief more often from men (Bond, 1979). Similarly, physicians are perceived as providing stronger recommendations to attend cardiac rehabilitation programmes to male than to female patients (Ades *et al.*, 1992).

OUTCOME OF HEALTH SERVICES FOR USERS AND PROFESSIONALS

The attitudes and behaviour of health professionals are often influenced by expectations regarding individuals or health problems. Thus, a range of studies which have documented the underdiagnosis of mental health problems in patients with physical disorders and vice versa (Lopez, 1989) suggests a dualist understanding of physical and psychological health problems and illustrates that those with both types of problem may be underserved by the current approach of health professionals. More generally the literature on the placebo effect demonstrates how the attitudes of professionals to health service users and their health problems may be a powerful influence in accelerating or retarding recovery (Friedman, 1993). Health services may be withheld because of a range of attitudes and beliefs of health professionals; thus advice on management of diet to lower cholesterol levels may be withheld because physicians either believe that changing diet will not reduce the risk of heart disease or because they believe that they themselves are not capable of providing the appropriate advice (Schuker *et al.*, 1987). The attitude of the health professional may be expressed in his or her interactions and may thus influence the health outcome. In an early study, Milmoe *et al.*, (1967) demonstrated that the degree of hostility expressed in a physician's voice tone while talking about alcoholic patients was positively associated with physician failure in getting patients into treatment for alcohol problems.

FUTURE DIRECTIONS

The developing literature on attitudes of health professionals is complemented by a more rapidly expanding research focus on cognitive aspects of decision-making in health settings. From the work of Tversky and Kahneman (1981), a large literature on clinical decision-making has evolved (see 'Medical decision making'). Attention to the overlap between these two approaches, i.e. one which focuses on cognitive processes which are seen to be universal influences on health professional decision-making and the other which documents attitudes (affective processes) seen to be exhibited by particular individuals or groups of professionals, may lead to a greater understanding of the nature of health professional behaviour and to more effective methods of educating health professionals as active evaluators of their own influence on the practice of, and outcome from, their interventions. An illustration of work at this level is the evolution of work on adherence to health professional recommendations. Here, rather than searching for the 'non-compliant personality' of the 'patient', recent research has focused on the interaction between health professional and service user and on how characteristics of the health professional and the context influence levels of adherence to health recommendations. Another example of the likely application of a joint approach is the area of professional preferences where, for instance, professionals and service users are both influenced in their choice of treatment by a positive framing (survival rather than mortality data) of information (McNeil *et al.*, 1982). Here, the evaluation of affective influences on choice for individual professionals, e.g. the influence of exposure to the disorder in one's own family or the influence of a poor outcome for a previous case in one's care, could complement the documentation of these general cognitive processes as displayed in decision making.

Further study of the attitudes of health professionals may counterbalance previous attention only to the attitudes of service users. If included in a wider research agenda as suggested here, the findings should positively influence the individual professional's understanding and management of his or her role and thereby improve the delivery of health services in the future.

REFERENCES

Ades, P.A., Wildmann, M.L., Polk, D.M. & Coflesky, J.T. (1992). Referral patterns and exercise response in the rehabilitation of female coronary patients aged > 62 years. *American Journal of Cardiology*, 69, 1422–5.

Bond, M.R. (1979). *Pain*. Edinburgh: Churchill Livingstone.

Casas, J.M., Brady, S. & Ponterotto, J.G. (1983). Sexual preference biases in counselling: an information processing approach. *Journal of Counselling Psychology*, 30, 139–145.

Friedman, H.S. (1993). Interpersonal expectations and the maintenance of health. In P.D. Baanck (Ed.). *Interpersonal expectations. Theory, research and applications*, pp. 179–93. Paris: Cambridge University Press.

Johnston, M., Bromley, I., Boothroyd-Brooks, M., Dobbs, W., Ilson, A. & Ridout, K. (1987). Behavioural assessments of physically disabled patients: agreement between rehabilitation therapists and nurses. *International Journal of Research in Rehabilitation*, 10, 205–3.

King, K.B., Clark, P.C. & Hich, G.L. Jr. (1992). Patterns of referral and recovery in men and women undergoing coronary artery bypass grafting. *American Journal of Cardiology*, 69, 179–82.

Lopez, S.R. (1989). Patient variable biases in clinical judgment: conceptual overview and methodological considerations. *Psychological Bulletin*, 106, 184–203.

Margolies, R., Wachtel, A.B., Sutherland, K.R. & Blum, R.H. (1983). Medical students' attitudes towards cancer: concepts of professional distance. *Journal of Psychosocial Oncology*, 1, 35–49.

Marteau, T.M. & Johnston, M. (1990). Health professionals: a source of variance in patient outcomes. *Psychology and Health*, 5, 47–58.

Marteau, T.M. & Riordan, D.C. (1992). Staff attitudes towards patients: the influence of causal attributions for illness. *British Journal of Clinical Psychology*, 31, 107–10.

McGee, H.M. & Fitzgerald, M. (1991). The impact of hospital experiences during training on GP referral rates. *Irish Journal of Psychological Medicine*, 7, 22–3.

McNeil, B., Pauker, S., Sox, H. & Tversky, A. (1982). On the elicitation of preferences for alternative therapies. *The New England Journal of Medicine*, 306, 1259–62.

Milmoe, S., Rosenthal, R., Blane, H.T., Chafetz, M.L., & Wolf, I. (1967). The doctor's voice: postdictor of successful referral of alcoholic patients. *Journal of Abnormal Psychology*, 72, 78–84.

Schuker, B., Wittes, J.T., Cutler, J.A., Bailey, K., Mackintosh, D.R., Gordon, D.J., Haines, C.M., Mattson, M.E., Goor, R.S. & Rifkind, B.M. (1987). Changes in physician perspective on cholesterol and heart disease: results from two national surveys. *Journal of the American Medical Association*, 258, 3521–6.

Tversky, A. & Kahneman, D. (1981). The framing of decisions and the psychology of choice. *Science*, 211, 453–8.

Breaking bad news

PETER MAGUIRE

CRC Psychologist Medicine Group,
Christie Hospital, Manchester, UK

INTRODUCTION

Studies of doctors breaking bad news to patients have found that they tend to make assumptions about whether the patient should be told the truth or not, or are too influenced by relatives who persuade them not to tell the patient. Most patients already have some awareness that their illness is potentially serious. This may have provoked specific worries about what might be said. As patients hear the news, this may confirm their worries and provoke new ones. This should lead them to become emotionally upset and give verbal and non-verbal signs of this.

Recordings of bad news consultations have found that, instead of exploring these worries, doctors immediately give detailed information about the patient's illness and treatment (Maguire, 1985).

The immediate consequence of this avoidance of exploring the patients' concerns and associated feelings is that they remain preoccupied with these concerns which often derive from bad experiences of serious illness in others. Because they are so preoccupied, they fail to take in the offered information and advice. Instead, they selectively register negative phrases even when positive statements are also being made.

Thus, in one example, the surgeon told a lady who had just been diagnosed as having breast cancer, 'we will give you radiotherapy to mop up any residual cells. I am sure we will eradicate your cancer'. The patient only remembered the phrase 'residual' cells and took that to mean that her cancer was going to spread through her body. Consequently, she remained very distressed.

A longer-term consequence of this avoidance of exploring patients' concerns and emotions after the breaking of bad news is that there is a much greater risk that patients will later develop a generalized anxiety disorder or depressive illness. For, a follow up study of over 600 newly diagnosed cancer patients found that one of the strongest predictors of later anxiety and depression was the number and severity of the patients' unresolved concerns (Parle, Jones & Maguire, 1996).

So, a key question in considering the breaking of bad news is why doctors are so loathe to explore patients' concerns and feelings before moving into information and advice mode.

BARRIERS TO HANDLING EMOTION

Lack of training

Experienced doctors and nurses attending workshops to help them improve their communication skills commonly ask for help with the breaking of bad news. (Maguire & Faulkner, 1988). Few have had any formal training in strategies that would help them to break bad news in a way that facilitated psychological adaption.

Fear of damaging the patient

Health professionals tend to perceive their patients as vulnerable psychologically. They fear that probing patients' concerns and feelings will damage the patient emotionally. They fear that they may unleash strong emotions like despair and anger and will not be able to contain these. Exploring patients' concerns and feelings will also take too much time.

Lack of support

Doctors and nurses are more likely to explore patients' concerns and feelings if they perceive that they will be supported practically and emotionally by their colleagues (Wilkinson, 1991; Booth, 1993). So, if doctors and nurses are to break bad news effectively, they need to feel that they are working in an environment which will be supportive of their efforts especially when they encounter difficulties as a result of breaking bad news.

Personal survival

Breaking bad news is a hard and unpleasant task. Once patients assimilate the truth they usually become very upset. If patients are then encouraged to talk about their concerns and feelings, this brings doctors face to face with the reality of their patients' predicament and suffering. Doctors question whether they can afford to do this frequently since they have to survive emotionally.

Given these barriers, any account of how to break bad news must consider the strategies that can be used, how to avoid damaging patients psychologically, and how health professionals can get the necessary support and survive emotionally.

WAYS OF BREAKING BAD NEWS

Guiding principles

A patient's psychological adaptation to serious disease is proportional to the extent to which they perceive the information given was adequate to their needs. Too much or too little information is associated with a poor psychological adjustment (Fallowfield *et al.*, 1990). So, a key aim is to try and tailor the information given to what the patient wishes and is ready to hear.

The second principle is to avoid withholding information because a relative insists that the patient is unable to handle the bad news. Such collusion is associated with the later development of affective disorders in patients and poor control of symptoms like pain. The secrecy leads to the surviving relatives having much unfinished business practically and emotionally. They may also feel guilty about witholding the truth from the patient. These factors greatly increase the risk that their grief will remain unresolved and be a source of major psychiatric morbidity. So, it is best to prevent collusion at the outset.

Objectives of breaking bad news

The main aims are to ensure that patients assimilate accurately the information they are ready to hear without provoking denial or overwhelming emotional distress. It is also important to help patients disclose their concerns about the news and mention and express associated feelings. Strategies that enable the health professional to achieve these objectives will now be described.

Key steps

The first step is to check the patient's awareness. It is important to ask patients what they think might be causing their symptoms rather than ask them what a doctor has previously told them. It is then useful to check why patients think they have a particular disease or poor prognosis to confirm that they are correctly aware of their predicament. The health professional is then in the position of confirming that the patients' perceptions are correct. ('I am afraid you are right, we are not going to be able to cure it'.)

Some 80% of patients with cancer are aware of the nature of their disease even if they have not been told directly. So, breaking bad news in this context is a matter of confirming an existing awareness. A more difficult issue is how to handle the important minority of patients who have little or no awareness that they have a serious illness.

It is particularly important to avoid breaking bad news abruptly since that will push the patient into denial or cause emotional disorganisation. It is best to slow the bad news process down and do so in a way that allows patients time to signal if they do not wish to proceed. This can be done by using a hierarchy of euphemisms. Thus, the clinician should begin by firing a warning shot, 'I am afraid it is more serious than we thought' and then give patients time to indicate if they wish to proceed or move on to some other topic. The patient who wishes to proceed will ask, 'What do you mean serious?' instead of moving the doctor onto a topic like treatment with a question like, 'What are you going to be able to do about it'? When a patient developed a recurrence of lung cancer, the dialogue went as follows:

Doctor	The X-ray we did showed some new shadows.
Patient	New shadows?
Doctor	Yes, this suggests there is more tumour.
Patient	So, it is spreading?
Doctor	It looks like it, yes.

It is important to heed patients' signals about how far they want to go rather than ignore them.

Doctor	So, you realize that you have got cancer of the cervix then?
Patient	Yes, I realized it was serious.
Doctor	I think it important I put you fully in the picture. I believe people should know all about their illness these days.
Patient	I don't want to hear the details, I just want you to tell me what you can do.
Doctor	No, I think I should tell you exactly what is going on

so that you fully understand the nature of your illness and the treatment.

This insistence on giving her unwanted information led to her to present within 48 hours to the psychiatric service with severe depression.

After awareness is confirmed or news broken

The health professional should pause and allow the bad news to sink in for patients need time to assimilate what is being said. Inevitably, they will become distressed. It is very important to acknowledge this as soon as it becomes evident by saying, for example, 'I can see that what I have told you has made you very upset'. It is then helpful to explore the reasons for patients' distress even though these may seem obvious. This can be done by saying, 'could you bear to tell me what exactly is making you so upset'? This may seem a banal question but it gives patients permission to talk about their concerns and feelings. Otherwise these are likely to remain undisclosed (Heaven & Maguire, 1996). Reassurance and advice should not be offered until all the patient's concerns have been identified. Otherwise, the reassurance may be inappropriate.

Surgeon	I am sorry I have had to tell you that you have breast cancer. The good news is I am confident we are going to cure it. We will get you in soon and sort it out.
Patient	I am not very happy about it.
Surgeon	I wouldn't say we could help you unless I was confident.
Patient	That's what the doctor told my sister. She still died from her cancer.

Had the surgeon first established why the patient was upset, he would have found out about her experience of cancer in her sister who had been reassured similarly. He, could then have pitched his reassurance at an appropriate level ('Of course, I can understand why you are so worried about your own cancer, but I think we have caught your cancer at a much earlier stage').

Once the patient's concerns have been elicited, the patient should be asked to put them in priority order in case there isn't sufficient time to cover them all. Patients usually have two or three main concerns and these are susceptible to effective reassurance because something can be done about each of them (Harrison et al., 1994). Thus, the doctor might say, 'You mention that you are worried about whether we are going to be able to treat it, that you may end up having a stoma, and may be given chemotherapy which would make you sick. Which of these worries would you like to talk about first'?

When patients disclose their concerns, these should be summarized before asking if they have any other concerns in case they are holding an important one back. When working through their concerns, every effort should be made to pitch any reassurance appropriately. If someone has early cancer, it is helpful to say, 'I am very confident we can eradicate it'. If the disease has recurred, it may be more appropriate to say, 'I am pretty sure we can control it' while, if a patient has advanced disease, it may be best to say, 'I don't think we are going to be able to cure your illness but we can do our best to control any symptoms like the pain you are having'. Such reassurance gives patients some hope.

If bad news is broken in this way, patients' distress will usually remain within manageable limits and they will adjust psychologically.

Exploring feelings

There are an important minority of patients who do not like to talk about their feelings and can be made worse by being encouraged to do so (Maguire et al., 1980). It is important to check this before exploring a patient's reactions to the bad news ('I can see you are upset. Can you bear to talk about it?'). If the patient indicates she doesn't want to, her wish should be respected.

Even when patients agree to talk about their reactions, the health professional should monitor the effects.

If the patient seems to be getting too distressed, the health professional should try to check by saying, for example, 'I can see you are getting very distressed, does that mean it would be better if we stopped talking about your illness at this point'?

It is always possible to validate how the interview is going by asking the patient directly 'How are you feeling at this point'?

CONCLUSION

It is increasingly apparent that the way the bad news consultation is handled has a profound effect on the patient's appraisal of his predicament and later psychological adjustment. It is likely that if this is handled more effectively there will be much less psychiatric morbidity associated with the diagnosis and treatment of cancer. Moreover, it has been found that training can lead to marked improvement in health professionals, ability to break bad news.

REFERENCES

Booth, K. (1993). Helping patients with cancer: putting psychological assessment skills into practice. PhD Thesis, University of Manchester.

Fallowfield, L.J., Hall, A., Maguire, G.P. & Baum, M. (1990). Psychological outcomes of different treatment policies in women with early breast cancer outside a clinical trial. British Medical Journal, 301, 575–80.

Harrison, J., Maguire, P., Ibbotson, T., MacLeod, R. & Hopwood, P. (1994). Concerns, confiding and psychiatric disorder in newly diagnosed cancer patients: a descriptive study. Psychological Oncology, 3, 173–9.

Heaven, C.M. & Maguire, P. (1996). Training hospice nurses to elicit patients' concerns. Journal of Advanced Nursing Studies, 23, 280–6.

Maguire, P. (1985). Barriers to psychological care of the dying. British Medical Journal, 291, 1711–13.

Maguire, P. & Faulkner, A. (1988). How to improve the counselling skills of doctors and nurses involved in cancer care. 297, 847–9.

Maguire, G.P., Tait, A., Brooke, M., Thomas, C. & Sellwood, R. (1980). The effects of counselling on the psychiatric morbidity associated with mastectomy. British Medical Journal 281, 1454–6.

Parle, M., Jones, B. & Maguire, P. (1996). Maladaptive coping and affective disorders in cancer patients. Psychological Medicine, 26, 736–44

Wilkinson, S. (1991). Factors which influence how nurses communicate with cancer patients. Journal of Advanced Nursing, 16, 677–88.

Burnout in health professionals

CHRISTINA MASLACH

Department of Psychology, University of California, Berkeley, USA

Burnout is a type of prolonged response to chronic emotional and interpersonal stressors on the job (Kleiber & Enzmann, 1990; Schaufeli, Maslach & Marek, 1993). As such, it has been an issue of particular concern for human services occupations where: (a) the relationship between providers and recipients is central to the work, and (b) the provision of service, care, treatment, or education can be a highly emotional experience. These criteria certainly apply to health professions, which have long been recognized as stressful occupations (Cartwright, 1979). Indeed, much of the earliest research on burnout was conducted in the area of health care (Maslach 1982; Maslach & Jackson, 1982).

THE MULTIDIMENSIONAL MODEL OF BURNOUT

Burnout has been conceptualized as an individual stress experience that is embedded in a context of social relationships, and thus involves the person's conception of both self and others. The operational definition that is most widely used in burnout research is a three-component model of emotional exhaustion, depersonalization, and reduced personal accomplishment (Maslach & Jackson, 1986; Maslach, Jackson & Leiter, 1996). Emotional exhaustion refers to feelings of being emotionally overextended and depleted of one's emotional resources (it has also been described as wearing out, loss of energy, depletion, debilitation, and fatigue). Depersonalization refers to a negative, callous, or excessively detached response to other people, who are usually the recipients of one's service or care (depersonalization has also been described as negative or inappropriate attitudes towards patients, loss of idealism, and irritability). Reduced personal accomplishment refers to a decline in one's feelings of competence and successful achievement in one's work (it has also been described as reduced productivity or capability, low morale, withdrawal, and an inability to cope).

These three components of burnout can be illustrated by the experiences of health-care professionals (Maslach & Jackson, 1982). Clearly, there are significant emotional experiences linked to the caregiving relationship between health worker and patient. Some of these experiences are enormously rewarding and uplifting, as when patients recover because of the worker's efforts. However, other experiences are emotionally stressful for the health practitioner, such as working with difficult or unpleasant patients, having to give 'bad news' to patients or their families, dealing with patient deaths, or having conflicts with coworkers or supervisors. These emotional strains are sometimes overwhelming and lead to emotional exhaustion.

To protect themselves against such disruptive feelings, health professionals may moderate their compassion for patients by distancing themselves psychologically, avoiding over-involvement, and maintaining a more detached objectivity (a process known as 'detached concern'; Lief & Fox, 1963). For example, if a patient has a condition that is upsetting to see or otherwise difficult to work with, it is easier for the practitioner to provide the necessary care if he or she thinks of the patient as a particular 'case' or 'symptom' rather than as a human being who is suffering. However, the blend of compassion and emotional distance is difficult to achieve in actual practice, and too often the balance shifts toward a negative and depersonalized perception of patients. A derogatory and demeaning view of patients is likely to be matched by a decline in the quality of the care that is provided to them.

Many health professionals have not had sufficient preparation for the emotional reality of their work and its subsequent impact on their personal functioning. Thus, the experience of emotional turmoil on the job is likely to be interpreted as a failure to 'be professional' (i.e. to be non-emotional, cool, and objective). Consequently, these health workers begin to question their own ability to work in a health career and to feel that their personal accomplishments are falling short of their expectations. These failures may be as much a function of the work setting as of any personal shortcomings; providing good health care may be difficult to accomplish in the context of staff shortages, poor training, or inadequate resources. Nevertheless, health workers may begin to develop a negative self-evaluation, which can impair their job performance or even lead them to quit the job altogether.

Burnout has often been described in terms of such symptoms as exhaustion, fatigue, loss of self-esteem, problems in concentration, irritability, and negativism, as well as a significant decrease in work performance over a period of several months. Burnout appears to last for some time, underscoring the notion that its nature is more chronic than acute. Unlike depression, which is considered to be context free and pervasive across all situations, burnout is regarded as job related and situation specific. It is usually assumed that burnout symptoms manifest themselves in 'normal' persons who do not suffer from prior psychopathology or an identifiable organic illness. However, there is not, as yet, a reliable method for diagnosing burnout at the individual level (Maslach & Schaufeli, 1993).

In terms of outcomes, burnout can lead to a deterioration in the quality of care or service provided to clients or patients. It appears to be a factor in job turnover, absenteeism, and low morale, and seems to be correlated with various self-reported indices of personal dysfunction, including poor physical health, insomnia, increased use of alcohol and drugs, and marital and family problems (Maslach & Jackson, 1986).

The multidimensional model of burnout has important theoretical and practical implications. It provides a more complete understanding of this form of job stress by locating it within its social context and by identifying the variety of psychological reactions that different workers can experience. Such differential responses may not be simply a function of individual factors (such as personality), but may reflect the differential impact of situational factors on the three burnout dimensions. For example, certain job characteristics may influence the sources of emotional stress (and thus emotional exhaustion), or the resources available to handle the job successfully (and thus personal accomplishment). This multidimensional approach also implies that interventions to reduce burnout should be planned and designed in terms of the particular component of burnout that needs to be addressed. That is, it may be more effective to consider how to reduce the likelihood of emotional exhaustion, or to prevent the tendency to depersonalize, or to enhance one's sense of accomplishment, rather than to use a more general approach.

KEY RISK FACTORS IN HEALTH PROFESSIONS

The context of the job setting defines the nature of health professionals' relationships with their patients. Inherent in the structure of this relationship are factors that can promote the risk of burnout because they either increase the level of emotional stress, produce negative perceptions of the care recipients, or reduce the workers' sense of efficacy. Given the centrality of this caregiving relationship in the aetiology of burnout, it is not surprising that research has found that job factors are more strongly predictive of burnout than are demographic or personality variables. Within health professions, the most critical job factors seem to be those that affect patient care, personal control, and social support.

Patient care

Health professionals are trained to provide cures and improve patient health. Thus the most 'desirable' health problems to work with, in terms of the greatest likelihood of success, are those that are non-chronic and remediable. However, there are many instances in which the health outcomes are not successful; treatments are ineffective, and patients either fail to improve or die. Health professionals' sense of personal accomplishment and competence can be seriously threatened in the face of inevitable failure to heal all of their patients or bring about long-term progress. In addition to (or instead of) blaming themselves for their apparent failures, health professionals may also deal with their frustrations by blaming the patient for not getting better or for contracting the disease in the first place.

Both the quantity and quality of the contact between health professional and patient are important risk factors. Burnout is associated with more time spent in direct care of patients, as opposed to other professional tasks, and with a greater intensity of patient contact. This intensity is a function of the physical and psychological demands involved in caring for particular patients, and these demands will vary with the health worker's job responsibilities and expectations. In terms of physical demands, professionals providing direct care for patients with highly debilitating health problems may have to work harder and do more than they would for patients with other problems. In addition to greater time and effort, many of these care-giving tasks may be quite difficult or upsetting to perform because they involve responding to multiple, severe, disfiguring and/or uncontrollable disease symptoms.

Increased psychological demands can also arise from having to deal with the emotional reactions of the patients themselves. Patients may express a wide range of feelings about their health problems and the procedures they have to undergo, including fear, anxiety, embarrassment, anger, and denial. They may have difficulty communicating with the health professional, they may complain and cause problems regarding their care, and they may even be rude or obnoxious in their personal style. Furthermore, some patients may be experiencing depression or other severe psychological problems. Health professionals without psychological training may feel that they are ill-equipped to respond to the emotional needs of their patients. The severity and unpredictability of these symptoms may increase the likelihood that the health professional will depersonalize the patient.

The emotional strain of working with any one patient can be multiplied by the need to deal with the patient's family as well. Family members may be upset or frightened by what is happening to the patient, they may be impatient and demanding in their actions on the patient's behalf, and so forth. Even when the needs of the family are well recognized, providing supportive care for these people can be an additional burden for the practitioner.

Other patient characteristics can exacerbate the emotional stress experienced by health workers. Anything that reminds practitioners of their own loved ones (such as a parent or child), or that causes them to identify with the patient, will increase the emotional strain of working with that patient. In particular, work with young patients who are terminally ill poses a greater risk of burnout for health professionals.

From another perspective, identification or solidarity with some patients can serve to provide an enhanced sense of meaning or purpose to professionals' work. Health workers may legitimately envision themselves as fighting on the scientific or political front lines in the battle against major diseases, such as AIDS, and providing critical services to people in dire need.

Control and ambiguity

Being able to control, or at least predict, outcomes is a critical aspect of human functioning. When opportunities for control are absent and people feel trapped in an environment that is neither controllable nor predictable, both psychological and physical health are likely to suffer (Janis & Rodin, 1979). In a related way, when workers experience ambiguity and uncertainty about what they are expected to accomplish and whether they are doing it sufficiently well, then they are likely to experience greater stress and their job performance suffers (McGrath, 1976).

Burnout is consistently linked to job factors in the health-care setting which entail greater ambiguity and less control (Maslach & Jackson, 1982). Some of these factors were mentioned earlier: the limitations of modern medicine, and the difficulties in working with patients. However, relationships with colleagues are a critical source of problems concerning control and ambiguity. Health professionals must often work closely and interdependently with each other, but may differ in status and power (as in the case of physicians and nurses). Consequently, some workers have little control over the decisions that determine their daily activities and may receive little feedback about the results of their efforts. In some cases, health workers have no influence on institutional policies that govern the hours and conditions of their work, and few opportunities for creativity and autonomy in carrying out their job tasks.

Although some of the factors that produce less control and more ambiguity are inevitable parts of the job, there are others that are amenable to change. Thus, for example, the development of more participative decision-making procedures or better methods of providing meaningful feedback and recognition have the potential to improve the job environment and thus reduce the risk of burnout. Improved job training should include preparation for difficult and stressful work-related situations, as well as essential medical skills. Such training is particularly important for those jobs that are judged to be 'purely technical', which means that the psychological stresses of the work often go unrecognized.

Accentuating the positive aspects of the job and finding ways to make ordinary tasks more meaningful are additional methods for gaining greater self-efficacy and control. A health worker's personal sense of control can also be strengthened by a feeling of participation in a larger community or movement. Such involvement in action-orientated groups or communities (and even small victories in the political or social arena) can counteract the helplessness and pessimism that are commonly evoked by the absence of long-term solutions to the problem.

Social support

Because involvement with people is central to the experience of burnout, it is not surprising that the role of other individuals is central to coping effectively with it. Social support and feedback, particularly from one's peers, is predictive of a lower risk of burnout (Leiter & Maslach, 1988; Maslach & Jackson, 1982). Peers can reduce stress by helping the worker to withdraw from a difficult situation and gain some perspective on it, by giving comfort and emotional support, by sharing their own feelings and alternative responses to similar problems, and by providing positive feedback.

Given the sources of stress and burnout inherent in the health-care setting, it is important for health professionals to develop and utilize support systems within that setting (as well as outside of it, in the sense of social support from family and friends). Such support can be the critical difference in enabling health professionals to deal effectively with such difficult issues as ambivalence towards patients, fear of infection, death anxiety, and burnout.

CONCLUSION

The practice of medicine has long been regarded as one of the noblest of occupations. To cure illness, repair injury, promote health, and even forestall death are skills that are highly esteemed in all societies. Although the personal rewards and satisfactions of a health career are many, it is not without its hazards, including that of burnout. However, recent research has improved our understanding of the dynamics of this syndrome, and provides many insights into possible solutions to this important problem.

REFERENCES

Cartwright, L.K. (1979). Sources and effects of stress in health careers. In G.C. Stone, F. Cohen & N.E. Adler (Eds.). *Health psychology*, pp. 419–445. San Francisco: Jossey-Bass.

Janis, I.L. & Rodin, J. (1979). Attribution, control, and decision making: social psychology and health care. In G.C. Stone, F. Cohen & N.E. Adler (Eds.), *Health psychology*, pp. 487–521. San Francisco: Jossey-Bass.

Kleiber, D. & Enzmann, D. (1990). *Burnout: 15 years of research: an international bibliography*. Gottingen: Hogrefe.

Leiter, M.P. & Maslach, C. (1988). The impact of interpersonal environment on burnout and organizational commitment.

Journal of Organizational Behavior, 9, 297–308.

Lief, H.I. & Fox, R.C. (1963). Training for 'detached concern' in medical students. In H.I. Lief, V.F. Lief & N.R. Lief (Eds.). *The psychological basis of medical practice*. New York: Harper & Row.

McGrath, J.E. (1976). Stress and behavior in organizations. In M.D. Dunnette (Ed.). *Handbook of industrial and organizational psychology*. Chicago: Rand McNally.

Maslach, C. (1982). *Burnout: the cost of caring*. Englewood Cliffs, NJ: Prentice-Hall.

Maslach, C. & Jackson, S.E. (1981/1986). *The Maslach Burnout Inventory*. Palo Alto, CA: Consulting Psychologists Press.

Maslach, C. & Jackson, S.E. (1982). Burnout in health professions: a social psychological

analysis. In G. Sanders & J. Suls (Eds.). *Social psychology of health and illness*. Hillsdale, NJ: Erlbaum.

Maslach, C., Jackson, S.E. & Leiter, M.P. (1996). *The Maslach Burnout Inventory* 3rd edn. Palo Alto, CA: Consulting Psychologists Press.

Maslach, C. & Schaufeli, W.B. (1993). Historical and conceptual development of burnout. In W.B. Schaufeli, C. Maslach & T. Marek (Eds.). *Professional burnout: recent developments in theory and research*. Washington, DC: Taylor & Francis.

Schaufeli, W.B., Maslach, C. & Marek, T. (Eds.). (1993). *Professional burnout: recent developments in theory and research*. Washington, DC: Taylor & Francis.

Compliance among health professionals

MARY K. O'BRIEN

Allegheny University of the Health Sciences,
Division of Medical Education,
USA

INTRODUCTION

Patient compliance with medical regimens has been reviewed, studied, and intervened with for decades. Research in a wide range of studies indicates that a high number of patients do not comply fully with prescribed medical treatments (Ley, 1988; Meichenbaum and Turk, 1987). While compliance among health-care professionals has seldom received the same attention as patient compliance, research indicates that noncompliance among health care professionals is also high. Efforts have intensified in this area of research more recently because it has been recognized as a health problem for patients and professionals alike. The concern for infection control in light of the HIV virus and AIDS as well as an increase in litigation in the health care field have resulted in the desire for more strict compliance with the health care delivery process. Although professional non-compliance behaviours can refer to health protective behaviours such as complying with medical treatment, quitting smoking, healthy eating, flossing teeth, exercising, and completing annual physical exams (Meichenbaum & Turk, 1987), the focus of this chapter is to look at types of professional non-compliance with health-care procedures, why these behaviours occur, and what can be done to improve professional compliance.

DEFINITION AND EXTENT OF PROFESSIONAL NON-COMPLIANCE

Professional non-compliance has been described as any departure by health professionals (including doctors, nurses, pharmacists and dentists) from guidelines for appropriate and satisfactory health and medical care (Ley, 1988). Non-compliance may cover a broad range of behaviours from improper procedures for infection control in hospitals to inappropriately prescribing medications.

In a review of professional non-compliance, Ley (1988) described a range of behaviours with which doctors sometimes fail to comply. For example, a number of studies have investigated how doctors prescribed medications. Estimates of the percentage of doctors who are non-compliant with antibiotic prescriptions in particular typically vary between 12% and 76% (Ley, 1988). Several studies found that up to 66% of patients received antibiotics when none was needed or in other inappropriate ways.

Doctors also appear to have low rates of compliance with providing information about the medications they prescribe. In general, about 50% of patient usually do not receive the information they should, although Ley (1988) reported that, in some studies, patients received no information at all. Ironically, doctors also fail to provide themselves with information. Even though most professional organizations require members to regularly attend continuing education seminars and complete refresher courses, 37–43% fail to do so. Research suggests that non-compliance with attending continuing education or refresher courses can be as high as 45% and non-compliance with providing enough information about the medical treatment ranges between 25 and 100%.

Other non-compliance behaviours by doctors include the inappropriate use of injections, not following up with appointments and treatment for patients with high blood pressure, not providing adequate information for other treatment components, and not completing appropriate diagnostic or preventative tests. For example, in a study of general practitioner's compliance with a number of recommended cancer screening tests, Osborn et al. (1991) found that there was an overall low level of compliance with six of seven cancer screening tests. There were exceptions, however. For instance, the higher the percentage of visits that were scheduled for preventative reasons, the more likely mammograms were ordered and pelvis and breast exams were conducted. In addition, the more often doctors reported reading journals and keeping up to date with recent trends in medicine and medical research, the more often stool occult blood tests, sigmoidoscopies and pap smears were ordered. Osborn et al. also found that female doctors were more likely to order pap smears and initiate preventative care medical visits with their patients.

Doctors are also required, in some places in the US for example, to report possible cases of child abuse to the proper authorities. One study found that, of nurses, doctors, ministers and psychologists, doctors were one of the groups most likely to be non-compliant with this regulation (Williams, Osborn & Rappaport, 1987). However, Williams et al. also found that overall knowledge of, and compliance with, the Louisiana mandatory child abuse reporting laws was low by all four groups of professionals. Nurses and ministers were more likely to report suspected cases of abuse than doctors and psychologists.

Compliance by doctors with universal precautions in a hospital environment also appears to be low. In one study, it was reported that, even though medical staff and medical students believed that they were at more risk at work than in their private lives, most of the medical students and about one-half of the staff did not comply with universal precautions for working with patients with AIDS in a hospital environment (Elford & Cockcroft, 1991). Future research could explore whether or not medical staff who perceive that they are at risk for HIV infection would have better compliance rates with precautions (Gerberding, 1991).

Nurses also have surprisingly low rates of compliance with infection control procedures in hospitals and with issuing medications to patients in hospitals. Wheeless, Wheeless and Riffle (1989) found that nurses were more likely to be compliant with hospital guidelines for proper care when rules were flexible and when the doctors appeared to be more responsive to nurses in discussions about patient treatment. The more doctors were responsive, the more nurses were compliant and the less they were apt to make quick and inappropriate decisions.

Weingarten et al. (1989) found that compliance with a flu vaccine by nurses and doctors in a hospital was low (2%). Of 108 nurses and 85 doctors, 35% experienced a flu when an influenza virus was isolated in the hospital. Of these, 76.6% continued to care for patients even when ill. The medical staff reported not complying with a flu vaccine because they wanted to avoid medications and any adverse reactions that be associated with the vaccine and because the process was inconvenient.

Non-compliance with isolation precautions by nurses in a hospital setting is widespread (Pettinger & Nettleman, 1991). The compliance rate for strict isolation behaviours in one study was 65% and with wound and skin infections was 40%. Compliance with isolation

precautions involving excretion/secretion problems was even lower (36%). In fact, Pettinger and Nettleman found that visitors' compliance with isolation precautions was significantly higher than nurses' and other health-care workers' compliance (88% versus 41%, respectively, $p < .01$). Perhaps the increased demands placed on nurses and doctors in order to contain health-care delivery costs affect the ability to comply with isolation precautions and other procedures.

Dentists have low compliance rates with their own professional guidelines such as protecting themselves and their patients from X-rays by providing shields and wearing eye protection, gloves, masks and disposable gowns. A review of the literature showed that 66–92% of patients receiving dental X-rays were not provided with protective shielding during the X-ray procedure (Ley, 1988). In a study looking at the incidence and type of accidents and non-compliance behaviours in the dental industry, a high rate of accidental parenteral inoculations with sharp instruments occurred to dentists (94%), dental hygienists (95%) and dental assistants (97%) (Klein et al., 1988). Klein et al. found that 69% of dentists did not always use gloves and 61% never wore disposable gowns. Non-compliance with wearing gloves was equally high for dental assistants (92%) but not as high for hygienists (27%).

Much like doctors, pharmacists have low rates of compliance with providing information about medications. Compliance with regulations to inform patients about medications and warn patients of potentially harmful contraindications or possible side-effects ranged from 36–57%. This included providing adequate instructions for taking the medication as well as giving patients information about the make-up of the drug in some sort of take-home pamphlet form.

In addition, pharmacists are often non-compliant with keeping records on patients or checking with patients at the time of purchase what other medications they may be taking. The range of compliance with this procedure has been as low as 8–17%. This health-care delivery policy is recommended so that pharmacists can avoid providing medications that are contraindicated with certain illnesses or with other drugs that are currently being taken.

VARIABLES ASSOCIATED WITH PROFESSIONAL NON-COMPLIANCE

There appear to be two categories of variables that contribute to professional noncompliance with health care delivery procedures. Non-compliance with the rules and regulations of administering medical care by professionals appears to occur intentionally and unintentionally. Lack of knowledge, forgetfulness, or lack of familiarity with the current technology are associated with, and are considered unintentional causes of, professional non-compliance. For example, Osborn et al. (1991) found that, if general practitioners understood the benefits of the screening tests and the ease with which they could be conducted, compliance with suggesting the tests could be higher. Williams et al. (1987) suggested that compliance with reporting suspected child abuse cases could increase if knowledge about the system was increased and if health-care professionals were regularly reminded.

Unintentional barriers to professional compliance also include issues to do with job satisfaction and the availability of resources. That is, if the health-care professional cares about his or her job, then attendance at refresher or continuing education courses may be higher than for those who are not as interested. The off-shoot of attending classes, of course, is the increase in the likelihood of proper health care such as more appropriate prescriptions or medical tests.

Space and time limitations, available personnel for assistance, the difficulty of having to handle multiple tasks are also considerations for compliance behaviours. These were found to be the unintentional obstacles that contributed to non-compliance by medical staff with existing regulations for the handling of chemotherapeutic drugs in an office setting. In addition, the cost-effectiveness of safety equipment for medical staff protection was unclear, thus compliance with obtaining the necessary equipment was low. Valanis, McNeil and Driscoll (1991) found that the use of protective garments and equipment by nurses, pharmacists and doctors was low when handling antineoplastic drugs. However, non-compliance in this case was associated with what the staff believed was important rather than policy content. The medical staff did not believe in the proposed dangers associated with handling antineoplastic agents and therefore actively chose not to use the protective gear.

This latter study illustrates variables that are regarded as intentional rather than unintentional causes of noncompliance among health-care professionals. Intentional variables usually include beliefs and attitudes of the professional. Savage *et al.* (1987) found that subjective norms such as beliefs about specific rules and attitudes towards doctors and patients contribute to nurses' compliance with do-not-resuscitate orders in a neonatal unit. Nurses were more compliant with those orders if they agreed that the infant should not be resuscitated and also if the parents agreed to these orders. Nurses respected the wishes of the parents when making decisions about resuscitation in this study. However, social pressures have also been reported as variables that contribute to non-compliance (nurses in particular) with hospital rules. That is, nurses may defer to doctors' decisions even though these decisions may result in noncompliance with health care delivery regulations.

Finally, Meichenbaum and Turk (1987) have described health-care professional inertia as a predominant variable contributing to non-compliance among these professionals. The seeming difficulty of a particular medical task (such as providing information when there is little time to discuss this information) as well as a belief that there is no direct benefit to the professional for compliance with certain regulations are some of the reasons for this inertia. This professional inertia may also result from job dissatisfaction and lack of knowledge about how or when to comply. However, there are a number of ways to overcome professional inertia as well as improve compliance with medical procedures and regulations. Improvements in the quality of service, saving time, financial benefits, and establishing long-term relationships with patients are just some of the benefits for professionals from improving the quality of health-care delivery through compliance with its procedures.

IMPROVING PROFESSIONAL COMPLIANCE

Two main approaches have been used to improve compliance among health-care professionals with some success: education and behaviour modification programmes. The goal of education programmes has been to increase the professional's knowledge by providing guidelines, training, or written information. It has been noted that it is difficult to evaluate the effects of education programmes on professional compliance because of the subjectivity of the information and difficulty in measuring professional compliance (Gerberding, 1991; Ley, 1988; Meichenbaum & Turk, 1987). In studies that have attempted to examine the effects of education programmes, many of the education programmes have failed to successfully increase long-term compliance. Even a simple information procedure such as informing medical staff of patients' diagnosis (e.g. those with AIDS or who were HIV positive) failed to increase compliance with precautions such as accidental exposures to blood and other body fluids or inadvertent injections (Gerberding, 1991). Campbell *et al.* (1991) found that education intervention alone appears not to have altered nursing staff's performance with geriatric patients urinary incontinence. However, they suggested that education programmes be used in conjunction with behaviour modification techniques in future professional compliance studies.

Behavioural strategies used to improve compliance include monitoring, feedback, and prompting. Memory prompts, reminder cues on the back of prescription forms or in patients' charts, behavioural feedback and performance contingencies are additional strategies used to encourage compliance. Hawkins *et al.* (1992) found that individual feedback and written feedback significantly increased the number of assigned prompted voidings of geriatric patients by geriatric nursing assistants. That is, behaviour modification techniques improved the compliance of nursing staff in encouraging patients to void. Another study reported that performance feedback increased nurses' compliance with wearing gloves with AIDS patients (DeVries, Burnette & Redmon, 1991).

Future strategies used to improve professional compliance may involve a combination of education programmes and behavioural techniques, but they may also include machines. For example, Bell (1991) suggested that preventing exposure to HIV positive patients could some day become dependent on engineering controls not requiring professional compliance.

CONCLUSIONS

Health-care professionals face patient non-compliance as a norm in everyday medical practice. The literature suggests a number of techniques that, when incorporated into normal clinical practice and routines, are likely to increase patient compliance. One cannot say the same about professional non-compliance with health-care guidelines. However, there appears to be more recent recognition in the literature that professional compliance is an important field in its own right and worthy of attention. Some significant advances have been made in this area of compliance research. Definitions, measurement systems, and criteria for compliance behaviours are becoming more clear and precise for health-care professionals. Variables that contribute to professional compliance, such as social pressures and lack of resources, continue to be identified and examined. While some descriptive research has taken place, more is required that is empirical theory-based research. In turn, this research may result in the development of practical interventions that successfully improve professional compliance.

REFERENCES

Bell, D.M. (1991). Human Immunodeficiency Virus transmission in health care settings: Risk and risk reduction. *American Journal of Medicine*, **91**, 294–300.

Campbell, E.B., Knight, M., Benson, M. & Colling, J. (1991). Effect of an incontinence training program on nursing home staff's knowledge, attitude, and behavior. *Gerontologist*, **31**, 788–94.

DeVries, J.E., Burnette, M.M. & Redmon, W.K. (1991). Improving nurses' compliance with glove wearing through performance feedback. *Journal of Applied Behaviour Analysis*, **24**, 705–11.

Elford, J. & Cockcroft, A. (1991). Compulsory HIV antibody testing, universal precautions and the perceived risk of HIV: a survey among medical students and consultant staff at a London teaching hospital. *AIDS Care*, **3**, 151–8.

Gerberding, J.L. (1991). Does knowledge of Human Immunodeficiency Virus infection decrease the frequency of occupational exposure to blood? *American Journal of Medicine*, **91**, 308–11.

Hawkins, A.M., Burgio, L.D. Langford, A. & Engel, B.T. (1992). The effects of verbal and written supervisory feedback on staff compliance with assigned prompted voiding in a nursing home. *Journal of Organizational Behavior Management*, **13**, 137–50.

Klein, R.S., Phelan, J.A., Freeman, K., Schnabl, C., Friedland, G.H., Trieger, N. & Steigbigel, N.H. (1988). Low occupational risk of human immunodeficiency virus infection among dental professionals. *New England Journal of Medicine*, **318**, 86–90.

Ley, P. (1988). *Communicating with patients: improving communication, satisfaction, and compliance*. London: Chapman & Hall.

Meichenbaum, D. & Turk, D.C. (1987). *Facilitating treatment adherence. A practitioner's guidebook*. New York: Plenum Press.

Osborn, E.H., Bird, J.A., McPhee, S.J. & Rednick, J.E. (1991). Cancer screening by primary care physicians: can we explain the difference? *Journal of Family Practice*, **32**, 465–71.

Pettinger, A. & Nettleman, M.D. (1991). Epidemiology of isolation precautions.

Infection Control and Hospital Epidemiology, **12**, 303–7.

Savage, T.A., Cullen, D.L., Kirschhoff, K.T. *et al.* (1987). Nurses' responses to do-not-resuscitate orders in the neonatal intensive care unit. *Nursing Research*, **36**, 370–3.

Valanis, B., McNeil, V. & Driscoll, K. (1991). Staff members' compliance with their facility's antineoplastic drug handling policy. *Oncology Nursing Forum*, **18**, 571–6.

Wheeless, V.E., Wheeless, L.R. & Riffle, S. (1989). The role of situation, physician communicator style, and hospital rules climate on nurses; decision styles and communication satisfaction. *Health Communication*, **1**, 189–205.

Weingarten, S, Riedinger, M., Bolton, L.B., Miles, P. & Ault, M. (1989). Barriers to influenza vaccine acceptance. A survey of physicians and nurses. *American Journal of Infection Control*, **17**, 202–7.

Williams, H.S., Osborne, Y.H. & Rappaport, N.B. (1987). Child abuse reporting law: Professionals' knowledge and compliance. *Southern Psychologist*, **3**, 20–4.

Compliance among patients

PHILIP LEY

University of Sydney, Australia

DEFINITION AND MEASUREMENT

Non-compliance (or non-adherence) is broadly defined as patients not following the advice they are given by health-care professionals. This advice might concern medication regimens, habit and lifestyle changes (eg. quitting smoking, losing weight), or advice about preventive measures (using car seat belts). Often compliance involves a complex or series of behaviours, each in themselves subject to non-compliance. For example, in the case of medication the first step is to obtain the medicine, then start taking it in the appropriate dose, at the appropriate intervals, for the appropriate time. In addition, it is sometimes necessary to abstain from particular foods or other drugs which might interfere with the effectiveness of the treatment.

Methods used to assess non-compliance have included: the patient's report; pill counts, blood tests; urine tests; mechanical devices, which record the time when a container is opened; direct observation (e.g. attendance at clinic); physician's estimate; and outcome (e.g. drop in blood pressure, weight loss). The most frequently used measure is patient's report, used alone in about 44%, and in conjunction with another method in further 23% of studies (Caron,

1985). Patient's report correlates reasonably well with other methods of assessment, the average correlation being about + 0.47 (Ley, 1988). The poorest method seems to be clinician's estimate which has an average correlation of about + 0.21 with other methods. Clinicians are also poor estimators of future compliance by their patients (Sackett, 1979).

In clinical practice, patient's report is likely to be a major factor in assessing compliance. Unfortunately, although it correlates with other measures, it is possible that it leads to over-estimates of compliance. In summarizing a small sample of nine studies which compared patients' reports with more objective methods, Ley (1988) reported that while, on average, 78% of patients reported themselves to be compliant, the more objective methods estimated the percentage to be 46.

However, sets of standard questions and questionnaire measures of self-reported compliance have been and are being developed and show early promise, e.g. Morisky, Green and Levine (1986), Di Matteo *et al.* (1993). For example, the questions used by Morisky *et al.* successfully predicted compliance over a five year period. The questions were as follows.

Do you ever forget to take your medicine?

Are you careless at times about taking your medicine?

When you feel better, do you sometimes stop taking your medicine?

Sometimes when you feel worse do you sometimes stop taking your medicine?

MAGNITUDE AND COSTS OF THE PROBLEM

The extent of non-compliance

Reviewers have computed averages of the percentage of patients reported as complying with medication advice in published studies. Illustrative data are shown in Table 1. Despite the differences in their publication dates, the three reviews from which these data were taken show a remarkable consistency in their findings (as do other reviews of non-compliance in the treatment of specific diseases). Despite the high level of interest that the problem has attracted in the past two to three decades, patient non-compliance seems to be as hardy as ever.

Similarly, compliance with regimens for the treatment of smoking, alcohol, and drug abuse, as measured by relapse rates, remain similar to those reported by Hunt, Barnett, and Branch (1971), with about 20 to 40% still abstinent after a year. In the treatment of obes-

Table 1. *Mean percentage (and range) of patients* not *complying with health-related advice.*

Type of advice	Ley (1976)	Dept. of Health, Education and Welfare (1979)	Meichenbaum & Turk (1987)
Medication			
Anti-tubercular	38 (8–76)	42 (28–53)	
Antibiotics	49 (11–92)		
Penicillin		45 (11–95)	
Other antibiotics		52 (37–71)	
Anti-psychotic	39 (11–51)	42 (19–63)	
Anti-hypertensive		43 (24–83)	
Anti-epilepsy			35 (20–75)
Other medicines	48 (9–87)	52 (25–89)	
Diet	49 (20–84)		
Other advice (attending antenatal classes, child care)	55 (30–79)		(30–94)
Patient groups			
Elderly			55 (43–62)
Paediatric			50 (34–82)

ity, drop-out rates vary considerably with the treatment package used, averaging between 10 and 13% over 8 to 13 weeks in controlled trials of behaviour therapy (Brownell & Wadden, 1986), ranging from 42 to 48% over 10 to 16 weeks in clinical work-site programme, and 30 to 70% in commercial weight loss programme over a similar period (Stunkard, 1986). However, as these habit and lifestyle changes are discussed in more detail elsewhere in this volume, the emphasis here will be on compliance with medication regimens.

Costs

The costs associated with non-compliance, apart from prolongation of the suffering caused by the illness, include: extra visits to the doctor, longer recovery times, extra time off work, and avoidable hospitalization. The Department of Health and Human Services (1980) estimated that, on average, non-compliance might lead to 10 to 20% requiring an otherwise unnecessary prescription refill; 5 to 10% having a further visit to the doctor; 5 to 10% needing an extra one or two days off work; and between a 0.25% and 1% requiring 1 to 3 days in hospital. Using these assumptions, it was estimated that, in 1979 US dollars, the costs of non-compliance with regimens for ten then commonly used drugs (ampicillins, benzodiazepines, cimetidine, clofibrate, digoxin, methoxsalen, propoxythene, phenytoin, thiazides, warfarin) would be between 400 and 800 million dollars. In today's dollars they would be considerably higher.

CORRELATES OF NON-COMPLIANCE

While no major sociodemographic variables or personality characteristics have been found to be associated with non-compliance (Haynes, Taylor & Sackett, 1979), the variables of the Health Belief Model do show such associations. Patients' perceptions of their vulnerability to an illness, their perceptions of the severity of that illness, their perceptions of the likely effectiveness of the treatment, and their perceptions of the costs and barriers to treatment, are all related to compliance with the recommended treatment or advice (Janz & Becker, 1984).

The main consultation related variable consistently associated with compliance is the patient's satisfaction with the consultation (Ley, 1988). Satisfied patients are more likely to comply. Other consultation variables (consultation style, communication style) have been suggested as important, but at present results of investigations into their relationship to compliance are not compelling (O'Brien, Petrie & Raeburn, 1992).

Finally, treatment characteristics also exert an effect. The simpler the treatment schedule, and the shorter its duration, the greater is compliance.

TECHNIQUES FOR REDUCING NON COMPLIANCE AND THEIR EFFECTIVENESS

Altering aspects of the regimen

The first of these is simplification of the regimen. If it were possible to treat illnesses with a single dose of a single drug, compliance problems would be much reduced. Although this ideal is currently unattainable, it should be kept in mind when prescribing. The clinician should strive to reduce the number of tablets to be taken on any occasion and to reduce the number of times a day that the medicine has to be taken. If multiple drugs are prescribed, if possible they should be scheduled to be taken at the same time, and so on.

Sometimes, because of pattern of life or the nature of the working environment, there will be times of day or occasions when it would be very difficult for a patient to follow treatment advice. In such cases, the regimen should be 'tailored' to fit in with the patient's pattern, and avoid the non-compliance likely to ensue from incompatibilities between regimen and life.

'Mechanical' aids might help, and mechanical barriers should be avoided. Such aids include packages and containers in which the medicines to be taken at a given time on a given day are grouped together. Avoidance of mechanical barriers involves considering the difficulties that the patient might have in using the medicine. For example, many elderly patients cannot cope with childproof containers, but continue to be given medicines packed in them (Burns *et al.*, 1992)

Counselling and educational methods

At their simplest 'counselling and educational' interventions involve ensuring that the patient clearly understands instructions for the amount and timing of doses, duration of the treatment, and its rationale. It is important to tell the patient what to do if a dose is missed. Where possible, written information should be provided for later reference and amplification of what has been said in the consultation. Other educational aids might also be used for patients with chronic conditions. The question of any difficulties encountered in complying with the regimen should be raised at follow-up, and solutions found.

The patient's health beliefs should also be investigated and misconceptions cleared up. Does the patient correctly perceive their vulnerability to the consequences of not taking the treatment properly? Is the seriousness of the condition properly appreciated? Does the patient believe that the treatment will be effective? Are there any costs (financial or other) and barriers which reduce the probability of compliance?

Behavioural methods

Behavioural methods include cueing and prompting, provision of feedback, and contingency management. Prompts and cues include tailoring the regimen so that events in the patients day will serve as reminders that it is medicine time, telephoned reminders, and medicine containers which provide an auditory signal when a dose should be taken.

Feedback to the patient can be in the form of self-monitoring: the patient keeps a record of their medicine taking. In addition patients might monitor their symptoms. For example, patients might use home blood pressure monitors. Feedback is also provided by the clinician at follow-up visits.

Contingency management involves finding ways of reinforcing (rewarding) patients for compliance. It ranges from simply inquiring specifically about compliance at follow-up and expressing clear approval when it has occurred, to much more complicated packages which reward patients for compliance or fine them in some way for non-compliance. Needless to say, these methods are devised and used with the patient's consent and often involve a written behavioural contract.

The involvement of significant others (spouse, relative or friend) in the treatment programme has also been advocated (e.g. Levy, 1986). This involvement can be of a general nature, with the supporter simply sitting in on the consultation so that they will be aware of what the treatment regimen is. Alternatively, the supporter can be an active part of a behavioural package for the patient, serving, for example, as a monitor, or as a dispenser of reinforcement.

More detailed guidance on the use of these techniques can be found in Meichenbaum and Turk (1987).

Effectiveness of these interventions

No single technique has shown consistent effectiveness when used alone, but in general methods using behavioural techniques have proved superior to educational techniques. The best results have been obtained by combining a number of techniques (Haynes, Wang & da Mota Gomes, 1987). The expected increase in compliance with medication regimens from the use of mixtures of these techniques averages at about an absolute increase of 20 to 25% or so. This is a relative improvement of 40 to 50% on the average compliance figure of 52% (Haynes *et al.*, 1987; Ley, 1988). In a case where compliance is absolutely essential but remains a problem, a clinical psychologist should be consulted to design a behavioural package specifically for that patient.

PRACTICAL STEPS THE CLINICIAN CAN TAKE TO IMPROVE COMPLIANCE

Practical advice based on the review above can be summarized as follows.

1. Make the treatment regimen as simple and short in duration as possible.
2. Find out what the patient's health beliefs are. Does the patient have an accurate perception of the seriousness of the condition? Does the patient believe that they are at risk of any of the adverse consequences treatment is designed to prevent? Does the patient believe that the treatment will cure them? Does the patient believe that on balance the advantages of following the treatment regimen outweigh its disadvantages? If there are problems try to solve them. Use an alternative treatment if necessary.
3. Tailor the regimen to fit in with the patient's pattern of behaviour. The aims of this tailoring should always include (a) the use of significant daily events as cues or reminders about medicine taking or other treatment routines, and (b) reducing the perceived disadvantages of following the regimen.
4. Make sure that the patient is satisfied with the amount of information given about the treatment.
5. Make sure that the patient clearly understands the amount, frequency, timing, and duration of treatment.
6. Make sure that the patients understands enough of the rationale of treatment to see why the regimen is as it is.
7. Where possible provide written back-up. This will help reduce forgetting, and help with other problems.
8. If appropriate, consider the involvement of a significant other person in the patient's life.
9. At follow-up ask the patient about any problems they have encountered in following the regimen, and any doubts they have about it. Find solutions to these problems and doubts. If necessary, change the regimen.
10. Provide feedback about progress. Consider advising the use

[283]

of self-monitoring. This can be as simple as asking the patient to keep a record, or could involve recommending the use of a home blood pressure measuring device. If the patient is to be asked to keep a record, make it easier to do so by providing prepared charts and checklists. As a request that the patient provide self-monitoring data relies on the patient's compliance, all of the above recommendations apply to this as well.

REFERENCES

Brownell, K.D. & Wadden, T.A. (1986). Behavior therapy for obesity: Modern treatment and better results. In K.D. Brownell & J.P. Foreyt (Eds.). *Handbook of eating disorders*. New York: Basic Books.

Burns, J.M., Sneddon, I., Lovell, M., McLean, A. & Martin, B.J. (1992). Elderly patients and their medication: a post-discharge follow-up study. *Age and Ageing*, 21, 178–81.

Caron, H.S. (1985). Compliance: the case for objective measurement. *Journal of Hypertension*, 3, *(Suppl. 1)*, 11–17.

Department of Health and Human Services (1980) Prescription drug products: patient package insert requirements. *Federal Register*, 45, 6075–817.

Department of Health, Education and Welfare (1979). Prescription drug products: patient labelling requirements. *Federal Register*, 44, 40016–41.

Di Matteo, M.R., Hays, R.D., Gritz, E.R., Bastani, R., Crane, L., Elashoff, R., Ganz, P., Heber, D., McCarthy, W. & Marcus, A. (1993). Patient adherence to cancer control regimens: scale development and initial validation. *Psychological Assessment*, 5, 102–12.

Haynes, R.B., Taylor, D.W. & Sackett, D.L. (1979). *Compliance in health care*. Baltimore: Johns Hopkins University Press.

Haynes, R.B., Wang, E. & da Mota Gomes, M. (1987). A critical review of interventions to improve compliance with prescribed medications. *Patient Education and Counselling*, 10, 155–66.

Hunt, W.A., Barnett, L.W. & Branch, L.G. (1971). Relapse rates in addiction programs. *Journal of Clinical Psychology*, 27, 455–6.

Janz, N.K. & Becker, M.H. (1984). The health belief model a decade later. *Health Education Quarterly*, 11, 1–47.

Levy, R.L. (1986). Social support and compliance: salient methodological components in compliance research. *Journal of Compliance in Health Care*, 1, 189–198.

Ley, P (1976). Psychological studies of doctor patient communication. In S. Rachman (Ed.) *Contributions to medical psychology*. Oxford: Pergamon Press.

Ley, P. (1988) *Communicating with patients*. London: Chapman and Hall.

Luscher, T.F. & Vetter, W. (1990). Adherence to medication. *Journal of Human Hypertension*, 4, 43–6.

Meichenbaum, D. & Turk, D.C. (1987). *Facilitating treatment adherence*. New York: Plenum Press.

Morisky, D.E., Green, L.W. & Levine, D.M. (1986). Concurrent and predicted validity of a self-reported measure of patient adherence. *Medical Care*, 24, 67–74.

O'Brien, M.K., Petrie, K. & Raeburn, J. (1992). Adherence to medication regimens: updating a complex medical issue. *Medical Care Review*, 49, 435–54.

Sackett, D.L. (1979). A compliance practicum for the busy practitioner. In R.B. Haynes, D.W. Taylor & D.L. Sackett (E.d.s) *Compliance in health care*. Baltimore: Johns Hopkins University Press.

Stunkard, A.J. (1986). The control of obesity: social and community perspectives. In K.D. Brownell & J.P. Foreyt (Eds.). *Handbook of eating disorders*. New York: Basic Books.

Doctor–patient communication

JOHN WEINMAN

UMDS (Guy's Campus), University of London, UK

The consultation between the patient and the doctor lies at the heart of all medical practice. The information which is transmitted during the consultation is very often critical in the formulation of diagnoses and in the organization of treatment. Thus effective communication is necessary to ensure not only that the patients' problems and concerns are understood by the doctor but also that relevant information, advice and treatment is received and acted upon by the patient. Communication is a two-way process which relies on verbal and non-verbal information. The non-verbal behaviour of the patient may provide important information about their underlying mood or concerns, and the non-verbal responses of the doctor can provide clear messages to patients about their level of interest and empathy which, in turn, can then influence what is revealed during the consultation.

The consultation has been the object of considerable research, particularly since there has been consistent evidence that the process and outcome are often not satisfactory for patients. Early research revealed quite high levels of patient dissatisfaction which was often associated with insufficient information, poor understanding of the medical advice and subsequent reluctance or inability to follow recommended treatment or advice (Korsch & Negrete, 1972). The development of relatively unobtrusive audio and video-recording techniques allowed researchers to get inside the consultation and many studies have analysed the process of the consultation and attempted to relate process variables or characteristics to outcome. However, these studies, while identifying important themes, have not always been successful in making clear links between process and outcome (Stiles, 1989). One reason for this is that patients vary in their expectations and preferences. As a result current frameworks for understanding doctor–patient communication tend to be based on the relations between inputs (ie the attitudes, beliefs, expectations, etc, which patient and doctor bring to the consultation), process (the nature of the encounter) and outcome (the short and longer-term effects on the patient). Each of these will now be examined.

INPUT FACTORS IN COMMUNICATION

Input factors which influence the consultation include not only aspects of the doctor and patient but also the context and setting in which the consultation occurs. For example, for many primary care consultations in the UK, patients are booked in for 10-minute appointments, whereas similar consultations in other countries may typically last two to three times longer. Although longer consultations do not inevitably result in better patient outcomes (Morrell *et al.* 1986), the resulting process may well be different.

A number of studies have shown that patients cope with health threats in diverse ways and show consistent differences in the extent to which they want to be involved in the health care process (Krantz, Baum & Wideman *et al.*, 1980) as well as in the amount of information which they would like to receive about their health problem. Similarly, a distinction has been made by Miller, Brody and Summerton (1987) between 'monitors' and 'blunters', with the former being more inclined to need and seek out information about their problem and treatment, whereas the latter group prefer consultations in which relatively limited information is provided.

There is also consistent evidence that patients have differing expectations for specific consultations. Contrary to medical opinion, patients do not always want or expect diagnosis or treatment since they may be looking to the consultation to gain more understanding of their health problem or may be hoping for support or understanding from their doctor. These prior expectations can be important in determining outcomes since consultations in which patient expectations are met result in greater satisfaction and an increased willingness to follow advice or treatment (Williams *et al.* 1995). Thus an important starting point for any consultation is to identify the patients' own expectations, as well as their own preferences and beliefs.

Before completing this brief overview of the nature of 'input' factors, it is important to acknowledge that doctors can vary considerably in the attitudes and beliefs, which they have not only about their own and the patient's role, but also about the function and conduct of the consultation. Doctors have been categorized in various ways according to their role perceptions and the extent to which they concentrate on the technical or more psychosocial aspects of patient care, as well as their beliefs about whether patients should be actively involved in the consultation and in decision-making about the management of the clinical problem (eg Grol *et al.*, 1990). Inevitably these broad attitudinal differences are reflected in differences in the way in which the consultation is conducted.

THE CONSULTATION PROCESS

There are a range of methods and frameworks for analysing and describing the process of the consultation. One of the broadest distinctions made has been between consultations which are described as patient centred and those which are doctor centred, reflecting the extent to which the doctor or patient determines what is discussed (Grol *et al.*, 1990). Doctor-centred consultations are ones in which closed-questions are used more often and the direction is determined by the doctor, typically with a primary focus on medical problems. In contrast, patient-centred encounters involve more open-ended questions with greater scope for patients to raise their own concerns and agendas. Related to this are consistent differences in the extent to which the doctor responds to the emotional agendas and the non-verbal cues of the patient. Although there has been a tendency to consider the more patient-centred/emotion-focused approach as preferable, what appears to be more important is for doctor and patient to be in agreement over the nature of the problem and the best course of action (Starfield *et al.*, 1981).

A number of specific methods have been developed for carrying detailed analyses of the social interaction between doctor and patient based on audio or videotapes or transcripts of the consultations. One of the earliest of these was the Bales' process analysis system which distinguishes verbal statements into those which are task or emotion-focused and then into more specific categories from transcripts and this approach has been adapted and extended by a number of other investigators (see Roter & Hall, 1989). An alternative approach has been developed by Stiles *et al.*, (1979) and which classifies each statement made by doctor and patient into one of eight basic categories (eg questions; giving interpretations, etc). Good overviews of these different approaches are available elsewhere (eg Roter & Hall, 1989) and attempts have been made to define a number of more general ways of classifying doctor–patient interactions. For example, one can distinguish between verbal and non-verbal information and within the verbal domain, six broad categories can be defined (information-giving; information-seeking; social conversation; positive talk; negative talk; partnership building). From a meta-analysis of these broad categories (Roter, 1989) it has been found that for the doctor, information-giving occurs most frequently (approximately 35% of the doctor's communication) followed by information-seeking (approximately 22%), positive talk (15%), partnership building (10%), social conversation (6%) and negative talk (1%). In contrast, the main type of patient communication consists of information giving (approximately 50%) with less than 10% involving question-asking.

A more specific approach to process analysis is found in the studies of Ley and colleagues (Ley, 1988), who concentrated on the informational content of the consultation and the quality of information provided by the doctor. In particular, they analysed the content in terms of its level of complexity, comprehensibility and the extent to which the information was organized. They and others have found that medical information may be too detailed or complex with the result that important information may not be understood or retained by the patient. There is even evidence that patients and doctors may interpret the same information in different ways and this communication gap can occur around anatomical information or other technical terms which are used to describe illness or treatment.

These various ways of conceptualizing and analysing the consultation process have given rise to a large number of indices or categories which have been related to outcome, often in quite a limited fashion. Outcomes, such as patient satisfaction or adherence to treatment are likely to be determined by a range of factors, reflecting

[285]

a complex interaction of input, process and situational variables. Hence it is not surprising that attempts to derive simple process, outcome models have been disappointing in their predictive value (Stiles, 1989). Moreover, there are various ways of defining outcomes, and it is very likely that different process variables will effect different outcome indicators.

OUTCOMES OF THE CONSULTATION

The most widely used outcome measure used in doctor-patient communication research is patient satisfaction (see Fitzpatrick, this volume). Although this can provide a useful general indicator of the patient's experience, there are some associated problems with its use, since many measures appear to be insensitive to variations in patient satisfaction and often do not distinguish between different categories of satisfaction. In his studies of the quality of information transmission Ley and colleagues have used patient knowledge and recall as outcome measures and these do show a clearer relation with process variables, such as the complexity and level of organization of the information presented (Ley, 1988). Moreover, their interventions to improve the clarity or comprehensibility of the information consistently resulted in better recall and understanding (see below). Despite this, there is still abundant evidence that patients often emerge from consultations with insufficient information or understanding of their problems, and as a result, forget a great deal of what they have been told. Some studies have also examined patients' beliefs before and after the consultation, and again these indicate that the consultation often has relatively little effect on these, often because they were not explicitly discussed. Patient satisfaction, understanding and beliefs can play a major role in influencing another important and widely studied outcome variable, namely compliance or adherence with treatment or advice. This is discussed in detail elsewhere in this volume and is obviously an important outcome in situations where non-adherence results in adverse health consequences. There is evidence of high levels of non-adherence and this can clearly affect other outcomes including health and well-being. The latter have not often been studied as communication outcomes but there are a few studies which demonstrate positive effects on patients' health and well-being arising from positive experiences in medical consultations. These have focused on psychological states such as anxiety as well as changes in specific physical variables such as blood pressure and blood glucose control. Some of the most impressive findings here have been found in the patient intervention studies, which are described below.

IMPROVING DOCTOR–PATIENT COMMUNICATION

In addition to increasing our understanding of doctor – patient communication and its central role in health-care delivery, some research findings have also provided insights for developing interventions to improve the quality of communication. The majority of these have been aimed at improving the communication skills of medical students or doctors at various stages of training, but a few have been targeted at patients, to enable them to get what they want from a consultation. Both types of intervention approach will be outlined.

In medical school, communication skills training is now regarded as a fundamental part of the curriculum but this varies considerably in terms of the amount and type of teaching and the stage at which it is taught. Typically, students are provided with an overview of the basic skills of 'active' listening, which facilitate patient communication. At a basic level these include the importance of developing good rapport and the use of open-ended questions early in the consultation, appropriate eye-contact and other facilitatory responses to help the patient talk, together with the ability to summarize and arrive at a shared understanding of the patients' problem. These skills can be taught in a number of ways, but the successful courses inevitably involve active learning, using role-plays with simulated patients as well as real patient interviews. Feedback is important to identify problem areas and directions for improvement and increasing use is made of videotape for this purpose. There is now consistent evidence that this type of training can result in clear improvements in basic communication skills which are maintained for a number of years. In addition to these basic packages, it is also necessary for students to learn how to communicate about sensitive or difficult areas of medical practice, including dealing with distressed patients or relatives and giving 'bad news'. Given the intrinsic difficulties in many of these areas, training packages have made good use of role play often involving the use of actors, for developing these skills (see Kendrick in this volume for more detailed account).

In recent years, there have been a number of interesting interventions aimed at patients. Generally, these have involved brief training packages for patients prior to a consultation in order to increase their level of participation, particularly to ensure that their own concerns are dealt with and that information provided by the doctor is clearly understood. A successful development of this approach can be seen in the work of Greenfield and colleagues (1985) who used a preconsultation intervention lasting 20 minutes for hospital outpatients who were helped to identify their main questions and encouraged to ask these in the consultation. These patients participated more actively in the consultation, and this was also associated with better long-term health outcomes.

Finally, mention should be made of two specific patient-based approaches which have been very successful. The first by Ley and colleagues (see Ley, 1988) involved hospital patients and an additional short visit which allowed them to ask for any information to be clarified. Compared with control groups these patients had a much higher level of satisfaction with communication, indicating that effective interventions need not be complex or time-consuming. In the more difficult area of the 'bad news' consultation, Hogbin and Fallowfield (1989). describe a simple yet effective intervention which consisted of tape-recording the consultation and allowing patients to keep the tape. Since this type of consultation is often very distressing, patients may often find it very difficult to take in all the information. Thus it was found that patients welcomed the use of these tapes as something which they could go back to, and which others could also listen to.

THE BENEFITS OF GOOD COMMUNICATION

One of the most widely reported effects of good medical communication is a higher level of patient satisfaction which also brings other benefits, such as increasing adherence to advice or treatment, for a number of reasons (Ley, 1988). First, effective communication should result in increased patient understanding recall of the information given in the consultation. Second, if the patient feels that the doctor understands their concerns and is empathic towards them, then there may be more confidence in the advice which is offered. Furthermore, empathic communication may result in reduced levels of patient anxiety, which may not only facilitate recall of information but also promote better coping with the problem. With chronic conditions, improved self-management resulting from a greater involvement in the consultation has also been shown to lead to improved health outcome (Greenfield et al., 1985-; Stewart, 1995).

Effective medical communication may be crucial in the many situations where patients are required to make important decisions relating to their own or another's health. For example, in genetic counselling, individuals may be required to process quite complex risk information which is often couched in terms of probabilities and may be difficult to take in. However, since the information may relate to the individual's long-term health prospects or may influence reproductive decisions, it is clearly vital not only that communication is clear but also that it takes account of the beliefs, expecta-

tions and needs of the individual in order that these major decisions can be taken in an informed way.

A final example of a situation in which effective communication can be beneficial is prior to stressful medical procedures or investigations. There is now considerable evidence that the provision of clear sensory and procedural information about an impending medical procedure can be extremely beneficial in helping patients cope with the procedure as well as promoting better recovery (Johnston & Vogele, 1993).

In view of the many problems which have been identified in doctor – patient communication and the documented benefits arising from effective communication, it is not surprising that communication teaching is now regarded as a critical component of medical training. The evidence from the detailed studies of input, process and outcome components of communication can provide an excellent basis for this training and for improving the quality of patient care.

REFERENCES

Greenfield, S., Kaplan, S. & Ware, J.E. (1985). Expanding patient involvement in care: effects on patient outcomes. *Annals of Internal Medicine*, **102**, 520–28.

Grol, R., de Maeseneer, J., Whitfield, M. & Mokkink, H. (1990). Disease-centred versus patient-centred attitudes: comparison of general practitioners in Belgium, Britain and the Netherlands. *Family Practice*, **7**, 100–4.

Hogbin, B. & Fallowfield, L.J. (1989). Getting it taped: the bad news consultation with cancer patients *British Journal of Hospital Medicine*, **41**, 330–3.

Johnston, M. & Vogele, C. (1993). Benefits of psychological preparation for surgery: a meta-analysis. *Annals of Behavioural Medicine*, **15**, 245–56.

Korsch, B.M. & Negrete, V.F. (1972). Doctor – patient communication *Scientific American*, **227**, 66–74.

Krantz, D., Baum, A. & Wideman, M. (1980). Assessment of preferences for self treatment and information in health care.

Journal of Personality and Social Psychology, **39**, 977–90.

Ley, P. (1988). *Communicating with patients*. London: Croom Helm.

Miller, S.M., Brody, D.S. & Summerton, J. (1987). Styles of coping with threat: implications for health *Journal of Personality and Social Psychology*, **54**, 142–8.

Morrell, D.C., Evans, M.E., Morris, R.W. & Roland, M.O. (1986). The five minute consultation: effect of time constraint on clinical content and patient satisfaction. *British Medical Journal*, **292**, 870–3.

Roter, D. (1989). Which facets of communications have strong effects on outcome: a meta-analysis. In M. Stewart & D. Roter (Eds.). *Communicating with medical patients*. pp. 283–196. Newbury Park: Sage.

Roter, D. & Hall, J.A. (1989). Studies of doctor – patient interaction. *Annual Review of Public Health*, **10**, 163–80.

Starfield, B., Wray, C., Hess, K., Gross, R., Birk, P.S. & D'Lugoff, B.C. (1981). The influence of patient – practitioner agreement on outcome of care. *American Journal of Public Health*, **71**, 127–31.

Stewart, M.A. (1995). Effective physician–patient communication and health outcomes: a review. *Canadian Medical Association Journal*, **152**, 1423–33.

Stiles, W.B. (1989). Evaluating medical interview process, components: null correlations with outcomes may be misleading. *Medical Care*, **27**, 212–20.

Stiles, W.B., Putnam, S.M., Wolf, M.H. & James, S.A. (1979). Verbal response mode profiles of patients and physicians in medical screening interviews. *Journal of Medical Education*, **54**, 81–9.

Williams, S., Weinman, J., Dale, J. & Newman, S. (1995) Patient expectations: what do primary care patients want from the GP and how far does meeting patient expectations affect patient satisfaction? *Family Practice*, **12**, 193–201.

Health-care work environments

RUDOLF H. MOOS

and

JEANNE A. SCHAEFER

Center for Health Care Evaluation Department of
Veterans Affairs and Stanford University Medical
Centers, Palo Alto, California, USA

INTRODUCTION

Over the past 70 years, organization theorists have formulated three main conceptual frameworks to examine the relationship between employees and their work environment. An emphasis on employee productivity in the 1920s led to Taylorism and the scientific school of management, which focused on specifying conditions to maximize task efficiency and production. Scientific management sees the work environment as a set of task-relevant reinforcers that can be used to control employees; there is little regard for interpersonal issues or individual differences.

The human relations approach was shaped by concern about employee alienation and the conviction that a narrow focus on productivity might lead to poorer job performance. This approach emphasizes the value of individual and small group relationships and focuses special attention on organizational development and the quality of work life. Most recently, proponents of the sociotechnical school have focused on both the technological or task attributes of a job as well as the interpersonal and organizational context in which it is performed.

These three approaches provide a gradually evolving perspective on the work environment and its connections to personal character-

istics and work outcomes. We use these ideas here by describing a systems perspective that considers job-related and personal factors, the key dimensions and impacts of health-care work environments, and how staff morale and performance can influence the quality of patient care and treatment outcome.

AN INTEGRATED SYSTEMS FRAMEWORK

The model shown in Fig. 1 depicts the health-care system (Panel I) as composed of organizational structure and policies, patient and task factors, and work climate. The personal system (Panel II) encompasses characteristics of individual staff members such as job position and work role, level of experience, demographic factors, and personal resources such as self-confidence.

The model posits that the link between health care system factors (Panel I) and work morale and performance (Panel V) is affected by the personal system (Panel II), as well as by specific work stressors (Panel III) and coping responses (Panel IV). Work stressors (Panel III) and the organizational and personal factors (Panels I and II) that contribute to them can shape coping responses (Panel IV) and staff morale and performance (Panel V). In turn, these staff outcomes ultimately affect the quality of care and patient outcomes (Panel VI). As the bidirectional paths in the model indicate, these processes are transactional; feedback can occur at each stage.

THE HEALTH-CARE SYSTEM

Health-care system variables can be classified into physical features, organizational structure and policies, patient and task factors, and work climate. The work climate is linked to specific work stressors that affect employees directly; the work climate and work stressors transmit and alter the influence of other sets of health-care system factors.

Work climate and work stressors

Based on research in a variety of work settings, the underlying facets of work climates and specific work stressors can be organized into relationship, task, and system maintenance dimensions. Relationship dimensions measure the extent to which employees and supervisors are involved with and supportive of one another. Relationship stressors arise from interactions with coworkers, supervisors, and other facility staff, and typically include communication problems, lack of teamwork, and conflicts with coworkers.

The second set of dimensions covers the goal and task aspects of the work setting, such as the level of autonomy, task orientation and

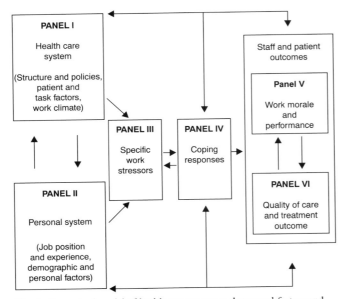

Fig. 1. Conceptual model of health care system and personal factors and staff and patient outcomes.

work pressure. Task stressors stem from the duties that staff confront in their job and how well prepared they are to handle them. Some key task stressors are caring for dying, chronically ill, or uncooperative patients and lack of knowledge and competence.

System maintenance dimensions assess the amount of structure, clarity, and openness to change that characterize the workplace. System stressors are related to the management of the work unit or facility and to the resources available to staff. Staff frequently cite heavy workload and understaffing as major stressors. Other system stressors arise from scheduling problems, lack of equipment and supplies, and inadequacies in the physical environment, such as too little space and too much noise.

Extensive research on health care employees points to special problems in their work settings. Compared with employees in non-health-related work settings, health-care employees report less job involvement and less coworker cohesion and supervisor support. Moreover, health-care settings are seen as lacking in autonomy and clarity, as less physically comfortable, and as placing more emphasis on work demands and managerial control (Moos, 1994).

As the model indicates, the overall work climate is associated with specific work stressors. Thus, a difficult work climate is likely to be associated with more relationship and task stressors; that is, staff in less involving, supportive, and clear work units with more work pressure report more relationship and task stressors. In addition, less involving, supportive, and clear workplaces that are low on managerial control and have more work pressure are associated with more stressors in the areas of workload and scheduling and facility design and maintenance (Schaefer & Moos, 1993).

DETERMINANTS OF WORK CLIMATES AND WORK STRESSORS

Health-care work settings vary widely in the quality of interpersonal relationships, the amount of task stressors and work demands, and the adequacy of clarity and management control. Two key sets of factors account for these differences: organizational structure and policies, and patient characteristics and related task factors.

Organizational structure and policies

With respect to organizational factors, staffing and the amount of contact with patients are related to work climate. Compared with hospital personnel in well-staffed units, for example, personnel working in poorly staffed areas tend to see their workplace as lower on the quality of coworker and supervisor relationships, less independent and clear, and more demanding. Employees who spend more time in direct contact with patients tend to rate their workplace as less innovative and higher on managerial control; they also report more alienation from their patients.

The overall policy perspective of a health-care organization can affect the workplace. Compared with health care facilities that follow a professional model, those with a bureaucratic model are likely to have more centralized decision making and formalized jobs, which are associated with a lack of support and autonomy, ambiguity about work-related policies, and high work demands and managerial control. In contrast, participative leadership helps to foster a clearer, more task focused, and more innovative work climate.

The organization of nursing services also influences the work environment. In primary nursing, each nurse is responsible for the care of specific patients; in team and functional nursing, however, each nurse performs specific delimited tasks for a group of patients. The head nurse retains overall responsibility for patient care. Nurses in primary nursing units tend to report more involvement, cohesion, and support than their team and functional nursing counterparts. Being accountable for specific patients may enhance nurses' job commitment and working relationships with coworkers and supervisors. Primary nurses also report more autonomy and less management control, probably because they have more independent responsibility for patients (Thomas, 1992).

Patient and task factors

The primary task performed by health care personnel can influence the workplace. For example, staff involved in patient care, such as nurses and nurses' aids, tend to report less cohesion, support, autonomy, and clarity and experience their work as more demanding than staff not involved in patient care, such as dietitians and laundry workers (Moos, 1994).

Consistent with the sociotechnical perspective, both patient care task and social systems factors, such as authority patterns and the division of labour, affect nurses' work-related attitudes and distress. Thus, the specialized nature of the primary tasks in intensive care units (ICUs) may create a particular work climate. For example, nurses in medical–surgical ICUs reported more involvement, supervisor support, and task orientation than did nurses working in general medical–surgical units (Hipwell, Tyler & Wilson, 1989). These findings imply that social systems factors such as a supportive work milieu can reduce the perception of high work demands and that, in an involving and task-focused workplace, high demands may contribute to team spirit and a sense of accomplishment.

Specialized tasks do not necessarily lead to more cohesive and independent work environments, however. For example, some special care units resemble a scientific laboratory with infants in incubators and large banks of automated monitoring equipment. The highly technical nature of these units and the structured tasks and set procedures may contribute to a lack of autonomy and innovation; dependence on experts for technical guidance can inhibit the development of cohesion and support (Spinks & Michaelson, 1989).

THE IMPACT OF WORK CLIMATES AND WORK STRESSORS

Aspects of health-care work climates are predictably linked to employee morale and performance. Staff who report high job autonomy and task orientation show better job morale and performance; staff who see their work milieu as supportive and innovative have a greater sense of personal accomplishment. Good communication with supervisors and cohesive work groups are also related to higher job satisfaction. In contrast, staff who report a lack of support and clarity in the job, and a lack of influence in decision making, are more likely to experience poor morale and detachment (Blegen, 1993; Moos & Schaefer, 1987).

Leadership styles may be especially important when complex and specialized treatment procedures are used, such as in ICUs. In this vein, Shortell and his colleagues (1991) found that ICU work cultures oriented toward team satisfaction, effective communication, and problem-solving approaches were associated with staff members' perceptions that they provided better quality of care and were better able to meet family members' needs, and with less nursing turnover.

Work stressors are also predictably associated with job morale and performance. In general, staff who experience more work stressors tend to report less job satisfaction and have high turnover. Importantly, however, task stressors may be associated with more job satisfaction and better performance. Staff who are challenged by, and successfully manage, task stressors may put more effort into their work and perform better. In turn, competent staff who perform well are likely to be given more patient care tasks and responsibilities (Schaefer & Moos, 1993).

The interplay of relationship, task, and maintenance domains

These findings highlight the value of considering the interplay of relationship, task, and management factors in examining the impact of work settings. Work groups characterized by strong task orientation and the opportunity for independent action tend to promote morale and performance. In contrast, the combination of high job demands and lack of freedom has a detrimental influence on employee health and satisfaction. However, challenging work can compensate for an unfavourable organizational climate.

Management factors can promote task orientation and job performance. Clear job tasks and policies, adequate performance feedback and moderate structure all contribute to satisfaction and effectiveness. In the relative absence of these factors (that is, ambiguous job roles, sparse feedback, and lax organizational policies), staff experience health and morale problems. There is a growing recognition of the importance of personal relationships in changing these associations. In general, cohesive coworker and supervisor relationships can amplify the influence of autonomy and task orientation and moderate the problematic consequences of demanding and constrained work settings.

As the model indicates, health-care system factors, work climates, and associated staff outcomes can affect the quality of patient care. Thus, a highly centralized, hierarchical organization may be associated with routinized, impersonal patterns of care. In turn, these custodial practices tend to make patients more passive. A decentralized or participative organization, in which decisions are made by staff in close contact with patients, promotes more individualized patterns of care. More generally, high staff morale facilitates better patient functioning, which, in turn, promotes positive staff work attitudes and staff and patient involvement in treatment.

IMPROVING HEALTH-CARE WORK SETTINGS

The framework we have described can be useful to health-care managers and staff who wish to improve the quality of their work settings. In this respect, Shinn and her colleagues (1993) have proposed a tripartite model of coping with work stressors. There are coping strategies used by individuals (setting limits on one's activities, focusing on the positive aspects of work), strategies undertaken by groups of individuals to aid one another (mutual support groups), and strategies initiated by agencies themselves (changing job designs, providing recreational facilities). Many of the stressors staff confront are linked to the overall organization of the health-care system and are beyond the control of individual employees.

Thus, management interventions to improve group and agency coping may be especially effective.

Implementing and monitoring change

One type of intervention is to provide supervisors and staff with information about the work climate and work stressors and use it to increase communication among them. In one ICU, for example, staff were quite dissatisfied and were showing dysfunctional reactions that seemed to stem from high work demands, role ambiguity, and lack of autonomy and support. The feedback process was used to identify target areas for change and a number of innovations were instituted: group discussions clarified areas of responsibilities for staff, work shifts were altered to better match staff preferences, and regular times were set up for nurses and physicians to meet. Staff felt that the work climate improved; they reported increased involvement and cohesion, more autonomy and clarity, and less work pressure (Koran et al., 1983).

Staff mutual support groups can also use feedback about the workplace to make changes. Such information can help to focus discussions on key themes, identify major problem areas such as lack of staff communication and confusion about work procedures, and guide staff problem-solving efforts. In one example, information about the work climate enabled a staff support group to increase clarity and organization closer to the levels staff members preferred (Tommasini, 1992). Overall, survey feedback and process consultation can help make health-care work settings more satisfactory for their employees.

Consultants and programme evaluators can also use information about work climate and work stressors to help assess changes in health care, such as initiating quality assurance programmes, reorganizing hospital nursing services, and implementing organizational development programmes. For example, Sinclair and Frankel (1982) reported an increase in supervisor support and a decline in managerial control when a new quality assurance programme was initiated. In another project, staff who participated in a Total Quality Management programme reported higher job satisfaction than did non-participants (Counte et al., 1992). Overall, studies in this area show that staff involvement in decision-making and team problem-solving can improve the work climate, reduce job stressors, and promote better individual and organizational outcomes.

FUTURE DIRECTIONS

Work stressors are likely to intensify as health-care staff encounter new medical technologies and the ethical dilemmas associated with them, more acutely ill patients, cost containment efforts and competition, and quality assurance programmes that demand ever greater accountability and perfection. To cope with these changes, Dueiren and Adams (1993) highlight the need for staff empowerment; that is, the development of responsive organizations in which health-care staff can participate actively in improving the workplace and health-care services. Such a development can enhance the work climate and contribute to better staff performance and patient outcomes.

ACKNOWLEDGEMENTS
Preparation of this manuscript was supported by Department of Veterans Affairs Health Services Research and Development Service research funds and by NIAAA Grant AA06699.

REFERENCES

Blegen, M.A. (1993). Nurses' job satisfaction: a meta-analysis of related variables. *Nursing Research* , **42**, 36–41.

Counte, M.A., Glandon, G.L., Oleske, D.M. & Hill, J.P. (1992). Total Quality Management in a health care organization: how are employees affected? *Hospital and Health Services Administration*, **37**, 503–18.

Dueiren, G.F. & Adams, K.L. (1993). Empowering health care improvement: an operational model. *Journal on Quality Improvement*, **19**, 222–3.

Hipwell, A.A., Tyler, P.A. & Wilson, C.M. (1989). Sources of stress and dissatisfaction among nurses in four hospital environments. *British Journal of Medical Psychology*, **62**, 71–9.

Koran, L., Moos, R., Moos, B. & Zasslow, M. (1983). Changing hospital work environments: an example of a burn unit. *General Hospital Psychiatry*, **5**, 7–13.

Moos, R.H. (1994). *Work Environment Scale manual: third edition*. Palo Alto, CA: Consulting Psychologists Press.

Moos, R. & Schaefer, J. (1987). Evaluating health care work settings: a holistic conceptual framework. *Psychology and Health*, **1**, 97–122.

Schaefer, J. & Moos, R. (1993). Relationship, task, and system stressors in the health care workplace. *Journal of Community and Applied Social Psychology*, **3**, 235–42.

Shinn, M., Morch, H., Robinson, P.E. & Neuner, R.A. (1993). Individual, group, and agency strategies for coping with job stressors in residential child care programs. *Journal of Community and Applied Social Psychology*, **3**, 313–24.

Shortell, S.M., Rousseau, D.M., Gillies, R.R., Devers, K.J. & Simons, T.L. (1991). Organizational assessment in Intensive Care Units (ICUs): construct development, reliability, and validity of the ICU Nurse–Physician Questionnaire. *Medical Care*, **29**, 709–26.

Sinclair, C. & Frankel, M. (1982). The effect of quality assurance activities on the quality of mental health services. *Quality Review Bulletin*, **8**, 7–15.

Spinks, P. & Michaelson, J. (1989). A comparison of the ward environment in a special care baby unit and a children's orthopaedic ward. *Journal of Reproductive and Infant Psychology*, **7**, 47–50.

Thomas, L.H. (1992). Qualified nurse and nursing auxiliary perceptions of their work environment in primary, team, and functional nursing wards. *Journal of Advanced Nursing*, **17**, 373–82.

Tommasini, N.R. (1992). The impact of a staff support group on the work environment of a specialty unit. *Archives of Psychiatric Nursing*, **6**, 40–7.

Medical accidents: adverse events in medical treatment

CHARLES VINCENT

Department of Psychology,
University College London,
UK

Medical accidents, sometimes referred to as 'adverse events', are occasions on which patients are unintentionally injured by medical treatment. Iatrogenic disease is a broader term, encompassing all adverse effects of medical treatment including, for example, known and predictable drug side-effects.

Very few errors, and only a proportion of accidents, involve negligence. Where an injury is due to negligent treatment, in that care fell below an accepted standard, patients and their relatives can seek compensation through legal action. The rising rate of litigation during the 1980s in both the UK and the USA (Dingwall & Fenn, 1991) was an important factor in stimulating research on the causes and prevention of medical accidents. Ideally, however, studies of medical accidents are a form of quality assurance. The aim is to improve the quality of care, not simply to reduce litigation, important though that is (Vincent, Ennis & Audley, 1993).

THE NATURE AND FREQUENCY OF MEDICAL ACCIDENTS

Medical accidents are much more common than is generally realized. In the Harvard Medical Practice Study (Hiatt *et al.*, 1989) a random sample of 30 195 records of patients admitted to hospitals in New York state were screened for adverse events. These included death, increased length of stay, readmission to the hospital, fever at discharge and unplanned transfer to the intensive care unit. Of admissions, 1133 (3.7%), involved an adverse event. Errors in management were identified in over half the cases and in 1% of admissions care was judged to be negligent. For 70% of patients the resulting disability was slight or short-lived, but in 7% it was permanent, and 14% of patients died in part as a result of their treatment. There were about seven times as many adverse events as claims for compensation, and about 14 adverse events for every paid claim. In the USA, and almost certainly in other countries as well, there is a potential for still higher levels of malpractice litigation (Leape, Brennan & Laird, 1991).

Serious medical accidents occur against a background of more frequent minor incidents and errors. Occurrence screening is a process in which medical records are reviewed for specific instances of poor quality care. Adverse occurrences include adverse events, but the screening criteria are much broader. Readmission for incomplete previous management, unplanned return to operating theatre, cardiac or respiratory arrest and abnormal results not accessed by the physician are all included. A British study found that over half of admissions included an adverse occurrence; many were trivial but over a third were clinically relevant (Bennett & Walshe, 1990). Studies of the accuracy of tests and clinical procedures also suggest that errors are common. High rates of error have been found in detecting the clinical signs of cyanosis, interpreting electrocardiograms and radiographs, taking a history and assessing biopsy speci-

[291]

mens in the laboratory. Even basic skills such as resuscitation have been found to fall well short of the expected standard; experience of resuscitation apparently increases confidence, but not skill (Vincent, 1989).

UNDERSTANDING MEDICAL ACCIDENTS

Few studies focus directly on adverse outcomes, but a number of different types of research shed some light on the various factors involved.

Confidential enquiries into maternal and postoperative deaths have revealed problems with supervision of junior staff and a higher mortality from surgeons operating outside their own speciality. Critical incident studies, which analyse potentially dangerous incidents reported by staff, have identified other common themes. Cooper, Newbower and Kitz (1984) examined anaesthetic incidents such as breathing circuit disconnections, drug-syringe swaps and losses of gas supply. Failure to check equipment, unfamiliarity with the equipment, inattention and haste were frequently implicated. A number of recommendations for improved technical training, supervision and the increased use of protocols were made.

A further line of enquiry, which concentrates on incidents where there is a *prima facie* likelihood of substandard care, is the analysis of closed claims. For instance, Ennis and Vincent (1990) summarized the findings of expert obstetricians in claims involving a stillbirth, perinatal or neonatal death, severe handicap or maternal death. Three major areas of concern were identified: inadequate fetal monitoring, in that staff were often unable to recognize abnormal fetal heart traces; mismanagement of forceps (undue traction, too many attempts; lack of involvement of senior staff) inexperienced doctors were left alone for long periods and could not get help when difficulties arose. Such serious incidents are very rare but further studies showed that training in fetal heart monitoring and the use of forceps was generally inadequate.

THE EVOLUTION OF AN ACCIDENT

Studies of accidents in industry, transport and military spheres have led to a much broader understanding of accident causation, with less focus on the individual who makes the error and more on pre-existing organizational factors. Human decisions and actions play a major part in nearly all accidents contributing in two main ways: through active failures and latent failures (Reason, 1993).

Active failures are unsafe acts committed by those at the 'sharp end' of the system (pilots, air-traffic controllers, anaesthetists, surgeons, nurses, etc.) whose actions can have immediate adverse consequences. These unsafe acts or omissions include memory lapses, slips during actions, mistakes due to ignorance or misreading a situation. Deliberate violations of procedures may also occur often simply as short-cuts or to save time. In medicine, most attention has been paid to the active failures. Legal arguments in medical negligence claims usually turn, often unfairly, on the actions of the staff involved rather than background conditions such as inadequate staffing levels.

Latent failures arise from fallible decisions often taken by people not directly involved in the workplace. Their damaging consequences may lie dormant for a long time becoming evident only when they combine with local triggering factors (e.g. unusual events). These latent failures provide the conditions in which unsafe acts occur: high workload and fatigue; inadequate knowledge, ability or experience; poor equipment design; inadequate supervision or instruction; a stressful environment; rapid change within an organization. Violations are encouraged by lack of safety culture, poor morale, macho attitudes and poorly expressed rules. Behind these error and violation-producing conditions may lie a further set of wider organizational problems such as incompatible goals (e.g. conflict between profit and safety), inadequate communications and deficient training.

The bones of this abstract formulation can be fleshed out with an example of an analysis of the death of a patient who vomited under anaesthesia (Reason, 1993). The following is an abbreviated account:

> *A urologist was due to carry out a cystoscopy on a 72-year-old man. Because the operation was to be carried out under local anaesthetic, the patient was not assessed by an anaesthetist beforehand. The urologist discovered that he had been double-booked in the operating theatre. Shortly before the operation he contacted a colleague who agreed to carry out the operation but decided on a general anaesthetic.*
>
> *The anaesthetist was unaware that the patient had not been assessed previously. The first time he saw the patient was in the operating theatre; the patient was belligerent, confused and unable to give a coherent history. The nursing notes showed that the patient had fasted for 24 hours. The records also showed that the patient was suffering metastatic cancer in the lungs and the liver, renal insufficiency and anaemia. After the patient was anaesthetized he regurgitated two litres of undigested food and fluids. The vomit was sucked from his mouth and he was immediately transferred to the Intensive Care Unit. Large quantities of fluid were found in the bronchi and he died some days later.*

Reason's analysis reveals a complex web of factors which ultimately lead to the patient's death. Only a few are given here. Unsafe acts included the first urologist incorrectly suggesting a local rather than a general anaesthetic and the anaesthetist assuming that a confused patient had fasted for 24 hours, as the nursing notes indicated, and only making a cursory preoperative assessment. There were, however, many other contributory factors: double-booking in the operating theatre (leading to a substitution by a second urologist, who did not know the patient); poor communication, so that the anaesthetist was unable to carry out a full preoperative assessment; a nurse's observations of the patient vomiting not being added to the patient's chart. General safety problems were also highlighted concerning the communication of information within the hospital, deficiencies in the operating theatre booking system, design and operation of the computerized record system. None of these failures would have been sufficient individually to cause an accident, but together the outcome was catastrophic.

Analysis of medical accidents often reveals a series of errors combined with a set of unusual circumstances which, together, lead to a catastrophic outcome. This kind of analysis has the potential to reveal deep-rooted unsafe features of organizations that are both inefficient and potentially dangerous. A full analysis, backed with a theoretical framework, makes injury to patients a rather less surprising phenomenon. Consider the range of factors involved. Training is often informal, the assumption often being that observation is sufficient, and the learning of key skills not assessed. Combine trial and error learning with a lack of supervision and the risks become apparent. Add work overload, lack of sleep, lack of awareness of hazardous situations, a degree of over-confidence stemming perhaps from a desire to prove oneself, and the potential for major disasters becomes apparent.

PREVENTING ACCIDENTS

In the USA, and to a lesser extent elsewhere, hospital risk management programmes are regarded by many as one of the most promising responses to the medical malpractice crisis. They are increasingly demanded by hospital insurers. Such programmes aim to: (i) reduce the frequency of preventable adverse events; (ii) reduce the chance of a claim being made after an adverse event and (iii) control the costs of claims that are made. At the heart of most programmes are methods for early identification of adverse events, using either staff reports or a systematic screening of records. Similar systems are already in operation in respect of drugs and the safety of medicines. Reports of serious incidents are made before claims are initiated, and while memories are still fresh. The reports are used to create a database to identify common patterns and prevent future incidents. Ideally patients and relatives are also informed about adverse incidents and action is taken to minimize both the physical and psychological trauma (Vincent, 1995).

Such programmes take years to establish and their effects only become gradually apparent. Evaluation of risk management is in its infancy. Nevertheless, at least some elements of risk management seem to be effective. Key elements in programmes are: educating clinicians about their role in risk management, formalizing channels of communication to enable early intervention with patients and their families after adverse incidents and establishing a strong organizational structure for dealing with the findings of reviews of adverse events. The involvement and personal commitment of senior clinicians is crucial (Morlock & Malitz, 1991).

Formal risk management programmes are desirable but more specific changes are also needed. Improvements in training and supervision are clearly important. Many senior doctors, and probably hospital management, may be unaware of the extent to which junior doctors are called upon to act beyond their competence. Poor communication between professions is another source of errors and lost information. Linked to the need for better training and supervision is the question of error-producing working conditions, particularly the excessive hours that junior staff are still required to work in Britain and many other countries. It is a curious paradox that it illegal to drive a coachload of healthy passengers without regular rest, yet it is considered acceptable to care for a ward full of desperately sick patients when close to exhaustion (Vincent, Ennis & Audley, 1993).

Another important theme that emerges from analyses of accidents is that many aspects of medical practice must rely less on an individual doctor's memory and clinical judgement and make greater use of guidelines and formal protocols. Protocols can be perceived as limiting clinical freedom or restricting innovation, but when flexibly applied they can allow clinical freedom while still setting limits on safe practice (Drife, 1993). They may be especially important in emergencies and unusual situations. An experienced doctor can react quickly, while a junior may flounder in the absence of an already rehearsed emergency drill. The complexity of many medical decisions, especially when they involve assessing both the probabilities and likely outcomes of different courses of action, means that computer – assisted diagnosis and the use of other formal decision – making aids may be needed to reduce some of the uncertainty and associated risks to patients.

THE COSTS OF INJURY TO PATIENTS

The financial costs of litigation, and the associated insurance premiums, have attracted great attention. In the USA malpractice costs were over one billion dollars per annum by 1985 and were continuing to rise (Dingwall & Fenn, 1991). There are, however, many other costs associated with medical accidents, both human and financial.

Many patients suffer increased pain and disability and psychological trauma. They may become depressed, angry and bitter, and their problems are often compounded by a protracted adversarial legal process. They may experience their treatment as a terrible betrayal of trust, and it is possible that this degree of feeling impedes recovery and is damaging in itself (Vincent, Pincus & Scurr, 1993). Staff may experience shame, guilt and depression after making a mistake. Feeling responsible for injuring a patient appears to be one of the main sources of stress for young doctors (Firth-Cozens & Morrison, 1989). Litigation imposes an additional burden, in that doctors may feel unfairly attacked and blamed.

Injury to patients means increased use of hospital resources and additional time with staff. A doctor whose confidence has been impaired will probably work less effectively and efficiently. At the worst they may abandon medicine as a career. Most importantly, in financial terms, there are huge costs in the form of increased disability payments and other benefits which are likely to far outweigh the costs to individual hospitals. The financial cost of adverse events is therefore many times greater than the immediate costs of litigation and compensation.

The cost, delays and unfairness of the various legal systems have led many to propose that compensation for medical injury should be awarded on a 'no-fault' basis. Usually, this means that a government backed scheme compensates victims simply on the grounds that medical treatment caused their injuries. This appears to be a simple and attractive option. However, there are several variants of the basic scheme and many potential problems. No-fault schemes potentially reduce the accountability of hospitals and their staff; the costs are usually unknown, and very much dependent on other benefits available; and, finally, establishing causation, which is often very difficult, is still necessary (Fenn, 1993).

WHEN ACCIDENTS DO OCCUR: CARING FOR THE INJURED PATIENT

When a patient is injured by treatment, compensation may be both justified and necessary. However, compensation is not the only motive for legal action. Patients may blame doctors not so much for the original mistakes as for a lack of openness or willingness to explain them after the event. A valuable feature of the legal system, seldom remarked on but much appreciated by patients, is that their case is reviewed by a truly independent expert instructed by their lawyer. Many patients find that a clear and sympathetic report or interview is a relief, whether or not it suggests that care was actually negligent. Simply knowing the truth brings some peace of mind.

Many injured patients wish to ensure that other patients do not suffer in the same way, and this is often one of their reasons for taking legal action. If useful changes are made they may feel that some good as come of their bad experiences which may also help them cope with the trauma involved. The accounts of injured patients are easily dismissed as angry, unbalanced and a great deal of useful information is lost.

Counselling for injured patients is often necessary. The counsellor needs a knowledge of medical practice as well as the skills required for the treatment of trauma and depression (Vincent &

Robertson, 1993). Mediating and supporting both patients and staff after adverse events is an important function of risk management staff. After major incidents, staff too may need help, and signs of stress in such situations should not be taken as weakness. For staff to attempt to cope regardless of the consequences to themselves and their patients is dangerously irresponsible. Senior staff and those involved in risk management need to be aware that the effects of serious incidents may be felt throughout the department and, on occasions, throughout the hospital.

REFERENCES

Bennett, J. & Walshe, K. (1990). Occurrence screening as a method of audit. *British Medical Journal*, **300**, 1248–51.

Cooper, J.B., Newbower, R.S. & Kitz, R.J. (1984). An analysis of major errors and equipment failures in anaesthesia management: considerations for prevention and detection. *Anaesthesiology*, **60**, 34–42.

Dingwall, R. & Fenn, P. (1991). Is risk management necessary? *International Journal of Risk and Safety in Medicine*, **2**, 91–106.

Drife, J.O. (1993). Errors and accidents in obstetrics. In *Medical accidents*, pp. 34–51, Oxford: Oxford University Press.

Ennis, M. & Vincent, C.A. (1990). Obstetric accidents: a review of 64 cases. *British Medical Journal*, **300**, 1365–7.

Fenn, P. (1993). Compensation for medical injury: a review of policy options. In Vincent, C.A., Ennis, M. & Audley, R.J. (Eds.). *Medical Accidents*, pp. 198–208, Oxford: Oxford University Press.

Firth-Cozens, J. & Morrison, L.A. (1989). Sources of stress and ways of coping in junior house officers. *Stress Medicine*, **5**, 121–6.

Hiatt, H.H., Barnes, B.A., Brennan, T.A., Laird, N.M., Lowthers, A.G., Leape, L.L., Localio, A.R., Newhouse, J.P., Peterson, L.M. & Thorpe, K.E. (1989). A study of medical injury and medical malpractice: an overview. *New England Journal of Medicine*, **321**, 480.

Leape, L.L., Brennan, T.A., Laird, N.M., Lowthers, A.G., Localio, A.R., Barnes, B.A., Hebert, C., Newhouse, J.P., Weiler, P.C. & Hiatt, H.H. (1991). The nature of adverse events and negligence in hospitalized patients. *Iatrogenics*, **1**, 17.

Morlock, L.L. & Malitz, F.E. (1991). Do hospital risk management programs make a difference?: relationships between risk management program activities and hospital malpractice claims experience. *Law and Contemporary Problems*, **54**, 1–22.

Reason, J.T. (1993). The human factor in medical accidents. In Vincent, C.A., Ennis, M. & Audley, R.J. (Eds.). *Medical accidents*, pp. 1–16, Oxford: Oxford University Press.

Vincent, C.A. (1989). Research into medical accidents: a case of negligence? *British Medical Journal*, **299**, 1150–3.

Vincent, C.A. (ed.). (1995). *Clinical risk management*. London: BMJ Publications.

Vincent, C.A., Ennis, M. & Audley, R.J. (Eds.). (1993). *Medical accidents*. Oxford: Oxford University Press.

Vincent, C.A., Pincus, T. & Scurr, J.H. (1993). Patient's experience of surgical accidents. *Quality in Health Care*, **2**, 77–82.

Vincent, C.A. & Robertson, I. (1993). Recovering from a medical accident: the consequences for patients and their families. In Vincent, C.A., Ennis, M. & Audley, R.J. (Eds.). *Medical accidents*, pp. 150–166, Oxford: Oxford University Press.

Medical decision-making

PETER AYTON
City University, London,
UK

GEORGE WRIGHT
Strathclyde Graduate Business School, Scotland,
UK

GENE ROWE
University of Surrey,
UK

INTRODUCTION

Doctors constantly make decisions that affect the health and lives of other people. They gather evidence by interpreting the signs and symptoms of the patient, conducting examinations and determining appropriate tests. Using such evidence they may form a diagnosis and conclude what, if anything, is to be done. All of these actions imply the use of judgement and decision-making. Many of these decisions will be based on clear evidence from the patient, and tried and tested methods drawn from the doctor's medical knowledge and may seem quite straightforward. However, very often, simple medical principles and rules will not be available. The evidence may be uncertain: signs and symptoms can be ambiguous and tests results are rarely 100% accurate. Tests and treatments can involve adverse

side-effects or a risk of permanent damage or even death. In the absence of a clear rule for such situations, doctors will be obliged to apply their judgement.

A number of questions then naturally arise: How do doctors make their judgements? How good is medical judgement? How does it develop? Can it be improved? This chapter provides a brief review of some of the answers to these questions that are emerging from the psychological research.

CLINICAL VERSUS STATISTICAL DECISIONS

Research investigating medical decision-making has a fairly short but intense history. The first significant development was Meehl's (1954) book which evaluated clinical judgement. Meehl compared the intuitive clinical judgements made by experts (e.g. is this patient schizophrenic?) with those that could be made by a statistical formula using the same information. The statistical decisions were based on a 'linear model'. A linear model summarizes the relationship between a set of predictor variables and some criterion value (the outcome to be predicted). For example, if predicting the chances of survival from major surgery, relevant predictor variables may be the age, weight and general fitness of the patient. The linear model is constructed in such a way as to maximize the statistical relationship between the predictor variables and the criterion to be predicted. The value of each of the predictor variables is differentially weighted according to the strength of its diagnostic relationship to the criterion, and then all the variables are summed.

In approximately 20 studies, which compared clinical decisions with statistical decisions, Meehl found that the statistical model provided more accurate predictions or the two models tied. Over the years since, there have been many more studies comparing clinical and statistical judgement in an enormous range of areas of judgement. The superiority of the statistical method over clinical judgement has been replicated in all of these studies. Meehl (1986) commented: 'There is no controversy in social science which shows such a large body of qualitatively diverse studies coming out so uniformly in the same direction as this one.'

Despite this claim, the effect of the research on the practice of clinical judgement has been limited; according to Dawes (1988) it is 'almost zilch'. Dawes argues that this is because the findings are a challenge to the self-perceptions of experts. It is difficult for highly trained clinicians to accept that they cannot outperform a procedure which simply adds up the cues in favour of each judgement and picks the one with the highest score. This resistance may well be stiffened by the knowledge that the statistical method will not be perfect. There is evidence that resistance to the use of simple decision rules, which (given present knowledge) cannot be outperformed, increases with expertise and the importance of the decision. Doctors may find it unacceptable to settle for the given number of errors implied by the statistical approach when they feel that their judgement might do better. Moreover, when the statistical decision conflicts with the doctor's decision, the statistical decision may be seen as risky while their own judgement is seen as safe, quite opposite to the conclusion drawn from research.

So why is statistical judgement superior? Of course, the statistical approach relies on all the relevant evidence being coded in a quantitative fashion, something which may itself require considerable clinical skill but which would not ordinarily be performed in clinical situations. The statistical model will, moreover, utilize this evidence in an entirely consistent fashion. The statistical model will not be influenced by fatigue and boredom or distracted by spurious factors as human judgement is. A large number of studies have discovered inconsistency in medical judgements. Studies reviewed by Schwartz and Griffin (1986) have shown that doctors will show substantial disagreement with each other when interpreting chest X-rays, electrocardiograms and electroencephalograms as well as more global quantities such as severity of depression. They will also sometimes disagree with their own previous judgements. One study that asked pathologists to examine the same tissue sample on two different occasions found that the conclusions (malign or benign) differed 28% of the time.

PSYCHOLOGICAL ACCOUNTS OF MEDICAL JUDGEMENT

The statistical modelling approach of Meehl and others makes no claims to investigate how medical judgements are actually made. However, other studies of medical judgement have sought to examine the extent to which descriptive theories of human judgement developed in the psychological laboratory apply in medical contexts. One theoretical approach to judgement assumes that, because human information processing capacity is limited, people do not judge under uncertainty using systematic strategies. Instead, they use mental heuristics (rules of thumb) to judge uncertainties (Kahneman, Slovic & Tversky, 1982). One such heuristic is representiveness. This heuristic determines how likely it is that an event is a member of a category, according to how similar or typical the event is to the category. For example, people may judge the likelihood that a given individual is employed as a librarian by the extent to which the individual resembles a typical librarian. This may seem a reasonable strategy but it neglects consideration of the relative prevalence of librarians. When base-rates of different categories vary, judgements may be correspondingly biased.

Another heuristic used for probabilistic judgement is availability. This heuristic is invoked when people estimate likelihood or relative frequency by the ease with which instances can be brought to mind. Instances of frequent events are typically easier to recall than instances of less frequent events so availability will often be a valid cue for estimates of likelihood. However, availability is affected by factors other than likelihood. For example, recent events and emotionally salient events are more easy to recollect. It is a common experience that the perceived riskiness of air travel rises in the immediate wake of an air disaster. Judgements made on the basis of availability then are vulnerable to bias.

The literature reporting investigations of expert medical judgement provides several instances of poor judgement attributable to heuristic processing, some of which have serious potential consequences. Eddy (1982) set a sample of physicians the task of estimating the likelihood that a patient had cancer given that, prior to the X-ray, their examination of the patient indicated a 99% probability that the lesion was benign but that the X-ray test was positive and had indicated it was malignant. They were told that research into the accuracy of the test showed that 79.2% of malignant lesions were correctly diagnosed, and 90.4% of benign lesions were correctly diagnosed by the test. Applying a probability rule known as Bayes' theorem to this evidence allows us to consider the diagnosis as a statistical inference and calculate that the probability of cancer, in the light of the positive test, is nearly 8%.

However, most of the physicians misinterpreted the information about the reliability of the test and estimated the likelihood of cancer to be about 75%. When asked about their reasoning, the physicians report that they assumed that the probability of cancer given a positive test result [p(cancer/positive)] is equal to the probability of a positive X-ray in a patient with cancer [p(positive/cancer)]. They seem to have used a representativeness heuristic in that they judged the likelihood of cancer in patients with a positive test in terms of how typical (or representative) they were of patients with cancer. They failed to properly consider the impact on the outcome of the very low incidence of the disease together with the tendency of the test to (falsely) show positive test results.

Confirmation that real decisions are taken on the basis of such misunderstandings is provided by Dawes (1988). He cites a case of a doctor performing mastectomy operations on women judged to have high risk of breast cancer. The surgery was justified on the grounds that 'one in two or three DY (highest-risk) women will develop it between the ages of 40 and 59'. It turns out that the conclusion was based on the probability that a woman with cancer will have DY breasts [p(DY/cancer)]. However, the relevant probability [p(cancer/DY)] is approximately one in eight.

In order to make a clinical diagnosis, the doctor must make an inference that involves assessing the probability that a patient has the disease given some pattern of symptoms [p(disease/symptoms)]. However, according to Eddy and Clanton (1982), medical knowledge is not organized to assist this process. Most medical texts discuss the probability that patients will present a certain pattern of symptoms given that they have the disease [p(symptoms/disease)]. This information is not sufficient for making a diagnosis and the focus on it may well encourage the false notion that p(disease/symptoms) is the same as p(symptoms/disease). The confusion between the two probabilities may be further engendered by the type of instruction that trainee physicians receive. On ward rounds, patients with certain diseases are examined, and the co–occurrence of symptoms is noted. But, people with the same symptoms but without the disease (healthy people not in hospital and patients with similar symptoms and different diseases) will not be subject to the same scrutiny. As a result, the diagnostic significance of a given set of symptoms may be overestimated.

Christensen-Szalanski et al. (1983) discovered an availability bias in physicians' estimates of the risk (mortality rate) of various diseases. They studied physicians and students and found that both groups overestimated the risks. In general physicians were more accurate than the students, but the estimates of both groups were found to be biased by actual encounters with people with the disease.

Another worrying judgement phenomenon is hindsight bias. This is the experimentally demonstrated tendency for people to give higher subjective likelihoods to events once they know that they have occurred (in hindsight) than they would to the same events if they don't know the outcome (Fischhoff, 1975). Arkes et al. (1981) asked physicians to read a case history and then assign likelihoods to each of four possible presented diagnoses. One group was told nothing about the correct diagnosis while the others were told that one of the presented diagnoses was the correct one. Knowledge of the supposedly correct diagnosis increased the subjective probability of that diagnosis; hence the probabilities for the diagnoses were influenced by hindsight.

The doctors in the hindsight conditions of the experiment were in a similar situation to that which will frequently occur in their education and training, examining a patient with a known diagnosis and reviewing the relationship with the symptoms. If, because of the hindsight bias, doctors fail to experience surprise when they learn of outcomes they may assume that their ability to gauge the likelihood of outcomes is more accurate than it actually is. This would cause overestimates of the diagnosticity of symptoms and result in overconfidence.

Evidence that physicians overconfidently diagnose is provided by Christensen-Szalanski and Bushyhead (1981) who explored the validity of the probabilities given by physicians to diagnoses of pneumonia. They found that their probability judgements were inaccurate; the proportion of patients who turned out to have pneumonia was far less than their probability statements implied. These authors had previously established that the physicians' estimates of the probability, of a patient having pneumonia was significantly correlated with clinically significant actions such as their decision to give a patient a chest X-ray and to assign a pneumonia diagnosis.

PRESCRIPTIVE APPROACHES TO MEDICAL DECISION-MAKING

The prescriptive approach to decision-making seeks to identify the ideal method by which decisions should be made. According to Expected Utility theory, the major theory defining rational decisions, choice of actions should reflect both probabilities and utilities. The approach prescribes evaluation of different courses of action in order to choose the best. Each option is evaluated in terms of the probabilities of achieving all of the possible outcomes that may ensue from it and their relative value. For each option these two quantities are multiplied together to determine the expected utility. Accordingly, the option which has the highest expected utility is chosen.

For example, consider contemplating risky surgery which has a chance of complete success and a chance of death, but without the operation you will be blind for the rest of your life. In order to determine the best option, quantification of the values associated with these outcomes and their likelihood is required. The values associated with the possible outcomes here may well vary for different individuals so Decision Analysis, the term given to the application of Expected Utility theory, encourages the expression of values that reflect individual patient's utilities for the outcomes. The method can thereby be used as a means for involving patients in decisions about their own treatment (important when informed consent is required) and it has been developed as a counselling technique to help pregnant women make decisions about risky tests for foetal abnormalities. The approach can also accommodate problems of allocation of limited resources and decisions about administering tests given that costs and risks are involved.

The strategy of decision analysis is to decompose what may be very complex decisions involving many considerations into basic components. Using a decision tree, the components are then evaluated so that the attractiveness of each option can be determined. The appeal of the procedure is that it represents a systematic attempt to analyse all relevant considerations and give them their appropriate weight. Studies of decision analysis used in real clinical settings indicate that the procedure results in different decisions being made to those that would have been made intuitively; doctors are sometimes surprised by the recommendations of the analysis (Sonnenberg & Pauker, 1986), which is one reason why they may be reluctant to accept the result. To this extent then the procedure is clearly not redundant, but does it produce *better* decisions? The decomposition rationale would suggest that it prevents information overload and permits consideration of more factors than unaided intuition would allow.

Elstein et al. (1986) studied decisions regarding oestrogen replacement therapy, a treatment for osteoporosis which entails an increased risk of cancer, for a sample of women with varying levels of cancer risk, fracture risk and symptom severity. They compared intuitive decisions made by the doctors with those made by decision analysis where the same doctors provided their own estimates of all the relevant probabilities and utilities for all the possible outcomes. The decision analysis recommended the treatment far more often than the clinicians' intuitions. Intuitively the clinicians appeared to give far too much weight to the risk of cancer. Calculations indicated that, as very poor outcomes are so rare, the increased risk was heavily outweighed by the powerful benefits of the therapy. The idea that the doctors' component probabilities and utilities were somehow in error was rejected. In general, the component estimates of likelihood were accurate and sensitivity analysis on the values used showed that any reasonable set of values entered in the decision analysis recommended treatment. Decisions therefore appeared to hinge on the suboptimal way different bits of information were combined, not on (un)awareness of specific risks and benefits. Doctors may also feel more troubled by harm that may be caused by their actions than that which 'just happens'. Decision analysis evaluates outcomes independently of their causes but bad outcomes judged as caused by intervention may intuitively be considered worse than equally bad outcomes caused by inaction (Baron, in press).

One difficulty for any method of deciding is that quite arbitrary ways in which risky dilemmas are described can strongly influence decisions. Tversky and Kahneman (1981) argue that, when contemplating benefits, people are 'risk averse' and will prefer certain gains to gambles. However, when contemplating losses people will be 'risk seeking' inasmuch as they will take risks to avoid certain losses. They presented physicians with the problem of deciding what to do in the event that a new disease threatened to kill 600 people. Programme A would save 200 people while programme B would give a 1/3 chance that all 600 would be saved and a 2/3 chance that none would be saved. Here the description of the problem refers to the lives that can be saved and the majority of respondents chose programme A. However, if the same problem was described in terms of the lives that will be lost then the majority chose B. Doctors have also been found to have different preferences for risky therapies for cancer depending on whether the probabilities refer to mortality or survival McNeil et al. (1982).

CONCLUSION

Traditionally, medical training has been largely concerned with the biomedical sciences. Increasingly, however, competence in the decision sciences is being seen as vital to good medical practice. The methods for making a decision become crucial when the physician is uncertain through incomplete or ambiguous information or when risks are involved. The growing mass of psychological research investigating medical decision-making present a strong argument for the view that these decisions may not always be optimal and that, with the application of developing methods, they can be improved. (See also 'Risk perception and health behaviour', 'Stress management', 'Written communication').

REFERENCES

Arkes, H.R., Saville, P.D., Wortmann, R.L. & Harkness, A.R. (1981). Hindsight bias among physicians weighing the likelihood of diagnosis. *Journal of Applied Psychology*, 66, 252–4.

Baron, J. (1994) Non-consequentialist decisions. *Behavioral and Brain Sciences*, 17, 1–42.

Christensen-Szalanski, J.J.J. & Bushyhead, J.B. (1981). Physicians use of probabilistic information in a real clinical setting. *Journal of Experimental Psychology, Human Perception and Performance*, 7, 928–35.

Christensen-Szalanski, J.J.J., Beck D.E., Christensen-Szalanski, C.M. & Koepsell. T.D. (1983). Effects of expertise and experience on risk judgements. *Journal of Applied Psychology*, 68, 278–84.

Dawes, R.M. (1988). *Rational Choice in an uncertain World*. Orlando: Harcourt.

Eddy, D. M. (1982). Probabilistic reasoning in clinical medicine: problems and opportunities. In Kahneman. D., Slovic, P. & Tversky, A. (Eds.) *Judgement under uncertainty: heuristics and biases*. Cambridge: Cambridge University Press.

Eddy, D.M. & Clanton. C.H. (1982). The art of clinical diagnosis: solving the Clinicopathological exercise. *The New England Journal of Medicine*, 306, 1263–8.

Elstein, A.S., Holzman, G.B., Ravitch, M.M., Metheny, W.A, Holmes, M.M, Hoppe, R.B, Rothert, M.L. & Rovner, D.R. (1986). Comparisons of physicians' decisions regarding estrogen replacement therapy for menopausal women and decisions derived from a decision analytic model. *American Journal of Medicine*, 80, 216–58.

Fischhoff, B. (1975). Hindsight foresight: the effect of outcome knowledge on judgement under uncertainty. *Journal of Experimental Psychology: Human Perception and Performance*, 1, 288–9.

Kahneman, D., Slovic, P. & Tversky, A. (1982). *Judgement under uncertainty: heuristics and biases*. Cambridge: Cambridge University Press.

McNeil, B.J., Pauker, S.G., Sox, H.E. & Tversky, A. (1982). On the elicitation of preferences for alternative therapies. *New England Journal of Medicine*, 306, 1259–62.

Meehl, P.E. (1954). *Clinical versus Statistical Prediction: a theoretical analysis and a review of the evidence*. Minneapolis: University of Minnesota Press.

Meehl. P.E. (1986). Causes and effects of my disturbing little book. *Journal of Personality Assessment*, 50, 370–5.

Schwartz, S. Griffin, T. (1986). *Medical thinking: the psychology of medical judgement and decision making*. New York: Springer Verlag.

Sonnenberg, F.A. & Pauker, S. G. (1986). Elective pericardiectomy for tuberculous pericarditis: should the snappers be snipped? *Medical Decision Making*, 6 110–23.

Tversky, A. & Kahneman, D. (1981). The framing of decisions and the psychology of choice. Science, 211, 453–8.

Nurse–patient communication: nursing assessment and intervention for effective pain control

VERONICA (NICKY) THOMAS

and

JILL MACLEOD CLARK

School of Life, Medical and Health Sciences,
King's College London, UK

INTRODUCTION

A number of factors in the health-care systems in the United Kingdom (UK) and elsewhere, have brought about a greater recognition of the need for nurses to communicate effectively with their patients. Over the past two decades the patient's role has changed from a predominantly passive dependent one to a more active, motivated role which assumes greater responsibility and involvement in care. Nurses' roles are also changing from a focus on caring for dependent patients to that of partnerships with clients in providing care. Perceptions of the illness role itself are changing with increased emphasis on the psychological and social aspects of illness (Bradley & Edinberg, 1982).

The parameters of nursing practice are thus continuously expanding and changing but there seems to be a consensus that nursing is a profession concerned with developing relationships which support the highly dependent, whilst helping others to achieve maximum independence in an area of health care. Good communication between the nurse and the patient or client is essential to this process.

The purpose of communication is to ensure effective social contact and interaction. In the context of nursing, this includes developing and maintaining relationships, making accurate assessments, giving information and advice and offering opportunities for the expression of preferences, feelings and emotions. Such interactions will only be effective and therapeutic if nurses possess and utilize appropriate communication skills and strategies. A considerable amount of research has been undertaken over the past three decades, which has illuminated the need to enhance the quality of nurse–patient communication in health care (Cartwright, 1964; Macleod Clark, 1982; Seers, 1986; Corney *et al.*, 1992; Field *et al.*, 1992).

Over the same period there has been a greatly increased emphasis on the development of communication skills during nurse education (Davis, 1987; Burnard, 1992). However, in spite of this clear recognition of the importance of this issue, the Ombudsmen annual review (Audit Commission, 1993) in the UK, continues to demonstrate that a significant proportion of patients' complaints focus on deficits in communication.

Assessment is a key nursing activity underpinning the process of executing an analysis of physical and psychosocial status, identifying problems, needs and priorities in care. Once an assessment has been skilfully completed, the emphasis shifts to the more therapeutic intention. Here, the nurse needs to use appropriate communication skills to ensure that any nursing intervention is indeed of benefit and that a trusting relationship is established. Different types of patients will have very different needs and there are huge variations in problems of both a psychological and physical nature that are encountered.

These all require a range of assessment and intervention skills and strategies. The focus of this chapter is on the common problem of acute pain after surgery to exemplify the advantages of effective communication. Pain is a psychophysiological problem that is frequently manifested across all nursing specialities and all contexts in hospital and the community. Expression of pain is an important means of communication.

COMMUNICATION IN EFFECTIVE PAIN ASSESSMENT

Pain is a multidimensional experienced that has sensory–discriminative, motivational–affective and cognitive–evaluative components (Melzack & Wall, 1988). Thus pain intensity, sensation and affect are all influenced by the unique qualities of the person. These include age (Belville *et al.*, 1971; Kaiko, 1980; Foley, 1985) gender (Miller & Shuter, 1984; Taenzer, Melzack & Jeans, 1986) cultural background (Miller & Shuter, 1984; Thomas & Rose, 1991) neuroticism (Taenzer *et al.*, 1986; Thomas, 1991) state and trait anxiety (Seers, 1986; Taenzer *et al.*, 1986; Thomas, 1991) and coping style (Miller & Mangan, 1983; Thomas, 1991). The nurse in the assessment of patients' pain should be aware that these patients' variables are likely to influence the manner in which pain is communicated.

The management of postoperative pain is a social transaction between the patient and the nurse, i.e. the patient reports the pain and the nurse acts on the report. Therefore, successful assessment and relief is dependent on establishing a positive therapeutic relationship between the nurse and patient. As stated earlier, patient-centred care is of central importance within all aspects of nursing care but the need to listen to what the patient says becomes absolutely paramount when assessing pain. According to McCaffrey (1972) 'pain is whatever the experiencing person says it is and exists whenever he says it does'. This definition highlights the subjectivity of the experience which is accessible to the patient only. Although the management of pain is problematic, nurses in general subscribe to this philosophy.

The mainstay of postoperative pain assessment should be the patients' self-report (AHCPR, 1992). There are a number of pain self-assessment tools available which include numerical rating, visual analogue and verbal rating scales. For a full discussion of pain assessment scales currently available, the reader is referred to Turk & Melzack, (1992). The patient's self-report is the most reliable indicator of the presence of pain and its associated distress and it is arguable that neither behaviour nor vital signs should be used instead (Beyer, McGrath & Berde, 1990). Patients may, in fact, be experiencing severe pain even while smiling and using laughter as a coping mechanism (Fritz, 1988).

Patients unable to communicate effectively in order to convey the fact that they have pain require special considerations for pain assessment, e.g. neonates and children, developmentally delayed persons and non-English speaking patients. Modified pain assessment scales have been developed and are used commonly among children and the developmentally delayed (Turk & Melzack, 1992). Translators or relatives of non-English speaking relatives should be utilized to ascertain from the patients' perspective the most convenient and appropriate manner in which to assess his pain.

Since it is well known that the preoperative period is often immensely stressful (Thomas, 1991; Wilson-Barnett 1979) and that this anxiety heightens pain experience, the assessment of pain in the surgical situation should begin before the actual operation. The time and place of assessment can have an important influence. Many patients find lack of privacy when communicating with nurses about their condition very stressful (French, 1979). The therapeutic environment is established when the patient feels able to talk to the nurse without fear of interruption or distraction and where the nurse has time to listen (Feely, 1994). This will enable the patient to speak freely and disclose more about the type and quality of pain which, in turn, will allow effective care to be planned.

During this assessment period the nurse attempts to minimize the degree of anticipated surgical pain by relieving the patient's apprehension. This is achieved by using appropriate questioning techniques and listening skills to elicit information about particular fears and to identify normal pain coping strategies. Open questions are most appropriate in this situation because a question such as 'tell me how you are feeling at this moment' is more likely to allow the patient to talk freely about fears and anxieties.

Nurses' assessment of pain is not a simple matter. Although they may make use of patients' verbal and non-verbal signals, these signals occur as part of an interaction and this may affect their perceptions. Patients may deny pain for a variety of reasons including cultural attitudes (the need to be stoical), fear of addiction to pain-relieving drugs, fear of injection or simply because they have low expectations of pain relief. When they do acknowledge their pain, some may be inhibited from their natural expression or, in their inability to endure and their desire to convince, may adopt modes of expression which are unacceptable to nurses (McCaffrey & Beebe, 1989). For example, patients may adopt pain behaviour which appears disproportionate to the physiological process. Those who give this unacceptable response easily become stereotyped and can be labelled as demanding and a complainer, which makes their task of convincing even more difficult. This breakdown in communi-

cation must be avoided in order to provide effective intervention. To achieve this, nurses must be aware at all times that pain assessment is a co-operative venture, and success depends not only on the assessment of the patient's expression but also on the management of their own reaction to that expression.

COMMUNICATION IN EFFECTIVE PAIN CONTROL INTERVENTION

Enhancing personal control through information

Within the postoperative pain situation patients are often helpless, attached to tubes and are dependent on the nursing staff for their most basic activities of living. Nurses can enhance patients' sense of control through effective communication by providing information and efficient patient teaching. To help patients to cope with pain effectively, the nurse explains fully the necessary preoperative procedures, the surgical course, the accompanying pain and the measures available for relief.

The provision of accurate information before surgery by nurses allows patients to interpret their surroundings and circumstances which helps them to anticipate events in the postoperative period. The importance of information in enhancing patients' sense of control, reducing pain and promoting recovery within the context of postoperative setting was highlighted first by the use of procedural information. In an early study, Hayward (1975) provided detailed procedural information preoperatively to surgical patients, and found that this group was less anxious and experienced less pain than an attention placebo control group.

Procedural information provided by nurses has been seen also to reduce the physiological indicators of stress. For example, Boore (1978) demonstrated that procedural information brought about a significant reduction in the amount of urinary hydroxicorticosteroids secreted and a reduction in infection rates. Although procedural information is of benefit, it seems that preoperative nurse–patient communication is more effective in enhancing patients' control if it focuses on the patient' sensory experience rather than on the objective nature of the procedure.

Sensory information is chronologically structured and include details of the common sensations that the patient will feel, see and hear. Terminology is derived from the patients themselves, their vocabulary reflecting both what is familiar and what is actually experienced. This is important because Byrne & Edeani (1983) found that several terms commonly used by nurses are not understood by patients.

'Sticking', 'pounding' and 'gurgling' are examples of sensory words commonly used by patients. Johnson (1983) considers that this type of information provides the patient with an imaginary map which minimizes pain because it reduces the incongruency between what the patient expects to experience and what he actually does experience.

NON-VERBAL COMMUNICATION: PROMOTING RECOVERY BY MEANS OF TOUCHING

Touch is an essential part of nursing since it is impossible to give a physical care such as a bedbath without touching patients. This kind of touch is referred to as procedural. Caring touch is that which does not involve physical care and is more sensitive than procedural touch (Bradley & Edinberg, 1982). Caring touch can be effectively used as a form of communication, conveying comfort, love, security and warmth and thereby enhance self-esteem (Mackereth, 1987).

Touch can overcome the potentially dehumanizing effect of the patient' stay in a hospital because it promotes trust, empathy as well as enhancing verbal communication. Research has demonstrated that caring touch is perceived by patients as a therapeutic gesture. Farrah (1979)(cited by Bradley & Edinberg, 1982) suggests that caring touch not only establishes and maintain openness of communication and the development of rapport, it often transcends oral communication and promotes contact with reality.

Receptors for pain and touch transmit both sensations at once but it has been found that caring touch of less than 1 second has enormous potential to make a person feel better (Doerhing, 1989). Therapeutic touch has been known for some time to have physiological benefits including pain relief, increased muscle flexibility, increased levels of haemoglobin and improved circulation (Horrigan, 1993). Such results are of particular advantage to the postoperative patient.

There are a number of nursing interventions where touch can be used therapeutically and also as an alternative to other less appropriate interventions (Boyek & Watson, 1994). For example, waking someone up by stroking the arm instead of shouting; holding a patient's hand while assisting him/her to walk to the lavatory or incorporating a gentle rub on the back during a bath. In addition to caring touch, there are a number of specific procedures which is slowly being introduced in the nursing repertoire for managing pain (Turton, 1989). For example, massage, reflexology and the laying on of hands. The warmth, care and non-verbal communication involved enables the patient to be more able to cope with the pain (Turton, 1989; Farrow, 1990).

The use of caring touch by nurses involves a certain element of risk because it can easily be misconstrued by patients. Nevertheless, caring touch in nursing encourages closeness, a sense of trust and reassurance (Bradley & Edinberg, 1982).

'Presencing' is also a form of non-verbal technique that is of value in helping patients to manage their pain. 'Presence' is more than simply being with the patient, it means behaving in a reassuring manner, that quietly and effectively communicates 'being there' (Benner & Wrubel, 1989). By being with patient in this way, some nurses are able to help reduce pain.

COMMUNICATION IN THE PRESENCE OF TECHNOLOGY

New technological advances are often being introduced into the clinical setting in an attempt to reform some aspect of patients' care. Within the context of postoperative pain, patient controlled analgesia (PCA) a method of analgesia that hands over the control of pain to the patient has been shown to be significantly more effective in controlling pain than nurse-administered analgesin (Thomas, Heath & Rose, 1990; Notcutt & Morgan; 1990; Thomas, 1991). However, successful use of PCA by the patient depends very much on good nurse – patient communication. It is essential that the nurse provides the patient with accurate information about its use, the basic principles and safety elements. In return the nurse is required to listen actively to what the patient says about how he or she is coping with this form of therapy. It is also extremely important to interact continually with patients whilst they are receiving this therapy in order to assess whether pain is being adequately controlled.

PCA provides patients with a great ability to control their level of pain. However, some patients have cause for dissatisfaction. Recent research (Koh & Thomas, 1994) has shown that some surgical patients using PCA would like more verbal interaction from nursing staff. This suggests that nurse–patient communication has an important role in enhancing pain relief and promoting patient satisfaction with care.

CONCLUSION

Currently the emphasis in nursing care is upon patient-centred care, and the standard of care is dependent upon the quality of the interpersonal relationship that the nurse has with her patient. This chapter has concentrated on communication as an effective way to the provide good quality holistic care in the context of postoperative pain management. Pain management in the past was framed around suspicion, i.e. was the pain real or severe enough for nursing intervention? This distrustful practice has been replaced by increasing the patient's control through effective communication and information exchange, various self-care pain relief strategies or through receiving pain relief via patient-controlled dosing.

Overall it seems that the responsibilities of the nurse are related to helping the patient cope with the stress related to (i) pain, its treatment and effort to maintain health and; (ii) the environment in which health care is provided.

REFERENCES

Audit Commission (1993). *What seems to be the matter: communication between hospitals and patients.* London: HMSO.

Agency for Health Care Policy and Research (AHCPR) (1992). Acute pain management: operative or medical procedures and trauma. Clinical Practice Guidelines. Public Health Service, US Department of Health and Human Services. AHCPR Pub. 92–0032. Rockville, MD.

Belville, W.I., Forest, W.H., Miller E. & Brown, B.W.R.Jr. (1971). Influence of age on pain relief from analgesics. A study of postoperative patients. *Journal of American Medical Association*, **217**, 1835–41.

Benner P. & Wrubel J. (1989). *The primacy of caring: stress and coping in health and illness.* California: Addison-Wesley.

Beyer, J.E.; McGrath, P.J. & Berde, C.V. (1990). Discordance between self-report and behavioural pain measures in children age 3–7 years after surgery. *Journal of Pain and Symptom Management*, **5**, 350–6.

Boore, J.R.P. (1978). *Information: a prescription for recovery.* London: Royal College of Nursing.

Boyek, K. & Watson, R. (1994). A touching story. *Elderly Care*, **6**, 20–1.

Bradley J.C. & Edinberg M.A. (1982). *Communication in the nursing context.* New York: Appleton-Century-Crofts.

Burnard, P. (1992). *Effective communications for health professionals.* London: Chapman & Hall.

Byrne, T.J. & Edeani, D. (1983). Knowledge of medical terminology among hospital patients. *Nursing Research*, 33, 178–81.

Cartwright, A. (1964) *Human relations and hospital care.* London: Routledge & Kogan.

Corney, R., Everett, H., Howells, A. & Crowther, M. (1992). The care of patients undergoing surgery for gynaecological cancer: the need for information, emotional support and counselling. *Journal of Advanced Nursing*, 17, 667–71.

Davis, K.J. (1987). Communication skills and learner nurses: a case study. Unpublished

MSc Thesis, University of Wales,
University College or Swansea.

Doerhing, K.M. (1989). Relieving pain
through touch. *Advancing Clinical Care*,
Sept/Oct, 32–3.

Farrow, J. (1990). Massage therapy and
nursing care, *Nursing Standard*, **14**, 17.

Feely, M. (1994) Know your patient: the
importance of assessment in care delivery.
Professional Nurse, **9**, 318–23.

Field, D., Dand, P., Ahmedzai, S. & Biswas.
B. (1992). Care and information received
by lay carers of terminally ill patients at
the Leicestershire Hospice. *Palliative
Medicine*, **6**, 237–45.

Foley, K.M. (1985). The treatment of cancer
pain. *New England Journal of Medicine*,
313, 84–95.

French, K. (1979). Some anxieties of elective
surgery patients and the desire for
reassurance and information. In D.J.,
Osborne, M.M. Gruneberg, & J.R. Eiser,
(Eds.). *Research in psychology and medicine.
Vol. 2: Social aspects; attitudes,
communication* care and training, pp, 336–
343. London: Academic Press.

Fritz, D.J. (1988). Non-invasive pain control
methods used by cancer outpatients
(Meeting Abstract) *Oncology Nursing
Forum*, Suppl. 108.

Hayward J. (1975). Information: a prescription
against pain. *The study of nursing care
project reports* series 2, no 5. London: Royal
College of Nursing.

Horrigan, C. (1993). Alternative nursing
interventions. In Carrol, D. & Bowsher, D.
(Eds.). *Pain management and nursing care*
pp, 136–145. Butterworth – Heinemann

Johnson, J.E. (1983). Preparing patients to cope
with stress. In: Wilson-Barnett, J. (Ed.).
*Patient teaching. Vol. 6, Recent advances in
nursing series*. Edinburgh: Churchill
Livingstone.

Kaiko, R.F. (1980). Age and morphine
analgesia in cancer patients with
post-operative pain. *Clinical Pharmacology
Therapeutics*, **28**, 823–6.

Koh, P & Thomas V.J. (1994). Patient
controlled analgesia: does time saved
improve patient satisfaction with care?
Journal of Advanced Nursing, **20**, 61–70.

McCaffrey, M. (1972). *Nursing management of
the patient with pain*. Philadelphia: J.B.
Lippincott.

McCaffrey, M. & Beebe, A. (1989). *Pain:
clinical manual for nursing practice*. St.
Louis: CV Mosby.

Mackereth, P.A. (1987). Communication in
critical care areas: competing for attention.
Nursing, **3**, 575–8.

Macleod Clark, J. (1982) Nurse – Patient
verbal interactions. PhD thesis, University
of London.

Melzack, R. & Wall, P.D. (1988). *The
challenge of pain*. Harmondsworth,
England: Penguin Books.

Miller, S.M. & Mangan, C.E. (1983). The
interacting effects of information and
coping style in adapting to gynaecologic
stress: should the doctor tell all? *Journal of
Personality and Social Psychology*. **45**, 233–
36.

Miller, J.F. & Shuter, R. (1984). Age, sex,
race affect pain expression. *American
Journal of Nursing*, August, 981.

Notcutt, W.G. & Morgan, R.J.M. (1990).
Introducing patient controlled analgesia for
postoperative pain control into a district
hospital. *Anaesthesia*, **45**, 1 401–6.

Rosenthal, C.J., Marshall. V.W.
Macpherson, A.S. & French, S.C.
(1980). Nurses, patients and families.
London: Croom Helm.

Seers, C. (1986). Talking to the elderly and its
relevance to care. Occasional Paper;
Nursing Times, **82**, 51–4.

Taenzer, P.A., Melzack, R., & Jeans, M.E.
(1986). Influence of psychological factors
on postoperative pain, mood, and analgesic
requirements. *Pain*, **24**, 331–42.

Thomas, V.J. (1991). Personality characteristics
of patients and the effectiveness of patient
controlled analgesia. PhD thesis.
Goldsmiths' College, University of
London.

Thomas, V.J. Heath, M.L. & Rose, F.D.
(1990). Effect of psychological variables
and pain relief system on postoperative
pain experience. *British Journal of
Anaesthesia*, **64**, 388–9.

Thomas, V.J. & Rose, F.D. (1991). Ethnic
differences in the experience of pain. *Social
Science and Medicine*, **32**, 1063–6.

Turk, D.C. & Melzack, R. (Eds.). (1992).
Handbook of pain assessment. Guilford New
York: Press.

Turton, P. (1989). Touch me, feel me, heal
me. *Nursing Times*, **85**, 42–4.

Wilson-Barnett J. (1979). *Stress in hospital:
patients' psychological reactions to illness and
health care*. Edinburgh: Churchill
Livingstone.

Patient satisfaction

RAY FITZPATRICK
Nuffield College, Oxford, UK

THE CONCEPT OF SATISFACTION

The concept of patient satisfaction is of fundamental importance for two reasons. First, it draws attention to the need to understand how patients respond to health care. In this sense patient satisfaction is a summary term that refers to the diverse range of patients' reactions to the experience of health care studied by psychology and other social sciences. Secondly, patient satisfaction is increasingly assessed in surveys of health care settings as a measure of the quality of care. In this applied use of the term, patient satisfaction is normally listed alongside five other dimensions whereby quality of health services should be assessed: access, relevance to need, effectiveness, equity, efficiency.

Despite being of importance to our understanding of the behavi-our of patients, it is remarkable how neglected patient satisfaction is in terms of theoretical discussion in psychology. A number of models have been proposed to explain available evidence regarding patient satisfaction. Thus satisfaction may be seen as the product of the discrepancies between patients' expectations of care and their perceptions of actual care received. Other approaches emphasize the anxiety and uncertainty that attends illness, and argue that satisfaction is determined by the extent of emotional support and reassurance that patients receive. However, to date, no model or theory has emerged that fully encompasses the range of available evidence and more effort has gone into refining measures of satisfaction and applying them in the context of pragmatic evaluations of the quality of care (Fitzpatrick, 1993). It is useful to consider patient satisfaction as an

Patient satisfaction

evaluation by the patient of a received service, where the evaluation contains both cognitive and emotional reactions.

A multidimensional construct

Patient satisfaction is best considered as a multidimensional construct. Patients may hold quite distinct views in relation to different aspects of their health care. Cleary and McNeil (1988) distinguish nine different dimensions of health care on which patients' views can be obtained: the 'art of care' (i.e. health professionals' interpersonal skills), technical quality, accessibility, convenience, finance, physical environment, availability, continuity and outcome. As will be evidenced below, the first category of influences, 'the art of care', contains elements of health care, such as health professionals' communication skills and sensitivity to patients' concerns, that have a particularly strong influence on patient satisfaction. Some evidence suggests that, so influential are such factors, patients are unable to distinguish between interpersonal skills on the one-hand and technical competence on the other hand (Ware & Snyder, 1975). It may be argued that such 'halo effects' reduce the value of patient satisfaction surveys, at least in assessing the quality of health care. However, there is sufficient evidence that, in response to well-designed questionnaires, patients are capable of distinguishing between technical and interpersonal aspects of the care that they receive (Fitzpatrick, 1993). It remains true that patients place great value on health professionals' empathic and communication skills, and value them as least as highly as technical proficiency. Moreover, patients are best convinced that the health professional's technical skills have been appropriately applied when they feel that effort has been made by the doctor personally to understand the patient.

RELATIONSHIP TO OTHER OUTCOMES

As well as being of primary importance as an objective of health care, patient satisfaction is also of importance because of its relationship to other outcomes of health care. In the first place it has been related to whether patients comply with their treatment regimen. In a study of a paediatric clinic in Los Angeles, mothers were interviewed by researchers immediately after their consultation and then visited at home a fortnight later (Korsch, Gozzi & Francis, 1968). Three-quarters of mothers had been satisfied with the consultation, the rest dissatisfied. The satisfied group were three times more likely eventually to have complied with the paediatrician's advice. The original paediatric consultations had been recorded and analysed. There was no relationship between the length of consultations and either satisfaction or compliance. The observation of a positive relationship between satisfaction and compliance has been noted in several other studies; for example, in a longitudinal study of patients attending a variety of neurological clinics in South East England, dissatisfaction with consultations was found to be a significant predictor of non-compliance with drug regimes one year later (Fitzpatrick & Hopkins, 1981).

A number of studies have also noted that satisfied patients are more likely to continue with their current health-care provider. Thus, Baker and Whitfield (1992) sent two patient satisfaction questionnaires to the patients of two general practices and also to patients who had recently changed surgeries without changing their home addresses. The two instruments assessed satisfaction with different aspects of the general practice and with consultations. Patients who

had changed their doctor produced poorer satisfaction scores on all dimensions of the two satisfaction instruments. A number of other studies have shown similar relationships to related variables such as reattendance at a given health-care facility, change to alternative provider or health plan, or resort to unorthodox medicine (Fitzpatrick, 1993).

Patient satisfaction and health status

The most intriguing evidence is of a relationship between patient satisfaction and health status: more positively satisfied patients report better health. Thus Cleary and colleagues (1991) carried out a telephone interview survey of 6455 adult patients recently discharged from medical or surgical services of 62 hospitals around the United States. Patients who reported their health as poor reported twice as many problems with regard to satisfaction with care as did those who rated their health as excellent. The same pattern was found when other indicators of health were used such as number of days in bed with ill-health. This relationship between satisfaction and poorer health status and dissatisfaction has now been reported for a wide range of inpatient, outpatient and primary care settings (Fitzpatrick, 1993). A number of quite different explanations are possible. Patients may express greater dissatisfaction because of their failure to make progress in response to treatment. Both satisfaction and health outcomes could be produced by higher quality care. Dissatisfied patients may comply less with treatment regimens, as a result of which they make less progress in terms of health. General psychological well-being could influence responses to both health status and satisfaction questionaires. In addition, there are a number of intervening non-specific or psychosomatic mechanisms that make it plausible that dissatisfaction may directly lead to poorer health. Longitudinal research designs are more likely to throw light on such processes. One such study examined the relationship between immediate satisfaction with consultations with a neurologist for headache and symptomatic change one year later (Fitzpatrick, Hopkins & Harvard-Watts, 1983). Patients who had expressed satisfaction with the neurological consultation were significantly more likely to report improvements in headaches one year later. Possible confounding variables such as severity of initial symptoms did not explain the relationship; nor were relationships due to intervening processes such as compliance. At present, it is not clear why relationships are consistently observed between satisfaction and health status. It is clear that satisfaction is positively related to a wide range of other desirable outcomes of health care.

FACTORS THAT INFLUENCE PATIENT SATISFACTION

A number of aspects of health care have been shown to influence patient satisfaction. Research evidence for such influences is most convincing when patient satisfaction has been measured by means of some standardized quantifiable instrument and measures have been obtained of the relevant component of health care independently of patients' reports. Roter (1989) carried out a meta-analysis of 41 such studies reporting aspects of doctors' behaviour and patient satisfaction. By far the most consistent influence upon patient satisfaction was found to be the doctor's information-giving. This overview confirms what is commonly assumed to be the case, that patients particularly appreciate receiving more information about their health problems and treatment. The importance of information-giving for patient satisfaction is confirmed by experimental as well as observational studies. Information needs to be appropriate and comprehensible to be fully appreciated by patients.

Effective communication between health professionals and patients is bidirectional; doctors need to be obtain medical histories and identify patients' main concerns as well as give information. Aspects of how doctors obtain information can also influence patient satisfaction. Thus Stiles *et al.* (1979) recorded the consultations of 19 doctors providing general medical care, and then interviewed their patients subsequently to assess satisfaction with consultations. The consultations were analysed by investigators rating the supposed intention of either the patient or doctor. Patients' satisfaction with the doctor was highest amongst those patients who had experienced consultations in which the doctor used a style of asking questions which invited patients to tell their stories in their own terms, what is often termed a 'patient-centred' rather than 'doctor-centred' form of history taking. Patients were more likely to feel, in response to this form of questioning, that the doctor had listened to them and understood their problem. In the meta-analysis of studies referred to above (Roter, 1989), a broad category of 'partnership building' processes had the biggest effect on patient satisfaction after information-giving. Roter includes in this category a wide range of behaviours by the doctor, including asking the patient's opinion, facilitating the patient's response or reflecting on statements by the patient. These may all be considered aspects of patient-centred communication and it is clear that such approaches have positive relationships with patient satisfaction. However, such effects are rarely large and not consistently found. Thus Henbest and Stewart (1990) studied the consultations of a sample of patients with six experienced family practitioners in Ontario. Consultations were recorded and rated in terms of a standardized four-point scale of 'patient centredness' and patients' views obtained with a follow-up questionnaire and interview. Some positive relationships were obtained in the predicted direction. Patient centred consultations were more likely to result in the patient feeling that the doctor knew why they had consulted. However, no significant effect could be found upon satisfaction scores. It may be that patient-centred forms of communication are only appropriate to certain presenting problems or patients' concerns and beneficial effects of this approach are less visible where all consultations are included in analysis.

A number of other factors measured independently of patients' opinions have been shown to influence patient satisfaction. Thus, DiMatteo and colleagues (1980) assessed 71 doctors in a New York hospital for their sensitivity to human emotions by rating their performance in interpreting non-verbal emotions expressed in films and also by their own ability to demonstrate a range of emotions in an experimental task. Patients consulting at the hospital were asked to assess the doctors via a patient satisfaction questionnaire. Patients' ratings of the doctors' interpersonal skills, but not of their technical skills, were found to correlate with the independently derived measures of doctors' interpersonal sensitivity. Such results are consistent with a wide range of evidence that patients are particularly aware of health professionals' interpersonal skills (Fitzpatrick, 1993). The study is also an example of how patient satisfaction questionnaires can be tested for discriminant validity. Other factors that have been independently measured and shown to

influence patient satisfaction include length of time of consultations, continuity in the doctor–patient relationship and accessibility and availability of doctors (Baker & Whitfield 1992; Fitzpatrick, 1993).

THE MEASUREMENT OF PATIENT SATISFACTION

There remain a number of measurement problems in the field of patient satisfaction. One difficulty is that several sociodemographic variables appear to exert consistent influence on patterns of response. In a meta-analysis of published patient satisfaction surveys Hall and Dornan (1990) found that the largest and most consistent variable to influence results was age with older patients reporting more positive satisfaction. A weaker but significant influence was that of education with less well-educated respondents expressing more favourable responses. Other sociodemographic variables were less consistent in effects. It is not clear why such influences occur, although it seems more likely that age effects are due to normative influences than real differences in the quality of health care received. Other influences already cited such as health status and psychological well-being are more difficult to interpret. It is at least clear that studies that fail to control for sociodemographic and other known influences should be interpreted with great caution. In particular, variations in satisfaction levels between different health-care providers may be due to other factors than the quality of care.

Results from satisfaction surveys tend to be positively skewed, with small minorities expressing dissatisfaction. Hall and Dornan (1988) carried out a meta-analysis of 68 published studies and found a median of 84% satisfied across surveys (range 43%–99%). It is not clear to what extent such skewness is due to methodological problems arising either from normative influences which inhibit patients expressing criticism of health-care providers and services or from limitations inherent in structured questionnaires. It is clear that the modest variability in satisfaction levels in some surveys make identifying explanatory factors from modelling of results implausible (Hall & Dornan, 1988).

Considerable effort has been put into improving measurement properties of some satisfaction instruments. Increasingly, views are assessed via scales rather than single items in order to improve reliability. Ware and Hays (1988) review a number of scales from patient satisfaction instruments that have internal reliability coefficients that exceed 0.90. Test–retest reliability of instruments is less commonly examined, but results are often very satisfactory (Fitzpatrick, 1993). Ware and Hays (1988) report a study to examine effects of alternative wording of questionnaires. Patients attending outpatient clinics were randomly assigned to receive satisfaction questionnaires after their visit that either involved six point ('very satisfied' to 'very dissatisfied') or five point response options ('excellent' to 'poor'). The five-point format consistently produced more variability and greater construct validity in that answers were more strongly related to other variables such as readiness to comply with medical regimen and whether respondents would recommend the doctor just visited to a friend.

Alternatives to the standardized questionnaire

Investigators remain concerned however that fixed-choice format questionnaires may not elicit patients' concerns fully or may not provide health-care providers with the kinds of feedback from patients that leads to improvements in services. An increasingly wide range of alternative forms of obtaining patients' views about their health care are available (Fitzpatrick & Hopkins, 1993). On the one hand, a number of standardized instruments are available which have reasonably well-established psychometric properties. On the other hand, a variety of more in-depth methodologies have also been developed. Critical incident analysis requires trained interviewers to obtain detailed narratives of their health-care encounters from which incidents which attract respondents' positive or negative reactions are abstracted for (largely) qualitative analysis. In a similar vein, non-schedule standardized interviews have been used to obtain detailed qualitatively rich accounts of medical encounters on which conventional quantitative analysis can be performed. Finally, focus

groups are increasingly used as a technique of eliciting patients' concerns and views in a way that is least contaminated by investigators' preconceptions. Examples of systematic approaches to these different methods exist but, to date, lacking are studies in which comparative advantages are directly compared (Fitzpatrick & Hopkins, 1993).

Ultimately, a large part of the purpose in assessing patient satisfaction is to provide evidence to health-care providers of the scope for improvement revealed by patients' views. It is not yet clear that the increasing sophistication observed in measurement systems is matched by practical arrangements within health-care organizations to respond constructively to evidence obtained from surveys. Increasingly, it will be necessary to examine the practical utility of alternative approaches to the assessment of patient satisfaction.

REFERENCES

Baker, R. & Whitfield, M. (1992). Measuring patient satisfaction: a test of construct validity. *Quality in Health Care*, 1, 104–9.

Cleary, P. & McNeil, B. (1988). Patient satisfaction as indicator of quality of care. *Inquiry*, 25, 25–36.

Cleary, P., Edgman-Levitan, S., Roberts, M., Moloney, T., McMullen, W., Walter, J. & Delbanco, T. (1991). Patients evaluate their hospital care: a national survey. *Health Affairs*, 10, 254–67.

DiMatteo, M., Taranta, A., Friedman, H. & Prince, L. (1980). Predicting patient satisfaction from physicians' non-verbal communication skills. *Medical Care*, 18, 376–87.

Fitzpatrick, R. (1993). Scope and measurement of patient satisfaction. In R. Fitzpatrick & A. Hopkins (Eds.). *Measurement of patients' satisfaction with their care*. pp. 1–17, London: Royal College of Physicians of London.

Fitzpatrick, R. & Hopkins, A. (1981). Patients' satisfaction with communication

in neurological outpatient clinics. *Journal of Psychosomatic Research*, 25, 329–34.

Fitzpatrick, R. & Hopkins, A. (Eds.). (1993). *Measurement of Patients' satisfaction with their care*. London: Royal College of Physicians of London.

Fitzpatrick, R., Hopkins, A. & Harvard-Watts, O. (1983). Social dimensions of healing: a longitudinal study of outcomes of medical management of headache. *Social Science Medicine*, 17, 501–10.

Hall, J. & Dornan, M. (1988). Meta-analysis of satisfaction with medical care: description of research domain and analysis of overall satisfaction levels. *Social Science Medicine*, 27, 637–44.

Hall, J. & Dornan, M. (1990). Patient sociodemographic characteristics as predictors of satisfaction with medical care: a meta-analysis *Social Science Medicine*, 7, 811–18.

Henbest, R. & Stewart, M. (1990). Patient-centredness in the consultation. 2:

Does it really make a difference? *Family Practice*, 7, 28–33.

Korsch, B., Gozzi, E. & Francis, V. (1968). Gaps in doctor–patient communications. I: Doctor–patient interaction and patient satisfaction. *Pediatrics*, 42, 855–71.

Roter, D. (1989). Which facets of communication have strong effects on outcome – a meta analysis. In M. Stewart & D. Roter (Eds.). *Communicating with medical Patients*, pp. 183–196. Newbury Park, CA: Sage Publications.

Stiles, W. Putnam, S., Wolf, M. & James, S. (1979). Interaction exchange structure and patient satisfaction with medical interviews. *Medical Care*, 17, 667–79.

Ware, J. & Snyder, M. (1975). Dimensions of patients' attitudes regarding doctors and medical care services. *Medical Care*, 13, 669–79.

Ware, J. & Hays, R. (1988). Methods for measuring patient satisfaction with specific medical encounters. *Medical Care*, 26, 393–402.

Psychological problems: detection

PETER BOWER

National Primary Care Research and Development Centre, University of Manchester, UK

In a number of countries around the world primary care is crucial for the delivery of mental health services to the community (Goldberg & Huxley, 1992). This is especially true in the United Kingdom where general practitioners (GPs) occupy a key role in controlling access to specialist mental health services (Dowrick, 1992; Goldberg & Huxley, 1992).

GPs and other primary health-care staff encounter a wide range of emotional problems in their everyday clinical practice, from obvi-

ous manifestations of mental illness to psychological responses to physical illness and various difficulties with normal function that cause distress (Markus *et al.*, 1989). Appropriate management requires that these conditions are accurately recognized and diagnosed. This chapter summarizes research concerning the detection of psychiatric and psychological disorders in primary care settings and the factors and processes which influence the accuracy of diagnosis.

Research on the detection of emotional disorders in general practice has focused on minor psychiatric disturbance, but it is important to note that the scope of the terms psychological and psychiatric are not equivalent (Salmon, 1984). Disorders in the former category range from anxiety and stress through habit disorders, interpersonal problems and psychological adjustment (Kincey, 1974) and the level of agreement between GPs and psychologists as to the presence of psychological disturbance is far from perfect (McPherson & Feldman, 1977; Salmon, Stanley & Milne, 1988).

Disorders present in general practice populations lack the sharp boundaries between both illness and health and between more specific categories of disorder. The dimensional models preferred in psychology may be more suitable in primary care than the traditional categorical models utilized in hospital psychiatry (Mirowsky & Ross, 1989; Goldberg & Huxley, 1992). Specifically, two highly correlated symptom dimensions comprising anxiety and depression seem to underlie most minor psychiatric morbidity in general practice (Goldberg et al., 1987).

Measuring the diagnostic accuracy of GPs requires a comparison between their subjective ratings of patient distress and an objective 'gold standard'. Although standardized psychiatric interviews are the preferred 'gold standard', considerations of time and economy mean that self-administered screening questionnaires are often used e.g. the General Health Questionnaire (Goldberg & Williams, 1988). Although these scales have demonstrated adequate sensitivity when compared with interviews, the requirement that they identify all psychiatric cases results in a relatively high false-negative rate and the estimates of prevalence may be inflated unless appropriate corrections are made (Markus et al., 1989). The GHQ uses a threshold to divide respondents into 'probable cases' and 'probable normals'. The threshold is the point at which the probability of 'caseness' according to standardized interview is 50%, with increasing scores indicating increasing probability of psychiatric diagnosis.

The complex and undifferentiated nature of many problems in general practice means that diagnosis tends to be concerned with the exclusion of serious disease rather than with precise categorization (McWhinney, 1972). In comparing GP assessment with screening questionnaires, doctors are normally required to use a simple scale of psychological distress rather than a precise diagnostic formulation.

There is wide variation in estimates of prevalence of emotional problems depending on the diagnostic criteria, time frame and population studied. Nevertheless, it is estimated that 30% of people in the United Kingdom are experiencing symptoms of depression or anxiety at any one time (Huppert, Roth & Gore, 1987) and up to 40% of consulting patients have a probable psychiatric disorder (Goldberg & Huxley, 1992).

GP detection of distress can be assessed using a number of indices. The identification index is a modified sensitivity measure ranging from 0 to 1.0 which represents the proportion of cases detected by the GP from among those probably present in the population according to the screening instrument. A large study of 91 GPs in Manchester (Marks, Goldberg & Hillier, 1979) found a mean identification index of 0.54. Doctors in South London had a mean of 0.36 (Boardman, 1987). Other indices use the correlation between the GP rating and the patient's total score on the screening test. These procedures have also been used with other health professionals such

as nurses, and the results have generally indicated similar levels of recognition (e.g. Briscoe, 1986).

The procedure described above is in effect bringing specialist psychiatric standards into the primary care setting and thus the rates of non-recognition given above may be based on criteria that are not appropriate to the clinical situation in general practice (Verhaak, Wennink & Tijhuis, 1990). Additionally, measures of diagnostic accuracy based on single consultations ignore the ongoing nature of the GP-patient relationship and GPs' use of time as a diagnostic aid to differentiate transient disorders from more enduring problems (Dowrick, 1995). Nevertheless, some GPs exhibit accuracy indices close to unity which suggests these criteria can be met.

Whatever the status of the identification index as an absolute measure of diagnostic accuracy, it also serves as a useful measure of the relative ability of GPs and a number of factors have been measured in relation to the index. Shorter consultations are associated with less consideration of psychosocial issues (Howie et al., 1991), although the proportion of variance in accuracy accounted for by time factors is low (Marks et al., 1979).

Various GP interview behaviours and communication skills (e.g. eye contact, clarification of complaint, picking up verbal and non-verbal cues, asking about social situation) have been shown to be associated with diagnostic accuracy (Goldberg et al., 1982; Marks et al., 1979). Furthermore, given patients suffering from equal distress, GPs demonstrating such communication skills elicit more verbal and non-verbal cues of emotional distress from their patients, (Davenport, Goldberg & Millar, 1987). Communication skills such as these have been successfully imparted to GPs using video based feedback and individual teaching, and the skills have been shown to persist over time (Goldberg et al., 1980; Gask, 1992).

GP attitude and personality variables related to greater diagnostic accuracy include greater perceived importance of psychosocial factors in disease (Marks et al., 1979), openness towards the patient and tolerance for risk-taking (Wilmink et al., 1989). Scores on these factors tend to be inter-related and it has been suggested that there is an underlying dimension of doctor- versus patient-centredness (Verhaak, 1986) which may in turn reflect underlying personality characteristics or cognitive styles (McWhinney, 1985). Such characteristics might include tolerance for ambiguity, intuition and empathy.

Patient factors have also been found to be important. Various constellations of demographic characteristics have been shown to be important influences on the probability of a psychiatric diagnosis being applied (Boardman, 1987; Marks et al., 1979). Some of these characteristics raise diagnostic rates and are confirmed by objective data (e.g. middle-aged housewife) while some artificially lower rates in contradiction of objective findings (e.g. young single male). GPs' background knowledge of patients (e.g. previous psychiatric history, social situation) and the patient's current illness behaviour (e.g. frequency of consultation or multiple symptom patterns) also act as cues to the presence of emotional distress (Hjortdahl, 1992; Howe, 1996; Wilmink et al., 1989).

The mode of presentation of disorder seems to be a crucial determinant of recognition. There is an inverse relationship between the severity of co-existing physical illness and rates of recognition of major depression (Tylee, Freeling & Kerry, 1993).

Somatization serves to complicate matters further. The various types of somatization described in specialist psychiatric manuals such as *DSM-IIIR* (APA, 1987) are of less relevance in general practice. Kirmayer and Robbins (1991) distinguished between three types of relevant somatization: functional somatic syndromes (reporting medically unexplained symptomatology); illness worry (high levels of distress in response to mild physiological disturbances); and somatized clinical presentations (the tendency to deny or ignore psychological symptoms and attend to somatic distress). The first two types of somatization served to increase rates of recognition of emotional disorder. Increasing levels of somatic presentation, measured by the patient's unwillingness to consider psychosocial factors as important, first spontaneously and then in response to probes, are associated with decreasing recognition rates (Kirmayer *et al.*, 1993).

Bridges and Goldberg (1985) distinguish between two types of somatized clinical presentations. Facultative somatization occurs when the presentation to the GP is physical in nature, but the patient will admit to the relevance of psychosocial factors in a psychiatric interview. Although the exact cause of this type of somatization is unclear, patient attitudes to the role of the GP (Cartwright & Anderson, 1981; DelVecchio-Good, Good & Cleary, 1987), the stigma associated with mental illness (Bhugra, 1989), the time available in the consultation and negative attitudes toward psychotropic drugs (Royal College of Psychiatrists, 1992) may all be involved. Educational initiatives such as the Defeat Depression campaign in the United Kingdom (Priest, 1991) are seeking to encourage the public to view the GP as a suitable resource for psychological problems which may lessen the prevalence of this form of illness behaviour.

True somatization is similar to the facultative form in that the presentation of the disorder is in terms of physical symptoms. However, these patients attribute the cause of their symptoms to a physical disorder; between 10 and 30% of patients with psychiatric disorders have been found to persistently deny any connection between somatic symptoms and psychological disturbance (Bridges & Goldberg, 1985; Kirmayer, Robbins & Paris, 1994). A variety of factors are associated with a somatic rather than psychological presentation (Kirmayer, Robbins & Paris, 1994): negative attitudes to mental illness; less depressed mood; less social stress; previous inpatient medical care (Bridges *et al.*, 1991); somatic attributional style; and lower likelihood of a previous psychiatric history (Robbins & Kirmayer, 1991*a*, *b*).

GP and patient characteristics may also interact. Somatized presentations that are legitimized by the GP ordering physical tests and investigations may validate the patient's erroneous attribution and make the disorder more resistant to re-framing in terms of psychological disorder (Goldberg, Gask & O'Dowd, 1989). There is also the increased risk of iatrogenic illness (Katon, Kleinman & Rosen, 1982). The GP's ability to tolerate the risk of missing rare but serious disease may be an important influence on patient presentation behaviour (Grol *et al.*, 1990).

In conclusion, accurate recognition of psychological problems in general practice is crucial for the proper delivery of care to the community (Goldberg & Huxley, 1992). Although levels of recognition are far from optimal, research has highlighted a number of professional and patient psychological characteristics associated with diagnostic error which may be amenable to change.

REFERENCES

American Psychiatric Association (APA). (1987). *Diagnostic and statistical manual* 3rd Ed. revised, Washington DC.

Bhugra, D. (1989). Attitudes towards mental illness. *Acta Psychiatrica Scandinavica*, **80**, 1–12.

Boardman, A. (1987). The General Health Questionnaire and the detection of emotional disorder by general practitioners: a replicated study. *British Journal of Psychiatry*, **151**, 373–81.

Bridges, K. & Goldberg, D. (1985). Somatic presentation of DSM III psychiatric disorders in primary care. *Journal of Psychosomatic Research*, **29**, 563–9.

Bridges, K., Goldberg, D., Evans, B. & Sharpe, T. (1991). Determinants of somatisation in primary care. *Psychological Medicine*, **21**, 473–83.

Briscoe, M. (1986). Identification of emotional problems in postpartum women by health visitors. *British Medical Journal*, **292**, 1245–7.

Cartwright, A. & Anderson, R. (1981). *General practice revisited. A second study of patients and their doctors.* London, Tavistock Publications.

Davenport S., Goldberg, D. & Millar, T. (1987). How psychiatric disorders are missed during medical consultations. *Lancet*, ii, 439–41.

DelVecchio Good, M., Good, B. & Cleary, P. (1987). Do patient attitudes influence physician recognition of psychosocial problems in primary care? *The Journal of Family Practice*, **25**, 53–9.

Dowrick, C. (1992). Improving mental health through primary care. *British Journal of General Practice*, **42**, 382–6.

Dowrick, C. (1995). Case or continuum? Analysing general practitioners' ability to detect depression. *Primary Care Psychiatry*, **1**, 255–7.

Gask, L. (1992). Training general practitioners to detect and manage emotional disorders. *International Review of Psychiatry*, **4**, 293–300.

Goldberg D., Steele J., Smith, C. & Spivey, L. (1980). Training family doctors to recognize psychiatric illness with increased accuracy. *Lancet*, ii, 521–3.

Goldberg, D., Steele, J., Johnson, A. & Smith, C. (1982). Ability of primary care physicians to make accurate ratings of psychiatric symptoms. *Archives of General Psychiatry*, **39**, 829–33.

Goldberg, D., Bridges, K., Duncan-Jones, P. & Grayson, D. (1987). Dimensions of neuroses seen in primary-care settings. *Psychological Medicine*, **17**, 461–70.

Goldberg, D. & Williams, P. (1988). *A user's guide to the general health questionnaire*, Windsor: NFER-Nelson.

Goldberg, D. & Huxley, P. (1992). *Common mental disorders: a biosocial model.* London: Routledge.

Goldberg, D., Gask, L. & O'Dowd, T. (1989). The treatment of somatisation: teaching techniques of reattribution. *Journal of Psychosomatic Research*, **33**, 689–95.

Grol, R., Whitfield, M., de Maeseneer, J. and Mokkink, H. (1990). Attitudes to risk taking in medical decision making among British, Dutch and Belgian general practitioners. *British Journal of General Practice*, **40**, 134–6.

Hjortdahl, P. (1992). The influence of GP knowledge about their patients on the clinical decision making process. *Scandinavian Journal of Primary Health Care*, **10**, 290–4.

Howe, A. (1996). 'I know what to do, but it's not possible to do it' – general practitioners perceptions of their ability to detect psychological distress. *Family Practice*, **13**, 127–32.

Howie, J., Porter, A., Heaney, D. & Hopton, J. (1991). Long to short consultation ratio: a proxy measure of quality of care for general practice. *British Journal of General Practice*, **41**, 48–54.

Huppert, F., Roth M. & Gore M. (1987). *Health and lifestyle survey, preliminary report*. London: Health Promotion Research Trust.

Katon, W., Kleinman, A. & Rosen, A. (1982). Depression and somatisation: a review (part 1). *American Journal of Medicine*, **72**, 127–35.

Kincey, J. (1974). General practice and clinical psychology – some arguments for a closer liaison. *Journal of the Royal College of General Practitioners*, **24**, 882–8.

Kirmayer, L. & Robbins, J. (1991) Three forms of somatisation in primary care: prevalence, co-occurrence and sociodemographic characteristics. *Journal of Nervous and Mental Disease*, **179**, 647–55.

Kirmayer, L., Robbins, J., Dworkind, M. & Yaffe, M. (1993). Somatisation and the recognition of depression and anxiety in primary care. *American Journal of Psychiatry*, **150**, 734–41.

Kirmayer, L., Robbins, J. & Paris, J. (1994) Somatoform disorders: personality and the social matrix of somatic distress. *Journal of Abnormal Psychology*, **103**, 125–36.

McPherson, J. & Feldman, M. (1977). A preliminary investigation of the role of the clinical psychologist in the primary care setting. *Bulletin of the British Psychological Society*, **30**, 342–6.

McWhinney, I. (1972). Problem solving and decision making in primary medical practice. *Proceedings of the Royal Society of Medicine*, **65**, 934–8.

McWhinney, I. (1985) Patient-centred and doctor-centred models of clinical decision making. In M. Sheldon, J. Brook, & A. Rector (Eds.). *Decision making in general practice*, London: Stockton.

Marks, J., Goldberg, D. & Hillier, V. (1979). Determinants of the ability of general practitioners to detect psychiatric illness. *Psychological Medicine*, **9**, 337–53.

Markus, A., Murray Parkes, C., Tomson, P. & Johnston, M. (1989). *Psychological problems in general practice*, Oxford: Oxford University Press.

Mirowsky, J. & Ross, C. (1989). Psychiatric diagnosis as reified measurement. *Journal of Health and Social Behaviour*, **30**, 11–25.

Priest, R. (1991). A new initiative on depression. *British Journal of General Practice*, **41**, 487.

Robbins, J. & Kirmayer, L. (1991*a*). Attributions of common somatic symptoms. *Psychological Medicine*, **21**, 1029–45.

Robbins, J. & Kirmayer, L. (1991*b*). Cognitive and social factors in somatisation. In: L. Kirmayer, & J. Robbins, (Eds.). *Current concepts of somatisation: research and clinical perspectives*, Washington DC: American Psychiatric Press.

Royal College of Psychiatrists. (1992). Research study conducted for the 'Defeat Depression' campaign. Unpublished manuscript: Royal College of Psychiatrists.

Salmon, P. (1984). The psychologist's contribution to primary care: a reappraisal. *Journal of the Royal College of General Practitioners*, **34**, 190–3.

Salmon, P., Stanley, B. & Milne, D. (1988). Psychological problems in general practice patients: two assumptions explored. *British Journal of Clinical Psychology*, **27**, 371–9.

Tylee, A., Freeling, P. & Kerry, S. (1993). Why do general practitioners recognize major depression in one woman patient yet miss it in another? *British Journal of General Practice*, **43**, 327–30.

Verhaak, P. (1986). Variations in the diagnosis of psychosocial disorders: a general practice observation study. *Social Science and Medicine*, **23**, 595–604.

Verhaak, P., Wennink, H. & Tijhuis, M. (1990). The importance of the GHQ in general practice. *Family Practice*, **7**, 319–24.

Wilmink, F., Ormel, J., Giel, R., Krol, B., Lindeboom, E., Van Der Meer, K. & Soeteman, J. (1989). General practitioners' characteristics and the assessment of psychiatric illness. *Journal of Psychiatric Research*, **23**, 135–49.

Psychological support for health professionals

VALERIE SUTHERLAND

Manchester School of Management, University of
Manchester Institute of Science and Technology,
UK

The importance of psychological support in the health and well-being of clients and patients is well documented and acknowledged by health-care professionals. However, the role of social support in reducing work stress and maintaining the health of these 'carers' received relatively scant attention until recent enforced changes prompted investigations on the impact of stress among health-care professionals. This chapter describes the concept of social support as a mediator and moderator of the stress response and explores some of the ways in which social support systems for health-care professionals might be improved. The effects of social support and the types and different sources of social support are considered.

Evidence is growing that stress is becoming more prevalent, pervasive and pernicious (Elkin & Rosch, 1990). It is a major problem for individuals, organizations and society, and the real costs of mismanaged stress are probably incalculable. Jobs in human services share many of the sources of stress present in other jobs, but also are characterized by the potential strain of intense involvement in the lives of others which requires a caring commitment and empathetic responding, often in a high demand situation. These conditions are optimal for 'burnout', that is, 'emotional exhaustion', which has deleterious consequences for both the health professional and the patient. Persons working in health-care occupations continually have their competence on trial in a highly visible environment, where the costs of mistakes are enormous. Thus, the job of the health-care professional is inherently stressful. It is suggested (Sutherland & Cooper, 1990) that health-care professionals will perform more effectively if they understand the role of stress and social support in their own lives and the impact that it might have on patients, clients, colleagues and staff.

A CONCEPTUAL FRAMEWORK FOR SOCIAL SUPPORT

Dunkel-Schetter and Bennett (1990) provide a framework to guide our understanding of the concept of social support which is based on the following assumptions.

1. Social support is defined in functional terms as an interpersonal transaction. Therefore, a distinction is made between the existence of social relationships (social integration), the structure of social relationships (social networks) and the function of social interactions/relationships. Although some authors believe that the term 'social support' should be reserved for this latter interpretation, research evidence indicates the importance of social integration, i.e. the existence of social relationships. For example, Knox *et al.* (1985) found that the actual number of contacts and acquaintances was one of the significant factors which was inversely related to elevated blood pressure among young, male hypertensives.

2. It is also necessary to differentiate between the availability of social support and the activation of it. The interactive model of stress defines a state of stress as an imbalance between perceived demand and perceived ability to meet that demand. The processes that follow are the coping process and the consequences of the coping strategy applied. This means that stress is a subjective experience contingent upon the perception of a situation. Likewise, it is the belief about social support available, if needed, rather than the actual support available, which influences one's cognitive appraisal of the situation and is the determinant of effective coping and crucial to health protection. It is this assumption that provides a rationale for the interchangeable usage of the terms 'social support' and 'psychological support'.

3. Individual differences in terms of needs, desires and social support seeking behaviour will have an impact on the activation, receipt of, and perceived satisfaction with social support. Chay (1993) suggests that personality dispositions interact to influence the appraisal of a situation and supportive relationships, affects one's readiness to seek help from others, influences the need for sociable and intimate interaction, and one's response to feedback from others. Chay (1993) found that higher levels of perceived availability of support were associated with a combination of trait extraversion, internal locus of control, and a high need for achievement among self-employed individuals and small business owners, suggesting that individual differences played a role in the utilization of support services. Since the term 'health-care professional' embraces a very wide range of employee groups working under quite different contractual arrangements, including both self-employed and employed status, it is important to include these factors in any operational model of social support for this occupational group.

TYPES OF SOCIAL SUPPORT

It is also necessary to acknowledge that different types of social support exist which will have a variable impact on strains and pressures. These have been described in various ways, although it would seem that the four classifications proposed by House (1981) tend to include recent citations.

Emotional support

Emotional support which involves providing love, caring, empathy and trust, is regarded by House as the most crucial because individuals tend to think of 'being supportive' in terms of emotional support. Research evidence suggests that dentists tend to experience high levels of stress at work because of the nature of the job. However, it is the routine problems in dentistry associated with time pressures, high case load and falling behind with schedules that cause most concern. These pressures are probably exacerbated because dentists tend to work in isolation from their peers and interact with clients who would, perhaps, rather not attend the surgery. The provision of effective emotional support would thus seem to be important for this occupational group.

Instrumental support

This involves actual assistance through an intervention. It refers to behaviour that directly helps the person in need. For example, to physically take over some aspect of a task for someone is instrumental support; it is also described as 'material or tangible aid'. Many health-care professionals have described work overload conditions and time pressures as the most stressful aspects of their job (Sutherland & Cooper, 1990, 1993, Tyler & Cushway, 1992). Having someone to physically provide help would alleviate these pressures, but financial constraints do not permit this simple solution to a stressful situation and the individual is usually left to cope with the strain and pressure of work overload conditions.

Informational support

This means providing a person with information that can be used in the coping process. The information itself is not viewed as instrumental support because it is usually aimed at helping the individuals to help themselves. For example, tutoring or coaching a person to help them to reach a desired goal. Beehr, King and King (1990) found evidence for the supportive value of informational and emotional support from supervisors among occupational, registered nurses. Both positive job-related and non-job-related communications (versus negative job related communications) were associated with the perception of the supervisor as supportive, and this had a positive, main effect on individual job strain. Evidence for a buffering effect (i.e. the interaction between social support and job stressors to reduce the strength of the stressor-strain relationship) was also found for non-job-related communication as a form of social support.

Appraisal support

This involves the transmission of self-evaluation information. Feedback from the environment, i.e. social comparison, is derived from information supplied directly and indirectly by the people around us. For example, we gauge our own work performance either from being told by significant others, or by interpreting what we see. At exam time, medical students all face the same challenge and potential threat. Knowing that everyone is in the same circumstance has an impact on the way in which that situation is perceived. An increased understanding of the role of social support will enable an organization to maximize support networks in the work place, especially during the times when strains and pressures are greatest (for example, threats to jobs, restructuring and during examinations, etc.). Research evidence also suggests that there are psychological and physical health benefits, in terms of better immune function and blood pressure, associated with self disclosure, including the sharing of personal secrets and disclosure of traumatic events (Kennedy, Kiecolt-Glaser & Glaser, 1990). Therefore, reciprocity in the transmission of appraisal and informational support would seem to be the most beneficial support strategy. However, many health-care professionals tend to feel that they do not have other people around them to provide this form of support. Although general practitioners and dentists rarely operate in single practice surgeries and increasingly find themselves working as part of a multidisciplinary team with other autonomous professionals, the working structure and climate often does not facilitate the supportive environment which is beneficial to the health and well-being of these carers. Some authorities are attempting to overcome such problems by providing counselling services and/or employee assistance programmes for health care professionals. Nevertheless, there is also scope for improvement in the levels of social support within a group-practice or team of health professionals, and the quality of interpersonal relationships at work is an area which would typically be addressed by a stress management intervention. Toloczko (1989) reports on the effectiveness of social support training on burnout and improving working relationships among nurses. Measures taken following a six-week training programme (one $2\frac{1}{2}$ hour session per week) showed significant reductions in emotional exhaustion and depersonalization, compared to a no-training control group of nurses, even though measures of total life experiences remained consistent for both groups.

SOURCES OF SOCIAL SUPPORT

In addition to the existence of different types of social support, it must also be acknowledged that sources of social support have a varying effect on outcomes, i.e. a specific source of support (e.g. a nurse manager) may buffer the effects of a specific source of stress (e.g. work overload) on a job related strain (eg. job dissatisfaction) and/or mental or physical health outcomes for a student nurse. Investigating these relationships is complex. For example, Tyler and Cushway (1992) found that having a friend, a partner, or a member of the family to whom nurses could talk about problems at work had a small but beneficial effect on mental well-being. However, levels of anxiety and insomnia were higher in single/un-partnered people if they could talk to a partner, but higher in married/partnered people if they could not. This highlights the need to consider:

(i) Perceptions held about the skill of the support givers (i.e. a partner may be there to help but is unable to engage in any clinically orientated discussion about a stressful experience at work, or understand the situation).

(ii) Stress experiences may be more acute when expectations of

support are too high and therefore, are not realized. Support providers may feel unable to help or to meet the continual demands made which might elicit emotional reactions such as fear, embarrassment, discomfort or helplessness (Dunkel-Schetter & Bennett, 1990). Indeed, it is suggested that informal support providers may experience the same burnout and emotional exhaustion that occurs when professional care providers are overextended. The outcome tends to be physical and/or psychological withdrawal, i.e. avoidance and detachment.

These results highlight the importance of having supportive work colleagues (or perceiving them to be supportive), because they share similar experiences and can help each other in a reciprocal manner. A formal way to maximize this form of social support is the introduction of co-counselling in the workplace. However, it is likely that much of this is already available informally. For example, Fletcher, Jones & McGregor-Cheers (1991) found that 87% of health visitors screened (N=124) believed that support and encouragement from work colleagues made the job easier most or all of the time. Performance feedback from colleagues and the ability to talk to colleagues during breaks were perceived as supportive in the work environment, and were ranked higher than support from the spouse and family. However, for individuals who work in isolation from other health care workers, social support from a spouse/partner, the family or friends is clearly desirable. In a prospective study of case managers hired to work with seriously and persistently mentally ill clients, Koeske, Kirk & Koeske (1993) found control coping strategies (which included talking to spouse, family and friends about the problems) facilitated the workers' ability to deal with a difficult and challenging work obligation. Workers who relied on avoidance coping strategies showed significantly poorer outcomes three months after starting the job (e.g. this included, keeping my feelings to myself, avoided being with people in general, drinking more, etc).

THE EFFECTS OF SOCIAL SUPPORT

Much of the literature on the effectiveness of social support has focused on two sorts of health effects, main effects, and buffer effects. The way in which social support works has generated considerable disagreement, but many of the differences in the findings appear to arise from the variation in the conceptual definition of the concept, the way in which it is operationalized, and the reliance on cross sectional research designs (Thoits, 1986). However, evidence exists to support the various hypotheses proposed, but the findings may be affected by the actual source and type of support studied, and the stressor(s), outcome measure(s) and the person variables measured (e.g. gender, age and socioeconomic status). For example, Sutherland and Cooper (1993) found that reported use of social support as a stress coping strategy was a significant predictor of job satisfaction among general practitioners. Low use of social support was a predictor of depression among this occupational group, and female general practitioners were significantly more likely to use this as a coping strategy than the males, who also evidenced a poorer level of psychological well-being than their female counterparts.

It is suggested that social support works in the following ways. Perceived social support can have a main effect on perceived job stress, job-related strain and/or mental and physical health. It can lessen the effect of perceived job stress on job-related strain, moderates job stress on mental and physical health, and ameliorates the effects of job related strain on mental and physical health. Some authors have suggested that a 'coping' hypothesis best explains their findings, and believe that social support is a coping mechanism that individuals use under stressful conditions. Thoits (1986) described similarities between social support and coping with stress:

(i) Instrumental support was identified with problem-focused coping strategies. This implies direct action on the environment or self to remove or alter the circumstances perceived of as a threat.

(ii) Emotional support was identified with emotion-focused coping in that cognitive appraisal is used to control the undesirable feelings that result from a stressful situation.

(iii) Informational support is identified with perception focused coping, which consists of cognitive attempts to alter the meaning of a situation so it is perceived as less threatening. Therefore, both support and coping act to change the situation, change the emotional reaction to the situation and/or the meaning of the situation. Indeed, it has been suggested that knowing help is available, but coping with one's problems without using outside assistance leads to the best outcomes in terms of confidence in one's own capabilities (i.e. self-confidence, a sense of mastery and high self-esteem).

CONCLUSION

Overall, change seems to be a consistent theme for many health-care professionals. This includes changes to systems and practice as medical research advances, changes brought by legislation and government which bring new roles for health carers, and the changes in society which alter the structure of social support networks in our environment. In order to adapt to change, we need to be flexible in our use of coping strategies. An improved understanding of the role of social support as a stress coping strategy will help us to adapt to these changes which are an inevitable part of life as a health-care professional. It is vital if we are to stay in the job, maintain a higher level of physical and psychological well-being and deliver a higher quality of service to clients.

REFERENCES

Beehr, T.A., King, L.A. & King, D.W. (1990). Social support and occupational stress: talking to supervisors. *Journal of Vocational Behaviour*, 36, 61–81.

Chay, Y.W. (1993). Social support, individual differences and well-being. A study of small business entrepreneurs and employees. *Journal of Occupational and Organizational Psychology*, 66, 285–302.

Dunkel-Schetter, C. & Bennett, T.L. (1990). Differentiating the cognitive and behavioural aspects of social support. In B.R. Sarason, I.G. Sarason & G.R. Pierce (Eds). *Social support: an international view*. USA: John Wiley.

Elkin, A.J. & Rosch, P.J. (1990). Promoting mental health at the workplace. *Occupational Medicine: State of the Art Reviews*, 5, 739–54.

Fletcher, B.C., Jones, F. & McGregor-Cheers, J. (1991). The stressors and strains of health visiting: demands, supports, constraints and psychological health. *Journal of Advanced Nursing*, 16, 1078–89.

House, J.S. (1981). *Work stress and social support*. USA: Addison-Wesley.

Kennedy, S., Kiecolt-Glaser, J.K. & Glaser, R. (1990). Social support, stress and the immune system. In B.R. Sarason, I.G. Sarason & G.R. Pierce (Eds.). *Work stress and social support*. USA: Addison-Wesley.

Knox, S.S., Theorell, T. Svensson, J. & Walker, D. (1985). The relation of social support and working environment to medical variables associated with elevated blood pressure in young males: a structural model. *Social Science and Medicine*, 21, 525–31.

Koeske, G.F., Kirk, S.A. & Koeske, R.D. (1993). Coping with job stress: which strategies work best? *Journal of Occupational and Organisational Psychology*, 66, 319–35.

Sutherland, V.J. & Cooper, C.L. (1990). *Understanding stress: a psychological perspective for health professionals*. UK: Chapman and Hall.

Sutherland, V.J. & Cooper, C.L. (1993). Identifying distress among general practitioners: predictors of psychological ill-health and job dissatisfaction. *Social Science and Medicine*, 37, 575–81.

Thoits, P.A. (1986). Social support as coping assistance. *Journal of Consulting and Clinical Psychology*, 54, 416–23.

Toloczko, A.M. (1989). The effects of social support training and stress inoculation training on burnout in nurses. PhD Thesis, Lehigh University.

Tyler, P. & Cushway, D. (1992). Stress, coping and mental well-being in hospital nurses. *Stress Medicine* 8, 91–8.

Quality of life assessment

RACHEL ROSSER

Department of Psychiatry, Medical School
University College London, UK

INTRODUCTION

The measurement of health-related quality of life (HQoL) is traced through the history of health service evaluation during the past 30 years. This chapter covers the concepts of need, demand and supply. Global health indicators and profiles are described leading to HQoL measures and cost per QALY league tables. These tools have in common a set of descriptors of states of health or HQoL and a scale of values (i.e. a utility scale) used to sum states and changes in individuals over time.

The term health-related quality of life and the concept that this can be quantified is relatively new. It implies that changes in people's quality of life can be attributed to health care separately from other planned quality-enhancing activities, e.g. education, recreation, the arts, housing, transport and military defence. This bold concept has yet to be operationally defined. A brief review of its recent origins may therefore be useful.

HISTORICAL ORIGINS

Supply and demand

With the increasing effectiveness of medical interventions as a result of scientific and technological advances, medical treatments were perceived as a necessity, which should be made accessible to all. In Britain, this idea was enshrined in the Beveridge Report recommending the radical development of a National Health Service offering medical care to all, free at the point of delivery irrespective of financial status. In other so-called 'developed' countries, other systems were introduced, e.g. reimbursement or means testing.

Beveridge, making recommendations at a time when poverty excluded many of the population from access to medical care, assumed that there would be a short-term increase in the need for medical care, followed by a reduction due to the improved health of the nation. Such an assumption now appears naive. It is recognized that demand increases as the supply of treatment increases. Further demand may or may not reflect need, some need is not expressed as demand, and some apparent needs, i.e. genuine morbidity, are not curable, emotional and practical support being the only help available.

From this observation followed the idea that priorities had to be set, since demand was potentially infinite and would increase with medical advances. This was all the more alarming since it became apparent that the old-established habit of self-medication with over-the-counter drugs and neighbourly and family advice was continuing and that, as these habits changed with changing expectations, more people would approach the Health Service.

The concept of quality of medical care followed; priority would be given to professionals and institutions providing the best quality of care. How then could quality be measured? For 20 years, research, audit and health-care evaluation internationally emphasized the process of care. This trend encouraged caution among health-care professionals and discouraged early discharge, with the effect of rapidly rising costs particularly in the hospital sector. The modern responses to this include cost-containment (which may be somewhat arbitrary) and community care, which requires evaluation as it expands.

Working against this main-stream was a small but expanding research community which emphasized the importance of outcome of care and questioned the relationship between this and cost, i.e. input and process, i.e. how resources are used.

These early pioneers paved the way for the development of health status indicators in the 1960s and 1970s, and the explosive growth of measures of quality of life in the 1980s and 1990s.

Outcome measurement

Diagnostically specific measures of change gradually evolved as the discipline of statistics provided rigour in clinical trials. The majority were biological indicators of interest to specialist clinicians. These were necessary, but on their own, unsuitable for setting priorities. Needed in addition were measures reflecting patients' experiences and changes in these during and after treatment. If these could be measured and generalized across diagnostic states, outcomes could be compared, costs could be included and information relevant to policies about Health Service priorities could become available.

To statistics was added the new discipline of operational research, an approach which in the 1960s by means of highly theoretical models laid down the framework for global health indicators. Regrettably and fortuitously, most of these were never converted into applicable instruments, i.e. operationalized and applied. An exception was the Q index (Miller, 1970) used to measure the state of health of North American Indians for whom a special health service was provided. Thus the thrust behind the first quantifiable global health indicator, which had the crucial characteristics of crossing diagnostic and age-groups and summing to a single figure, was the assessment of health status in a deprived ethnic minority.

The next ten years produced enormous advances in health status measurement. In 1976 Torrance (1972) identified 14 different mathematical approaches to health status measurement. Four of the groups established in the late 1960s continued to flourish (Torrance in Hamilton, Ontario; Fanshel and Bush, followed by Kaplan in San Diego, California; Williams and Culyer in York, UK; and Rosser in London, UK). Each was based on standard descriptions of patients' states to each of which was added a valuation, referred to by economists as a utility, expressing the importance or advantage of each state relative to every other state. Most research groups have used more than one method of obtaining relative values for different states. Various types of category rating, which is an easy and quick exercise, are perhaps the most popular. Others include time trade off which requires subjects to choose the durations of a severe state compared with a milder one; magnitude estimation which asks questions about the ratio between different states; and the standard gamble which requires people to define the maximum risk they would be prepared to take when choosing a treatment which might restore them from a particular mild or moderate state to perfect health with the possibility of either death or a much more severe state ensuing.

There is also discussion about whether people can estimate the values of states which are composite, e.g. a state comprising different levels of pain, immobility, mood disturbance and loss of function, and whether they can provide a better set of values by scaling separately along different dimensions or attributes which are combined at a second stage (multi-attribute scaling).

However, although these instruments were potentially useful for measuring and comparing the states of target populations and the effect on them of various interventions and health programmes, they were criticized by some epidemiologists, clinicians and sociologists as oversimplistic.

This provided the stimulus for the design of health profiles. Each profile had different characteristics. Best known were the symptom impact profile (SIP) designed by Bergner (1993), the Nottingham Health Profile (NHP) designed by McEwen and developed by Hunt (1993) and the McMaster Index designed by Chambers & Sackett (1993).

The SIP (translated into UK English by Patrick to form the

Functional Limitation Profile, FLP) contained 136 descriptive items edited from a large data set obtained from substantial samples of the general population. Only items which could be defined in observable behavioural terms were included. Values were elicited by a method known as category scaling (assigning states to one of a limited number of levels of severity). The items were grouped ultimately into 12 subscales which were valued again relative to one another. Hence the state of individuals' health could be expressed in various levels of detail depending on the needs specified by any particular study.

The NHP was derived in a similar manner but used both behavioural and subjective descriptors. It was simpler, consisting of six scales (section A) and a more narrative part (section B). Unlike the SIP no provision was made for summarizing section A into a single number, not because this would be technically difficult, but because the authors took the view that it was conceptually unjustifiable to assume that different scales, e.g. mobility, pain and fatigue, could all be expressed as a single number. This is a crucially controversial point. In practice the issue did not determine the many applications of these two profiles, the SIP being used more frequently in North America and the NHP attracting more interest in the UK.

By contrast, the McMaster Index, comprising subjective descriptive items all receiving an arbitrary score of 1, has not been so widely applied, but remains a viable alternative.

Some of the issues which followed included first, a return to diagnostically specific instruments, which could only be used for comparisons of the severity of single conditions in different populations at different times or of changes in state over time (e.g. Guyatt et al. 1987). Secondly, there was a swing towards even greater simplicity by discarding specifically designed health indicators or profiles and instead choosing a set of standard measures of severity for different applications in different conditions, e.g. hypertension (Cox et al., 1992).

PRESENT INSTRUMENTS
The approach used in the SIP, which provides the detail of a profile and the simplicity of an index has retained its popularity in more recent measures, e.g. the Index of Health Related Quality of Life (IHQL, Rosser et al., 1993)

There is increasing concern that individuals should be able to choose the set of descriptors or domains which are of greatest importance to them and to place their individual values on personal scales which can subsequently be aggregated to produce a single scale for that group of individuals. This complex method has been pioneered by McGee et al. (1991).

The most important modern development is the use of internationally and cross-culturally designed scales. These all draw on similar approaches to those described above but involve international debate at every stage, e.g. Short Form (SF36 & SF20; 1992); the EuroQol (EuroQol Group, 11) and WHOQol (Sartorius, 1993). The EuroQol is a five-dimensional linkage tool (Brook & EuroQol group). WHOQol produces scores across six domains and 24 subdomains (Herrman et al., 1996).

The oscillation between such measures, all complex in different ways, and much simplified measures such as the abbreviated and specialized versions of the IHQL, reflect the demand for briefer, more comprehensible and more transparent techniques in which the method of obtaining values for different states is easily apparent to the user.

QUALITY OF LIFE: ITS EVOLUTION
The previous section obscured the transition from the concept of health states to the more comprehensive notion of health-related quality of life.

This development naturally accompanied the growing complexity of profiles and the quest for cross-cultural applicability. Such factors resulted in the inclusion of more abstract attributes, e.g. spirituality, harmony; fulfilment; and many more.

Health status indicators acquired new labels as their underlying conceptual frame extended, e.g. Kaplan's group in California developed their health status index into a measure of the Quality of Well-being (QWB).

The term 'Quality of Life' (QoL) is now most popular but it still remains an elusive and ill-defined concept. Descriptive components are selected either by groups of 'experts' (e.g. EuroQol and WHOQOL) or by surveys of random population samples or selected groups of individuals who respond to questions about how they think that their quality of life might be affected by impairment in health. In either case, large numbers of descriptors have to be reduced by editing procedures.

One of the earliest uses of the term was derived from the highly contentious and original QALY league tables and the even more contentious step in which the costs of treatment are included to produce cost per QALY tables (QALY stands for quality adjusted life year) (Table 1). How these should be used in policy decisions is the subject of continuing technical and ethical arguments, particularly in view of the points listed below. This important debate has stimulated much of the recent work on health-related quality of life. The simplicity of the approach has appealed particularly to economists, although some have reservations (Gerrard & Mooney, 1993), and has provoked other health professionals into discussions about the restriction of clinical judgement, and rationing by management based on such data. The discussion becomes all the more important in the UK with the development of an internal market since providers of health services might compete to sell their achievements in terms of such league tables to purchasers, e.g. general practices and health authorities. Alternative approaches are now under debate by economists, e.g. the concept of a healthy year equivalent (HYE) or disability adjusted year (DALYS). This discussion is based on fundamental economic assumptions which are confusing to many members of other disciplines!

CURRENT ISSUES
Present uncertainty revolves around some of the issues mentioned above and others which are the subject of relatively little published work (in a field generating some 1000 papers per year). Major areas of discussion include the following.

Choice of descriptors
There is no consensus on whether experts can be used as 'surrogate' members of the general public to choose items for inclusion in the measurement of HQoL or whether the prolonged and expensive stage of population surveys must be followed. Population returns in

	QALYs gained per patient (discounted at 5%)	Annual cost per patient	Total cost (discounted at 5%)	Cost per QALY
Continuous ambulatory peritoneal dialysis (4 years)	3.4	12 866	45 676	13 434[b]
Haemodialysis (8 years)	6.1	8 569	55 354	9 075[b]
Treatment of cystic fibrosis with ceftazidime (over 22 years)	0.4	250	3 290	8 225[b]
Kidney transplant (lasting 10 years)	7.4	10 452	10 452	1 413[a]
Shoulder joint replacement (lasting 10 years)	0.9	533	533	592[a]
Scoliosis surgery idiopathic adolescent	1.2	3 143	3 143	2 619[a]
neuromuscular illness	16.2	3 143	3 143	194[a]

[a]Represents one-off costs per case, and benefits discounted over life of case.

[b]Represents recurring annual costs and annual QALYs per case.

Reproduced with permission from Gudex, C. QALYs and their use by the Health Service, University of York, Centre for Health Economics. Discussion Paper No. 20, October 1986.

percentages at any stage of instrument design are disappointingly low and unacceptable to many epidemiologists. This means that cheap and quick postal surveys which yield from 30% to 60% returns must be replaced by interviews. Even this is likely to bias the population towards the elderly, housewives, domestic employees and home-based workers unless household surveys are conducted in the evenings or at weekends. But refusals, some hostile, may come from hard working people looking for relaxation at home, and financial incentives are irrelevant to those on high salaries. In urban centres the population may be so mobile that census data cannot be used for drawing samples, the lack of community cohesiveness can be a problem and there are language and translation problems if a high proportion of the population comprises immigrants.

Scaling

There is no agreement about the best method of obtaining values of QoL states from samples either of the general population or of health professionals. Transformation between scales derived from different experimental methods is difficult. Also there is no agreement as to whether it is better to use a simple set of descriptors which can be administered to a total sample or whether methods such as the 'balanced incomplete block design' should be used, permitting different subsamples to place values on a limited number of the total set of descriptors with an overlap between descriptors scaled by the subsamples and some descriptors common to all.

Time factors

Relatively little work is available on the important question as to whether duration is perceived linearly (e.g. a week in a state is seven times as severe as one day). Furthermore this may not be the same for all descriptors, e.g. pain may be rated worse with longer duration whereas disability may be rated as progressively less important as time permits adjustment. Such effects could be obscured if composite states combining, e.g. disability and pain are rated by duration. The question casts doubt on the assumption that time is valued in a linear manner by raters. Could the apparent simplicity and comparability of the time trade off method be obscuring a forced assumption of linearity?

Even more complex is the issue of prognosis, first tackled by Fanshel & Bush. Techniques such as the QALY league table assume either that impaired QoL in future years is not discounted or an arbitrary discount rate is used. However, there is little empirical information on this issue, and there is some evidence that, in developed countries, placing emphasis on health education and prevention at the cost of foregone pleasures, may actually be preferred to delayed problems in the future.

Instrumental properties

A great deal of effort has been devoted to establishing the reliability and validity of some classical instruments, e.g. the QWB and the SIP. Newer instruments await empirical data and statistical analysis to ascertain these properties. Standardization and sensitivity are yet to be clearly defined in this field. Specificity and validity are difficult to assess in the absence of a 'gold standard' for comparison.

Cultural questions

As indicated above, cross-cultural comparisons are a major matter under current investigation. This is a problem with measures such as the EuroQol which are being applied outside the Northern European countries of origination. But thorough attempts to achieve a meticulous cross-cultural translation, especially with the SIP and its derivative the FLP, seem to be underused. Yet without rigorous efforts, literal translations are sometimes used even without reference to the originators of an instrument. Computerized data bases containing up to date critiques of instruments and information on the location of their originators should be a protection against this as should major handbooks (e.g. I.5.) (Patrick & Erickson, 1993). However, the aim of obtaining good translations, as in the new WHOQOL designed by experts from multiple cultures, may be the best solution.

Arising from cross-cultural work, there is new debate about the importance of including abstract descriptors in addition to focusing exclusively on behavioural ones which may not satisfy all cultures.

Another unresolved issue with cross-cultural implications is the value assigned to death relative to all living states. Being dead may be the most valued state, the least valued state, or may fall anywhere in between these two extremes. It seems likely that cultural factors, especially religion, are influential here.

Philosophical issues

The uses of QoL measures especially in determining health service policies from national level to that of the individual patient has attracted a much broader debate. The principal issues are semantic, cognitive and ethical.

The semantic issue is concerned with the wording of descriptors and the question of how individuals understand the intended sense either in scaling experiments or when evaluating their own QoL.

Close to this are questions of cognition. What are the mental processes involved at every stage, especially in providing numerical valuations?

The ethical questions include doubts about the validity of the techniques used to derive QoL measures, particularly in the light of discrepant results from studies applying two or more instruments.

There is even more controversy about the ethics of how the instruments are used. The issues include fairness (equal distribution of benefits between individuals without discrimination against the old, those without dependents and those with severe states for which treatment is palliative but costly); justice (consistent with allocation of resources according to the highest benefit : cost ratio) and desert. The principle of desert questions whether people who have neglected or abused their health through theoretically avoidable habits, e.g. smoking, excessive drinking, should have the same entitlements as those who have made every sacrifice of immediate pleasure to prevent future illness (Lockwood, 1986; Griffin, 1986). This principle is already being implemented by clinicians with managerial support.

Those people who have not stopped smoking, may be deprived of coronary artery bypass and those who still drink may miss out on anything from anti-depressants to liver transplants. (Deception is, of course, the obvious route: patients may decide not to trust their doctors.) Inconsistently, there is no explicit discrimination against suicide attempts or other forms of deliberate self-harm, despite covert discrimination by health-service professionals.

One of the most important contributions of the cost per QALY and more recent related methods has been the provocation of debate about these crucial issues.

CONCLUSIONS

Quality of life is an ill-defined concept, although it is now receiving much research attention. Its origins have been traced in this chapter from the recognition that outcomes of medical interventions must be measured so as to set priorities in health service policy decisions, resulting in global health status indicators, profiles and ultimately QoL instruments. These are now used in clinical trials and may well be incorporated into routine medical audit in the future. Despite 25 years of research, and more than 400 instruments, thorny issues have yet to be defined relating to the design and application of measures of the abstract term 'quality of life', and its relationship to medical care and state of health.

ACKNOWLEDGEMENT

The author wishes to thank Green College, Oxford for accommodating her for her research scholarship during the Michaelmas Term, 1993.

REFERENCES

Bergner, M. (1993). Development, testing, and use of the sickness impact profile. In S. Walker and R.M. Rosser (Eds.). *Quality of life assessment: key issues in the 1990s*. pp. 95–110. Kluwer Academic Publishers.

Brazier, J.E., Haper, R., Jones, N.M.B. *et al.* (1992). Validating the SF-36 health survey questionnaire: new outcome measure for primary care. British Medical Journal. **305**, 160–4.

Brooks, R. with the Eurqol Group (1996). Eurqol: the current state of policy. *Health Policy*, 37, 53–72.

Chambers, L.W. (1993). The McMaster Health Index Questionnaire: an update. In S. Walker & R.M. Rosser *Quality of life assessment: key issues* pp. 131–150.

Cox, D.R., Fitzpatrick, R., Fletcher, A.E., Gore, S.M., Spiegelhalter D.J. & Jones, D.R. (1992). Quality of life assessment: can we keep it simple? *Journal of the Royal Statistics Society*, 155, 353–93.

The EuroQol Group. (1990). EuroQol – a new facility for the measurement of health-related quality of life. *Health policy*, **16**, 199–208. North Holland: Elsevier.

Gerrard, K. & Mooney, G. (1993). Qaly league tables: handle with care. *Health Economics*. **2**, 59–64.

Griffin, J.G. (1986). *Well being. Its meaning, measurement and moral importance*. Oxford: Clarendon Press.

Guyatt, G., Berman L., Toronsend M. *et al.* (1987). A measure of quality of life for clinical trials in chronic lung disease. *Thorax*, **42**, 773–7.

Lockwood, M. (1988). Quality of life and resource allocation. In J.M. Bell & S. Mendus (Eds.). *Philosophy and medical welfare*. pp. 33–55. Cambridge: Cambridge University Press.

McEwen, J. (1993). The Nottingham health profile. In S. Walker & R.M. Rosser (Eds.). *Quality of life assessment: key issues in the 1990s*, pp. 95–110, Kluwer Academic Publishers

McGee, H.M., O'Boyle, C.A., Hickey, A. *et al.* (1991). Assessing the Quality of Life of the Individual: the SEIQOL with a Healthy and a Gastroenterology Unit Population. *Psychological Medicine*, **21**, 749–59.

Miller, J. (1970). An indicator to aid management in assigning program priorities. *Public Health Reports*, 85, 725–8.

Orley, J. (1996). Quality of life: the WHOQol. *European Psychiatry*, 11, 228s.

Patrick, D.L. & Erickson, P. (1993). *Health status and health policy. Allocating resources to health care*. New York: Oxford University Press.

Rosser, R.M., Allison, R., Butler, C., Cottee, M., Rabin, R. & Selai, C. (1993). The index of health-related quality of life (IHQL): a new tool for audit and cost-per-QALY analysis. In S. Walker & R.M. Rosser *Health policy*, pp. 179–184, North Holland: Elsevier.

Sartorius, N. (1993). A WHO method for the assessment of health related quality of life. In S. Walker & R.M. Rosser (Eds.). *Health policy* vol. 16, pp. 201–207, North Holland: Elsevier.

Torrance, G.W., Thomas, W.H. & Sacket, D.L. (1972). A utility maximisation model for evaluation of health care programs. *Health Services Research*, 7, 118–33.

Recall by patients

PHILIP LEY

University of Sydney, Australia

AMOUNT REMEMBERED

Studies of what patients remember of what they are told have been conducted in a variety of hospital and general practice settings. The material involved has consisted of the clinician's conclusions about the illness, its treatment, investigation and prognosis, and advice to the patient, or of some subset of this material, or of informed consent information. Analogue studies have also been conducted. In these, healthy volunteers have been presented with material, which might have been said to a real patient, and asked to recall it. Patients frequently forget much of the information given to them. Table 1, based on the review by Ley (1988), summarizes the results of several studies of such forgetting.

There is one investigation which yielded results which are very different from those summarized in Table 1. Tuckett, Boulton and Olson (1985) reported that only 10% of the patients they studied failed to remember all of the 'key points' made to them by their general practitioner. The 'key points' were those considered most important, and it is well established that patients remember better what they consider to be most important (Ley & Spelman, 1967; Ley, 1972). This, and other factors to be discussed below (such as the use of probed recall) probably explain why Tuckett *et al.* obtained such discrepant results.

Investigations have differed considerably in methodology (Ley, 1988), and in the samples studied. In addition to differences in content of the communication already mentioned, the patients involved in some studies have been making their first attendance with a particular illness, while other studies have taken all comers including those making a repeat attendance with their illness. The use of first attenders allows better experimental control. If repeat attenders are studied, there is no control over what they will have been told on previous visits. However, it has been argued that the use of samples which include repeat attenders has greater ecological validity, because those attending at clinics and other consultations usually include a proportion of repeat attenders (Bartlett *et al.*, 1984).

The method of assessing recall has also varied. Some investigations have used free recall, ie. patients are simply asked to state what they were told. Others have used cued recall. In these, patients are asked what they were told about the diagnosis, what they were told about the treatment, what they were told about investigations, etc. Yet other studies have used probed recall in which the investigator continues to probe the patient's recall, usually with prompting questions until sure that the patient can recall no more. Finally, some of the investigations of memory for informed consent materials have used a multiple choice recognition task. It is not known which of these methodological variants yields the most valid predictor of patients' memory outside the experimental situation.

Another complication is that, at least for common illnesses, patients will have expectations of what is likely to be said. For example, the expectations of a mother taking a school-aged child with a sore throat to a general practitioner will probably include: that the child has tonsilitis, that an antibiotic will be prescribed, that it should be taken four times a day, that plenty of fluids should be provided, that the child should be kept off school for a few days, and possibly have to stay indoors for a day or two. In many cases, some or all of these expectations will be met, thus making it easier to remember what has been said. Similarly, many general practitioners will give the same lifestyle advice about weight, smoking habits and exercise to particular patients on each encounter. This predicability would be expected to apply less to visits to a less familiar clinician in an outpatient clinic. These complications should be kept in mind when considering studies of forgetting (Ley, 1988).

PATIENT CHARACTERISTICS AND RECALL

Findings in relation to patient characteristics can be summarized as follows:

(i) No consistent relationship between age and recall has been found (Ley, 1988).

(ii) Intellectual level has shown a low but consistent relationship to recall, the correlations ranging from 0.18 to 0.26 (Ley, 1988).

(iii) The higher the patient's medical knowledge, the better is recall (Ley, 1988).

(iv) Anxiety is related to recall, but not in the curvilinear fashion reported by Ley and Spelman (1967), the more common finding being that the more anxious the patient, the more is recalled, (Kupst *et al.*, 1975; Anderson *et al.*, 1979; Leeb, Bowers & Lynch, 1976).

With regard to anxiety it is also worth noting that the clinician's level of anxiety might also affect patient's recall. In an analogue study, patients recalled less of the information given if the physician appeared worried rather than unworried (Shapiro *et al.* 1992).

Table 1. *Summary of the results of clinical and analogue studies of memory for medical information*

Type of sample	Number of samples	Mean percentage recalled	Range
(a) Hospital patients	8	54	40–70
(b) General practice patients	6	65	50–88
(c) Patients given informed consent materials	9	47	29–72
(d) Analogue subjects	10	47	28–64

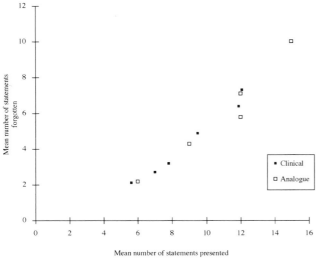

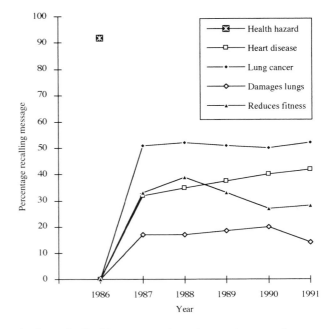

Fig. 1. Relationship between mean number of statements presented and mean number forgotten in hospital out-patient and analogue studies.

Fig. 2. Recall of health messages and warnings on cigarette packs.

EFFECTS OF THE CONTENT AND STRUCTURE OF THE COMMUNICATION ON MEMORY.

Characteristics of the material presented also affect recall. The main finding are as follows:

(i) There is a primacy effect in recall of medical information, material presented first is better recalled (Ley & Spelman, 1967; Ley, 1972, 1982).

(ii) Statements which are perceived as important are better recalled than those which are seen as less important (Ley & Spelman, 1967; Ley, 1972).

(iii) The greater the number of statements the smaller is the mean percentage recalled (Ley, 1979, 1982, 1988). The relationship between number of statements presented and the number forgotten is shown in Figure 1. The drop in percentage recalled is linear in studies of free recall by new outpatients, and in analogue studies. Note, however, that the absolute amount recalled does not fall with increased amount of information presented. Surprisingly, forgetting by out-patients and by analogue subjects is almost identical. The fact that the information is true and personally relevant seems to make no difference.

(iv) Also surprisingly, there seems to be no tendency for forgetting to increase with the passage of time. What patients can recall shortly after the consultation they tend to retain for a considerable time (Ley, 1982, 1988).

RECALL OF PASSIVELY PRESENTED HEALTH MESSAGES

Sometimes health information is presented passively. Active messages are those oral or written communications aimed at a particular individual in circumstances where it can normally be assumed that the individual will hear or read the message. This is the situation in clinical consultations and in letters sent to a patient as an individual. Passively presented health information includes information where no personal contact is involved. Examples include posters, package inserts and health warnings on products. Investigations of recall of passively presented material usually simply ask subjects to state what message or messages were present in the passively presented material. As there is no guarantee that subjects will have noticed or read the information, these studies are only partly studies of recall. In general such investigations show that many people are unable to state the content of messages to which they have been passively exposed. A good example is provided by Centre for Behavioural Research in Cancer (1992). Following the introduction in Australia a quarterof four new health warnings presented in rotation on cigarette packs, annual surveys were conducted to ascertain the percentage of smokers who could state what the warnings were. Previously there had only been one warning, which 92% of smokers recalled. Recall of the new warnings showed no improvement after the first year of exposure and stabilized at much lower recall levels than the single warning. The results of these surveys are summarized in Figure 2. Over half of the samples recalled one or fewer messages, with about a quarter recalling none. When there was only one warning, only 8% could not say what it was. When there were four warnings, about a quarter of smokers could recall none of them. (For more discussion of written health related information and warnings see 'Written communication'.)

IMPROVING RECALL

Techniques useful in increasing recall (and which sometimes also increase satisfaction as well) are listed below. Also given are the absolute changes in recall found in key studies of the techniques.:

Two techniques affect which part of the message will be best recalled:

(i) use of primacy effects: telling patients first the information that it is most important for them to remember (increased recall by 36%, Ley, 1972);

(ii) stressing importance of key parts of the information by saying something like: 'It's very important for you to remember what I am going to say next' (increased recall by 15%, Ley, 1972).

Other techniques increase the total amount recalled. These are:

(iii) simplification: use of shorter words and shorter sentences (increased recall by 13%, Bradshaw, *et al.*, 1975);

(iv) explicit categorization: categorizing the material, listing the category names to the patient before presenting the information, and then repeating the appropriate category name before each category of information is presented. For example:

'Now I am going to tell you:

what is wrong with you;

what tests and investigations will be needed;

what the treatment will be;

what you must do to help yourself;

and what the outcome will be.

Firstly, what I think is wrong with you . . .

Secondly, what tests and investigations will be needed . . .'

and so on.

(Use of this technique increased recall by 9 – 18%, Ley, 1979; Ley, *et al.*, 1973; Reynolds, *et al.*, 1981);

(v) repetition (recall increased by 14–19%, Kupst, *et al*, 1975; Bertakis, 1977; Ley, 1979; satisfaction also increased, Bertakis, 1977);

(vi) use of specific, concrete statements, rather than general, more abstract statements, for example 'Go for an hour's walk three times a week' rather than 'Make sure you take regular exercise' (increased recall by 35%, Bradshaw *et al*, 1975);

(vii) mixtures of the above techniques (increased recall by 9–21%, Ley *et al.* 1976).

As none of these techniques is anywhere near totally effective, it is always desirable to provide written back up material whenever possible (See 'Written Communication').

Phoned and mailed reminders (in a sense a form of repetition) have been used to increase compliance in appointment-keeping. In studies reviewed by Ley (1988) the mean absolute increase in percentage of patients keeping their appointments was 17.1% (s.d. 7.2%). This effect is probably due at least in part to increased recall, but other explanations are possible (Levy & Loftus, 1983; Ley, 1988). (See also 'Stress management', 'Written communication', 'Medical decision-making'.)

REFERENCES

Anderson, J.L., Dodman, S., Kopelman, M. & Fleming, A. (1979). Patient information recall in a rheumatology clinic. *Rheumatology and Rehabilitation*, 18, 18–22.

Bartlett, E.E., Grayson, M., Barker, R., Levine, D.M., Golden, A. & Libber, S. (1984). The effects of physician communications skills on patient satisfaction, recall, and adherence. *Journal of Chronic Diseases*, 37, 755–64.

Bertakis, K.D. (1977). The communication of information from physician to patient: a method for increasing retention and satisfaction. *Journal of Family Practice*, 5, 217–22.

Bradshaw, P.W., Ley, P., Kincey, J.A. & Bradshaw, J. (1975). Recall of medical advice: comprehensibility and specificity. *British Journal of Social and Clinical Psychology*, 14, 55–62.

Centre for Behavioural Research in Cancer (1992). *Health warnings and contents labelling on tobacco products.* Melbourne: Centre for Behavioural Research in Cancer.

Kupst, M.J., Dresser, K., Schulman, J.L. & Paul, M.H. (1975). Evaluation of methods to improve communication in the physician–patient relationship. *American Journal of Orthopsychiatry*, 45, 420–9.

Leeb, D., Bowers, D.G. & Lynch, J.B. (1976). Observations in the myth of informed consent. *Plastic and Reconstructive Surgery*, 58, 280–2.

Levy, R.L. & Loftus, G.R. (1983). Compliance and memory. In P. Morris (Ed.). *Everyday memory* London: Academic Press.

Ley, P. (1972). Primacy, rated importance and the recall of medical information. *Journal of Health and Social Behavior*, 13, 311–17.

Ley, P. (1979). Memory for medical information. *British Journal of Social and Clinical Psychology*, 18, 245–56.

Ley, P. (1982). Studies of recall in medical settings. *Human Learning*, 1, 223–33.

Ley, P. (1988). *Communicating with patients.* London: Chapman and Hall.

Ley, P. & Spelman, M.S. (1967). *Communicating with the patient.* London: Staples Press.

Ley, P., Bradshaw, P.W., Eaves, D. & Walker, C.M. (1973). A method for increasing patients' recall of information presented by doctors. *Psychological Medicine*, 3, 217–20.

Ley, P., Whitworth, M.A., Skilbeck, C.E., Woodward, R., Pinsent, R.J.F.H., Pike, L.A., Clarkson, M.E. & Clark, P.B. (1976). Improving doctor–patient communication in general practice. *Journal of the Royal College of General Practitioners*, 26, 720–4.

Reynolds, P.M., Sanson-Fisher, R.W., Poole, A.D., Harker, J. & Byrne, M.J. (1981) Cancer and communication: information-giving in an oncology clinic. *British Medical Journal*, 282, 1449–51.

Shapiro, D.E., Boggs, S.R., Melamed, B.G. & Graham-Pole, J. (1992). The effect of varied physician affect on recall, anxiety, and perceptions in women at risk for breast cancer: an analogue study. *Health Psychology*, 11, 61–6.

Tuckett, D.A., Boulton, M. & Olson, C. (1985). A new approach to the measurement of patients' understanding of what they are told in medical consultations. *Journal of Health and Social Behaviour*, 26, 27–38.

[317]

Shiftwork and health

EMMA TAYLOR

Unit of Psychology, Guy's Medical School, UMDS
at Guy's Campus, University of London, UK

Shiftwork involves either continuous or discontinuous staffing of a work place by teams of employees who work at different times, with work often occurring outside the normal day work hours of 7.00 to 18.00 (eg Kogi, 1985; Scott & Ladou, 1990).

Shiftworkers typically live in a society orientated towards day work, so that they face disruption to their social patterns, including their family and domestic lives (Kogi, 1985). Evidence suggests that shifts also disrupt biological rhythms. Most human functions have a rhythm with peaks and troughs that occur in a 24 to 26–hour period. It is suggested that these circadian rhythms, geared toward activity during the day and rest at night, never completely adjust during the course of night work. Shiftwork leads to the circadian system splitting into components, causing temporal disorder amongst physiological functions. This internal desynchronization leads to a general malaise including headaches, loss of appetite, fatigue, difficulty with bowel movements and inability to sleep (eg Scott & Ladou, 1990; Waterhouse, 1993). Social and circadian disruption may interact with sleep problems to produce deleterious effects on the general psychological and physical well-being of shiftworkers (Scott & Ladou, 1990).

There are numerous methodological problems which beset research on the shiftworker's well-being. Studies use self-selected shiftworkers, leading to a 'healthy worker effect' with robust people applying for, and remaining in, shiftwork. There is also a preponderance of self-report studies using non-standardized measures, and a reliance on cross-sectional designs that exclude analysis of the causal role shiftwork may play in disease. However, there is a wide body of research which indicates that shiftwork is a risk factor in health problems. This has led to the claim that 5% to 20% of shiftworkers have disproportionate symptoms of illness after starting shiftwork, labelled shift maladaptation syndrome (SMS). SMS consists of sleep disturbance and chronic tiredness; gastro–intestinal complaints; alcohol or drug abuse; higher rates of accidents; depression, mood disturbance and interpersonal relationship difficulties (Scott & Ladou, 1990).

Gastrointestinal complaints are amongst the most frequent problems of shiftworkers. For instance, Segawa *et al.* (1987) medically screened employees for a period of four years. They found significant differences in the prevalence of duodenal ulcer between 2269 night workers and 6525 day workers. The proportion of gastric ulcers and all peptic ulcers was also greater amongst ex-shiftworkers than day workers. In a retrospective cohort study, Angersbach *et al.* (1980) reported that, in an 11-year period, 46% of 370 shiftworkers, on 12-hour rotating shift compared with 37% of 270 day workers consulted the occupational health service for transient gastrointestinal complaints. The risk of suffering from a gastrointestinal disease

for the first time increased amongst shiftworkers, but not day workers, after 5 years of work. Compared with day workers and permanent shiftworkers, these diseases were most prevalent amongst shiftworkers who eventually left shiftwork for medical reasons. These findings suggest a cumulative effect of shiftwork on gastrointestinal disease, with the people who suffer adversely choosing to transfer to day work but not fully recovering after the switch.

There is also evidence of a cumulative effect of shiftwork on cardiovascular complaints. In a longitudinal, retrospective cohort study spanning 15 years, incidence of coronary heart disease (CHD) was examined in 504 male day and shiftworkers on a three-shift rota (Knutsson *et al.*, 1986). Knutsson *et al.* (1986) reported a dose – response relationship between experience of shiftwork and CHD in the first two decades. After 20 years, the risk of CHD was reduced due to 60% of shiftworkers with CHD transferring to day work. Knutsson, Anderson and Berglund (1990) investigated the reasons for this high prevalence of CHD amongst shiftworkers. Risk factors in heart disease were examined before employment and after 6 months of work in 12 shiftworkers, on a three-shift rotation, and 13 day workers. A change was found in the ratio of serum lipoproteins in shiftworkers but not in day workers. Shiftworkers also significantly reduced their intake of dietary fibre and increased their intake of saccharose. However, although some risk factors increased with experience of shiftwork, these were still within normal levels.

While the above results suggest that shiftwork is a risk factor in CHD, the number of studies in this area is small. Studies also suffer from methodological flaws such as not matching for job type and work demands. We can therefore only conclude that shiftwork may be one risk factor in cardiovascular disease. For whom, and how, have yet to be determined.

Findings from longitudinal research imply that shiftwork is also a causal or aggravating agent in psychological problems. Bohle and Tilley (1989) examined general psychological distress in two groups of nurses from their induction to a year after starting shifts. One group stayed on a three-shift system throughout the study, whilst the other switched to a two-shift system after 6 months. There was a rise in distress with experience in shiftwork for both groups interpreted as the negative impact of shiftwork. Healy, Minors and Waterhouse (1993) also looked at nurses from the time of starting 3 months of night work to the week after this block of nights. They reported an increase in feelings of loss of control, loss of energy and loss of interest, and concluded that shiftwork produces changes typical of depression.

To summarize, psychologists have found an association between shiftwork and gastrointestinal complaints, coronary heart disease and mental health problems. Not all shiftworkers will experience these complaints, but a sizeable number suffer the cumulative effects of shiftwork that do not appear to subside completely after transferring to day work. Several interventions have been recommended to deal with shift-related problems, including changing shift systems; education in coping skills; medical surveillance; imposing selection criteria; bright light and melatonin therapy (Rosa *et al.*, 1990). Psychologists are now calling for more work on the practical implications of research on shiftwork as a risk factor in health problems.

REFERENCES

Angersbach, D., Knauth, P., Loskant, H., Karvonen, M.J., Undeutsch, K. & Rutenfranz, J. (1980). A retrospective cohort study comparing complaints and diseases in day and shiftworkers. *International Archives of Occupational Environmental Health*, 45, 127–40.

Bohle, P. & Tilley, A.J. (1989). The impact of night work on psychological well being. *Ergonomics*, 32, 1089–99.

Healy, D., Minors, D.S. & Waterhouse, J.M. (1993). Shiftwork, helplessness and depression. *Journal of Affective Disorders*, 29, 17–25.

Knutsson, A., Akerstedt, T., Jonsson, B.G. & Orth-Gomer, K. (1986). Increased risk of ischaemic heart disease in shiftworkers. *Lancet*, 12, 89–93.

Knutsson, A., Anderson, H. & Berglund, U. (1990). Serum-lipoproteins in day and shiftworkers: a prospective study. *British Journal of Industrial Medicine*, 47, 132–4.

Kogi, K. (1985). Introduction to the problems of shiftwork. In S. Folkard & T.H. Monk (Eds.). *Hours of work: temporal factors in work scheduling*. pp. 165–183. Chichester: John Wiley.

Rosa, R.R., Bonnet, M.H., Bootzin, R.H., Eastman, C.I., Monk, T., Penn, P.E., Tepas, D.I. & Walsh, J.K. (1990). Intervention factors for promoting adjustment to night work and shiftwork. *Occupational Medicine: State of the Arts Review*, 5, 1177–93.

Scott, A.J. & Ladou, J. (1990). Shiftwork: effects on sleep and health with recommendations for medical surveillance and screening. *Occupational Medicine: State of the Arts Reviews*, 5, 273–99.

Segawa, K., Nakazawa, S., Tsukamoto, Y., Kurita, Y., Goto, H., Fukui, A. & Takano, K. (1987). Peptic ulcer is prevalent among shiftworkers. *Digestive Diseases and Sciences*. 32, 449–53.

Waterhouse, J. (1993). Circadian rhythms. *British Medical Journal*, 306, 448–51.

Stress in health professionals

JENNY FIRTH-COZENS

Department of Psychology,
University of Leeds, UK

Over the last decade, the subject of stress in health professionals has become of major interest, not just to researchers (Payne & Firth-Cozens, 1987) but also to hospital and community service managers (Seccombe & Buchan, 1993) who may know that the levels of stress in their staff are contributing to the quality of care they offer their patients, to the number of complaints and legal actions they have to face, and to the absence data and turnover of staff. This chapter will look at the levels of stress and other stress-related conditions in health workers, at the sources of these studied at both an individual and an organizational level, and at the ways that stress has been tackled within the organization.

STRESS LEVELS IN HEALTH WORKERS

There is no doubt that the proportion of health workers who are showing symptoms of stress at levels indicative of being at risk for psychiatric problems is high. For example, studies have shown that around one-third of nurses (Tyler & Cushway, 1992; West Jones & Savage, 1988) are suffering at these levels using the General Health Questionnaire (GHQ: Goldberg, 1978) as an estimate of potential psychiatric caseness. Nursing, in addition, has the one of the highest rates of suicide among professional groups and they also lead in psychiatric outpatient referrals (Gillespie & Gillespie, 1986). Within the mental health field, for both nurses and psychiatrists, there is evidence that the levels may be even worse (Jones, 1987; Margison, 1987). In other groups such as dentists, paramedics, laboratory workers, and managers, levels have been shown to be equally high.

In doctors, studies have considered not just general stress, but also depression and alcoholism, the two psychological conditions that seem most prevalent for this profession. For example, again using the GHQ, studies have shown caseness levels of almost 50%, with 28% indicating clinical depression during the first postgraduate year (Firth-Cozens, 1987). In the States, Reuben (1985) has shown that around a third of new doctors are depressed, compared to 15% using the same instrument in community samples, but this falls over subsequent years, perhaps as their hours become more reasonable and their confidence grows. Nevertheless, there are some specialties where the rates remain abnormally high; for example, Reuben found prevalence of 37% in ICU second year postgraduates compared to 22% overall.

Stress and depression are sometimes seen as related to raised alcohol rates, though some studies show that there is no such correlation, certainly when subjects are young (Firth-Cozens, 1987). It is the long-term use of alcohol that causes concern (Brooke, Edwards & Taylor, 1991) and that can harm the health of both the professionals and their patients (Firth-Cozens, 1993). In this regard and in relation to physical disorders which are seen as stress-related, much more is known about doctors than about other professional groups. Nevertheless, the US National Institute for Occupational Safety showed nurses to have a relatively high prevalence of conditions such as hypertension, peptic ulcers and coronary heart disease (Heim, 1991).

It is clear from most studies, including those reported above, that health workers generally do show high levels of stress, depression, and stress-related disorders when compared to the community samples on which the measures are validated. However, we have less knowledge of how they compare with other occupational groups facing some of the same environmental factors both inside and outside the workplace. A large study by Rees & Cooper (1992) addressed this issue by studying health workers across all professions, but also comparing them with non-health workers. In terms of the various occupational groups within the health field, there were few differences in mental or physical health, apart from general managers scoring much more positively than the other groups on both counts. Ancillary staff and scientists and technicians in particular had very low levels of job satisfaction and high sickness absence, both of which are significantly related to stress.

However, the health-care workers reported fewer symptoms of mental ill-health and similar levels of job satisfaction to those not in the non-health sector. In other words, what we might be looking at is not so much a population with elevated stress levels when compared to other workers, but one which suffers in similar ways but perhaps acts differently as a result. For example, recent reports by the Industrial Society (1993) and the Confederation of British Industry (1993) concluded that employee absence in the NHS is higher than in most other job sectors, and the managers in the study by Seccombe & Buchan (1993) reported that nurse absence was on the increase. Because of this, recognizing the perceived stressors becomes an important step in attempting to reduce the symptoms.

THE CAUSES OF STRESS

In the measures they used, Rees & Cooper (1992) found no significant differences in the sources of stress reported by the various types of health professionals, though nurses reported the highest levels of pressure in their jobs (workload, lack of variety, rates of pay, promotion prospects, role conflict, and so on), compared especially to general managers who reported the lowest. Similarly, health workers in general felt significantly more pressures than did the controls, despite this not being made apparent in higher symptom levels.

It is certainly true that, when you ask doctors what causes them stress, and get them to complete pre-constructed questionnaires, they see overload as being the main cause of their problems (Firth-Cozens, 1987). However, when you ask them to write about what stressed them most over the past month, they talk primarily about incidents concerning death and dying, followed by difficult relationships with their senior doctors, and by personally making mistakes (Firth-Cozens & Morrison, 1989). This tendency to use reports of overload to mask stressors which are actually much more anxiety-provoking, such as death and suffering, intimacy, and madness has been commented upon by other writers (for example, Mumford, 1983) and has been noted by the psychoanalyst Isobel Menzies-Lyth (1988) in her studies of nurses in the fifties. She described the organizational strategies (such as uniforms to distinguish the well from the sick, and long hierarchies to reduce the stress of responsibility) which are designed to reduce this anxiety, even though they may not be ultimately for the good of the patient. Handy (1986) has used similarly qualitative methodology (though more from a sociological viewpoint than psychoanalytic) to describe the sources of conflict that surround issues of patient control, for example, and which cause stress in psychiatric nursing. Certainly she and others in the field have criticized the more usual methodologies which involve the completion of questionnaires designed usually from previous literatures. The complexity of stressors for health workers can be seen in the following descriptions of stressful events a general practitioner and an A&E doctor by (Firth-Cozens, 1994).

It was the sudden death of a patient – unexpected. I had to deal with the anger of the relatives. Also discussing death with coroner and issuing a death certificate when not 100% certain of cause, in order to avoid postmortem (not wanted by family). Feelings of guilt that I could have done more to prevent death – probably unrealistic. This occurred when my partner was on holiday, I had no locum and there was a flu epidemic in full swing! Slight worries about litigation.

A patient with chest pain (probably dyspepsia) was accompanied by his two sons who were verbally aggressive: 'If anything happens to my father, I'll get you.' I threatened them with calling the police which made the situation worse. It was a busy Saturday and I was alone except for a female receptionist. I was worried in case I came across them in the street at another time. I felt vulnerable and scared.

These accounts show the difficulty of being able to identify with any precision the job-related stressors that health workers have to face. Although overload or a lack of support may not be the overt stressor, it underlies many of the incidents that people report, as it does here. Other underlying facts are the increasing threat of litigation, and the reduction in status and respect with which health workers (and perhaps all professionals) are held, something that perhaps once compensated for the long hours they worked and difficult situations they faced.

INDIVIDUAL FACTORS IN EXPERIENCING STRESS

Over the last ten years or more, the growth of a dispositional model of stress has gained favour from a number of writers (for example, Costa McCrae & Zonderman 1987). This argues that there is some personality factor, often called negative affectivity, which makes some people stressed or dissatisfied across any number of situations. Such a trend has great implications, of course, for what organizations decide to do about their stress problems, and this will be discussed in the last section of the chapter. However, it also puts the focus back on the individual and captures the idea which most lay people would recognize, that 'one man's meat is another man's poison' – in other words, that the experience of stress is very individual and that we need to search for the factors that will make some jobs particularly difficult for some people.

Psychoanalysts such as Malan (1979) have told us that those who work in professions such as health and social services are likely to have backgrounds which predispose them to a particular form of distress which he called 'helping profession syndrome'. This is seen as arising from early experience of having a poorly functioning parent or parents (for example, depressed, alcoholic, or simply in conflict) and being as a child unable to make this better. The adult then attempts to rectify these early experiences by choosing a helping profession where he or she feels it is possible to make up for the past. Certainly there is evidence that doctors have had more illnesses in their close early family than lawyers who likewise have had more legal actions (Paris & Frank, 1983). Moreover, one of the key predictors of choosing a medical career that brought you very close to patients (psychiatrists and general practitioners) rather than distant (public health doctors, pathologists) was a guilty anxious relationship with one's mother (Firth-Cozens, unpublished observations).

So, it may be that one chooses a health service career to make good, but that the job itself often fails to allow the person to do that and so the sense of failure for some people continues and causes adult stress and depression. One of the key personality variables in this chain is self-criticism which has been shown to be the best predictor (along with the same guilty, anxious relationship with the mother) of stress and depression in junior house officers (Firth-Cozens, 1992 and in senior doctors 10 years later (Brewin & Firth-Cozens, in press). These individual factors far outweighed the influence of job-related variables such as hours worked, bed responsibility, and so on. In this longitudinal study, following 170 medical students into their preregistration year, a discriminant analysis of those stressed on both occasions compared to those never stressed revealed that the groups could be distinguished as students with 80% success using the variables of: self-criticism, the relationship to mother scale referred to above and a similar one to father, older fathers, a perception of father as strict, powerful and hard to please, and dissatisfaction with their role as students. Similarly, those who had lost their mothers when young were severely depressed as junior doctors, although they had shown no sign of it as students, perhaps indicating that it takes the environmental stressors of death and responsibility to bring out earlier traumas. The importance of self-criticism and of early family experience in the perception of chronic stress was very clear with these analyses. Certainly in a profession where occasional mistakes or failure to cure is not just inevitable but is often denied right from early training, then being self-critical is likely to be one of the most destructive personality factors for health workers to have.

INDIVIDUAL COPING
Another area of research on the ways that individual factors might contribute to stress involves how they cope with the inevitable difficulties of health-related jobs. In particular, there has been some interest in palliative coping in nurses (Ogus, 1992), and some sug-

gestion that these might be less effective than strategies which confront or attempt to change the stressor (Pines & Kafry, 1981). Tyler and Cushway (1992) reported that negative mental health outcomes in hospital nurses were predicted by perceptions of high workload and their use of avoidance as a coping strategy. Similarly, the use of denial and avoidance was found to be the only significant difference in coping styles in the longitudinal study referred to earlier when doctors who were highly stressed on each testing were compared with those who were consistently low scoring (Firth-Cozens & Morrison, 1989). It seems that, when faced with some of the distressing and often uncontrollable events that take place within health care, trying to put them out of your mind is certainly not a useful coping strategy. Although not significant, there was a strong suggestion in the doctors' study that those consistently healthy talked much more to others as a means of support.

ORGANIZATIONAL TACTICS
A number of health services now have counselling services for their staff, and this type of job-related short-term counselling in organizations has been shown to be very effective, not just in reducing symptoms but also in improving job attitudes and even changing traits such as anxiety which might be seen as factors in the dispositional negative affectivity referred to earlier (Firth-Cozens & Hardy, 1992). Certainly it matters that hospital services do tackle the individual and organizational causes of stress: absence levels and turnover are unacceptably high in most services and there is strong evidence too that complaints, medication errors and litigation suits are highly related to the stress levels of staff (Jones et al., 1988). In this study, the simple introduction of stress management workshops reduced the incidence of litigation claims in 22 hospitals from a yearly average of 31 claims down to 9, compared to the matched control group of hospital where claims stayed almost the same.

CONCLUSION
Stress levels in health workers are high, though perhaps no higher than those in other organizational groups. Nevertheless, the cost in terms of the worker, the organization and the patient make the levels particularly unacceptable. Their causes are complex, but individual personality factors such as high self-criticism as well as various early experiences are likely to play as strong a part as organizational stressors. The need to tackle stress levels is paramount, and counselling services and stress management courses have both been shown effective in protecting health professionals and their patients.

REFERENCES
Brewin, C.R. & Firth-Cozens, J. (1997). Predicting depression in junior doctors. Journal of Occupational Health (in press).
Brooke, D., Edwards, G. & Taylor, C. (1991). Addiction as an occupational hazard: 144 doctors with drug and alcohol problems. British Journal of Addiction, 86, 1011–16.
Confederation of British Industry (1993). Too much time out. London: CB 1.
Costa, P.T., McCrae, R.R. & Zonderman, A.B. (1987). Environmental and dispositional influences on well-being: longitudinal follow-up of an American

national sample. British Journal of Psychology, 78, 299–308.
Firth-Cozens, J. (1987). Emotional distress in junior house officers. British Medical Journal, 205, 533–6.
Firth-Cozens, J. (1992). The role of early experiences in the perception of organizational stress: fusing clinical and organizational perspectives. Journal of Occupational and Organizational Psychology, 65, 61–75.
Firth-Cozens, J. (1993). Stress, psychological problems and clinical performance. In C. Vincent, M. Ennis & B. Audley (Eds.).

Medical accidents. Oxford: Oxford University Press.
Firth-Cozens, J. (1994). Stress in doctors. Repeat to the NHSE R & D, Northern & Yorkshire.
Firth-Cozens, J. & Hardy, G. (1992). Occupational stress, clinical treatment and changes in job perceptions. Journal of Occupational and Organizational Psychology, 65, 81–8.
Firth-Cozens, J. & Morrison, L.M. (1989). Sources of stress and ways of coping in junior house officers. Stress Medicine, 5, 121–6.

Gillespie, C. & Gillespie, V. (1986). Reading the danger signs. *Nursing Times*, 30 July, 24–7.

Goldberg, D. (1978). *Manual of the general health questionnaire*. Windsor: NFER.

Handy, J.A. (1986). Considering organisations in organisational stress research: a rejoinder to Glowinski & Cooper and to Duckworth. *Bulletin of the British Psychological Society*, **39**, 205–10.

Heim, E. (1991). Job stressors and coping in health professionals. *Psychotherapy and Psychosomatics*, **55**, 90–9.

Industrial Society (1993). *Wish you were here*. Edgbaston: Society. Industrial.

Jones, J.G. (1987). Stress in psychiatric nursing. In R.L. Payne & J. Firth-Cozens (Eds.). *Stress in health professionals*. Chichester: John Wiley.

Jones, J.W., Barge, B.N., Steffy, B.D., Fay, L.M., Kunz, L.K. & Wuebker, L.J. (1988). Stress and medical malpractice: organizational risk assessment and intervention. *Journal Applied Psychology*, **4**, 727–35.

Malan, D.H. (1979). *Individual psychotherapy and the science of psycho-dynamics*. London: Butterworths.

Margison, F.R. (1987). *Stress in psychiatrists*. In R.L. Payne & J. Firth-Cozens (Eds.). *Stress in health professionals*. Chichester: John Wiley.

Menzies-Lyth, I. (1988). *Containing anxiety in institutions*. London: Free Associations Press.

Mumford, E. (1983). Stress in the medical career. *Journal of Medical Education*, **58**, 436–7.

Ogus, E.D. (1992). Burnout and coping strategies: a comparative study of ward nurses, *Journal Social Behavior and Personality*, **7**, 111–24.

Paris, J. & Frank, H. (1983). Psychological determinants of a medical career. *Canadian Journal of Psychiatry*, **28**, 354–7.

Payne, R.L. & Firth-Cozens, J. (Eds.). (1987). *Stress in health professionals*. Chichester: John Wiley.

Pines, A. & Kafry, D. (1981). Coping with burnout. In J.W. Jones (Ed.). *The burnout syndrome Park Ridge*, Il: London House Management Press.

Rees, D. & Cooper, C.L. (1992). Occupational stress in health service workers in the UK. *Stress Medicine*, **8**, 79–90.

Reuben, D.B. (1985). Depressive symptoms in medical house officers: effects of level of training and work rotation. *Archives of International Medicine*, **145**, 286–8.

Seccombe, I. & Buchan, J. (1993). High anxiety. *Health Service Journal*, **103**, 22–4.

Tyler, P. & Cushway, D. (1992). Stress, coping and mental wellbeing in hospital nurses. *Stress Medicine*, **8**, 91–8.

West, M., Jones, A. & Savage, Y. (1988). Stress in health visiting: a quantitative

Teaching communication skills

TONY KENDRICK

Division of General Practice and Primary Care,
St George's Hospital Medical School, London,
UK

INTRODUCTION

In the field of health and medicine, communication skills are important in several contexts. These include not only communication between health professionals and their clients, individually, in groups, or through the media, but also communication between one health professional and another. In practice, most communication skills teaching relates to encounters between health professionals and individuals seeking their help. In this chapter I shall focus on the teaching of consultation skills to medical students and practising doctors.

The need for consultation skills teaching

Research has shown that doctors commonly fail to elicit patients' problems and concerns, and fail to make important diagnoses. For example, emotional problems are common in general medical practice, but treatable depression is missed in up to 50% of cases (Freeling *et al.*, 1985). Perhaps it is not surprising therefore that many patients do not comply with the treatments they are offered. Improved communication leads to better health outcomes for patients (Simpson *et al.*, 1991).

Power and roles

Presiding as they do over matters of life and death, doctors have traditionally been accorded great respect and invested with authority.

This means that, in most doctor–patient encounters, the balance of power is most definitely shifted towards the doctor. However, to detect a patient's problems and concerns accurately, and to enable a patient to comply with treatment and advice, the doctor must recognize that the patient is a partner in the process whose own perceptions and ideas need to be taken into account. Szasz and Hollender (1956) described three basic models of the doctor–patient relationship:

(i) Activity–Passivity
(ii) Guidance–Cooperation
(iii) Mutual participation.

The doctor-active, patient-passive model may be appropriate in certain situations, such as the emergency resuscitation of an unconscious person. The second model assumes that the doctor uses knowledge and skill to guide a sick patient who co-operates in order to regain health, the power remaining largely in the doctor's hands. However, many encounters may not proceed successfully unless the third model is adopted. This is more likely, for example, when the best choice of treatment is not clear-cut, or if the solution to the patient's problem lies in changing behaviour or lifestyle, or learning to adapt to disability.

Increasingly, complaints and litigation against doctors cite poor communication as an important element. This may have played a part in fuelling the proliferation of consultation skills teaching in undergraduate medical training.

SKILLS TRAINING

Theory

Much consultation skills teaching is based on a social skills training model derived from learning theory (Argyle, 1983). The model assumes that successful consultations depend on the use of particular behaviours which are learned. These include specific types of questions but also non-verbal behaviour such as posture and eye-contact. It follows that a relatively unskilled subject can become more skilled by learning to use the correct behaviours.

Tasks and processes

The first stage in skills training must be to define the task to be accomplished. For the doctor, the central task of the consultation is to solve the patient's problem. The Royal College of General Practitioners' (1972) working party on vocational training for general practice formulated a six-stage problem-solving model of the consultation (see Table 1).

Given that the doctor should cede power to the patient in many consultations, for the reasons outlined above, it follows that successful problem-solving may involve a number of processes. These include: helping patients to identify and articulate their problems and concerns, both overt and covert; defining and agreeing problems with the patient; giving information and dealing with worries and concerns; generating, exploring and agreeing possible solutions; and committing patients to implement the solutions agreed (Pendleton et al., 1984). The doctor may have to complete these tasks within a limited time.

Microbehaviours

The next step is to identify the behaviours which are most effective in accomplishing these tasks, those which are most efficient in terms of the time taken, and which behaviours are counter-productive. Ideally, these should be derived from the observation of professionals with a whole range of skills in carrying out the tasks, although this is time-consuming and difficult. In practice, desirable behaviours may be specified by 'expert' opinion, or through discussion in consensus groups.

There have been some good observational studies, however. Byrne and Long (1976) studied audiotaped consultations in general practice and identified a range of interviewing styles from extreme 'patient-centredness' to extreme 'doctor-centredness', with most doctors somewhere in the middle. Patient-centredness involved listening, allowing silences and reflecting, clarifying and interpreting the patient's concerns, while doctor-centredness involved more information gathering and analysing, probing for symptoms of particular concern to the doctor. What was remarkable was the consistency of the style of most doctors, despite the broad range of illness presented, from the purely organic through to psychosomatic illness, and despite a wide range of verbal ability of the patients.

Extreme doctor-centredness was associated with spending little time with patients, five minutes or less, a distinct preference for the first symptoms offered, and an apparent unwillingness to discuss feelings or enter into any real relationship with patients. The

Table 1. *A problem-solving model of the consultation (Royal College of General Practitioners 1972).*

A Problem(s) stated
B Problem(s) examined
C Problem(s) defined
D Solution(s) generated
E Solution(s) examined
F Solution(s) selected

researchers pointed out that such a style may be appropriate for entirely physical problems but is unlikely to aid the exploration of emotional problems.

Goldberg et al. (1980) studied the interviewing styles of family doctors in training and measured their accuracy in detecting emotional disorders in their patients, compared to the results of a standardized psychiatric interview for such problems. They found that a number of interviewing behaviours were related to increased accuracy (Table 2).

An open-ended question is one which allows a whole range of possible responses, such as 'How are you?'. A closed question is one to which there are only a limited number of possible answers, such as 'Do you wake early in the morning?' ('Yes or no'). Open questions are most useful at the beginning of a consultation, allowing the patient to set the agenda and map out the areas of concern, rather than closing down prematurely on one area of particular interest to the doctor. Closed questions are more useful later on, when homing in and carefully defining the problem. Therefore moving through 'open-to-closed cones' is efficient interviewing behaviour.

Often, patients do not volunteer all their concerns immediately, especially when their underlying problems are emotional in origin and they are unsure of how receptive the doctor may be. Therefore sensitivity to verbal cues ('I'm so tired all the time') and non-verbal cues (such as anxious looks and clenched fists) are important in detecting such problems.

Empathy means imaginatively entering into another's feelings. Telling patients that you can see how the world must look to them usually encourages them to tell more about how they feel, as does repeating the patient's last few words, plus non-verbal facilitation including nods, smiles and giving eye-contact, and 'para-verbal' behaviours such as grunts and murmurs.

Ley et al. (1976) studied the giving of information and advice in consultations and found that patients' recollection of such information was improved by teaching family doctors to adopt the behaviours listed in Table 3.

Giving important information early on in the interview, and repeating it towards the end, utilizes primacy and recency effects to improve recall, by reducing retroactive and proactive inhibition of storage into memory. Stressing the importance of what is about to be said ensures that the patient's attention is raised to receive information.

Explicit categorization means arranging the information to be given into clear categories ('First I'm going to tell you what I think is wrong with you, then I'm going to tell you what you can do to help yourself, then I'll tell you about the medicines I want you to take'). Specific advice is recalled better than general recommendations

Table 2. *Ten aspects of a family doctor's interview style which are related to accuracy in detecting emotional problems (Goldberg et al., 1980)*

Outset:
1. Gives eye-contact at outset
2. Clarifies presenting complaint
3. Uses directive questions for physical complaints
4. Uses 'open-to-closed cones'

Interview style:
5. Empathic comments (frequency)
6. Sensitive to verbal cues
7. Sensitive to non-verbal cues
8. Doesn't read notes while taking the history
9. Can deal with over-talkativeness
10. Asks fewer questions about past history

Table 3. *Aspects of giving information which increase patients' recollection (Ley et al., 1976)*

1. Giving instructions and advice early in the interview
2. Stressing the importance of the advice given
3. Using short words and short sentences (avoiding jargon)
4. Explicit categorization
5. Repeating advice
6. Giving specific detailed advice rather than general recommendations
7. Encouraging the patient to ask questions, and answering them.

('You should walk briskly for twenty minutes three times a week', rather than 'Take more exercise').

Millar and Goldberg (1991), in a study of trainee general practitioners, found that those who were better at detecting emotional problems in their patients were also better at giving information and advice. They were more likely than poor detectors to negotiate management with the patient, explain the effects and side-effects of treatment, and check the patient's understanding. It seems that good consultation skills are indicative of a generally higher standard of medical practice.

Modelling

The third stage in skills training is to inform learners of which behaviours are effective and efficient. This will usually involve giving them lists of desirable and undesirable behaviours, on a handout for example. Videotaped or live demonstrations may be shown to illustrate their use in practice. Such teaching gives learners an anatomy of the consultation on which to base understanding of its function (Kendrick & Freeling, 1993). Tutors may portray 'ideal' consultations, perhaps with simulated patients played by actors instructed to respond as required.

Feedback

The final stage involves giving learners practice in using the desired behaviours, and feedback on their performance. Such practice may include role-playing, mock consultations with simulated patients, or encounters with patients with real problems. Playing the role of patients themselves may give learners insights into how it feels to be interviewed and into the effects of particular behaviours. Simulated

Table 4. *Interview skills of young doctors shown to be improved five years after feedback training as medical students (Maguire et al., 1986)*

Clarification of patients' statements
Using open questions
Noticing verbal clues to patients' problems
Inquiring about patients' psychosocial problems
Preventing needless repetition
Keeping patients to the point
Verbal and visual encouragement
Getting precise information
Using brief questions
Reducing use of jargon

patients can be asked to present particular types of problems in a predetermined fashion, and can be relied upon to give the learner feedback from the patient's perspective.

The traditional apprenticeship method of teaching medical students history-taking involves asking them to interview several patients and then discussing the abstracted histories that they obtain in seminars or on ward rounds. Maguire and colleagues (1978) demonstrated a clear advantage in giving medical students detailed feedback about their interviewing skills compared with such traditional teaching. The students' ability to elicit accurate and relevant information was improved significantly by giving them handouts on the skills to be used, practice with patients, feedback on their performance and discussion with a tutor. Videotape and audiotape feedback were more successful than direct feedback from an observer.

Evaluation

Ideally, the success of such skills training should be measured in terms of improved health outcomes for patients. In practice, it is often assumed to be sufficient to measure changes in the frequencies of behaviours in consultations before and after training, to demonstrate that learning has taken place.

Maguire, Fairbairn and Fletcher (1986) demonstrated clear increases in the frequencies of desirable behaviours used by medical students after interviewing skills feedback training, compared to a traditionally taught control group, which persisted after they had qualified and were working as doctors five years later (Table 4).

Gask et al. (1988), also using videotape feedback, have demonstrated similar improvements in the interviewing skills of trainee psychiatrists, family doctors in training, and established general practitioners.

A PSYCHODYNAMIC APPROACH

The skills training approach has been shown to improve learners' knowledge and skill in using desirable consulting behaviours, at least when they are being observed. However, such an approach may not in itself be sufficient to change behaviour in everyday practice. Psychodynamic approaches stress the prime importance of the doctor's attitudes and feelings towards the patient, which must be favourable if the learner is to be motivated to use the knowledge and skills.

Psychodynamic theory suggests that observable behaviour depends on underlying pervasive psychological mechanisms, which may be unconscious. Byrne and Long's extreme doctor-centred style could for example, be interpreted as a defence mechanism to protect the doctor from uncomfortable involvement with patients.

The psychoanalyst Michael Balint (1957) made a major contribution to thinking about the doctor–patient relationship and provided a method by which attitudes could be explored and developed. He stressed that the doctor's feelings and reaction to the patient (counter-transference) are an important source of information in defining the patient's problem, that is in reaching a diagnosis. Furthermore, feeding back and interpreting such feelings may help the patient gain insight into the nature of the problem and so aid treatment.

Adapting the model of case supervision in psychotherapy, Balint suggested that doctors could become more sensitive to their own and to their patient's feelings using supervised group discussion of cases with their peers, through a 'limited but considerable change in the doctor's personality'. Doctors who have taken part seem convinced of the value of Balint training, and some continue to attend such groups for many years.

CONCLUSION

Consultation skills teaching must address learners' knowledge, skills and attitudes. The behavioural approach has proved successful in increasing consulting knowledge and skills. To motivate them to use the skills acquired however, medical students and doctors must be helped to understand the purposes of the consultation, the roles of doctor and patient and the importance of the interaction between them, if they are to help their patients respond to their problems most effectively.

REFERENCES

Argyle, M. (1983). Doctor–patient skills. In J. Hasler & D. Pendleton, (Eds.). *Doctor–patient communication*, pp. 57–74. London: Academic Press.

Balint, M. (1957). *The doctor, his patient and the illness*. London: Pitman.

Byrne, P.S. & Long, B.L. (1976). *Doctors talking to patients*. London: HMSO.

Freeling, P., Rao, B.M., Paykel, E.S., Sireling, L.I., & Burton, R.H. (1985). Unrecognized depression in general practice. *British Medical Journal*, **290**, 1880–3.

Gask, L., Goldberg, D., Lesser, A.L., & Millar, T. (1988). Improving the psychiatric skills of the general practitioner trainee. An evaluation of a group training course. *Medical Education*, **22**, 132–8.

Goldberg, D.P., Steele, J.J., Smith, C., & Spivey, L. (1980). Training family doctors to recognize psychiatric illness with increased accuracy. *Lancet*, **ii**, 521–3.

Kendrick, T., & Freeling, P. (1993). A communication skills course for preclinical medical students: evaluation of general practice based teaching using group methods. *Medical Education*, **27**, 211–17.

Ley, P., Whitworth, M.A., Skilbeck, C.E., Woodward, R., Pinsent, R.J.F.H., Pike, L.A., Clarkson, M.E. & Clark, P.B. (1976). Improving doctor-patient communication in general practice. *Journal of the Royal College of General Practitioners*, **26**, 720–4.

Maguire, P., Roe, P., Goldberg, D., Jones, S., Hyde, C., & O'Dowd, T. (1978). The value of feedback in teaching interview skills to medical students. *Psychological Medicine*, **8**, 695–704.

Maguire, P., Fairbairn, S., & Fletcher, C. (1986). Consultation skills of young doctors: I – Benefits of feedback training as students persist. *British Medical Journal*, **292**, 1573–6.

Millar, T. & Goldberg, D. (1991). Link between the ability to detect and manage emotional disorders: a study of general practitioner trainees. *British Journal of General Practice*, **41**, 357–9.

Pendleton, D., Schofield, T., Tate, P. & Havelock, P. (1984). *The consultation. An approach to learning and teaching*. Oxford: Oxford University Press.

Royal College of General Practitioners (1972). *The future general practitioner: learning and teaching*. London: RCGP.

Simpson, M., Buckman, R., Stewart, M., Maguire, P., Lipkin, M., Novack, D. & Till, J. (1991). Doctor–patient communication: the Toronto consensus statement. *British Medical Journal*, **303**, 1385–7.

Szasz, T.S. & Hollender, M.H. (1956). A contribution to the philosophy of medicine. *Archives of Internal Medicine*, **97**, 585–92.

Training and the process of professional development

COLIN COLES

Institutes of Health and Community, Studies, Bournemouth University, UK

THE PROBLEMS OF PROFESSIONAL EDUCATION

Most professional education is divided into two distinct phases: a relatively brief initial qualifying period leading to some kind of professional registration, followed by postregistration specialist education with an extensive period of continuing professional development. This pattern is no more clearly seen than in medicine which will form the focus for this chapter. Educating doctors, whilst having specific features, has much in common with other professions, particularly in health care.

Initial training in medicine, largely coinciding with an undergraduate qualification, is conventionally divided into pre-clinical and clinical parts. During the preclinical course, students are presented with information thought to be relevant to medical practice, largely comprising biological and behavioural-science teaching. Traditionally, academic disciplines, and more recently topics reflecting bodily systems, are formally presented through lecture programmes by staff who also teach degree level students of their own. The preclinical course conventionally ends with an examination of students' so-called 'basic' knowledge, leading to clinical attachments mainly to hospital departments though increasingly in general practice. Clinical education is largely experiential, supplemented by lectures. By the end of the undergraduate phase students will have been examined on their clinical knowledge and some practical skills such as history taking and physical examination.

Successful medical graduates enter a short period of practical training (which currently in the United Kingdom comprises one year of salaried hospital posts to receive official registration by the General Medical Council), and are then free to pursue a specialty career of their choice, which over several more years will involve a number of training posts together with study for higher specialist examinations. Once they become a hospital consultant or a principal in general practice they face up to 35 years of medical practice with little formalized continuing medical education.

The problems medical students and trainees face have been well documented elsewhere (Coles, 1985a; Dowling & Barrett, 1991; Grant, Marsden & King, 1989). Briefly, the picture is this: Undergraduates feel overloaded with content, lose their early motivation, find it difficult to see the relevance of much of what they are taught especially in the early years, commit vast amounts of information to memory to pass examinations and then quickly forget what they have learnt. Many are unable to apply their knowledge in their clinical attachments. They see even less relevance in the behavioural sciences they are taught, coming to believe at this stage that medicine is a technological (if not technical) profession, concerned more with biology than behavioural science. Once qualified, they must balance heavy service demands with the need to pursue their own specialist education, usually in their spare time, and may or may not receive adequate supervision from their seniors. As they themselves assume more senior posts the nature of their professional work changes (they deal less with clinical matters and more with managerial ones) but they are ill-prepared for these changes and give little attention to their continuing professional development.

HOW DO PROFESSIONALS WORK?

It has been suggested that professionals face both well-defined and ill-defined problems (Elstein, Schulman & Sprafka, 1978). Well defined problems can often be dealt with through agreed procedures. Ill-defined problems, which form the bulk of professional work, do not. Slight differences in these problems can lead to very large differences in their management, and much professional practice has been characterized as problem-defining rather than problem-solving.

The relatively few well-defined problems professionals tackle can be dealt with at a technical level (Oakeshott, 1962) and require the professional to have what has been described as propositional knowledge (Eraut, 1985): the professional knows what to do. However, ill-defined problems can rarely be addressed by the use of propositional knowledge, and require what has been called process knowledge (Eraut, 1985); professionals know how (Ryle, 1949) to proceed, even though they may not know precisely what needs to be done.

An example of this is the management of diabetes. The proposi-

tional knowledge taught to medical students and trainees largely emphasizes the pathophysiology of the disease and the pharmacology of the various treatments. In practice, rather different knowledge is needed. The diagnosis of diabetes is relatively straightforward from the patient's history and symptoms, and can be confirmed with a simple laboratory test carried out even in a general practitioner's surgery. However, once the diagnosis has been made and the treatment prescribed, day-to-day management of diabetes passes from the health professional into the hands of the diabetic and possibly relatives and friends. Whether or not the management is successful depends on how well the health professional can hand over control. Clinical management is a partnership between the patient and the professional who requires a considerable amount of process knowledge: knowledge of people and how to deal with them; knowledge of situations and what to do in certain circumstances. Rarely is this process knowledge taught to medical students and trainees. Health professionals must acquire it, usually covertly, through their professional development. It is acquired tacitly (Polanyi, 1966) through experience, or not at all.

Schon (1983) suggests professionals reflect-in-action with 'on-the-spot experimentation'. They use high grade skills to monitor their performance and adjust it in accordance with the nature of the problem as it unfolds, using novel or up to then untried means for addressing it. They utilize a considerable amount of personally acquired 'implicit theory', not the 'espoused theory' (Argyris & Schon, 1976) that forms the basis for much of their more formalized professional education.

Eraut (1985, 1994) supports this claim. He suggests that, while the propositional knowledge professionals are taught might help them understand problems, it does not help deal with them. Indeed propositional knowledge is not 'applied' by professionals but 'interpreted' by them in practice. Thus, any prior knowledge professionals acquire is rarely 'used' in a professional context. Rather it is transformed in action by its new use. The implications are:

- Professional knowledge is actually 'created' in the practice setting.
- Professionals learn while doing.
- Knowledge created in one professional context is not necessarily 'available' for use in some other situation.
- If the same problem is tackled in a new and slightly altered context it will require further interpretation of the professional's existing knowledge.
- Each professional therefore has a unique knowledge store.
- The education of professionals should recognize these principles, but in reality often does not.

PROFESSIONAL SOCIALIZATION

It is generally recognized that, whatever formalized education professionals receive, most of their development occurs through a process of professional socialization which is largely passive and learned on-the-job (Schon, 1987). This has its strengths. Senior professionals can inspire their junior colleagues. The educational costs are relatively low. Young professionals carry out service work whilst receiving training, frequently at a lower cost than if the work were carried out by their more senior colleagues. But there are dangers. Professional socialization can perpetuate poor practice, and restrict opportunities for change. Because the professionalisation process is rarely articulated, it does not guarantee that personal development will occur, and it rarely leads to the related development of professional services.

A further danger of professional socialization being largely covert is that it often involves 'rites of passage'. 'Hurdles' are put in the path of the juniors' development, sometimes rationalized by seniors as being 'good for them' because 'we did it ourselves' Frequently these rites of passage have little to do with the normal functioning of professional life, can be damaging to morale, and are often associated more with 'control' than professional development.

Yet another danger in professional socialization is that different agencies can have different agendas which can be in conflict. In undergraduate medical education, for example, academic departments might perpetuate educational practices so as to maintain departmental funding and existing staffing levels than for any reasoned argument that they provide an appropriate preparation for professional service.

THE NATURE OF PROFESSIONAL DEVELOPMENT

It has been suggested (Benner, 1984) that professionals develop through a number of stages:

- Novices utilize prescribed modes of operation.
- Advanced beginners recognize that these prescriptions do not work in all situations but that appropriate actions are contextually related.
- Competent professionals make conscious choices about what to do. Their practice is self-managed and self-regulated.
- Proficient professionals work at an intuitive level, utilizing considerable amounts of 'know-how', and seeing professional practice in a holistic way.
- Experts practise in such a way that they and the tasks they are performing are inseparable.

Most professionals reach the competent stage relatively quickly. However, further progress can be difficult, protracted and not guaranteed. The challenge of professional education is to ensure that competence is reached effectively and efficiently, and that continuing development occurs.

THE PROCESS OF PROFESSIONAL EDUCATION

Seeing professional education as a continuing process raises several questions. What should be the balance between initial and in-service education? What should constitute the content and educational process? What is the role of academic education in professional development? What should be the contribution of practitioners? When and how should professionals be examined, accredited and possibly reaccredited?

Eraut (1994) formulates three principles for initial professional education:

(i) If knowledge is not used for a professional purpose within the programme itself, it should not be included.

(ii) If the time gap between the introduction of such knowledge and its first use is too large, it is being introduced at the wrong point in the sequence.

(iii) The objectives for the theoretical aspects of professional education programmes should be defined . . . in terms of knowledge use in professional contexts.

Barnett, Becher & Cork (1987) suggest a partnership model for professional education, and formulate five principles:

1. Professional education has three inter-related facets:
   (a) the initial development of practical skills;
   (b) the ability to analyse and reflect on such skills;
   (c) hence, the ability to continue to learn throughout one's professional career.
2. Theory has to be seen as a body of knowledge directly related to and illuminating practice.
3. It follows that practical experience has primacy, but this has to be accompanied by metapractice (reflection and analysis).
4. There is a need for academics to address practical problems and be conversant with professional realities.
5. There is a need for practitioners to be full partners in the enterprise of initial professional education.

In medical education, one attempt to resolve these challenges has been problem-based learning (Walton & Matthews, 1989), where from the very beginning of the curriculum students are presented with clinical problems, often in the form of 'paper-and-pencil cases', which they attempt to solve, utilizing previously prepared study resources to enable them to acquire relevant knowledge for the solution of these problems.

While problem-based learning has been shown to be associated with the development of appropriate study approaches (Coles, 1985b), the longer-term effects on medical practice are much less clear. This is perhaps understandable in the light of the arguments presented above. Problem based learning, while helping students understand clinical problems, allowing considerable educational autonomy, and developing self study skills, does not necessarily focus on knowledge creation. Rather students acquire their professional knowledge often away from the practice setting.

An alternative might be for initial professional education to be more firmly grounded in students' actual experience of professional practice. In medicine this might also involve settings outside hospitals such as general practice, reflecting where the bulk of health care occurs. Developments like this, loosely called 'community-based' medical education, have been seen in developing countries, and have recently been encouraged in the United Kingdom by proposals from the General Medical Council (GMC 1993, para 45, page 17).

Turning to postinitial professional education, it should be recognized that this is a complex phenomenon requiring different forms of learning at different levels (Calderhead, 1991; Schon, 1987). Currently in medical education the emphasis is on acquiring propositional knowledge in the context of specialist examinations. Process knowledge or 'know-how' is acquired tacitly 'on-the-job'. This has meant that process knowledge has not been accorded a high status, and its codification (let alone research base) is virtually non-existent (Eraut, 1985). Consequently its profile remains low and its introduction in formal professional development under represented in relation to its importance for professional practice.

Once formal postregistration qualifications have been obtained, professionals enter an extended period of continuing development. Again, learning here is largely on-the-job. In some areas of health care the notion of reaccreditation is being actively discussed. Without this, professionals are left to 'develop' themselves according to their own perceived needs. One approach advocated by the Royal College of General Practitioners (1993) is portfolio-based learning, comprising the collection of evidence to demonstrate the personal learning needs have been fulfilled, facilitated by a 'mentor' (see Chapter on 'Training educators'). Nursing education now accepts accreditation for prior experiential learning (APEL), particularly for obtaining credits that count towards higher professional qualifications at academic institutions.

CONCLUSIONS

The nature of professional development is now more clearly understood. The implications need to influence educational programmes.

Professional development at present largely comprises formal education in propositional knowledge in academic settings, and tacit on-the-job learning of process knowledge. In future it should more and more be seen as an interactive partnership between academics and practitioners. There should be a planned continuum of professional development from a student's entry into an initial training course through professional qualification to continuing professional development in-service. The balance between initial and in-service education needs further consideration, as does the relationship between the relative teaching (and especially learning) of propositional knowledge and process knowledge, with the role of 'know-how' being afforded a much higher status than at present. Examinations of professional competence should be seen in a strategic manner contributing towards someone's professional development, and not as a series of one-off 'hurdles' to be surmounted. Moreover, links between the individual's development and that of the professional service need to be explored.

REFERENCES

Argyris, C. & Schon, D.A. (1976). *Theory in practice: increasing professional effectiveness*, San Francisco: Jossey-Bass.

Barnett, R.A., Becher, R.A. & Cork, N.M. (1987). Models of professional preparation: pharmacy, nursing and teacher education. *Studies in Higher Education*, 12, 51–63.

Benner, P. (1984). *From novice to expert: excellence and power in clinical nursing practice*, California: Addison-Wesley.

Calderhead, J. (1991). The nature and growth of knowledge in student teaching. *Teaching and Teacher Education*, 7, 531–5.

Coles, C.R. (1985a). A study of the relationships between curriculum and learning in undergraduate medical education. PhD thesis, University of Southampton.

Coles, C.R. (1985b). Differences between conventional and problem-based curricula in their students' approaches to studying, *Medical Education*, 19, 4.

Dowling, S. & Barrett, S. (1991). *Doctors in the making. The experience of the preregistration year*. Bristol University, Bristol: SAUS publications.

Elstein, A.S., Schulman, L.S. & Sprafka, S.A. (1978). *Medical problem solving: an analysis of clinical reasoning*. Boston, Mass: Harvard University Press.

Eraut, M. (1985). Knowledge creation and knowledge use in professional contexts. *Studies in Higher Education*, 10, 117–33.

Eraut, M. (1994). *Developing professional knowledge and competence*. London: The Falmer Press.

GMC (1993). *Recommendations on undergraduate medical education*. London: GMC Education Committee.

Grant, J., Marsden, P. & King, R.C. (1989). Senior House Officers and their training, *British Medical Journal*, 299, 1263–8.

Oakeshott, M. (1962). *Rationalism in politics: and other essays*. London: Methuen.

Polanyi, M. (1966). *The tacit dimension*. New York: Doubleday.

RCGP (1983) *Portfolio learning*. Occasional paper. London: Royal College of General Practitioners.

Ryle, G. (1949). The concept of mind. London: Hutchinson.

Schon, D.A. (1983). *The reflective practitioner: how practitioners think in action*. San Francisco: Jossey-Bass.

Schon, D.A. (1987) *Educating the reflective practitioner: towards a new design for teaching and learning in the professions*. San Francisco: Jossey Bass.

Walton, H.J. & Matthews, M.B. (1989) *Essentials of problem-based learning*. ASME Medical Education Research Booklet 23, Dundee: Association for the Study of Medical Education.

Training educators

COLIN COLES

Institute of Health and Community Studies,
Bournemouth University, UK

EDUCATORS AND EDUCATING

Before looking at how people learn to educate, we should first look at what educating involves. The task of an educator covers a multitude of actions: one-to-one communication, small group working, as well as lecturing; educators counsel, help people with learning difficulties, and deal with reluctant and difficult learners; then there is the assessment of others, whether to help people learn or to judge their performance.

Educators have other less obvious functions: assisting with the development of courses and the curriculum; policy discussions concerning educational strategy; management of educational situations and other educators; resource management and development;

the training of other educators; educational research; and educational writing ranging from professional publications to academic journals.

Clearly, within this range of activities, there can be a conflict of roles. Lecturing and one-to-one teaching are quite different. Counselling can be incompatible with making judgements about people. Curriculum development is long term while face-to-face teaching has more immediate demands. The different tasks require different skills and frames of reference. They might be better suited to some people and not others.

Education is a complex and often unpredictable task. Educators must adapt to situations in which they find themselves, monitor their own actions, and be responsive to changes as they occur. Education has a number of different aims: preparation, socialization, personal and moral development, and the inculcation of standards and values. It is concerned with drawing out people's self, as well as developing their intellectual and social skills.

LEARNING TO EDUCATE

Outside of school teaching very few educators have formally learnt to educate. Many rely on previous experience of education, particularly as a learner, and are influenced by the attitudes, assumptions, values and expectations they hold concerning the nature of education, not all of them helpful (Calderhead, 1991).

Educators, like other professionals, develop through a series of stages from novice to expert which often happens passively by a process of professional socialization. Because this process is largely tacit, developing educators must weave their way through a maze of complex interactions with other professionals and the professional environment, often in an unsupported manner, sometimes identifying with certain groups but finding difficulties in identifying with others.

Learning to educate is often depicted as a matter of developing certain 'competencies'. The novice educator might clutch at tips-for-teachers to make sense of the complex world of education (Berliner, 1987). However, this can limit the educator's development. The novice will tend to make simple, common-sense interpretations of educational situations, and be less able than the expert to anticipate possibilities and act accordingly (Calderhead, 1991).

Educators must relearn their subject to teach it (Calderhead, 1991). For example, behavioural scientists teaching medical students about communication must learn how to teach not just facts but how to communicate effectively. This needs 'know how' (Ryle, 1949) about helping people acquire ways of communicating. In addition, they will have to learn how to plan a curriculum, how to work with colleagues in collaborative teaching, to cope with difficult people (learners and colleagues), and to deal with their own anxieties about teaching.

Being an educator exposes one's personality in a way that other professions do not (Calderhead, 1991). It is concerned in part with performance. There is a need to become aware of one's strengths and weaknesses; to recognize affective and ethical aspects of education, to see that one is not just teaching a subject, or even another person, but communicating one's values, and exposing one's attitudes towards others and their development. There is a need to develop self-knowledge, sometimes called metacognition, and above all appropriate self-confidence.

Learning to educate thus needs different forms of learning, making the process a complex one.

EDUCATING EDUCATORS

In common with other professions, the relationship between academic (propositional) knowledge about education and knowledge of professional educational practice (process knowledge) is far from straightforward (Eraut, 1985; Schon, 1987). Certainly the case for 'front loading' the education of educators with educational theory prior to its application is questionable but so too is an entirely practice-based training. The education of professionals has been discussed elsewhere in this book (see Chapter on 'Training and the process of professional development'). Applying these principles to the education of educators suggests:

1. It is essential to start the education of educators where people are, and for them to discover where they are regarding their current approaches to education, their knowledge and experience, and their assumptions and views. However, some who are starting to educate may not know where they are at the start, nor recognize that they have a particular approach to education that might be problematic. They will need help to do so.

2. The education of educators should begin in a concrete manner rather than with educational theory. First hand experience of relevant examples and illustrations is needed before considering conceptual information. People must reflect on their educational experiences, where possible directly observing themselves in action such as for example watching video recordings of themselves educating.

3. Educators also need to learn the theoretical principles underpinning good educational practice. These principles should be derived as much from their own analysis of practice as from received wisdom about education. This will mean educators in part deriving the criteria of education for themselves, directly from analysis of their own and others' educational practice, and a close interactive partnership between academics and educational practitioners.

4. People learning to educate should be closely involved in determining their own educational objectives. Having said this, what they perceive themselves as having to learn (their learning wants) may differ from what others consider they ought to learn (their learning needs). Any differences must be articulated and possibly negotiated.

5. People must be active participants in their own education as educators. As they learn to educate they will acquire knowledge and know-how, and so build up a more and more complex understanding concerning education. In other words, they will elaborate their knowledge. They must learn too that their personal knowledge about education will subtly differ from other educators. These differences should be acknowledged and discussed.

6. People who educate educators should be facilitating their learning rather than telling them about education. Educating educators should model good educational practice. There should be a supportive environment, thus

addressing people's social, emotional and physical needs as well as their intellectual ones.

7. Educators must learn to assess their own development. Knowing about one's progress is essential to effective learning. Identifying one's strengths clarifies the criteria of good practice. Identifying weaknesses indicates the problems to be addressed. Assessment should help rather than hinder the learning process. If examinations have to be summative (accredit someone's achievements) they should also contribute constructively to the learning process.

In summary, educators will learn to educate best when they are allowed to reflect on their practice, help to define their own problems, acknowledge and accept their strengths and weaknesses, decide on a course of action for themselves, and evaluate the consequences of their decisions. Those who educate them should adopt a facilitative role, that is to arrange appropriate experiences and to create a constructive environment, so that the educators can learn to educate for themselves. Educating educators should balance academic knowledge and practical know-how. It should be a partnership between academics and practitioners (Barnett, Becher & Cork, 1987).

SUPPORTING THE TRAINING OF EDUCATORS

The complex developmental process of learning to educate requires support. Sadly, many educators remain unsupported and their problems unrecognized. Frequently, the role of education has been thrust upon them, one can experience 'culture shock' when starting to educate others.

Mentors are a way of supporting educators (Calderhead, 1991; RCGP, 1983). This role is very varied (friend, guide, instructor, facilitator) and requires a number of skills. Mentors must communicate effectively. Most educator training has either been academic or trial-and-error without a language for talking about education that reflects the complexity of the tasks in hand or the skills to support and facilitate development. Mentors themselves need educating.

A second form of support is through the institution. Academics must teach in addition to carrying out research. Clinicians who teach also have busy clinical practices. The institution must value people's different contributions, and acknowledge the range of complex professional skills involved. This valuing should be both personal and practical. Personal support should recognize the stressful nature of educating and possible conflicts of interest, and make available time for learning to educate and provide peer support. Practical help from institutions should recognize people's educational contributions through the conferment of posts, promotions, and salary increments. Unless, and until, education is accorded the same status and rewarded in the same way as people's research effort or service contribution, it will never be taken seriously.

RESEARCHING EDUCATOR TRAINING

Educational research has been afforded a low priority in professional education. Surprisingly little research has been published concerning the education of educators (Coles & Tomlinson, 1994).

What characterizes this form of professional development? What interventions are most valuable? What constitutes appropriate mentoring? How should mentors be selected and trained? In what ways can and should institutions value the educational contributions of its members?

The role of educational theory in educational practice needs to be explored further. What is the relationship between good educational practice, and the practitioners' theoretical knowledge and understanding? How can educational theory help people practise effectively?

One of the challenges of this research agenda directly relates to the people carrying out this research and their research methods. What is their background? How can they best be recruited and trained? What constitutes effective research methodology?

Finally, there is a need to rationalize and coordinate the research being undertaken. Collaboration and co-operation between research groups is essential. People must publicize their findings so others with shared interests can comprehend, and so the practice of educator training can itself develop. Ultimately, the success of educational research will lie not in studies undertaken, data collected and academic journal articles published, but in the dissemination of findings, the discussing of results, and the implementation of conclusions.

REFERENCES

Barnett, R.A., Becher, R.A. and Cork, N.M. (1987). Models of professional preparation: pharmacy, nursing and teacher education, *Studies in Higher Education*, **12**, 51–63.

Berliner, D.C. (1987). Ways of thinking about students and classrooms by more and less experienced teachers, In J. Calderhead (Ed.). *Exploring teachers' thinking*, London: Cassell.

Calderhead, J. (1991). The nature and growth of knowledge in student teaching, *Teaching and Teacher Education*, **7**, 531–5.

Coles, C.R. & Tomlinson, J M (1994) Teaching student-centred educational approaches to general practice teachers, *Medical Education.*, **28**, 234–8.

Eraut, M. (1985). Knowledge creation and knowledge use in professional contexts. *Studies in Higher Education*, **10**, 117–33.

RCGP (1983). *Portfolio learning*, Occasional paper, London: Royal College of General Practitioners.

Ryle, G. (1949). *The concept of mind*, London: Hutchinson.

Schon, D.A. (1987). *Educating the reflective practitioner: towards a new design for teaching and learning in the professions*. San Francisco: Jossey Bass.

Written communication

PHILIP LEY

University of Sydney, Australia

TYPES OF WRITTEN INFORMATION AND THE REQUIREMENTS FOR ITS EFFECTIVENESS

Written information has several uses in clinical practice and in health care generally. It can provide (a) a reminder of what has been said in the consultation; (b) further and more detailed information about illness than that given in the consultation; (c) information about medication and other treatments, e.g. dietary advice; (d) warning about dangers in treatment use; (e) warning about potential dangers of everyday products, eg cigarettes; (f) information about forthcoming clinical investigations, surgical procedures, or hospitalization; (g) health educational and health promotional advice, e.g. urging regular pap smears, taking exercise; (h) information necessary for informed consent.

The minimum conditions required for written information to effectively fulfil these functions are that it has to be (a) noticed, (b) legible, (c) read, (d) understood, (e) believed, and (f) (sometimes) remembered.

HOW WELL DOES WRITTEN INFORMATION MEET THESE REQUIREMENTS

Is it always noticed?

Noticeability is mainly a problem with warnings and text printed on the outside of packages. For example, a median of 58% of users did not notice warnings and other health messages, in the ten studies reviewed by Ley (1995).

There seems to be little direct evidence about how often written materials about prescribed medication are noticed, probably because it is assumed that they always are. Moreover, the extent to which they are noticed can be inferred to some extent from the frequency with which patients claim to have read them (see below). By this criterion, it appears that such information is usually noticed.

Is it always legible?

The size of print is sometimes too small for patients to read. This is especially likely to be true of elderly patients (e.g. Zuccollo & Liddell, 1985). Other factors making text difficult to read include printing all of the text in capital letters or in italics; insufficient contrast between text and background; making lines of text too short or too long; and not allowing the right hand margin of the text to be ragged (unjustified).

Is it always read?

Research studies have reported that 49 to 97% of recipients claim to have read written information about their medication (Ley, 1988). A major US study by the RAND Corporation of leaflets concerning erythromycin, oestrogens, and nitrazepam, found that across vari-ous samples an average of 72% (s.d. 9%) claimed to have read the leaflets issued with their medication (Kanouse *et al.*, 1981). This investigation also provided data on the frequency with which patients kept and referred to their leaflets. Of those receiving the erythromycin, nitrazepam, and oestrogen leaflets, the percentages claiming to have kept them for future reference were 54, 57, and 45%; and claiming to have read them on more than one occasion were 32, 22, and 29%.

A series of British studies reported that 88% patients given a leaflet about penicillin or non-steroidal anti-inflammatory drugs (NSAIDs), claimed to have read their leaflet. It was further reported that, in other samples, 97% of patients receiving a leaflet about NSAIDs, β-adrenoceptor antagonists, or inhaled bronchodilators claimed to have read it (Gibbs, Waters & George 1987, 1989*a*, 1989*b*, 1990).

Is it always understood?

One approach to assessing whether a message is understandable is to see whether the words used in it are understood by the intended audience. When such investigations are undertaken it is often found that at least some of the words will not be understood by some of the intended readers. For example, warnings on tobacco products have as one of their main targets teenage presmokers. Centre for Behavioural Research in Cancer (1992) asked samples of young teenagers to define words used or intended for use in tobacco warning messages. Understanding was measured by both free response and multiple choice tests. Well over half of the words were understood by fewer than half of the teenagers. Included amongst these words were 'addictive', 'cavity', 'chronic', 'fatal', 'hazard', 'pollution', and 'premature'.

A second method used to assess the understandability of text is to ask people to answer questions about it. Jolly *et al.* (1993) asked patients questions about information contained in discharge forms commonly used in US hospital emergency departments. Patients had the forms to refer to, but were unable to answer many of the questions.

Another alternative is to use the Cloze procedure, which presents subjects with the passage to be assessed with every fifth word replaced by a blank. The score is the percentage of missing words that the subject can guess absolutely correctly. A Cloze score of 35% is approximately equal to getting 75% correct on a multiple choice comprehension test, a score of 55% is approximately equal to 90% correct.

A different approach to assessing the likely understandability of a piece of written information is to use a 'readability formula'. (For further discussion of readability formulae commonly used with health-related materials see Ley & Florio, 1996.) Many studies

Table 1. *The interpretation of Flesch Reading Ease Scores*

Reading ease score	Classification	Typical text	Grade level required to understand text	Percentage likely to understand text at this level or higher
90–100	Very easy	Comics	5	85%
80–90	Easy	Pulp fiction	6	
70–80	Fairly easy	Slick fiction	7	
60–70	Standard	Digests	8–9	60%
50–60	Fairly difficult	Quality	10–12	
30–50	Difficult	Academic	13–16	
0–30	Very difficult	Scientific	College graduate	

using readability formulas were reviewed by Ley (1988) who found that in general written materials were too difficult for their intended audience. For example, informed consent documents were frequently found to be written in very difficult language, and this continues to be true. Other investigations since Ley's review have found *inter alia* that leaflets about AIDS, arthritis, cancer, cholesterol management, condom use, and radiological investigation commonly require a level of reading ability well above that of the ordinary person (Ley & Florio, 1996).

The easiest way to compute a readability measure is to enter the text into one of the several computer word processing programs, containing the option of applying one or more readability formulae. If such an option is not available, two easily calculated formulas are the SMOG Index and the Flesch Reading Ease Formula.

The SMOG Index (McLaughlin, 1969) involves taking three groups of ten consecutive sentences, one group from the beginning, one from the middle, and one from the end. The estimated reading grade required for understanding is given by the formula:

SMOG Grading = 3 + the square root of the number of words of three or more syllables in the 30 sentences.

The Flesch Reading Ease Formula (Flesch, 1948) requires selection of a number of passages about 100 words in length. (With medication leaflets and other shorter pieces it is preferable to use the whole of the text). The formula is:

Reading ease = $206.835 - 0.846W - 1.015S$

where:

W = number of syllables per 100 words

S = average number of words per sentence.

Table 1 provides some guidance on the interpretation of Reading Ease Scores.

Current evidence suggests that (a) for many hospital and clinic samples text should be written at the 4th or 5th Grade level (if not lower), (b) there is a gap of 4 years or so between reading ability and years of school completed, (c) it is possible that nearly half of the adult population read at Grade 8 or lower (Ley & Florio, 1996). These factors should be borne in mind when deciding on an acceptable level of difficulty for text.

A readability formula should always be applied to written information intended for patients. If the result indicates that the material is too difficult, re-write it using shorter words, shorter sentences and more common words. Explain any technical terms used. Ideally, the final version should be field tested using either the Cloze procedure or a comprehension test.

Other factors which make text hard to understand include the use of (a) passive sentences, (b) negative sentences, and (c) abstract rather than concrete words. The passive voice should not be used in situations where it is not demonstrable that there is not a less undesirable alternative. So, don't use the passive voice unless you have to.

Is it always believed?

It seems to be assumed (probably quite correctly) that most health-related messages are believed. However, sometimes large proportions of key target groups do not find warning messages believable. For example, Centre for Behavioural Research in Cancer (1992) investigated the believability to teenagers of 36 tobacco health warnings. Fifteen of them were not believed by half or more of the sample, and only six were believed by more than 75%. Believability of written information for general use should obviously be assessed.

Is it always remembered?

Patients often forget written material (Ley & Morris, 1984). In the small number of investigations reviewed the mean percentage recalled ranged from 28 to 74%, with an overall mean of 60%. This is a similar rate of forgetting to that for orally presented information. However, as we have seen, such written information can be, and often is, kept and referred to more than once.

Techniques for increasing recall of written materials include increasing understandability, use of specific rather than general instructions, repetition, and explicit categorization (Ley, 1988). Further description of these methods is given in the chapter *Recall by patients*.

EFFECTIVENESS OF WRITTEN INFORMATION

From what has been said it will be apparent that much of the written material for patients is likely to be less effective than it could be. Despite this, the use of such material has frequently been shown to have beneficial effects on patients' knowledge; patients' compliance with treatment and health-related advice; levels of satisfaction with the care received; anxiety and distress caused by investigative and surgical procedures; and even on the outcome of treatment. Thus, Ley and Morris (1984) reported that the provision of written information about medication increased patients' knowledge in over 90% of investigations, increased compliance in about 60%, and improved outcome in four out of seven. Gibbs, Waters and George (1989a, 1989b, 1990) in three large-scale studies also found that medication leaflets increased both patients' knowledge and levels of satisfaction. The mean percentage completely satisfied with the

Table 2. *Content and format factors likely to increase the effectiveness of written information*

Desirable feature of message	Psychological packaging feature(s) likely to help	Physical packaging feature(s) likely to help

that it be noticed	Verbal symbol: e.g.
	  'Warning';
	  'Danger';
	  'Hazard'
	Graphic symbol
	Novelty
		Highlighting by use of:
		  colour
		  borders
		  space
		  different typeface
		  larger typeface
		  pointers
		Size
		  the larger the area the more likely it is that the text will be noticed
		Position
		  on front of package near top
		Interactive packaging

that it be legible		Contrast
		  Where possible use matt, non-glossy, non-reflective surfaces
		  Black letters on white backgrounds are easiest to read
		Size of type
		  Print should be at least 8 point, and preferably 10 point
		  Avoid text all in capitals
		Spacing
		  Leading of 1 or 2 points, depending on letter size and line length.
		Line length
		  Keep line length appropriate to print size.
		Italics
		  Italic text is harder to read.

that it be read	Ensure high 'readability'
	  use short words
	  use words familiar to the reader
	  use short sentences
	  avoid negatives
	Specify vulnerable groups
	Personalize message by use of 'you'
	Vary wording and content.
		High legibility

that it be understood	Ensure high 'readability' Explain technical terms Use active rather than passive sentences Be specific in any instructions Use headings where possible.	High legibility

that it be believed to be true	Cite sources for the message who are likely to be seen as high in:
	  credibility
	  expertness
	  attractiveness
	Use two-sided communications	

that it be believed by its target audience to be relevant to them	Explicitly mention target groups Deal with likely counter-propaganda	
that it be remembered if necessary	Ensure high 'Readability' Use repetition Use specific/concrete statements Use explicit categorization Use primary effect	Highlighting parts of message which need to be remembered

amount of information provided was 37% in the groups receiving leaflets, but only 30% in the control groups.

Examples of benefit in other areas of health care include reduced anxiety, distress, and length of stay in patients undergoing hysterectomy (Young & Humphrey, 1985); reduced distress in gynaecological outpatients (Wallace, 1986); and increased attendance for follow-up mammography in those with a prior abnormal result (Lerman *et al.*, 1992). For further examples see Ley (1988).

IMPROVING WRITTEN INFORMATION
It is possible to increase the effectiveness of written information by optimizing its psychological (mainly content) and physical presenta-

tion. A listing of possible improvers is given in Table 2. As the following examples will show the expected improvement from use of the suggested methods does not always occur, but harmful effects are virtually non-existent.

One example of a usually effective psychological method of improvement is simplification, i.e. rewriting the material in shorter words and shorter sentences. Ley (1988) reviewed 13 comparisons of the effects of simplification on recall of written information. In ten of these recall increased significantly. Mean increase in recall was approximately 55%. In addition simplification was found to increase reading speed in an elderly sample, and to increase accuracy of medicine taking in psychiatric patients.

More complicated attempts at improvement have not proved so successful. Ley (1978) found that a package consisting of simplification, explicit categorization and repetition led to increased weight loss in only one of three experiments. Kanouse *et al.* (1981), used a set of rules for improving written communications based on findings of laboratory studies of comprehension and memory. These included: avoiding the use of negatives, using the active rather than the passive voice, and using concrete nouns and sentences, simplification, and filling subject verb and object positions with important words rather than fillers. The ensuing package had no greater effect on knowledge nor on compliance than the usual procedure.

Other attempts to improve written information have involved the use of illustrations, cartoons, colour, and highlighting of certain sorts of content, which it is desired to emphasize. No consistent findings seem to have emerged from this array of investigations. (Ley & Morris 1984; Ley, 1988).

It is worth repeating that the factors listed in Table 2 should be regarded as potential improvers. Whether they actually work in a given situation can only be found out by trying them. More detailed reviews of many of them can be found in Ley and Morris (1985), Ley (1988), and Ley (1995). These sources also contain more detailed bibliographies.

Finally, the probability that written information will be noticed or read can be adversely affected by both previous exposure to the message, and previous experience of the activity or product referred to (Wright, Creighton & Threlfall, 1982; Ley, 1995). It is even possible that frequent exposure to warning messages might have counter-productive effects. For example, Skilbeck, Tulips and Ley (1977) reported that obese women who were exposed daily over a

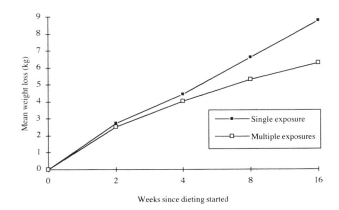

Fig 1. The effects on weight loss of a single exposure versus multiple exposures to fear arousing messages about the dangers of obesity.

several week period to messages about the dangers of obesity lost less weight than women who were only exposed once to such warnings. This effect is shown in Fig. 1.

The negative effects of exposure on noticing and reading written information and warnings are often of little importance provided that the information has been absorbed on previous occasions. However, if new information, instructions or warnings are incorporated into the message, then steps should be taken to emphasize that the message differs from previous ones. The use of the techniques suggested for increasing noticeability and likelihood of reading becomes essential. (See also 'Stress management', 'Medical decision-making'.)

REFERENCES

Centre for Behavioural Research in Cancer (1992). *Health warnings and contents labelling on tobacco products.* Melbourne: Centre for Behavioural Research in Cancer.

Flesch, R. (1948). A new readability yardstick. *Journal of Applied Psychology,* **33,** 221–33.

Gibbs, S., Waters, W.E. & George, C.F. (1987). The design of prescription information leaflets and the feasibility of their use in general practice. *Pharmaceutical Medicine,* **2,** 23–33.

Gibbs, S., Waters, W.E. & George, C.F. (1989*a*). The benefits of prescription information leaflets (1). *British Journal of Clinical Pharmacology,* **27,** 723–39.

Gibbs, S., Waters, W.E. & George, C.F. (1989*b*). The benefits of prescription information leaflets (2). *British Journal of Clinical Pharmacology,* **28,** 345–51.

Gibbs, S., Waters, W.E & George, C.F. (1990). Communicating information to patients about medicine. Prescription information leaflets: a national survey. *Journal of the Royal Society of Medicine,* **83,** 292–7.

Jolly, B.T., Scott, J.L., Feied, C.F. & Sanford, S.M. (1993). Functional illiteracy among emergency department patients: a preliminary study. *Annals of Emergency Medicine,* **22,** 573–8.

Kanouse, D.E., Berry, S.H., Hayes-Roth, B., Rogers, W.H. & Winkler, J.D. (1981). *Informing patients about drugs: summary report.* Santa Monica, Ca: RAND Corporation.

Lerman, C., Ross, E., Boyce, A., Gorchov, P.M., McLaughlin, R., Rimer, B. & Engstrom, P. (1992). The impact of mailing psychoeducational materials to women with abnormal mammograms. *American Journal of Public Health,* **82,** 729–30.

Ley, P. (1978). Psychological and behavioural factors in weight loss. In G. Bray (Ed.). *Recent advances in obesity research: II,* pp. 86–100, London: Newman Publishing.

Ley, P. (1988). *Communicating with patients.* London: Chapman and Hall.

Ley, P. (1995). *Effectiveness of label statements for drugs and poisons.* Canberra: Australian Government Publishing Service.

Ley, P. & Florio, T. (1996). The use of readability formulas in health care. *Psychology, Health and Medicine,* **1,** 7–28.

Ley, P. & Morris, L.A. (1985). Psychological aspects of written information for patients. In S. Rachman (Ed.). *Contributions to medical psychology.* vol. 3. Oxford: Pergamon Press.

McLaughlin, H. (1969). Smog grading: a new readability formula. *Journal of Reading,* **22,** 639–46.

Ridout, S., Waters, W.E. & George, C.F. (1986). Knowledge of and attitudes to medicines in the Southampton community. *British Journal of Clinical Pharmacology,* **21,** 701–11.

Skilbeck, C.E., Tulips, J.G. & Ley, P. (1977). Effects of fear arousal, fear position, fear exposure, and sidedness on compliance with dietary instructions. *European Journal of Social Psychology,* **7,** 221–39.

Wallace, L.M. (1986). Communication variables in the design of pre-surgical preparatory information. *British Journal of Clinical Psychology,* **25,** 111–18.

Wright, P. Creighton, P. & Threlfall, S.M. (1982). Some factors determining what instructions will be read. *Ergonomics,* **25,** 225–37.

Young, L. & Humphrey, M. (1985). Cognitive methods of preparing women for hysterectomy: does a booklet help? *British Journal of Clinical Psychology,* **24,** 303–4.

Zuccollo, G. & Liddell, H. (1985). The elderly and the medication label: doing it better. *Age and Aging,* **14,** 371–6.

PART III **Medical topics**

This part contains a series of brief chapters on specific illnesses, treatments and prophylaxes. In some cases the boundaries between health psychology and clinical psychology or psychiatry can become blurred. However, this simply reflects the fact that, although the primary domains of these disciplines are distinguishable, there is overlap between them. In some cases decisions had to be made about the level of generality to treat important topics (e.g. cancer). We have tried in these cases to cover general issues in one chapter and deal with specific aspects of sub-topics in separate chapters.

Decisions about which topics to include or exclude were made partly on the basis of whether there appeared to be interesting and non-obvious psychological findings relevant to these topics. Thus some important illnesses may be omitted if we could find little that was novel to report. We may also have omitted illnesses if the issues concerning these appeared to be very close to those arising from related conditions that have been covered. Although we canvassed widely to try to make the selection as informed as possible, it is likely that at least some areas have been incorrectly omitted. In some cases, general principles concerning psychological factors related to such conditions may be found in Part II. However, the reader would be advised also to conduct an on-line search if possible to check on current research in that area.

Abortion

Accidents: psychological influences

AIDS

Alcohol abuse/alcoholism

Allergies to drugs

Allergies to food

Allergies: general

Amnesia

Amputation and phantom limb pain

Anaesthesia

Androgens

Anorexia nervosa and bulimia

Antenatal care

Aphasia

Asthma

Atopic dermatitis

Battering and other violence against women

Benzodiazepine dependency

Beta-blockers: psychological effects

Blindness and visual disability

Blood transfusion and donation

Breast cancer

Breastfeeding

Bronchitis (chronic) and emphysema

Burns

Cardiac surgery

Carotid artery stenosis and endarterectomy

Child abuse and neglect: prevention of

Chromosomal abnormalities

Chronic fatigue syndrome

Cleft lip and palate

Cold, common

Colour blindness

Complementary medicine

Contraception

Coronary heart disease: impact

Coronary heart disease: treatment

Cystic fibrosis

Deafness and hearing loss

Dementias

Dental care and hygiene

Diabetes mellitus

Dieting

Digestive tract cancer

Drug dependence: opiates and stimulants

Dyslexia

Dyslexia and dysgraphia: acquired

Dysmorphology and facial disfigurement

Encopresis

Endoscopy and bronchoscopy

Enuresis

Epidemics

Epilepsy

Epstein-Barr virus infection

Fetal alcohol syndrome

Foetal well-being: monitoring and assessment

Gastric and duodenal ulcers

General cancers

Genetic counselling

Glaucoma

Growth retardation

Gynaecological cancers

Haemophilia

Head and neck cancers

Head injury

Headache and migraine

Hodgkin's disease and Non-Hodgkin's
lymphoma

Huntington's disease

Hyperactivity

Hyperhidrosis

Hypertension

Hyperthyroidism

Hyperventilation

Hypochondriasis

Hysterectomy

Iatrogenesis

Immunization

Incontinence

Infertility

Inflammatory bowel disease

Irritable bowel syndrome

Lactose and food intolerance

Lead: health effects

Leprosy

Leukaemia

Low back pain

Lung cancer

Malaria

Mastalgia

Meningitis

Menopause and postmenopause

Menstrual abnormalities

Motor neurone disease

Multiple sclerosis

Munchausen's syndrome

Myasthenia gravis

Neurofibromatosis

Osteoarthritis

Osteoporosis

Parkinson's disease

Pelvic pain

Plastic and cosmetic surgery

Post-traumatic stress disorder

Postpartum depression

Pre-menstrual syndrome/Late luteal phase
disorder

Pregnancy and childbirth

Premature babies

Radiation

Radiotherapy

Rape and sexual assault

Renal failure, dialysis and transplantation

Repetitive strain injury

Rheumatoid arthritis

Road traffic accidents

Rubella

Self-examination: breast, testicles

Sexually transmitted diseases

Sickle cell disease

Skin cancer

Spina bifida

The spinal cord injury

Sterilization and vasectomy

Steroids

Stigma

Stroke

Stuttering

Suicide

Tetanus

Tinnitus

Tobacco smoking

Torticollis

Transplantation

Transsexual surgery

Vertigo and dizziness

Voice disorders

Volatile substance abuse

Vomiting and nausea as side-effects of drugs

Well woman/well man clinics: the Australian
context

Abortion

PAULINE SLADE

Department of Psychology, University of Sheffield,
UK

Although induced and spontaneous abortion both involve the death of a foetus, there are important differences in these experiences. In the former, pregnancy ends through an individual's choice while in the latter, it occurs not because of, but often in spite of, the woman's and professionals' best efforts to save the baby. Women who have miscarried are often distressed by staff usage of the term spontaneous abortion as this carries an unpleasant connotation, and this will not be used further.

MISCARRIAGE

Up to 20% of recognized pregnancies end in miscarriage, defined as a pregnancy loss up to 24 weeks of gestation. Studies suggest that anxiety symptoms may be elevated for many months afterwards and a proportion of women may show depressive symptoms (Slade, 1994). Miscarriage has been compared to bereavement but the process of coping may be complicated by the abstract nature of the loss and the absence of memories of an individual. The loss is often hidden as many women will not have shared news of their pregnancy at such an early stage, and support that unpleasant events often generate may be absent. Our society lacks ritual acknowledgement of miscarriage and the prevailing view is often as exemplified by the phrase 'it was for the best'.

In addition to the aspect of loss, the process of the event may be traumatic, involving pain, blood loss, rapid hospitalization and operation. These are the features of fear inducing situations that may lead to subsequent anxiety symptoms. The woman may also have fears about her future fertility, and there is evidence that anxiety symptoms are elevated in subsequent pregnancies, even though the risk of a further miscarriage is not itself increased (Statham & Green, 1994).

Many of the assumptions that staff and lay persons make about who will be most distressed as a result of miscarriage are unsubstantiated by the literature. There is little evidence that demographic factors such as age or parity exert any impact. Findings concerning the effects of gestational age, previous miscarriage or infertility are equivocal. The personal meaning of the event appears to be important, and there are also suggestions that the quality of care received may exert some impact although further investigation of this issue is still required (Slade, 1994).

A major issue of concern is the quality of psychological care for women experiencing a miscarriage. One difficulty concerns the gross mismatch of perceptions of the significance of the event between the staff and patients. For many women this is undeniably an important distressing life experience. For medical staff it is often viewed as a frequent, routine, trivial and medically insignificant event allowing little potential for useful intervention and which is generally dealt with by the most junior staff (Moohan, Ashe & Cecil, 1994; Friedman, 1989). Where such disparate perceptions of the same event occur, it is unsurprising that many women complain of insensitive care.

One aspect of care that seems to be particularly important is that women should be given the news about the viability or non-viability of their pregnancy as soon as this is available, that is at the scan, rather than after a protracted wait. (See 'Breast cancer', for more on this issue.) They should be given the news in circumstances of privacy, in a sensitive manner, and also be provided with an opportunity to talk with appropriately trained staff about their feelings and concerns. In addition, women express a need for information about potential physical and emotional consequences together with an opportunity to discuss these issues at a follow-up appointment two to three weeks after the event. A referral service to clinical psychology should be available for the very small percentage showing extreme psychological distress (Slade & Wills, 1993). Unfortunately, few of the current services offer this quality of care.

INDUCED ABORTIONS

In the USA the legal situation is extremely complex. The fundamental right to terminate a pregnancy was established in 1973 by the US Supreme Court. However, since they there have been numerous attempts to limit access to abortion services which have differed on a statewise basis. These have involved incorporating mandatory delays, requirements to consult parents, limits on the use of public funding and even prohibition of the performance of abortion in public hospitals. However, any state law affecting previability abortions (as defined by viability tests) must be 'necessary in order to protect a woman's health'. After viability the law must be shown 'to further the state's interests in protecting maternal health or promoting potential life'.[1]

The legal situation in Britain is now governed by the 1990 amendment of the 1967 Abortion Act. This provides an upper time limit of 24 weeks' gestation for most abortions, but there is no time limit if there is a risk to life of the mother, risk of grave permanent injury or serious fetal handicap. The process of care varies with stage of gestation and, with pregnancies less than 13 weeks, typically involves a general anaesthetic and evacuation of the contents of the womb by suction. At later stages this may involve a hormonally induced labour throughout which the woman is conscious. Many of the later induced abortions occur because of detection of

---

[1] The status of a Woman's Right to choose Abortion in Reproductive Freedom in the States from the Centre for Reproduction Law and Policy, 120 Wall Street, New York.

abnormality in the foetus through the use of blood tests and amniocentesis. As the motivation is different, this may be an important subgroup in terms of psychological issues raised. Recently, medical methods for early terminations have been introduced. These involve the administration of prostaglandins to trigger contractions of the uterus. The woman is conscious throughout the process and may see the foetus. The nature of this experience and its consequences may differ significantly from the surgical method, and these issues are currently under exploration.

The literature suggests that the emotional consequences of induced abortion, in general, are unremarkable with many women at least initially showing a sense of relief. There is little evidence of significant negative emotional responses although so-called long-term follow-ups rarely extend beyond two years and in reality are short term (Adler *et al.*, 1990). It appears to be important that the woman should feel that she has made the decision herself and that she has not been coerced by partner or parent. Whilst follow-ups of cohorts have not indicated evidence of emotional distress, there have been criticisms that the more distressed may absent themselves from studies thereby biasing findings. Certainly some individuals do report unpleasant psychological repercussions and the term 'post-abortion syndrome' has been coined (Speckhard & Rue, 1992).

Again, there are issues about the quality of care for women undergoing induced abortions in that censorious attitudes or insensitive care from staff may enhance guilt and may negatively affect emotional outcome. It is important that staff involved in such care provision examine their own attitudes and values, and are aware of their own potential for influencing adjustment in a positive or negative way.

REFERENCES

Adler, N.E., Henry, P., Major, B.N., Roth, S.H., Russo, N.G. & Wyatt, G.F. (1990). Psychological responses after abortion. *Science*, 24, 41–4.

Friedman, T. (1989). Women's experiences of General Practitioner management of miscarriage. *Journal of the Royal College of General Practitioners*, 39, 456–8.

Moohan, J., Ashe, R.G. & Cecil, R. (1994). The management of miscarriage: results from a survey at one hospital. *Journal of Reproductive and Infant Psychology*, 12, 17–19.

Nichols, K.A. (1993). *Psychological care in physical illness.* 2nd edn, London: Chapman & Hall.

Slade, P. (1994). Predicting the psychological impact of miscarriage. *Journal of Reproductive and Infant Psychology*, 12, 5–16.

Slade, P. & Wills, G. (1993). Improving the quality of psychological care for women experiencing early miscarriage. Report to the Northern General Hospital Trust.

Speckhard, A.C. & Rue, V.M. (1992). Postabortion syndrome: an emerging public health concern. *Journal of Social Issues*, 48, 95–119.

Statham, H. & Green, J.M. (1994). The effects of miscarriage and other 'unsuccessful' pregnancies on feeling early in a subsequent pregnancy. *Journal of Reproductive and Infant Psychology*, 12, 45–54.

Accidents: psychological influences

ROBERT G. FRANK

College of Health Professions, University of Florida, Health Sciences Center, Gainesville, Florida, USA

Injury is a leading cause of death and disability for America's young adults and children. It is the fourth leading cause of death for all Americans and the second leading cause of death for those from age 1 to 45 (Spielberger & Frank, 1992). Injuries are associated with higher treatment cost than the other three leading causes of death. Traffic accidents are the leading cause of severe brain injury including most paraplegic and quadraplegic cases (Spielberger & Frank, 1992).

For many years, injuries were viewed as 'accidents' that were inevitable and not responsive to prevention efforts. Injury events tended to be attributed to human error or misaction; individuals died or were injured due to driving while intoxicated or a leg was broken when someone failed to watch their step. This psychological model of injury was related to the emergence of the concept of 'accident-proneness' during the 1930s and 1940s. In this approach, accidents occurred to individuals as a function of unconscious wishes or desires (Waller, 1994).

Injury events were also attributed to human error or misaction because they often involved relatively rare events that were perceived as unpredictable. Even now, many data systems tend to record only 'single' causes of injury, negating the idea that a crash may occur both because the driver is impaired by alcohol and because the roadway geometry at the crash location is inadequate (Waller, 1994). Rarely did anyone examine the overall frequency of injuries to determine if higher risk existed under certain circumstances. For example, lacking statistics, the crash risk at a particular bend in a roadway may go unrecognized. Only when examined, will the 1 per 250 000 vehicle risk achievable with improved roadway design, compared to the existing crash risk of 1 per 50 000, be recognized (Waller, 1994).

CURRENT MODELS OF INJURY CONTROL
In 1959 James J. Gibson, an experimental psychologist, recognized that injury was caused by energy interchange which occurred at the

moment and subsequent to the incident. Gibson suggested the most effective method of classifying sources of energy is the form of the physical energy involved (Rosenberg & Fenley, 1992). Gibson's observation became the lifework of Dr William Haddon, Jr, an engineer and public health physician. Haddon narrowed the potential agents to five forms of physical energy: kinetic, chemical, thermo, electrical and radiation. Haddon also recognized 'negative agents' for injuries produced by the absence of critical elements such as oxygen or heat. Haddon labelled these agents as vectors and the vehicles as energy forms. He divided injuries into three phases: (i) a preinjury; (ii) a very brief injury phase; and (iii) a postinjury phase.

During the preinjury phase, the control of the energy source is lost. The preinjury phase includes everything that determines whether a crash will occur (e.g. driver ability, vehicle functioning, seat-belt usage). The injury phase typically lasts less than a second and transfers energy to the individual causing damage. The postinjury phase determines whether the injuries and consequences could be reduced with subsequent prevention of further disability (e.g. speed, inefficiency of first responders). During the postinjury phase, attempts are made to retain physiological homeostasis and repair damage. Haddon also observed that injuries can often be prevented by attending to the vector (Rosenberg & Fenley, 1992; Waller, 1994).

Using this model, Haddon developed an innovative plan to intervene upon injury events by: (i) preventing or limiting energy build-up; (ii) controlling the circumstances of energy to prevent unlimited release; (iii) modifying the energy in transfer phase to limit damage; and (iv) improving emergency, acute, and rehabilitative care to affect recovery (Waller, 1994).

Haddon's model led to the development of the Haddon Matrix. Haddon's 'phase-factor matrix' is actually a series of matrices developed for different purposes. The Haddon matrix emphasizes the preventive value of the epidemiological approach to injury control. In the matrix, the host, agent (vector), and environment are seen as factors that interact over time to cause injury.

Haddon's work led to the recognition that, during each of the three phases, preinjury, injury and postinjury, injury likelihood can be reduced by changes in the driver (in the case of vehicular injury), the agent (or vehicle), or the environment. Previous models of injury prevention have emphasized psychological factors, thereby allowing only one intervention point. In contrast, the Haddon matrix creates nine cells, each of which offers an opportunity for intervention. While behaviour is undeniably an important factor in injury causation, the Haddon matrix demonstrates it is only one of several areas where intervention may be effective. In determining the appropriate intervention, it is important to recognize that injury prevention is not necessarily based upon the most obvious cause of contributing factors. Interventions may occur at a number of points in the chain of events that can lead to injury (Williams & Lund, 1992). Adoption of an energy control strategy to injury prevention led to discarding the term 'accident'. The connotation of chance, fate, and unexpectedness has been replaced by descriptions of injuries and physical and chemical injuries involved (Williams & Lund, 1992).

PSYCHOLOGICAL FACTORS AND INJURY CONTROL

Human behaviour remains an important factor in injury control. This view has been reinforced in recent years as psychologists and others have begun to contribute to our understanding of the behavioural and social causes. Within the field of injury prevention, a dialectic has developed between proponents of individually directed interventions and those who support public health models (Frank *et al.*, 1992). These approaches to prevention have been characterized as active versus passive or individual versus population. Active individual injury prevention requires action by the individual to reduce risk (e.g. wearing a seat belt, using a motorcycle helmet, exercising or maintaining proper diet). Active or individual approaches reflect the legacy of health psychology, with its emphasis upon individuals assuming responsibility for their own behaviour (Frank *et al.*, 1992).

The passive intervention model, derived from public health approaches, emphasizes altering health behaviours at the population level (Frank *et al.*, 1992). In this approach, intervention is designed to automatically affect all individuals. Passive intervention models are viewed as most effective because they avoid difficulties associated with individuals making consecutive decisions regarding health and safety behaviours. Examples of the passive or population approach include automatic seat belts, mandatory air bags, locking systems to prevent drunken driving, and air safety restraints.

Most often, active and passive approaches have been viewed as mutually exclusive. Others have suggested that active and passive approaches to injury reflect a continuum (Frank *et al.*, 1992). Recent models of health psychology have included a broader emphasis upon the health of communities (Winett, King & Altman, 1989). Roberts (1987) has suggested that a multilevel approach is the most effective approach to injury control. In this approach, the active individual model congruent with health psychology is viewed as one end of a continuum, while the passive approach that matches public health models anchors the other end of the continuum.

Although many opportunities exist for psychologists in the community approach to prevention of injury, the traditional niche occupied by health psychologists with its emphasis upon the individual has most often been the focus of the profession. Because injury most often affects individuals under age 24, a disproportionate emphasis has been placed upon injury prevention among children and adolescents.

Recently, the prevention of childhood injuries has become a major research area (Peterson & Roberts, 1992). It is now clear that the parents whose children are most at risk (poor, undereducated, disturbed, or from single parent families), are least likely to utilize safety precautions. Often, even middle-class parents lack a strong sense of risk factors for their children. Many parents do not appreciate, or are indifferent to, factors that may contribute to injury. Children are rarely taught safety behaviours (Peterson & Roberts, 1992). Too often, injury prevention is based upon single presentations of safety material in classrooms. Peterson and Roberts (1992) observed that educators would never consider teaching maths by working arithmetic problems before children for one hour, or teaching spelling by having the teacher discuss spelling. These methods often serve as a safety curriculum in schools. Parents greatly overestimate their children's safety knowledge, and when asked where the child acquired these presumed skills, parents most frequently cite visits of police or fire officials to the class (Peterson & Roberts, 1992).

Injury prevention in children includes a wide variety of interventions. As has been the case with adult and adolescent populations, the two predominant methods have been legislation and education. Legislative changes have often been directed at product manufacturers. In contrast, educational efforts are most often directed at children's caregivers and may be direct, utilize weak contingencies (such as suggestion that a low probability negative event may be prevented) or immediate rewards (such as a lottery ticket or prize to a child). In general, the stronger the contingency, the more effective the intervention (Peterson & Roberts, 1992).

The most frequently cited legislative success, aimed directly at the injury vector, was a 1973 mandate requiring child-resistant packaging and limiting the amount of a drug contained in any one package (Peterson & Roberts, 1992). Although legislation can be very successful, the large number of products known to cause injury to children are inadequately controlled for a variety of reasons. Many known hazards to children, such as guns, have political connotations making legislation problematic. In other cases, items directly marketed to children are hazardous, but have not been prohibited. For example, as many as 42% of accidental injuries to children under one year of age may be due to 'baby walkers' (Peterson & Roberts, 1992) which offer no developmental advantage to children. Underinflated or uninflated balloons also pose a high risk to small children. Failure to regulate these items may stem from the perception that injury is as much a function of poor parental supervision as it is of the product alone. Thus, regulation may not be sufficient.

Persuasion to behave differently through mass media campaigns, enhanced product availability, and social sanctions may rival legislative change. For example, the first child restraint law in Tennessee was accompanied by extensive publicity and media coverage. The eventual success of this legislation may reflect the publicity as much as the legislation (Peterson & Roberts, 1992).

Efforts to use education to prevent injury have yielded an uneven history. Most successful have been recent programmes that target caregivers with simple interventions requiring minimal consumer effort. When safety products are freely available, or available at a reduced cost in exchange for safety behaviour, education is effective. For example, smoke detectors, lightweight rails to guard windows, or programmes providing individualized attention rewards for decreasing hazards have all shown to be highly effective (Peterson & Roberts, 1992). How mass media tends to influence children's safety has rarely been evaluated. Programmes aimed directly at children have had some success (Peterson, 1989). Young children can successfully learn a variety of skills ranging from bicycle safety, management of small emergencies like house fires and serious cuts, to the preparation of safe snacks if provided intensive modelling, rehearsal, and use of clear, positive consequences (Peterson, 1989).

Because adolescence is a time of particular risk for injury, as well as the period when many patterns of behaviour are established, it has been a developmental epoch that has been the target of many intervention efforts. Although it is a critical developmental period for the consolidation of cognitions, behaviour, and learning, many common adolescent beliefs make intervention particularly problematic. Teens have strong beliefs of personal immortality and invulnerability. Adolescence is a period of increased testing of autonomy and growing identification with peers. Risky behaviours are common, and peer pressure may increase risk-taking activities. Even when the risk of injury is understood, avoiding danger may be less important

than obtaining peer approval. Attempts by adults to minimize this behaviour may simply increase peer pressure to engage in such activities.

The highest rate of fatalities and injuries in traffic crashes is among young men from ages 15 to 24 years. Because young drivers are involved in the disproportionate number of traffic injuries and fatalities, many prevention programmes have focused on altering the behaviour of the driver. The most common example of these are driver education programmes which have been implemented throughout high schools in the United States. Unfortunately, these educational programmes, at best, have had limited success. There is no evidence that driver education programmes result in a reduction of the number of crashes (Robertson, 1986).

An alternative approach designed to increase safe behaviours among adolescents utilizes behavioural and/or mass media approaches to increase use of seat belts. Behaviour approaches have been criticized by authors such as Robertson (1986), who note that while contingencies are in effect, there is an increase in seat belt behaviour use. However, when rewards are withdrawn, seatbelt use declines. What has often been ignored is that decline typically does not return to baseline, but nets a gain in overall belt usage. Similar improvements have been reported in other behavioural interventions to reduce injury risk, such as high noise environments and child restraint programmes (Frank et al., 1992).

The high personal and emotional cost of catastrophic injuries, such as head and spinal cord injuries, have resulted in the proliferation of programmes designed to change behaviours associated with injury risk. Many hospitals have viewed these prevention programmes as an attractive way to provide a public service while marketing their name. Schools are particularly eager to endorse such programmes (Frank et al., 1992). These programmes have often utilized a 'shotgun' approach which includes education, modelling, and persuasion. Evaluation of the efficacy of these programmes has been problematic for a number of reasons. First, the injuries their programmes are designed to prevent are low frequency events. The number of injuries occurring in any area covered by a prevention programme is likely to be small, thus complicating statistical inferences. Secondly, the proliferation of prevention programmes combined with public media efforts has resulted in a barrage of prevention type interventions. Adolescents are often exposed to a variety of such messages, making it virtually impossible to find an unexposed sample of teenagers.

As was discussed with regard to child injury prevention efforts, adolescent injury prevention programmes are often provided in a single presentation. There is little reason to believe that, regardless of the emotional or educational content of the programme, a single presentation will be sufficient enough to alter the complex and diverse behavioural factors involved in injury in adolescents. In general, evaluation of injury prevention programmes is demonstrated by increased knowledge and improved attitudes regarding safe behaviours in students who are exposed to the programme. Students exposed to prevention programmes show long-term maintenance of improved knowledge, better attitudes and more safe behaviours than children not exposed to programmes. However, specific analysis after exposure to a prevention programme does not demonstrate improved driving habits or increased perceived vulnerability to injury either immediately after exposure to the prevention programme or at a one month follow-up (Bouman, 1992). Taken together, it appears that prevention programmes influence attitudes and knowledge, but may have little effect upon behavioural change. Again, expectations of behavioural changes after exposure to a single programme are naive.

In general, altering of adolescent injury risk is more complex than most studies to date have recognized. Evaluation of the multiple determents, the gradual nature of behavioural change, assessment of the individual's current behaviour, beliefs, social support, and alternative responses, as well as the maintenance of behaviour, are all essential steps (Frank *et al.*, 1992). Most injury prevention programmes have addressed only one or two of these issues. Successful implementation of safe behaviours will require cognizance of the individual, the community, and national health priorities. Interventions must recognize an altered perceived vulnerability to injury, as well as social support factors.

CONCLUSIONS

Injury is the leading cause of death in Americans under age 44. Narrow prevention interventions designed to assess or alter injury, based on unidimensional concepts, whether psychological, behavioural, or environmental have been shown to rarely succeed. Successful prevention of injury is more likely to occur when injury is viewed from an epidemiological perspective with multiple causations. Recognition of the interaction between these causal factors and development of multiple interventions is critical to successful prevention of injury. Psychological factors comprise one element of the matrix leading to injury. Psychologists and other researchers interested in preventing injury have been most successful when they designed interventions targeting the individual, the community, and state and national policy.

REFERENCES

Bouman, D.E. (1992). Examination of a traumatic injury prevention program: Adolescent's reactions and program efficiency. Unpublished doctoral dissertation. University of Missouri-Columbia.

Frank, R.G., Bouman, D.E., Cain, K. & Watts, C. (1992). Primary prevention of injury. *American Psychologist*, **47**, 1045–9.

Peterson, L. (1989). Latchkey children's preparation for self-care; overestimated, underdeveloped and unsafe. *Journal of Clinical Child Psychology*, **18**, 36–43.

Peterson, L. & Roberts, M.C. (1992).

Complacency, misdirection and effective prevention of children's injuries. *American Psychologist*, **47**, 1040–4.

Roberts, M.C. (1987). Public health and health psychology: two cats of Kilkenny? *Professional Psychology Research and Practice*, **18**, 145–9.

Robertson, L.S. (1986). Injury. In B.A. Edelstein & L. Michelson (Eds.). *Handbook on Prevention* pp. 343–360, New York: Plenum Press.

Rosenberg, M.L. & Fenley, M.A. (1992). The federal role in injury control. *American Psychologist*, **47**, 1031–5.

Spielberger, C.D. & Frank, R.G. (1992). Injury control: a promising field for psychologists. *American Psychologist*, **47**, 1029–30.

Waller, J.A. (1994). Reflections on a half century of injury control. *American Journal of Public Health*, **84**, 664–70.

Williams, A.F. & Lund, A.K. (1992). Injury control: what psychologists can contribute. *American Psychologist*, **47**, 1036–9.

Winett, R.A., King. A.C. & Altman, D.G. (1989). *Health psychology and public health: an integrative approach.* New York: Pergamon Press.

AIDS

ROBERT BOR

Medical Counselling Unit, Psychology Department, City University, London, UK

Fifteen years have elapsed since AIDS was first reported in 1981. On 5 June 1981 the US Centers for Disease Control (CDC) reported five cases of a rare pneumonia among young homosexual men living in Los Angeles (CDC, 1981). A month later, CDC reported a further ten cases of Pneumocystis carinii pneumonia and 26 cases of Kaposi's sarcoma in New York, San Francisco and Los Angeles. By the end of 1981, the number had reached 257. Fourteen years on, that figure has increased more than 1000-fold, and cases of AIDS have been reported in almost every country. There are over a million cases of AIDS worldwide, and by the middle of the next century, this number will have risen to 18.3 million (Chin, Sato & Mann, 1990) affecting both men and women as well as heterosexual and homosexuals. Human immunodeficiency virus (HIV) infection is a slow, progressive, immunological disorder, and psychological research has contributed an understanding of a number of relevant issues. These include the primary prevention of transmission (including and understanding of lifestyle and risk behaviour), coping and adjustment, assessment and treatment of AIDS-associated psychological and neurological disorders, and the effects on social and professional caregivers. Alongside the rapid advances over the decade in the fields of epidemiology, virology, immunology, clinical management, nursing care, clinical therapy and prophylaxis, there has been a concerted effort to translate this knowledge into preventive counselling and psychological support for those affected.

Primary prevention of AIDS

In the absence of a vaccine, the prevention of the spread of HIV will, for many people, require changes in risk-taking behaviour. This entails the use of condoms during penetrative sexual intercourse (see also 'Contraception') or clean equipment when injecting drugs. Health promotion efforts in many countries have been modeled on a belief that behaviour can be changed by providing those at risk of HIV with information and by challenging prevailing beliefs or attitudes about risky sexual activities. This gave rise to a spate of 'Knowledge–attitude–behaviour' (KAB) studies of AIDS in the 1980s. While KAB studies continue to be reported in the literature, there is increasing recognition that behaviour modification strategies depend on an appreciation of the complexities of social context, risk and relationships, as well as some impediments to discussing sex and negotiating safer sex practices. This includes an understanding of self-efficacy and social support as sexual behaviour is not necessarily the outcome of a consensual and rational decision (Wight, 1992). There are four factors that should to be considered:

1. What is a sexual encounter? People may have different views as to a definition of what counts as sex.

2. Do health–care workers feel comfortable talking to their patients about sex? Research confirms that many health care workers feel embarrassed about talking to their patients about sex, and lack the necessary training to do so (Merrill, Laux & Thornby, 1990).

3. Do people always adhere to safer sex guidelines when they have access to condoms? Availability and use of condoms before and during a sexual encounter may reduce the risk of transmission, but it is no guarantee that they will be used. People sometimes make judgements about risk based on false assumptions, such as a sexual partner's physical appearance.

4. Is there consistency in relationships in adhering to safer sex practices over time? Trust between partners may build up in a long-term relationship, leading to a change from the use of barrier forms of contraception to the use of the contraceptive pill. The continued use of condoms in long-term relationships during intercourse may undermine the assumption of trust in monogamous relationships. By way of contrast, there may not be open discussion between the couple about current or past sexual relationships outside of the dyadic relationship. In some cases, this may place the index case and his or her partner at risk of acquiring HIV or other sexually transmitted diseases (Holland *et al.*, 1991).

Negotiating safer sex prior to the commencement of sexual activity may place sexual partners in double jeopardy. Not only is there a premium in sex attached to a level ambiguity and mystery surrounding the sexual intentions of each partner (Wight, 1992), but there is no clearly defined language or terminology which can best serve this purpose. Recent health education initiatives have identified some impediments to talking about sex and attempted to portray as sexy 'safer sex' and negotiating sexual activity. Hopefully this will introduce to young people a language for discussing sex, in the same way as health care professionals have had to come to terms with being more open with their patients about intimate matters in the era of HIV (Silverman, Perakyla & Bor, 1992).

Negotiating risk as it pertains to sex presupposes that both (or however many) partners are equally empowered to consent to sex and to make decisions pertaining to risk. While this may be to some

extent valid in same-sex relationships, there may be gender determined patterns of relationships and role expectations between heterosexual partners (Wight, 1992). Many women report that their first sexual experience (and indeed, subsequent one's) involved their male partner coercing them to have intercourse (Holland *et al.*, 1992). Although the female partner may be 'invested' with the prime responsibility for ensuring proper contraception, she may not be empowered to insist that her male partner use a condom. Female sex workers have reported that it is difficult to persuade some clients to use condoms because they are drunk and potentially violent (Wilson *et al.*, 1989), while there is sometimes an incentive not to use condoms as clients will pay more for unprotected sex.

At one level, 'advice to keep to safer sex' in the era of HIV addresses 'risky behaviour' which in some circumstances may need to change in order to reduce the number of new HIV transmissions. At another level, there are 'risky situations' (Zwi & Cabral, 1991) which need to be identified if the factors which give rise to risk-taking behaviour are to be properly addressed. Economic deprivation, migrancy, gender determined relationships and cultural rules about marriage and procreation may, in part, determine the nature and extent of impediments to negotiating or adhering to safer sex guidelines.

PSYCHOLOGICAL IMPACT OF AIDS

Physical illness has an impact on the individual as well as those around him or her. The psychological consequences of HIV disease are directly linked to the social context of AIDS-related illness and the meaning this holds, the nature of the disease and the clinical manifestations associated with it. In some cases, neurological, psychiatric or behavioural problems may be the presenting symptom of HIV infection, while a proportion of those diagnosed will at some stage receive treatment for major affective disorders or psychosis. A comprehensive assessment is needed to determine the extent of organic involvement in psychological problems.

The relationship between HIV disease and psychological morbidity has been studied by many researchers. Early reports suggested that psychiatric problems were common in patients with HIV infection. Findings from recent research, however, indicate that the rates of persistent psychiatric problems in this population are comparable with other life-threatening conditions. Adjustment disorders are the most commonly presenting problems, particularly around the time of HIV antibody testing (Perry *et al.*, 1993). While psychological treatment, and in particular cognitive–behavioural therapy, is usually effective in many cases, there is a definite risk of suicide in these patients. Factors which increase risk for suicide include social stigma, withdrawal of family and social support, loss of employment and housing, disfigurement, increased dependence on carers, as well as depression and psychosis. (See also 'Suicide'.)

Psychological problems may extend to people who have an exaggerated or unremitting fear of contracting HIV and to those who have a delusional conviction that they have AIDS (Munchausen's Syndrome). The former often refuse to undergo HIV testing or are not reassured by a negative HIV antibody test result. The latter may thrive on the attention of medical staff and, in some cases, relish the prospect of undergoing medical tests and investigations. In both cases, patients' irrational beliefs may thwart medical management.

The prognosis is generally good where patients receive treatment for their underlying psychological problem.

As the natural history of HIV infection unfolds, the experience of long-term survivors can be studied. The median survival period for people diagnosed with AIDS is three years, although up to 10% of AIDS patients in developed countries are alive at least six years after their diagnosis. Some face problems in their personal relationships as a consequence of the uncertainty of the prognosis (Bor & Elford, 1994). Results of preliminary studies suggest that the majority of long-term survivors are optimistic and resilient. The extent to which psychological well-being affects the immune system is relevant in this regard. Researchers in the field of psychoneuroimmunology have contributed to an understanding of the relationship between stress, lifestyle, mood, diet, sleep patterns and exercise on psychological morbidity and mortality.

IMPACT OF AIDS ON THE FAMILY

Since the beginning of the epidemic, AIDS has been viewed as a social problem that has repercussions for relationships by virtue of the social stigma and isolation experienced by those affected, as well as the fact that HIV is transmitted through sexual contact. By way of contrast, most published research in the 1980s described the implications of HIV disease for the individual rather than the family or other social systems. Even though gay men in the West were most affected by HIV in the first decade, the absence of family-related research may have perpetuated a stereotype that gay men are not connected to families. Yet, for every person infected with HIV, there is a family or social support system that will also be affected. The advent of AIDS has prompted a redefinition of 'the family', and some contemporary definitions include extended kin networks as well as non-conventional family constellations, such as same-sex couples.

It is common knowledge that people react differently to illness. What is striking about families affected by HIV is that they usually face the additional problem of social stigma. Disclosure of the diagnosis in the family may confront its members with revelations about lifestyle or behaviour. Non-infected family members may themselves suffer stigma and may experience rejection from friends, loss of jobs and harassment, as well as more subtle gestures such as neighbours not visiting and children not being invited to parties. There may be secrets between family members and between the family and those around them. While secrets may serve to protect people from the effects of stigma, such as rejection, they can also have hazardous consequences, as in the case of an HIV-infected person who refuses to inform or protect a sexual partner during intercourse (by using a condom).

Parents' disclosure of their diagnosis to their children, and children being told of their own illness are some of the most challenging problems in the care of people with HIV in the 1990s. As yet, there is little research to guide parents as to whether, how and when to tell children. In almost all cases, the effects of AIDS will alter the family structure and roles; normal developmental patterns are reversed. Children may die before their parents, while grandparents become carers at a time when they would expect to be taken care of (Bor & Elford, 1994).

There may be no respite for the survivors after a family member has died from AIDS. The bereaved may continue to experience rejection and other forms of stigma. Children may become orphans and suffer emotional and practical deprivation. Some of the survivors may themselves be infected with HIV and face terminal illness. The experience of multiple losses, resulting in complicated bereavement reactions, are increasingly common and those affected may require psychological therapy.

The problems for surviving partners when the HIV infected partner dies are complex. HIV-infected surviving partners experience high levels of anxiety in their grief, most likely linked to fantasies relating to their own mortality and a feeling of an inability to have a new relationship (Bor, Miller & Goldman, 1992). Most common is the fear of loneliness, having to face their own illness and the possibility of dying alone with no partner to care for them. The surviving partner may express anger at their partners betrayal by dying first. After initial grieving, a sense of relief can also be recognized where the surviving partner is HIV negative. It may become possible for the negative partner to begin to build a new life and find a new partner. However fears of being 'tarnished' by having had a positive partner may make exploring new relationships in the least, extremely difficult. (See also 'Bereavement'.)

REACTIONS TO TESTING FOR HIV AND AN AIDS DIAGNOSIS

How patients react to a positive HIV antibody test result or to an AIDS diagnosis is inextricably linked to prevailing biomedical knowledge. Many studies in which reactions to HIV testing are described were carried out on cohorts of homosexual men. It is difficult to control for other relevant variables in this group such as social stigma, marginality, social isolation and previous experience of personal loss through AIDS.

There are several clinical and social issues which may increase an HIV infected patient's susceptibility to stress, anxiety and other psychological symptoms. These include uncertainty and unpredictability about course of illness and the future, risk (and consequently some constraints) in sexual activities, and secrecy and confidentiality-related problems.

For those who decide to be tested for HIV, there is the fear of receiving a positive result. The next fear may be of developing symptoms and having an AIDS-defining illness, such as *Pneumocystis carinii* pneumonia. Bad news for those patients attending for regular monitoring may be a falling CD4 count (a marker of immune system functioning), or a fear that resistance might develop to a drug being used to treat them where there is no substitute or alternative treatment. A fear of Kaposi's sarcoma (a disfiguring skin condition) or extreme weight loss, which many patients regard as obvious or tell-tale signs of HIV disease to other people, features prominently among the fears of patients. The news that a child is infected or that the infection has been transmitted to a sexual partner can be devastating. Symptoms of HIV-related neurological impairment may be especially frightening to patients and carers.

Patients' psychological responses to a fear of these conditions are mediated by a number of factors. In the case of Kaposi's sarcoma, for example, patients may respond differently depending on the location, size or contour of the lesion. Social and cultural factors may determine the extent to which patients are distressed by their changing physical appearance. Some patients find that psychological problems become more pressing after they have been discharged

AIDS

[345]

from hospital to convalesce as the hospital provides a protective social environment for patients. Similarly, the signs and symptoms of neurological disease can impair patients' functions in a number of ways and therefore have different implications for them. These range from apathy, social withdrawal, impaired handwriting, headaches, to memory loss, seizures, dysphasia, hemiparesis and even coma.

It should be borne in mind that not all patients diagnosed with AIDS develop psychological problems. For some, they may experience relief at being told the diagnosis which may end a period of uncertainty or doubt about clinical signs and symptoms. In the case of HIV disease, we must conclude that patients are at risk psychologically not only because of the stress associated with having to cope with a life-threatening medical condition, but also because of their marginality as a social group, although these factors will contribute to varying degrees.

THE IMPACT OF HIV ON HEALTH-CARE STAFF

No illness occurs in a vacuum. Treatment and care take place in a particular setting with designated staff at a certain point in the evolution of a health care or medical service. HIV has had a profound impact on health-care services. Many health-care staff themselves have concerns about being infected by patients. In spite of what appears to be a low occupational risk for HIV transmission, these fears persist. Anxiety and concern about working with patients infected with HIV may also be associated with negative perceptions of patients and homophobia (Treiber, Shaw & Malcolm, 1987). Large-scale studies of occupationally-related stress and burnout in health-care staff caring for people with HIV disease have recently commenced. The results of these studies will provide more detailed information about the psychological impact of HIV on health care staff.

ACCESS TO HIV SERVICES

The medical, psychological and social care and management of HIV infected people in the 1990s is both complex and challenging. In the 1980s it was predominantly gay men (in the West) who were most affected and consequently medical and social support services developed to meet their needs. As the natural history of the disease unfolds, new demands and challenges are placed on existing services. In the 1990s, this will entail a shift in emphasis in care from an acute to a chronic medical condition. An important new emphasis will be on developing appropriate services for the increasing number of women infected with HIV, the majority of whom will be young and of childbearing age.

Outpatient HIV care services in the UK are mainly situated in sexually transmitted diseases (STD) clinics. These clinics have been at the forefront of HIV testing initiatives, offering a confidential service to those who use them. While it is possible to provide follow-up care for most patients in these clinics, they operate on an outpatient basis and therefore patients have to be transferred to hospital-based physicians when symptoms occur. HIV infected women, especially those with children, may feel that they do not fit with an STD-based service, particularly because of the absence of child-care facilities and the lack of gynaecological care in STD clinics. HIV disease may exacerbate gynaecological problems, and issues pertaining to fertility, reproduction, childbearing and childrearing may need to be dis-

cussed. As a consequence, HIV infected women have expressed a need for special care and support services to enable them to attend regularly at hospitals.

The medical system may also inadvertently discriminate against women with HIV disease. Not only is an infected man at slightly higher risk of infecting a woman during intercourse than the other way around, but women with AIDS have been found to have a shorter survival time than men (Rothenberg et al., 1987). A number of methodological and clinical reasons for these trends have been put forward. None the less, there are also important social reasons for the observed increase in vulnerability of woman to AIDS. Women may delay seeking medical attention due to poverty or pressure by the partner or family to provide care in the home (Bury, Morrison & McLachlan, 1992). The clinical system of classification for people with HIV disease may also exclude some women who may be infected and suffer with gynaecological conditions closely associated with advanced HIV disease. Without an AIDS diagnosis, these women may be denied social, medical and practical benefits and support. They may also be excluded from entry into controlled experimental trials of drugs not only because of this anomaly in the case definition of AIDS, but also because of pregnancy. In the 1990s, there is likely to be a shift in emphasis in HIV care to include improved services for women, children and families.

THE CHALLENGE TO THE TRADITIONAL DOCTOR–PATIENT RELATIONSHIP

There is wide diversity in views among professionals about treatments, drug trials and approaches to care. At times, this gives rise to confusion and conflict in patient management. The advent of AIDS has challenged some of the traditional perceptions of the hierarchical doctor–patient. In the 1990s, there is renewed debate in medical journals about informed consent, accountability and quality of life. Patients have formed pressure groups (for example, ACT UP) which have sometimes successfully challenged the policies and practices of pharmaceutical companies, health ministries and the medical profession. They have campaigned to make experimental treatments available at an earlier stage than might usually be the case. On their own initiate, some patients on experimental treatments have sought to 'break the code' of the trials by having their blood or urine analysed to determine whether they are on the treatment or placebo arm of the trial. In desperation, illicit supplies of new or experimental drugs have been obtained by patients.

A wide range of health-care professionals have had to learn to talk openly with some of their patients about intimate sexual activities, recreational drug use and profound uncertainties about illness, its course and outcome. Patients have succeeded in redressing some of the imbalance in the doctor–patient relationship by becoming active in designing and delivering health care, and in assessing the effectiveness of services.

CONCLUSIONS

The rapid advances in knowledge about AIDS and HIV infection have been paralleled by a growing body of literature describing the psychosocial impact of HIV disease on individuals, families, communities and health-care services. In the west, and in many developing countries, these descriptions emanate from a social context in which HIV/AIDS is co-terminus with fear, ostracism and marginalization of those infected or affected. It is not surprising that some people with HIV disease, or with associated fears, may develop psychological problems ranging from neurotic symptoms to psychosis.

What direction will psychosocial research take in the 1990s? Will it be sustained? Current trends reveal an established imbalance in medical research. There is a decline in the amount of research into HIV prevention and control, inspite of the growing number of cases worldwide and reports of relapse among those who have previously adopted safer sex practices (Elford, Bor & Summers, 1991). The changing emphasis in medical care for people with HIV disease in the 1990s from crisis management to monitoring and early interven-

tion will be replicated in psychosocial care. Long-term psychological support (and the problems that it will bring), and more specialized care for different subpopulations affected will need to be developed. More rigorous research is needed into issues relating to gender and power in relationships, be they in the personal lives of those affected by HIV disease, or between patients and their carers. Questions about the impact of the changing social context on psychological morbidity on patients, their contacts and family, also merit further study. In the absence of a cure or vaccine, behavioural research into HIV prevention must take precedence on the list of research priorities. In so doing, we will come to learn more about the social context of HIV disease.

REFERENCES

Bor, R. & Elford, J. (1994). *The family and HIV*. London: Cassell.

Bor, R., Miller, R. & Goldman, E. (1992). *Theory and Practice of HIV Counselling*. London: Cassell.

Bury, J., Morrison, V. & McLachlan, S. (1992) *Working with Women and AIDS*. London: Routledge.

Centres for Disease Control (CDC). (1981). Pneumocystis pneumonia – Los Angeles. *Morbidity and Mortality Weekly Report*, 30, 250–2.

Chin, J., Sato, P. & Mann, J. (1990). Projections of HIV infection and AIDS cases to the year 2000. *Bulletin of the World Health Organization*, 68, 1–11.

Elford, J., Bor, R. & Summers, P. (1991). Research into HIV and AIDS between 1981 and 1990: the epidemic curve. *AIDS*, 5, 1515–19.

Holland, J., Ramazanoglu, C., Scott, S., Sharpe, S. & Thomson, R (1991). Between embarrassment and trust: young women and the diversity of condom use. In P. Aggleton, P. Davies & G. Hart (Eds.). *AIDS: responses, intervention and care*. Basingstoke: Falmer Press.

Merrill, J., Laux, L. & Thornby, J. (1990). Why doctors have difficulty with sex histories. *Southern Medical Journal*, 83, 613–17.

Perry, S., Jacobsberg, L., Card, A., Ashman, T., Frances, A. & Fishman, B. (1993). Severity of symptoms after HIV testing. *American Journal of Psychiatry*, 150, 775–9.

Rothenberg, R., Woelfel, M., Stoneburner, R., Milberg, J., Parker, R. & Truman, B. (1987). Survival with AIDS. *New England Journal of Medicine*, 317, 1297–302.

Silverman, D., Perakyla, A. & Bor, R. (1992). Discussing safer sex in HIV counselling: assessing three communication formats. *AIDS Care*, 4, 69–82.

Treiber, F., Shaw, D. & Malcolm, R. (1987). AIDS: psychological impact on health care personnel. *Journal of Nervous and Mental Disease*, 175, 496–9.

Wight, D. (1992). Impediments to safer heterosexual sex: a review of research with young people. *AIDS Care*, 4, 11–21.

Wilson, D., Chiroro, P., Lavelle, S. & Mutero, C. (1989). Sex worker, client sex behaviour and London use in Harare, Zimbabwe. *AIDS Care*, 3, 269–80.

Zwi, A. & Cabral, A. (1991). Identifying 'high risk situations' for preventing AIDS. *British Medical Journal*, 303, 1527–9.

Alcohol abuse/alcoholism

MICHAEL A. SAYETTE
and
MICHAEL R. HUFFORD
University of Pittsburgh, USA

Alcohol has been consumed by people in all parts of the world for thousands of years. Most people who routinely consume alcohol generally do not develop drinking problems. Nevertheless, the millions of people who do develop problems associated with alcohol create enormous social, economic, and medical costs for society. Complications resulting from chronic alcohol problems include liver damage, peripheral neuropathy, and memory loss, as well as a host of negative life events. Although the term 'alcoholism' is used widely in both the lay and professional communities, its lack of specificity and moralistic overtones have led to use of terms such as alcohol abuse and alcohol dependence in recent diagnostic formulations.

In the most recent edition of the *Diagnostic and statistical manual of the mental disorders* (*DSM-IV*: American Psychiatric Association, 1994), alcohol dependence includes biological, psychological, and social components. Most importantly, alcohol dependence involves difficulty controlling alcohol consumption and continued drinking despite aversive consequences. Edwards (1986) notes an increase in the salience of drinking, with alcohol taking on an increasingly dominant role in a drinker's life, as an important element in the alcohol dependence syndrome. Although none of the following is required for diagnosis, alcohol dependence symptoms include: tolerance (a diminished effect of alcohol, usually accompanied by increased consumption); withdrawal symptoms following reduced consumption;

consumption of larger amounts or for a longer time period than was intended; persistent desire or unsuccessful efforts to cut down or control drinking; excessive time spent obtaining, consuming, or recovering from the effects of alcohol; reduction of important activities due to drinking; and continued drinking despite knowledge that it is causing or exacerbating a physical or psychological problem.

Alcohol abuse is conceptualized by DSM-IV as a maladaptive drinking pattern (i.e. continued drinking despite knowledge that it is causing or exacerbating a problem). Individuals diagnosed with alcohol abuse must meet the criteria for alcohol dependence and manifest at least one of the following: recurrent drinking despite its interference with the execution of major role obligations; continued drinking despite legal, social, or interpersonal problems related to its use; and recurrent drinking in situations where intoxication is dangerous. Data from the recent Epidemiological Catchment Area study (Robins & Reiger, 1991) indicated a lifetime prevalence rate for either alcohol abuse or dependence of 13.8%, with men being significantly more likely than women to develop drinking problems.

For heuristic purposes, this chapter will use the term 'alcoholism' to denote alcohol abuse or dependence. Alcoholism is a heterogeneous disorder that is multiply determined by both genetic and psychological factors. Support for a genetic aetiology for alcoholism is derived from adoption, twin, and family studies, as well as animal studies in which rodents are bred for sensitivity to alcohol's effects and alcohol seeking behaviour. Both twin studies and research identifying cultural and occupational differences in alcoholism rates reveal that environmental and psychological factors also contribute to the development of alcoholism (see Sher, 1991 for review of both genetic and environmental influences). From a psychological perspective, alcoholism can be considered to be a disorder of behavioural excess, a maladaptive habit that has developed through powerful reinforcement contingencies, rather than a biomedical disease (Marlatt & Gordon, 1985).

A number of psychological theories have been developed to understand alcohol use and alcoholism (Blane & Leonard, 1987). Generally, these theories state that people drink alcohol to increase pleasant feelings (positive reinforcement) or to decrease unpleasant feelings (negative reinforcement). Often, these theories lead to predictions about which people will be most sensitive to these reinforcing effects, and thus will be at greatest risk for developing alcoholism.

Many people, including both those who treat and those who suffer from alcoholism, believe that alcohol is consumed because it reduces anxiety. This tension reduction hypothesis has spawned more than 40 years of experimental research. Although the data have been mixed, it appears that, under certain conditions, alcohol does provide anxiolytic effects and that anxiety symptoms can sometimes precipitate drinking or relapse. Recent models have attempted to explore the mechanisms underlying these anxiolytic effects. These include models positing direct pharmacological effects of alcohol on the nervous system and the notion that anxiolytic effects are mediated by alcohol's effects on information processing (Sayette, 1993). This latter position is represented in a number of recent social–cognitive models.

Hull (1987) has proposed that alcohol's anxiolytic properties are cognitively mediated. By impairing the encoding of information in terms of self-relevance, intoxication decreases self-awareness. The inhibition of encoding processes reduces performance-based self-evaluation – which, in situations where such evaluation is unpleasant, increases the probability of drinking. Alternatively, intoxication may interfere with self-evaluation rather than self-awareness of one's vulnerabilities. That is, we may know that we were judged unfavourably by another, but this information does not adversely affect the way that we view ourselves. Other cognitive mechanisms proposed to account for alcohol's anxiolytic effects include effects on attentional capacity, and initial appraisal of stressful information (see Sayette, 1993 for a review of the preceding theories).

Although alcohol's effects on anxiety have received the most scrutiny, other negatively reinforcing effects have also been investigated. For example, alcohol has been consumed to cope with a variety of life events or situations. From this social learning perspective, alcoholism may result when one becomes overwhelmed by the demands of a situation. An opponent processing theory posits that alcohol is used to alleviate unpleasant emotional states associated with withdrawal. An attributional *self-handicapping* model asserts that alcohol can be used in some cases as an excuse for undesirable behaviour or negative outcomes. This approach maintains self-perceptions of competence by providing external attributions (e.g. 'I was drunk') for the behaviour. (See edited volume by Blane & Leonard (1987) for detailed accounts of these different theories.) A recent biopsychological account posits that drinking alcohol serves to replenish depleted endorphin levels following a stressful event (Volpicelli, 1987). This latter model argues that alcohol is most effective as an anodyne, and is most likely to be consumed, following a stressful experience.

In addition to these negative reinforcing effects, alcohol often is consumed in order to produce positive effects such as enhanced arousal and positive mood. For example, alcohol can enhance feelings of power. The euphoric effects of alcohol generally appear while blood alcohol concentrations are rising and are thought to be important in decisions concerning drinking, as people's beliefs about drinking will be most affected by the most immediate consequences of alcohol consumption (Marlatt, 1987).

VULNERABILITY TO ALCOHOLISM

Children of alcoholics are at heightened risk to develop alcoholism compared with children without this background (Sher, 1991). Considerable research is underway to explore the genetic and environmental moderators and mediators of this relationship. Individuals at risk for alcoholism due to a family history of the disorder tend to show stronger effects of alcohol during the ascending limb of the blood alcohol curve yet weaker effects on the descending limb than those without familial risk (Newlin & Thomson, 1990). Although the evidence is mixed, some investigators have observed that alcohol's anxiolytic effects are enhanced among children of alcoholics (Sayette, 1993; Sher, 1991). Research also has documented relationships between certain personality traits such as impulsivity and habituation to stimuli and the development of alcoholism. Because alcoholism is now recognized to be a heterogenous disorder, current personality theories of alcoholism have shifted away from identifying a unitary alcoholic personality and instead focus on specific personality dimensions, such as behavioural undercontrol or negative emotionality, that may place an individual at increased risk (Sher, 1991).

PSYCHOLOGICAL CONTRIBUTIONS TO THE TREATMENT OF ALCOHOLISM

Approaches to alcoholism treatment are becoming increasingly integrated with attempts to address biological, psychological, and social aspects of the disorder. A number of pharmacological treatments continue to be developed to treat alcoholism. Disulfiram (Antabuse) has long been used to deter persons from drinking. When alcohol is consumed, disulfiram produces an accumulation of the toxic metabolite acetaldehyde, causing nausea and hypotension. If disulfiram is reliably used, these extremely unpleasant sensations often can deter an individual from drinking. Other drugs, such as Fluoxetine and Naltrexone have been posited to reduce alcohol craving and drinking. In addition to these pharmacological agents, a number of psychosocial interventions have been developed, which are summarized below.

Relapse prevention

Because the majority of alcoholics who quit drinking relapse, a trend in alcoholism treatment has been on maintaining treatment gains rather than focusing entirely on initial cessation. Alan Marlatt (Marlatt & Gordon, 1985) has developed a model of relapse prevention that focuses on factors that can promote relapse. This model posits that particular situations, and not just personality traits, can precipitate a return to drinking. Marlatt argues that initial drinking following attempted abstinence (a lapse) leads to full-blown relapse due to the shame involved in violating abstinence. This Abstinence Violation effect is treated psychologically by helping patients recognize the situational precipitants of the lapse, rather than interpreting the lapse as indisputable evidence that they are treatment failures. Thus, treatment focuses on anticipating high-risk situations that might jeopardize abstinence and identifying coping strategies. Should a lapse occur, however, relapse prevention seeks to prevent it from developing into a full-blown relapse. In this case, treatment involves exploring the events and experiences that triggered the lapse. Interest in understanding the variables that can precipitate relapse has led to a number of psychological strategies that are used in treatment programmes.

Skills training

The ability to cope effectively with high risk situations is related to effective treatment and is believed to prevent relapse. Certain situations appear to pose a high risk for relapse, including interpersonal anger and frustration, social pressure, negative emotional states, and stimulus-elicited craving (Marlatt & Gordon, 1985). Communication difficulties also have been implicated as a problem for many alcoholics. Deficient areas that often are targeted in coping skills interventions include assertiveness, initiating conversations, listening skills, giving and receiving compliments and criticism, and enhancing close relationships. Particular attention is paid to developing skills specific to drinking situations. For example, drink refusal training permits modelling and practising of skills needed to cope with offers to drink by peers. In addition, receiving criticism about drinking and enhancing non-alcoholic support networks are targeted in skills treatment. These coping-skills training programmes have reduced alcohol consumption and increased work days after treatment (Monti et al., 1993).

Cue exposure

Both clinical observations and experimental research suggest that exposure to alcohol cues can precipitate relapse. For example, being around alcohol at a party may lead to a return to drinking. Individuals in this situation may become physiologically aroused, experience a craving for alcohol, and ultimately act on their urge and drink. Treatments have been developed in which patients are repeatedly exposed to alcohol cues (e.g. sniffing their favourite drink) but are not permitted to drink the beverage. Initially, patients experience heightened reactions such as intense cravings for the drink, increased physiological arousal, and increased salivation. With repeated exposure to the drink over several sessions, however, patients' responses to the cues diminish. In conditioning terms, cue exposure attempts to extinguish or attenuate the strength of association between alcohol cues and drinking behaviour. From a social learning perspective, cue exposure permits modification of one's beliefs concerning both the reinforcing aspects of drinking (positive outcome expectancies) and the perceived ability to cope with, or resist, the urge to drink (self-efficacy judgements). Regardless of its underlying mechanisms, cue exposure treatment has shown promising results in conjunction with skills training in improving treatment success (e.g. Monti et al., 1993).

Couples therapy/family therapy

The emphasis on determining triggers for drinking has led to increased focus on the patient's spouse or family members in understanding the aetiology of alcoholism. Although family and relationship issues are generally not the primary cause of alcoholism, they often contribute to the maintenance of alcohol problems. Thus, among individuals with alcoholism, marital and family conflict can precipitate drinking. Further, the non-alcoholic spouse and family members may reinforce problem drinking by providing financial and emotional support during times of heavy consumption. These factors have led to the use of couples and family therapy as an adjunct to individual treatment. Specifically, treatment has effectively improved (a) patients' initial motivation to quit, (b) treatment gains during the year following initiation of therapy, and (c) maintenance of treatment gains during long-term recovery (O' Farrell, 1992).

Alcohol expectancies

An individual's alcohol expectancies (i.e. beliefs about the effects of alcohol on affect, behaviour and cognition) predict drinking behaviour over time as well as treatment outcome (Goldman, 1994). Furthermore, it appears that individuals at increased risk for alcoholism, due to a personality marked by behavioural undercontrol or negative affectivity, or a family history of alcoholism, show differential patterns of alcohol expectancies relative to individuals who are not considered to be at risk. These expectancies may in turn predict drinking (Goldman, 1994; Sher, 1991). Expectancies about alcohol's effects may provide a common pathway that permits other factors such as personality variables or reactivity to alcohol's effects to influence the initiation and maintenance of alcohol use and alcoholism. Developments in the alcohol expectancy domain hold promise for providing a theoretical foundation for conceptualizing advances in the prevention of alcohol problems (Goldman, 1994).

Motivation enhancement

Alcoholism treatment failure often has been attributed to poor motivation to recover on the part of the alcoholic. Recently, the ability to enhance one's motivation to quit has become a therapeutic goal. Simple interventions designed to improve motivation have produced significant changes in an individual's willingness to accept treatment. Research by Miller and colleagues (Miller, 1992) have begun to identify dispositional variables, such as locus of control, that can moderate an individual's motivation for a particular type of treatment.

Self-help groups

Many alcoholics have derived benefit from self-help groups such as Alcoholics Anonymous (AA) or Rational Recovery. Self-help group meetings involve discussion by members of their experiences abstaining from alcohol. These groups can serve a number of important functions. Members gain a nondrinking support network, discuss their fears and concerns about relapse, and perhaps most importantly, realize that their struggle with alcohol is shared by others. More than one million people throughout the world attend AA meetings annually. AA relies on a 12-step treatment approach that emphasizes a belief in a higher power to combat what is viewed as an incurable but arrestable illness. Despite its widespread appeal, systematic evaluations of AA's effectiveness have not been conducted. Rational Recovery offers a non-spiritual treatment alternative that appeals to those who are uncomfortable with AA. Currently, efforts are under way to begin to gauge the impact of AA and associated groups.

Patient/treatment matching

Traditionally, patients being treated for alcoholism would receive the particular treatment package implemented by that agency. The degree of individualization of treatment often has been minimal (Miller, 1992). Currently, a large multisite randomized clinical trial known as 'Project Match' is comparing responses to a 12-step, a cognitive–behavioural, and a motivational enhancement approach to treatment. The principal objective of Project Match is to determine which type of treatment works best for different types of individuals (matching patients to treatments using characteristics such as social support and degree of dependence). Once such relationships emerge, further research aims to demonstrate that patients matched to the 'appropriate' treatment will manage better than those patients who are unmatched or mismatched (Miller, 1992).

ALCOHOLISM: CONTEXTUAL ISSUES

Understanding the aetiology of alcoholism requires an appreciation for a host of other psychological disturbances that may face the patient. Two such issues are comorbid psychiatric disorders and polydrug use. Affective, anxiety, and personality disorders are examples of psychiatric conditions often comorbid with alcoholism. Exploring the nature of these relationships is important for understanding risk factors as well as for developing effective treatment strategies for these individuals.

Polydrug use among alcoholics is increasingly becoming the rule rather than the exception. Because many alcohol treatment facilities and research projects have excluded polydrug users, important information regarding these subjects has until recently been lacking. Generally, polydrug patients present with more severe problems than those whose problems are exclusive to alcohol. The nature of these differences has just begun to be explored. Research is needed to determine whether cessation is indicated for all drugs simultaneously or, if not, what the sequence of cessation ought to be. This concern typifies the current view of alcoholism that recognizes the importance of understanding the disorder within a broader biopsychosocial context.

ACKNOWLEDGEMENTS

Supported by the National Institute on Alcohol Abuse and Alcoholism (1 R29 AA09918–01). We thank Chris Martin for his feedback on a previous draft.

REFERENCES

American Psychiatric Association. (in press). *Diagnostic and statistical manual of mental disorders* (4th edn.). Washington, DC: Author.

Blane, H.T. & Leonard, K.E. (Eds.). (1987). *Psychological theories of drinking and alcoholism*. New York: Guilford.

Edwards, G. (1986). The alcohol dependence syndrome: the concept as stimulus to inquiry. *British Journal of Addiction*, 81, 71–84.

Goldman, M.S. (1994). The alcohol expectancy concept: applications to assessment, prevention, and treatment of alcohol abuse. *Applied and Preventive Psychology*, 3, 131–44.

Hull, J.G. (1987). Self-awareness model. In H.T. Blane & K.E. Leonard (Eds.). *Psychological theories of drinking and alcoholism*, pp. 272–304. New York: Guilford.

Marlatt, G.A. (1987). Alcohol, the magic elixir: stress, expectancy, and the transformation of emotional states. In E. Gottheil, K. Druley, S. Pasko & S. Weinstein (Eds.), *Stress and addiction*, pp. 302–322. New York: Brunner/Mazel.

Marlatt, G.A. & Gordon, J.R. (Eds.). (1985). *Relapse prevention*. New York: Guilford Press.

Miller, W.R. (1992). Client/treatment matching in addictive behaviors. *The Behavior Therapist*, 15, 7–8.

Monti, P.M., Rohsenow, D.J., Rubonis, A.V., Niaura, R.S., Sirota, A.D., Colby, S.M., Goddard, P. & Abrams, D.B. (1993). Cue exposure with coping skills treatment for male alcoholics: a preliminary investigation. *Journal of Consulting and Clinical Psychology*, 61, 1011–19.

Newlin, D.B. & Thomson, J.B. (1990). Alcohol challenge in sons of alcoholics: a critical review and analysis. *Psychological Bulletin*, 108, 383–402.

O'Farrell, T.J. (1992). Families and alcohol problems: an overview of treatment research. *Journal of Family Psychology*, 5, 339–59.

Robins, L. & Reiger, D. (Eds.). (1991). *Psychiatric disorders in America: the Epidemiological catchment area study*. New York: Macmillan.

Sayette, M.A. (1993). An appraisal–disruption model of alcohol's effects on stress responses in social drinkers. *Psychological Bulletin*, 114, 459–76.

Sher, K.J. (1991). *Children of alcoholics: a critical appraisal of theory and research*. Chicago: University of Chicago Press.

Volpicelli, J.R. (1987). Uncontrollable events and alcohol drinking. *British Journal of Addiciton*, 82, 381–92.

Allergies to drugs

MARY BANKS GREGERSON
Psychology Department,
The George Washington University, USA

FEATURES

Allergies to drugs have become well-accepted phenomena. These sensitivities are often termed 'side-effects' since they are epiphenomenal to the drug's intended effect. Although this phrase's connotations implies lesser importance to these non-intentional effects, this terminology does not diminish their intensity nor impact. These adverse reactions are real, and can be life-threatening. The phrase 'concurrent effects' better describes these effects.

The physical sequelae of an allergy to drugs can vary widely. Symptoms may be as benign as simple mild skin rashes, or as threatening as potentially fatal anaphylactic reactions. Anaphylaxis, a constriction of smooth muscles, results in a reddening and swelling of affected areas. If the breathing passages are swollen, suffocation can occur.

Particular antibiotics termed beta-lactams often cause allergic reactions. Allergy to penicillin is quite common. On the other hand, concurrent effects from macrolides seldom produce hypersensitivity.

Three different types of drug allergies have been detailed (Pichler, 1993). First, classic drug allergies are over-reactions to the medication itself. Secondly, an immune reaction occurs but is not mediated by other immune substances. Thirdly, an autoimmune reaction can occur when the drug invokes an immune reaction to autologous structures.

DIAGNOSIS

Diagnosis is difficult for drug allergies (Sabbah & Caradec, 1992). Skin tests and lymphoblast transformation tests may imitate the drug-invoked allergic reaction or merely indicate sensitivity. A prevalent test to determine allergy to drugs is the leukocyte migration inhibition test. A recent simplification of this test proved 66% effective (Tarasov, Zherdev & Shuvalov, 1991). Another common test assesses for basophil degranulation against the exposition. Some evidence exists that this latter test, although more risky, is quicker, simpler, and more useful with more specificity (Rangel *et al.*, 1991).

The most definitive test is a provocation test showing the drug's elicitation of the allergic reaction (see 'Allergies: general' for more on provocation tests).

MEDICAL TREATMENT

Use of the drug causing the allergic reaction is contraindicated. Other related drugs in that same class may also need to be avoided. For instance, discontinuance of histamine-releasing drugs is usually advised, although some question exists concerning this practice (Moss, 1993).

Additional concern, based on clinical evidence, exists for indirect exposure from secondary trace sources. Although injection is the most potent dosage method, oral ingestion can produce reactivity, especially if the allergen is undiluted, although for trace form, for instance, in an antibiotically treated animal's meat, researchers continue to examine ingestion's potency. Investigations have scrutinized allergic reactions to residues in foods such as dairy products and meats (for a review see Dewdney *et al.*, 1991). Although no conclusion can be drawn at this point, caution is warranted regarding ingestion or inhalation of the allergen or its derivatives in trace amounts. Those with a prior allergic history especially need to carefully monitor for traces of antibiotic residuals.

BEHAVIOURAL AND PSYCHOLOGICAL ASPECTS

Presenting symptoms may seem psychological, at first blush. When no fore-knowledge of medication use is available, allergic reactions may appear as a panic attack (Jasnoski, Bell & Peterson, 1994). Psychological sequelae may include hyperarousal, hyperactivity, feelings of impending doom, scattered cognitions, uncontrollability, and 'unreasonable' fear.

Adverse reactions to medications need to be ruled out before diagnosing panic attack as the primary symptom rather than as a secondary response to the allergic reaction.

REFERENCES

Dewdney, J.M., Maes, L., Raynaud, J.P., Blanc, F., Scheid, J.P., Jackson, T., Lens, S. & Verschueren, C. (1991). Risk assessment of antibiotic residues of beta-lactams and macrolides in food products with regard to their immuno-allergic potential. *Food and Chemical Toxicology*, **29**, 477–83.

Jasnoski, M.B.L., Bell, I.R. & Peterson, R. (1994). What associations exist between shyness, hay fever, anxiety, anxiety sensitivity, and panic disorder? *Anxiety, Stress, and Coping*, **2**, 1–15.

Moss, J. (1993). Are histamine-releasing drugs really contraindicated in patients with a known allergy to drugs? *Anesthesiology*, **79**, 623–4.

Pichler, W.J. (1993). Diagnostic possibilities in drug allergies. *Schweizerische Medizinische Wochenschrift, Journal Suisse de Medecine*, **123**, 1183–92.

Rangel, H., Montero, P., Espinosa, F. & Castillo, F.J. (1991). Leukocyte migration inhibitory factor and basophil degranulation in drug reactions. *Revista Alergia Mexico*, **38**, 105–9.

Sabbah, A. & Caradec, J. (1992). Measurement of mediators in drug allergies. Preliminary study. *Allergie et Immunologie (Paris)*, **24**, 2899–902.

Tarasov, A.V., Zherdev, A.V. & Shuvalov, L.P. (1991). A modification of the leukocyte migration inhibition test in vivo. *Laboratornoe Delo (Moskva)*, **12**, 38–40.

Allergies to drugs

Allergies to food

MARY BANKS GREGERSON

*Psychology Department, The George Washington
University, USA*

FEATURES

Food allergies are immunological hyper-reactions to ingested substances. This immune dysfunction may create gastrointestinal, respiratory, or dermatological symptoms like migraine, gluten enteropathy, Crohn's disease, eczema, wheeze, urticaria, irritable bowel syndrome, or abdominal pain, and, in extreme cases, systemic anaphylactic shock (Del Rio Navarro & Sienra-Monge, 1993). Besides producing discomfort and disease, these allergies can be fatal, and need serious consideration.

Food allergy is different from food intolerance and aversions (Ferguson, 1992). Allergy requires an immune over-reaction, typically with elevated immunoglobulin E (IgE). Intolerance simply cannot absorb food by catabolism, resulting in sensitivity. Aversion is a taste preference without physical problems.

Food allergic reactions depend upon the patient's age and amount of substance ingested and the nature of the substance (Estaban, 1992). Food allergens, or sensitizing substances, have been reported to various fruits, nuts, vegetables, dairy products, and meats (Gluck, 1992). Fruit allergy usually centralizes in throat and mouth reactions like lip or tongue swelling, hoarseness, and uncontrollable throat clearing. Nuts and vegetables, though, produce a more systemic acute attack with symptoms like laryngeal oedema, asthma, urticaria, and even anaphylactic shock. Meat or fish reactions often result in asthma.

INCIDENCE

Prevalence numbers can only be considered estimates since no conceptual agreement and diagnostic procedures are consensually accepted (Estaban, 1992). Of the population 1–3% may evidence food allergies (Del Rio Navarro & Sinera-Monge, 1993). This prevalence rate varies with age and country. Children have more food allergies than adults. For children under 3, 8% have food allergies, which dissipate after reaching 1 to 3 years of age. Tolerance appears to grow with age and exposure, yet food allergies can also appear initially in adulthood. Nationality differences, like a diminishing infant rate in Spain, may be an epiphenomena of either differential diagnostic criteria or other, more relevant criteria like breast-feeding, or different dietary patterns.

DIAGNOSIS

Allergies to food have only recently been accepted because diagnostic techniques lacked scientific rigour and full clinical acceptance (Finn, 1992). Clinical skill and history taking have been the basis for many past diagnoses. More recently cutaneous tests for immediate hypersensitivity and response to specific IgE antibodies (RAST, ELISA) have proved useful, although disagreement exists on their reliability.

A careful diagnostic evaluation would include medical history, a dietary diary, a physical exam, and various *in vitro* and *in vivo* tests (Burks & Sampson, 1992). Standardized skin-prick tests and radio-allergosorbent (RIA) assays may be used for screening, but their high rate of false positives require further confirmation with the 'gold standard', a double-blind, placebo-controlled food challenge. This rigorous approach eliminates psychological confounds that continue to influence patients' dietary practices when they think they have food allergies (Wisocki & King, 1992). Other techniques include the basophil release assay, intestinal mast cell histamine release, intragastric provocation under endoscopy, and intestinal biopsy after allergen elimination and feeding.

TREATMENT

Subcutaneous injections have been ineffective with food allergies (Evans, 1992). The primary standard treatment programme consists of elimination diets as well as challenge tests (Ferguson, 1992). Elimination simply requires systematic abstinence from the suspected allergen. Then, if signs and symptoms disappear, the allergen is reintroduced and confirmed in the most rigorous fashion with a double-blind placebo-controlled provocation test. If and when symptoms re-appear would determine the subsequent treatment plan.

Although their scientific validation is only now commencing, some alternative approaches have treated food allergies (Kay & Lessof, 1992). Treatments that have been used with clinical success are clinical ecology, acupuncture, homeopathy, hypnosis, and herbalism. Again, even though case studies have verified effectiveness, the mechanisms and limits to these treatments are little known. Caution is warranted, though, since many of the evaluative findings are not currently available.

BEHAVIOURAL AND PSYCHOLOGICAL ASPECTS

Psychologists need to concern themselves most with the proper diagnosis of a food allergy and subsequent adherence to a diet regime. Those reporting food allergies which objective tests do not confirm have a hypochondriacal and hysteric profile compared to those tests that do confirm (Parker *et al.*, 1991). Whether undiagnosed food allergies cause these problems or the reported 'allergies' stem from a psychological disturbance is unclear.

Food allergies produce physical symptoms like migraine headaches that are perhaps misdiagnosed as psychological. Food allergies also needs checking in psychological syndromes like attention deficit disorder (Burks & Sampson, 1992). Attention to other physical symptoms indicating allergies should assist in proper diagnosis. Biofeedback has actually been used to uncover food sensitive persons (Laird, 1986).

Avoidance of allergy-producing foods concerns adherence (Burks & Sampson, 1992). Skill education is for label reading, menu planning, and food abstinence. Elimination diets work for about one-third of those with food allergies (see Allergies: general).

REFERENCES

Burks, A.H. & Sampson, H.A. (1992). Diagnostic approaches to the patient with suspected food allergies. *Journal of Pediatrics*, 121, S64–S71.

Del Rio Navarro, B.E. & Sienra-Monge, J.J. (1993). Food allergy. *Boliva Medical Hospital Infant Mexico*, 50, 422–9.

Estaban, M.M. (1992). Adverse food reactions in infancy and childhood. *Journal of Pediatrics*, 121.

Evans, R. III (1992). Environmental control and immunotherapy for allergic disease. *Journal of Allergy and Clinical Immunology*, 90, 462–8.

Ferguson, A. (1992). Definitions and diagnosis of food intolerance and food allergy: Consensus and controversy. *Journal of Pediatrics*, 121, S7–11.

Finn, R. (1992). Food allergy – fact or fiction: a review. *Journal of the Royal Society of Medicine*, 85, 560–4.

Gluck, U. (1992). Neglected allergens. *Therapeutische Umschau*, 49, 669–73.

Kay, A.B. & Lessof, M.H. (1992). Allergy. Conventional and alternative concepts. A report of the Royal College of Physicians Committee on Clinical Immunology and Allergy. *Clinical and Experimental Allergy*, 22, 1–44.

Laird, D. (1986). Using biofeedback to uncover food sensitive persons. *Journal of Orthomolecular Medicine*, 1, 78–83.

Parker, S.L., Garner, D.M., Leznoff, A., Sussman, G.L. *et al.* (1991). Psychological characteristics of patients with reported adverse reactions to foods. *International Journal of Eating Disorders*, 10, 433–9.

Wisocki, P.A. & King, D.S. (1992). The construction of a food-behavior inventory to measure beliefs about the behavioral effects of food. Paper presented at the annual conference of the American Psychological Association, San Francisco, CA.

Allergies: general

MARY BANKS GREGERSON

Department of Psychology, The George Washington University, USA

FEATURES

Allergies are an immediate immune hypersensitivity called Type I. The genetic basis of allergies is commonly accepted. Even with similar genetic risk, some persons either never get allergic symptoms or theirs disappear, while others continually experience allergies. Family transmission of allergy has been acknowledged since 1920. If two parents have Type I Hypersensitivity, offspring have a 50% chance to manifest atopy, and with one parent, almost a 30% chance. These individual differences in responsiveness and the interruption of Mendelian genetic transmission makes psychological and behavioural treatment factors important considerations in allergies.

Allergies result from an immune over-reaction to a specific agent called an allergen or antigen. Typically, but not always, allergies have an abnormal elevation of the protein immunoglobulin E (IgE). This elevation results in distinct clinical features for a myriad of diseases, that is, asthma, eczema, rhinitis (perennial and seasonal, which is commonly called hay fever), and urticaria. The umbrella term for these symptoms is atopy.

Allergies cause physical and psychological discomfort, and, sometimes, death. In hay fever, the mucous membranes in the nasal passages swell; in eczema, the skin inflames with wheals and flares; in asthma, the bronchial passages constrict severely, and in anaphylaxis the smooth muscles vasodilate and constrict causing vasculature collapse because there is no blood pressure. Also, allergies are associated with a number of psychological symptoms (see Bell *et al.*, 1991; Jasnoski, Bell & Peterson, 1994). Specifically, depression, shyness, panic, and anxiety have been connected to allergies. Concomitant allergies have been observed frequently in other diseases, like eating disorders such as bulimia, schizophrenia, and systemic lupus erythematosus. Left-handedness and cerebral dominance have equivocal evidence indicating a connection to allergies. The direction of causality is in question in these circumstances. *Other, more controversial syndromes perhaps or perhaps not connected to immune substrates include chronic fatigue syndrome, Alzheimer's syndrome, seasonality, and multiple chemical sensitivities. The plausibility of a shared third aetiological variable looms in these cases. More future systematic investigations need to investigate the relationship between psychology and allergies.*

MECHANISMS

People with atopy evidence higher levels of circulating IgE (up to 12 micrograms/ml) compared to normals (approximately 0.3 micrograms/ml). IgE's heat sensitivity could explain why rapid temperature or humidity changes and drafts often increase allergic nasal obstruction. IgE further degranulates histamine which produces positive immediate wheal and flare skin reactions.

In a classical conditioning phenomena, sometimes histamine itself can produce allergic reactions without the involvement of IgE. Total IgE levels are elevated in only 30% to 40% of those with allergic rhinitis. A residual histamine priming could, even in the absence of IgE elevation, conceivably result in an allergic response, thus accounting for those with allergic symptoms that do not evidence higher IgE levels.

DIAGNOSIS

Double-blind, placebo-controlled provocation tests often discount IgE mediation for as many as 60% of those with a history of allergies (Jarvis, 1993). In some instances, a 'placebo' allergic reaction has been evoked when the patient thought the allergen was present and it was not. For instance, pictures of hayfields or misrepresented 'placebo' liquids have actually caused a full allergic attack. The question arises, though, what causes an allergic response to trigger histamine priming or other provocations of the allergic response? In the absence of physiological answers, psychological and behavioural factors are implicated, even in the methods to determine the existence of allergies implicates psychological factors.

Interestingly, one research study (for review see Jemmott & Locke, 1984) distinguished between clinical symptoms and cellular changes. A 'placebo' non-allergic mixture represented as the allergic substance elicited symptoms and cellular changes, while the allergic mixture represented as non-allergic also elicited cellular changes, but not symptoms. Other work has shown a conditioned allergic response elicited by the colour of the vial and not the substance in the vial. This growing body of evidence heavily implicates psychological factors in allergic clinical manifestations.

Skin tests, radioallergosorbent tests (RASTs) and relevant provocation tests have been effective in diagnosing allergies. Skin prick tests and enzyme allergosorbent test usually screen for allergy specificity. Then the 'gold standard' provocation test confirms the allergy. A small percentage of disagreement may exist between these tests. Both false positives and negatives are possible.

TREATMENT

Besides allergen avoidance, immunotherapy is the main pharmacological treatment available. This treatment desensitizes the person with allergies by creating a tolerance. A number of well-designed studies have corroborated immunotherapy's effectiveness to reduce symptoms for allergies like hay fever and allergic asthma.

Antihistamines can be used to curtail the intensity of allergic symptoms. This treatment interferes with the late phase following the immediate allergic response. Often this late phase correlates with severity. This approach, though, controls symptoms without decreasing hypersensitivity.

With time and with change, allergies can disappear without pharmacological treatment. A relevant, well-accepted aspect of allergies is their responsiveness to adaptive patterns and changes in life situation. Therefore, psychological and behavioral treatments are sensible adjunctives to medical treatment for those experiencing allergic symptoms.

PSYCHOLOGICAL AND BEHAVIOURAL TREATMENTS

Emotional treatment and behavioural medicine approaches (Schmidt-Traub & Bamler, 1992) have proved effective in diminishing allergies. Other alternative approaches have included hypnosis (for review see Jemmott & Locke, 1984) and nutrition (Van Flandern, 1985). The ubiquitous issue of adherence/compliance with allergy treatments has responded to behavioral intervention (Finney et al., 1990).

Allergies also have a strong body of research addressing the effects of the mother–child relationship and family environment upon symptom severity. For example, one study identified parent dyadic patterns that predicted allergy risk level in children (Faleide et al., 1988). Other work found that higher support, independence, and organization as well as lower religiosity predicted lesser atopic dermatitis symptom severity in children (Gil et al., 1987). Family therapy compared to conventional medical treatment has resulted in significant relief of asthmatic symptoms (Gustafsson, Kjellman & Cederblad, 1986).

CONCLUSION

Allergies, or Type I Hypersensitivity, are widely accepted as a psychosomatic phenomenon. Psychological and behavioural factors are implicated heavily. The role of these non-physiological factors may be found in any disease stage such as aetiology, maintenance, and treatment efficacy. Aetiologically, personal and family circumstances many precipitate allergy occurrences, and may also guard against realization of an inherited propensity. The continuation of allergic responses even to non-allergens, may be explained with classical conditioning principles resulting in developed associations, to non-physiological stimuli like pictures and also to non-IgE based allergic responses. When other than physiological factors cause disease, psychological factors may intervene to avert or curb disease manifestation. A diathesis-stress model crisply conceptualizes the widely accepted understanding of how allergies develop, continue, and abate. It is questionable whether allergies are ever truly cured. Genetic engineering may change allergic haplotypes, or gene configurations, found in the major histocompatibility complex. If this occurs, then cure may be possible. Otherwise, management is central, with psychology a key mechanism in prevention and treatment.

REFERENCES

Bell, I.R., Jasnoski, M.L., Kagan, J. & King, D.S. (1991). Depression and allergies: survey of a nonclinical population. *Psychotherapy and Psychosomatics*, **55**, 24–31.

Faleide, A.O., Galtung, V.K., Unger, S. & Watten, R.G. (1988). Children at risk of allergic development: the parents' dyadic relationship. *Psychotherapy and Psychosomatics*, **49**, 223–9.

Finney, J.W., Lemanek, K.L., Brohy, C.J. & Cataldo, M.F. (1990). Pediatric appointment keeping: improving adherence in a primary care allergy clinic. Special Issue: adherence with pediatric regimens. *Journal of Pediatric Psychology*, **15**, 571–579.

Gil, K.M., Keefe, F.J., Sampson, H.A., McCaskill, C.C., Rodin, J. & Crisson, J.E. (1987). The relation of stress and family environment to atopic dermatitis symptoms in children. *Journal of Psychosomatic Research*, **31**, 673–84.

Gustafsson, P.A., Kjellman, N-I.M. & Cederblad, M. (1986). Family therapy in the treatment of severe childhood asthma. *Journal of Psychosomatic Research*, **30**, 369–74.

Jarvis, W.T. (1993). Allergy related quackery. *New York State Journal of Medicine*, **93**, 100–4.

Jasnoski, M.B.L., Bell, I.R. & Peterson, R. (1994). What associations exist between shyness, hay fever, anxiety, anxiety sensitivity, and panic disorder? *Anxiety, Stress, and Coping*, **7**, 1–15.

Jemmott, J.B. III & Locke, S.E. (1984). Psychosocial factors, immunologic mediation, and human susceptibility to infectious diseases: how much do we know? *Psychological Bulletin*, **95**, 78–105.

Schmidt-Traub, S. & Bamler, K.J. (1992). The psychoimmunological relationship among allergies, panic disorder, and agoraphobia. *Zeitschrift für Klinische Psychologie, Psychopathologie und Psychotherapie*, **40**, 325–45.

Van Flandern, B.A. (1985). Last chance. *Journal of Orthomolecular Psychiatry*, **14**, 251–6.

Amnesia

BARBARA A. WILSON

MRC Applied Psychology Unit, Cambridge, UK

Amnesia and organic memory impairment are commonly seen after many types of brain injury including degenerative disorders, head injury, anoxia and infections of the brain. If severe, amnesia is usually more handicapping in everyday life than severe physical problems.

People with the classic amnesic syndrome show an anterograde amnesia (AA), i.e. they have great difficulty learning and remembering most kinds of new information. Immediate memory, however, is normal when this is assessed by forward digit span or the recency effect in free recall. There is usually a period of retrograde amnesia (RA), that is a loss of information acquired before the onset of the amnesia. This gap or period of RA is very variable in length and may range from a few minutes to decades. Previously acquired semantic knowledge about the world and implicit memory (remembering without awareness or conscious recollection) are typically intact in amnesic subjects. Other cognitive skills, apart from memory, are normal or nearly normal. As the majority of patients with severe memory disorders present with additional cognitive problems such as attention deficits, word finding problems or slowed information processing, those with a classic amnesic syndrome are relatively rare.

Nevertheless, people with a 'pure' amnesic syndrome and people with more widespread cognitive deficits tend to share certain characteristics. In both cases immediate memory is reasonably normal; there is difficulty in remembering after a delay or distraction; new learning is difficult and there is a tendency to remember things that happened a long time before the accident or illness better than things that happened a short time before.

Although precise figures are not available, there are considerable numbers of memory impaired people in society. Some 10% of people over 65 years have dementia and some 36% of people with severe head injury will have permanent memory impairments. Add to these figures those whose memory deficits result from Korsakoff's syndrome, encephalitis, anoxia, AIDS and so forth, and one can begin to appreciate the enormity of the problem.

Assessment of memory should include both neuropsychological and behavioural measures as it is important to identify cognitive strengths and weaknesses and to identify the everyday problems arising from memory impairment. Neuropsychological tests should include general intellectual functioning, language, perception and executive functioning as well as detailed memory assessments. Immediate and delayed memory, visual and verbal memory, recall and recognition, semantic and episodic memory, implicit memory (remembering without awareness) and new learning will all need to be assessed (see Lincoln & Brooks, 1992 for further discussion). More functional and behavioural measures will identify everyday problems causing concern and distress. These measures include observations in real life settings, interviewing patients, their relatives and care staff and the collection of information from such self report measures as diaries, checklists, questionnaires and rating scales (Wilson & Staples, 1992 and Wilson et al., 1989).

Restoration of memory functioning or retraining of memory following brain damage appear to be unachievable goals although some recovery may occur for a period of years (Wilson, 1991). Consequently, rehabilitation for memory impaired people focuses on environmental adaptations, compensatory strategies, improving learning and helping people make better use of their residual skills. For those who are very severely intellectually impaired, structuring the environment to reduce the need to remember, is probably the most effective method. Examples include labelling doors, cupboards and drawers, drawing coloured lines from one place to another and positioning material so it cannot be missed. External memory aids are probably the most beneficial of all therapeutic approaches although many memory impaired people find it difficult to use these aids efficiently and it requires considerable ingenuity to teach their use (Sohlberg & Mateer, 1989). Kapur (1995) and Glisky (1995) cover aspects of external and compensatory aids in some detail. One of the recent developments for improving learning in amnesic subjects is the errorless learning approach (Baddeley & Wilson, 1994; Wilson et al., 1994) whereby it was shown that preventing errors during the learning process led to improved learning by amnesic subjects. Helping people to make better use of their residual, albeit damaged, memory skills can be achieved through the use of mnemonics and study or rehearsal strategies (see Wilson, 1995 for a discussion).

Finally, many memory impaired people are anxious and isolated; so too are their families. Rehabilitation should address these anxieties through anxiety management programmes, information and counselling and perhaps through groups for patients and/or their relatives. Wilson (1995) addresses these issues and other aspects of rehabilitation for people with amnesia.

REFERENCES

Baddeley, A.D. & Wilson, B.A. (1994). When implicit learning fails: amnesia and the problem of error elimination. *Neuropsychologia*, **32**, 53–68.

Glisky, E. (1995). Computers in memory rehabilitation. In A.D. Baddeley, B.A. Wilson & F. Watts (Eds.). *Handbook of memory disorders*. Chichester: Wiley.

Kapur, N. (1995). Memory aids in rehabilitation of memory disordered patients. In A.D. Baddeley, B.A. Wilson & F. Watts (Eds.). *Handbook of memory disorders*. Chichester: Wiley.

Lincoln, N.B. & Brooks, N. (1992). Assessment for rehabilitation. In B.A.

Wilson & N. Moffat (Eds.). *Clinical management of memory problems*, pp. 32–58. London: Chapman & Hall.

Sohlberg, M.M. & Mateer, C.A. (1989). Training use of compensatory memory books. *Journal of Clinical and Experimental Neuropsychology*, **9** 871–91.

Wilson, B.A. (1991). Long term prognosis of patients with severe memory disorders. *Neuropsychological Rehabilitation*, **1**, 117–34.

Wilson, B.A. (1995). Management and remediation of memory problems in brain injured adults. In A.D. Baddeley, B.A. Wilson & F. Watts (Eds.). *Handbook of memory disorders*. Chichester: Wiley.

Wilson, B.A. & Staples, D. (1992). Working with people with physical handicap. In J. Marzillier & J. Hall (Eds.). *What is Clinical Psychology?* 2nd pp 142–198, Oxford: Oxford University Press.

Wilson, B.A., Cockburn, J., Baddeley, A.D. & Hiorns, R. (1989). The development and validation of a test of everyday memory. *Journal of Clinical and Experimental Neuropsychology*, **11**, 855–70.

Wilson, B.A., Baddeley, A.D., Evans, J.J. & Shiel, A. (1994). Errorless learning in the rehabilitation of memory impaired people. *Neuropsychological Rehabilitation*, **4**, 307–26.

Amputation and phantom limb pain

RONALD MELZACK

Department of Psychology, McGill University, Montreal, Canada

JOEL KATZ

Department of Psychology, Toronto Hospital/General Division, Toronto, Canada

Phantom limbs occur in 95–100% of amputees who lose an arm or leg. The phantom is usually described as having a tingling feeling and a definite shape that resembles the somatosensory experience of the real limb before amputation. It is reported to move through space in much the same way as the normal limb would move when the person walks, sits down, or stretches out on a bed. At first, the phantom limb feels perfectly normal in size and shape, so much so that the amputee may reach out for objects with the phantom hand, or try to step on to the floor with the phantom leg. As time passes, however, the phantom limb begins to change shape. The arm or leg becomes less distinct and may fade away altogether, so that the phantom hand or foot seems to be hanging in mid-air. Sometimes, the limb is slowly 'telescoped' into the stump until only the hand or foot remain at the stump tip (Solonen, 1962). However, the neural basis of the phantom does not disappear. Injury of the stump years or decades after fading or telescoping may suddenly produce a phantom as vivid and full-sized as that felt immediately after amputation (Cohen, 1944).

Amputation is not essential for the occurrence of a phantom. After avulsion of the brachial plexus of the arm, without injury to the arm itself, most patients report a phantom arm (the 'third arm') which is usually extremely painful (Wynn-Parry, 1980). Even nerve destruction is not necessary. About 95% of patients who receive an anesthetic block of the brachial plexus for surgery of the arm report a vivid phantom, usually at the side or over the chest, which is unrelated to the position of the real arm when the eyes are closed but 'jumps' into it when the patient looks at the arm (Melzack & Bromage, 1973). Similarly, a spinal anesthetic block of the lower body produces reports of phantom legs in most patients (Bromage & Melzack, 1974), and total section of the spinal cord at thoracic levels leads to reports of a phantom body including genitalia and many other body parts in virtually all patients (Bors, 1951; Conomy, 1973; Melzack & Loeser, 1978).

PHANTOM LIMB PHENOMENA

The most astonishing feature of the phantom limb is its incredible reality to the amputee (Simmel, 1956), which is enhanced by wearing an artificial arm or leg; the prosthesis feels real, 'fleshed out'. Amputees in whom the phantom leg has begun to 'telescope' into the stump, so that the foot is felt to be above floor level, report that the phantom fills the artificial leg when it is strapped on and the phantom foot now occupies the space of the artificial foot in its shoe (Riddoch, 1941). Patients who have undergone a cleavage of the forearm stump muscles, to permit them to hold objects, report that the phantom hand also has a cleavage and lies appropriately in the stump (Kallio, 1950).

The remarkable reality of the phantom is reinforced by the experience of details of the limb before amputation (Katz & Melzack, 1990). For example, the person may feel a painful bunion that had been on the foot or even a tight ring on a phantom finger. Still more astonishing is the fact that some amputees who receive drugs that produce the tremor of tardive dyskinesia report a tremor in the phantom (Jankovic & Glass, 1985).

Phantoms of other body parts feel just as real as limbs do. Heusner (1950) describes two men who underwent amputation of the penis. One of them, during a 4-year period, was intermittently aware of a painless but always erect phantom penis. The other man had severe pain of the phantom penis. Phantom bladders and rectums have the same quality of reality (Bors, 1951; Dorpat, 1971). The bladder may feel so real that patients, after a bladder removal, sometimes complain of a full bladder and even report that they are urinating. Patients with a phantom rectum may actually feel that they are passing gas or faeces. Menstrual cramps may continue to be felt after a hysterectomy. A painless phantom breast, in which the nipple is the most vivid part, is reported by about 25% of women after a mastectomy and 13% feel pain in the phantom (Kroner et al., 1989).

The reality of the phantom body is evident in paraplegics who suffer a complete break of the spinal cord. Even though they have no somatic sensation or voluntary movement below the level of the break, they often report that they still feel their legs and lower body (Bors, 1951; Burke & Woodward, 1976). The phantom appears to inhabit the body when the person's eyes are open and usually moves co-ordinately with visually perceived movements of the body. Initially, the patient may realize the dissociation between the two when he sees his legs stretched out on the road after an accident yet feels them to be over his chest or head. Later, the phantom becomes co-ordinate with the body, and dissociation is rare.

Descriptions given by amputees and paraplegics indicate the range of the qualities of experience of phantom body parts (Bors, 1951; Katz & Melzack, 1987, 1990). Touch, pressure, warmth, cold and many kinds of pain are common. There are also feelings of itch, tickle, wetness, sweatiness, and tactile texture. Even the experience of fatigue due to movement of the phantom limb is reported (Conomy, 1973). Furthermore, male paraplegics with total spinal sections report feeling erections and paraplegic women describe sexual sensations in the perineal area. Both describe feelings of pleasure, including orgasms (Bors, 1951; Money, 1960; Verkuyl, 1969).

One of the most striking features of the phantom limb or any other body part, including half of the body in many paraplegics, is that it is perceived as an integral part of one's self. Even when a phantom foot dangles 'in mid-air' (without a connecting leg) a few inches below the stump, it still moves appropriately with the other limbs and is unmistakably felt to be part of one's body-self. So, too, the multiple phantoms sometimes felt after an amputation are all part of the self (Lacroix et al., 1992). The fact that the experience of 'self' is subserved by specific brain mechanisms is demonstrated by the converse of a phantom limb, the denial that a part of one's body belongs to one's self. Typically, the person, after a lesion of the right parietal lobe or any of several other brain areas (Mesulam, 1981) denies that a side of the body is part of himself and even ignores the space on that side (Denny-Brown, Meyer & Horenstein, 1952). From these cases, it is evident that the brain processes that underlie the experience of our bodies must impart a special signal that provides the basis for experience of the self. When these brain areas are lost, the person denies that a part of the body belongs to the self. Even when a hand, for example, is pinched hard so that the patient winces or cries out, he still denies that the hand is his.

There is convincing evidence that a substantial number of people who are born without all or part of a limb (congenital limb deficiency) feel a vivid phantom of the missing part. These phantoms are reported by children (Poeck, 1964; Weinstein, Sersen & Vetter, 1964) as well as by adults (Saadah & Melzack, 1994), and possess all the properties of phantoms described by amputees. Furthermore, the phantom may sometimes not appear until maturity, usually after a minor injury or surgery of the deficient limb (Saadah & Melzack, 1994).

The innate neural substrate implied by these data does not mean that learning experience is irrelevant. Learning obviously underlies the fact that people's phantoms often assume the shape of the prosthesis, and people with a deformed leg or a painful corn often report, after amputation, that the phantom is deformed or has a corn. That is, sensory inputs play an important role in the experience of the phantom limb. Heredity and environment clearly act together to produce the phenomena of phantom limbs.

These observations can be summarized in the form of four propositions (Melzack, 1989) which derive from the data:

1. The experience of a phantom limb has the quality of reality because it is produced by the same brain processes that underlie the experience of the body when it is intact.
2. Neural networks in the brain generate all the qualities of experience that are felt to originate in the body; inputs from the body may trigger or modulate the output of the networks but are not essential for any of the qualities of experience.
3. The experience of the body has a unitary, integrated quality which includes the quality of the 'self', that the body is uniquely one's own and not that of any other individual.
4. The neural network that underlies the experience of the body-self is genetically determined but can be modified by sensory experience.

A HYPOTHESIS FOR PHANTOM LIMBS: THE NEUROMATRIX

The anatomical substrate of the body-self, Melzack (1989) proposes, is a network of neurons that extends throughout widespread areas of the brain. He has labelled the network, whose spatial distribution and synaptic links are initially determined genetically, and are later sculpted by sensory inputs, as a 'neuromatrix'. Thalamocortical and limbic loops that comprise the neuromatrix diverge to permit parallel processing in different components of the neuromatrix and converge repeatedly to permit interactions between the output products of processing. The repeated cyclical processing and synthesis of nerve impulses in the neuromatrix imparts a characteristic pattern or 'neurosignature'.

The neurosignature of the neuromatrix is imparted on all nerve impulse patterns that flow through it; the neurosignature is produced by the patterns of synaptic connections, which are initially innate and then modified by experience, in the entire neuromatrix. All inputs from the body undergo cyclical processing and synthesis so that characteristic patterns are impressed on them in the neuromatrix. Portions of the neuromatrix are assumed to be specialized to process information related to major sensory events (such as injury) and may be labelled as neuromodules which impress subsignatures on the larger neurosignature.

PHANTOM LIMB PAIN

About 70% of amputees suffer burning, cramping and other qualities of pain in the first few weeks after amputation. Even seven years after amputation, 50% still continue to suffer phantom limb pain (Krebs et al., 1985). Why is there so much pain in phantom limbs? Melzack (1989) proposes that the active neuromatrix, when deprived of modulating inputs from the limbs or body, produces an abnormal signature pattern that subserves the psychological qualities of hot or burning, the most common qualities of phantom limb pain. Cramping pain, however, may be due to messages from the neuromatrix to produce movement. In the absence of the limbs, the messages to move the muscles may become more frequent and 'stronger' in the attempt to move a part of the limb. The end result of the output message may be felt as cramping muscle pain. Shooting pains may have a similar origin, in which the neuromatrix attempts to move the whole limb and sends out abnormal patterns that are felt as pain shooting down from the groin to the foot. The origins of these pains, then, lie in the brain. Sensory inputs, however, clearly contribute to the phantom: stimulation of the stump or other body sites often produces sensations referred to the phantom limb (Katz & Melzack, 1987).

Surgical removal of the somatosensory areas of the cortex or thalamus generally fails to relieve phantom limb pain (White & Sweet, 1969). However, the new theory conceives of a neuromatrix that extends throughout selective areas of the whole brain, including the somatic, visual and limbic systems. Thus, to destroy the neuromatrix for the body-self which generates the neurosignature pattern for pain is impossible. However, if the pattern for pain is generated by cyclical processing and synthesis, then it should be possible to block it by injection of a local anesthetic into appropriate discrete areas that are hypothesized to comprise the widespread neuromatrix. Data obtained in rats have shown that localized injections of lidocaine into diverse areas, such as the lateral hypothalamus (Tasker et al., 1987), the cingulum (Vaccarino & Melzack, 1989), and the dentate gyrus (McKenna & Melzack, 1992) produce striking decreases in experimentally produced pain, including the pain in an animal model of phantom limb pain (Vaccarino & Melzack, 1991).

REFERENCES

Bors, E. (1951). Phantom limbs of patients with spinal cord injury. *Archives of Neurology and Psychiatry*, **66**, 610–31.

Bromage, P.R. & Melzack, R. (1974). Phantom limbs and the body schema. *Canadian Anesthetists' Society Journal*, **21**, 267–74.

Burke, D.C. & Woodward, J.M. (1976). Pain and phantom sensation in spinal paralysis. *Handbook of Clinical Neurology*, **26**, 489–99.

Cohen, H. (1944). The mechanism of visceral pain. *Transactions of the Medical Society of London*, **64**, 65–99.

Conomy, J.P. (1973). Disorders of body image after spinal cord injury. *Neurology*, **23**, 842–50.

Denny-Brown, D., Meyer, J.S. & Horenstein, S. (1952). The significance of perceptual rivalry resulting from parietal lesion. *Brain*, **75**, 433–71.

Dorpat, T.L. (1971). Phantom sensations of internal organs. *Comprehensive Psychiatry*, **12**, 27–35.

Heusner, A.P. (1950). Phantom genitalia. *Transactions of the American Neurological Association.* **75**, 128–31.

Jankovic, J. & Glass, J.P. (1985). Metoclopramide-induced phantom dyskinesia. *Neurology.* **35**, 432–5.

Kallio, K.E. (1950). Phantom limb of forearm stump cleft by kineplastic surgery. *Acta Chirurgica Scandinavica*, **99**, 121–32.

Katz, J. & Melzack, R. (1987). Referred sensations in chronic pain patients. *Pain*, **28**, 51–9.

Katz, J. & Melzack, R. (1990). Pain 'memories' in phantom limbs: review and clinical observations. *Pain*, **43**, 319–26.

Krebs, B., Jensen, T.S., Kroner, K., Nielsen, J. & Jorgensen, H.S. (1985), Phantom limb phenomena in amputees seven years after limb amputation. In H.L. Fields, R. Dubner, & F. Cervero, (Eds.). *Advances in pain research and therapy*, vol. 9, pp.425–429, New York: Raven Press.

Kroner, K., Krebs, B., Skov, J. & Jorgensen, H.S. (1989). Immediate and long-term phantom breast syndrome after mastectomy: incidence, clinical characteristics and relationship to pre-mastectomy breast pain. *Pain*, **36**, 327–34.

Lacroix, R., Melzack, R., Smith, D. & Mitchell, N. (1992). Multiple phantom limbs in a child. *Cortex*, **28**, 503–7.

McKenna, J.E. & Melzack, R. (1992). Analgesia produced by lidocaine microinjection into the dentate gyrus. *Pain*, **49**, 105–12.

Melzack, R. (1989). Phantom limbs, the self and the brain. *Canadian Psychology*, **30**, 1–16.

Melzack, R. & Bromage, P.R. (1973). Experimental phantom limbs. *Experimental Neurology*, **39**, 261–9.

Melzack, R. & Loeser, J.D. (1978). Phantom body pain in paraplegics: evidence for a central 'pattern generating mechanism'. *Pain*, **4**, 195–210.

Mesulam, M.M. (1981). A cortical network for directed attention and unilateral neglect. *Annals of Neurology*, **10**, 309–15.

Money, J. (1960). Phantom orgasm in the dreams of paraplegic men and women. *Archives of General Psychiatry.* **3**, 373–82.

Poeck, K. (1964). Phantoms following amputation in early childhood and in congenital absence of limbs. *Cortex*, **1**, 269–75.

Riddoch, G. (1941). Phantom limbs and body shape. *Brain*, **64**, 197–222.

Saadah, E.S.M. & Melzack, R. (1994). Phantom limb experiences in congenital limb-deficient adults. *Cortex*, **30**, 479–85.

Simmel, M. (1956). On phantom limbs. *Archives of Neurology and Psychiatry*, **75**, 69–78.

Solonen, K.A. (1962). The phantom phenomenon in amputed Finnish war veterans. *Acta Orthopaedica Scandinavica, Suppl. 54*, 7–37.

Tasker, R.A.R., Choinière, M., Libman, S.M. & Melzack, R. (1987). Analgesia produced by injection of lidocaine into the lateral hypothalamus. *Pain*, **31**, 239–48.

Vaccarino, A.L. & Melzack, R. (1989). Analgesia produced by injection of lidocaine into the anterior cingulum bundle of the rat. *Pain*, **39**, 213–19.

Vaccarino, A.L. & Melzack, R. (1991). The role of the cingulum bundle in self-mutilation following peripheral neurectomy in the rat. *Experimental Neurology*, **111**, 131–4.

Verkuyl, A. (1969). Sexual function in paraplegia and tetraplegia. *Handbook of Clinical Neurology*, **4**, 437–65.

Weinstein, S., Sersen, E.A. & Vetter, R.T. (1964). Phantoms and somatic sensation in cases of congenital aplasia. *Cortex*, **I**, 276–290.

White, J.C. & Sweet, W.H. (1969). *Pain and the neurosurgeon*. Springfield, Illinois: CC Thomas.

Wynn-Parry, C.B. (1980). Pain in avulsion lesions of the brachial plexus. *Pain*, **9**, 41–53.

Anaesthesia

KEITH MILLAR

Behavioural Sciences Group, University of
Glasgow, UK

PSYCHOLOGY AND ANAESTHESIA

Psychology has made significant contributions to two particular fields of anaesthesia research. The first is the assessment of recovery of cognitive and psychomotor functions after anaesthesia. The second is the problem of conscious awareness during the anaesthetic and subsequent memory for surgical events.

Recovery from anaesthesia: method

Some two million general anaesthetics are administered annually in the UK, with 35–40% being suitable for day-care treatment where the patient is admitted, treated and discharged home on the same day. In such cases, it is vital to ensure that recovery from anaesthesia is complete before discharge. Consequently, the tasks and methodological principles derived from decades of human performance research have been applied to assess the degree and duration of anaesthetic impairment (Klepper, Sanders & Rosen, 1991).

The typical methodology for assessment of recovery employs a battery of tests to assess a range of cognitive functions such as vigilance, reaction speed and memory. Prior to anaesthesia and surgery, the patient practises on the tests in order to stabilize performance. A baseline measure is taken to represent the patient's 'normal' performance and with which to compare the postanaesthetic performance. Upon recovering consciousness, the patient performs the tests at regular intervals for between one and four hours: when baseline and postanaesthetic performance do not differ significantly, it is assumed that recovery is complete.

There is, however, a risk that this routine underestimates residual impairment because performance may continue to benefit from practice in the postanaesthetic period. Recovery to the level of performance attained at the preanaesthetic baseline is then an unreliable indicator of 'normal' performance. It is therefore important that a control group of comparable patients, who do not receive anaesthesia, perform the tests at identical intervals to the anaesthesia group to account for improvement in performance with practice. It should be noted that many studies are inconclusive because they fail to attain an adequate methodological standard (see critical reviews by Hindmarch and Bhatti, 1987; Millar, 1992).

Recovery from anaesthesia: test duration and complexity

Duration

The factor of 'time-on-task' is an important determinant of the sensitivity of the task to impairment. Only when performance extends perhaps for 15 to 20 minutes may adverse effects be seen. On short tasks, even when sedated or fatigued, patients can probably pull themselves together sufficiently to perform adequately for a few minutes, and this may give the misleading impression that their faculties have returned to normal.

Many assessments of recovery may have been inaccurate because tasks lengths were too short. Some studies used performance periods of only 60 seconds and bear no resemblance to the real-life conditions encountered by patients when discharged after day-case treatment. While the hospital environment obviously constrains the nature and degree of performance testing, a useful strategy might be to concentrate upon extended performance of one or two tasks, rather than the commonly used battery of assessments.

Complexity and attentional demand

Just as brief tasks may be insensitive so, too, may tasks which are very simple and undemanding. Tasks which require sustained attention may be particularly effective because they provide no opportunity for respite. The demands of complex tasks may also permit the use of relatively shorter performance periods without loss of sensitivity to impairment.

Tasks

These assess primary cognitive and psychomotor abilities relevant to efficient and safe performance of everyday activities. Unfortunately, however, most tasks tend to measure several cognitive functions simultaneously so that, when performance is impaired, it may be unclear which function is affected. Therefore, the lack of a reliable taxonomy of performance tasks can make it difficult to draw conclusions from an individual study or to compare it with other studies.

The tasks applied in recovery studies are legion and a comprehensive review has been provided by Hindmarch and Bhatti (1987). Here, for reasons of space, a summary of important tasks is given in Table 1. Broadly, the tasks assess functions of attention, vigilance and reaction time. Particular note may be made of dual tasks which require patients to divide their attention. Patients may be able to perform the primary task efficiently, but residual impairment is reflected in lengthy responses to the secondary task. The relevance of the task to driving is obvious.

Memory

The problem in summarizing the impairment of memory after anaesthesia derives from a recent review which has shown much of the published research to be of dubious reliability (Ghoneim, Ali & Block, 1990). Few studies include control groups (only 42% of studies reviewed), few are double-blind (only 47%) and very few take

[359]

Table 1. *Commonly used performance tasks in anaesthetic recovery research*

Task	Function/s assessed	Performance
'Dual task': Primary tracking and Secondary reaction time (RT)	Visuo-motor co-ordination Divided attention Reaction speed	Time on target and reaction time to secondary task. When recovering tracking may be maintained but secondary RT is slower, implying reduced attentional capacity.
Digit-symbol substitution (DSST)	Perceptual and motor speed Short-term memory function	From code given on stimulus page, subject substitutes appropriate symbol for digit in rows of digit stimuli. Performance is slower and prone to error during recovery etc.
Reaction time (RT): 1. Simple 2. Choice: serial or discrete	Simple RT: attention and motor speed Choice RT: attention, decision and motor speed	RT is usually slower during early recovery phase. Serial choice RT may be more sensitive because task demands continuous performance and provides no respite.
Letter deletion	Attention and vigilance Memory	Subject scans rows of random letters for designated target. Slower in early recovery
Number matching	Attention and vigilance Memory	Digits are presented at rate of 80/min with designated target to be detected. May be sensitive to impairment even 4 h after anaesthesia.
Maze drawing tracing, co-ordination and dexterity, tapping and 'postbox' test	Visuo-motor co-ordination	Some evidence of impairment in early recovery period, but many studies afflicted by methodological flaws which obscure conclusions

baseline control measures (only 23%). The conceptual approach has yet to encompass current theorizing in working memory.

The typical approach is to use tasks of short-term recall employing verbal or visual material. Whilst many studies do report significant impairment of memory after anaesthesia, it is unclear whether this is a secondary consequence of impaired attentional ability. There is also evidence that poor memory performance may be partly a function of the methodology and stimuli employed. Whilst patients often have poor recall of the contrived materials of conventional memory tests, they may have good recall of salient surgical events and information regarding their immediate clinical circumstances. The implication then is that conventional memory tests may have limited sensitivity in assessing amnesic effects of anaesthesia.

There is reliable evidence, however, concerning the amnesic effects of benzodiazepine drugs which are often administered for sedative or anaesthetic purposes (for review see Ghoneim & Mewaldt, 1990). Such drugs have an anterograde amnesic effect and impair episodic memory, but seem to spare short-term and semantic memory.

Typical recovery profiles

These indicate, hardly surprisingly, that maximal impairment is found in the first 30 to 90 minutes after recovery of consciousness. Whilst modern intravenous anaesthetics have fast recovery characteristics when compared with earlier intravenous and inhalational agents, the recovery of cognitive function may take longer than the supposed 90 minutes. Indeed, some studies show continuing impairment even at 4 hours. It is sobering to note that studies employing 30-minute performance periods in a driving simulator have shown impairment for some 6 to 8 hours after recovering from thiopentone. The few studies that have

extended assessment for several days after surgery have also reported residual impairment of reaction time and attention which may have serious implications for driving safely after anaesthesia. Moreover, as most studies assess average or mean performance of groups of patients, they neglect the fact that some individuals may remain impaired long after the group average performance has apparently returned to normal.

Future studies of recovery might benefit from systematic research to establish a reliable battery of tasks whose sensitivities are catalogued under varying anaesthetic regimes and performance conditions. Moreover, patients should be monitored after discharge to their home in order to monitor everyday cognitive function.

Memory and awareness

A recent report cites the incidence of awareness during non-obstetric anaesthesia to be some 0.2%. This refers to occasions where the patient, upon recovery from the anaesthetic, makes a spontaneous report of memory for incidents such as conversations or incisions and other procedures which occurred during the period when they were ostensibly unconscious. In other words, the patient has an explicit memory for the event of awareness. Such explicit memories may occur because of inadequate anaesthesia due to human error or equipment failure. The extensive literature on the 'ergonomics of anaesthesia' cannot be covered here but is reviewed by Weinger and Englund (1990).

Whilst explicit memories are rare, they may underestimate the true occurrence of intra-operative awareness. It has been proposed that some patients, even when adequately anaesthetised, may register auditory stimuli and retain unconscious memories of intra-operative events. Although inaccessible to conscious recall, it is supposed that such memories may affect the patient's mood and behaviour in an unconscious manner. Clinical case reports have

Table 2. *The nature and outcome of implicit memory tasks commonly used in assessing memory for anaesthesia*

Task	Performance	Evidence of memory for anaesthesia	Result +	−
Stimulus preference	Patient chooses preferred one of several stimuli (eg. musical passages)	Patient prefers stimuli previously presented during anaesthesia	1	2
Word priming				
1. Stem/fragment completion	1. Patient completes word stem e.g. 'our-' or fragment e.g. '—1–d–y'	1. Stems and fragments completed with words given during anaesthesia	3	1
2. Homophones	2. Patient spells spoken homophone (e.g. 'pain' *vs.* 'pane')	2. Patient gives less common spelling according to the context in which homophone was presented during anaesthesia.		
Word production				
1. Category generation	1. Patient names as many instances of category as possible in time limit	1. Intra-anaesthetic presentation of category examplers increases chance of generation	6	10
2. Free association	2. Patient responds to stimulus word with first that comes to mind	2. As above		
Familiarity				
1. General knowledge	1. Patient answers general knowledge questions whose answers were previously presented during anaesthesia	1. Prior presentation of information increases chance of correct answer	1	2
2. 'Famous' names	2. Patient makes judgements of 'fame' or familiarity of names (truly non-famous) presented during anaesthesia	2. Prior presentation of names increases judgements of fame or familiarity.		

Figures in the 'Results' column indicate the number of studies reporting positive ('+') and negative ('−') results for each task.

recorded neurotic disorders supposedly deriving from an unrecognized traumatic episode of intra-operative awareness.

The possibility that the anaesthetized brain may be capable of recording experience has provoked considerable research to determine the reliability of the supposed phenomenon and how it might be prevented (for review see Andrade, 1994). Current theorizing suggests that intra-operative memories (if they exist at all) may be so faint that very subtle retrieval tasks might be required to elicit them. Such tasks assess 'implicit' or 'indirect' memory and have been shown effective in demonstrating unconscious memories in organic amnesic patients. Hitherto, such patients had been thought, erroneously, to be amnesic for previous learning episodes when tested with conventional explicit memory tasks. Indirect memory tests do not depend upon patients having any conscious recall of a previous learning episode. Rather, memory and its retrieval are evidenced by a change in behaviour (often verbal) which indicates the influence of previous exposure to the material in the learning session. Thus prior exposure to a list of words may increase their probability of being given as instances when patients 'free associate' to a category name, or perform word-completion tasks. Table 2 describes implicit memory tasks which have been used in anaesthetic research. Whilst such tests may have been effective in demonstrating unconscious memory in organic amnesic patients, success has been more elusive in anaesthetics studies.

Table 2 also shows the number of positive and negative findings (as determined by the researchers) associated with each test as known to the present author in January 1994. Note that not all the results derive from studies published in peer-reviewed journals, and many of the conclusions have been questioned in critical reviews.

Another approach has presented 'positive suggestions' to the anaesthetised patient that their postsurgical recovery will be rapid and without complications. The intention is to implant an uncon-

scious memory that will influence recovery behaviour. The effectiveness of the suggestions is inferred from differences between control and 'suggestion groups' on measures such as complications and days spent in hospital. Of 19 studies, 12 have reported positive effects, but many of these have been criticized methodologically, and the generality of the effects needs to be replicated. Negative results may be unreliable because of the small sizes of patient samples.

The variable results of psychological assessments of memory for anaesthesia can be ascribed to three primary failings. The cardinal failing has been the omission of a measure of the depth or adequacy of anaesthesia. Positive results may be due to light anaesthesia where the patient is in an analgesic state and in a twilight state of consciousness. Although conscious at the time when auditory stimuli are presented, patients may subsequently be amnesic for the intra-operative events. They may then have no explicit memory but show implicit recall for the material. The misleading conclusion is then drawn that the memory was established during adequate anaesthesia and full unconsciousness.

The second fundamental difficulty lies in establishing absolutely the anaesthetic state. Physiological signs and gross EEG are insensitive. However, recent studies of the brain's cortical auditory evoked response (AER) during anaesthesia have shown great promise. They indicate that at certain concentrations of a given anaesthetic drug, the sensitivity of the brain to auditory events is reduced. Memory for such events would therefore seem less likely. A very recent study has shown great ingenuity in employing a recognition memory test during states of increasing anaesthesic concentration to demonstrate that memory function is lost as the drug concentration increases and the AER shows decreasing responsivity.

The latter finding is important in light of the third factor which underlies variable results. In a review, Merikle and Rondi (1993) have widely criticized previous studies for their methodological and conceptual inadequacies regarding memory and unconscious processes. The reader will find an excellent model for future research in their review.

Research into the phenomenon of memory and awareness in anaesthesia offers fascinating insights to the ability of the sedated brain to conduct complex processing of verbal material. Continuing studies which are employing electrophysiological and behavioural measures may establish whether the fully anaesthetized brain has similar abilities.

REFERENCES

Andrade, J. (1994). Learning during anaesthesia: a review. *British Journal of Psychology*, 86, 479–506.

Ghoneim, M.M. & Mewaldt, S.P. (1990). Benzodiazepines and human memory: a review. *Anesthesiology*, 72, 926–8.

Ghoneim, M.M., Ali, M.A. & Block, R.I. (1990). Appraisal of the quality of assessment of memory in anesthesia and psychopharmacology literature. *Anesthesiology*, 73, 815–20.

Hindmarch, I. & Bhatti, J. (1987). Recovery of cognitive and psychomotor function following anaesthesia. A review. In I. Hindmarch, J.G. Jones & E. Moss (Eds.). *Aspects of recovery from anaesthesia*, pp. 113–165. Chichester: John Wiley.

Klepper, I.D., Sanders, L.D. & Rosen, M. (1991). *Ambulatory anaesthesia and sedation: impairment and recovery*. Oxford: Blackwell.

Merikle, P.M. & Rondi, G. (1993). Memory for events during anesthesia has not been demonstrated: a psychologist's view. In P.S. Sebel, B. Bonke & E. Winograd (Eds.). *Memory and awareness in anesthesia*, pp. 476–497, Englewood Cliffs NJ: Prentice Hall.

Millar, K. (1992). The effects of anaesthetic and analgesic drugs. In A.P. Smith & D.M. Jones (Eds.). *Handbook of human performance: Volume 2, Health and performance*. pp. 337–385. London: Academic Press.

Weinger, M.B. & Englund, C.E. (1990). Ergonomic and human factors affecting anesthetic vigilance and monitoring in the operating room environment *Anesthesiology*, 73, 995–1021.

Androgens

JOHN ARCHER

Department of Psychology, University of Central Lancashire, Preston, UK

Androgen is the general name for hormones whose action stimulates the development of male characteristics, including the male reproductive system, general somatic features (such as muscle development, via an anabolic effect on protein metabolism), secondary sexual characteristics (such as body hair) and behaviour. The main androgen secreted by the testes is testosterone, although there are smaller amounts of other hormones with weaker androgenic action, such as androstenedione and dehydroepiandrosterone. Larger quantities of these hormones are secreted by the adrenals of both sexes and by the ovaries, both of which also secrete small amounts of testosterone. For example, 5% of plasma testosterone in the human male comes from the adrenal cortex.

In foetal life, the testis (under the influence of the Y chromosome) produces testosterone, which stimulates the development of the male internal organs (at around three months after conception): a little later, the androgen dihydrotestosterone stimulates the development of the external genitals. There are also a marked increase in testosterone secretion in the months following birth, but its significance is unknown. It is known that foetal or early neonatal androgens influence the central nervous system in rodents and non-human primates, one result of which is that males and females show different levels of rough-and-tumble play (as do humans); another is that the nervous system is primed so that various physiological and behavioural changes occur at puberty under the influence of testosterone. Such delayed actions of early hormones are called 'organizing' effects, to distinguish them from more direct actions, or activational effects.

The direct actions of androgens on behaviour are much better understood in certain rodents, primates and ungulates than they are in humans, where there is much speculation and debate, and preliminary evidence concerning sexuality, aggression, personality and cognition.

Studies measuring circulating testosterone levels and self-reported sexual activity have found inconsistent results, although there is clear evidence of an association in a pubertal sample and in one of older men (Hubert, 1990). Where penile tumescence was measured, a clear association with testosterone levels was found within the normal range. There is also evidence of an increase in frequency of sexual thoughts among low androgen men treated with exogenous testosterone (O'Carroll, Shapiro & Bancroft, 1985; O'Carroll & Bancroft, 1984). Several studies have shown an association between circulating testosterone levels and measures of female sexuality, although there is no association between estrogens and female sexuality (Hubert, 1990).

There is clear evidence for a causal link with aggression for several animal species, but the evidence linking testosterone and aggression for humans is correlational. A meta-analysis of studies involving ratings by other people showed a weighted mean of 0.38 (Archer, 1991). Since success in competitive and aggressive encounters produces increased testosterone levels, the correlation could have arisen from testosterone being increased as a consequence of being aggressive rather than causing aggressiveness (Archer, 1994).

There is also evidence for an association between testosterone and spatial ability in young men, although there are also failures to confirm this (Hubert, 1990). Animal studies have linked testosterone with persistence in a motivated task. Several studies have reported an increase in positive mood after androgen administration, and this is consistent with correlational studies. There is also preliminary data indicating a lower emotional response to stress among young males with higher testosterone levels (Hubert, 1990).

A large-scale study of US military veterans (Dabbs & Morris, 1990) has found that testosterone levels were associated with a history of physical aggression, having many sexual partners, and drug and alcohol use, fitting other findings linking testosterone to sensation seeking (Daitzman & Zuckerman, 1980). In the same sample, testosterone was inversely correlated with occupational status (Dabbs, 1992), suggesting that high testosterone levels may in some way inhibit occupational achievement.

REFERENCES

Archer, J. (1991). The influence of testosterone on human aggression. *British Journal of Psychology*, 82, 1–28.

Archer, J. (1994). Testosterone and aggression: a theoretical review. *Journal of Offender Rehabilitation*, 21, 1–25.

Dabbs, J.M. Jr. (1992). Testosterone and occupational achievement. *Social Forces*, 70, 813–24.

Dabbs, J.M. Jr. & Morris, R. (1990). Testosterone, social class, and antisocial behavior in a sample of 4,462 men. *Psychological Science*, 1, 209–211.

Daitzman, R. & Zuckerman, M. (1980). Disinhibitory sensation seeking, personality and gonadal hormones. *Personality and Individual Differences*, 1, 103–10.

Hubert, W. (1990). Psychotropic effects of testosterone. In E. Nieschlag & H.M. Behre (Eds.). *Testosterone – action, deficiency, substitution*, pp. 51–69. Berlin, Heidelberg & New York: Springer-Verlag.

O'Carroll, R. & Bancroft, J. (1984). Testosterone therapy for low sexual interest and erectile dysfunction in men: a controlled study. *British Journal of Psychiatry*, 145, 146–51.

O'Carroll, R., Shapiro, C. & Bancroft, J. (1985). Androgens, behavior and nocturnal erection in hypogonadal men: the effects of varying the replacement dose. *Clinical Endocrinology*, 23, 527–38.

Anorexia nervosa and bulimia

JANE WARDLE

University College London,
Health Behaviour Unit
Department of Epidemiology and Public Health,
UK

DIAGNOSIS

There are a number of different classification systems for eating disorders, but the American Psychiatric Association's diagnostic criteria (the *Diagnostic and Statistical Manuals, DSM*), in the third revision (American Psychiatric Association, 1987), have come to be the most widely used. The DSMIIIR diagnostic criteria for anorexia nervosa include (i) refusal to maintain body weight above 85% of the expected level, (ii) intense fear of weight gain, (iii) disturbance of body image and (iv) amenorrhoea for at least three months. A classification into subtypes of anorexia, characterized by the presence or absence of bulimic episodes, is proposed in the latest revision of DSM (*DSMIV*). The DSMIIIR criteria for a diagnosis of bulimia nervosa include (i) at least two bulimic episodes a week for at least 3 months, (ii) lack of control over eating, (iii) behaviour designed to avoid weight gain and (iv) persistent over-concern about weight. As is apparent from the core clinical features, anorexia and bulimia have a number of common psychopathological features. Intense concern about weight and fear of weight gain are characteristic of both disorders, as is the use of extreme weight control behaviours (strict dieting, laxatives, vigorous exercise). Bulimic episodes are also reported by 40–50% of anorexic patients. Clearly, it is possible for an individual to meet criteria for both disorders if they are both underweight and binge, but this is resolved in DSMIV by giving primacy to anorexia nervosa; a diagnosis of bulimia nervosa will require that the patient should not meet the criteria for anorexia nervosa. Psychiatric diagnoses are usually based on a clinical interview, but the Eating Disorder Examination, which is a structured interview designed to assess the present state of eating disorder pathology, includes objective criteria to generate the DSM diagnoses (Fairburn & Cooper, 1993).

EPIDEMIOLOGY

Eating disorders represent one of the most common psychiatric diagnosis in young women in western countries. In a study of case registration in primary care in The Netherlands, an annual incidence of 6.3 per 100 000 for anorexia and 9.9 per 100 000 for bulimia was reported (Hoek, 1991), with the highest rates in young women from urban environments. Eating disorders are unique among psychiatric conditions in having a very strong gender bias. Both clinical case series and community studies suggest a 10 : 1 ratio of women to men. Eating disorders are also unusual in being more common among higher social class groups, although there is some evidence for a progressive diminution of the social class bias. The other unusual characteristic is that there appears to have been a substantial increase in the incidence of anorexia over this century, although some of this apparent increase may be attributable to changes in diagnostic practices. Bulimia nervosa, was only identified as a distinct disorder in 1979 (Russell, 1979), so extensive data on historical trends are not available. Nevertheless, it seems likely that, if bulimia nervosa had always been as prevalent as it is today, it would have been described earlier. Finally, cross-cultural studies suggest that westernization is associated with substantially higher rates of eating disorders.

AETIOLOGY

Aetiological theories of eating disorders have ranged from the purely biological (an underlying hypothalamic disorder), through the psychodynamic and family systems approaches, to the purely social (eating disorder as an expression of the cultural meaning of thinness). There are well-established biological abnormalities associated with both anorexia and bulimia connected with both the low body weight and the abnormal eating and vomiting practices. Disturbances at all levels of the hypothalamic–pituitary–adrenal axis have been identified in patients with anorexia nervosa, and similar, although often smaller, changes have been associated with bulimia. Changes in adrenergic, dopaminergic and neuropeptide systems have also been observed. It has proved difficult to establish the role of neuro-endocrine abnormalities in the aetiology of eating disorders, but the consensus is that they are secondary to the weight loss and caloric restriction, and as such are effects, rather than causes, of eating disorders.

There has always been a stronger emphasis on a sociocultural aetiology for eating disorders than for most other psychiatric disorders. This has stemmed in part from the epidemiological findings; biological causes, it is argued, neither distribute themselves in such a fashion across gender, class or culture, nor change rapidly enough to cause the observed increases in eating disorders. The sociocultural hypothesis has also been supported by observations of continuities between the clinical features of eating disorders and the weight dissatisfaction reported by many normal women. In the most 'at risk' age-group (young adult women), extreme dietary restriction is quite customary, while binge-eating and even self-induced vomiting, are not uncommon. However, most authorities recognize a disjunction between weight-preoccupied women and eating disordered women, both in the specific psychopathology of eating and the associated features of depression, anxiety, and obsessional features (Garner *et al.*, 1984). Feminist analyses of eating disorders have also supported the sociocultural view, with an emphasis on dieting and binge-eating as understandable responses by women to the constraints of women's social roles and to the cultural ideals of female beauty (Orbach, 1986). However, feminist writings have represented self-starvation in terms of both extreme compliance with the cultural ideals of femininity (aspiring to the thin physique) and rejection of the female sexual role (refusal to maintain a womanly physique), leaving uncertainty as to which of these analyses offers the most useful insights.

One difficulty with the sociocultural analysis derives from uncertainty over what information would cause it to be rejected. Other disorders such as heart disease show gender, social class, and cul-

tural variation, as well as changes in prevalence over time. Nevertheless, while it is acknowledged that roles and cultures provide the context which influences behaviour and hence risk factors and disease, the aetiology is usually analysed at the level of biological processes.

In practice, most aetiological accounts of the development of eating disorders draw on social, behavioural and biological factors in a dynamic process. The changes in fat distribution in adolescent girls, particularly among those who have a larger build, provide the foundations for dissatisfaction. A social and family environment in which there is an emphasis on the desirability of slimness, foster weight dissatisfaction. At the individual level, certain personality constellations (e.g. perfectionism) combined with stressful life events, may further the decision to diet. Once food restriction and weight loss begin, new and different biological and psychological factors come into play. Starvation and loss of fat stores result in a range of metabolic and neuroendocrine responses, which can be associated with physical and psychological changes. Once weight loss has occurred, many patients become more, not less, weight-phobic as they adapt to a new body shape in which the skeleton is prominently visible. Any fatness comes to be regarded with horror and some patients seek ever lower weights to provide a margin of safety. In some cases appetite is reduced, but many patients experience stronger urges to eat, creating a new fear of loss of control. If binge eating develops, the patient's focus usually shifts to preoccupation with what is experienced as an increasingly out-of-control appetite. Self-induced vomiting, if it is part of the pathology, is usually initiated after the onset of binge-eating, and often as a temporary solution to the effects of overeating. However, through learned modifications of appetite, vomiting can come to perpetuate binge-eating and has been associated with an increase in binge size.

TREATMENT OF EATING DISORDERS

A range of treatments have been used for eating disorders, ranging from force-feeding to family therapy. Most authorities now agree that treatment must address both the eating behaviour and the attitudes towards weight and shape which perpetuate the disorder. The APA has prepared practice guidelines (American Psychiatric Association, 1992) which are not a treatment manual, but a set of evidence-based recommendations for good practice in the management of eating disorders.

Restoration of normal body weight is always a priority in anorexia, and many of the biological and psychological disturbances are diminished after re-feeding. When body weight is low enough to be life threatening, a hyper-caloric regimen may be imposed, resulting in rapid weight gain, but this is no longer widely recommended. In the classic behaviour-modification approaches, weight restoration was reinforced through increasing access to privileges or, in the case of in outpatient programmes, through avoidance of hospitalization. However, these stringent regimes have tended to be replaced with the provision of a more supportive 'milieu', using staff who are both experienced with, and sympathetic to, eating disordered patients. This kind of approach appears to be associated with equally rapid weight restoration (Eckert *et al.*, 1979). In parallel with weight restoration, treatment directed towards helping the patient to accept a normal body weight and to develop a more positive body image is provided. Cognitive or 'psychoeducational' approaches have become the most widely used method for modification of attitudes both for anorexia and bulimia (Garner & Bernis, 1985; Garner *et al.*, 1985).

Where binge eating is a major feature of the disorder, the treatment must usually encompass both the dietary restriction which could perpetuate the binge eating (i.e. the patient must learn to be less restrictive) and the binge eating itself, which, along with self-induced vomiting may have become a self-sustaining practice. Several different cognitive–behavioural approaches have been used, including exposure to food with prevention of excessive eating, exposure to overeating with prevention of vomiting, and training in self-management (i.e. avoidance of food cues, high risk situations).

The contribution of pharmacological treatments to the management of eating disorders is controversial. Some authorities have argued that antidepressant treatment could achieve fundamental correction of a basic neurochemical abnormality and hence offer a valuable therapeutic tool. Most, however, regard pharmacological treatment as essentially supplementary, addressing secondary depression or comorbid conditions.

TREATMENT OUTCOME

There are few controlled trials of the outcome of treatment for anorexia primarily because it is a comparatively rare disorder, but also because consensus was reached early on as to the basic elements of treatment. However, although in the shorter term most treatment approaches can achieve weight restoration, the high relapse rate and poor long-term outcome suggests that better treatments are still required (Hsu, 1980). Many anorexic patients lose weight again as soon as they are discharged and readmission rates exceed 50%. Longer-term follow-up studies show that the majority of anorexic patients, even those whose weight is restored to normal levels, have persistent preoccupation with food and weight, and many have obsessional, social or mood disturbances. No more than 50% of the patients in most longer-term follow-up series achieve a good clinical outcome, and there is substantial mortality associated with cardiovascular complications and suicide. Superior treatment outcomes are associated both with less severe disorders and a better level of general adjustment and family support, but there are no specific indicators of a good prognosis. The symptoms which persist are those which are specific to eating disorders (*e.g.* fear of fatness), which suggests that current treatment approaches are not adequate to the task of modifying the fundamental dysfunctional attitudes. Consequently, there is scope for considerable improvement in treatment efficacy and a need for careful studies of the predictors of treatment outcomes.

There have been many more controlled trials of the treatment of bulimia nervosa, which is both more prevalent, and was initially considered to be more difficult to treat. The predominant treatment approach has been cognitive–behavioural and improvements in attitudes towards eating and weight and binge frequency are almost always reported in the short term. Comparisons between cognitive–behavioural and other treatment approaches (usually other forms of psychotherapy) have not always found differential efficacy, but there is often common ground in the treatments. When treatment communalities are reduced to a minimum, there is evidence for a significantly better outcome for cognitive–behavioural compared with psychodynamic treatments (Wilson & Fairburn, 1993), but non-specific aspects of treatment are still contributing substantially to the outcome. As is the case for treatment for anorexia, longer-term evaluations have not produced entirely favourable results, and complete remission of symptoms is the exception.

REFERENCES

American Psychiatric Association (1987). *Diagnostic and statistical manual of mental disorders* (3rd edn rev). Washington, DC: American Psychiatric Association.

American Psychiatric Association (1992). Practice guidelines for eating disorders. *American Journal of Psychiatry*, 150, 207–28.

Eckert, E.D., Goldberg, S.C., Halmi, K.A., Casper, R.C. & Davis, J.M. (1979). Behavior therapy and anorexia nervosa. *British Journal of Psychiatry*, 134, 55–9.

Fairburn, C.G. & Cooper, Z. (1993). The eating disorder examination. In *Binge eating: nature, assessment and treatment.* New York: Guilford.

Garner, D.M. & Bernis, K.M. (1985). Cognitive therapy for anorexia nervosa. In D.M. Garner & P.E. Garfinkel (Eds.). *Handbook of psychotherapy for anorexia nervosa and bulimia* pp. 107–146. New York: The Guilford Press.

Garner, D.M., Olmsted, M.P., Polivy, J. & Garfinkel, P.E. (1984). Comparison between weight-preoccupied women and anorexia nervosa. *Psychomatic Medicine*, 46, 255–60.

Garner, D.M., Rockert, W., Olmsted, M.P., Johnson, C. & Coscina, D.V. (1985). Psychoeducational principles in the treatment of bulimia and anorexia nervosa. In D.M. Garner & P.E. Garfinkel (Eds.). *Handbook of psychotherapy for anorexia nervosa and bulimia* pp. 107–146. New York: The Guilford Press.

Hoek, H.W. (1991). The incidence and prevalence of anorexia nervosa and bulimia nervosa in primary care. *Psychological Medicine* 21, 455–60.

Hsu, L.K.G. (1980). Outcome of anorexia nervosa. *Archives of General Psychiatry*, 37, 1041–6.

Orbach, S. (1986). *The anorexic's struggle as a metaphor for our age.* New York: W W Norton.

Russell, G. (1979). Bulimia nervosa; an ominous variant of anorexia nervosa. *Psychological Medicine*, 9 429–48.

Wilson, G.T. & Fairburn, C.G. (1993). Cognitive treatments for eating disorders. *Journal of Consulting and Clinical Psychology*, 61, 261–9.

Anorexia nervosa and bulimia

Antenatal care

JENNY HEWISON

Department of Psychology, University of Leeds,
UK

The main purpose of antenatal care is to monitor the course of pregnancy, and to manage any problems that arise. In the UK, blood and urine samples are analysed at regular intervals, blood pressure measurements are taken, the baby's heartbeat is monitored, and ultrasound scans are performed. Diet and smoking are discussed. Prenatal screening and diagnostic testing may be offered, and at a later stage, plans are made for the delivery and care of the baby. Antenatal classes are usually available, and health professionals of different kinds (midwives, general practitioners, obstetricians) provide information and support in hospital or community settings.

Most pregnancies are normal and have a wholly satisfactory outcome for mother and baby. Although it is often argued that this is the result of antenatal care, this is very hard to prove. Women cannot be obliged to attend for antenatal care, and even within the UK, the minority of women who do not attend, or who attend late, have more pre-existing risk factors (e.g. smoker, very young mother) than those who attend from early in pregnancy. After adjusting for such risk factors, no relationship was found in a large UK birth cohort study between delayed attendance (after 28 weeks of pregnancy) and any important indicator of pregnancy outcome (Thomas, Golding & Peters, 1991). Scientific evaluation of the various components of antenatal care has shown many of them to be 'of dubious value' (Steer, 1993). None the less, women in Britain continue to have an average of 15 antenatal checks during pregnancy. It is likely that no more than five are necessary, plus simple blood pressure checking in the last three months. To quote Steer (a professor of obstetrics and gynaecology): 'Why then has such a pattern of largely ineffective ritual persisted in antenatal care?' Steer thinks the answer is psychological: women are believed to like the present arrangements and find them reassuring, and doctors and midwives are thought to be afraid of missing something if they fail to conform to the expected pattern of care, essentially unchanged from that specified by Dame Janet Campbell in the 1920s.

Even if antenatal care is of limited value for most women, its screening function does result in the identification of a small proportion of pregnancies in which there are problems, e.g. diabetes of pregnancy, or a genetic abnormality in the foetus. Over the last 40 years, antenatal care has become more and more clearly devoted to identifying such problem pregnancies. It is probably fair to say, as many midwives as well as social scientists have said, that the social and psychological needs of women, especially the great majority who are low risk, have been neglected in pursuit of this goal (Garcia, 1982). Not only, it seems, have women been persuaded that 15 antenatal checks are necessary, they have also been persuaded that a medically oriented and often impersonal style of care is the price to be paid for the surveillance that they require.

This picture is currently changing. An influential report has recommended that the maternity services become more woman centred (Department of Health, 1993). A greater role is envisaged for midwives, care is to be shifted from hospital to community services, and efforts are to be made to provide more continuity of care. These changes are being justified not only on the grounds that women would prefer the new kind of care but also that it would be more supportive, and would lead to improved pregnancy outcomes.

The change in the service is too recent to be reflected in the evaluation literature. However, a meta-analysis (Elbourne, Oakley & Chalmers, 1989) of the results of controlled trials carried out prior to 1989 suggested that women who received enhanced support were less likely than controls to feel unhappy, nervous and worried during pregnancy, and more likely to feel 'in control' during their pregnancy, to be satisfied with their care, and to report that they had enjoyed a worry-free labour. After delivery, they were less likely to be unhappy, and more likely to be breastfeeding and to feel 'in control'. Their partners were also more likely to be involved in the baby's care.

It has sometimes been claimed that physical indicators such as preterm delivery and low birthweight could also be changed as a result of enhanced social and psychological support during pregnancy. These claims have not been supported in meta-analyses (Elbourne *et al.*, 1989), or in a large recent study of pregnancies at high risk due to poor psychosocial circumstances (Villar *et al.*, 1992), but other studies have found modest effects, or effects confined to subgroups of women (Oakley, Rajan & Grant, 1990).

Non-experimental studies have repeatedly shown an association between social background factors, stress, and reproductive outcomes (Elbourne *et al.*, 1989). In a sample of predominantly white middle class women, Wadhwa *et al.* (1993) found that, independently of medical risk factors, life event stress was negatively correlated with infant birthweight, and that women who reported high levels of pregnancy-related anxiety were more likely to have a preterm baby. In a large Danish study, after allowing for other confounding factors, psychological distress in late pregnancy was found to be associated with an increased risk of preterm delivery (Hedegaard *et al.*, 1993). The physiological mechanisms mediating the relationships between psychological distress and birth outcomes are not understood (Wadhwa *et al.*, 1993).

Psychological distress in the antenatal period is also a predictor of postnatal distress (Green, 1990). Further research is needed into how antenatal care might help to reduce distress, both as an end in itself, and as a potential means of improving the physical and the psychological outcomes of pregnancy.

Providing more supportive antenatal care is time consuming.

Providing proper counselling for women about the screening tests now available is time consuming too, as is encouraging them to stop smoking. The reorganization of maternity services provides an opportunity for midwives and doctors to omit much of the routine weighing and measuring from antenatal care, and spend the time saved on interventions such as these, which have real potential for improving pregnancy outcomes for both mothers and babies (Steer, 1993).

REFERENCES

Department of Health (1993). *Changing childbirth: report of the expert maternity group.* London: HMSO.

Elbourne, D., Oakley, A. & Chalmers, I. (1989). Social and psychological support during pregnancy. In M. Enkin, M.J.N.C. Keirse & I. Chalmers, (Eds.). *Effective care in pregnancy and childbirth*, pp. 221–236. Oxford: Oxford University Press.

Garcia, J. (1982). Women's views of antenatal care. In M. Enkin & I. Chalmers (Eds.). *Effectiveness and satisfaction in antenatal care*, pp. 81–91. London: William Heinemann Medical Books.

Green, J.M. (1990). 'Who is unhappy after childbirth?': antenatal and intrapartum correlates from a prospective study. *Journal of Reproductive and Infant Psychology*, 8, 175–83.

Hedegaard, M., Henriksen T.B., Sabroe, S. & Secher, N.J. (1993). Psychological distress in pregnancy and preterm delivery. *British Medical Journal*, 307, 234–9.

Oakley, A., Rajan, L. & Grant, A. (1990). Social support and pregnancy outcome. *British Journal of Obstetrics and Gynaecology*, 97, 155–62.

Steer, P. (1993). Rituals in antenatal care – do we need them? *British Medical Journal*, 307, 697–8.

Thomas, P., Golding, J. & Peters, T.J. (1991). Delayed antenatal care: does it affect pregnancy outcome? *Social Science and Medicine*, 32, 715–23.

Villar, J., Farnot, U., Barros, F., Victora, C., Langer, A. & Belizan, J.M. (1992). A randomized trial of psychosocial support during high risk pregnancies. *The New England Journal of Medicine*, 327, 1266–71.

Wadhwa, P.D., Sandman, C.A., Porto, M., Dunkel-Schetter, C. & Garite, T.J. (1993). The association between prenatal stress and infant birth weight and gestational age at birth: a prospective investigation. *American Journal of Obstetrics and Gynecology*, 169, 858–65.

Aphasia

CHRIS CODE

*Brain Damage and Communication Research,
School of Communication Disorders, University of
Sydney, Australia*

Aphasia is the generic term used to describe the common range of language impairments which can follow left hemisphere brain damage that can be described in terms of disorders of the core components of a linguistic model: features like semantics, syntax, morphology, phonology. Neurological damage can also cause a range of communication problems which do not directly effect straight linguistic aspects of language, such as right hemisphere language impairments and dysarthria (i.e. articulation impairment). This chapter will outline the recovery from, psychosocial adjustment to, and therapy for, aphasia.

RECOVERY

Most research into recovery from aphasia has been without reference to any theoretical model. Group studies have shown that most aphasic people make some recovery, yet most studies have used operational definitions, based on a groups' improved performance on a test battery (Basso, 1992; Code, Rowley & Kertesz, 1994).

Such operational definitions, like change in an Overall Score or Aphasia Quotient on a psychometric battery are used widely, but do not help improve understanding of the cognitive processes which underlie recovery. One hypothesis (Le Vere, 1980) is that recovery is best seen as neural sparing and distinguishes between 'losses' which simply cannot be recovered, and behavioural deficits which are the result of attempts to shift control to undamaged neural systems. Real recovery requires the sparing of the underlying neural tissue. Behavioural deficits, the characteristics or symptoms of aphasia for instance, are compensatory. Recovery for an individual therefore may occur through a combination of restitution of lost cognitive functions or compensation for lost functions.

There have been three basic approaches to predicting recovery. A range of prognostic factors have been identified but reviews complain (Code, 1987; Basso, 1992) that on many of them there is disagreement. Such factors as severity, aphasia type, site and extent of lesion, presence of dysarthria and bilateral damage, are clearly interrelated and probably interdependent (Code, 1987). There is considerable controversy as to whether some are useful theoretical constructs (e.g. type of aphasia). For several, such as age, sex and handedness there is considerable disagreement between studies regarding their prognostic value (Basso, 1992). Some recovery studies have included very heterogenous groups of patients, including a wide range of ages and aetiologies. Very young subjects have been grouped with 90-year olds and closed head injuries grouped with stroke. Some have used basic clinical ratings to determine severity, some standardised tests.

A second approach involves classification into aphasia type. If type is known then some prognosis can be made. However, up to 30% of patients are not classifiable, many change type with recovery and many do not recover in predictable ways. Fundamentally, milder types ('Conduction', 'Transcortical', 'Anomia') have the best prognosis and severe types ('Global', 'Broca's', 'Wernicke's') have the least hopeful. However, type correlates highly with severity.

Thirdly, Porch *et al.* (1980) developed a statistical approach to predict a likely recovery entailing detailed analysis of scores on the *Porch Index of Communicative Abilities* (the PICA) (Porch, 1967), a standardized aphasia test. Using multiple regression, they demonstrated that PICA scores at 1 month postonset could predict an overall PICA score at 3, 6, and 12 months postonset with correlations ranging from .74 to .94. Code *et al.* (1994) have examined the application of neural networks to predicting recovery, and initial results suggest that this method is superior to standard statistical approaches, and offers the possibility of comparing a range of possible models of aphasia through 'lesioning'

Clinicians and patients are not just interested in psychometric recovery but also in ability to cope, to get by, to function; which is what really matters to the patient and family. Recovery of these aspects of communication have hardly been researched at all.

THERAPY

Generally treatment aims either for restitution (or re-establishment) of lost functions or compensation (or substitution) for lost functions (Code & Muller, 1989a). Therapists may employ specific re-organizational methods to achieve re-establishment or compensation. Aphasia therapy utilizes aspects of education, learning theory, counselling, linguistics, neuropsychology and cognitive psychology. Following Howard and Hatfield (1987), we can classify approaches into several main methodologies, although in practice most clinicians adopt a fairly eclectic approach. Didactic methods aim to reteach language utilizing traditional and intuitive educational methods from child and foreign-language teaching. Overlapping didactic methods are essentially atheoretical behavioural methods like imitation and modelling, prompting and cuing, and the use of reinforcement. These techniques are universally used by therapists who would take offence at being called 'behaviourists'. They are utilised in some hierarchically organised therapy approaches for apraxia of speech and contemporary computer based methods use systematic behavioural methods (see chapters in Code & Muller, 1989b, 1995, Helm-Estabrooks & Albert, 1991).

Language stimulation is also universally used. On this view language functions are not seen to be lost but inaccessible. Language performance is impaired but language competence has survived. Therapy involves facilitating and stimulating language use. If improvement occurs, it is because the patient does not relearn lost vocabulary or syntactic forms, but facilitates and integrates what he or she already knows. Intense auditory stimulation, maximum response from the patient and repetition, facilitation and various types of cuing are general features. The widely used facilitation techniques of repetition and phonemic cuing (i.e. providing the patient with the first phoneme of a target word) have a marked immediate effect on naming, but the effect wears off within minutes and the patient's naming is just as poor as before the stimulation (Code & Muller, 1989b).

Luria's (1970) neuropsychological model forms the basis for an approach to the re-organisation of function. Intact functional sub-systems can substitute for impaired subsystems. For instance, 'articulograms', which are drawings of the lips producing particular com-

binations of speech sounds, have been developed for severe apraxia of speech. Here the patient makes use of an intact visual route into the speech production system.

Approaches exist based on surviving right hemisphere processing, which are mostly reorganizational and aim to compensate for lost functions (Code, 1987, 1994a, b). Melodic Intonation Therapy (Helm-Estabrooks & Albert, 1991), for instance, tries to re-establish some speech in patients with apraxic problems by reorganization of the speech production process using intoned speech. Artificial languages have been developed made up of arbitrary visual shapes and symbols. Significant success is claimed with globally impaired patients being able to use such systems for propositional communication. Heightening of right hemisphere visual imagery and the use of hypnosis have also been advocated in aphasia therapy. There have also been attempts to directly influence right hemisphere processing and stimulate latent right hemisphere language using dichotic listening, and divided visual field techniques (Code, 1994a, b).

For most patients, linguistic levels are affected with pragmatic and functional language often spared. For patients whose problems are so severe that they fail to make progress with restitution, therapists have developed compensatory methods for lost functions. The PACE (promoting aphasics communicative efficiency) approach (Davis & Wilcox, 1985; Carlomagno, 1994) has a large following where the emphasis is on successful communication, not correct oral naming or grammar. PACE mainly entails (i) therapist and patient participating equally as message sender and receiver; (ii) therapeutic interactions involve the exchange of new information; (iii) patients choose the communication modality or methods; (iv) feedback is based on success in communicating the message. Typically writing, gesture, drawing, pointing, are encouraged; in fact any available means to communicate the message. There are a range of treatment studies using gesture and drawing (Helm-Estabrook & Albert, 1991) and studies of the efficacy of PACE (Carlomagno, 1994). Group therapy is often considered relevant for functional communication (see chapters in Chapey, 1987, 1994; Code & Muller, 1989b, 1995).

The neurolinguistic approach covers methods which grew from the developments in linguistics in the 1960s. At this time linguistic characterizations of aphasia began to be taken seriously. Many studies of treatment have concentrated on linguistic characterizations of the patient's problems and targeted specific impaired linguistic features. In practice this has meant linguistically inspired treatment for the various manifestations of grammatical impairment, and examples can be found in Code and Muller (1989a, b 1995), Helm-Estabrooks and Albert (1991), and Howard and Hatfield (1987).

The progress of cognitive neuropsychology has strongly influenced development of an hypothesis-driven single case assessment process, based on an information processing model. The contention is that standardized assessment can provide only inadequate information on the specific deficits underlying individual impairment. Hypotheses concerning impairments must be tested using psycholinguistically controlled tests, and such resources have been developed (Kay, Lesser & Coltheart, 1992). The alternative view is that standardized and reliable tests should provide a baseline against which to measure change (Shallice, 1979). Batteries may be best seen as standardized and reliable screens providing a basic profile and to pinpoint areas for detailed investigation.

Howard and Patterson (1990) outline three strategies for therapy inspired by the cognitive neuropsychological model: (i) reteaching of the missing information, missing rules or procedures based on detailed testing; (ii) teaching a different way to do the same task; (iii) facilitating the use of impaired access routes. Research suggests that patient- and deficit-specific treatment can improve performance in patients which can not be accounted for in terms of spontaneous recovery or non-specific effects (Howard & Hatfield, 1987).

PSYCHOSOCIAL AND EMOTIONAL ADJUSTMENT

Research is beginning to show that recovery and response to rehabilitation in aphasia are probably significantly influenced by emotional and psychosocial factors.

There are three broad factors to consider concerning the emotional and psychosocial effects of brain damage on the individual with aphasia. The direct effects of neurological damage on the neurophysical and neurochemical substrate of emotional processing, the indirect effects, which we should see as natural reactions to catastrophic personal circumstances, and the pre-existing psychological balance, constitution and the ways of coping that the individual can harness. While our knowledge of the significance of the first two factors is improving, little is known about the interaction of the third factor.

Psychosocial refers to the social context of emotional experience. Most emotions are closely associated with our interactions with society and this is what produces most of our happiness, sadness, anxiety, etc. Psychosocial adjustment to aphasia entails coming to terms with a unique constellation of life events. Because the aphasia affects others too, it has implications for the individual's whole social network, especially the immediate family (Code & Muller, 1992; Wahrborg, 1991). The disability as experienced by the patient, rather than the impairment itself, is of particular importance. Studies investigating how psychosocial adjustment to aphasia is perceived have concluded that aphasic people and their families suffer from considerable stressful changes resulting from professional, social and familial role changes, reductions in social contact, depression, loneliness, frustration and aggression. The value dimensions of psychosocial factors in our lives, like health, sexuality, career, creativity, marriage, intelligence, money, family, etc. are markedly affected by aphasia for patients and relatives (Herrmann & Wallesch, 1989).

Traditional clinical observation has identified the two main mood states following brain damage as a negative catastrophic reaction or a positive indifference reaction. There has been increased attention to direct emotional disorders recently as interest in the cerebral representation of emotion and its relationship to language impairment has grown (for review see Code, 1986, 1987; Starkstein & Robinson, 1988). Unfortunately, several conflicting models exist including the anterior-posterior (or front-back) and the right-left, both models which were born out of clinical observation (Code, 1986; Davidson, 1993). The catastrophic reaction – indifference reaction division is simply too narrow to adequately characterize the emotional state of the individual with brain damage. Research has identified three different forms of depression following brain damage: catastrophic reaction, major poststroke depression and minor poststroke depression (Starkstein & Robinson, 1988). Post-stroke depression correlates highly with anterior lesions but does not appear to correlate with aphasia type. However, research also shows that, with time since onset, there is an increase in the interaction between extent of cognitive and physical impairment and depression Robinson *et al.*, 1986).

But there has been very little research which has sought to identify reactive emotional states following brain damage and to separate them from direct effects. Herrmann Bartells & Wallesch (1993) found no differences in overall depression between acute and chronic aphasic groups, but acute patients showed significantly higher ratings for physical signs of depression and disturbances of cyclic functions (e.g. sleep), generally considered direct effects and an association between severity of depression and anterior lesions close to the frontal pole. Further, patients with major depression (all acute) shared a common subcortical lesion. This suggests that the symptoms of depression in acute patients may be caused more by the direct effects of the damage. At later times postonset it is a more reactive depression which emerges.

One approach has been to view the depression accompanying aphasia within the grief model (Tanner & Gerstenberger, 1988). On this model, individuals grieving for the loss of the ability to communicate move through stages of denial, anger, bargaining, depression and acceptance. The extent to which patients work through the stages of the model has not been systematically investigated. However, it has served as a framework for counselling. The psychological processing of denial, bargaining, acceptance, are not amenable to more objective forms of measurement but have been investigated in aphasic persons through interpretive assessments like personal construct therapy techniques by Brumfitt (1985, p.93) who argues that the impact of becoming aphasic is seen as an event of such magnitude as to affect core-role construing and that the grief the aphasic individual feels concerns loss of the essential element of oneself as a speaker. Brumfitt's (1985) subjects were all constricted construers so it is difficult to know to what extent the inner world glimpsed through adapted PCT techniques is truly representative or reflects severe expressive impairment.

Studies of depression following brain damage have used factors considered symptomatic of depression, like diminished sleep and eating, restlessness and crying. These are the factors included in depression questionnaires, although these symptoms may be caused by physical illness, anxiety, hospitalization directly unrelated to mood state (Starkstein & Robinson, 1988). While the most reliable method of gaining information on the emotional state of people seems to be to ask them, language plays a special role in the problem of identifying and measuring mood for aphasic individuals. The intersection of language is further problematic because mood manifests itself externally through facial expression, voice quality, rate and amount of speech, gesture and posture, as well as linguistic expression and comprehension, all of which can be affected in impaired mood and all can be affected by neurological damage. In addition, it is far from clear whether the apparent emotional deficit of right hemisphere-damaged patients is an impairment of emotional processing, or reflects impairment in the actual communication of emotion (Code, 1987).

Using self-report depression questionnaires with brain-damaged individuals has been popular, but raises well-known problems (for review see Code & Muller, 1992; Wahrborg, 1991). From the point of view of their use with the communicatively impaired, questionnaires which do not involve self-report have the advantage in that the clinician completes the assessment through questioning and observation (Hamilton, 1960; Alexopoulos *et al.*, 1988). Relatives and friends can also assist to verify accuracy. Nevertheless, determining mood in an individual with aphasia presents many problems, and one approach to tapping inner feelings is to use the non-verbal *Visual Analogue Mood Scale* (VAMS). Despite its simplicity the VAMS has been shown to be reliable and valid (Folstein & Luria, 1973). The VAMS can be made more meaningful to severely aphasic patients by substituting schematic faces for words (Stern & Bachman, 1991). Facial expression is the most direct method of communicating emotion and an ability that should be preserved in most aphasic individuals, for both the expression and comprehension of facial expressions.

Normally the best way to find out how someone feels is to ask them. Although aphasia is a barrier to gaining insight into emotional and psychosocial state, there are options for asking patients, and relatives, how they feel. The comprehension abilities of the patient determines to a large extent the reliability of any of them.

REFERENCES

Alexopoulos, M.P., Abrams, R.C., Young, R.C. & Shamoian, C.A. (1988). Cornell scale for depression in dementia. *Biological Psychiatry*, **23**, 271–84.

Basso, A. (1992). Prognostic factors in aphasia. *Aphasiology*, **6**, 337–48.

Brumfitt, S. (1985) The use of repertory grids with aphasic people. In N. Beail (Ed.). *Repertory grid techniques and personal constructs*. London: Croom Helm.

Carlomagno, S. (1994). *Pragmatic and communication therapy in aphasia*. London: Whurr.

Chapey, R. (Ed.). (1987). *Language intervention strategies in adult aphasia*. 2nd edn. Baltimore: Williams & Wilkins.

Chapey, R. (Ed.). (1994). *Language intervention strategies in adult aphasia*. 3rd edn. Baltimore: Williams & Wilkins.

Code, C. (1986). Catastrophic reactions and anosognosia in anterior–posterior and left–right models of the cerebral control of emotion. *Psychological Research*, **48**, 53–5.

Code, C. (1987). *Language aphasia and the right hemisphere*. Chichester: Wiley.

Code, C. (1994*a*). Mechanisms underlying recovery from aphasia. Keynote Address, German Aphasiology Society Conference, Magdeburg, Germany, October.

Code, C (1994*b*). The role of the right hemisphere in the treatment of aphasia, In R. Chapey (Ed.). *Language intervention strategies in adult aphasia*. 3rd edn Baltimore: Williams & Wilkins.

Code, C. & Muller, D.J. (1989*a*). Perspectives in aphasia therapy: an overview. In C. Code, & D.J. Muller (Eds.). *Aphasia therapy*. 1st edn. London: Edward Arnold.

Code, C. & Muller, D.J. (1989*b*). (Eds.). *Aphasia therapy*. London: Whurr.

Code, C. & Muller, D.J. (1992). *The Code-Muller protocols: assessing perceptions of psychosocial Adjustment to aphasia and related disorders*. London: Whurr.

Code, C. & Muller, D.J. (1995). (Eds.). *The treatment of aphasia: from theory to practice*. London: Whurr.

Code, C. Rowley, D.T. & Kertesz, A. (1994). Predicting recovery from aphasia with connectionist networks: preliminary comparisons with multiple regression. *Cortex*, **30**, 527–32.

Davis, A. & Wilcox, J. (1985). *Adult aphasia rehabilitation: applied pragmatics*. Windsor: NFER-Nelson.

Davidson, R.J. (1993). Cerebral asymmetry and emotion: conceptual and methodological conundrums. *Cognition and Emotion*, **7**, 115–38.

Folstein, M.F. & Luria, R. (1973). Reliability, validity, and clinical application of the visual analogue mood scale. *Psychological Medicine*, **3**, 479–86.

Hamilton, M. (1960). A rating scale for depression. *Journal of Neurology, Neurosurgery and Psychiatry*, **23**, 56–87.

Helm-Estabrooks, N. & Albert, M.L. (1991). *Manual of aphasia therapy*. Austin, TX.: Pro-Ed.

Herrmann, M. & Wallesch, C-W (1989). Psychosocial changes and adjustment with chronic and severe nonfluent aphasia. *Aphasiology*, **3**, 513–26.

Herrmann, M., Bartells, C. & Wallesch, C-W. (1993). Depression in acute and chronic aphasia: symptoms, pathoanatomical–clinical correlations and functional implications. *Journal of Neurology, Neurosurgery, and Psychiatry*, **56**, 672–8.

Howard, D. & Hatfield, F.M. (1987) *Aphasia therapy: historical and contemporary issues*. London: Lawrence Erlbaum Associates.

Howard, D. & Patterson, K. (1990). Methodological issues in neuropsychological therapy. In X. Seron & G. Deloche (Eds.). *Cognitive approaches in neuropsychological rehabilitation*. London: Lawrence Eribaum Associates.

Kay, J., Lesser, R. & Coltheart, M. (1992). *Psycholinguistic assessments of language processing in aphasia*. Hove: Lawrence Eribaum Associates.

Le Vere, T.E. (1980). Recovery of function after brain damage: a theory of the behavioural deficit. *Physiological Psychology*, **8**, 297–308.

Luria, A.R. (1970). *Traumatic aphasia*. The Hague: Mouton.

Muller, D.J. (1992). Psychosocial aspects of aphasia. In G. Blanken, J. Dittmann, H. Grimm, J.C. Marshall, & C-W. Wallesch, (Eds.). *Linguistic disorders and pathologies: an international handbook*. Berlin: Gruyer & Co.

Muller, D.J. & Code, C. (1989). Interpersonal perceptions of psychosocial adjustment to aphasia. In C. Code & D.J. Muller (Eds.). *Aphasia therapy* 2nd edn. London: Whurr.

Porch, B.E. (1967). *The porch index of communicative ability*. Palo Alto: Consulting Psychologists Press.

Porch, B.E., Collins, M., Wertz, R.T. & Friden, T.P. (1980). Statistical prediction of change in aphasia, *Journal of Speech and Hearing Research*, **23**, 312–21.

Robinson, R.G., Bolla-Wilson, K., Kaplan, E., Lipsey, J.R. & Price, T.R. (1986). Depression influences intellectual impairment in stroke patients. *British Journal of Psychiatry*, **148**, 541–7.

Shallice, T. (1979). Case study approach in neuropsychological research. *Journal of Clinical Neuropsychology*, **1**, 183–211.

Starkstein, S.E. & Robinson, R.G. (1988) Aphasia and depression. *Aphasiology*, **2**, 1–20.

Stern, R.A. & Bachman, D.L. (1991). Depressive symptoms following stroke. *American Journal of Psychiatry*, **148**, 351–6.

Tanner, D.C. & Gerstenberger, D.L. (1988). The grief response in neuropathologies of speech and language. *Aphasiology*, **2**, 79–84.

Wahrborg, P. (1991). *Assessment and management of emotional and psychosocial reactions to brain damage and aphasia*. London: Whurr Publishers.

Asthma

AD A. KAPTEIN

Medical Psychology, Department of Psychiatry,
Leiden University, The Netherlands

Shortness of breath, wheezing and coughing are the most prominent symptoms in asthma. Asthma may be defined as a disease characterised by wide variations over short periods of time in resistance to airflow in intrapulmonary airways (Rees & Price, 1995; Scadding, 1983). The prevalence of asthma is estimated to be at least 10% and is rising (Newman Taylor, 1995). Age of onset of asthma tends to be by the age of 8 to 12. At a young age, asthma has a male/female ratio of about 2 to 1. Contrary to popular belief, most children do not outgrow their asthma. Having asthma is associated with an increased risk of developing chronic bronchitis and/or emphysema (see 'Chronic bronchitis and emphysema').

The consequences of asthma are considerable. Asthma is the most important cause of school absenteeism in children (Friday & Fireman, 1988). Restrictions of daily activities (e.g. work, sexuality, social life) and hospitalization are common in patients with asthma. Asthma can be lethal: in the UK some 2000 persons die each year because of acute, severe asthma (status asthmaticus) (Burney, 1986).

The psychological consequences of asthma have been studied extensively and can be described as substantial. Patients report feelings of anxiety, panic, irritability and fatigue in relation to asthma symptoms (Kinsman *et al.*, 1973). It is often hard for the patient to predict when, why and how the symptoms of asthma will appear. Feelings of anger, shame and betrayal are mentioned by patients, especially when appropriate preventative actions have been taken (e.g. sanitation of the home environment, taking adequate prophylactic medication) and asthma attacks are still occurring.

As for most chronic disorders, the general practitioner is the main provider of medical care for asthma patients. The quality of this care has been criticized in the past decade: under-diagnosis, under-treatment and inadequate patient education being the three areas which were identified (Weiss & Budetti, 1993). The development of asthma guidelines in which diagnosis, management and patient education are outlined was prompted by these criticisms (e.g. BTS, 1994).

Asthma is not a psychosomatic disorder. There is no evidence that psychological factors cause asthma (Creer *et al.*, 1992). Patients with asthma do not exhibit a high degree of psychopathology. However, many patients, physicians, psychologists and other health professionals still seem to harbour sympathies with psychosomatic theories of asthma expressed by Alexander and Dunbar some 50 years ago (Alexander, 1952). Explaining to mothers with children who have asthma, and to the patients themselves, that asthma is 'not in

the head' quite often has relieving effects. As in any somatic disorder, psychological factors shape the response of the patient to the illness. This response (illness behaviour) is currently the focus of psychological assessment and interventions in asthma patients.

The research by Kinsman and colleagues in Denver, USA, demonstrated that anxiety, panic and shame ('stigma') predicted the medical outcome in asthma patients to a large extent. Two patterns of illness behaviour, overly focusing on and extreme denial of respiratory symptoms, were found to be associated with more frequent and longer episodes of hospitalization (Kinsman, Dirks & Jones, 1982). The research findings from the Denver group contributed to the development of psychological interventions in asthma patients. Relaxation training, systematic desensitization and biofeedback training were applied in order to improve pulmonary function and help asthma patients to cope better with the respiratory symptoms. The effectiveness of these intervention methods, however, turned out to be low. More recent psychological interventions focus on improving the self-management skills of asthma patients. Creer and his colleagues developed elaborate self-management training programmes for children and adults. These programmes generally have positive effects regarding frequency and severity of episodes of shortness of breath, hospitalization, absenteeism from school or work, and psychological concomitants of asthma (e.g. self-efficacy) (Creer & Bender, 1993).

In self-management training programmes patients learn, individually or in a group setting, to recognize and perceive signs of beginning periods of shortness of breath, how to avoid situations or triggers that may provoke an asthma attack, how to take adequate action (e.g. increase medication, go to a physician) when an attack sets in, and how to cope with the social and psychological consequences of the disorder. Increasingly, these programmes are being incorporated into the regular medical care for asthma patients with encouraging results (Evans, 1993). Recently, measuring pulmonary function by the patients themselves via peak flow meters, and training of symptom perception, were added as ingredients in asthma self-management training programmes (Stout, Kotses & Creer, 1993).

Increasingly, patients, physicians and psychologists are co-operating in developing, refining and evaluating integrated asthma care, recognising that the management of a chronic disorder such as asthma requires the combination of optimal medical care with the active participation of the patients themselves.

REFERENCES

Alexander, F. (1952). *Psychosomatic medicine*. London: Allen & Unwin.

BTS British Thoracic Society. (1994). Guidelines on the management of asthma. *Thorax*, **48**, S1–S24.

Burney, P.G.J. (1986). Asthma mortality in England and Wales: evidence for a further increase, 1974–84. *Lancet*, August 9, 323–6.

Creer, T.L. & Bender, B.G. (1993). Asthma. In R.J. Gatchel & E.B. Blanchard (Eds.). *Psychophysiological disorders*, pp. 151–203. Washington, DC: American Psychological Association.

Creer, T.L., Stein, R.E.K., Rappaport, L. & Lewis, C. (1992). Behavioral consequences of illness: childhood asthma as a model. *Pediatrics*, **90**, 808–15.

Evans, D. (1993). To help patients control asthma the clinician must be a good listener and teacher. *Thorax*, **48**, 685–7.

Friday, G.A. & Fireman, P. (1988). Morbidity and mortality of asthma. *Pediatric Clinics of North America*, **35**, 1149–62.

Kinsman, R.A., Dirks, J.F. & Jones, N.F. (1982). Psychomaintenance of chronic physical illness. In T. Millon, C. Green & R. Meagher (Eds.). *Handbook of clinical health psychology*, pp. 435–466. New York: Plenum Press.

Kinsman, R.A., Luparello, T., O'Banion, K. & Spector, S. (1973). Multidimensional analysis of the subjective symtomatology of asthma. *Psychosomatic Medicine*, **35**, 250–67.

Newman Taylor, A.J. (1995). Environmental determinants of asthma. *Lancet*, **345**, 296–9.

Rees, J. & Price, J. (1995). *ABC of asthma*. London: BMJ Publishing Group.

Scadding, J.G. (1983). Definition and clinical categories of asthma. In: T.J.H. Clark & S. Godfrey (Eds.). *Asthma*, pp. 1–11. London: Chapman and Hall.

Stout, C., Kotses, H. & Creer, T.L. (1993). Improving recognition of respiratory sensations in healthy adults. *Biofeedback and Self-Regulation*, **18**, 79–92.

Weiss, K.B. & Budetti, P. (1993). Examining issues in health care delivery for asthma. *Medical Care*, **31**, MS9–19.

Atopic dermatitis

DENISE CHARMAN
Department of Psychology, Victoria University, Australia

DAVID DE L. HORNE
Department of Psychiatry, University of Melbourne, Australia

Atopic dermatitis (AD), or eczema, is probably the most common of the atopy diseases (eczema, asthma and rhinitis) to come to the attention of psychologists and psychiatrists for treatment, although asthma has also received considerable attention. AD may co-exist with other atopy disorders in up to 48% of cases (Diepgen & Fartasch, 1992). However, AD has the earliest onset, 50% of sufferers having skin lesions before the age of 2 years. Early onset of AD also, seems an important predictor for asthma.

Other skin conditions, e.g. psoriasis (which may affect up to two percent of the population) have found psychological treatment to be beneficial, but the evidence for this is less clear cut than for AD, being heavily based on case studies involving hypnotherapy, biofeedback, group therapy, relaxation and behaviour therapy.

Rajka (1986) defined AD as 'a specific dermatitis in the abnormally reacting skin of the atopic, resulting in itch (often extreme) [current authors' words in parenthese] with sequelae as well as inflammation' (p.3). It is in many cases a lifelong disease where the typical pattern is of a labile course resulting in some uncertainty and insecurity.

Atopy, in general, has a prevalence rate of 20–25%, with the prevalence of AD, in particular, varying from 5 to 17% (e.g. Kuehr *et al.*, 1992). Reasons for the variance in prevalence estimates are a lack of consistency in measures of AD and the use of varying age-groups and different sampling procedures, in studies of the disease. However, there is some evidence that prevalence of atopy has doubled over recent decades. Approximately two-thirds of all AD cases have a family history of atopy (Rajka, 1986).

Prognosis of AD has been examined, mainly, via cross-sectional studies of risk factors, plus a limited number of longitudinal or follow-up studies. The most famous of these is that by Vickers (1980) who studied 2000 children for 2 to 21 years, with excellent response rates to his surveys. He found that for this sample, that AD cleared up in about 90 percent of cases and only recurred in about 7 percent. Such factors as severity of AD, birth order, method of infant feeding, ichthyosis, rhinitis or urticaria had no prognostic value. Early onset, seborrhaeic pattern, and being male seemed to be good prognostic signs. Late onset, 'reversed pattern' (AD in the antecubital and popliteal fossae, on the knees and elbows, and perhaps the dorsum of the wrists and hands), comorbid asthma and poor social environment seem to adversely affect prognosis. Why this should be so is not immediately apparent, and no adequate theoretical framework has been developed to account for such findings.

Specific features of the typical AD patient on presentation, are the itch, the erythema and sleeping problems. Itch is the main parameter to describe AD and its effective control is a major prognostic sign. Various events, immunological and non-immunological, can affect the itch threshold. The scratching response has been well studied by Jordan and Whitlock (1974) who demonstrated that AD sufferers develop conditioned itch–scratch responses more readily than controls and these responses were slow to extinguish.

Sleep disturbances may be an issue in 'resistant' or 'severe' AD, and certainly itchy patients do tend to have a pattern of light, broken sleep. There has been debate as to why this sleep pattern develops but, recently, one study argued that scratching behaviour itself (in response to the itch?) arouses AD sufferers from deeper stages of sleep (Aoki et al., 1991). On the other hand, the sleep pattern described is similar to that associated with depression and general emotional constriction (Tantum, Kalvey & Brown, 1982).

PREDISPOSING FACTORS

Multidisciplinary research has endeavoured to relate presence or severity of AD to a range of other features, e.g. immunological status, level of cortisol, growth patterns, sleep patterns, family coping style, personality, etc. (e.g. Koblenzer & Koblenzer, 1988, in children; White, Horne & Varigos, 1990, in adults). Essentially, for AD children, there may be a 'lack of attunement' between the child and mother or 'emotional unavailability of the mother', and, in adults, difficulty in expressing emotion, particularly anger. Such phenomena raise questions about masked depression, with patients attempting, possibly not very successfully, to achieve more control in their lives. Certainly families with AD sufferers have been reported as having more hassles, regardless of number of life events, and a perceived lack of personal resources to cope (Charman, 1996).

Psychosomatic patients, in general, describe bodily sensations as strange, frightening, confusing such that no adaptive action can be taken. Some AD patients do seem to 'over-value' some signs and symptoms, e.g. a red face. Moreover, in our experience in treating patients with eczema, we have noted that some patients describe their skin as though it had a mind of its own! The need for control and frustration at the skin's unwillingness to respond may be significant factors in psychological treatment. Some patients may be difficult to help because they have difficulty in accepting that their emotions may affect the condition of their skin, but paradoxically, they may be hypersensitive to emotional issues.

Thus, predisposing factors consistently appear to be the quality of the skin and role of affect in the lives of the patients. Studies generally reveal reports of a background of chronic life stress (rather than major life events). However, at present, the mediating variables of the experiences of stress on AD are ill-defined.

PRECIPITATING FACTORS

Allergens may be external or internal. For example, food allergies, and even emotional stress and strain, might be thought of as allergens. Self-monitoring of correlates with the condition of the skin is usually poor in both AD patients and their families, and hence recall of events associated with flare-ups can be scanty. However, recurrences are often coincidental with significant transition points in the life-span, e.g. commencing school, anticipating marriage, during the honeymoon period, a period of grief, etc. These stressful experiences may result in a reduction of the immunological system's ability to cope (e.g. Teshima et al., 1982).

PERPETUATING FACTORS

Psychological variables may maintain or exacerbate AD (Faulstich and Williamson, 1985) by eliciting poor compliance and/or scratching behaviours. For example, a general attitude of negative affectivity can make it difficult to develop and maintain rapport and adherence to treatments. The role of conditioning in developing an itch-scratch habit has been clearly demonstrated (Jordan &

Whitlock, 1974). Also, as a chronic disease, AD has psychosocial implications and to some extent a self-perpetuating course.

PROTECTIVE FACTORS

Little is known about protective factors. Why do so many young children get better (up to 90% by the age of 5 years) but a minority do not? Few, if any, medical explanations are proffered, but some psychological hypotheses have been canvassed. Male gender and absence of atopy in either parent appear to be protective factors but why and how remains a mystery. These features may influence adherence to treatment regimes. For example, parents may be more responsive to distress or comorbidities as they are expressed in their male children and thereby present them more frequently to the doctor for treatment. Possibly, if atopy or chronic illness is not a familiar experience for a family, they will be more inclined to attempt to actively seek treatment for eczema. Psychological considerations include maturational factors which may enable individuals to comprehend both how their disease is manifested and also how to deal with stress in their environment. With maturation, individuals may develop a capacity for intimacy which better meets their emotional needs and increases their ability to self-monitor their lives and to develop improved capacity for self-management of experienced stress.

MEDICAL TREATMENT

Treatment from a medical viewpoint is multifaceted and places heavy reliance upon the use of both oral and topical steroids and emollient creams. Certainly the usefulness of steroids is not to be underestimated and when there is a severe flare up of AD symptoms, control is often quickly restored via medication such as prednisone. However, prolonged use of steroids is a problem, even for topical treatments using steroid creams, because of unwanted side-effects, such as general immunosuppression and damage to the skin. Also, there is some evidence that drug therapy produces permanent improvement in only about 50% of cases (Faulstich & Williamson, 1985) and most medications are purely palliative.

PSYCHOLOGICAL INTERVENTIONS

Research into psychological aspects of atopic disease has fluctuated over time. Early research was in line with early psychodynamic formulations of psychosomatic medicine and did not seem to be particularly useful, although more recent research (see above) has confirmed the importance of strong emotions in AD sufferers (e.g. Horne, White & Varigos, 1989). The two contemporary strands of psychology that seem to offer something active in managing AD, and the other atopy disorders and psoriasis, appear to be developmental psychology/family systems research (particularly with child patients) and cognitive – behavioural theory and therapeutic intervention. There is beginning to be evidence that combining either or both of these with conventional medical treatments can certainly ameliorate symptoms, both physical and psychological, and enhance future management and therefore, the ultimate prognosis for many sufferers.

SYSTEMS APPROACH

Parents handle their children differently depending upon the sex of the child. This in turn, may impinge upon presentation to the

[373]

doctor and on compliance. Research generally estimates that AD affects females more frequently than males, yet males present more frequently to the clinics and have a better prognosis. Males may also more frequently have comorbid asthma (Vickers, 1980). Alexithymic personality features (Tantum, Kalvey & Brown, 1982), the quality of attachment in children and the experience of chronic stress due to AD, clearly can have implications for how a family functions.

Thus, a systems perspective can provide the clinician with insights into the health utilization patterns of their patients. Where and when a patient opts to attend for treatment may serve as a guide to co-morbidities. Those who attend hospital-based specialty clinics and seek additional services have been reported as experiencing more stress, less emotional support and significantly more depression, anger, anxiety and subjective distress than those attending a general dermatology clinic or private practitioner. At this stage of our knowledge, the impact of psychosocial issues in terms of disease complexity and utilization of health facilities is not well understood, but they could be critical in determining effective long-term treatment (Charman, 1996).

COGNITIVE–BEHAVIOURAL

Cognitive–behavioural therapy has been reported as useful in several studies over the past 25 years. As with the psychodynamic reports, most such studies are on small groups of patients and lacking in controls. These cognitive behavioural studies include the use of biofeedback, relaxation, habit-reversal and so on. However, recent research has shown that training in self-monitoring of symptom severity and change associated with environmental effects (both internal, such as the patient's own feelings (especially of itchiness) and thoughts; and external such as specific stressful situations at work or home) combined with habit-reversal (e.g. closing hands for three minutes to prevent scratching when feeling itchy) can be effective. Relaxation training also seems to be of benefit, especially when combined with self-monitoring and habit-reversal. One of the authors (DH) uses these three elements regularly in treating adult AD patients and has found relaxation using guided imagery to produce some interesting soothing imagery from patients, often involving a gentle breeze over water, such as a lake or the sea.

A controlled trial of self-monitoring and habit reversal currently under way (Borge, 1994) shows these two elements, in combination, can be effective in breaking the itch – scratch habit for a significant proportion of AD patients. However, some patients do not respond adequately to this simple treatment procedure and further psychological investigation, in our experience, shows that they have more profound emotional problems and require more intensive therapy, e.g. along the line described in an earlier paper (Horne *et al.*, 1989).

When the patient is a child, family intervention may be required to reduce scratching behaviours by, for example, activity scheduling and non-contingent attention. Gil *et al.* (1988) found that parent responses, i.e. contingent physical touching and/or contingent attention to scratching behaviour in children were important predictors of scratching behaviour even after controlling for demographic and medical status variables. Contingent attention by nursing staff has also been used very effectively in an in-patient setting.

Whilst cognitive behavioural treatments tend to be more active or operant than psychodynamic therapies, it would appear patients do gain an important understanding of the relationships between stressors in their lives and flare-ups in their skin. This combined with the effective prevention of scratching the skin through habit reversal, does seem to allow AD patients to both lower their baseline levels of scratching (and it is scratching that can make the difference between experiencing acute episodes and chronic AD) and to take immediate, effective ameliorative measures when a flare-up does occur. Certainly, the present authors have treated numerous patients who prior to cognitive – behavioural therapy were on long-term steroid medication and required occasional hospitalization. Subsequently oral steroids usage is vastly reduced as is dependence on steroid creams and inpatient admission has been unnecessary.

The collaboration of dermatologists and clinical psychologists has been crucial to building up the present writers' clinical and research expertise in treating this distressing disorder.

CONCLUSIONS

Clinical judgements of disease severity tend to be contaminated by other clinical observations, based upon the patient's age, gender and estimated compliance. These judgements seem to influence decisions about treatment. Occasionally, the negative interactions, characteristic of some AD patients, can be a feature of the doctor – patient relationship. Hence guidelines for clinicians using a systems approach, may help overcome some treatment resistance difficulties.

The first step in therapy is to reassure the AD sufferer that they have a real bodily illness with real discomfit, but also to help them realize that the body and mind are not disconnected.

Self-monitoring of factors leading to increased itchiness and scratching appears to be extremely effective in increasing awareness of symptoms and their relationship to the patient's life. The addition of habit-reversal and relaxation training, once a self-monitoring baseline has been established, appears to be a powerful therapeutic intervention. However, for patients who do not respond to this 'package', more intensive psychological treatment may be warranted.

The role of psychological factors in understanding and treating people with skin disorders has made some progress in the last 20 years but generally the research is limited to case studies or small groups of patients. More needs to be done.

ACKNOWLEDGMENTS

The authors wish to acknowledge the on-going collaboration and encouragement provided by Dr George Varigos, the Senior Dermatologist at the Royal Melbourne Hospital, Australia.

REFERENCES

Aoki T., Kushimoto H., Hishikawa Y. & Savin J.A. (1991). Nocturnal scratching and its relationship to the disturbed sleep of itchy subjects *Clinical and Experimental Dermatology*, **16**, 268–72.

Borge A. (1994). Behaviour therapy for skin disorders. MSc thesis, University of Melbourne, Australia.

Charman, D.P. (1996). Patterns in atopic dermatitis: developing models to predict hospital utilization patterns in young children. Unpublished PhD thesis, University of Melbourne, Australia.

Diepgen T.L. & Fartasch M. (1992). Recent epidemiological and genetic studies in atopic dermatitis. *Acta-Dermatologia Venerologia Suppl. Stockholm*, **176**, 13–18.

Faulstich M.E. & Williamson D.A. (1985). An overview of atopic dermatitis: toward a bio-behavioural integration. *Journal of Psychosomatic Research*, **29**, 647–59.

Gil K.M., Keefe A., Sampson H.A., McCaskill C.C., Rodin J. & Crisson J.E. (1988). Direct observation of scratching behaviour in children with atopic dermatitis. *Behaviour Therapy*, **19**, 213–27.

Horne D.J. de L., White A.E. & Varigos G.A. (1989). A preliminary study of psychological therapy in the management of atopic eczema. *British Journal of Medical Psychology*, **62**, 241–8.

Jordan J.M. & Whitlock F.A. (1974). Atopic dermatitis anxiety and conditioned scratch responses in cases of atopic dermatitis. *British Journal Dermatology*, **86**, 574–85.

Koblenzer C.S. & Koblenzer P.J. (1988). Chronic intractable atopic eczema. *Archives of Dermatology*, **124**, 1673–7.

Kuehr J., Frischer T., Karmaus W., Meinert R., Barth R. & Urbanek R. (1992). Clinical atopy and associated factors in primary-school pupils. *Allergy Diseases*, **47**, 650–5.

Rajka G. (1986). Natural history and clinical manifestations of atopic dermatitis. *Clinical Review Allergy*, **4**, 3–262.

Tantum D., Kalvey R. & Brown D.G. (1982). Sleep, scratching and dreams in eczema. *Psychotherapy Psychosomatic*, **37**, 26–35.

Teshima H., Kubo C., Kihara H., Imada Y., Nagata S., Ago Y. & Ikemi Y. (1982). Psychosomatic aspects of skin diseases from the standpoint of immunology. *Psychotherapy Psychosomatic*, **37**, 165–75.

Vickers C.H.F. (1980). The natural history of atopic eczema. *Acta Dermatologia Venereologia Suppl.*, **92**, 113–15.

White A., Horne D.J. de L. & Varigos G.A. (1990). The psychological profile of the atopic eczema patient. *Australasian Journal of Dermatology*, **31**, 13–16.

Battering and other violence against women

MAUREEN C. McHUGH

and

IRENE H. FRIEZE

Women's Studies, Indiana University of Pennsylvania, 350 Sutton Hall, Indiana, USA

Department of Psychology, University of Pittsburgh, USA

Estimates are that 1/4 to 1/3 of US marriages involve at least one incident of physical assault. Annually domestic violence will result in serious injury to more than 3.4 million US women (Frieze & Browne, 1989). Dating violence is as extensive as marital violence, and violence is at similar levels in gay and lesbian relationships (McHugh, Frieze & Browne, 1993).

Battering by an intimate often results in serious injury. Injuries typically involve bruises, lacerations, and/or broken bones to the head, chest, abdomen, and/or extremities. Battered women also experience stab and/or bullet wounds. Violence is more likely to occur on weekends, in the evenings and in warm summer months. Over 60% of battered women report beatings during pregnancy. The violence generally escalates in frequency and severity over time. In some cases a spouse is murdered.

Domestic violence is believed to be an under-reported crime. Yet, research suggests that battered women do report the beatings to help sources. Women report the incidents to friends, family, police, lawyers, physicians, ministers, counsellors, and social service agencies. The help-givers typically do not effectively address the violence (Gondolf & Fisher, 1988).

Large numbers of battered women are not being identified by health care personnel (Kurtz, 1987). Evidence of old injuries and injuries inconsistent with the 'story' given are clues to identification of battering. The battered woman may be depressed and/or suicidal, abuse alcohol and/or drugs, and report psychosomatic complaints. Physicians are instructed to: ask the woman about the origin of her injuries; document the injuries on her chart; determine the woman's safety; alert her to the danger of returning to the abuser; and make referrals to shelters or other agencies and programmes (Kurtz, 1987).

Although 65% of abused women have received psychiatric care, most of their therapists failed to inquire about violence. Advocates have called for a proactive approach by therapists to assess for violence, even when it is not the presenting complaint. Battered women frequently present with problems of anxiety, depression, and somatic complaints. Intake interviews and schedules should include questions about interpersonal violence. Corroborating evidence, when available, suggests that battered women tend to underestimate both the frequency and the severity of the violence they experience. Forgetting and minimizing are two coping strategies used by battered women (McHugh *et al.*, 1993).

Recent research (Hansen & Harway, 1993) indicates that therapists fail to identify the importance of reported physical violence, and fail to generate appropriate interventions. Cessation of the violence should be the treatment goal. To date, most intervention strategies focus on the victim. This perspective is increasingly seen as both victim-blaming and counter-productive (Yllo & Bograd, 1988). Previously, much of the literature and treatment was based on the model proposed by Walker (1984) that battered women suffer from learned helplessness, a series of behavioural, cognitive, and motivational deficits resulting from the randomness and aversiveness of the beatings. Newer approaches emphasize the help-seeking and coping mechanisms of battered women, viewing them as survivors rather than victims (e.g. Gondolf & Fisher, 1988).

Psychotherapy for battered women typically addresses the following themes: isolation, self-esteem, expression of anger, life choices and decision-making, grief and loss, and termination issues. Alternatively, Hansen and Harway (1993) recommend that appropriate treatment for the battered woman include the following: an assessment including questions regarding the lethality of the situation and the client's safety; crisis intervention and provision of immediate protection to the victim; education including information about battering; and referrals (e.g. to shelters, and legal resources).

Research indicates that women remain at risk for violence and homicide even after terminating the relationships and physically relocating. Also, men who batter in one relationship are likely to batter in subsequent relationships. Thus, it is imperative to intervene legally or therapeutically with the batterer.

Treatments for male batterers have been developed (Sonkin & Dutton, 1988). The treatment approaches stress the need to challenge the abuser's rationalizations and excuses. Batterers are more likely than men in general to abuse drugs and alcohol. Interventions with batters frequently take the form of batterers' groups. Most treatment groups attempt to identify and confront ingrained beliefs: general attitudes towards women: beliefs about power in intimate relationships; and beliefs about male dominance. A principal component of most batterers' treatment is anger management. When batterers are in treatment, their partners may be imperiled while falsely believing that the abuser is cured. It should be made clear to batterers and their partners that the risk of violence still exists. Therapists need to provide resources for safety and support of the partner, and monitor the situation for reoccurrence of violence. Indications of potentially lethal violence include: serious depression, drug and alcohol use, threats, and available firearms; these indications warrant warnings (to the spouse) and intervention (Hansen & Harway, 1993).

REFERENCES

Frieze, I.H. & Browne, A. (1989). Violence in marriage. In L. Ohlin & M. Tonry (Eds.). *Family violence.* pp. 163–218. Chicago: The University of Chicago Press.

Gondolf, E. & Fisher (1988). *Battered women as survivors: an alternative to treating learned helplessness.* Lexington, MA: Lexington Books.

Hansen, M. & Harway, M. (1993). *Battering and family therapy: a feminist perspective.* London: Sage Publications.

Kurtz, D. (1987). Emergency department responses to battered women: resistance to medicalization. *Social Problems,* 34, 69–81.

McHugh, M. C., Frieze, I. H. & Browne, A. (1993). Research on battered women and their assailants. In F. Denmark & M. A. Paludi (Eds.). *Psychology of women: a handbook of issues and theories.* pp. 513–552. Westport, Conn: Greenwood Press.

Sonkin, D. & Dutton, D. G. (Eds.). (1988). Special issue on wife assaulters. *Violence and Victims,* 3.

Walker, L. (1984). *The battered woman syndrome.* New York: Springer.

Yllo, K. & Bograd, M. (Eds.). (1988). *Feminist perspectives on wife abuse.* Newbury Park, CA: Sage.

Benzodiazepine dependency

HEATHER ASHTON

School of Neurosciences, Division of Psychiatry,
The Royal Victoria Infirmary, Newcastle upon
Tyne, UK

Drug dependence has always been difficult to define. This complex condition, which may develop after repeated use of some psychoactive drugs, involves variable combinations of at least three interacting factors: (i) an *emotional state* consisting of a craving or compulsion to continue taking the drug, either for its directly rewarding (reinforcing) properties or to avoid the discomfort of its absence, (ii) a *behaviour* consisting of compulsive drug-taking or drug-seeking, and (iii) a *physical state* which may include drug tolerance and an abstinence syndrome with somatic and/or psychological symptoms. A drug-dependent individual eventually becomes enmeshed in a self-replicating loop upon which many other factors impinge (Fig. 1).

TYPES OF BENZODIAZEPINE DEPENDENCE

In the case of benzodiazepines the definition becomes doubly difficult for there are at least two types of benzodiazepine dependence: (i) *low dose dependence* on medically prescribed benzodiazepines and (ii) *high dose dependence* on illicitly obtained benzodiazepines. In low dose dependence, patients receive long-term prescriptions from their doctors in clinically recommended oral doses, often over periods of 20 years or more. There is a slight tendency to escalate dosage over the years but prescriptions usually remain within therapeutically recommended limits. The drugs are used initially for their anxiolytic or hypnotic properties and later to prevent perceived or anticipated withdrawal effects. Such patients

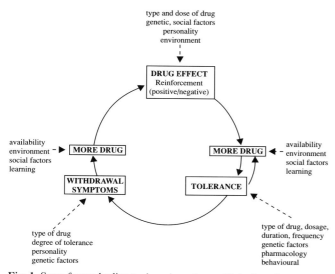

Fig. 1. Some factors leading to drug dependence. (Only those factors directly relevant to the pharmacological actions of benzodiazepines are discussed in the text).

do not abuse other drugs and only a minority over-indulge in alcohol.

High dose benzodiazepine dependence is often combined with abuse of other drugs. Most polydrug abusers throughout the world today also abuse benzodiazepines. These individuals take benzodiazepines irregularly, often in doses ten times or more greater than 'therapeutic' users and may inject intravenously (particularly temazepam in the UK).* The drugs are used recreationally to obtain a 'high', to increase the 'high' obtained from other recreational drugs, and/or to alleviate the abstinence syndrome from other drugs of abuse (opiates, cocaine, amphetamine). For some of these individuals, benzodiazepines were initially prescribed by doctors.

Although the two types of benzodiazepine dependence generally involve different populations, there is (iii) an *intermediate group* in which individuals may have started on prescribed benzodiazepines but have escalated their dosage, take more than their prescribed doses and drift from doctor to doctor or visit hospital casualty departments in order to obtain increased supplies which they self-prescribe. Sometimes, though not always, this group combines benzodiazepine misuse with excessive consumption of alcohol.

The different populations of benzodiazepine-dependent persons manifest various degrees of 'addictive' features. All exhibit drug-seeking behaviour: prescribed dose users by regular visits to their doctors to obtain repeat prescriptions; high dose abusers by prescription forgeries, theft or purchase from illegal suppliers. All, manifest psychological dependence on their drugs in that they become anxious if a ready supply is not available. Therapeutic dose users often carry their tablets around with them and not uncommonly take an extra dose before an anticipated stressful event or, in the case of hypnotic users, a night in a strange bed. They make sure to obtain the next prescription before the previous supply has run out. Higher dose users concoct ingenious stories in order to obtain prescriptions: some personally experienced examples include 'taken

* The capsule form of this drug (commonly used for intravenous injection) was withdrawn in the UK in 1996, but tablets are still available.

by teenage daughter'; 'put in garbage bin by mistake just before bin collected'; 'stolen with purchases in shopping centre'; 'left in flat from which subject ejected', etc.

Such behaviour is evidence of a strong desire or perceived 'need' for the drugs in all types of dependent users.

EXPERIMENTAL STUDIES OF DEPENDENCE POTENTIAL

Reinforcement

The reinforcement potential of a drug is judged by its ability to maintain or increase the frequency of drug-taking or drug-seeking behaviour. Positive reinforcement is assumed to be associated with some 'rewarding' or hedonic effect directly exerted by the drug, while negative reinforcement is associated with a drug's ability to alleviate aversive or 'punishing' states such as anxiety or withdrawal symptoms.

Positive reinforcement by benzodiazepines has been hard to demonstrate in animals or man. In animals, strongly reinforcing drugs such as amphetamines or cocaine are readily and repeatedly self-administered after suitable priming and are preferred to placebo. Such self-administration of benzodiazepines has not been consistently demonstrated in animals. Indeed, in an extensive review of the literature Woods, Katz & Winger (1992) state that 'across a wide range of conditions, benzodiazepines generally do not maintain appreciable self-administration behaviour' (p. 168). In certain experimental situations benzodiazepines can maintain self-administration, but much less potently than barbiturates and other drugs of dependence. On the other hand, there is much evidence that benzodiazepines provide negative reinforcement. They reverse the behavioural inhibition produced by electric shocks paired with food reward, the Geller–Seifter procedure, and that produced by several anxiogenic procedures in rodents (File & Baldwin, 1989). Whether or not self-administration is increased in aversive situations, especially in withdrawal states in benzodiazepine-dependent animals is at present not clear.

The avidity with which animals will self-administer drugs shows some parallels with drug preference and 'liking' scores in human subjects (Warburton, 1988). In drug preference tests the subject, after previous experience of taking a range of drugs and placebo in colour-coded capsules, chooses which capsule to take over several occasions in constant experimental conditions. The tests are usually combined with subjective ratings of mood and of hedonic or euphoriant effects ('liking' scores). In line with animal studies, normal subjects and anxious volunteers show no preference or increased liking compared with placebo for a variety of benzodiazepines in several doses within the therapeutic range. In contrast, amphetamine (5 mg) is significantly preferred by normal subjects, though not by anxious volunteers. Among abusers of other recreational drugs liking scores for benzodiazepines are low compared to other drugs (Fig. 2) and scores for drugs of abuse in general correlate with their potency as positive reinforcers in animals.

Nevertheless, reinforcing effects of benzodiazepines are apparent in particular human populations: (i) In patients with psychoneurotic disorders to whom benzodiazepines are available on demand, the amount of drug requested is related to the degree of anxiety, and anxious subjects seeking treatment prefer benzodiaze-

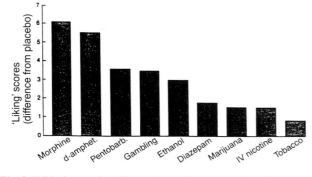

Fig. 2. 'Liking' scores for different drugs. (Scores plotted as difference from placebo) From Warburton (1988).

pines to placebo; (ii) patients undergoing abrupt benzodiazepine withdrawal show a preference for benzodiazepines and self-administer them when available; (iii) insomniac subjects express significantly increased liking for benzodiazepines over placebo when offered as an aid to sleep; (iv) subjects with a history of sedative drug abuse show preference and increased liking scores for benzodiazepines, especially in high doses; (v) benzodiazepines also have greater reinforcing effects in subjects with a history of alcohol abuse compared to non-alcohol abusers and in normal subjects with a history of moderate alcohol consumption compared to those with low levels of alcohol consumption.

Thus both human and animal studies show that benzodiazepines in therapeutic doses have little potency as positive reinforcers; they do however act as negative reinforcers, alleviating anxiety and withdrawal states. As argued elsewhere (Ashton, 1989) benzodiazepines act essentially as 'depunishing' rather than as directly rewarding drugs. High doses (in the range of 100 mg diazepam or more) may have positive reinforcing effects in some subjects, notably abusers of other sedative drugs, a finding in agreement with the testimony of intravenous temazepam users. These individuals and those with a history of excessive alcohol use are at particular risk of developing high dose benzodiazepine dependence, while anxious patients with certain dependent personality traits are at risk of low dose dependence (Tyrer, 1987; Ashton, 1989).

TOLERANCE

Dependence on many drugs of addiction is linked with the development of tolerance, an adaptive state which develops on repeated administration such that larger doses are required to elicit the original effect. Tolerance to the actions of benzodiazepines, including anxiolytic effects, has been demonstrated in animals (File & Baldwin, 1989). In man, a remarkable degree of tolerance can develop in high dose benzodiazepine users. For example, a patient taking 240 mg diazepam and 240 mg oxazepam daily (confirmed by blood concentrations) regularly rode a bicycle and also passed a written English examination with merit. The patient was still highly anxious, suggesting tolerance to the anxiolytic as well as to the hypnotic and ataxic effects of the benzodiazepines. Patients on therapeutic doses rapidly develop tolerance to hypnotic effects of benzodiazepines; tolerance to anxiolytic effects seems to develop more slowly but may lead to dosage escalation or 'break-through' anxiety on fixed doses.

The mechanisms of benzodiazepine tolerance are not fully understood but may involve down-regulation of affinity or density of gamma-aminobutyric acid (GABA)/benzodiazepine receptors in the brain (Nutt, 1986), or possibly alterations in activity of putative endogenous benzodiazepine-like substances (File & Baldwin, 1989). There is little doubt that chronic use of benzodiazepines causes profound adaptive changes in the brain. Such changes may be largely responsible for withdrawal effects on drug cessation, and clinical experience suggests that long-term users take benzodiazepines more to prevent withdrawal effects than to alleviate the condition for which they were originally prescribed.

PHARMACOLOGICAL DEPENDENCE: WITHDRAWAL EFFECTS

Pharmacological (or physiological) dependence is defined as a state which develops during chronic drug treatment in which cessation of the drug (or administration of a pharmacological antagonist) elicits an abstinence reaction which is time limited and is reversible by renewed administration of the drug. Animal studies have consistently shown that all benzodiazepines are capable of inducing physiological dependence after chronic administration. Withdrawal signs differ between species and the intensity and duration of the withdrawal syndrome depends on drug dosage, duration of administration, and to some extent on type of benzodiazepine. It is not clear to what degree withdrawal effects are influenced by the extent of previous drug tolerance.

It has been known for some time that high doses of benzodiazepines produce pharmacological dependence in man and that abrupt cessation after chronic use can cause severe withdrawal phenomena such as convulsions and psychotic reactions. The existence of dependence in long-term therapeutic dose users was established by placebo-controlled clinical studies (Petursson & Lader, 1981; Owen & Tyrer, 1983) and the human benzodiazepine withdrawal syndrome was described. This syndrome, which is similar to the abstinence syndrome of other sedative/hypnotic drugs and of alcohol, consists of a large constellation of somatic and psychological symptoms. The clinical picture is mainly that of anxiety, but certain symptoms such as sensory hypersensitivity and perceptual distortion appear to be especially prominent. The non-specific nature of the symptoms and the fact that anxiety is often present before withdrawal makes definition of the syndrome difficult (Ashton, 1991). 'Pseudowithdrawal' anxiety may occur in patients who believe their benzodiazepines are being withdrawn and a distinction is traditionally made between psychological and pharmacological dependence. However, anxiety in the face of anticipated drug deprivation is itself a feature of dependence (and involves physiological changes in CNS activity), and treatment is the same whether the symptoms are 'true' or 'pseudowithdrawal' symptoms.

The incidence of the withdrawal syndrome is not clear. Estimates vary, depending on factors such as definition and measures of withdrawal symptoms, selection of patients, and rate of withdrawal. Such estimates do not usually take account of dropouts (often due to severe withdrawal symptoms) or of those who decline to undergo withdrawal (50–100% of eligible patients in some studies). In general a withdrawal syndrome is believed to occur in 30–45% of patients who have used regular therapeutic doses of benzodiazepines for more than a few months, but the incidence varies between less than 20% and 100% in different studies. It is not clear why some chronic users apparently do not become dependent; and if not dependent why they continue drug use over many years. However, drug dependence is not an absolute; it can exist in many different degrees.

The duration of the withdrawal syndrome is also debatable. Classically symptoms subside to prewithdrawal levels within 4–6 weeks, but some symptoms may decline more slowly, merging into a period of increased vulnerability to stress which may be partly a consequence of learned behaviour related to drug taking (Ashton, 1991; Owen & Tyrer, 1983). Certain potent, rapidly metabolized benzodiazepines (alprazolam, triazolam, lorazepam) have been associated with more severe withdrawal symptoms, possibly because of their greater potency. Because of their short half-lives, the onset of withdrawal is also more acute and withdrawal symptoms may occur between doses (inter-dose anxiety). Dosage (within the therapeutic range) and duration of benzodiazepine use (above 6–12 months) do not appear to affect the incidence or severity of withdrawal, but anxious and passive-dependent personality types (Owen & Tyrer, 1983) and alcohol-dependent subjects may be especially vulnerable. High dose benzodiazepine abusers are at almost certain risk of withdrawal symptoms unless dosage tapering is extremely slow.

BENZODIAZEPINE CONSUMPTION
Consumption of benzodiazepines is still enormous worldwide (for a review of the epidemiology, see Woods *et al.*, 1992). Although prevalence of benzodiazepine use has recently declined in many countries, 10.9% of the US population surveyed in 1990 reported having used benzodiazepines during the previous year. In the UK prevalence, as thus defined, fell from 11.2% in 1981 to about 3.3% in 1986 (lower than in most European countries). These decreases resulted mainly from changes in tranquillizer use; hypnotic use has remained relatively stable since 1981 (Table 1 shows benzodiazepines marketed as tranquillizers and hypnotics).

Meanwhile sales of benzodiazepines have risen markedly in the US and most European countries, except the UK where sales have fallen. The discrepancy between general trends in prevalence of use and sales of benzodiazepines suggests the existence of a growing cohort of long-term regular benzodiazepine users, as presaged by Owen and Tyrer in 1983. Population surveys support this interpretation, and about 2% of the adult populations of the US (*ca.* 4 million people) and of the UK (*ca.* 1 million people) appear to have used benzodiazepine hypnotics or tranquillizers regularly for 12 months or over; 50% of these for 5–10 years or more. A high proportion of these users must be assumed to be at least to some degree dependent on benzodiazepines.

Amongst the chronic benzodiazepine users, females outnumber males by 2 : 1 and use is related to age. Frequency of use of anxiolytic benzodiazepines increases up to 50–65 years of age, while hypnotic use continues to rise to a peak at 65 years or over. Such use may be related to the higher prevalence of anxiety disorders in younger age groups and of insomnia amongst the elderly, but it should be noted that the pharmacological actions, dependence potential and incidence and type of withdrawal symptoms is similar for all benzodiazepines, whether marketed as hypnotics or as anxiolytics. Prevalence of physical and psychological ill-health and scores for trait and state anxiety are significantly higher amongst

Table.1 *Benzodiazepines marketed as tranquilizers (anxiolytics) and as hypnotics*

Tranquillizers	Hypnotics
Alprazolam	Flurazepam
Chlordiazepoxide	Loprazolam
Clorazepate	Lormetazepam
Diazepam	Nitrazepam
Lorazepam	Temazepam
Oxazepam	Triazolam[a]
Prazepam	

Note: The pharmacological actions of all benzodiazepines are similar; the distinction between tranquilizers and hypnotic preparations is based on commercial, not pharmacological, grounds
[a]Withdrawn UK in 1991.

chronic benzodiazepine users than in the general population. The extent to which benzodiazepines are prescribed and used for sociological reasons and as psychological coping strategies is discussed by Gabe (1991).

Prevalence of benzodiazepine use as primary recreational drugs is claimed to be trivial compared with other drugs of abuse (Woods *et al.*, 1992), but reports from many countries show that a large proportion (30–90%) of polydrug abusers, especially opiate abusers, also abuse benzodiazepines. Benzodiazepines used orally for recreational purposes include diazepam, alprazolam, temazepam, flunitrazepam and, to a lesser extent, triazolam and lorazepam. Temazepam is also injected intravenously and its use in combination with the opiates buprenorphine and dihydrocodeine appears to be particularly common amongst intravenous drug abusers in Scotland. The population of recreational benzodiazepine users is perhaps a tenth of that of chronic prescribed users, but probably amounts to some hundreds of thousands in the US and UK, and may be increasing.

ADVERSE EFFECTS OF LONG-TERM BENZODIAZEPINE USE
Growing experience with benzodiazepines in the 1980s led many patients and professionals to question the value of long-term use. Disadvantages of chronic benzodiazepine use include psychomotor, cognitive and memory impairment, interactions with other sedative drugs such as alcohol, emotional clouding, depression, and sometimes paradoxical excitement and aggressiveness. Sociological costs may include increased risk of traffic and other accidents, falls and fractures in the elderly, shoplifting (due to amnesia) and violent behaviour (due to paradoxical effects). Furthermore, dependence and withdrawal reactions make it difficult for many long-term users to stop taking benzodiazepines despite adverse effects.

RATIONAL USE OF BENZODIAZEPINES
Although benzodiazepines are highly effective in short-term treatment for anxiety and insomnia, in long-term use the risks of dependence and other adverse effects outweigh the benefits (Tyrer, 1987). Most authorities in the UK, recommend that the use of benzodiazepines should be limited where possible to short-term (maximum 4 weeks) or intermittent courses, in minimal effective doses, prescribed only when symptoms are severe (Committee on

Safety of Medicines, 1988; Royal College of Psychiatrists, 1988; Consensus Conference, 1992; Drug and Therapeutics Bulletin, 1990). It is recognized that psychological treatments (sometimes combined with antidepressants) are more appropriate in the longer term for most patients with anxiety disorders.

The management of patients already dependent on benzodiazepines is described in detail elsewhere (Ashton, 1994). Essentially it consists of gradual, individualized and patient-controlled dosage reduction (usually over a period of months) combined with individual psychological support. Adjuvant drugs such as beta-blockers, carbamazepine, buspirone and others have not been found to be generally helpful, but antidepressants may be indicated if depression is severe. Animal studies (and limited clinical experience) suggest a potential use for drugs which act as partial agonists or antagonists at benzodiazepine receptors. The outcome of withdrawal for therapeutic dose users who are motivated to withdraw is good: abstinence rates 1–5 years after withdrawal vary between 54% and 92% in different studies, and there is no evidence of increased alcohol use or psychiatric morbidity in those who withdraw successfully. For patients unwilling to withdraw continued prescribing in minimal doses may be necessary. Long-term follow-up information on high dose abusers is scarce but withdrawal failures and relapse rates appear to be higher than in therapeutic dose users.

THE FUTURE

With rational prescribing, benzodiazepines are likely to remain useful drugs for short-term use. Prevalence of use should continue to decline as the number of chronic users decreases and fewer new patients become dependent. The medical profession should be cautious in prescribing new non-benzodiazepine anxiolytics and hypnotics now appearing on the market. Such successors to benzodiazepines, if used as chronic treatments, may not be without a dependence potential similar to that of benzodiazepines.

REFERENCES

Ashton, H. (1989). Risks of dependence on benzodiazepine drugs: a major problem of long-term treatment. *British Medical Journal*, **298**, 103–4.

Ashton, H. (1991). Protracted withdrawal syndromes from benzodiazepines. *Journal of Substance Abuse Treatment*, **8**, 19–28.

Ashton, H. (1994). The treatment of benzodiazepine dependence. *Addiction*, **89**, 1535–41.

Committee on Safety of Medicines (1988). Benzodiazepines, dependence and withdrawal symptoms. *Current Problems*, 21.

Consensus Conference. (1992). Guidelines for the management of patients with generalised anxiety. *Psychiatric Bulletin*, **16**, 560–5.

Drug and Therapeutics Bulletin. (1990).

The treatment of insomnia. *Drug and Therapeutics Bulletin*, **28**, 97–9.

File, S.E. & Baldwin, H.A. (1989). Changes in anxiety in rats tolerant to, and withdrawn from, benzodiazepines: behavioural and biochemical studies. In P. Tyrer, (Ed.). *The psychopharmacology of anxiety*, pp. 28–51. Oxford: Oxford University Press.

Gabe, J. (1991). Personal troubles and public issues: the sociology of long-term tranquilliser use. In J. Gabe (Ed.)., *Understanding tranquilliser use: the role of the social sciences*, pp. 31–47, London: Tavistock/Routledge.

Nutt, D. (1986). Benzodiazepine dependence in the clinic: reason for anxiety? *Trends in Pharmacological Sciences*, **7**, 457–60.

Owen, R.T. & Tyrer, P. (1983). Benzodiazepine dependence: a review of the evidence. *Drugs*, **25**, 385–98.

Petursson, H. & Lader, M.H. (1981). Benzodiazepine dependence. *British Journal of Addiction*, **76**, 133–45.

Royal College of Psychiatrists. (1988). Benzodiazepines and dependence: a College statement. *Bulletin of the Royal College of Psychiatrists*, **12**, 107–8.

Tyrer, P. (1987). Benefits and risks of benzodiazepines. In H. Freeman & Y. Rue (Eds.). *The benzodiazepines in current clinical practice*, pp. 3–11, London: Royal Society of Medicine Services.

Warburton, D.M. (1988). The puzzle of nicotine use. In M. Lader (Ed.). *The psychopharmacology of addiction*, pp. 27–49, Oxford: Oxford University Press.

Woods, J.H., Katz, J.L. & Winger, G. (1992) Benzodiazepines: use, abuse and consequences. *Pharmacological Reviews*, **44**, 151–338.

Beta-blockers: psychological effects

DAVID S. KRANTZ

Department of Medical and Clinical Psychology,
Uniformed Services University of the Health
Sciences, Bethesda, USA

Beta-blockers are a class of drugs that selectively compete for and inhibit binding at the beta-adrenergic subset of receptors of the sympathetic, nervous system (Middlemiss, Buxton & Greenwood, 1981; Patel & Turner, 1981). Beta-adrenergic receptors are primarily located in the heart and in the smooth muscle of the blood vessels and the lungs, but also exert metabolic and other effects. The beta-blockers are structurally similar to the body's adrenergic neurotransmitters, norepinephrine and epinephrine, and they exhibit their greatest effects during periods of intense sympathetic nervous system (SNS) activation. Therefore, the most common clinical use of these drugs is for the treatment of cardiovascular disorders, including hypertension and manifestations of ischaemic heart disease such as angina pectoris and cardiac arrhythmias (Frishman, 1980; Weiner, 1985; Patel & Turner, 1981).

However, since the introduction of these drugs and their wide therapeutic use, a variety of both desirable and unwanted psychological effects have been observed. One of the most frequently noted beneficial effects has been the reduction of reported anxiety by individuals in certain acutely stressful situations (e.g. performing before an audience, or dental surgery) that are normally accompanied by several somatic manifestations of arousal (Frishman et al., 1981; Noyes, 1982). There have also been some reports that chronic beta-blocker therapy might lessen some manifestations of the Type A or 'coronary-prone' behaviour pattern (Schmeider et al., 1983; Krantz & Durel, 1983). In addition to these psychological effects – some of which may be considered to be beneficial) – unwanted psychological and behavioural effects of beta-blockers have also been noted. These include side-effects such as fatigue, depression, nightmares and disturbances of sleep and sexual function (Patel & Turner, 1981; Weiner, 1985; Moss & Procci, 1982). This chapter will provide a brief overview of the psychological and behavioural effects of beta-blocking drugs.

PSYCHOLOGICAL EFFECTS

Reduction of chronic anxiety

The anxiolytic (anxiety-reducing) effects of beta-blockers in chronically anxious patients was first reported by Granville-Grossman and Turner for the drug propranolol (Granville-Grossman & Turner, 1966). However, when compared with other anxiolytic drugs such as the minor tranquilizers (e.g. benzodiazepines), beta-blockers are probably most effective in patients whose anxiety is characterized by bodily complaints (Tyrer, 1976). In other words, when patients experience their anxiety more in terms of palpitations and tremor than as worry or mental tension, their anxiety is likely to be reduced by a beta-blocker. When psychic symptoms predominate, beta-blockers are considered much less effective than benzodiazepines.

Effects during situational stress

Considerable evidence has shown that beta-blockers can be useful in decreasing anxiety in certain acute stress situations. In healthy subjects, and in patients with cardiovascular disease, these drugs blunt the increases in cardiovascular activity and anxiety that accompany certain stressful activities such as public speaking, racing car driving, musical performance, and oral surgery (Middlemiss et al., 1981; Suzman, 1981; Krantz et al., 1982; Neftel et al., 1982). Anxiolytic effects have been reported for a variety of beta-blockers regardless of whether they have pharmacological properties that enable them to readily cross the blood – brain barrier.

Effects on Human Performance

Less consistent are the effects of beta-blockers on human performance during stress and non-stressful circumstances. Some reviewers conclude that these drugs exert their anxiolytic effects without significant impairment in cognitive or physiological performance (Turner, 1983; Landauer et al., 1979), whereas others report poorer performance or increased variability with some beta-blockers on tests of reaction time or memory (Broadhurst, 1980; Solomon et al., 1982). Still others have concluded that the occasionally observed decrement in several psychomotor functions is indicative not of a depressant effect on central nervous system function but of an action on skeletal muscle (Middlemiss et al., 1981). In this regard, when situational stress leads to a decrement in performance, which in turn, increases anxiety further (e.g. tremor experienced by some musicians during public performance), reduction of anxiety or tremor by beta-blockade apparently leads to improved performance (Neftel et al., 1982). There is also evidence that there may be mild performance deficits that result from disease states such as hypertension that are improved by drug treatment (e.g. with beta-blockers) (Miller et al., 1984).

MECHANISM OF BETA-BLOCKER EFFECTS ON ANXIETY

It is not entirely clear whether the anti-anxiety effects of beta-blockers result from their direct effects in the central nervous system or whether these effects result from the peripheral effects of these drugs. A central site of action is often assumed, especially when effects on mood or behaviour are associated with a beta-blocker that readily penetrates into the brain (Cruickshank, 1980). However, various drugs in this class vary in the extent to which they penetrate the CNS, and anti-anxiety effects in acute stress situations are evident even for those beta-blockers that do not readily penetrate the brain (Neftel et al., 1982).

It has therefore been suggested that the peripheral effects of beta-blockers are sufficient to account for their anxiolytic effects, and that this involves the role of information processing concerning peripheral sympathetic responses on the subjective experience of emotion (Tyrer, 1976; Durel et al., 1985). Peripheralist views of emotion (e.g. James–Lange, Schachter–Singer) suggest that the subjective experience of anxiety is a result of a sequence of physiological events beginning with sympathetic nervous system stimulation leading to arousal manifestations, such as palpitation and tremor. The perception, cognitive interpretation, or automatic processing of these responses acts to heighten the psychological aspects of anxiety based on this interpretation, beta-blockade inhibits peripheral physiological responses (e.g. rapid heart rate, tremor), interrupts the somatic–psychic interaction, and thus reduces anxiety (Tyrer, 1976; Durel et al., 1985).

EFFECTS OF BETA-BLOCKERS ON TYPE A BEHAVIOUR

Several studies (Schmeider et al., 1983; Krantz et al., 1982; Krantz & Durel, 1983) suggest that, among patients with hypertension or coronary disease, chronic administration of beta-blockers may reduce behavioural manifestations of Type A or so-called 'coronary-prone behaviour'. More recent studies suggest that these effects may be confined to beta-blockers that penetrate the brain, and are only evident among a subset of individuals (Krantz et al., 1988).

SUMMARY AND CONCLUSION

Beta-adrenergic blocking drugs, such as propranolol and atenolol, have utility in reducing the peripheral manifestations of anxiety and acute stress. These beneficial effects are most pronounced among individuals with somatic manifestations of anxiety. Effects of these drugs on performance and memory are less consistent, and chronic use of these medications have occasionally been associated with unwanted side-effects such as fatigue and depression.

REFERENCES

Broadhurst, A.D. (1980). The effect of propranolol on human performance. *Aviation Space Environmental Medicine*, **51**, 176–9.

Cruickshank, J.M. (1980). The clinical importance of cardioselectivity and lipophilicity in beta blockers. *American Heart Journal*, **100**, 160–8.

Durel, L.A., Krantz, D.S., Eisold, J.F., et. al. (1985). Behavioral effects of beta blockers: Reduction of anxiety, acute stress, and type A behavior. *Journal of Cardiopulmonary Rehabilitation*, **5**, 267–73.

Frishman, W.H. (1980). *Clinical pharmacology of the beta-adrenoreceptor blocking drugs.* New York: Appleton Century-Crofts.

Frishman, W.H., Razin, A., Swencionis, C., *et al.* (1981). Beta-adrenoreceptor blockade in anxiety states: New approaches to therapy? *Cardiovascular Rev Rep*, **2**, 447–59.

Granville-Grossman, K. & Turner, P. (1966). The effect of propranolol on anxiety. *Lancet*, **i**, 788.

Krantz, D.S., Contrada, R.J., Durel, L.A., et. al. (1988). Comparative effects of two beta-blockers on cardiovascular reactivity and type A behavior in hypertensives. *Psychosomatic Medicine*, **50**, 615–26.

Krantz, D.S. & Durel, L.A. (1983). Psychobiological substrates of the type A behavior pattern. *Health Psychology*, **2**, 393–411.

Krantz, D.S., Durel, L.A., Davia, J.E., et. al. (1982). Propranolol medication among coronary patients: Relationship to type A behavior and cardiovascular response. *Journal of Human Stress*, **8**, 4–12.

Landauer, A.A., Pocock, D.A. & Prott, F.W. (1979). Effects of atenolol and propranolol on human performance and subjective feelings. *Psychopharmacology*, **60**, 211–15.

Middlemiss D.N., Buxton D.A., Greenwood D.T. (1981). Beta-adrenoceptor antagonists in psychiatry and neurology. *Pharmacol Therapy*, **12**, 419–37.

Miller, R.E., Shapiro, A.P., King, H.E., et. al. (1984). Effect of antihypertensive treatment on the behavioral consequences of elevated blood pressure. *Hypertension*, **6**, 202–8.

Moss, H.B. & Procci, W.R. (1982). Sexual dysfunction associated with oral hypertensive medications: a critical survey of the literature. *General Hospital Psychiatry*, **4**, 121–9.

Neftel, K.A., Adler, R.H., Kapelli, L., et. al. (1982). Stage fright in musicians: a model illustrating the effect of beta-blockers. *Psychosomatic Medicine*, **44**, 461–9.

Noyes, R. (1982). Beta-blocking drugs and anxiety. *Psychosomatics*, **23**, 155–70.

Patel, L. & Turner, P. (1981). Central action of beta-adrenoceptor blocking drugs in man. *Medical Research Review*, **1**, 387–410.

Schmeider, R., Friedrich, G., Neus, H., et. al. (1983). The influence of beta-blockers on cardiovascular reactivity and type A behavior pattern in hypertensives. *Psychosomatic Medicine*, **45**, 417–23.

Solomon, S., Hotchkiss, E., Saravay, S.M., et. al. (1982). Impairment of memory function by antihypertensive medication. *Archives of General Psychiatry*, **40**, 1109–12.

Suzman, M.M. (1981). Use of beta-adrenergic receptor blocking agents in psychiatry. In G.C. Palmer (Ed.). *Neuropharmacology of central nervous system and behavioral disorders*, pp.340–391. New York: Academic Press.

Turner, P. (1983). Beta-adrenoceptor blocking drugs and the central nervous system in man. In P. Turner & D. Shand, (Eds.). *Recent advances in clinical pharmacology*, pp.223–234. London: Churchill and Livingston.

Tyrer, P.J. (1976). *The role of bodily feelings in anxiety*. London: Oxford University Press.

Weiner, N. (1985). Drugs that inhibit adrenergic nerves and block adrenergic receptors. In A.G. Goodman-Gilman, L.S. Goodman, A. Gilman (Eds.). *Goodman and Gilman's The pharmacological basis of therapeutics* (Edn. 7), pp.181–214. New York: Macmillan.

Blindness and visual disability

LINDA PRING

Psychology Department, Goldsmiths' College,
University of London, UK

According to the Royal National Institute for the Blind (1991) there are about 20 000 children and about 1 million adults who are blind or partially sighted in the UK. The age at which the visually impaired experience sight loss, and the length of time over which they experience deteriorating eyesight, are both important factors in their ability to adjust. It can be useful to distinguish between the sudden, traumatic loss of vision, which is relatively uncommon; about 14% across the whole age range, the onset at birth; where about 30% of the under 60 year-old-age-group have had problems, and the large majority, 86%, of visually impaired people who experience a progressive deterioration in their eyesight. The over 75 year-old age-group make-up 66% of the population who are blind. For adults, cataracts, glaucoma, general ill-health and diabetes can be singled out as commonly reported causes of eye problems, these in addition to the eye conditions developing from birth including retinopathy of prematurity and coloboma.

From a psychological perspective, the important questions have been related to the consequences of loss of vision for general development (Lewis, 1987), the role of vision in our understanding of space, and the related question of how far our senses provide independent, unitary or complementary information (Schiff & Foulke, 1982). These perspectives have meant that relatively little research has concentrated on the psychological correlates of visual impairment for those who go blind after childhood. Often, it is hard to determine the exact role that visual impairment plays in the experiences of these groups. In the older age-group, the complete loss of sight can lead to grief responses in the individual, but in addition, the situation may be compounded by other events caused simply by old age, such as widowhood or loss of mobility.

In terms of early development, we find that total blindness from birth causes the greatest problems for the young infant; some of these can be significantly diminished if the total loss of sight is delayed by just a few months. Early blind, before the age of two years for example, suffer more problems than those who go blind later. Many forget what it was like to see. Retaining some sight, however limited, provides a substantial advantage in nearly all aspects of development. Retaining enough sight to gain a partial sight status can still be misleading, since they may still recognize friends by voice in preference to their face. Although exceptional musical ability is associated with some types of congenital blindness, in general, blindness does not have consistent psychological consequences. Fraiberg (1977) noted this and also referred to autistic tendencies, such as problems with symbolic play, pronoun reversal in language and a preference for 'aloneness' with respect to social contact. For parents to discover that their newborn child is blind causes a range of emotional reactions from shock, helplessness and anger to guilt, depression and even revulsion. Certainly it would be surprising if such anxiety states did not affect the relationship between the child and the mother. Social smiling, in babies who are blind, occurs later in development than with the sighted and may be elicited more from tactile stimulation than the mother's voice, also, the repertoire of facial expressions in blind infants decreases during early development connected to the failure of reinforcement. The responses of caregivers to similar behaviours in infants who are blind and those who are sighted differ. This may be caused, in part, by the anomalous communication pattern seen in the mother/child interactions, where the infant may show less initiation of communication, less vocalizations and fewer positive responses to the mother. Thus, the loss of sight in this regard has effects on the consistency and therefore predictability of pattern of non-verbal communication between the infant and mother. Also, throughout childhood there is a tendency for parents to be over-protective towards their visually impaired child, leading perhaps to less exploratory and more dependent behaviour by the child.

In terms of motor development, there is likely to be a delay of most milestones but these appear to be affected both by a lack of experience with the world as well as the failure to 'see' the world. It is interesting to note that infants who are blind and those who are sighted will reach out, in the dark, towards a sound source at the same point in development, while reaching for an object, crawling and walking may be substantially delayed. 'Blindisms' is a label for the often strange movements displayed by children who are blind with no obvious communication role e.g. arm flapping or pressing the eyes, and often suppressed in adults.

Mobility and the use of spatial codes may be problematic for the visually impaired. The fact that vision is specialized for picking up information about the relation between external objects and planes means that forms of coding which depend on this information will be more difficult to acquire by the visually impaired, but should not be impossible provided the information is communicated by some other means (Millar, 1990). The visually impaired do use spatial imagery since vision is not the only sense that can supply spatial information. There is overlap in the information sight and touch can provide and thus the loss of vision cannot always be ascribed directly to a loss of spatial concepts. Research has sometimes been misguided, therefore, in trying to look at where the spatial concepts of blind and sighted individuals differ. However, certainly those who are blind do tend to use fewer external reference cues in some forms of spatial imagery than do the sighted, but the differences tend to reflect differences in strategy rather than imagery.

Some aspects of language may be delayed in those who are blind, but most are not. Although it has been noted that, as with autism, children who are blind can suffer problems of pronoun reversal, that is using the terms 'I' and 'you' incorrectly. If the child can make up for the experiences lost through impaired sight by the use of other channels, many aspects of delay can, in time, be compensated for. This may explain why there are few accounts of genuinely deviant or divergent psychological processes or behaviours amongst the visually impaired in adulthood. Nevertheless, the influence of an early impoverishment to the understanding of some concepts and word meanings may be difficult to completely correct. This can lead to flaws in communication and has, at times, been blamed for the failure of standardized tests to measure accurately, due to a misunderstanding of the instructions followed. Finally, a word needs to be said about 'verbalisms' a term used to describe a child's tendency to use words for which she does not have a first-hand sensory experience. At first, this was considered rather bizarre behaviour but more recently has emerged as often being meaningful ('I see', can mean 'I perceive with my dominant sensory channel').

Psychological issues within the area of visual impairment have tended to look for cognitive inabilities caused by the loss of vision. As I have reported already, these do exist but have surprisingly little impact, especially where residual sight can provide a spatial framework in which to place touch/haptic experience. O'Connor and Hermelin (1978) compared many aspects of handicap from a cognitive point of view, and by comparing autistic and intellectually less able children with individuals who are blind and deaf, they have made an invaluable contribution. For them, one important aspect of visual impairment was the emphasis on sequential processing of information available in language and perception which in turn, influenced cognitive style. Thus sequential rather than parallel, 'gestalt-like' processing may be emphasized in those who are blind. They, amongst others, have argued that there is very little evidence to suggest that being blind can lead to more sensitivity in other areas such as hearing. Sadly, loss of experience will rarely lead to advantages elsewhere.

Educational issues including a concern with reading, drawing and memory have been the focus of a great deal of research (Tobin, 1979; Millar, 1975; Pring, 1992; Kennedy, 1982). Interestingly, children with little or no residual sight can draw human figures that can be said to be indistinguishable from the drawings of some sighted children. However, the figure a child who is blind draws is often lying down or at an angle to the vertical. This indicates that the vertical and horizontal anchors play a less natural role for them.

The consequences of blindness for adults are often social isolation and an increase in depression and anxiety. Some research suggests that help with social cognition in young children may also have positive outcomes. Society has often failed to recognise the real needs of those adults and children with visual impairment. Rehabilitation in terms of occupational training and in terms of mobility play crucial roles in the lives and psychological health of those who go blind after school age. Increasingly, technology has

impacted on the lives of the visually disabled providing both jobs and communication aids and future psychological research is more targeted towards these issues than ever before.

REFERENCES

Fraiberg, S. (1977). *Insights from the blind.* London: Souvenir Press.

Kennedy, J.M. (1982) Haptic pictures. In W. Schiff & E. Foulke (Eds.). *Tactual perception: a source book.* Cambridge: Cambridge University Press.

Lewis, V. (1987). *Development and handicap.* Oxford: Blackwells.

Millar, S. (1975). Visual experience or translation rules? Drawing the human figure by blind and sighted children. *Perception,* **4**, 363–71.

Millar, S. (1990). Imagery and blindness. In P.J. Hampson, D.F. Marks & J.T.E. Richardson (Eds.) *Imagery: current developments.* London: Routledge.

O'Connor, N. & Hermelin, B. (1978). *Hearing and seeing and space and time.* New York: Lawrence Erlbaum and Associates.

Pring, L. (1992). More than meets the eye. In R. Campbell (Ed.) *Mental lives.* Oxford: Blackwell.

Royal National Institute for the Blind (1991). *Blind and partially sighted adults in*

Britain: the RNIB survey. London: HMSO.

Schiff, W. & Foulke, E. (1982). *Tactual perception: a source book.* Cambridge: Press. Cambridge University.

Tobin, M.J. (1979). *A longitudinal study of blind and partially sighted children in special schools in England and Wales.* University of Birmingham: Research Centre for the Education of Visually Handicapped children. School of Education.

Blood transfusion and donation

ROBERT WEST

and

OLGA EVANS

Psychology Department, St George's Hospital Medical School, London, UK

Blood transfusions are an essential part of medical practice. There is a continuing requirement for blood donation, which in most developed countries is normally able to be met by willing donors, although occasional shortages do occur.

Most blood is obtained from donors who give on a regular basis. It appears that being a blood donor forms an integral part of their personality and that contributes to their continued beneficence (Piliavin, 1992). Habit or simple inertia may also play a role (Piliavin, 1991). It is not clear what factors lead individuals into blood donation in the first place but, as would be expected, altruistic attitudes appear to play a role (Piliavin & Callero, 1991). There is also evidence of peer influence and to a lesser extent family influence (McCombie, 1991).

There is interest in ways of increasing donation practices within communities. Research suggests that approaches that involve modelling and use of social norms are more effective than conventional educational approaches (Sarason *et al.*, 1991).

Potential blood donors are questioned about illnesses and activities that might compromise the safety of their donation. Such questioning probably cannot be relied upon to ensure safety (Chiavetta, Nusbacher & Wall, 1989). However, direct and explicit questioning

about high risk activities appears to be acceptable to potential donors and to improve self-screening (Silvergleid, Leparc & Schmidt, 1989).

There is concern among potential recipients that HIV infection can be acquired from blood transfusions. Concern over HIV also appears to have been responsible for a sharp decline in blood donation in the US (Surgenor, Wallace, Hao & Chapman, 1990). However, the risk of this is small compared with other possible complications including haemolytic transfusion reaction. The possibility of complications, and concerns over the need to conserve blood stocks, has led to increased interest in autologous blood transfusion, where an individual receives his or her own blood which is pre-donated or salvaged during surgical procedures (Slater, 1992).

It is widely assumed that clinical decisions concerning transfusions are relatively straightforward. However, research shows that transfusion practices can vary widely and the proportion of actual transfusions that audit and physician review shows to be acceptable varies between hospitals and can be as low as 48% (Salem-Schatz, Avorn & Soumerai, 1993). The same study showed that knowledge of transfusion indication and receptiveness to advice from colleagues was associated with a high quality of transfusion practice.

REFERENCES

Chiavetta, J.A., Nusbacher, J. & Wall, A. (1989). Donor self-exclusion patterns and human immunodeficiency virus antibody test results over a twelve month period. *Transfusion*, 29, 81–3.

McCombie, R.P. (1991). Blood donation patterns of undergraduate students: family and friendship correlates. *Journal of Community Psychology*, 19, 161–5.

Piliavin, J.A. (1991). Is the road to helping paved with good intentions? Or inertia? In J. Howard & P. Callero (Eds.). *The self-society dynamic: cognition, emotion and action*, pp. 259–279. New York: CUP.

Piliavin, J.A. (1992). Role identity and organ donation: some suggestions based on blood donation research. In J. Shanteau & R. Harris (Eds.). *Organ donation and transplantation: psychological and behavioral factors*, pp. 150–158. Washington DC: APA.

Piliavin, J.A. & Callero, P.L. (1991). *Giving blood*. Baltimore: Johns Hopkins University Press.

Salem-Schatz, S.R., Avorn, J. & Soumerai, S.B. (1993). Influence of knowledge and attitudes on the quality of physicians' transfusion practice. *Medical Care*, 31, 868–78.

Sarason, I.G., Sarason, B.R., Pierce, G.R. & Shearin, E.N. (1991). A social learning approach to increasing blood donation.

Journal of Applied Social Psychology, 21, 896–918.

Silvergleid, A.J., Leparc, G.F. & Schmidt, P.J. (1989). Impact of explicit questions about high risk activities on donor attitudes and donor deferral patterns, results in two community blood centres. *Transfusion*, 29, 362–4.

Slater, N.G. (1992). Autologous blood transfusion today. *British Journal of Clinical Practice*, 46, 193–7.

Surgenor, D.M., Wallace, E.L., Hao, S.H. & Chapman, R.H. (1990). Collection and transfusion of blood in the United States: 1982–1988. *New England Journal of Medicine*, 322, 1646–51.

Breast cancer

LESLEY FALLOWFIELD

*Department of Oncology, University College
London Medical School, London, UK*

Many women regard breast cancer with dread, and consider it one of the most distressing diseases. They know that, despite the millions of pounds spent annually in attempts to find a cure, breast cancer is the biggest killer of western women in their middle years. No matter how reassuring their clinicians may be, most women know through articles in magazines and newspapers that their future is uncertain. With over 24 500 newly diagnosed cases and over 15 000 dying each year in the United Kingdom, many women will also have had a friend or relative who succumbed to the disease. These grim statistics, together with the personal experience of knowing someone with breast cancer, further fuels a woman's own anxieties and her feelings of vulnerability. The many controversies concerning the most appropriate management of breast cancer feature prominently not only in the scientific literature but also in the lay press and the issues are aired with monotonous regularity on radio and television. Against such a backdrop of fear and uncertainty (and often misinformation), it is hardly surprising that the discovery of a lump and a diagnosis of breast cancer causes considerable psychological distress, social and sexual dysfunction. Nor is this psychosocial toll avoided by breast conserving therapies (Fallowfield, Baum & Maguire, 1986; Fallowfield *et al.*, 1990a). Whatever treatment modality chosen, a woman still has to confront the fact that she has a life-threatening disease, and these fears may severely disrupt the quality of her life.

Much of the psychosocial morbidity experienced by women can be prevented or at least ameliorated through effective communication skills and professional counselling (Fallowfield, 1991). In this chapter, I shall discuss the aetiology of psychosocial dysfunc-

tion at different stages of the disease trajectory and consider some of the ways in which clinicians can help reduce the psychological trauma.

PSYCHOLOGICAL ASPECTS OF SCREENING

One means of reducing long-term psychological distress may be to identify the disease at an early stage when treatment might be more beneficial. However, the advent of the national mammographic screening programme in Britain which commenced in 1988 following the Forrest Report (HMSO, 1986) poses many important and interesting psychological, social and ethical questions. The actual benefits that may accrue to an individual woman, as opposed to a screened population of women, are probably few and have to be weighed against the many potential disadvantages such as time off work, anxiety, the discomfort of the procedure, the small, but uncertain hazards of repeated exposure to radiation every three years from the age of 50, wasted time and unnecessary stress if the quality of the mammogram leads to further investigations, etc. Some women will never accept screening on the seemingly irrational grounds that one should not go looking for trouble (Fallowfield, Rodway & Baum, 1990b). Any woman who does accept the offer of screening must feel sufficiently motivated to do so and there are a wide variety of sociodemographic and psychological reasons why certain women would be more likely than others to attend. The health beliefs model of Rosenstock (1974) provides a useful outline of some of the attitudes that may influence behaviours such as breast self-examination (BSE) or attendance at mammographic screening clinics. Inconsistencies between these beliefs provide some explanation as to why certain women decline screening or BSE. For example, some women may be well aware of their susceptibility to the disease and recognize the seriousness of it, but beliefs that treatments are ineffective (especially if one has witnessed a friend or relative dying following unsuccessful treatment) would militate against such women feeling motivated to participate in schemes aimed at early detection. One of the most powerful motivating factors is the positive influence of a woman's general practitioner (French *et al.*, 1982). Unfortunately, not all GPs have adequate information about modern breast cancer treatment to provide good positive education and encouragement to patients and some studies have shown that they harbour as many doubts and uncertainties and have as inadequate knowledge about breast cancer as their patients (Cockburn *et al.*, 1989).

Regular BSE (see also self-examination) is a good predictor of attendance for mammographic screening, but at best only 40% of women perform this regularly. Even women at high risk to breast cancer do not practise it any more frequently than those at low risk (Alagna *et al.*, 1987). Amongst the population who do claim to practise it regularly, few feel confident that they perform it correctly (Fallowfield *et al.*, 1990b) and, furthermore, studies have shown that even women who do it correctly and regularly are just as likely to delay seeking prompt medical attention as those who rarely self-examine. Until such time as a really effective treatment for breast cancer is found, it is doubtful, despite the cajoling by health educationalists and others, that mammographic screening and BSE will be acceptable to large numbers of women.

Results from studies, to date, have failed to support fears that mammographic screening would induce psychological problems. It could, for example, encourage neurotic hypervigilant monitoring of the breasts or an anxious preoccupation with fear about developing breast cancer. Little work has been done as yet on the psychological impact of a woman finding a breast lump herself in comparison to having one found during screening. It is worth remembering that, in general, women are asymptomatic and attend for screening expecting confirmation of themselves as fit and healthy. Their psychological adjustment is likely to be rather different from that of a woman who knows that she has a breast lump.

REACTIONS TO FINDING A LUMP (see also 'General cancer')

Although few women practise BSE regularly, the majority of breast lumps are discovered by women themselves and most women recognize the potentially sinister significance straight away, as the following quotations show:

'I was turning over in bed and I thought, oh no – I knew exactly what it was. I woke up my husband and I said to him 'I've got cancer''.'

'I was having a bath and I felt the lump. I felt sick and shook all over – my Mum died of breast cancer, so I guessed straight away what it was.'

quoted from Fallowfield & Clark, 1991

Denial is one means individuals employ to help cope with crises of any nature and as many as 20% of patients with symptoms delay seeking advice for three months or more. However, the majority of women see their doctor as soon as possible and most report that the

period between discovering a breast lump and having a diagnosis of cancer confirmed is the most stressful part of the whole experience (Fallowfield, Baum & Maguire, 1987).

'It was a living nightmare, that three weeks – knowing what it was but not knowing for sure. Nothing that has happened since – the mastectomy or the treatment sessions – were so bad as that time. Thinking it might be cancer and it spreading everywhere was all that I could do night and day.'

quoted from Fallowfield & Clark, 1991

One study (Scott, 1983) measured the anxiety and cognitive functioning of women awaiting breast biopsy and then six weeks later after confirmation of benign disease. The impairments to critical thinking, concentration and elevation of anxiety rates were significantly higher prior to the diagnosis.

Much of the early work done examining the psychological impact of breast cancer suggested that fear of breast loss was the primary reason for distress following discovery of a breast lump, but recent work by Fallowfield *et al.* (1990a) found that only 12% of their sample of 269 women reported that fear of losing a breast was their primary focus of concern, with 59% more concerned at the thought of having cancer (a life-threatening disease).

BREAKING THE BAD NEWS (See also 'General cancer')

Women may react in a wide variety of ways to the news that they have breast cancer and how they cope depends on many factors, such as individual personality characteristics and the level of social support available. Morris & her colleagues (Morris, Steven-Greer & White, 1977) described essentially five primary styles: denial, fighting spirit, stoic acceptance, anxious/depressed acceptance and helpless/hopelessness.

Some women claim to experience relief when told they have cancer, as at last the uncertainty is over and they can marshal all their energies into adjusting and coping. Particularly important at this time are the consultation skills of a woman's medical carers, especially those of the surgeon who breaks the bad news.

Clinicians who provide their patients with clear, accurate information in a sensitive, empathetic and unhurried manner can greatly enhance the ability of women to take in the news and to find something positive and hopeful. Remember that many will have imagined all manner of depressing scenarios, mutilating surgery, debilitating chemotherapy, inevitably followed by a lonely, painful and undignified death. 'I imagined the worst – no chest, no hair and dying anyway.' Awareness that lay populations are likely to have very pessimistic ideas of the five-year survival statistics gives the clinician an opportunity to provide some more hopeful and honest reassurance.

The presence of a trusted partner, spouse, friend or relative when the diagnosis is discussed can help long-term adaptation. Fallowfield *et al.* (1987) reported that the presence of a close ally during the bad-news consultation appeared to reduce the incidence of anxiety and/or depression at 12 months following surgery. This is probably due to the fact that many patients feel so shocked, confused and anxious when they learn the diagnosis that they fail to assimilate all the information given by the doctor which leads to further uncertainty and anxiety. The presence of a partner may also allow the patient to discuss what was said at a later time when she feels less emotionally distressed.

Hogbin & Fallowfield (1989) reported a novel method of helping patients being told their diagnosis of cancer. They gave audio-tape recordings of their consultations to 46 patients, 35 of whom were women with breast cancer. These tapes contained an explicit statement of the diagnosis and descriptions of the tests and treatment available. Follow-up questionnaires revealed that patients found the tapes beneficial for many reasons: they helped them to recall forgotten information, made them more confident, helped them trust the doctor more and assisted them in breaking the bad news to their family and friends. Social support from these sources is vital in helping women to recover from the physical and mental trauma of breast cancer and its treatment, so providing the close family and/or friends of patients with clear accurate information should not be overlooked.

PSYCHOLOGICAL MORBIDITY FOLLOWING TREATMENT

The psychological distress following treatment for breast cancer have been well documented since the early 1950s (Bard & Sutherland, 1955; Renneker & Cutler, 1952). The largely anecdotal, but nevertheless seminal, papers published at that time described anxiety, depression, physical and sexual impairments as common sequelae to mastectomy. Later studies (Morris *et al.*, 1977; Maguire *et al.*, 1978) compared the psychiatric morbidity experienced by women following mastectomy with that of women found to have benign breast disease and reported significantly more distress amongst the women with breast cancer. It was assumed that in a western culture in which breasts were regarded as such potent symbols of femininity and sexuality, the amputation of a breast because of cancer so profoundly and negatively affected self-esteem and body image that psychological and sexual dysfunction was an almost inevitable consequence. With the advent of breast conserving procedures, it was hoped that the psychosocial toll would be significantly reduced. However, the 17 published studies (Table 1) comparing the psychological outcome of mastectomy versus lumpectomy show few substantial differences between treatments. Some studies show a small advantage to some women in terms of improved body-image following lumpectomy rather than mastectomy, but approximately 35% of women develop moderate to severe anxiety and/or depression whatever surgical treatment is performed. As mentioned earlier in this chapter, most women are more worried about having cancer than about losing a breast. This diagnosis which many women regard as inevitably fatal, together with their worries that they will endure rejection, be stigmatised and die a lonely, painful and undignified death, are issues that confront all women, whatever their primary surgical therapy.

Recognition that the woman who undergoes a breast conserving procedure may experience substantial psychological morbidity despite retaining her breast also highlights the need to ensure that all women have access to effective counselling whatever treatment they are given. Consider the plight of the woman in the following quotation:

What I couldn't understand was why the nurses didn't have any thought for what I was going through the night before the operation.

They were all terribly concerned and kind to another lady on the ward who had to have her breast removed, but no-one came and talked to me. I was really scared; all sorts of awful things were going through my mind, but I got the feeling that I was meant to be grateful to someone that I wasn't having the breast off, so I shouldn't make a fuss.'

quoted from Fallowfield & Clark, 1991

Some women who have a lumpectomy experience guilt that they feel anxious and depressed post-treatment. The role of a sick person is acceptable while in hospital and during radiotherapy treatment, but thereafter as time passes with few overt signs of physical problems there is an unwritten convention in our culture that demands stoicism in the face of both physical and emotional pain. I have argued (Fallowfield *et al.*, 1987) that for the woman who has had a mastectomy a flat chest wall in some way 'legitimizes' continuation of the sick role. However, removal of 'just a little lump' imputes that, as surgery was relatively 'trivial', the patient should be pleased at retaining her breast and return to normal psychological and physical functioning quite quickly. She may feel guilty about her difficulty in adjustment and attempt to repress her unexpected anxiety and unhappiness. An inability to do so increases feelings of inadequacy and worthlessness and may lead to depression. Another underestimated problem for these patients is the enervating effect of radiotherapy which in itself can cause depression. In one study almost one-third of patients were still complaining of excessive tiredness a year after treatment (Fallowfield *et al.*, 1986) (See also 'General cancer' (section on surgery)).

THERAPEUTIC BENEFITS OF COUNSELLING

As well as worries about the treatment that they must embark upon, women with breast cancer ask themselves many other questions (see Table 2). They profit from an opportunity to discuss these issues with an empathic person who could be the doctor, but more often is a specialist nurse or oncology counsellor. Although evidence that counselling can reduce psychiatric morbidity remains equivocal, patients attest to the benefits of having received good counselling from the specialist nurses and oncology counsellors who are employed increasingly in breast cancer clinics. There are several reasons why it is difficult to show a clear benefit from studies of counselling. These include such things as small patient samples, inappropriate outcome measures, vaguely defined counselling techniques and/or an inadequately trained counsellor (Fallowfield, 1988). Counselling is only as good as the person doing it, and benefits are linked to the skills, training and supervision of the counsellor. In a recent survey (Roberts & Fallowfield, 1990) specialist oncology nurses were found to be undertrained, overworked, undervalued and under-supervised. Few had any recognizable formal counselling qualifications or used any particular counselling model.

Detailed descriptions of the counselling needs pre- and post-operatively and during chemotherapy or radiotherapy can be found in a recently published book by Fallowfield and Clark (1991). They conclude that, instead of offering a prophylactic service aimed at preventing distress, most counsellors are only able to operate a 'casualty-based system offering mainly crisis counselling'. An interesting study of women with breast cancer has shown how it is

Table 1. *Psychological outcome of mastectomy (Mx) vs. breast conservation (BC)*

Authors	Patients	Derivation of sample	Outcome
Sanger & Reznikoff (1981)	40 Mx (20) BC (20)	Diverse sources: non-comparable treatment groups	No difference between groups in psychosocial morbidity. Greater overall 'body satisfaction' in BC group
Schain et al. (1983)	38 Mx (20) BC (18)	Randomized clinical trial	No significant psychosocial differences, but less negative body image in BC group
Steinberg, Juliano & Wise (1985)	67 radical Mx (46) BC (21) ($\frac{1}{2}$ chose BC)	Retrospective study: non-comparable treatment groups. No information on how sample was selected from those eligible	No significant differences between groups in psychosocial morbidity. BC group less self-conscious
Ashcroft, Leinster & Slade (1985)	40 Mx ? BC ? (numbers unknown)	Some women randomized and some women chose treatment (numbers not given): prospective study of consecutive cases	Little difference between groups on psychosocial measures but better body satisfaction in BC group
de Haes, van Oostrom & Welvaart (1986)	39 Mx (18) BC (21)	Randomized clinical trial. Retrospective psychological assessment	Less negative body image in BC group. No differences in sexual or psychological functioning, or in fear of recurrence or death
Bartelink, van Dam & van Dongen (1985)	172 Radical Mx (58) BC (114)	Retrospective study of consecutive patients	Less negative body image and less fear of recurrence in BC group
Fallowfield, Baum & Maguire (1986)	101 Mx (53) BC (48)	Randomized clinical trial. Retrospective study	No difference in psychiatric morbidity between groups, but more overt concern with cancer in BC group
Lasry et al. (1987)	123 Mx (43) BC+RXT (36) BC (44)	Randomized clinical trial. Retrospective study no information on how sample was selected from those eligible	Depression highest in BC+RXT group. Better body image in BC group. Fear of recurrence greatest amongst patients receiving chemotherapy.
Wolberg et al. (1987)	206 Mx (no choice) 96 Mx (choice) 56 BC (choice) 54	Prospective study: consecutive patients	Psychosocial data reported from only 39 eligible patients. Advantage in terms of anxiety and depression to women who chose BC
Ganz et al. (1992)	50 Mx (31) BC (19)	Consecutive patients assessed approx. 1 month postoperatively	No differences in psychological morbidity or sexual dysfunction
Kemeny, Wellisch & Schain (1988)	52 Mx (27) BC (25)	Randomized clinical trial. Retrospective study	No significant difference in psychological morbidity between groups. Less 'sadness when first viewing breast surgery' in BC group
Morris & Royle (1988)	30 Mx (no choice) 10 Mx (choice) 7 BC (choice) 13	Prospective study: consecutive patients	No difference in psychological morbidity between Mx & BC but less morbidity in patients offered choice
Meyer & Aspergren (1996)	58 Radical Mx (30) BC (28)	Sample drawn from consecutive patients No other details: retrospective study	No differences in psychological morbidity between groups. Less negative body image in BC group
Maunsell, Brisson & Deschenes (1989)	227 Mx (147) BC (80)	Consecutive patients assessed at 3 and 18 months	Significantly more psychological morbidity in BC group at 3 months. No differnce at 18 months although psychological morbidity high (35%) in both
Holmberg et al. (1989)	99 Mx (62) BC (37)	Consecutive patients randomized to participation: assessed at 4 and 13 months	No statistically significant differences in adjustment except in sexual relationships. BC patients significantly more dysfunction
McArdle, Hughson & McArdle (1990)	119 Mx (52) BC (67)	Prospective consecutive patients	Depression highest amongst Mx patients

Table 1. (cont.)

Authors	Patients	Derivation of sample	Outcome
Fallowfield *et al.* (1990)	269 MX (154) BC (115) Choice Sgns Pts: (118) Real Choice No Choice 62 56 Mx (19) BC (43)	Prospective non-randomized study	No differences in psychological morbidity or sexual interest between treatments. Psychological morbidity lowest in patients treated by surgeons who offered choice where possible

Table 2. *Questions women with breast cancer ask themselves*

1. Why me?
2. What caused it?
3. Will I die?
4. Which treatment?
5. Will it return?
6. What will I look like?
7. What will others do?

possible for a motivated general surgeon to be trained in Rogerian counselling techniques which proved to be of great benefit to his patients by preventing and ameliorating psychological distress (Burton & Parker, 1988).

PSYCHOLOGICAL REACTIONS TO RECURRENCE (See also 'General cancer')

There is a dearth of research in the area of psychosocial response during recurrent disease in contrast to the copious amount of work reported on early stage disease. Intuition would lead one to predict that the emotional impact of discovering that the cancer had returned (or never gone away) would be devastating. Clinical experience, however, shows that reactions to the news are rarely uniform. Many are distressed but others treat the news with equanimity and claim that they had always felt that they were living on borrowed time and that the cancer would return. These women usually adopt a stoical or practical approach and worry about the distress that the news will cause their loved ones, as the following quotation shows:

> *I suppose in my heart of hearts I'd always expected it to come back in spite of what they'd told me. I didn't really cry or anything. I just made an appointment to see my GP and wondered what I should tell the family.*
>
> *quoted from Fallowfield & Clark, 1991*

Holland (1977) suggests that recurrence leads to more psychological despair than that found in newly diagnosed cancer patients and another study (Weisman & Worden, 1986) of 102 mixed cancer patients which included women with breast cancer reported that 30% found recurrence less emotionally traumatic than the original diagnosis. Anecdotal observations based on interviews with patients convey an impression of distress, concern about further treatment

and renewed worries about long-term survival. However, the majority of women do appear prepared for the cancer to return and, provided that the support systems marshalled together in the earlier stages of their breast cancer remain intact, then most seem to cope fairly well (Fallowfield & Clark, 1991).

ADVANCED DISEASE

When advanced disease is discovered, the only criterion of benefit from treatment should be palliation or symptom control which can improve the quality of the life left. A lack of good psychological support at this time for the patients and their families makes women easy prey for the pedlars of quack cures and remedies. Unless the patient and her family are convinced that active therapy is no longer appropriate and are confident that everything possible will be done to control symptoms, then they may seek out unorthodox, alternative therapies. Good supportive care is imperative at this time and should include good quality counselling. A recently published paper (Hall, Fallowfield & A'Hern, 1996) reported that 50% of 38 women with recurrence of their breast cancer were anxious and/or depressed. Only eight women had been offered any extra supportive counselling at this stressful time.

THE FUTURE

Some of the understandable anxiety and depression associated with breast cancer could be alleviated if current treatments were less toxic and more effective. Hopefully, with improved pharmacological preparations the need for surgery may disappear altogether, and the use of drugs such as tamoxifen give us a realistic possibility of preventing or delaying the expression of disease in the women identified as being at high risk to breast cancer.

In the meantime, there is still much that the clinician can offer patients in terms of good psychological support that may make the psychosocial distress caused by the diagnosis and treatments more bearable. This can only come about if adequate attention is given to the training of medical and surgical oncologists in effective communication and counselling skills. Furthermore, much more thought needs to be given to means of resourcing the provision of psychological support for the whole medical team who deal with women with cancer. We cannot really expect health-care professionals working in high stress areas to get closer to the psychological needs of their patients if they have no opportunities to obtain support themselves.

Breast cancer

REFERENCES

Alagna, S.W., Morokoff, P.J., Bevett, J.M. *et al.* (1987). Performance of breast self-examination by women at high risk for breast cancer. *Women's Health*, **12**, 29–46.

Ashcroft, J.J., Leinster, S.J. & Slade, P.D. (1985). Breast cancer – patient choice of treatment: preliminary communication. *Journal of the Royal Society of Medicine*, **78**, 43–6.

Bard, M. & Sutherland, A.M. (1955). Psychological impact of cancer and its treatment. *Cancer*, 8, 656–72.

Bartelink, H., van Dam, F. & van Dongen, J. (1985). Psychological effects of breast conserving therapy in comparison with radical mastectomy. *International Journal of Radiation Oncology and Biological Physics*, 11, 381–5.

Burton, M.V. & Parker, R.W. (1988). A randomised controlled trial of pre-operative psychological preparation for mastectomy: a preliminary report. In M. Watson, S. Greer, & C. Thomas (Eds.). *Psychosocial oncology*. Oxford: Pergamon.

Cockburn, J., Irwig, L., Turnbull, D., Simpson, J.M., Mock, P. & Tattersall, M. (1989). Encouraging attendance at screening mammography: knowledge, attitudes and intentions of general practitioners. *Medical Journal of Australia*, 151, 391–6.

de Haes, J.C.J.M., van Oostrom, M.A. & Welvaart, K. (1986). The effect of radical and conserving surgery on the quality of life of early breast cancer patients. *European Journal of Surgical Oncology*, 12, 337–42.

Fallowfield, L.J. (1988). Counselling for patients with cancer. *British Medical Journal*, 297, 727–8.

Fallowfield, I.J. (1991). Counselling patients with cancer. In H. Davis & L. Fallowfield (Eds.). *Counselling and communication in health care*. Chichester: John Wiley & Sons.

Fallowfield, L.J., Baum, M. & Maguire, G.P. (1986). Effects of breast conservation on psychological morbidity associated with diagnosis and treatment of early breast cancer. *British Medical Journal*, 293, 1331–4.

Fallowfield, L.J., Baum, M. & Maguire, G.P. (1987). Adressing the psychological needs of the conservatively treated breast cancer patient: discussion paper. *Journal of the Royal Society of Medicine*, 80, 696–700.

Fallowfield, L.J., Hall, A., Maguire, G.P. & Baum, M. (1990). Psychological outcomes of different treatment policies in women with early breast cancer outside a clinical trial. *British Medical Journal*, 301, 575–80.

Fallowfield, L.J. & Clark, A.W. (1991). *Breast cancer*. London: Routledge.

Fallowfield, L.J., Hall, A., Maguire, G.P. & Baum, M. (1990a). Psychological outcomes of different treatment policies in women with early breast cancer outside a clinical trial. *British Medical Journal*, 301, 575–80.

Fallowfield, L.J., Rodway, A. & Baum, M. (1990b). What are the psychological factors influencing attendance, non-attendance and re-attendance at a breast screening centre? *Journal of the Royal Society of Medicine*, 83, 547–51.

French, K., Porter, A.M.D., Robinson, S.E., McCallum, F.M., Howie, J.G. & Roberts, M.M. (1982). Attendance at a breast screening clinic: a problem of administration or attitudes. *British Medical Journal* 285, 617–20.

Ganz, P.A., Coscarelli Schag, C.A., Lee, J.J., Polinsky, M.L. & Tan, S-J. (1992). Breast conservation versus mastectomy. *Cancer*, 69, 1729–38.

Hall, A., Fallowfield, L.J. & A'Hern, R.P. (1996). When breast cancer recurs: a 3-year prospective study of psychological morbidity. *The Breast Journal*, 2, 197–203.

HMSO (1986). *Breast cancer screening*. London: (Forrest Report). Department of Health & Social Security

Hogbin, B. & Fallowfield, L.J. (1989). Getting it taped: the 'bad news' consultation with cancer patients. *British Journal of Hospital Medicine*, 41, 330–3.

Holland, J.C. (1977). Psychological aspects of oncology. *Medical Clinics of North America*, 61, 737–48.

Holmberg, L., Omne-Ponten, M., Burns, T., Adami, H.O. & Bergstrom, R. (1989). Psychosocial adjustment after mastectomy and breast-conserving treatment. *Cancer*, 64, 969–74.

Kemeny, M.M., Wellisch, D.K. & Schain, W. (1988). Psychosocial outcome in a randomised surgical trial for treatment of primary breast cancer. *Cancer*, 62, 1231–7.

Lasry, J-C.M., Margolese, R.G., Poisson, R., Shibata, H., Fleischer, D., Lafleur, D., Legault, S. & Taillefer S. (1987). Depression and body image following mastectomy and lumpectomy. *Journal of Chronic Diseases*, 40, 529–4.

McArdle, J.M., Hughson, A.V.M. & McArdle, C.S. (1990). Reduced psychological morbidity after breast conservation. *British Journal of Surgery*, 77, 1221–3.

Maguire, G.P., Lee, Eg., Bevington, D.J., Küchemann, C.S., Grabhee, R.J. & Comell, C.E. (1978). Psychiatric problems in the year after mastectomy. *British Medical Journal*, i, 963–5.

Maunsell, E., Brisson, J. & Deschenes, L. (1989). Psychological distress after initial treatment for breast cancer: A comparison of partial and total mastectomy. *Journal of Clinical Epidemiology*, 42, 765–71.

Meyer, L. & Aspergren, K. (1996). Long term psychological sequelae of mastectomy and breast conserving treatment for breast cancer. *Acta Oncologia* in press.

Morris, T. & Royle, G.T. (1988). Offering patients a choice of surgery for early breast cancer. *Social Science Medicine*, 26, 583–5.

Morris, T., Steven-Greer, H. & White, P. (1977). Psychological and social adjustment to mastectomy (a 2-year follow-up study). *Cancer*, 40, 2381–7.

Renneker, R. & Cutler, M. (1952). Psychological problems of adjustment to cancer of the breast. *Journal of the American Medical Association*, 148, 833–9.

Roberts, R. & Fallowfield, L.J. (1990). Who supports the cancer counsellors? *Nursing Times*, 86, 32–4.

Rosenstock, I. (1974). The health belief model and preventative health behaviour. *Health Education Mono*, 2, 354.

Sanger, C.K. & Reznikoff, M. (1981). A comparison of the psychological effects of breast-saving procedures with the modified radical mastectomy. *Cancer*, 48, 2341–6.

Schain, W., Edwards, B.K., Gorell, C.R., de Moss, E.V., Lippman, M.E., Gerber, L.H. & Lichter, A.S. (1983). Psychosocial and physical outcomes of primary breast cancer therapy: mastectomy vs excisional biopsy and irradiation. *British Cancer Research Treatment*, 3, 377–82.

Steinberg, M.D., Juliano, M.A. & Wise, L. (1985). Psychological outcome of lumpectomy versus mastectomy in the treatment of breast cancer. *American Journal of Psychiatry*, 142, 34–9.

Scott, D.W. (1983). Anxiety, critical thinking and information processing during and after breast biopsy. *Nursing Research*, 32, 24–9.

Weisman, A.D. & Worden, J.W. (1986). The emotional impact of recurrent cancer. *Journal of Psychosocial Oncology*, 3, 5–16

Wolberg, W.H., Tanner, M.A., Romsaas, E.P., Trump, D.L. & Malec, J.F. (1987). Factors influencing options in primary breast cancer treatment. *Journal of Clinical Oncology*, 5, 68–74.

Breastfeeding

ANTONY MANSTEAD

Department of Social Psychology, University of Amsterdam, The Netherlands

Research on the psychological aspects of breastfeeding tends to focus on one of two general issues: (i) the factors that determine a mother's choice of infant feeding method (breast vs. bottle) and (ii) the consequences of the adopted feeding method for the cognitive development of the child. This entry will summarize the conclusions that can be drawn from research addressing each of these issues.

MATERNAL ATTITUDES TO AND BELIEFS ABOUT BREASTFEEDING

In western industrialized countries the present century has witnessed a steady decline both in the proportion of mothers who elect to breastfeed their infants, and in the duration of breastfeeding among those mothers who do choose this feeding method. Because the consensus of medical opinion on this issue is that breastfeeding is better for a baby's health, a number of investigators have studied maternal attitudes to, and beliefs about, breastfeeding in order to establish why some mothers elect to breastfeed whereas others do not. An example is the large-scale study reported by Jones (1986), who interviewed 1525 mothers in hospital, shortly after delivery, and the mothers who chose to breastfeed their babies (*n*=649) again 12 months later. The majority of mothers who breastfed reported that they had received sufficient advice about breastfeeding, that they had found breastfeeding enjoyable and satisfying, that they would breastfeed their next child, and that they would encourage their friends to breastfeed. Among those who did not find breastfeeding enjoyable or satisfying, the majority reported having experienced physical problems such as sore breasts or cracked nipples. There was a significant tendency for mothers having their first baby to report having more of these problems. There was also a consistently negative relationship between enjoyment and satisfaction, on the one hand, and degree of embarrassment experienced when breastfeeding in front of other persons, on the other. How embarrassed a mother reported feeling was negatively associated with how long she continued to breastfeed. On the other hand, embarrassment was not often cited as a reason for not wanting to breastfeed a next child, if the mother were to have one. Instead, problems with sore nipples were cited most frequently. Among the reasons for wanting to breastfeed a next baby, the most commonly cited ones were that it is better for the baby and that it is enjoyable and satisfying for the mother. To summarize, in this research (like others of its type) it was found that the mothers' attitudes to breastfeeding were closely associated with the duration of breastfeeding.

In Jones' study the direction of causality in the relationship between attitudes and behaviour necessarily remained ambiguous, in that mothers who initially had negative attitudes to breastfeeding might have experienced more problems, or mothers who experienced more problems in trying to breastfeed might have later developed negative attitudes. It is clear from other research on this issue, however, that antenatal attitudes to infant feeding methods do help to determine which feeding method is chosen. For example, Manstead, Proffitt and Smart (1983) found that attitudes to infant feeding methods as measured during the last trimester of pregnancy were strongly predictive of which infant feeding method mothers elected to use. Mothers who breastfed during the first six weeks of the baby's life were significantly more likely than bottlefeeding mothers to believe that breastfeeding provides better nourishment for the baby, is good for the mother's figure, protects the baby against infection, and establishes a close bond between mother and baby. Mothers who bottlefed throughout the first six weeks of the baby's life were significantly more likely than breastfeeding mothers to believe that bottlefeeding is a convenient feeding method, is a trouble-free feeding method, and makes it possible for the father to be involved in feeding. Because these beliefs were assessed antenatally and were significantly associated with postnatal behaviours, it is reasonable to interpret these associations as reflecting the causal impact of beliefs on behaviours.

BREASTFEEDING AND CHILD DEVELOPMENT

Several researchers have examined the claim that there is a relationship between breastfeeding and cognitive development. An example is the study reported by Morrow-Tlucak, Haude and Ernhart (1988). They compared three groups of children, namely those who had been bottlefed, those who had been breastfed for four months or less, and those who had been breastfed for more than four months. The researchers first compared these three groups on a large number of potential confounding variables. Where the groups were found to differ significantly, the influence of these variables was statistically controlled in the main analyses, in which the Mental Development Index of the Bayley scales served as the primary dependent measure. Children were assessed on this index at 6, 12, and 24 months. At each age, the observed MDI scores of the three groups fell in the same order: the highest scores were those of the group breastfed for more than 4 months, followed by the group breastfed for 4 months or less, followed by the bottlefed group. The difference between the three groups was significant at 12 and 24 months, even after controlling for the effects of potentially confounding variables. Such findings can be interpreted as supporting the hypothesis that breastfeeding has a directly beneficial effect on cognitive development. However, the causal mechanisms responsible for such an effect are unclear, and the possibility remains that these findings reflect the influence of maternal, social or environmental factors that were either uncontrolled or insufficiently controlled.

With respect to causal mechanisms, it has been suggested that differences between formula milk and breast milk, with respect to osmotic load or protein and lipid concentrations, might account for the findings. It has also been suggested that the observed effects might be mediated by risk of infection or by qualitative differences in mother–child interaction. In short, although it has often been reported that breastfed children exhibit higher scores on measures of cognitive development by comparison with bottlefed children, it is by no means clear that this relationship between feeding method and cognitive development is a genuinely causal one; and even if it were established to be causal, the nature of the responsible mechanism(s) is as yet unclear.

REFERENCES

Jones, D.A. (1986). Attitudes of breast-feeding mothers: a survey of 649 mothers. *Social Science and Medicine*, 23, 1151–6.

Manstead, A.S.R., Proffitt, C. & Smart, J.L. (1983). Predicting and understanding mothers' infant feeding intentions and behavior: testing the theory of reasoned action. *Journal of Personality and Social Psychology*, 44, 657–71.

Morrow-Tlucak, M, Haude, R.H. & Ernhart, C.B. (1988). Breastfeeding and cognitive development in the first 2 years of life. *Social Science and Medicine*, 26, 635–9.

Bronchitis (chronic) and emphysema

AD A. KAPTEIN
Medical Psychology, Department of Psychiatry,
Leiden University, The Netherlands

Chronic, irreversible shortness of breath and coughing up of sputum are the two central symptoms in patients suffering from chronic bronchitis and/or emphysema. Chronic bronchitis is defined as 'the condition of subjects with chronic or recurrent excess mucus secretion into the bronchial tree' (ATS, 1987, p. 226). 'Chronic' refers to 'occurring on most days for at least three months of the year for at least two successive years' (ATS, 1987, p. 226). Emphysema is defined as 'a condition of the lung characterized by abnormal permanent enlargement of the airspaces distal to the terminal bronchiole, accompanied by destruction of their walls, and without obvious fibrosis' (ATS, 1987, p. 225). Increasingly, chronic bronchitis and emphysema are subsumed under the category chronic obstructive pulmonary disease (COPD), defined as 'a disorder characterized by abnormal tests of expiratory flow that do not change markedly over periods of several months observation. The qualification is intended to distinguish COPD from asthma' (ATS, 1987, p. 255); (see 'Asthma'). Chronic bronchitis may lead to emphysema although this is a debated issue.

EPIDEMIOLOGY

The prevalence of COPD in the industrialized countries is 5%. Men form the majority of COPD patients. Increased smoking rates in women will lead to an increased prevalence of COPD in this group. Tobacco smoking is the most important behavioural risk factor for COPD. Genetic and environmental factors are also involved in the development of COPD in susceptible persons. The prevalence of COPD is rising.

COPD accounts for 4% of the mortality in the western world. The morbidity due to COPD is not only reflected in restrictions in daily activities but especially in absenteeism from work, hospitalization and forced retirement (Higgins, 1993).

BEHAVIOURAL AND PSYCHOLOGICAL CONCOMITANTS

Increased levels of feelings of depression, anxiety and social isolation and problems with sexuality and sleep are the predominant psychological consequences of COPD (McSweeny & Labuhn, 1990). In a study by Kinsman *et al.* (1983) on symptoms and experiences in patients with chronic bronchitis and emphysema, the most frequently reported symptoms were dyspnea, fatigue, sleep difficulties, congestion and irritability. Indicators of the objective severity of the illness (e.g. pulmonary function measures) were not related to the symptoms experienced.

The impact of COPD on the daily lives of patients has been assessed in research which falls under the heading 'quality of life'. A study by Schrier *et al.* (1990) is particularly illuminating as it described the negative consequences of COPD in a group of patients in a general practice setting, i.e. with a relatively mild degree of COPD. The sickness impact profile (SIP) was used to assess the impact of the illness in the patients, and SIP scores were compared with those of healthy controls of similar age. The COPD patients experienced significantly more negative consequences in the areas of ambulation, communication, emotional behaviour, sleep and rest, eating, home management, and employment. Similar to Kinsman *et al.*'s findings, pulmonary function was not related to SIP scores, indicating that quality of life was not determined by the medical severity of COPD but was related to a large extent by the coping behaviour of the patients.

Two areas which appear to be of major importance, judging from clinical experience, but which have rarely been studied by physicians or psychologists, are sexuality and the increased strain for partners of COPD patients. The available data indicate that sexual function of patients with COPD is severely impaired (Hanson,

1982), and that the well-being of wives of COPD patients is reduced because of the caregiving tasks they perform (Cossette & Lévesque, 1993).

PSYCHOLOGICAL INTERVENTIONS IN COPD

Psychological interventions in patients with COPD focus on psychological treatment ('secondary prevention') and pulmonary rehabilitation ('tertiary prevention', including smoking cessation). Primary prevention concerns preventing people taking up smoking tobacco (see 'Tobacco Smoking').

Psychological treatment.

The first studies by psychologists on patients with COPD pertained to assessing personality characteristics (DeCencio, Leshner & Leshner, 1968) and to alleviating the feelings of depression associated with COPD by way of psychotherapeutic interventions (Rosser *et al.*, 1983). Currently, more modern approaches, e.g. self-management training, patient education and home rehabilitation programmes are being applied. In a review of the effectiveness of these approaches, it was concluded that dyspnea, feelings of depression and anxiety, and limitations in daily activities were reduced by behavioural interventions (Kaptein, 1997).

The most elaborate study evaluating psychological interventions in COPD-patients was done by Atkins *et al.* (1984). Patients were randomly assigned to one of five conditions: (i) behaviour therapy, (ii) cognitive modification, (iii) combined cognitive–behavioural modification, (iv) attention control, and (v) no-treatment control. In the experimental conditions (i), (ii) and (iii), principles of behaviour modification and cognitive modification were explained to the patients and they were motivated to apply them in their homes. Self-control, self-monitoring of daily walking and self-statements, relaxation and breathing exercises comprised the elements of the interventions.

After the intervention, patients in the combined cognitive–behavioural modification group spent significantly more time walking, their exercise tolerance was significantly higher, and their scores on scales which assessed self-efficacy and well-being were significantly higher than in the attention control or no-treatment control group. Substituting negative self-statements ('I can't walk very far without getting short of breath, so what's the use') with more positive ones ('This walking is uncomfortable, but I can handle it. Soon I will be able to walk farther', p. 544) is an illustration of the cognitive modification condition.

Pulmonary rehabilitation programmes

In pulmonary rehabilitation programmes, traditional medical interventions such as physiotherapy, graded exercise, breathing exercises, are combined with coping skills training and patient education (about medication, smoking, physical activity), which have a group therapy format with the spouses attending in order to facilitate carry-over effects. Physicians, nurses, dieticians and psychologists make up the staff of such programmes. Recent studies indicate that pulmonary rehabilitation programmes have positive effects on psychological factors (e.g. anxiety, depression, self-efficacy) and health care utilization (e.g. hospitalization) (Kaplan, Eakin & Ries, 1993). Smoking cessation usually is a part of pulmonary rehabilitation programmes.

SOME CLOSING REMARKS

Psychological treatment of patients with COPD tends to be hampered by at least three problems which appear to be quite specific for this disease. First, COPD patients tend to be unexperienced and rather unwilling to discuss emotional and behavioural problems. The 'non-YAVIS' character of many COPD-patients coupled with therapeutic pessimism in the medical or psychological expert, is at least one reason why COPD is an area which does not enjoy as much interest from psychologists as, for example, cancer or cardiovascular disease. Secondly, many intervention programmes for patients with COPD. medical or psychological, tend to suffer substantial drop-out rates (as high as 80%). Thirdly, further research should focus on identifying those patients who are most likely to benefit from what component in intervention programmes, irrespective of whether these programmes are embedded in a pulmonary rehabilitation setting (Williams, 1993).

If every cigarette smoker gave up the habit today, the offices of pulmonary physicians would be a lot emptier. Primary prevention, therefore, is the most rational intervention, for medical and behavioural professionals. Smoking cessation, psychological treatment, optimal medical care and pulmonary rehabilitation programmes are the next stage in caring for patients with COPD. The decline in lung function is a serious and potentially lethal threat for smokers susceptible for COPD. Psychological interventions will barely help in slowing down this decline in lung function. However, research, often combining medical and psychological expertise, makes it increasingly clear that the application of behavioural interventions in COPD patients does impact on the central outcome of health care, i.e. behavioural health outcomes (Kaplan, 1990).

REFERENCES

Atkins, C.J., Kaplan, R.M., Timms, R.M., Reinsch, S. & Lofback, K. (1984). Behavioral exercise programs in the management of chronic obstructive pulmonary disease. *Journal of Consulting and Clincial and Psychology*, **52**, 591–603.

ATS (American Thoracic Society). Standards for the diagnosis and care of patients with chronic obstructive pulmonary disease (COPD) and asthma. (1987) *American Review of Respiratory Disease*, **136**, 225–44.

Cossette, S. & Lévesque, L. (1993). Caregiving tasks as predictors of mental health of wife caregivers of men with chronic obstructive pulmonary disease. *Research in Nursing and Health*, **16**, 251–63.

DeCencio, D.V., Leshner, M. & Leshner, B. (1968). Personality characteristics of patients with chronic obstructive pulmonary emphysema. *Archives of Physical and Medical Rehabilitation*, **49**, 471–5.

Hanson, E.I. (1982). Effects of chronic lung disease on life in general and on sexuality: Perceptions of adult patients. *Heart and Lung*, **11**, 435–41.

Higgins, M. (1993). Epidemiology of obstructive pulmonary disease. In R. Casaburi & T.L. Petty (Eds.). *Principles and practice of pulmonary rehabilitation*, pp. 10–17. Philadelphia: Saunders.

Kaplan, R.M. (1990). Behavior as the central outcome in health care. *American Psychologist*, **45**, 1211–20.

Kaplan, R.M., Eakin, E.G. & Ries, A.L. (1993). Psychosocial issues in the rehabilitation of patients with chronic obstructive pulmonary disease. In R. Casaburi & T.L. Petty (Eds.). *Principles and practice of pulmonary rehabilitation*, pp. 351–365. Philadelphia: Saunders.

Bronchitis and emphysema

Kaptein, A.A. (1995). Behavioural interventions in COPD: A pause for breath. *European Respiratory Review*, 7, special issue.

Kinsman, R.A., Yaroush, R.A., Fernandez, E., Dirks, J.F., Schocket, M. & Fukuhara, J. (1983). Symptoms and experiences in chronic bronchitis and emphysema. *Chest.*, 83, 755–61.

McSweeny, A.J. & Labuhn, K.T. (1990). Chronic obstructive pulmonary disease. In B. Spilker (Ed.). *Quality of life assessments in clinical trials*, pp. 391–417. New York: Raven Press.

Rosser, R., Denford, J., Heslop, A., Kinston, W., Macklin, D., Minty, K., Moynihan, C., Muir, B., Rein, L. & Guz. A. (1983). Breathlessness and psychiatric morbidity in chronic bronchitis and emphysema: a study

of psychotherapeutic management. *Psychological Medicine*, 13, 93–110.

Schrier, A.C., Dekker, F.W., Kaptein, A.A. & Dijkman, J.H. (1990). Quality of life in elderly patients with chronic nonspecific lung disease seen in family practice. *Chest*, 98, 894–9.

Williams, S.J. (1993). *Chronic respiratory illness*. London: Routledge.

Burns

JOHN WEINMAN

UMDS (Guy's Campus), University of London,

UK

Burns are relatively common and potentially life-threatening injuries which arise from a number of causes. The latter include accidents and trauma over which the individual has had no control, as well as injuries which may have been preventable and those arising from deliberate self-harm. Burn injuries vary greatly in their extent and are usually described in terms of the degree and percent of the body surface area affected. Survival rates following burn injury have increased significantly in recent years as the result of advances in medical care. The medical treatment of patients with burn injuries comprises three phases, each with different treatment demands and stresses for the patient. The initial emergency phase is concerned with the immediate stabilization of the patient and with such tasks as the maintenance of fluid and electrolyte balance. The acute phase follows this, and is usually when the highest levels of pain are experienced with treatments involving dressing changes, topical medications and skin grafting. The rehabilitation phase involves a range of specific self-care practices and may include repeated hospitalization for reconstructive or cosmetic surgery. Rehabilitation and adaptation from burns is influenced by a variety of psychosocial processes within the patient and their social support systems (Browne *et al.*, 1985).

In considering psychological aspects of burns a number of separate issues will be considered. First, there will be a general overview of the psychological effects of burns and this will be followed by an examination of the psychosocial effects in children and their families. The final section will examine the extent to which burns survivors experience post-traumatic disorders. A number of reviews have documented the psychological and social effects of burn injuries (e.g. Browne *et al.*, 1985; Tucker, 1987). One salient finding to emerge from these studies is that a significant number of adult burn patients have prior psychological or social problems, which are particularly prevalent in those with self-or-other-inflicted burns (e.g. Hammond, Ward & Pereira, 1988). Thus the subsequent psychological effects may not be solely attributable to the injury and trauma.

In the acute phase of burns treatment, raised levels of anxiety are

relatively common, especially in those with premorbid difficulties. For these reasons, early psychological intervention is recommended and this is discussed in more detail below.

More long-term studies are now emerging and, although earlier studies indicated high rates of continuing psychological problems, more rigorous studies tend to show that these are only found in about 10–15% of patients (Knudson-Cooper, 1984). Again, these are more likely to be found in those with pre-existing psychological difficulties. Contrary to earlier expectations, no direct correlations have been found between the degree of long-term psychological distress and the extent of the burns injury. Psychological distress can be just as common in those with relatively minor burns, particularly if these have caused visible disfigurement to the face and limbs. The critical factors in determining the more persistent effects are therefore associated with the patient's perception of the problems and their patterns of coping and social support (Shenkman & Stechmiller, 1987). The effects of facial disfigurement are discussed by Rumsey elsewhere in this section (see 'Dysmorphology and facial disfigurement'), and these are of particular relevance in understanding the longer-term impact on individuals and their immediate social supports. The patient's own cognitions are important in determining their coping with the pain and possible disfigurement, as well as with the continuing treatment. Higher levels of internal control and self-efficacy facilitate rehabilitation and recovery, including return to work and resumption of full social activities (Achterberg-Lawliss, 1983), whereas self-blame and guilt can serve to interfere with recovery (Kiecolt-Glaser & Williams, 1987).

Children are at particular risk for burn injuries and, although deaths from burns are now relatively rare (approximately 4 per 100 000), two-thirds of all fatalities occur in children. With severe, non-fatal burn injuries children experience long, often repeated periods of hospitalization as well as considerable pain and discomfort from the injury and treatment. The hospitalization, treatment and associated distress can have adverse, acute psychological effects particularly in younger children (see 'Hospitalization in Children') and psychological interventions may be very helpful for preparing children for specific stressful procedures. Moreover, many child burns survivors have to live with permanent disfigurement and physical disability.

A number of studies have investigated the acute and longer-term psychological impact of burns on children and their families and these have been reviewed by Tarnowski *et al.* (1991). As this review shows, it is difficult to draw clear conclusions from these studies since they vary greatly in methodology and in the findings which emerge. The evidence from earlier studies seemed to show that high levels of long-term psychological distress were common in children with burns, but there are many methodological flaws in these. In contrast to these older studies which were often small-scale and uncontrolled, more recent investigations, based on more psychometrically sound measures in larger and more carefully selected samples, have revealed much lower levels of psychological distress in children and adolescents as the result of burn injuries. Following the considerable initial disruption and distress associated with hospitalization and related treatments, a relatively small proportion of children experience longer-term social and psychological disruption. A number of studies provide evidence that re-entry back into the school and social environment can be difficult, particularly for pre-adolescents and adolescents who may also be more likely to have lower levels of self-esteem. Self-esteem and adjustment have been related to the degree and visibility of burn injuries and, in some studies, positive findings have been obtained (e.g. Love *et al.*, 1987), but these are not consistent and one study has found a positive association between increased burn severity and better post-burn adjustment (Byrne *et al.*, 1986).

Inevitably major childhood health problems such as burns need to be related to family functioning since there will be short- and longer-term effects on families and the extent of these will also depend on various premorbid family characteristics. Although there is relatively little work on this, there have been studies of maternal adjustment and some of these do indicate high rates of maternal disturbance which may be greater than the effects on the children. Indeed, one recent methodological study has shown that, if self-assessments and parental assessments of child burn survivors' psychological responses are compared, then parents are more likely to report that their children are experiencing difficulties in psychological adjustment (Meyer *et al.*, 1995). In this study, children tended to report good psychological and social adjustment, as did their teachers, but the parents rated their children as having significantly more psychosocial difficulties. This is an important finding in the light of the fact that many studies of adjustment of child burn survivors have been based on parental reports. Nevertheless, there is also evidence that maternal adjustment can have direct effects on children's responses to burn injuries. In particular, responses such as self-blame and avoidant coping can serve to create an emotional climate which will not be helpful for the child's own adjustment.

More recently the psychological responses to burn injury have been described and diagnosed as a type of post-traumatic stress disorder (PTSD) using DSM III-R Criteria (American Psychiatric Association, 1987). PTSD is described in more detail in a separate chapter and includes re-experiencing of the trauma (e.g. flashbacks), avoidance behaviour and arousal symptoms. A number of studies have shown that, while many burns survivors may report single PTSD symptoms such as re-experiencing, only about one-third are found to meet the full DSM III-R Criteria. Some of these studies indicate that those experiencing PTSD are more likely to have more extensive burns, but were less likely to have been responsible for their burn injury. However, these findings are not consistent and it has been suggested that the term 'continuous Traumatic Stress Disorder' should be applied to burns survivors since there is ongoing trauma associated with the hospitalization and longer-term rehabilitation (Gilboa, Friedman & Tsur, 1994).

Just as psychological approaches, particular cognitive therapies, have been found to be useful in the management of PTSD, these are also used in treating burns patients. These therapies allow the patient to talk about, and make sense of, the trauma and to identify and use coping strategies that have worked in the past in order to regain a sense of mastery and control in the recovery process. Avoidant coping may be helpful particularly during the painful, acute phase (e.g. Cahners & Bernstein, 1979) but, in the longer-term, regaining control and mastery is important in rehabilitation since self-blame and guilt have been found to interfere with adjustment (Kiecolt-Glaser & Williams, 1987).

Over the past 30 or so years there have been major advances in the care of patients with extensive burns with the result that survival rates have increased dramatically. This has resulted in increasing attention to the psychological impact of burn injuries and the role of psychological interventions in the rehabilitation process. Many patients make excellent recoveries from extensive burn injury but some have major problems in post-treatment adaptation. There is a continuing need to be able to identity these patients at an early stage and to develop psychological interventions to facilitate their recovery.

REFERENCES

Achterberg-Lawliss, J. (1983). Health beliefs: predictive factors of burn rehabilitation. *Journal of Burn Care and Rehabilitation*, 4, 437–41.

American Psychiatric Association (1987). *Diagnostic and statistical manual of mental disorders*. 3rd edn. Washington, DC: American Psychiatric Press.

Browne, G., Byrne, C., Browne, B., Pennock, M., Streiner, D., Roberts, R., Eyles, P., Truscott, D. & Dabbs, R. (1985). Psychological adjustment of burn survivors. *Burns*, 12, 28–35.

Byrne, C., Love, B., Browne, G., Brown, B., Roberts, J. & Streiner, D. (1986). The social competence of children following burn injury: a study of resilience. *Journal of Burn Care*, 7, 247–52.

Cahners, S.S. & Bernstein, N.R. (1979). Rehabilitating families with burned children. *Scandinavian Journal of Plastic and Reconstructive Surgery*, 13, 173–5.

Gilboa, D., Friedman, M. & Tsur, H. (1994). The burn as a continuous traumatic stress: implications for emotional treatment during hospitalisation.

Journal of Burn Care and Rehabilitation, 15, 86–94.

Hammond, J.S., Ward, C.G. & Pereira, E. (1988). Self inflicted burns. *Journal of Burn Care and Rehabilitation*, 9, 178–9.

Kiecolt-Glaser, J.K. & Williams, D.A. (1987). Self-blame, compliance and distress among burn patients. *Journal of Personality and Social Psychology*, 53, 187–93.

Knudson-Cooper, M.L. (1984). The antecedents and consequences of children's burn injuries. *Advances in Developmental and Behavioural Pediatrics*, 5, 33–74.

Burns

Love, B., Byrne, C., Roberts, J., Browne, G. & Browne, B. (1987). Adult psychosocial adjustment following childhood injury: the effect of disfigurement. *Journal of Burn Care and Rehabilitation*, 8, 280–5.

Meyer, W.J., Blakeney, P.E., Holzer, C.E., Moore, P., Murphy, L., Robson, M.C. & Herndon, D.N. (1995). Inconsistencies in psychosocial assessment of children after severe burns. *Journal of Burn Care and Rehabilitation*, 16, 559–68.

Shenkman, B. & Stechmiller, J. (1987). Patient and family perception of projected functioning after discharge from a burn unit. *Heart and Lung*, 16, 490–6.

Tarnowski, K.J., Rasnake, L.K., Gavaghan-Jones, M.P. & Smith, L. (1991). Psychosocial sequelae of pediatric burn injuries: a review. *Clinical Psychology Review*, 11, 371–98.

Tucker, P. (1987). Psychosocial problems among adult burn victims. *Burns*, 13, 7–14.

Cardiac surgery

STANTON NEWMAN

Unit of Health Psychology, Department of Psychiatry and Behavioural Sciences, University College London Medical School, UK

PSYCHOLOGICAL RESPONSES TO CARDIAC SURGERY

It has been suggested that a relatively high level of psychological morbidity follows cardiac surgery, but this has not been borne out in formal studies. Studies of general psychiatric morbidity, using standardized instruments, have shown a general reduction following surgery. For example, Magni *et al.* (1987) examined 99 patients undergoing a variety of cardiac surgical procedures and found a reduction in distress on all the subscales of the SCL 90 shortly after surgery and 12 months later. Other studies have produced similar findings and emphasize that the transient distress which may be apparent in some patients dissipates in the longer term. Patterns of anxiety are similar to those found in other forms of surgery with a significant increase in anxiety in the days immediately after surgery followed by a significant drop in the weeks and months following surgery (Strauss & Paulsen, 1990).

One possible reason for the belief that psychological morbidity is high after cardiac surgery is that patients who present for cardiac surgery may have a higher psychiatric morbidity and thus be atypical of the general population. For example, Mayou & Bryant (1987) found that the number of psychiatric cases in patients presenting for cardiac surgery was almost double the number that would be expected on the basis of population norms.

Predictors of mood state after surgery

It is not surprising that the most potent predictor of mood state after cardiac surgery is mood prior to surgery. For example, Magni *et al.* (1987) found depression scores preoperatively accounted for 34% of the variation in depressed mood postoperatively.

Other factors are, however, important. The effect of perceived social support on recovery from cardiac surgery has been examined by Coombs, Roberts and Crist (1989). Seventy-five coronary artery bypass graft (CABG) patients were assessed on their perceptions of practical and emotional support at the same time as assessing amongst other things, depression and health status. Assessments were performed within a few days of surgery and at 3, 6 and 12 months. Emotional social support was found to be highest in the days after surgery. Higher social support at 5 days and at 3 months was significantly associated with lower levels of depressed mood. This relationship, however, was not significant at the later assessments. These findings suggest that perceived social support has an effect on psychological well being in the immediate days following CABG but this dissipates in the long term.

The patients' perceptions of their own health has also been shown to be important in relation to mood state following cardiac surgery. Coombs *et al.* (1989) found that recurrence of chest pain and perceived health both contributed significantly to depressed mood when assessed 3 and 6 months after surgery. They attribute the importance of these findings to patients' increasing concerns regarding the success of the procedure.

Interventions

Interventions to reduce the anxiety most patients experience when having surgery or other stressful medical procedures are common. In cardiac surgery, Anderson (1987) examined the effects of information provision and information (delivered by video) combined with exercise training (delivered by video and tape recorder) as compared with standard hospital procedures. Both interventions significantly reduced preoperative anxiety, whilst the standard hospital procedures did not. In addition, nurses' ratings of recovery were higher in the two experimental groups. Whilst this study failed to show any differences between the two intervention procedures, it did establish that the provision of information yields wide ranging benefits in cardiac surgery.

At a more simple level Kulik & Mahler (1987) manipulated the rooming arrangements of patients. When preoperative patients were assigned to share with a postoperative patient, they exhibited lower presurgical anxiety, became physically active sooner after surgery and were discharged from hospital earlier. The authors interpret these findings as reflecting the calming and reassuring effects of being with somebody who has been through their operation successfully, the possible information imparted by the postoperative patients about the surgery and its effects, and the fact that visitors to the room mate are likely to have lower anxiety as they would no longer be as anxious about surgery.

CHANGES IN COGNITIVE FUNCTION

Changes in cognition as shown in the change in performance on neuropsychological tests from before to after surgery has been an area of considerable study in cardiac surgery. A significant deterioration in performance has been found to occur in the days shortly after surgery with the incidence of neuropsychological morbidity in these studies ranging from 12% to 79%. Differences in surgical practice, the number, type and sensitivity of neuropsychological tests used, the assessment of deficit and the nature of the patients selected for surgery are some of the reasons for the wide range of deficits found to occur (Newman, 1993).

These early assessments are likely to be contaminated by variations in general recovery from surgery, and consequently may not be a true reflection of persisting neuropsychological problems. In addition, recovery from brain damage may occur over the weeks and months after surgery. Consequently, it was seen as important to establish whether these deficits persist. Studies have examined patients up to 12 months after surgery and found persisting deficits in up to 29% (Newman, 1993).

The longer-term consequences of cardiac surgery have also been assessed by Sotainemi, Mononen & Hokkanen (1986) in a five-year follow-up of valve replacement surgery. He found that individuals who showed even a transient disturbance in early assessments were more likely to show cognitive disturbance at the follow-up assessment in contrast to individuals who had an uncomplicated recovery.

Some authors have suggested that the incidence of neuropsychological morbidity should vary according to the type of cardiac surgery. In particular, it has been suggested that valve replacement surgery, which is an open heart procedure, should show a higher incidence of neuropsychological problems than that observed in bypass grafting (Mills & Prough, 1991). To date, there are no published studies specifically comparing these two forms of surgery.

Factors influencing cognitive dysfunction

Patient-related factors

The impact of surgery on neuropsychological performance has been found to be worse for older patients in both valve and CABG procedures (Newman, 1993). Because of the reduced frequency of CABG surgery in women, few studies have specifically made comparison between males and females on neuropsychological performance. One study which examined the impact of valve surgery found that the female patients had a less favourable outcome in comparison to males (Sotainemi, Juolasmaa & Hokkanen, 1981).

Early research found that individuals with severe cardiac disease, evidenced by symptoms in excess of six months, were significantly more likely to develop neurological damage following CABG. Other research has also found a number of different measures of cardiac function such as left ventricular function to be related to the likelihood of developing neuropsychological deficits after surgery (Shaw et al., 1987).

The importance of assessing cerebrovascular disease and, where appropriate, performing either a prior or concurrent carotid endart-

erectomy with CABG surgery has been a common practice. The impact of cerebrovascular disease on neuropsychological deficits following cardiac surgery has been examined by studying the carotid arteries by means of digital subtraction angiography (Harrison et al., 1989). The incidence of patients with neuropsychological deficits was no different for those classified as having abnormal or normal angiograms.

Other co-morbidities have been found to be an important factor related to outcome in cardiac surgery. Diabetes has been identified as a potential important co-morbidity and has been suggested to be of importance in relation to neuropsychological functioning but, to date, no study has examined this question.

Per-operative factors

A number of studies have found the duration of bypass to be related to the incidence of neuropsychological deficit (Newman, 1993). These findings are consistent with an explanation for the neuropsychological deficits being related to extracorporeal circulation.

The level of arterial pressure during surgery was suggested to be an important aetiological factor for neuropsychological disturbance (Smith et al., 1986). Later studies in both CABG (Newman, 1989) and valve replacement surgery have, however, failed to confirm arterial pressure as an important factor.

Glucose control during surgery and its relation to neuropsychological changes has become an increasing area of interest. One technique has been to include dextrose in the priming solution. Griffin et al. (1992) examined the impact on neuropsychological functioning of 5% dextrose in the prime and found a tendency towards greater neuropsychological deficits in this group as compared to a control group receiving a standard priming solution.

It is most common for cardiac surgery involving extracorporeal circulation to involve hypothermia. Hypothermia has been considered to be a protection against ischaemic damage. Two techniques have been used to manage the effects of hypothermia on pH. In one, the fall in pH is corrected by adding CO_2 (pH Stat); in the other the CO_2 is kept constant (alpha stat). It has been demonstrated that alpha stat leads to fewer individuals with cognitive deficits (Patel et al., 1993).

Equipment used for extracorporeal circulation is constantly changing. A number of studies have examined whether newer forms of equipment lead to lower levels of neuropsychological problems. These include the method of oxygenation where membrane oxygenators have been found to produce less deficits than bubble oxygenators (Blauth et al., 1989) and the use of arterial line filters (see below)).

Relationship between neuropsychological deficit and putative mechanism of damage

The mechanisms contributing to post-CPB neuropsychological deficits are uncertain. However, two major inter-related aetiological factors, hypoperfusion and microemboli have been suggested. Microemboli in cardiac surgery may be either gaseous or particulate in nature. The candidates for particulate matter include artheromatous matter, fat, platelet aggregates, etc. Recent neuropathological studies have identified the occurrence of what has been termed small capillary arteriolar dilatations (SCADS) in the brains of both humans who have succumbed in cardiac surgery as well as dogs undergoing cardiopulmonary bypass, but not in those who have not been on extracorporeal circulation (Moody *et al.*, 1990).

In recent years both transcranial doppler detection at the middle cerebral artery and at the carotid have been applied to detect high frequency signals that appear to reflect either air or particulate matter going into the brain. Both of these techniques offer the ability to perform continuous measurement of emboli. It has been demonstrated that patients with neuropsychological deficits tend to have more emboli than those without deficits (Pugsley *et al.*, 1994). In addition, the introduction of a 40 micron filter on the arterial line has been shown to reduce both the number of emboli and the frequency of neuropsychological deficits.

ADJUSTMENT TO OUTCOME IN CARDIAC SURGERY

Physical health
It would be expected that, without the constraints of chest pain and breathlessness associated with cardiac disease, increased levels of physical activity would occur after surgery. The advice given to the patient frequently includes a recommendation for increased physical activity. Consequently, it is not surprising that studies on both valve replacement and CABG have found patients reporting the ability to perform at increased levels of physical activity following cardiac surgery (Stanton *et al.*, 1984, 1985; Mayou & Bryant, 1987).

Social activities
A number of studies have reported increases in social activities following cardiac surgery. Jenkins attributes these to increased physical mobility (Jenkins *et al.*, 1983). In contrast, Bunzel & Eckersberger (1989) retrospectively assessed the social and leisure activities of 94 patients 12 months after surgery and found most leisure behaviours showed little change. The increase that did occur was in more passive activities while more active and social behaviours tended to decline (inviting guests home, eating out and cinema visits). The authors suggest that patients after surgery re-evaluate their priorities and tend to withdraw setting limits to their activities.

Sexual functioning
Difficulties in sexual functioning amongst males is a frequent clinical report following cardiac surgery. Gundle *et al.* (1980) found 57% of cardiac surgery patients reported postoperative sexual dysfunction. Kornfeld *et al.* (1982) found a considerable decrease in sexual activity 9 months after surgery which persisted in many when followed up 3.5 years after surgery. This area of life may have important repercussions on relationships, but relatively little attention has been directed to it.

Return to work
The ability to return to work has been considered a useful and easily measured indicator of the success of a procedure (Walter, 1985). Its ease of assessment, however, belies the complexity of any interpretation, as the likelihood of return to work is dependent upon a number of factors including the nature of work, level of seniority, economic support available such as pensions, housing, etc., and the general level of economic activity. Return to work following cardiac surgery has produced findings ranging from 17% to 75% and studies have also failed to find any relationship between symptoms and likelihood of returning to work or the reasons for not seeking work.

Satisfaction with surgery
Kornfeld *et al.* (1982) performed a follow-up of 3.5 years on a group of 57 patients who underwent CABG. When asked whether they were pleased at having undergone the operation, 60% reported they were extremely pleased and only 4% reported displeasure. Self-reports have generally yielded a high frequency of positive responses with 71% reporting without qualification that they would undergo surgery again (Jenkins *et al.*, 1983) and 70% reporting that they were very pleased with the operation (Mayou & Bryant, 1987).

REFERENCES

Anderson, E.A. (1987). Preoperative preparation for cardiac surgery facilitates recovery, reduces psychological distress, and reduces the incidence of postoperative hypertension. *Journal of Consulting and Clinical Psychology*, **4**, 513–20.

Blauth, C., Smith, P., Newman, S., Arnold, J., Siddons, F., Harrison, M., Treasure, T., Klinger, L. & Taylor, K. (1989). Retinal microembolism and neuropsychological deficit following clinical cardiopulmonary bypass: comparison of a membrane and a bubble oxygenator; A preliminary communication. *European Journal of Cardio-thoracic Surgery*, **3**, 135–9.

Bunzel, B. & Eckersberger, F. (1989). Changes in activities performed in leisure time after open heart surgery. *International Journal of Cardiology*, **23**, 315–20.

Coombs, D., Roberts, R. & Crist, D. (1989). Effects of social support on depression following coronary artery bypass graft surgery. *Psychology and Health*, **3**, 29–35.

Griffin, S., Hothersall, J., Klinger, L., Newman, S., McLean, P. & Treasure, T. (1992). The effects of substrate load and blood glucose management on cerebral dysfunction following cardiopulmonary bypass. *Vascular Surgery*, **26**, 656–64.

Gundle, M., Reeves, B., Tate, S., Raft, D. & McLaurin, L. (1980) Psychosocial outcome following coronary artery surgery. *American Journal of Psychiatry*, **137**, 1591–4.

Harrison, M., Schneidau, R., Ho, R., Smith, P., Newman, S. & Treasure, T. (1989). Cerebrovascular disease and functional outcome after coronary artery bypass surgery. *Stroke*, **20**, 235–7.

Jenkins, C.D., Stanton, B., Savageau, J.A., Derlinger, P. & Klein, M.D. (1983). Coronary artery bypass surgery. Physical psychological, social and economic outcomes six months later. *Journal of the American Medical Association*, **250**, 782–8.

Kornfeld, D., Heller, S., Frank, K., Wilson, S., & Malm, J. (1982). Psychological and behavioral responses after coronary artery bypass surgery. *Circulation*, **66**, 24–8.

Kulik, J. & Mahler, H. (1987). Effects of preoperative roommate assignment on preoperative anxiety and recovery from coronary-bypass surgery, *Health Psychology*, **6**, 525–43.

Magni, G., Unger, H., Valfre, C., Polesel, E., Cesari, F., Rizzardo, R., Paruzzolo, P. & Galluci, V. (1987). Psychosocial outcome one year after heart surgery. *Archives of Internal Medicine*, **147**, 473–7.

Mayou, R. & Bryant, B. (1987). Quality of life after coronary artery surgery. *Quarterly Journal of Medicine*, **62**, 239–8.

Mills S. & Prough, D. (1991). Neuropsychiatric complications following cardiac surgery, *Seminars in Thoracic and Cardiovascular Surgery*, **3**, 39–46.

Moody, D.M., Bell, M.A., Challa, V.R., Johnston, W.E., & Prough, D.S. (1990).

Brain microemboli during cardiac surgery or aortography. *Annals in Neurology*, 28, 477–86.

Newman, S. (1989). The incidence and nature of neuropsychological morbidity following cardiac surgery. *Perfusion*, 4, 93–100.

Newman, S. (1993). Neuropsychological and psychological consequences of Cardiac Surgery. In K. Taylor & P. Smith (Eds.). *The brain and cardiac surgery*. Andrew Arnold.

Patel, R., Newman, S., Turtle, M.R.J. & Venn, G.E. (1993). Improved neuropsychological outcome following cardiopulmonary bypass using alpha stat acid base management. *Perfusion*, 8, 264.

Pugsley, W., Klinger, L., Paschalis, C., Treasure, T., Harrison, M. & Newman, S. (1994). The impact of microemboli in cardiopulmonary bypass on neuropsychological functioning. *Stroke*, 27, 1393–79.

Shaw, P.J., Bates, D., Cartlidge, N.E.F.,

French, J.M., Heavside, D., Julian, D.G. & Shaw, D.A. (1987). Neurologic and neuropsychological morbidity following major surgery: comparison of coronary artery bypass surgery and peripheral vascular surgery. *Stroke*, 18, 700–7.

Smith, P., Treasure, T., Newman, S., Joseph, P., Ell, P. & Harrison, M. (1986). Cerebral consequences of cardiopulmonary bypass. *Lancet*, i, 823–5.

Sotinemi, K.A., Juolasmaa, A. & Hokkanen, T.E. (1981). Neuropsychologic outcome after open-heart surgery. *Archives in Neurology*, 38, 2–8.

Sotainemi, K.A., Mononen, H., Hokkanen, T.E. (1986). Long-term cerebral outcome after open-heart surgery: a five year neuropsychological follow-up study. *Stroke*, 17, 410–16.

Stanton, B., Jenkins, C., Savageau, J. &

Thurer, R. (1984). Functional benefits following coronary artery bypass graft surgery. *Annals of Thoracic Surgery*, 37, 286–90.

Stanton, B., Jenkins, C., Goldstein, R., Vander-Salm, T., Klein, M. & Aucoin, R. (1985). Hospital readmissions among survivors six months after myocardial revascularisation. *Journal of the American Association*, 253, 3568–73.

Strauss, B. & Paulsen, G. (1990). Psychiatric methods of the international study: Hamilton depression and anxiety scales. In A. Wilner & G. Rodewald (Eds.). In A. Wilner & G. Rodewald (Eds.). *Impact of cardiac surgery on the quality of life*. New York: Plenum Press.

Walter, P. (Ed.) (1985) *Return to work after coronary artery bypass surgery*. Berlin: Springer–Verlag.

Carotid stenosis and endarterectomy

STANTON NEWMAN

Unit of Health Psychology, Department of Psychiatry and Behavioural Sciences, University College London Medical School, UK

Thrombo-embolism and haemodynamic ischaemia secondary to atheromatous stenotic disease of the carotid and vertebral arteries are important causes of ischaemic stroke. Detection of significant carotid or vertebral artery stenosis after a transient ischaemic attack (TIA) or stroke provides the opportunity for secondary preventive treatment of the stenosis to prevent a further stroke. The average risk of stroke following a TIA is about 8% in the first year and then 5% per annum, but, in patients with severe carotid stenosis, the risk in medically treated patients increases up to 28% over 2 years (NASCETC, 1991). The recent European Carotid Surgery Trial (ECSTCC, 1991) and the North American Symptomatic Carotid Endarterectomy Trial (Winslow *et al.* 1988) have convincingly demonstrated that this risk is significantly reduced by carotid endarterectomy in symptomatic medically fit patients with carotid stenosis of greater than 70%.

In some studies little deterioration and in some cases even an improvement in cognitive function have been reported following carotid endarterectomy surgery (CES; Bornstein, Benoit & Trites, 1981). Other studies have shown effects on the brain in a proportion of patients. In more recent studies which patients are affected has been shown to be related to the occurrence of microemboli as detected by transcranial doppler which are produced during carotid endarterectomy (Gaunt *et al.*, 1994; Jansen *et al.*, 1994). Gaunt *et al.* (1994) related the incidence of emboli to changes in cognition, and established that the detection of more than ten emboli during the initial carotid dissection was associated with an increased likelihood of postoperative cognitive deterioration. Jansen *et al.* (1994) demonstrated that the number of emboli produced in the dissection stage is related to the likelihood of infarcts as detected by MRI.

Trudel, Fabia & Bouchard (1984) found that activities of daily living were not particularly affected following CES. In contrast, there were marked restrictions in social and leisure activities. Salenius *et al.* (1990) examined the results of 44 surgically and 40 non-surgically treated patients with carotid stenosis documented by angiography in 1974–1976. During the follow-up period, the occurrence of cerebrovascular complications (death, stroke and/or TIA) was more frequent in the non operated than in the operated group. No differences were found in the quality of life between the two groups but the operated group expressed higher levels of satisfaction than the non-operated group. Sirkka *et al.* (1992) followed up patients 8–11 years after surgery and found that only those who had had two operations had a poorer quality of life than patients who did not have surgery.

Carotid artery stenosis

REFERENCES

Bornstein, R., Benoit, B.G. & Trites, R.L. (1981). Neuropsychological changes following carotid endarterectomy *Canadian Journal of Neurological Science*, 8, 127–32.

European Carotid Surgery Trialists Collaboration Group (ECSTCC) (1991) MRC European carotid surgery trial: interim results for symptomatic patients with severe (70–99%) or with mild stenosis (0–29%) carotid stenosis. *Lancet*, 337, 1235–43.

Gaunt, M.E., Martin, P.J., Smith, J.L., Rimmer, T., Cherryman, G., Ratliff, D.A., Bell, P.R.F., & Naylor, A.R. (1994). Clinical revelance of intraoperative embolization detected by transcranial Doppler ultrasonography during carotid endarterectomy: a prospective study of 100 patients. *British Journal of Surgery*, 81, 1435–9.

Jansen, C., Ramos, L.M.P., van Heesewijk, M.D., Moll, F.L., van Gijn, J. & Ackerstaff, R.G.A. (1994). Impact of microembolism and hemodynamic changes in the brain during carotid endarterectomy. *Stroke*, 25, 992–7.

North American Symptomatic Cartoid Endarterectomy Trial Collaborators (NASCETC) (1991) Beneficial effect of carotid endarterectomy in symptomatic patients with high grade carotid stenosis. *New England Journal of Medicine*, 325, 445–53.

Salenius, J.P., Harju, E., Kuukasjarvi, P., Haapanen, A. & Riekkinen, H. (1990). Late results of surgical and nonoperative treatment of carotid stenosis. Eighty-four patients documented by angiography in 1974–1976. *Journal of Cardiovascular Surgery: Torino*. 31, 156–61.

Sirkka, A., Salenius, J.P., Portin, R. & Nummenmaa, T. (1992). Quality of life and cognitive performance after carotid endarterectomy during long-term follow-up. *Acta Neurologica Scandinavica*, 85, 58–62.

Trudel, L., Fabia, J. & Bouchard, J.P. (1984). Quality of life of 50 carotid endarterectomy survivors: a long term follow up study. *Archives in Physical Medicine and Rehabilitation*, 65, 310–12.

Winslow, C.M., Solomon, D.H., Chassin, M.R., Kosecoff, J., Merrick, N.J. & Brook, R.H. (1988). The appropriateness of carotid endarterectomy. *New England Journal of Medicine*, 318, 721–7.

Child abuse and neglect: prevention

KEVIN BROWNE

School of Psychology, University of Birmingham, UK

In recent years, the problem of child abuse and neglect has received a great deal of attention worldwide (e.g. Finkelhor, 1994). Most countries have now considered the problem, and many have signed Article 19 of the UN Declaration on Children's Rights concerning Child Protection. However, what is the reality of the situation?

The findings from western countries suggest the majority of abused children cannot be expected to be proactive in preventing their abuse. In reality, four out of five child victims are unlikely to be able to use the phone or adopt other recommended protective strategies. Helplines, while excellent for teenagers, cannot be expected to prevent most of the abuse and neglect for younger children, and many children will be abused before they have the opportunity of being exposed to a school-based prevention programme. Therefore, professionals in 'Child Protection' must be proactive, rather than reactive, on their behalf.

The most important indicator that there is a need for early prevention is the level of fatal abuse and serious injury, the National Society for the Prevention of Cruelty to Children in the UK claim that three to four children die each week at the hands of their parents (NSPCC, 1985). For every child who dies there is another disabled for life, giving three to four children each week who are blind, deaf, brain damaged, etc., as a result of abuse or neglect. Therefore, whenever the need for prevention is discussed, it is important to remember the number of children who continue to die or who are disabled for life often because our interventions are too late or our preventative service inadequate.

Prevention is traditionally classified into three levels: 'primary' prevention which involves the whole population; 'secondary' prevention that involves identifying high risk populations to offer intervention before abuse occurs and finally 'tertiary' prevention or treatment given after abuse has occurred. For the dead or disabled child tertiary prevention comes too late. Tertiary prevention does not even work that well for children who do survive. In the USA and UK, physical re-abuse occurs in at least half of all cases referred to child protection agencies (Magura, 1981), and sexual abuse will recur in the majority of cases where the offender remains in the family (Bentovim, 1991). There is also some evidence that services available are insufficient to provide appropriate support and therapy to abused children and their families. In a study of 202 sexually abused children in London (Prior, Lynch & Glaser, 1994), 37% received no therapy; yet all these children had described contact abuse and there was a professional consensus that the abuse had occurred.

PRIMARY PREVENTION

Primary prevention techniques attempt a fundamental change across society. For example, public awareness campaigns that challenge misconceptions, and aim to increase people's understanding of the extent and nature of physical and sexual violence against women and girls. Such approaches to primary prevention are far from easy. The campaigners have to balance the need for a clear message against over simplifying the problem. For example, the claim that one in every two children will be sexually assaulted by the time they

PART III: Medical topics

Table 1. *Relative importance of screening characteristics for child abuse (as determined by stepwise discriminate function analysis)*[b]

Checklist: Characteristics	Abusing families	Non-abusing families
	(*n*=62)	(*n*=124)
	%	%
1. Parent indifferent, intolerant or over-anxious towards child	83.9	21.8*a*
2. History of family violence	51.6	5.6*a*
3. Socioeconomic problems such as unemployment	85.5	34.7*a*
4. Infant premature, low birth weight	24.2	3.2*a*
5. Parent abused or neglected as a child	43.5	6.5*a*
6. Step-parent or cohabitee present	35.5	4.8*a*
7. Single or separated parent	38.7	8.1*a*
8. Mother less than 21 years old at the time of birth	40.3	23.4*a*
9. History of mental illness, drug or alcohol addiction	61.3	21.8*a*
10. Infant separated from mother for greater than 24 hours postdelivery	17.7	5.6*a*
11. Infant mentally or physically handicapped	1.6	0.8
12. Less than 18 months between birth of children	22.6	15.3
13. Infant never breast-fed	46.8	40.3

[a] Significant difference < 0.05

[b] From Browne & Saqi (1988*a*).

reach adulthood is based on a broad definition of maltreatment, which includes non-contact abuse. Thus, individuals who think in terms of contact abuse will regard the message as exaggerated. In addition, for messages to appear clear sometimes they need to be very specific. Hence, some campaigns do not consider the sexual abuse of prepubertal boys who are often equally at risk.

An equally controversial approach to the primary prevention of sexual abuse promotes change through school education programmes for children. A New Zealand programme (Briggs & Hawkins, 1994) was effective because of teacher commitment, parental support and age appropriate material. One important ingredient of the programme described was the development of children's self-esteem. Research has shown that sex offenders target children with a low sense of self-worth who appear vulnerable and unsure of themselves, with a need to be cared for (Elliott, Browne & Kilcoyne, 1995). Thus, assertion training needs to go hand in hand with the development of self-esteem.

Children who have experienced family breakdown and separation are more likely to develop the emotional problems described above and therefore could be considered to be a high risk group. Secondary prevention involves professionals in interventions aimed at giving special attention to such groups before maltreatment occurs within or outside the family.

SECONDARY PREVENTION
Single-parent families and those with stepparents have been identified as 'at risk' for child abuse by a number of studies and some researchers have advocated these 'risk factors' be included for use in the screening out of high-risk populations (Browne, 1995). This approach to secondary prevention can be seen as controversial. However, as long as the intervention following screening is positive and empowering, the effects of any 'false positive' will be minimal. Another approach is to provide a service that allows parents to identify themselves as in need of parenting advice.

In the short term, intervention techniques aimed at the early prediction and identification of potential or actual abusing parents are more realistic than instigating changes in child-care practice for all parents (primary prevention). This secondary prevention can involve professionals in counselling, home visits and clinic, health centre or hospital care. Such professionals can be instructed routinely to screen for predicative characteristics in all families who come in contact with the service they are providing.

A number of articles have been written on the prediction of child abuse, many of which have presented a list of characteristics common to abusing parents and to abused children. For example, it has been suggested that an 'early warning system' could begin in the labour room and that abusing parents can be predicted with 76% accuracy from characteristics noted during the first 24 hours after birth (Gray *et al.*, 1977). However, a recent review of the relative value of these characteristics for the practical and routine monitoring of potential child abusing families has emphasized a need for caution (Browne, 1995).

Browne (1995) demonstrated the danger of predictive claims by evaluating a typical checklist completed by community nurses around the time of birth. The concept of the checklist was that, when applied to all families with a newborn child in a given locality, exceptional families with a high number of adverse risk factors were identified and visited more often. It was assumed that the higher the number of factors present, the greater the intervention required and the more 'at risk' the child. Evidence for the predominance of factors used for screening in abusing families had already been established (Browne & Saqi, 1988a).

Community nurses completed a 13-item checklist (see Table 1) on all children under five years for whom a case conference was called on child physical abuse and neglect in the past year. In total, information was collected on 62 case-conferred families. The community nurse concerned then identified two matched 'control' non-abusing families from the same district (i.e. 124 families) to whom the checklist was also applied.

The percentage of abusing and non-abusing families showing each risk factor is presented in Table 1. Most of the risk factors exhibit a significant difference between the two samples, with the abusing families invariably showing a higher percentage. The risk factors are presented in order of relative importance as determined by stepwise discriminant function analysis, which takes into account any confounding influences between factors. Thus, the contribution of each risk factor to discriminate between abusing (NAI) cases and their matched controls was determined. Table 1 shows that the observation of whether the parent was indifferent, intolerant or over-anxious was the best predictor, followed by family violence and socio economic problems.

Using discriminant function analysis, the optimum performance of the whole checklist as a screening instrument was established. It was found that fully completed checklists, with the relative weighting for each factor taken into account, could correctly classify 86% of cases, which is better than most studies (Starr, 1982). The screening procedure was sensitive to 82% of the abusing families and specified 88% of the control families as non-abusing. However, if the checklist of risk factors is used in this way it will miss 18% of the abusing families and incorrectly identify 12% of the non-abusing families as potential NAI cases. This has grave implications when such a checklist is applied prospectively to a population of births.

The low prevalence of child abuse, combined with even the most optimistic estimates of screening effectiveness, implies that a screening programme would yield large numbers of false positives. The checklist detection rate of 82% compared to 12% false alarms suggests that, for every 10 000 births screened, it would be necessary to distinguish between 33 true risk cases and 1195 false alarms. This would indicate the requirement of a second screening procedure, to be carried out only on the 1228 or so families labelled 'high risk' (Browne, 1989b).

A more lengthy assessment could be used on these high-risk families, based on the significant differences between abusing and non-abusing families found in parent – child interaction studies (e.g. Browne & Saqi, 1987, 1988b). Thus, a second screening could possibly distinguish the true potential NAI cases from the false positives by the use of behavioural indicators. A more difficult problem would be to distinguish the seven missed cases of potential child abuse from the 8765 correctly identified non-abusers, as they would be mixed up in a low-risk population of 8772 families.

When the checklist was applied prospectively to a sample of 14 252 births (Browne, 1995), it was found that 6.8% of families with a new-born had a high number of 'pre-disposing' factors for child abuse. On follow-up, only one in 12 (7.6%) of these 'high risk' families went on to abuse their child within five years of birth, in comparison to one in 391 (0.3%) for the low-risk families. Thus, it can be concluded that risk factors significantly predispose families to child abuse, but are not sufficient actually to cause violence in the vast majority (92%) of families under stress.

The chances of situational stressors (risk factors) resulting in child abuse and other forms of family violence are mediated by, and depend on, the interactive relationships within the family (Browne, 1988, 1989a). A secure relationship between family members will 'buffer' any effects of stress and facilitate coping strategies on behalf of the family. In contrast, insecure, or anxious relationships will not 'buffer' the family under stress and any overload, such as an argument or a child misbehaving, may result in a physical or emotional attack. Overall, this will have a negative effect on the existing interpersonal relationships and reduce any 'buffering' effects still fur-

ther, making it easier for stressors to overload the family system once again. This may lead to a situation where stress results in repeated physical assaults on the child.

Leventhal (1988) provides evidence from longitudinal cohort studies that suggests prediction is feasible. However, he concludes that improvements in the assessment of high-risk families are necessary, including the further development and use of a standardized clinical assessment of the parent-child relationship.

Browne (1989b) suggests that the behavioural responses of the parent and the infant to an observer/stranger will be similar to their reactions to a community worker. Thus, the precise determination of behavioural characteristics is considered to be of value, to provide indicators that will help to recognize families needing extra support and help in parenting. It is suggested that screening for child abuse should have at least three stages to eliminate false alarms (Browne & Saqi, 1988a,b).

1. All families with a newborn should be screened perinatally for stressful social and demographic characteristics of the child and its family. This will identify a target group for further screening. However, the remaining population cannot be considered immune to family stress and child abuse. Any change in family circumstances leading to increased stress should be assessed and, if applicable, the family added to the target group.
2. All parents in the target group should be screened for 3 to 6 months after birth on their perceptions of the newborn child and those aspects of parenting and family life they consider to be stressful.
3. Approximately, 9 to 12 months after birth the infants' attachment to the primary caregiver should be assessed, together with parental sensitivity to the infant's behaviour.

Those parents who are under stress with negative perceptions about the child's behaviour need help with parenting. Those parents who in addition have a poor relationship with their child, as measured the quality of attachment and their sensitivity to the child's behaviour, must be considered as a potential child abuser and professional support for the family should be given before any aggressive incidents occur. It is claimed, that given adequate intervention and resources, 80% of child maltreatment is preventable.

For social and background risk factors to be of use in the recognition and prediction of child abuse and neglect they must be considered with the context of the family's interpersonal network, which take into account poor parenting, family violence, social isolation, mental illness and chemical dependency. These factors have been shown by research to be strong predictors for child maltreatment. Indeed, families presenting with depression, withdrawal, low self-esteem and limited parenting skills and unrealistic expectations of their children are most unlikely to show change with home-based interventions. In the presence of family violence and chemical dependency there is a tendency for these families to deteriorate, and the child's safety must be carefully monitored.

INTERVENTION

Child maltreatment is a complex problem with no quick fix solutions. The majority of facets appear to respond better to prevention better than treatment and the research of Olds *et al.* (1986) in the

USA provides a good example of effective interventions in promoting parental confidence and self-confidence in the management and care of the child. These interventions have been shown to improve mother – child play and reduce physical punishment and the incidence of child abuse and neglect.

In the past 20 years there has been much debate on what services can be delivered to minimize the maltreatment of children. This debate has been limited by a poor understanding of intervention strategies for child abuse and neglect and of what constitutes a desirable outcome. Reviews on the causes of maltreatment (e.g. Browne, 1988) have emphasized a growing recognition that child abuse and neglect is a product of a poor parent/child relationship, which often occurs in the context of other forms of family breakdown. Therefore, child maltreatment is often associated with other forms of family violence which also need to be addressed (Stanley & Goddard, 1993; Browne, 1993; Carroll, 1994).

Wolfe (1993) observes that there have been promising developments in early interventions which address parental competency and family support to promote more positive parental knowledge, attitudes, skills and behaviour. Given that the prediction of child abuse and neglect in families has met with limited success and a high number of false alarms, such positively orientated interventions are preferable with the child remaining in the family.

Nevertheless, it should be recognized that some children are in danger if they remain in a violent family. Despite the costs to these children of being taken into care, their immediate safety must take precedence over intervention strategies. Hence, the careful and accurate assessment of the potential for change in family interactions and relationships is essential. Health and social service resources must be adequately provided to meet this need.

REFERENCES

Bentovim, A. (1991). Clinical work with families in which sexual abuse has occurred. In C. Hollin, & K. Howells, (Eds.) *Clinical approaches to sex offenders and their victims.* pp. 179–208. Chichester: Wiley.

Briggs, F. & Hawkins, R. (1994). Choosing between child protection programmes. *Child Abuse Review*, 3, 272–83.

Browne, K.D. (1988). The nature of child abuse and neglect: an overview. In K. Browne, C. Davies & P. Stratton (Eds.). *Early prediction and prevention of child abuse.* pp. 57–86. Chichester: Wiley.

Browne, K.D. (1989a). The naturalistic context of family violence and child abuse. In J. Archer & K. Browne (Eds). *Human aggression: naturalistic approaches.* London: Routledge.

Browne, K.D. (1989b). The health visitor's role in screening for child abuse. *Health Visitor*, 62, 275–7.

Browne, K.D. (1993). Violence in the family and its links to child abuse. *Ballière's Clinical Paediatrics*, 1, 149–64.

Browne, K.D. (1995). Preventing child maltreatment through community nursing. *Journal of Advanced Nursing*, 21, 57–63.

Browne, K.D. & Saqi, S. (1987). Parent–child interaction in abusing families: possible causes and consequences. In P. Maher (Ed.). *Child abuse: an educational perspective*, Oxford: Blackwell.

Browne, K.D. & Saqi, S. (1988a). Approaches to screening families high risk for child abuse. In K.D. Browne, C. Davies & P. Stratton (Eds) *Early prediction and prevention of child abuse*, Chichester: Wiley.

Browne, K.D. & Saqi, S. (1988b). Mother–infant interactions and attachment in physically abusing families. *Journal of Reproduction and Infant Psychology*, 6, 163–82.

Carroll, J. (1994). The protection of children exposed to marital violence. *Child Abuse Review*, 3, 6–14.

Elliott, M., Browne, K.D. & Kilcoyne, J. (1995). Child sexual abuse prevention: what offenders tell us. *Child Abuse and Neglect*, 19, 579–94.

Finkelhor, D. (1994). The international epidemiology of child sexual abuse. *Child Abuse and Neglect*, 18, 409–17.

Gray, J.O., Cutler, C.A., Dean, J. & Kempe, C.H. (1977). Prediction and prevention of child abuse. *Child Abuse and Neglect*, 1, 45–58.

Leventhal, J. (1988). Can child maltreatment be predicted during the perinatal period: evidence from longitudinal cohort studies. *Journal of Reproductive and Infant Psychology*, 6, 139–61.

Magura, M. (1981). Are services to protect children effective? *Children and Youth Service Review*, 3, 193.

National Society for the Prevention of Cruelty to children (1985). *Child abuse deaths. Information Briefing No.5*, London: NSPCC.

Olds, D., Henderson, C., Chamberlin, R. & Tatelbaum, R. (1986). Preventing child abuse and neglect: randomized trial of nurse home visiting. *Pediatrics*, 78, 65–78.

Prior, V., Lynch, M.A. & Glaser, D. (1994). *Messages from children.* London: NCH Action for Children.

Stanley, J. & Goddard, C. (1993). The association between child abuse and other family violence. *Australian Social Work*, 46, 3–8.

Starr, R.H. (1982). *Child abuse and prediction: policy implications.* Cambridge, Mass: Ballinger.

Wolfe, D.A. (1993). Child abuse prevention: blending research and practice. *Child Abuse Review*, 2, 153–65.

Chromosomal abnormalities

JEREMY TURK

Section of Child and Adolescent Psychiatry,
St. George's Hospital Medical School, University
of London, UK

INTRODUCTION

The influence of genes on cognition, behaviour and personality is well established. The usual interaction is between polygenic inheritance and environment. However, a number of genetic and chromosomal disorders seem to have characteristic behaviours or cognitive profiles.

The term behavioural phenotype refers to those aspects of an individual's behaviour (cognition and emotions included in the broadest sense) which can be attributed to underlying genetic disorder. Possibly the first published use of the term was by Nyhan (1972). He proposed an association between the inborn error of purine metabolism and the self-mutilatory behaviour in Lesch–Nyhan syndrome. Nyhan also commented on behaviours characteristic of Cornelia de Lange syndrome including self-injury, autistic-like features and hyperactivity.

Clinical considerations

Data on psychological and behavioural functioning can be categorized under the following headings:

- intellectual functioning
- speech and language
- attentional deficits
- social impairments
- other behavioural disturbances

Intellectual functioning

Intellectual abilities within a given condition vary widely. In Down's syndrome the average level of intellectual functioning is in the severe learning disability range yet some individuals have only mild learning difficulties. In fragile X syndrome mild-to-moderate learning disability is the rule but some subjects will be severely affected. The profile and natural history of intellectual disturbance is important too.

Speech and language

Speech and language assessment must consider level of intellectual functioning. Speech may be entirely absent as in Angelman syndrome (Jolleff & Ryan, 1993), may be described as having a particular quality as in fragile X syndrome (Ferrier *et al.*, 1991), or may be characterized by particular deficits such as the expressive language impairments in Klinefelter's syndrome (Mandoki *et al.*, 1991).

Attentional deficits

Attentional deficits range from mild inattentiveness and distractibility through to severe hyperactivity. Some conditions have specific associations, for example fragile X syndrome (Turk, 1994*a*) and Smith–Magenis syndrome (Colley *et al.*, 1990).

Social impairments

Social impairments are common in people with learning disabilities. Their significance is magnified by their association with language and communication disorders and ritualistic/obsessional tendencies, which may indicate autistic disturbances.

Other behavioural disturbances

Self-injurious behaviour (SIB) is surprisingly syndrome specific. Skin scratching, lip biting and knuckle gnawing characterize Lesch–Nyhan syndrome (Clements, 1987). In fragile X syndrome, SIB takes the form of hand biting usually over the base of the thumb, often in response to excitement or anxiety (Turk, 1991). In Prader–Willi syndrome, already delicate skin is aggravated by picking and scratching (Donaldson *et al.*, 1994). In Smith–Magenis syndrome (17p11.2, p11.2 deletion) particularly extreme forms of self-mutilation include pulling out finger and toe nails (onychotillomania) and inserting objects into body orifices (polyembolokoilomania) (Greenberg *et al.*, 1991). Smith–Magenis syndrome has also been reported as being associated with extreme sleep disturbance and hyperactivity. There may also be a co-occurrence with autism (McNaught & Turk, 1994).

A GENERAL REVIEW OF BEHAVIOURAL PHENOTYPES

Sex chromosome anomalies

Turner's syndrome

Turner's syndrome (45X) is usually associated with average intellectual functioning. However, there is a verbal/performance discrepancy with reasonable verbal skills but special needs in numeracy and visuospatial abilities (Silbert, Wolff & Lilienthal, 1977). Recent work suggests problems with gender role development (Downey *et al.*, 1989) and other areas including social anxiety, shyness, communication difficulties and inattentiveness (Skuse, Percy & Stevenson, 1994).

Klinefelter's syndrome (47XXY)

People with Klinefelter's syndrome tend to have speech and language impairments but relatively intact non-verbal intellectual skills (Ratcliffe, Butler & Jones, 1991). Speech development is often delayed with impairments in expressive language plus visual-motor and sensory integration problems (Mandoki *et al.*, 1991). It has been claimed that comparable studies in adult populations do not show such deficits and that pubertal maturation may eliminate them (Stewart et al., 1991). Decreased verbal IQ may depress full-scale IQ scores, but it appears that less than 20% have an IQ below 90, and performance scores have not been found to be significantly reduced, indicating absence of a predisposition to learning disability (Bolton & Holland, 1994). There have also been reports of XXY boys being introverted, less assertive, having lower levels of activity and tending to socially withdraw. Ratcliffe et al. (1982) found boys with Klinefelter's syndrome to be apprehensive and insecure with peer group relationship problems and less sexual interest in girls.

XYY syndrome

Up to half of people with XYY syndrome have language and reading difficulties. A similar proportion experience childhood psychiatric disturbance (Ratcliffe et al., 1991). Antisocial behaviour is rare though temper tantrums, impaired social relationships and oppositional or conduct disorders are common. Intelligence is mildly depressed in comparison with close relatives but within the normal range. Violent behaviour does not seem to be specifically associated with an extra Y chromosome (Schiavi et al., 1984) so another, unidentified, factor must act to cause such an excess.

Fragile X syndrome

Most recent research into behavioural phenotypes has related to the fragile X syndrome (Hagerman & Silverman, 1991). The condition is associated with an abnormal DNA enlargement just below the X chromosome's tip which can expand transgenerationally and interfere with protein transcription (Verkerk et al., 1991). Intellectual functioning is usually in the mild to moderate learning disability range (IQ 35–70) (Hagerman & Sobesky, 1989) with specific weaknesses in numeracy and visuospatial skills (Kemper, Hagerman & Altshul-Stark, 1988). The trajectory of intellectual development shows a characteristic profile with the rate of development remaining parallel to that of non-disabled peers up until puberty when the discrepancy widens (Hagerman et al., 1989). This is due to specific difficulties in sequential information processing (Hodapp et al., 1991). All the above intellectual anomalies are witnessed in female carriers, most of whom have average intellectual functioning (Miezejeski et al., 1986). Female carriers also often display difficulties with 'executive function' skills to do with planning ahead, attending, sustaining effort, generating problem-solving strategies, using feedback, self-monitoring and shifting responses (Mazzocco et al., 1992).

Speech and language in fragile X syndrome is almost always delayed to a varying degree (Newell et al., 1983). The style of talking has been described as jocular and litanic-like due to its humorous-sounding quality and up-and-down swings of pitch. Cluttering is also often evident. This consists of rapid speech with dysrhythmic elements (Hanson, Jackson & Hagerman, 1986).

Controversy persists as to whether hyperactivity and attentional deficits have a specific association with fragile X syndrome. These disturbances have been considered by some to be the most striking impairments experienced (Fryns et al., 1984). Hyperactivity has been reported as the presenting feature in non-learning disabled boys with fragile X syndrome (Hagerman, Kemper & Hudson, 1985). Recent research suggests that, whilst boys with fragile X are not generally more overactive than other children with similar learning disabilities, they do display poorer concentration spans with more restlessness and fidgetiness (Turk, 1995).

Autistic-like communicatory and ritualistic disturbances are associated with fragile X syndrome more than typical autism is. Fragile X syndrome accounts for no more than 2–3% of cases of typical autism (Bailey et al., 1993). The prevalence of typical autism in fragile X syndrome is probably no higher than in learning disabled populations generally (see Turk, 1992). It is the profile of social relationship disturbances which often typifies the condition. Echolalia may be immediate but is often delayed. Speech is very repetitive and perseverative and palilalia may also be demonstrated (repetition of phrases with increasing speed and diminishing volume) (Ferrier et al., 1991). Eye contact is often poor due to gaze aversion (Wolff et al., 1989) rather than gaze indifference, which is more often associated with typical autism. Other forms of sensory defensiveness occur, in particular tactile defensiveness and hyperacusis. There may be delayed development of symbolic and imaginative play, and individuals often show ritualistic and obsessional tendencies including hand flapping, hand biting and insistence on particular routines. It is often the paradoxical juxtaposition of a friendly and sociable, if somewhat shy or socially anxious personality, with certain autistic-like features which raises suspicions of fragile X syndrome.

Autosomal chromosomal disorders

Of the autosomal disorders, Down's syndrome stands out by virtue of relatively low rates of serious psychiatric disturbance such as autism and hyperactivity (Turk, 1994b). However, these do occur and can be severe (Pueschel, Bernier & Pezzullo, 1991). There is a well-established association of Down's syndrome with dementia of the Alzheimer type (Oliver & Holland, 1986) which may be mistaken for depression, 'challenging behaviour' or a psychological reaction to changes in life circumstances (Blackwood et al., 1988). Almost all people with Down's syndrome have the neuropathological changes typical of Alzheimer's dementia (Whalley, 1982), but clinically the disease is not so universally present. The possibility of a characteristic personality profile remains contentious.

Tuberous sclerosis

In tuberous sclerosis, autism and hyperactivity seem to occur more often and more severely than expected (Hunt & Dennis, 1987). Hyperactivity relates to the degree of cerebral damage and intellectual impairment. However, autistic tendencies seem to be dictated more by the presence and severity of the frequently associated hyperarrhythmic salaam attacks, a particularly serious and intractable form of epilepsy.

Williams syndrome

Speech and language abnormalities are universal in Williams syndrome (idiopathic hypercalcaemia). Many people with Williams syndrome exhibit superior verbal skills compared to their visuospatial and motor abilities (Udwin, Yule & Martin, 1987). Their verbal precociousness has been described as 'cocktail party chatter' due to lack of depth and meaning despite apparent sophistication. Speech is sometimes characterized by excessive use of cliches, perseverations and a habit of introducing irrelevant personal experiences into fluent chatter (Udwin & Yule, 1990). Hyperacusis (dislike of loud or intense sounds) is usually present, yet does not prevent sociable behaviours. Rates of behavioural disturbance are high, particularly hyperactivity, anxiety and eating and sleeping difficulties.

Angelman and Prader–Willi syndromes

Angelman's syndrome and Prader–Willi syndrome have strikingly different behavioural phenotypes despite relatively similar chromosome 15 long arm deletions. Prader–Willi syndrome individuals display marked obesity, hyperphagia and absence of satiety. Increased food intake is aggravated by reduced total energy expenditure attributable to reduced activity (Schoeller *et al.*, 1988). Decreased foetal movements herald hypotonia, poor feeding, abnormal weak or absent cry and sometimes failure to thrive. Expressive language and articulation problems occur. Hyperphagia and obesity develop throughout childhood. Behaviour problems include skin picking, stubbornness and temper outbursts in response to frustration combined with decreased sensitivity to pain. Intellectual abilities are uneven. Visuospatial skills seem good, yet numeracy, arithmetic and short-term memory processing present difficulties. By adolescence, obsessional tendencies often manifest as tantrums in response to trivial changes in routine (Donaldson *et al.*, 1994).

Angelman's syndrome individuals display a happy disposition with paroxysmal laughter, jerky ataxic gait, and a tendency towards an open mouth with tongue protrusion (Clayton-Smith, 1993). Learning disability is usually severe (Robb *et al.*, 1989). Autistic tendencies are common with substantially delayed social and communicatory skills (Sales & Turk, 1991). Individuals develop very few words and have difficulty in using gestural or sign systems (Jolleff & Ryan, 1993). Neonatal observations include feeding problems and an abnormal high-pitched cry (Clayton-Smith, 1993). Sleep requirements are reduced but do increase and some adolescents may even sleep longer than usual (Clayton-Smith, 1993).

Disorders with suspected but unascertained genetic aetiology

Many conditions have been described with behavioural profiles sufficiently characteristic to convince one of the presence of a behavioural phenotype. The best example is Rett's syndrome where its manifestation only in females could be explained by X-linked inheritance with lethality in males. Intellectual and social decline commences at 6–12 months with subsequent plateauing of abilities following a phase of apparently normal development (Trevathan & Naidu, 1988). There is associated loss of purposeful hand movements, replacement by midline hand wringing and hyperventilation, breath-holding, bruxism and tremulousness (Naidu *et al.*, 1986).

Sotos syndrome (Sotos *et al.*, 1964) has been recognized as having possible behavioural associations along with classic physical features of excessively rapid growth and non-progressive cerebral disorder with learning disability. Original case reports commented on hyperactivity, clumsiness and poorly articulated speech. Rutter & Cole (1991) suggest a common but variable behavioural pattern including social difficulties (solitariness, difficulty with peer relationships) and high rates of emotional and behavioural disturbance including tantrums, sexual precocity, sleep problems, object phobias and attention deficits.

THE IMPORTANCE OF DIAGNOSIS

The importance of recognizing behavioural phenotypes and diagnosing the underlying genetic disorder rests on the fundamental right of the individual and family to know the exact nature of their disabilities. Outdated notions that diagnostic labels produce negativism and suspension of efforts to help have been recognized as inappropriate. Indeed, it is individuals with learning disability for whom no cause can be found who seem to present the greatest emotional adjustment reactions for their families. This may be linked to the need to undergo a bereavement reaction for the anticipated, yet never realized, ideal child, and the coming to terms with the less than perfect offspring (Bicknell, 1983). Diagnosis facilitates familial relief from uncertainty and guilt and resolution of the grief reaction. While nobody would want bad news, it is still better than no news at all. Successful grief resolution enables focusing on the future, adjusting one's individual and family life accordingly, and planning ahead. Practical aspects, including genetic counselling for the extended family, can proceed following a diagnosis. Diagnostic awareness can also lead to more rational interventions relevant to the particular profile of strengths and needs. Possession of a diagnostic label also allows for membership of and identification with appropriate peer support networks.

REFERENCES

Bailey, A., Bolton, P., Butler, L., Le Couteur, A., Murphy, M., Scott, S., Webb, T. & Rutter, M. (1993). Prevalence of the fragile X anomaly amongst autistic twins and singletons. *Journal of Child Psychology & Psychiatry*, **34**, 673–88.

Bicknell, J. (1983). The psychopathology of handicap. *British Journal of Medical Psychology*, **56**, 167–78.

Blackwood, D.H.R., St Clair, D.M., Muir, W.J., Oliver, C.J. & Dickens, P. (1988). The development of Alzheimer's disease in Down's syndrome assessed by auditory event-related potentials. *Journal of Mental Deficiency Research*, **32**, 439–53.

Bolton, P. & Holland, A. (1994). Chromosomal abnormalities. In

M., Rutter, E. Taylor, & L. Hersov, (Eds.). *Child and adolescent psychiatry; modern approaches.* Oxford: Blackwell Scientific.

Clayton-Smith, J. (1993). Clinical research on Angelman syndrome in the United Kingdom: observations on 82 affected individuals. *American Journal of Medical Genetics*, **46**, 12–15.

Clements, J. (1987). Biological aspects of severe learning disabilities. In *Severe learning disability and psychological handicap.* London: Wiley.

Colley, A.F., Leversha, M.A., Voullaire, L.E. & Rogers, J.G. (1990). Five cases demonstrating the distinctive behavioural features of chromosome deletion 17 (p11.2 p11.2) (Smith – Magenis syndrome).

Journal of Paediatrics and Child Health, **26**, 17–21.

Donaldson, M.D.C., Chu, C.E., Cooke, A., Wilson, A., Greene, S.A. & Stephenson, J.B.P. (1994). The Prader–Willi syndrome. *Archives of Disease in Childhood*, **70**, 58–63.

Downey, J., Ehrhardt, A.A., Gruen, R., Bell, J.J. & Morishima, A. (1989). Psychopathology and social functioning in women with Turner syndrome. *Journal of Nervous and Mental Disorders*, **177**, 191–201.

Ferrier, L.J., Bashir, A.S., Meryash, D.L., Johnston, J. & Wolff, P. (1991). Conversational skills of individuals with fragile-X syndrome: a comparison with autism and Down syndrome. *Developmental Medicine and Child*

Neurology, 33, 776–88.

Fryns, J.P., Jacobs, J., Kleczkowska, A. & Van den Berghe, H. (1984). The psychological profile of the fragile X syndrome. *Clinical Genetics*, 25, 131–4.

Greenberg, F., Guzzetta, V., Montes-De-Oca-Luna, R., Magenis, R.E., Smith, A.C., Richter, S.F., Kondo, I., Dobyns, W.B., Patel, P.I. & Lupski, J.R. (1991). Molecular Analysis of the Smith-Magenis syndrome: a possible contiguous gene syndrome associated with del (17) (p11.2). *American Journal of Human Genetics*, 49, 1207–18.

Hagerman, R., Kemper, M. & Hudson, M. (1985). Learning disabilities and attentional problems in boys with the fragile X syndrome. *American Journal of Diseases of Children*, 139, 674–8.

Hagerman, R.J., Schreiner, R.A., Kemper, M.B., Wittenberger, M.D., Zahn, B. & Habicht, K. (1989). Longitudinal IQ changes in fragile X males. *American Journal of Medical Genetics*, 33, 513–18.

Hagerman, R.J. & Silverman, A.C. (1991). *Fragile X syndrome: diagnosis, research and treatment*. Baltimore: Johns Hopkins University Press.

Hagerman, R.J. & Sobesky, W.E. (1989). Psychopathology in fragile X syndrome. *American Journal of Orthopsychiatry*, 59, 142–52.

Hanson, D.M., Jackson, A.W. & Hagerman, R.J. (1986). Speech disturbances (cluttering) in mildly impaired males with the Martin–Bell/fragile X syndrome. *American Journal of Medical Genetics*, 23, 195–206.

Hodapp, R.M., Dykens, E.M., Ort, S.I., Selinsky, D.G. & Leckman, J.F. (1991). Changing patterns of intellectual strengths and weaknesses in males with fragile X syndrome. *Journal of Autism and Developmental Disorders*, 21, 503–16.

Hunt, A. & Dennis, J. (1987). Psychiatric disorder among children with tuberous sclerosis. *Developmental Medicine and Child Neurology*, 29, 190–8.

Jolleff, N. & Ryan, M.M. (1993). Communication development in Angelman's syndrome. *Archives of Disease in Childhood*, 69, 148–50.

Kemper, M.B., Hagerman, R.J. & Altshul-Stark, D. (1988). Cognitive profiles of boys with the fragile X syndrome. *American Journal of Medical Genetics*, 30, 191–200.

McNaught, A. & Turk, J. (1994). A girl with Smith–Magenis syndrome and autistic spectrum disorder misdiagnosed as parental emotional abuse. British Paediatric Neurology Association, Annual Meeting, Birmingham (poster presentation).

Mandoki, M.W., Sumner, G.S., Hoffman, R.P. & Riconda, D.L. (1991). A review of

Klinefelter's syndrome in children and adolescents. *Journal of the American Academy of Child & Adolescent Psychiatry*, 30, 167–72.

Mazzocco, M.M., Hagerman, R.J., Cronister-Silverman, A. & Pennington, B.F. (1992). Specific frontal lobe deficits among women with the fragile X gene. *Journal of the American Academy of Child & Adolescent Psychiatry*, 31, 1141–8.

Miezejeski, C.M., Jenkins, E.C., Hill, A.L., Wisniewski, K., French, J.H. & Brown, W.T. (1986). A profile of cognitive deficit in females from fragile X families. *Neuropsychologia*, 24, 405–9.

Naidu, S., Murphy, M., Moser, H.W. & Rett, A. (1986). Rett syndrome – natural history in 70 cases. *American Journal of Medical Genetics*, 24, 61–72.

Newell, K., Sanborn, B. & Hagerman, R. (1983). Speech and language dysfunction in the fragile X syndrome. In R.J. Hagerman & P.M. McBogg (Eds.). *The fragile X syndrome – diagnosis, biochemistry and intervention*. Dillon, Colorado: Spectra Publishing.

Nyhan, W.L. (1972). Behavioral phenotypes in organic genetic disease. *Pediatric Research*, 6, 1–9.

Oliver, C. & Holland, A.J. (1986). Down's syndrome and Alzheimer's disease: a review. *Psychological Medicine*, 16, 307–22.

Pueschel, S.M., Bernier, J.C. & Pezzullo, J.C. (1991). Behavioural observations in children with Down's syndrome. *Journal of Mental Deficiency Research*, 35, 502–11.

Ratcliffe, S.G., Bancroft, J., Axworthy, D. & McLaren, W. (1982). Klinefelter's syndrome in adolescence. *Archives of Disease in Childhood*, 57, 13–17.

Ratcliffe, S.G., Butler, G.E. & Jones, M. (1991). Edinburgh study of growth and development of children with sex chromosome abnormalities. IV. *Birth Defects: Original Articles Series*, 26, 1–44.

Robb, S.A., Pohl, K.R.E., Baraitser, M., Wilson, J. & Brett, E.M. (1989). The 'happy puppet' syndrome of Angelman: review of the clinical features. *Archives of Disease in Childhood*, 64, 83–6.

Rutter, S.C. & Cole, T.R.P. (1991). Psychological characteristics of Sotos syndrome. *Developmental Medicine and Child Neurology*, 33, 898–902.

Sales, J. & Turk, J. (1991). Angelman's syndrome; is there a behavioural phenotype? *Society for the study of behavioural phenotypes, annual workshop, London: abstracts*. Oxford: SSBP.

Schiavi, R.C., Theilgaard, A., Owen, D.R. & White, D. (1984). Sex chromosome anomalies, hormones and aggressivity. *Archives of General Psychiatry*, 41, 93–9.

Schoeller, D., Levitsky, L., Bandini, L.,

Dietz, W. & Walczak, A. (1988). Energy expenditure and body composition in Prader–Willi syndrome. *Metabolism*, 37, 115–20.

Silbert, A., Wolff, P.H. & Lilienthal, J. (1977). Spatial and Temporal Processing in patients with Turner's Syndrome. *Behavioral Genetics*, 7, 11–21.

Skuse, D., Percy, E. & Stevenson, J. (1994). Psychosocial functioning in the Turner syndrome: a national survey. *British Paediatric Association, annual meeting, University of Warwick: abstracts*. London: BPA.

Sotos, J.F., Dodge, P.R., Muirhead, D., Crawford, J.D. & Talbot, N.B. (1964). Cerebral gigantism in childhood. *New England Journal of Medicine*, 271, 109–16.

Stewart, D.A., Bailey, J.D., Netley, C.T. & Park, E. (1991). Growth, development, and behavioural outcome from mid-adolescence to adulthood in subjects with chromosomal aneuploidy: the Toronto study. *Birth Defects: Original Article Series*, 26, 131–88.

Trevathan, E. & Naidu, S. (1988). The clinical recognition and differential diagnosis of Rett syndrome. *Journal of Child Neurology*, 3, Suppl. S6–16.

Turk, J. (1991). Behavioural characteristics of children with fragile X syndrome. *Psychiatric Genetics*, 2, 98.

Turk, J. (1992). The fragile X syndrome: on the way to a behavioural phenotype. *British Journal of Psychiatry*, 160, 24–35.

Turk, J. (1994a). Attentional deficits in boys with fragile X syndrome: evidence for a characteristic developmental profile. *British Paediatric Association, annual meeting, University of Warwick: abstracts*. London: BPA.

Turk, J. (1994b). Profiles of autistic disturbances in children with genetically determined learning difficulties. *Royal College of Psychiatrists, winter meeting; conference abstracts*. London: Royal College of Psychiatrists.

Turk, J. (1995). The psychiatric, psychological and behavioural functioning of a British sample of boys with the fragile X syndrome. MD Thesis, University of London.

Udwin, O. & Yule, W. (1990). Expressive language of children with Williams syndrome. *American Journal of Medical Genetics*, Suppl. 6, 108–14.

Udwin, O., Yule, W. & Martin, N. (1987). Cognitive abilities and behavioural characteristics of children with idiopathic infantile hypercalcaemia. *Journal of Child Psychology and Psychiatry*, 28, 297–309.

Verkerk, A.J.M.H., Pieretti, M., Sutcliffe, J.S., Fu, Y.H., Kuhl, D.P.A., Pizzuti, A., Reiner, O., Richards, S., Victoria, M.F., Zhang, F., Eussen, B.E., van

Ommen, G.J.B., Blonden, L.A.J., Riggins, G.J., Chastain, J.L., Kunst, C.B., Galjaard, H., Caskey, C.T., Nelson, D.L., Oostra, B.A. & Warren, S.T. (1991). Identification of a gene (FMR-1) containing a CGG repeat coincident with a breakpoint cluster region

exhibiting length variation in fragile X syndrome. *Cell*, **65**, 905–14.

Whalley, L.J. (1982). The dementia of Down's syndrome and its relevance to aetiological studies of Alzheimer's disease. *Annals of the New York Academy of Sciences*, **396**,

39–53.

Wolff, P.H., Gardner, J., Paccia, J. & Lappen, J. (1989). The greeting behaviour of fragile X males. *American Journal of Mental Retardation*, **93**, 406–11.

Chronic fatigue syndrome

COLETTE RAY

Department of Psychology, Brunel University,
Uxbridge, Middlesex, UK

Chronic fatigue syndrome (CFS) is characterized by severe and debilitating fatigue which persists over time and which cannot be explained by a recognized medical diagnosis. Fatigue is typically worsened by exertion, and may be accompanied by a variety of other symptoms including myalgia, muscle weakness, and difficulties with concentration and memory. The causes of the illness have been much debated, and there is discussion too about how the patient should best cope with the condition in order to facilitate recovery. These uncertainties create difficulties for both the patient and practitioner.

Several case definitions have been proposed, with the aim of defining a relatively homogeneous group of patients for research purposes. Recently proposed criteria for CFS (Fukuda *et al.*, 1994) require that the fatigue should have a definite onset rather than be lifelong, and not be attributable to ongoing exertion. Symptoms should be present for at least six months and result in a substantial reduction in previous levels of occupational, educational, social or personal activities. This definition also proposes additional symptom criteria, but other definitions favour less restrictive criteria which focus upon fatigue and fatiguability without specifying accompanying symptoms.

The onset of illness may be acute or, less commonly, it may develop gradually. The majority of patients report that it began with an apparent infection, and a significant number report that they were under stress at the time (Komaroff & Buchwald, 1991). Various avenues of research have been pursued in the attempt to elucidate the aetiology of the disorder. There is evidence of persistent viral infection in a proportion of patients, and of immune system and neurohormonal dysfunction (Bock & Whelan, 1993); psychological factors have also been investigated, and it is likely that these interact with physical factors as causes of the disorder. CFS may be a multifactorial and heterogeneous condition, with some causes acting together to produce the syndrome and the salience of different aetiological factors varying with the individual patient.

The role of psychological factors in CFS is controversial. A relatively high percentage of patients fulfil criteria for psychiatric disorder, with depression being the most common diagnosis (Kendell, 1991). Parallels between the symptoms of CFS and depression have

been noted, with fatigue being a feature of both, and such similarities have led some to suggest that these disorders share a common pathology. The association between CFS and depression is, however, open to different interpretations. The fact that there is an overlap between their symptoms does not necessarily indicate a common origin, and others have pointed to differences between the two disorders. Anhedonia, weight loss, suicidal ideation, guilt, and low self esteem appear to be less common in CFS, while flu-like symptoms, muscle weakness and pain, and fatigue and myalgia brought on by physical effort are more common. To the extent that the patient experiences depression, and not all patients will fulfil criteria for this or other psychiatric disorder, this could be secondary to CFS. It could be due to some physiological effects or represent in part a reaction to malaise and functional limitations, and to the uncertainties associated with the nature, prognosis and management of the condition. Given that the role of emotional factors is ambiguous, disorders such as anxiety or depression are not regarded as grounds for excluding a diagnosis of CFS.

The pattern of the illness over time varies from patient to patient. A proportion report improvement or full recovery, while for others the illness may be constant or worsen, and others will experience a pattern of illness characterized by relapses and remissions (Dowsett *et al.*, 1990; Hinds & McCluskey, 1993). There is as yet no generally accepted drug regimen for CFS, and the emphasis thus falls upon recommendations for the management of the illness. Since exertion can exacerbate symptoms, many patients limit their activity. Various sources recommend appropriate rest and moderating activity to a level which can be tolerated, but the dangers of avoiding activity have also been highlighted. It has been suggested that avoidant behaviour may sustain symptoms by decreasing tolerance for activity, resulting in a vicious circle of avoidance, fatigue and demoralization. Cognitive – behavioural interventions designed to encourage tolerance of symptoms and activity and to modify maladaptive illness beliefs have produced improvement in a substantial proportion of patients (Butler *et al.*, 1991; Sharpe *et al.*, 1996). However, another evaluation of cognitive behaviour therapy, incorporating a graded exercise programme, found no evidence of gain compared with routine clinic attendance (Lloyd *et al.*, 1993).

Further studies of the consequences of different ways of coping with the illness, and of the effects of interventions to modify outcomes, are required, and advice should be tailored to the individual and his or her circumstances. Key factors in determining the appropriate response to the illness may be its stage, and the current pattern of symptoms in the context of the patient's own management approach. At the beginning of the illness, the patient's response may be to push him or herself in spite of symptoms, resulting in an increase in fatigue and malaise and a subsequent withdrawal from activity in order to recuperate. Some patients may continue with this approach of alternating exertion with rest, and experience a recurring cycle of relapse and recovery. Others may conclude that avoiding exertion is the best approach if symptoms are to be controlled, but achieve this at the cost of increased limitations in functioning (Ray *et al.*, 1993). Thus, both over-exertion and over-avoidance of activity may reinforce the experience of illness. A balanced and consistent approach to rest and activity may be the most appropriate strategy, with the emphasis first being placed on establishing a level of activity at which symptoms are not unduly exacerbated, and then attempting over time to achieve modest and gradual gains in functioning.

The patient with CFS may be disheartened by receiving a diagnosis which has become associated with the prospect of possible long-term illness, and may feel confused by the current lack of consensus about its causes and other related issues. These factors, together with the debilitating nature of the symptoms, will contribute to feelings of frustration and helplessness. The practitioner can help the patient to cope both practically and emotionally with the illness by undertaking an ongoing supportive role: acknowledging current uncertainties, while offering reassurance and encouragement, treatment of symptoms where appropriate, and advice aimed at improving well-being and functioning.

REFERENCES

Bock, G.R. & Whelan, J. (1993). *Chronic fatigue syndrome: Ciba Foundation Symposium 173*. Chichester: Wiley.

Butler, S., Chalder, T., Row, M. & Wessely, S. (1991). Cognitive behaviour therapy in the chronic fatigue syndrome. *Journal of Neurology, Neurosurgery and Psychiatry*, **54**, 153–8.

Dowsett, E.G., Ramsay, A.M., McCartney, R.A. & Bell, E.J. (1990). Myalgic encephalomyelitis – a persistent enteroviral infection? *Postgraduate Medical Journal*, **66**, 526–30.

Fukuda, K., Straus, S.E., Hickie, I., Sharpe, M.C., Dobbins, J.G. and Komaroff, A. (1994) Chronic fatigue syndrome: a comprehensive approach to its definition and study. *Annals of Internal Medicine*, **121**, 953–9.

Hinds, G.M.E. & McCluskey, D.R. (1993). A retrospective study of the chronic fatigue syndrome. *Proceedings of the Royal College of Physicians, Edinburgh*, **23**, 10–14.

Kendell, R.E. (1991). Chronic fatigue, viruses and depression. *Lancet*, **337**, 160–2.

Komaroff, A.L. & Buchwald, D. (1991). Symptoms and signs of chronic fatigue syndrome. *Reviews of Infectious Diseases*, **13**, 8–11.

Lloyd, A.R., Hickie, I., Brockman, A., Hickie, C., Wilson, A., Dwyer, J. & Wakefield, D. (1993). Immunologic and psychologic therapy for patients with chronic fatigue syndrome: a double-blind, placebo-controlled trial. *American Journal of Medicine*, **94**, 197–203.

Ray, C., Weir, W., Stewart, D., Miller, P. & Hyde, G. (1993). Ways of coping with chronic fatigue syndrome: development of an illness management questionnaire. *Social Science and Medicine*, **37**, 385–91.

Sharpe, M., Hawton, K., Simkin, S., Surawy, C., Hackmann, A., Klimes, I., Peto, T., Warrell, D. & Seagroatt, V. (1996). Cognitive behaviour therapy for the chronic fatigue syndrome: a randomised controlled trial. *British Medical Journal*, **312**, 22–6.

Cleft lip and palate

EMMA TAYLOR
Unit of Psychology, UMDS at Guy's Campus, University of London, UK

There are different forms of cleft conditions which affect the lip, alveolus, vomer, hard and soft palate and nose singly or in combination (Koch, Grzonka & Koch, 1995). Depending on the type and severity of the cleft, clefts are accompanied by several features that affect psychosocial development. Facial disfigurement is common. Macgregor (1990) emphasizes the importance of the face as a vehicle of verbal and non-verbal communication. A deviant facial appearance is central in impression formation, with attractiveness being important to psychological development and social relationships (Strauss & Broder, 1991). Given the social significance of the face, facial malformations may lead to adverse reactions in those with and without the disfigurement. Speech impairments are also associated with clefts. Peterson-Falzone (1995) examined speech outcomes in 110 adolescents with cleft lip and palates, and found that speech was normal in 22.7% of patients, with 66% of this population showing speech problems, and 10.9% showing habilitive failure. Clefts are also sometimes accompanied by hearing difficulties and other congenital anomalies. Having a cleft requires long-term care that includes surgery, hospitalization and follow-up. All these features may affect cognitive performance, self-concept and interpersonal relationships.

Children with clefts often have lower verbal intelligence scores than children without these conditions, which has been attributed to speech and hearing problems. In addition, hearing loss has been linked to visual–perceptual motor problems amongst children with clefts. Although these intelligence differences are not clinically significant (Richman & Eliason, 1982), children with clefts often under-achieve at school. Kapp (1979) found that 11–13 year-old girls with clefts reported less intellectual and school status than a matched sample of girls with no cleft condition. This poor school performance is linked to low parental and teachers' expectations and to general verbal and language difficulties (Richman & Eliason, 1982). Thus, studies that have assessed IQ and academic achievements show that children with clefts are at risk of delays (Strauss & Broder, 1991).

Poor self image has been found amongst people with cleft conditions (Strauss & Broder, 1991). While the self-concept of people with clefts is good, there is situational concern related to physical appearance (Richman & Eliason, 1982). For example, while Kapp (1979) found no differences on global self-concept between teenagers with and without cleft lip and palates, he reported that those with clefts reported less satisfaction with their physical appearance. This may particularly affect adolescents with clefts who are having to cope with integrating facial differences with a changing body image, and intimate relationships despite possible dissatisfaction with their appearance (Kapp-Simon, 1995).

Relationships may be affected by dissatisfaction with and reactions to facial malformations (see 'Dysmorphology and facial disfigurement'). Early studies of adolescents with cleft lips have found that psychological difficulties are mainly evident in the domain of social adjustment and competency, which many adolescents attribute to facial disfigurement (Kapp-Simon, 1995). Poor social competence may stem from trying to cope with reactions to a facial anomaly. Richman (1983) found that adolescents with cleft lips who were concerned about their facial appearance had higher scores on social introversion than those with less concern. Richman

and Eliason (1982) concluded that inhibition may be a positive adaptive response to having a cleft. However, this may also reduce social contact, and others' expectations of a person with adverse effects.

The treatment regimes for those with cleft palate have psychosocial impacts themselves. In one study, after hospitalization of on average a week or less, infants with clefts below the age of one showed greater avoidance toward their mother in the short term than a matched control group, with those hospitalized at a later age showing more negative behavioural changes than those hospitalized earlier (Koomen & Hoeksma, 1993). Medical treatment also affects adolescents who have to cope with both relating to medical staff and with surgeries that might alter facial appearance but still leave scarring (Canady, 1995; Kapp-Simon, 1995). Canady (1995) stated that those responsible for adolescent care should consider the emotional impact of a change in appearance following surgery; the impact of unsuccessful surgery and whether surgery is really wanted by the patient. The latter is particularly relevant when the teenagers' and their parents' views may conflict (Kapp-Simon, 1995). (See also 'Plastic Surgery'.)

These findings have been derived from self-report data; parent, teacher and peer reports; test results; observation and interviews. Despite this consistency, there are many weaknesses affecting research including lack of adequate sample sizes and control groups, and the confounding of different forms of clefts and different treatment regimes (Strauss & Broder, 1991). However, research does have treatment implications including the use of multidisciplinary team care. Psychosocial interventions have included education for the family and school; counselling, communication skills training; careful preparation for surgery including discussion of what the patient wants, of the risks and benefits of surgery and ensuring the patient and their family have realistic expectations of surgery (Canady, 1995; Kapp-Simon, 1995; Strauss & Broder, 1991).

REFERENCES

Canady, J.W. (1995). Emotional effects of plastic surgery on the adolescent with a cleft. *The Cleft Palate-Craniofacial Journal*, 32, 120–4.

Kapp, K. (1979). Self concept of the cleft lip and or palate child. *The Cleft Palate Journal*, 16, 171–6.

Kapp-Simon, K.A. (1995). Psychological interventions for the adolescent with cleft lip and palate. *The Cleft Palate – Craniofacial Journal*, 32, 104–8.

Koch, H., Grzonka, M. & Koch, J. (1995). Cleft malformation of lip, alveolus, hard and soft palate and nose: a critical review of the terminology, the diagnosis and gradation as a basis for documentation and

therapy. *British Journal of Oral and Maxillofacial Surgery*, 33, 51–8.

Koomen, H.M.Y. & Hoeksma, J.B. (1993). Early hospitalisation and disturbance of infant behaviour and the mother–infant relationship. *Journal of Child Psychology and Psychiatry*, 34, 913–17.

Macgregor, F.C. (1990). Facial disfigurement: problems and management of social interaction and implications for mental health. *Aesthetic Plastic Surgery*, 14, 249–57.

Peterson-Falzone, S.J. (1995). Speech outcomes in adolescents with cleft lip and palate. *The Cleft Palate – Craniofacial Journal*, 32, 125–8.

Richman, L.C. (1983). Self reported social, speech and facial concerns and personality adjustment of adolescents with cleft lip and palate. *The Cleft Palate Journal*, 20, 108–12.

Richman, L.C. & Eliason, M. (1982). Psychological characteristics of children with cleft lip and palate: intellectual achievement, behavioural and personality variables. *Cleft Palate Journal*, 19, 249–57.

Strauss, R.P. & Broder, H. (1991). Directions and issues in psychosocial research and methods as applied to cleft lip and palate and craniofacial anomalies. *The Cleft Palate – Craniofacial Journal*, 28, 150–6.

Cold, common

ANNA L. MARSLAND
Behavioral Physiology Laboratory University of Pittsburgh, USA

SHELDON COHEN
Department of Psychology Carnegie Mellon University, Pittsburgh, USA

ELIZABETH BACHEN
Behavioral Physiology Laboratory University of Pittsburgh, USA

Upper respiratory infections (URI) as a group are responsible for 50% of all acute illnesses, with the common cold syndrome being most familiar. Colds are caused by over 200 viruses and are characterized by sore throat, congestion, and mucus secretion. When exposed to viruses or other infectious agents, only a proportion of people develop clinical illness. Reasons for variability in response are not well understood and the possibility that psychological factors play some role in the aetiology and progression of infectious disease has received increased attention.

It is commonly believed that stressful life events influence the onset of URI by causing negative affective states (e.g. anxiety and depression) which, in turn, exert direct effects on biological processes or behavioural patterns that increase disease risk. The influence of stress on the immune system is considered the primary biological pathway through which stress can influence infectious disease susceptibility. While there is substantial evidence that stress is associated with changes in immune function (Herbert & Cohen, 1993), the implications of stress-induced immune changes for susceptibility to disease have not been established. To date, studies of stress and URI susceptibility have focused on establishing a link between stress and disease with little attention to pathways through which such an association might occur. The major findings of these studies are examined below.

There is consistent evidence that persons under stress report greater levels of URI symptoms, and that stress results in greater health-care utilization for URI (Cohen & Williamson, 1991). For example, Glaser et al. (1987) demonstrated that medical students report more infectious (mostly URI) illness during examination periods than at other times. Similarly, Stone, Reed & Neale (1987) found that, for 79 married couples followed over three months, daily life events rated as undesirable increased 3 to 4 days prior to onset of self-reported symptoms of URI, close in time to the incubation period of many common cold viruses. The self-reported symptoms of URI measured in these studies may tap underlying pathology; however, it is also possible that they reflect a stress-induced misinterpretation of physical sensations without underlying illness. The latter interpretation is supported by studies in which effects of stress on symptoms, but not verified disease, are observed, and by evidence that stress is associated with increased symptom reporting in general, not only with symptoms directly associated with infectious pathology (Cohen & Williamson, 1991).

Other investigators have verified the presence of pathology by physician diagnosis or biological methods. Several of these studies provide evidence that life stressors increase risk for verified upper respiratory disease. For example, Meyer and Haggerty (1962) followed 100 members of sixteen families for a 12-month period. Daily life events that disrupted family and personal life were four times more likely to precede than to follow new streptococcal and non-streptococcal infections (as diagnosed by throat cultures and blood antibody levels) and associated symptomatology. Similar results were reported in a study of viral URIs in 235 members of 94 families (Graham, Douglas, Ryan, 1986). Here, high stress, as defined by scores on reported major stressful life events, daily events and psychological stress, was associated with more verified episodes and more symptom days of respiratory illness. In sum, studies verifying infectious episodes suggest that stress increases risk for upper respiratory disease. However, community studies, like these, do not control for the possible effects of stressful events on exposure to infectious agents. Moreover, the literature on this topic is not entirely consistent; indeed, several studies have failed to find a relation between stress and upper respiratory disease (for review, see Cohen & Williamson, 1991).

Several prospective studies have eliminated the possible role of psychological effects on exposure by inoculating healthy volunteers with common cold viruses in attempts to determine whether psychological factors (measured prior to the viral exposure) influence susceptibility to URI. However, early viral inoculation studies were limited by a range of methodological weaknesses (Cohen & Williamson, 1991), including insufficient sample sizes and lack of control for factors known to influence susceptibility to viral infection (e.g. pre-existing antibodies to the infectious agent, gender, and age). Furthermore, the possible role of stress-elicited changes in health practices such as smoking and alcohol consumption was not considered. These limitations may account for failure of initial viral challenge studies to find consistent relations between stress and susceptibility to URI.

In contrast, Cohen, Tyrrell & Smith (1991, 1993) performed a large-scale viral inoculation study, including multiple controls for factors known to be independently associated with susceptibility to viral infection. In this prospective investigation, 420 healthy adults were assessed for degree of stress, and then experimentally exposed to one of five cold viruses or placebo. Increases in stressful life events, perceptions of current stress and negative affect were all associated with an increased risk of developing biologically verified URI. However, the investigators found that perceptions of stress and negative affect increased risk for illness through a different pathway than stressful life events. The former measures increased the probability of becoming infected (replicating virus), while the latter increased the probability of infected people developing clinical symptoms. A large group of control factors including age, sex, allergic status, body weight, season, and virus-specific antibody status before challenge, could not explain the increased risk of colds for

[411]

persons reporting greater stress. Smoking, alcohol consumption, diet, exercise, and sleep quality also failed to explain the association between stress and illness.

In a similar study, Stone *et al.* (1992) examined development of symptoms among persons infected with rhinovirus. They found that those with more life events were more likely to develop clinical colds, although perceptions of current stress and negative affect were unrelated to symptom development. In contrast to the study described earlier, this investigation included only infected persons and hence could not assess susceptibility to infection where Cohen

and colleagues found perceptions of stress and negative affect were related to susceptibility.

In sum, recent, well-controlled studies support prospective studies of community samples in indicating that psychological stress is associated with increased susceptibility to the common cold. In addition, there is consistent evidence for increased symptom-reporting under stress. A number of potential pathways exist through which an association between stress and infectious pathology might occur, including behavioural, hormonal and immune mechanisms. Future work is needed to explore these alternatives.

FURTHER READING

Cohen, S., Tyrrell, D.A.J. & Smith, A.P. (1991). Psychological stress and susceptibility to the common cold. *The New England Journal of Medicine*, 325, 606–12.

Cohen, S., Tyrrell, D.A.J. & Smith, A.P. (1993). Negative life events, perceived stress, negative affect, and susceptibility to the common cold. *Journal of Personality and Social Psychology*, 64, 131–40.

Cohen, S. & Williamson, G.M. (1991). Stress and infectious disease in humans. *Psychological Bulletin*, 109, 5–24.

Glaser, R., Rice, J., Sheridan, J., Fertel, R.,

Stout, J., Speicher, C. E., Pinsky, D., Kotur, M., Post, A., Beck, M. & Kiecolt-Glaser, J.K. (1987). Stress-related immune suppression: health implications. *Brain, Behavior, and Immunity*, 1, 7–20.

Graham, N.M.H., Douglas, R.B. & Ryan, P. (1986). Stress and acute respiratory infection. *American Journal of Epidemiology*, 124, 389–401.

Herbert, T.B. & Cohen, S. (1993). Stress and immunity in humans: a meta-analytic review. *Psychosomatic Medicine*, 55, 364–79.

Meyer, R.J. & Haggerty, R.J. (1962).

Streptoccocal infections in families. *Pediatrics*, 29, 539–49.

Stone, A.A., Reed, B.R. & Neale, J.M. (1987). Changes in daily event frequency precede episodes of physical symptoms. *Journal of Human Stress*, 13, 70–4.

Stone, A.A., Bovbjerg, D.H., Neale, J.M., Napoli, A., Valdimarsdottir, H., Cox, D., Hayden, F.G. & Gwaltney, J.M. (1992). Development of common cold symptoms following experimental rhinovirus infection is related to prior stressful life events. *Behavioral Medicine*, Fall, 115–20.

Colour blindness

JOHN MOLLON

The Psychological Laboratory, University of Cambridge, UK

Inherited deficiencies of colour vision are so common in western populations that some have supposed that these variant forms of human vision are maintained by a biological advantage; and certainly it is possible to show in the laboratory that a colour-blind observer can detect small variations in texture that are masked for the normal by uncorrelated variations in colour. Some 2% of Caucasian men are dichromats: to match all colours they require only two primary wavelengths, rather than the three needed by the normal. A further 6% of men are anomalous trichromats: they need three primaries in a colour-matching experiment but for most test lights they mix the primaries in different proportions from the normal. Anomalous trichromacy is commonly, but not invariably, associated with poorer colour discrimination than normal. Both dichromacy and anomalous trichromacy are usually sex-linked conditions: to exhibit a defect, a woman must normally inherit it from both parents. Thus frank colour blindness is seen in less than 0.5% of women, although some 15% of all women are carriers and can often be detected by subtle tests.

Normal colour vision depends on the presence in the retina of three classes of cone cell, with peak sensitivities respectively in the

violet (short-wave), green (middle-wave) and yellow-green (long-wave) regions of the spectrum. Embedded in the membranes of the cones are light-sensitive molecules, members of the superfamily of heptahelical molecules (the family also includes the dopaminergic and serotonergic receptors). It is differences in the amino acid sequences of these light-sensitive pigments that lend the cones their different spectral sensitivities. However, an individual cone cannot distinguish the photons of different wavelength that it absorbs, and so the visual system must neurally compare the quantum catches of different types of cone in order to distinguish colour from intensity.

The common forms of inherited colour blindness arise from alterations of either the long-wave or the middle-wave photopigment. The genes that code for these pigments lie in a cluster on the X-chromosome (at locus Xq28) and are thought to have arisen from duplication of a single ancestral gene at an early stage of primate evolution. The juxtaposition and the homology of the long- and middle-wave genes appear to encourage unequal crossing-over, giving rise to a rich variety of genotypes and phenotypes. The cluster may contain more than one copy of the normal genes as well as hybrid genes that draw part of their sequence from the long-wave

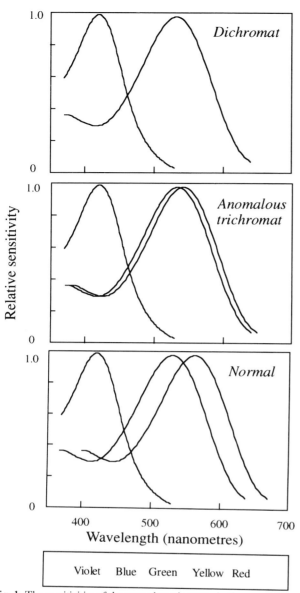

Fig. 1. The sensitivities of the cone photopigments, in the case of the normal eye and two types of colour deficiency.

dichromat can match any mixture of red and green to the orange. Those anomalous trichromats who require more red in the match than the normal are called protanomalous, those who require less, deuteranomalous. The clinical instrument for effecting the Rayleigh match, the anomaloscope, requires time and skill, and for occupational screening purposes the most efficient instruments are pseudo-isochromatic plates, such as those of Ishihara. The latter test is poor for classification, but, if administered under the correct illumination, seldom fails to detect even the mildest colour anomaly.

The gene for the short-wave photopigment is located on chromosome 7 and defects of this gene give rise to a third form of dichromacy, tritanopia. In its congenital form, the latter is very rare, but the short-wave cones (or the neurons that carry their signals) appear to be disproportionately vulnerable to toxins and to ocular and systemic conditions that affect the retina. Tritan-like impairments are thus often seen in glaucoma and in diabetes. Disorders of the optic nerve, such as optic neuritis, typically produce anarchic losses of colour discrimination, affecting the red–green axis of colour space, as well as the tritan (yellow–violet) axis. Lesions of the prestriate cortex can produce the condition of cerebral achromatopsia, where the subject can detect edges defined by a colour difference but cannot match or name colours.

Almost all countries exclude the colour deficient from occupations such as aviation, marine navigation, train driving and railway signalling. With increasing miniaturization of circuits, colour blindness has become less of an obstacle to work in electronics, although many firms still screen recruits. However, there are less obvious occupations where colour blindness remains a handicap, such as market gardening, butchery or hairdressing. Within medicine, the colour-deficient doctor should avoid the specialities of dermatology and anaesthesiology, since he or she may have reduced ability to detect erythema and cyanosis. Remarkably, in the UK, pharmacists are not required to pass a colour vision test, although colour coding is widely used in drug capsules and in labelling. Most police forces exclude colour-deficient recruits: whether or not an officer would be impaired in his actual duties, it would be easy for a defence barrister to discredit in court the perceptions of a colour-blind police witness.

In everyday life, the most celebrated difficulty experienced by colour-deficient people is in gathering red or orange fruit against a background of randomly varying foliage, a difficulty that suggests why trichromatic vision evolved in frugivorous primates. There are other inconveniences of colour blindness. For example, a colour-blind parent may not readily detect that his child is becoming sunburnt or has a rash. But, in general, the handicap is a slight one and many colour-deficient people do not recognize that their vision is abnormal until they are tested at school or they apply to enter a profession in which colour-coding is used. When reporting that a child or candidate is colour blind, the occupational psychologist should take care neither to rouse unnecessary anxiety in the client nor to cause the mother to feel guilt at passing on the trait. And, if a colour blind woman tells you her father was not colour blind, think twice before hastening to contradict her. *Pater semper incertus est.*

gene and part from the middle-wave gene. In dichromacy either the long-wave or the middle-wave gene is effectively lost, the former condition being called protanopia, the latter deuteranopia. The anomalous trichromat also lacks (or does not express) one of the normal genes, and his residual discrimination in the red–green range is thought to depend on the presence of two variant forms of one of the normal genes or on one normal and one hybrid gene.

The definitive test for classifying inherited colour deficiencies is the Rayleigh match, in which a red (669 nm) and a green (546 nm) light are mixed to match a monochromatic orange (589 nm). The

FURTHER READING

Foster, D.H. (Ed.). (1991). *Inherited and acquired colour vision deficiencies*, vol 7 In J.R. Cronly-Dillon (Ed.) *Vision and visual dysfunction*, Basingstoke: MacMillan.

Hunt, D.M., Dulai, K.S., Bowmaker J.K. & Mollon, J.D. (1995). *Science*, **267**, 984–8.
Mollon, J.D. (1989). *Journal of Experimental Biology*, **146**, 21–38.

Nathans, J. (1989). *Scientific American*, **260**, 28.
Viénot, F., Brettel, H., Oh, L., Ben M'Barek, A. & Mollon, J.D. (1995). *Nature*, **376**, 127–8.

Colour blindness

Complementary medicine

CHARLES VINCENT

Department of Psychology, University College
London, UK

The term complementary medicine embraces a wide range of diverse therapies and diagnostic methods. Previous terms have included fringe medicine, unconventional medicine, unorthodox medicine, natural medicine and, the most widely used, alternative medicine. Complementary medicine is now the preferred description as practitioners of these therapies now see them as supplementing rather than replacing orthodox medicine.

A British Medical Association report (Anon. 1986) listed 116 different types of complementary therapy and diagnostic aid. Their history, philosophy and methods are extremely diverse. The origins of some, for example, acupuncture, are ancient while osteopathy and homeopathy date from the nineteenth century. Some (acupuncture, homeopathy) are complete systems of medicine, while others are restricted to diagnosis alone (iridology) or to a specific therapeutic technique (massage). The range of treatments is equally diverse: diet, plant remedies, needles, minuscule homeopathic doses, mineral and vitamin supplements and a variety of psychological techniques. The theoretical frameworks and underlying philosophy vary in coherence, complexity, and the degree to which they could be incorporated in current scientific medicine. Complementary practitioners vary enormously in their attitude to orthodox medicine, the extent of their training and their desire for professional recognition.

THE MAJOR COMPLEMENTARY THERAPIES

The principal complementary therapies practised in Europe, the United States, and Australasia are acupuncture, homeopathy, herbalism, osteopathy, chiropractic and naturopathy. In some cases, such as acupuncture in China, the therapies have a central role in health care. Practitioners of these therapies usually belong to professional associations, have undertaken formal training and are often anxious to dissociate themselves from the wilder fringes of complementary medicine. The dedicated, skilled osteopath does not want to be bracketed with the fraudulent quack knowingly peddling dubious remedies for cancer, simply because both are unconventional forms of medicine.

The following brief descriptions give the flavour of the major complementary therapies.

Acupuncture

The human body is considered to be an energy system. The acupuncturist influences this energy flow by inserting and manipulating needles along the meridians of energy; restoring the balance of the energy flow restores health and harmony to the individual.

Herbalism

Plants have been used for medicinal purposes for at least 5000 years. Herbal remedies can provoke protective reactions within the body, act to stimulate the elimination of toxins and provide the body with a balance of nutrients and minerals. Herbalists would consider that complex combinations of actual plant material are more effective than the specific isolated compounds used in modern pharmacology.

Homeopathy

The homeopath stimulates the body's vital energies to prevent and treat disease. Diagnosis takes account of physical, emotional, mental and even moral factors. Homeopathic remedies would produce symptoms that are similar to those being treated. However they are frequently, but not always, diluted to the point where little if any of the original substance is left.

Manipulative therapies: Osteopathy and Chiropractic

Osteopaths and chiropractors are skilled in the examination, treatment and interpretation of abnormalities of function of the musculo-skeletal system. They hold that many common conditions are caused by, or at least aggravated by, misalignments or excessive strain placed on the vertebrae and other joints. They are primarily, but not exclusively, concerned with musculo-skeletal disorders.

Naturopathy

The task of the naturopath is to promote the conditions for healing, which relies on the stimulation of a vital curative force within the human organism. Naturopaths will use many conventional diagnostic techniques, such as blood tests, but will also rely upon iridology (eye diagnosis) and hair analysis. Treatment consists of prescribing a therapeutic regimen (diet, supplements, exercise, hydrotherapy) for the patient to follow. The naturopath is more of a guide or teacher than a therapist.

Each of these therapies is associated with a coherent and systematic theory of the functioning of the body, which is not to say that the theories are necessarily correct or empirically founded. Although there is considerable variety, they share some common features. Most embrace the idea that the body and emotions are maintained by an underlying energy or vital force and that the body is essentially self-healing. Specific symptoms are seen as a manifestation of a general imbalance or dysfunction affecting the whole system. The task of the practitioner is to assist the healing process, a fundamentally gentler approach to treatment than orthodox medicine (Fulder, 1984).

Complementary therapies aim to be preventative, to detect and treat subtle signs of disease and aim for an optimal state of physical and emotional health. Complementary practitioners aim to treat the whole person. In practice, this means that they will routinely enquire about emotional issues, lifestyle and other personal information. The emphasis on emotional factors may encourage an empathy and sensitivity in complementary practitioners, which is probably an important part of their appeal. However, orthodox practitioners may be equally 'holistic' in their approach to their patients.

Many medical and lay practitioners reject some or all of the traditional theories, yet still consider the technique to be useful. Some acupuncturists, for example, diagnose in conventional terms and consider that acupuncture will eventually be satisfactorily explained in neurophysiological terms. Generally, such practitioners consider that the scope of the therapy is more limited than the more traditionally oriented practitioners.

THE USE OF COMPLEMENTARY MEDICINE

Complementary therapies are extremely widely used. In the United States, Eisenberg, Kessler & Foster (1993) found that 34% of Americans had used at least one unconventional therapy or remedy in the past year, and a third of these people visited unconventional therapists. More visits were made to providers of unconventional therapy than to all US primary care physicians. The expenditure on unconventional therapies ($13.7 billion) was comparable to that spent on all hospitalizations in the US ($12.8 billion). Eisenberg included vitamin and mineral supplements, and relaxation techniques in their definition of unconventional therapy so these results exaggerate the use of complementary therapies as defined above.

In Europe, surveys also suggest that a third of people have seen a complementary therapist or used complementary remedies in any one year. In Britain, Fulder and Munro (1985) found that about 1.5 million people per annum (2.5% of the population) were receiving courses of complementary treatment. Common reasons for seeking complementary treatment are frustration or dissatisfaction with orthodox medicine (at least in relation to its effect on a particular complaint), the absence of iatrogenic effects and a more positive patient practitioner relationship. Consultations are longer and fees lower than for comparable orthodox treatments.

Patients tend to be female, well educated and of higher than average social class. There is little to support the view that complementary patients are especially gullible or naive, or have unusual personalities or value systems. They may differ in their beliefs about their illness. Some studies of cancer patients using complementary medicine have found that they were more likely to believe cancer was preventable through diet, stress reduction and environmental changes and to believe that patients should take an active role in their own health.

Complementary medicine is generally used for chronic conditions such as musculo-skeletal problems, arthritic conditions, respiratory disorders, skin conditions and psychological problems and they are sometimes used in more serious conditions. There have been some alarming reports of patients abandoning potentially life-saving orthodox treatment for dubious, if well intentioned, complementary therapies (Cassileth, 1989). However, it is now clear that cancer patients almost always use complementary therapies as an adjunct to conventional treatment not a substitute. Cancer patients do not hope for a cure from complementary therapies, but find that they enhance their quality of life and help them cope with the disease (Thomas *et al.*, 1991).

THE ATTITUDE OF DOCTORS TO COMPLEMENTARY MEDICINE

Although medical critics of complementary medicine can be vehement many doctors are extremely interested in complementary therapies. Wharton and Lewith (1986) found that 59% of British general practitioners believed that complementary therapies were useful; many were practising complementary techniques or intending to train. Almost all general practitioners considered manipulation useful, with acupuncture and homeopathy also scoring highly. Similar results have been reported elsewhere in Europe. Almost all of a sample of 360 doctors in the Netherlands reported referring patients to complementary practitioners and over a third viewed complementary medicine as 'something more than a placebo effect'. General practitioners take a pragmatic view and are willing to give a method the benefit of the doubt, even if its efficacy has not yet been established. They are even more willing to do so at the patient's request and when regular care has not shown sufficiently positive results (Visser & Peters, 1990).

THE EVALUATION OF COMPLEMENTARY MEDICINE

The major criticisms of complementary therapies have been either that they are not effective or, if they are, that it is nothing more than a placebo effect. These questions are most powerfully addressed by randomized controlled trials.

Complementary practitioners place great stress on an individual approach to each patient. Individual differences in diagnosis, treatment and response tend to be obscured in controlled trials. For this and other reasons some researchers have suggested that the classic experimental methodology of the randomized controlled trial does not do justice to complementary medicine. Most of these problems are not unique to complementary medicine. There are many difficulties in the interpretation, feasibility and ethics of controlled trials of many different types of intervention (Kramer & Shapiro, 1984). Some of these problems are, however, particularly acute in complementary medicine.

One major difficulty is that double-blind trials are not feasible for some types of therapy, namely those that require a skilled physical intervention, such as acupuncture, physiotherapy or surgery. A double-blind trial of acupuncture cannot be carried out, except under very artificial conditions, as the acupuncturist could not be unaware of the type to treatment s/he was giving. Finding an appropriate placebo control can also be difficult. In the case of drugs it is relatively straightforward to produce inert pills, identical in appearance to the true tablets. With treatments requiring a physical intervention (such as surgery or acupuncture) the definition of an appropriate placebo is extremely problematic. A further difficulty is that complementary practitioners may wish to use their own diagnostic system; in practice, however, most trials have used conventional diagnoses (Vincent, 1993).

RESULTS OF CONTROLLED TRIALS

Reviewing the outcome literature for complementary medicine would be a massive task; only a few major reviews are discussed here. All reviewers have commented on the poor quality of many of the studies, though it must be remembered that few conventional treatments have been properly evaluated. Complementary

[415]

practitioners, necessarily in private practice, do not generally have either the time or the expertise to mount studies, so most trials have been conducted by doctors and researchers with an interest in complementary therapies.

Acupuncture

Richardson and Vincent (1986) found good evidence for the short-term effectiveness of acupuncture for low-back pain, mixed results for headache, and some encouraging preliminary results for cervical pain and arthritis. The proportion of patients helped varied from study to study, but commonly fell in the region 50–80%. In a later and larger review Ter Riet and colleagues (1990) identified 51 controlled trials of acupuncture for chronic pain. Each study was scored on 18 methodological criteria, some weighted more heavily than others, with a maximum possible score of 100. Only 11 studies scored 50 or more points. Positive and negative results were approximately equally divided in the higher quality studies. The treatment for musculo-skeletal problems of the spine (mostly low-back pain) showed the most positive results. There is inconsistent evidence for the efficacy of acupuncture in the treatment of asthma and in the treatment of addictions (Vincent, 1993).

Homeopathy

The most comprehensive review is by Kleijnen, Knipschild & Ter Riet (1991), who made a Herculean effort to track down all known controlled trials of homeopathy. They identified 107 trials dealing with respiratory disorders, allergies, chronic pain, gastrointestinal complaints, hypertension, psychological problems and a variety of other diagnoses. Each study was blind-rated for methodological soundness by two of the authors. Of the 105 trials with interpretable results, 81 were positive when homeopathy was compared with (mostly placebo) controls. Mindful of the fact that more positive findings can be associated with poorer methodology the authors separated out the best studies: ten showed an advantage for homeopathy against four negative findings. Kleijnen and colleagues, who were initially extremely sceptical of the value of homeopathy, concluded that the evidence, although generally positive, was probably not sufficient for most people to form a definite view. They suggest that further large scale trials, under rigorous double-blind conditions are definitely warranted.

Manipulative therapies

The most comprehensive review of spinal manipulation (Koes *et al.*, 1991) followed the same methods of the Kleijnen review of homeopathy. Thirty-five randomized controlled trials were identified, but no trial scored over 60 points out of a possible 100. In 18 trials (51%) the authors reported better results for spinal manipulation than for the comparison treatment, usually physiotherapy (short-wave diathermy, massage, exercises) or drugs (generally analgesics) or placebo. In a further five studies, spinal manipulation was more effective in a subgroup of patients. There was a tendency for trials with lower methodology scores to be more likely to report positive findings. Four of eight studies involving a placebo comparison, usually detuned short wave diathermy, found a significant advantage for manipulation.

Overall, Koes and colleagues suggest that the results are promising, but not conclusive. In their own trial of manipulation for back pain, in which they tried to avoid the methodological flaws identified in their review, manipulation showed a slight advantage over physiotherapy, and both were superior to placebo and general practitioner treatment. It is noteworthy that patients receiving manipulation needed only half as many treatments as those receiving physiotherapy.

Herbal remedies

A review of trials of all herbal remedies would be an impossibility, given the vast number of medicinal plants and potential uses. Pharmacologists are devoting considerable efforts to analysing herbal remedies and identifying active ingredients. A large number of clinical trials of herbal remedies have been carried out. Recent examples include positive results of feverfew for migraine (Murphy, Heptinstall & Mitchell, 1988) and traditional Chinese herbal therapy for atopic dermatitis (Sheehan *et al.*, 1992). The efficacy of many herbs is not really in question as many widely used and evaluated drugs (e.g. digitalis) are derived from plant materials. The conventional approach is to identify the active ingredients and produce them in a purer form. The herbalist, on the other hand, holds that the interaction of different herbs in their natural form produces, in the long term, superior therapeutic effects. The crucial question is whether this, herbal, approach has any advantage over a conventional pharmacological approach. Few, if any, studies have addressed this question.

Naturopathy

The range of techniques employed by naturopaths precludes any overall review. Naturopathy emphasizes dietary changes, the use of exercise, identification of allergic reactions and stress reduction rather than the use of drugs. Evidence for the efficacy of these approaches is growing, whether or not they are described as naturopathic. There is evidence, for instance, that rheumatoid arthritis, hypertension, and otitis media respond to naturopathic approaches (Bergner, 1991). The Lifestyle Heart Trial (Ornish *et al.*, 1990) suggests that changes in diet and lifestyle can make profound differences to the rate of relapse of cardiac patients. Whether or not naturopathic theories are accepted, there is supportive evidence for several aspects of the approach.

MECHANISMS OF ACTION

There is a huge literature on the neurophysiology of acupuncture, the action of herbal remedies and disputed findings on a possible mechanism for homeopathy. A discussion of mechanisms is well beyond the scope of this paper. However one point must be made: the assessment of the results of clinical trials depends partly on whether there is, at least potentially, a scientifically plausible underlying mechanism. The theories underlying osteopathy may or may not be correct, but manipulation is certainly a plausible treatment for musculo-skeletal problems. The discovery that acupuncture provoked the release of endorphins and enkephalins did much to encourage its acceptance, even though the results of clinical trials are still equivocal. Conversely, the implausibility of very dilute homeopathic remedies having any effect undoubtedly hinders its acceptance, even though trial results are reasonably positive.

THE INFLUENCE OF COMPLEMENTARY MEDICINE

The dividing line orthodox and complementary medicine will always be changing. Some complementary therapies are probably destined to always remain outside conventional, scientifically based medicine. Others may gain acceptance and be no longer considered complementary, perhaps losing their unique character in the process. Acupuncture is widely used in pain clinics, but not in its traditional form. The influence of complementary medicine may be more pervasive and more important than any of its particular therapies. For many patients it represents a form of medicine that is more personal, less invasive and less risky, and which offers them more time and more opportunity to take an active part in their own treatment. Many of the major threats to health are primarily problems of lifestyle. Conventional medicine may have to become more complementary in method and in spirit, while not relinquishing its scientific base and insistence on a critical evaluation of all forms of therapy.

REFERENCES

Anon (1986). *Alternative therapy*. British Medical Association.

Bergner, P. (1991). *Safety, effectiveness and cost effectiveness in naturopathic medicine*. American Association of Naturopathic Physicians.

Cassileth, B.R. (1989). The social implications of questionable cancer therapies. *Cancer*, 63, 1247–50.

Eisenberg, D., Kessler, R.C. & Foster, C. (1993). Unconventional medicine in the United States. *New England Journal of Medicine*, 328, 246–52.

Fulder, S. (1984). *The handbook of complementary medicine*. London: Hodder and Stoughton.

Fulder, S.J. & Munro, R.E. (1985). Complementary medicine in the United Kingdom: patients, practitioners, and consultations. *Lancet*, 11, 542–5.

Kleijnen, J., Knipschild, P. & Ter Riet, G. (1991). Clinical trials of homeopathy. *British Medical Journal*, 302, 316–23.

Koes, B.W., Assendelft, W.J.J., van der Heijden, G.J.M.G., Bouter, L.M. &

Knipschild, P.G. (1991). Spinal manipulation and mobilisation for back and neck complaints: a blinded review. *British Medical Journal*, 303, 1298–303.

Kramer, M.S. & Shapiro, S.H. (1984). Scientific challenges in the application of randomized controlled trials. *Journal of the American Medical Association*, 252, 2739–45.

Murphy, J.J., Heptinstall, S. & Mitchell, J.R.A. (1988). Randomised double-blind placebo-controlled trial of feverfew in migraine prevention. *Lancet*, ii, 189–92.

Ornish, D., Brown, S.E., Scherwitz, L.W. Billings, J.H., Armstrong, W.T., Parts, T.A., Mclanahan, S.M., Kirkeeide, R.C., Brand, R.J. & Garld, K.L. (1990). Can lifestyle changes reverse coronary heart disease: the Lifestyle Heart Trial. *Lancet*, 336, 129–33.

Richardson, P.H. & Vincent, C.A. (1986). Acupuncture for the treatment of pain: a review of evaluative research. *Pain*, 24, 15–40.

Sheehan, M.P., Rustin, M.H.A., Atherton,

D.J., Buckley, C., Harris, D.J., Brostoff, J., Ostlere, L. & Dawson, A. (1992). Efficacy of traditional Chinese herbal therapy in adult atopic dermatitis. *Lancet*, 340, 13–17.

Ter Riet, G., Kleijnen, J. & Knipschild, P. (1990). Acupuncture and chronic pain: a criteria based meta-analysis. *Journal of Clinical Epidemiology*, 11, 1191–9.

Thomas, K.J., Carr, J., Westlake, L. & Williams, B.T. (1991). Use of non-orthodox and conventional health care in Great Britain. *British Medical Journal*, 302, 207–10.

Vincent, C.A. (1993). Acupuncture. In *Clinical research methodology*. London: Hodder & Stoughton.

Visser, G.J. & Peters, L. (1990). Alternative medicine and general practitioners in The Netherlands: towards acceptance and integration. *Family Practice*, 7, 227–32.

Wharton, R. & Lewith, G. (1986). Complementary medicine and the general practitioner. *British Medical Journal*, 292, 1498–500.

Contraception

BETH ALDER

Department of Epidemiology and Public Health
University of Dundee
Ninewells Hospital and Medical School, UK

The need to control human population growth and the demands of women for safe and reliable methods to control their fertility have driven developments in contraception. The psychological aspects of contraception, even in relation to sexuality, have been given less attention than medical aspects (Alder, 1993). Health psychologists have considered contraception in the context of preventing teenage pregnancies and condom use to reduce the spread of HIV infection. However contraception is practised by millions worldwide who are neither teenagers nor at risk of HIV infection.

ORAL CONTRACEPTION

Most women in the UK have relatively easy access to a range of contraceptive methods. In a study of women aged 35 in 1987/88 in the West of Scotland, Hunt (1990) found that 80% were using contraception. Over 90% had used the oral contraceptive pill at one time, although only 12% were currently using it. Reduced sexual interest and depression were among the side-effects reported in retrospective studies of the early high oestrogen oral contraceptive pills. Prospective studies are difficult to do because women who have side-

[417]

effects may stop using the pill and long-term users are less likely to report side-effects. Lack of compliance with pill taking may be the main cause of failure. We know that compliance with medication is often low, but we might expect it to be higher when lack of compliance may result in a pregnancy.

OTHER CONTRACEPTIVE METHODS

The disadvantages of using the pill may be the reason for choosing other methods of contraception. The most widely used method worldwide is sterilization. Vasectomies in men and laparasopic sterilization in women are safe and effective, although usually irreversible. In Hunt's (1990) sample of 35 year-old women, 53% relied on surgical sterilization. Early studies of female sterilization suggested a regret rate of up to 15%, but prospective studies find a much lower rate (Alder, 1984).

In the last decade there has been an increase in the use of condoms because of their protection against HIV infection. Female condoms have recently been introduced and appear to be acceptable. The male pill is another possibility but there is some doubt about whether women could trust men to take it regularly (Guillebaud, 1991)

MODELS OF CONTRACEPTIVE CHOICE

Several models of contraceptive decision making have been proposed. Lindemann (1977) described a contraceptive career in women as consisting of three stages. In the first 'natural' stage' sexual intercourse is relatively rare and unplanned. The woman does not perceive herself as a sexual being and she neither uses contraception nor takes responsibility for it. In the second 'peer prescription' stage, sexual activity is more frequent. There is a moderate acceptance of sexuality and she may seek information from friends. In the third, 'expert' stage, she accepts her sexuality and becomes willing to seek contraceptive advice.

In Fishbein's Model of Reasoned Action, people weigh up the costs and benefits of the expected outcomes and estimate the probability of occurrence of the outcomes. The probability of pregnancy and the probability of obtaining an abortion may be offset against the costs of obtaining contraception and its effect on the experience of intercourse and the dynamics of the relationship. This suggests a rational decision making process, but if the method requires an action such as putting on a condom (possibly in an emotionally charged sexual interaction), the actual behaviour may not match the intention.

Prochaska and DiClemente's Transtheoretical model of behaviour change suggests that people pass through a sequence of stages of precontemplation, contemplation, preparation, action and maintenance. In a study of 248 college students, Grimley et al. (1995) found that general contraceptive users were furtherest along the stages, followed by condom users. The model was effective in predicting patterns of contraceptive behaviour. Galavotti et al. (1995) looked at the use of condoms by women at high risk of HIV infection and found that self-efficacy increased across the stages.

Mahoney, Thombs and Ford (1995) tested the Health Belief Model in relation to condom use in college students. Sporadic users were distinguished from consistent users and non users in the number of sex partners in the previous year, the frequency of drunkenness during sexual intercourse, perceived susceptibility to infection, and self-efficacy. The model was effective in discriminating between non-users and consistent users, and could be used in health promotion programmes.

Whitley and Schofield (1986) compared adolescent contraceptive users and non-users in a meta-analysis of over 130 studies. They found strong support for the career model for women but not for men. Sexual self-acceptance was a major variable for both men and women, in addition to frequency of intercourse, age, self-esteem, and rejection of traditional roles. The decision model also received good support for women. Contraceptive use was strongly associated with the perceived risk of pregnancy. In women, positive attitudes to contraception and positive subjective norms were related to contraceptive use.

CONTRACEPTION AND SEXUALITY

Contraception, almost by definition, is used only when there is penetrative sexual intercourse and consequently it is only of relevance for couples at risk of pregnancy. There is much sexual activity that does not involve contraception, but contraceptive behaviour is always confounded with sexuality. Women who take the oral contraceptive pill are more sexually active than those who use other methods or no method at all. This could be because sexually active women choose the pill or because taking the pill allows relaxed spontaneous intercourse. Bancroft (1989) suggests that a positive effect of oral contraceptives on sexuality may be mediated by a positive effect on mood.

If either partner has been sterilized, they can have spontaneous and uninterrupted sexual activity, and in contrast to early retrospective reports' prospective studies suggest an increase in sexual activity and desire (Alder, 1993). Condoms may distract from the enjoyment of intercourse, although they can be used in foreplay. However, they may involve the couple in overt negotiation of responsibility for contraception and this may be difficult for inexperienced young people. Public awareness programmes have focused on the use of condoms in 'safer sex' and this may mistakenly imply that condoms will reliably prevent pregnancy. (See 'AIDS'.)

REFERENCES

Alder, E. (1984). Sterilisation. In A. Broome and L. Wallace (Eds.). *Psychology and gynaecological problems*. London: Tavistock

Alder, B. (1993). Contraception. In C. Niven & D. Carroll (Eds.). *The health psychology of women*. C. Reading: Harwood Academic Publishers.

Bancroft, J. (1989). *Human sexuality and its problems*. 2nd edn. Edinburgh: Churchill Livingstone.

Galavotti, C., Cabral, R.J., Lansky, A., Grimley, D.M., Riley, G.E. & Prochaska, J. (1995). Validation of measures of condom and other contraceptive use among women at high risk for HIV infection and unintended pregnancy. *Health Psychology*, **14**, 570–8.

Guillebaud, J. (1991). *The pill*. Oxford: Oxford University Press.

Grimley, D.M., Prochaska, J.O., Velicer, W.F. & Prochaska, G.E. (1995). Contraceptive and condom use adoption and maintenance: a stage paradigm approach. *Health Education Quarterly*, **22**, 20–35.

Hunt, K. (1990). The first pill taking

generation: past and present use of contraception among a cohort of women born in the early 1950's. *The British Journal of Family Planning*, **16**, 3–15.

Lindemann, C. (1977). Factors affecting the use of contraceptives in the non-marital context. In R. Gemme & C. Wheeler

(Eds.). New York: Plenum. *Progress in sexuality*.

Mahoney, C.A. Thombs, D.L. & Ford, O.J. (1995). Health belief and self efficacy models: their utility in explaining college student condom use. *AIDS Education and Prevention*, **7**, 32–49.

Scherran, P. White, D. & Phillips, K. (1992).

Premarital contraceptive use: a review of the psychological literature. *Journal of Reproductive and Infant Psychology*, **9**, 253–69.

Whitley, B.E. & Schofield, J.W. (1986). A meta analysis of research on adolescent contraceptive use. *Population and Environment*, **8**, 173–203.

Coronary heart disease: impact

PAUL BENNETT

Gwent Psychology Services and School of Psychology, University of Bristol, UK

DOUGLAS CARROLL

School of Sports and Exercise Sciences University of Birmingham, UK

A heart attack (myocardial infarction: MI) may be a devastating event. Its onset is sudden, painful, and potentially life-threatening. Not surprisingly, the psychological consequences of MI may be profound and persistent. Wiklund *et al.* (1984), for example, found that one year after their first MI, 74% of patients experienced frequent worries concerning their cardiac state and symptoms, while 58% reported they were protected from physical exertion by their friends or family, frequently as a consequence of anxiety rather than symptom severity.

Most research studying sequelae to MI has focused on the emotional impact of the event on the patient and their partner (focusing particularly on anxiety, depression, and denial), and indices of recovery such as the time taken to return to work. Fewer studies have focused on changes in risk behaviour, such as smoking and exercise levels.

THE EMOTIONAL IMPACT OF AN MI

Between 40 and 50% of MI patients report moderate to severe levels of anxiety while in hospital. Three to six months later this figure has typically dropped to about one-third of patients, and to about a fifth at one-year follow-up. Incidence rates for depression of between 20 and 30% are typical during the acute phase, rising slightly in the months following discharge, perhaps reflecting some patients' increased understanding of the implications of their illness.

Psychological distress may impact adversely on recovery. Mayou, Foster and Williamson (1978), for example, found baseline measures of depression were associated with poor outcomes on measures of physical symptoms, coping, quality of marriage, and leisure and work satisfaction at one-year follow-up; although the absence of premorbid or control group data (as in all similar studies) suggests the need for caution in attributing all these problems only to the MI. Trelawney-Ross and Russell (1987) found that depression in hospital, or ten days after discharge, was associated with the number of cardiac symptoms reported at six-month follow-up. Since cardiac damage was not so related, it can be inferred that poorer psychosocial outcomes cannot be attributed to depression mirroring physical

state. A number of studies have reported that people who report significant depression during the immediate rehabilitation period evidence earlier and higher levels of mortality than those who do not report such emotional distress. These effects can be extremely powerful. Nancy Frasure-Smith, for example, in an address to the 1994 Annual Conference of the Society of Behavioral Medicine, reported an eightfold difference in mortality rates over a period of 18 months between those who were, and were not, depressed in a large cohort of post-MI men. Unfortunately, in the absence of behavioural measures such as smoking or exercise in this study, and those relating to denial (see below), we can only speculate at the mediating factors between emotional state and disease progression.

There is, as yet, no consensus regarding the definition of denial in the context of heart disease. However, one of the more useful conceptual analyses is that provided by Havik and Maeland (1986) who distinguished three types: denial of illness, of affective consequences (impact), and suppression. Over a follow-up period of up to five years, they found denial of illness was unrelated to emotional outcome, return to work, use of drug or hospital facilities, and resumption of sexual activity. However, participants with higher denial scores reported more limitations during sexual intercourse due to fear of exertion, suggesting some recognition of disease, if not heart disease. Not surprisingly, as denial of impact is defined by an absence of emotional reaction to MI, high deniers reported less emotional upset throughout the study period. It was also associated with less use of psychoactive drugs during hospital stay and at six-month follow-up.

A few studies have attempted to address the issue of whether denial impacts on survival. Unfortunately, these have been confounded by severity of MI and age (Hackett, Cassem & Wishnie, 1968) or between group differences in the frequency of cardiac complications and differential follow-up periods (Havik & Maeland, 1988) and no firm conclusions can be drawn from their findings.

BEHAVIOURAL INDICES OF RECOVERY

Two major behavioural indices of recovery have been whether and when patients return to work and resume sexual relations. While these are important outcomes, they present some problems of interpretation as return to work is governed by macro- and microeconomic factors and measuring sexual activity is fraught with definitional and reporting problems.

Between 75 and 90% of MI-patients return to work. White collar, male, and young workers are most likely to retain their jobs. However, psychological factors are also predictive of outcome. A majority of studies suggest that depression during the acute phase is predictive of low rates of non–return as are expectations of reduced work capacity or autonomy. Smith and O'Rourke (1988) reported that patients who found their work stressful were least likely to return. In contrast, Abbott and Berry (1991) found that those who returned to work earlier were more likely to attribute their MI to occupational stress. They explain this apparent paradox in terms of job commitment. Those who considered work to be of central importance in their lives were more likely to return to their job as early as possible.

The percentage of post-MI patients to report returning to pre-MI levels of sexual activity varies across studies and time. Stern, Pascale and McLoone (1976) reported that by one year post-MI, 82% of patients had returned to 'previous or near previous levels of sexual functioning', 69% achieved this within 12 weeks of their infarction. In contrast, Trelawney-Ross and Russell (1987) found that 45% of their sample of 32 married men had not returned to previous levels of sexual activity by six-month follow-up. Somatic symptoms such as pain, breathlessness and fatigue were associated with lower sexual activity although anxiety and depression were not. Wiklund et al. (1984) reported that compared to two months prior to MI, at one-year follow-up only 35% of the participants in their study claimed they had experienced no change in their sexual activity, while 60% 'had noted a decline'. Five per cent reported that they had ceased sexual activity altogether. While fear was the predominant reason for reduced sexual activity at two-month follow-up assessment, impotency and loss of interest were the most frequent explanations one year after MI.

RISK FACTOR CHANGE
Smoking has been identified as the most important behavioural predictor of re-infarction. Accordingly, it is somewhat surprising that remarkably few studies have tracked smoking levels in post-MI patients. Schwartz (1987) noted that, though several studies have reported immediate cessation rates above 50%, many smokers resume smoking during the follow-up period. With some exceptions, most studies report cessation in about one-third of patients at one-year follow-up; those with the most severe infarctions are least likely to resume smoking (Baile et al., 1982). In addition, Scott and

Lamparski (1985) reported that only patients who believed that smoking contributed to their cardiac problems were likely to maintain abstinence. It should be noted that these data are based on self-report, and are likely to be overestimates of cessation. Ockene et al. (1992), for example, found a 17 to 20% misreporting of smoking cessation levels in control subjects in a smoking cessation intervention study.

A significant majority of people who experience an MI attribute its onset to some life stress. Anecdotal evidence also suggests that some people attempt to moderate these stresses subsequent to their MI. How many people who attempt to do so, and how successful they are, is not clear. However, data from the Recurrent Coronary Prevention Project suggests that about 10% of Type A men who have an infarction attempt and achieve significant behavioural change in the absence of any formal attempt to facilitate change (Friedman et al., 1986).

IMPACT OF MI ON PARTNERS
A frequently neglected issue in the clinical care of patients is the severity of distress experienced by the relatives of patients. These may be as great, or greater, than that experienced by the patients themselves, although the degree of distress signified by a patient may not be correlated with that of their spouse. Stern and Pascale (1979) found that the women at greatest risk of depression or anxiety were those married to men who denied their infarction. Many were overwhelmed by the infarct experience, the resulting family disequilibrium, and an unwillingness of their partner to discuss their health. Nevertheless, at least in some cases, this mismatch may have a positive effect on rehabilitation (Bar-On & Dreman, 1987).

Many wives inhibit aggressive and sexual feelings, and become overprotective of their husbands for at least one year post-MI. Whilst the impact of MI may exacerbate pre-existing marital problems, there are exceptions, and some relationships improve. Risk for re-infarction may be increased as a consequence of the extra burden on the cardiovascular system that results from stressful interpersonal episodes characteristic of marital discord (Brown & Smith, 1992).

A majority of partners experience an increase in household chores, although only a small percentage expressed dissatisfaction with this. They may also reduce their hours of working outside the house during the early rehabilitation phase, although, by one year, a small number of previously unemployed partners have started paid work to compensate for the loss of earnings consequent on their partner's redundancy. Older wives of blue collar workers are likely to experience a greater decrease in leisure activities and in life satisfaction.

REFERENCES

Abbott, J. & Berry, N. (1991). Return to work during the year following first myocardial infarction. *British Journal of Clinical Psychology*, **30**, 268–70.

Baile, W.F., Bigelow, G.E., Gottlieb, S.H., Stitzer, M.L. & Sactor, J.D. (1982). Rapid assumption of cigarette smoking following myocardial infarction: inverse relation to MI severity. *Addictive Behaviors*, **7**, 373–80.

Bar-On, D. & Dreman, S. (1987). When spouses disagree: a predictor of cardiac rehabilitation. *Family Systems Medicine*, **5**, 228–37.

Brown, P.C. & Smith, T.W. (1992). Social influence, marriage, and the heart: cardiovascular consequences of interpersonal control in husbands and wives. *Health Psychology*, **11**, 88–96.

Friedman, M., Thoresen, C.E., Gill, J.J.,

Ulmer, D., Powell, L.H., Price, V.A., Brown, B., Thompson, L., Rabin, D.D., Breall, W.S., Bourg, E., Levy, R. & Dixon, T. (1986). Alteration of type A behavior and its effect on cardiac recurrences in postmyocardial infarction patients: summary results of the Recurrent Coronary Prevention Project. *American Heart Journal*, **112**, 653–65.

Hackett, T.P., Cassem, N.H. & Wishnie,

H.A. (1968). The coronary-care unit. An appraisal of its psychological hazards. *New England Journal of Medicine*, 279, 1365–70.

Havik, O.E. & Maeland, J.G. (1986). Dimensions of verbal denial in myocardial infarction. *Scandinavian Journal of Psychology*, 27, 326–39.

Havik, O.E. & Maeland, J.G. (1988). Verbal denial and outcome in myocardial infarction patients. *Journal of Psychosomatic Research*, 32, 145–57.

Mayou, R., Foster, A. & Williamson, B. (1978). Psychosocial adjustment in patients one year after myocardial infarction. *Journal of Psychosomatic Research*, 22, 447–53.

Ockene, J., Kristeller, J.L., Goldberg, R., Ockene, I., Merriam, P., Barrett, S., Pekow, P., Hosmer, D. & Gianelly, R.

(1992). Smoking cessation and severity of disease: the Coronary Artery Smoking Intervention Study. *Health Psychology*, 11, 119–26.

Schwartz, J.L. (1987). *Review and evaluation of smoking cessation methods: the United States and Canada, 1978–1985.* 87–2940 Bethesda, Maryland: US Department of Health and Human Services.

Scott, R.R. & Lamparski, D. (1985). Variables related to long-term smoking status following cardiac events. *Addictive Behaviours*, 10, 257–64.

Smith, G.R. & O'Rourke, D.F. (1988). Return to work after a first myocardial infarction. *Journal of the American Medical Association*, 259, 1673–7.

Stern, M.J. & Pascale, L. (1979). Psychosocial

adaption postmyocardial infarction: the spouses' dilemma. *Journal of Psychosomatic Research*, 23, 83–7.

Stern, M.J., Pascale, L. & McLoone, J.B. (1976). Psychosocial adaption following an acute myocardial infarction. *Journal of Chronic Diseases*, 29, 523–6.

Trelawney-Ross, C. & Russell, O. (1987). Social and psychological responses to myocardial infarction: multiple determinants of outcome at six months. *Journal of Psychosomatic Research*, 31, 125–30.

Wiklund, I., Sanne, H., Vedin, A. & Wilhelmsson, C. (1984). Psychosocial outcome one year after a first myocardial infarction. *Journal of Psychosomatic Research*, 28, 309–21.

Coronary heart disease: treatment

DEREK W. JOHNSTON

School of Psychology,
University of St Andrews,
Scotland, UK

Psychological interventions in patients with clinically manifest coronary artery disease (CAD) or who have suffered a myocardial infarction (MI) have two broad aims, to minimize further deterioration in the patients cardiovascular health, or even to improve it, and to reduce the distress and interference with normal life associated with symptomatic heart disease. Coronary artery disease underlies many clinical conditions including angina pectoris, myocardial infarction, cardiac arrythmias, sudden death, and heart failure and is treated with complex medical and surgical procedures. However, most systematic treatment studies have been on patients with angina pectoris or MI. It is probable, but largely unproven, that some of the findings from these studies can be applied to patients with other manifestations of CAD or following procedures like angioplasty, coronary artery grafting or even heart transplantation.

ANGINA PECTORIS

Angina is usually experienced as a pain in the chest and/or left arm and is generally caused by stenosis in the coronary arteries restricting the blood supply to heart muscle so that it is ischaemic during periods of increased cardiac work, such as during exercise or emotion. Patients with angina are at increased risk of MI and stroke. Psychological interventions have been directed at either reducing coronary artery disease or anginal pain. Ornish (Ornish *et al.*, 1990) described a randomized control trial of a programme of stress management, exercise and a very low fat diet in patients with angina and unequivocally demonstrated CAD. A one-week intensive residential programme was followed by 12 months of regular, lengthy meet-

ings. At the end of that time, the experimental subjects experienced less severe angina and, most spectacularly, showed significant reversal of coronary artery stenosis. It is not clear which aspect of the programme led to these very impressive benefits. The Ornish programme is very demanding and it is doubtful if many patients would be able or willing to persist with such a regime. Bundy and colleagues (Bundy *et al.*, 1994) have reported a less daunting stress management programme with angina patients. An eight-week intervention led to an increase in exercise capacity, and a reduction in symptoms and medication usage. Lewin *et al.* (in press) in a larger study of a combined stress management and exercise programme found a reduction in angina, use of medication and an improvement in exercise tolerance. In addition, half of the patients who were awaiting coronary artery bypass grafting (CABG) were removed from the waiting list since, in the view of independent cardiologists, they no longer needed surgery. Most elective CABG for angina patients is done in the hope of reducing pain, and not, as is often thought, to lengthen life, hence it is reasonable to avoid surgery if the pain is no longer a major problem. Stress management, perhaps in combination with exercise has great appeal as a cost effective method of treating anginal pain.

Atypical chest pain

A related problem to angina occurs in patients with anginal-like symptoms but little CAD. As well as being distressing for the patient, atypical chest pain can be a management problem for physicians and can lead to unnecessary and repeated medical investi-

[421]

gations. Such pain has been successfully treated as a psychological problem and cognitive behavioural methods directed at symptom control and modification of inappropriate health beliefs has led to a reduction in chest pain, associated disability and distress (Klimes *et al.*, 1990).

MYOCARDIAL INFARCTION

Risk factor reduction

The same modifiable risk factors predict the recurrence of an MI as predict a first MI, although the relative importance of the factors may vary. Smoking, a sedentary life style, raised blood pressure and elevated cholesterol or some of the lipid fractions all increase the risk of recurrence. Smoking and exercise have been the primary concern of rehabilitation programme, although there is increasing interest in applying psychological principles to ensure that patients adhere to medical advice and take prescribed medication for blood pressure and lipid control (DeBusk *et al.*, 1994). Most smokers stop smoking after a MI, and those who do have a better prognosis. Recent randomized control trials of brief smoking cessation programmes have shown additional useful reductions in smoking (Taylor *et al.*, 1990). Exercise programmes have long been the mainstay of cardiac rehabilitation programmes. It is probable that such programmes improve cardiovascular fitness, at least in the short term, but it has proved difficult to demonstrate health benefits in individual studies. Meta-analyses of studies suggest that rehabilitation programmes that include exercise (but may also have other components) reduce the rate of recurrence of fatal MI by approximately 20% in the three years following the rehabilitation programme but have no effect on non-fatal MI (Oldridge *et al.*, 1988). This difference is unexplained.

Stress and stress-related behaviours are also considered probable risk factors for MI and recurrent MI. It has been argued that Type A behaviour, or some of its components such as hostility, predict recurrence of MI. In addition, depression and the closely related state of vital exhaustion predict recurrent MI and re-stenosis after angioplasty. A number of studies have shown that cognitive behavioural interventions can reduce Type A behaviour and hostility. In the most important of these studies, the recurrent coronary prevention programme (RCPP), almost 600 patients were randomly allocated to a group Type A change programme, while 300 received usual care plus group meetings directed at the problems associated with heart disease and its management (Friedman *et al.*, 1986). The Type A programme used a wide range of cognitive behavioural techniques to enable the patients to alter their environment, behaviour and thoughts. After a programme that ran for over four years, there were greater reductions in Type A behaviour and hostility in the Type A change group. More importantly, total cardiovascular mortality and morbidity were reduced by 50%, and this reduction was greatest in the patients showing the most Type A reduction. Recent Scandinavian studies have confirmed these findings.

Frasure-Smith and Prince (1989) adopted a simpler approach than the RCPP and assigned nurses to contact post-MI patients regularly for the year following their MI to determine in a standardized fashion if they were experiencing significant distress. If they detected distress, the nurses instigated what they considered the appropriate stress reduction procedure. In approximately half the instances, the nurses dealt with the problems themselves, in the remainder they referred the patient to other health professionals, such as cardiologists, psychologists and psychiatrists. A control group received normal care. Patients were followed up for seven years. While there are some problems with the randomization in this study, it appears to show that managing stress in this way reduced stress, and reduced sudden death in the short term and cardiac morbidity in the long term. It is probable that stress reduction procedures such as this could be introduced in many health care systems, possibly as part of a nurse organized care-management plan such as has been shown to be useful in the medical management of post-MI patients (DeBusk *et al.*, 1994).

Distress

A MI can cause substantial distress to both the patient and their family. While many patients make a good physical and psychological recovery from their MI and resume most of their previous activities, some remained impaired for a considerable time. Estimates of psychological distress following an MI are variable, possibly reflecting the different forms of care that are routinely available, but perhaps one third of patients (and their spouses) have significant anxiety and depression a year after the MI (see previous chapter). As well as being a problem in its own right stress and depression may increase the risk of reinfarction (see previous chapter).

After a long period of neglect, a major goal of many recent rehabilitation programmes is to reduce this distress and aid the patients return to a normal, perhaps healthier, lifestyle. Even the older exercise based rehabilitation programmes had, as their goal, distress reduction and improvement in quality of life. While experimental studies suggest that the relationship between exercise and mood is complex, a recent meta-analysis suggests that exercise based rehabilitation programmes reduce anxiety and depression by a small amount (Kugler, Seelbach & Kruskemper, 1994).

While exercise is still included in most rehabilitation programmes, research is now focusing on cognitive behavioural approaches to reducing the distress the patient, and possibly their spouse, experience. As we have already noted a nurse-based stress management procedure reduced distress 12 months after a MI (Frasure-Smith & Prince, 1989). Cognitive behavioural approaches have been shown to be more effective than exercise or educational approaches in reducing distress up to 12 months after a MI (Oldenburg, Allan & Fastier, 1989; Oldridge *et al.*, 1991). Such approaches can be very time consuming, however, e.g. Oldenburg describes a programme of 24 1.5 hour sessions, and this may be difficult to achieve in many centres. Lewin *et al.* (1992) have developed an apparently very cost effective approach. They compared an intervention based on a *Heart Manual* with routine care. The manual consisted of sections on exercise, relaxation (supplemented with tapes) and a stress management programme dealing with topics such as intrusive thoughts, anxiety and depression, and undue concern about health. There was also additional material for the patient's spouse. The manual was compared with a control condition based on general advice supplemented by literature on heart disease produced by various charitable bodies. Patients in both conditions had a similar amount of contact with a nurse, which, following a brief initial interview, largely entailed telephone contacts at 1, 3 and 6 weeks after discharge. In a sample of 176 patients this brief intervention reduced anxiety, depression and scores on measures of psychiatric caseness both when the six-week programme ended and 12 months later. The effects were particularly powerful in patients who had been significantly distressed when in hospital. Distressed control subjects were just as distressed 12 months after their MI as they had been at baseline, while treated subjects had returned to within normal limits. Patients receiving the *Heart Manual* were less likely to consult their GP in the subsequent year. This apparently very cost-effective form of intervention is now in widespread use in the UK

It is widely recognized that the family of patients who have suffered a MI experience considerable distress, but there have been very few systematic attempts to either study this or to alleviate it. Some studies (such as Lewin *et al.*) include the patient's spouse in the intervention but do not report if the spouse benefits. Thompson and Meddis (1990) describe a brief (three session) inpatient counselling programme for male MI patients and their wives. As well as confirming that the spouses are at least as distressed as the patients, they showed that both patient and spouse benefited from the programme and were less anxious even 6 months later than patients who had received normal care.

The use of psychological interventions after a myocardial infarction

Myocardial infarction is a very common condition and it is important that psychological interventions be applied effectively. The need to target interventions depends on the cost of the intervention. If an intervention is very expensive, for the health-care system or the patient, then it should be applied only to those likely to benefit. However, an inexpensive but effective intervention, with no or few side-effects, can be more liberally offered. There are great difficult-

ies in deciding who needs a psychological intervention after a MI. Some have argued that treatment should be offered to those who are distressed at discharge, and it has been shown that such patients benefit most, but distress is not necessarily maximal in hospital and the patient is often not the family member showing most distress. This suggests that cost-effective interventions could be offered routinely to all patients and their spouses following a MI. Results from Thompson and others suggest that such interventions can be given during the inpatient period but it is likely that interventions should continue when the patient returns home, when they and their families have to actually deal with the problems of returning to a normal work and social life. While many interventions claim to have a broad focus and attempt to deal with risk reduction, distress and return to normal activities, it is clear that different interventions have focused more on some aspects than others. This is unfortunate since all aspects of rehabilitation are important and broadly similar psychological principles apply to altering diet, stopping smoking, increasing exercise and reducing distress and worry. An integrated package that can be offered to all patients and their families both in hospital and after discharge has much to commend it.

CONCLUSION

Psychological interventions can reduce the symptoms, improve the exercise capacity and perhaps even lead to regression of the underlying pathology of patients with CAD to the extent that they may no longer need cardiovascular surgery. In patients following a MI a variety of interventions, some very cost effective, can reduce the distress associated with the MI, aid return to normal activities, reduce risk factors for CHD and there is encouraging evidence that psychological interventions can reduce the likelihood of a further MI.

REFERENCES

Bundy C., Carroll, D., Wallace, L. & Nagle, R. (1994). Psychological treatment of chronic stable angina pectoris. *Psychology and Health*, 10, 69–77.

DeBusk, R., Miller, N.H., Superko, R., Dennis, C.A., Thomas, R.J., Lew, H.T., Berger, W.E., Heller, R.S., Rompf, J., Gee, D., Kraemer, H.C., Bandura, A., Chandour, G., Clark, M., Shah, R.V., Fisher, L. & Taylor, C.B. (1994). A case-management system for coronary risk factor modification after acute myocardial infarction. *Annals of Internal Medicine*, 120, 721–9.

Frasure-Smith, N. & Prince, R. (1989). Long-term follow up of the Ischemic Heart Disease Life Stress Monitoring Program. *Psychosomatic Medicine*, 51, 485–513.

Friedman, M., Thoresen, C.D., Gill, J.J., Ulmer, D., Powell, L.H., Price, V.A., Brown, B., Thompson, L., Arbin, D.D., Breall, W.S., Bourg, E., Levy, R., & Dixon, T. (1986). Alteration of Type A behaviour and its effect on cardiac recurrences in post myocardial infarction patients: summary results of the recurrent coronary prevention project. *American Heart Journal*, 112, 653–65.

Klimes, I., Mayou, R.A., Pearce, M.J., Coles, L. & Fagg, J.R. (1990). Psychological treatment for atypical non-cardiac chest pain: a controlled evaluation. *Psychological Medicine*, 20, 605–11.

Kugler, J., Seelbach, H. & Kruskemper, G.M. (1994). Effects of rehabilitation exercise programmes on anxiety and depression in coronary patients: a meta-analysis. *British Journal of Clinical Psychology*, 33, 401–10.

Lewin, B., Robertson, I.H., Irving, J.B. & Campbell, M. (1992). Effects of self-help post-myocardial-infarction rehabilitation on the psychological adjustment and use of health services. *The Lancet*, 339, 1036–40.

Lewin, B., Cay, E., Todd, I., Soryal, I., Goodfield, N., Bloomfield, P., Elton, R., Watt, K., Metcalf, R., Cadogan, E., Spence, S., & MacDonald, L. (in press). The angina management programme: a rehabilitation treatment for chronic angina pectoris. *British Journal of Cardiology*

Oldenburg, B., Allan, R. & Fastier, G. (1989). The role of behavioral and educational interventions in the secondary prevention of heart disease. *Clinical Abnormal Psychology*, 27, 429–38.

Oldridge, N.B., Guyatt, G.H., Fischer, M.E. & Rimm, A.A. (1988). Cardiac rehabilitation after myocardial infarction: combined experience of randomized trials. *Journal of the American Medical Association*, 260, 945–50.

Oldridge, N., Guyatt, G., Jones, N., Crowe, J., Singer, J., Feeny, D., Mckelvie, R., Runions, J., Streiner, D. & Torrance, G. (1991). Effects on quality of life with comprehensive rehabilitation after acute myocardial infarction. *American Journal of Cardiology*, 67, 1084–9.

Ornish, D., Brown, S.E., Scherwitz, L.W., Billings, J.H., Armstrong, W.T., Ports, T.A., McLanahan, S.M., Kirkeeide, R.L., Brand, R.J. & Gould, K.L. (1990). Can lifestyle changes reverse coronary heart disease? *The Lancet*, 336, 129–33.

Taylor, C.B., Houston-Miller, N., Killen, J.D., & DeBusk, R.F. (1990). Smoking cessation after acute myocardial infarction: effects of a nurse management intervention. *Annals of Internal Medicine*, 113, 118–23.

Thompson, D.R. & Meddis, R. (1990). Wife's responses to counselling early after myocardial infarction. *Journal of Psychosomatic Research*, 34, 249–58.

Cystic fibrosis

CLAIRE A. GLASSCOE

Lewisham Park Child and Family Mental Health
Clinic, London, UK

NATURE OF THE DISEASE

Cystic Fibrosis (CF) is the most common fatal hereditary disease in the Caucasian population; 4–5% carry the recessive gene and 1 : 2000 live births are affected.

The disease is manifested by generalized dysfunction of the exocrine glands which produce excessively viscous mucus secretions. The pancreas and lungs are the main organs involved. Pancreatic insufficiency occurs in 85% of patients with malabsorption of fat and protein; and airways in the lungs become blocked leading to infections which are difficult to eradicate. The patient's fate is generally determined by the extent of the resulting pulmonary damage. Sterility occurs in 98% of males, whereas female fertility is near normal and puberty is generally delayed by 2 years in both sexes.

Treatment is mainly palliative, aimed at slowing or preventing some of the secondary effects of the disease, and includes:

(a) replacement of pancreatic enzymes and nutritional supplementation;
(b) antibiotics;
(c) chest physiotherapy, postural drainage and nebulization;
(d) lung transplantation in some cases.

The prognosis has improved largely because of the availability of specialist multidisciplinary CF centres, early diagnosis and treatment breakthroughs, while identification of the CF gene in 1989 brought real hope for an eventual cure. The median age of survival in the US was 28 years in 1990 and it is forecast that 50% of patients with CF will be adult by 1996. Cystic fibrosis is therefore no longer solely a childhood disease and efforts are currently focused on expanding adult services. (For a detailed account, see Geddes & Hodson (1994))

IMPACT ON PSYCHOSOCIAL FUNCTIONING

Patients

Some studies of the psychological effect of CF on patients have found no evidence of abnormality, while others have shown symptoms of anxiety, depression, and eating disorder. These differences have been attributed to variations in methodology. Thompson, Hodges & Hamlett, (1990) compared children aged 7–14 years, with psychiatrically referred and non-referred children. Those with CF showed no more psychological disturbance than non-referred children, although they reported equivalent levels of worry, anxiety and poor self-image to children referred to child psychiatry.

Pearson, Pumariega and Seilheimer (1991) examined differences in two age-groups, 8–15 years and 16–40 years and found both groups had elevated levels of disturbance. This was manifested by anorexic type eating disorder in younger patients (16.4%) and symptoms of anxiety (22.2%) and depression (42.4%) in the older age-group. These findings suggest a developmental progression with younger children possibly expressing distress through oppositional behaviour with food consumption as a control issue.

Parents

Variations in parental stressors and responses to CF have been found. In a study by Quittner *et al.* (1992), mothers indicated that fathers rarely assisted with medical routines. When specific stressors were examined in relation to parenting a child with CF, a strong association was found between role strain and depression for mothers but not for fathers, despite both reporting elevated levels of depression (64% of mothers, and 43% of fathers). Fathers acknowledged more difficulties in carrying out treatment routines and worried about the financial burden associated with CF.

In this same study, partners tended to rate their relationship between the norms for married and divorced couples, suggesting some degree of marital difficulty. There is, however, no evidence of a higher than average divorce rate amongst parents of children with CF.

Families

The interplay between the course of the disease, normal developmental processes and family life cycle events is often problematic. The dilemma for parents is to balance their child's growing need for independence and autonomy with the need for enforcing time-consuming and rigorous treatment regimes.

Families endeavour to contain the intrusion that CF makes on their lives with strategies such as routinizing tasks, compartmentalizing information, redefining normality, reassessing priorities and the future and avoiding reminders of the disease (Bluebond-Langner, 1991). In a two-year ethnographic study Bluebond-Langner observed these strategies being employed adaptively at salient points in the overall disease process, allowing families to live as normal a life as possible. However, these same strategies were also thought to create a climate where communication about the disease was at times precluded, leading to problems for patients, siblings and parents when they needed to talk.

EFFECT OF PSYCHOSOCIAL FUNCTIONING ON HEALTH STATUS

Early studies into the psychosocial aspects of families with a child with CF tended to emphasize dysfunction. Recent research has focused more on resilience, coping strategies and adaptation.

Patterson, McCubbin and Warwick (1990) used the family

adjustment and adaptation response (FAAR) model to examine the effects of family functioning on health changes. The variables of family stress, family resources and parental coping combined explained 22% of the variance in height and weight changes over a 15-month period. Although the relationship is undoubtedly reciprocal, this finding lends credence to the view that the whole family system needs to be considered with respect to the health of children with CF which has implications for intervention.

Factors known to promote positive adaptation in families are:

(i) fathers' early involvement with the care of the child with CF;
(ii) both parents involvement in activities that enhance self-esteem and provide social support
(iii) a trusting relationship with the child's paediatrician;
(iv) open communication within families and the attribution of meaning to the illness;
(v) maintainance of a hopeful outlook within an atmosphere of normality;
(vi) use of multiple strategies to meet family needs.

PROBLEMS OF ADHERENCE TO TREATMENT

Physiotherapy is crucial in preventing the onset of pulmonary disease, which is responsible for 90–95% of CF deaths, and yet it is the least complied with aspect of treatment; only 40% completely comply (Stark et al., 1987). Dietary management is also necessary to prevent pulmonary decline. The energy requirement needed to maintain optimum height and weight is 120–200% of the recommended dietary allowance (RDA) for healthy children, yet the average reported intake for children with CF is only 80% RDA (Stark et al., 1990).

Koocher, McGrath and Gudas (1990) argue that patients with CF do not all fail to follow medical advice for the same reasons. Three general categories are outlined: those who for a variety of reasons are misinformed about treatment requirements; those who for emotional or psychological reasons are resistant to treatment; and, those who have arrived at a rational decision to refuse treatment. The authors recommend each case be assessed in relation to these categories, and interventions tailored accordingly. In the first instance, a psychoeducational approach might be indicated, while, in the second, it would be more appropriate to offer individual, group or family therapy. In the final case, the patient's wishes should be respected and accommodated as far as possible.

INTERVENTIONS

In addition to the approaches already mentioned and those of anxiety management and genetic counselling, which are described elsewhere in this handbook, the following interventions have specific relevance to CF.

Behaviour therapy

Poor compliance with physiotherapy and dietary requirements has been shown to be amenable to individual behavioural contracting and a group behavioural approach (Stark et al., 1987, 1990).

Psychoeducation

Parents of children with CF are expected to perform complex and highly skilled medical tasks at home and monitor changes in their child's health. Such responsibility requires sound judgement and swift decision-making. A comprehensive health education programme for the self-management of CF, developed by Bartholomew et al. (1991), utilizes Social Learning Theory as a conceptual framework. It recognizes that acquisition of the complex skills required is not just a matter of information but also demands consideration of psychosocial adjustment factors. The approach thus emphasizes the development of coping strategies and effective communication skills within the context of CF self-management.

Interpersonal skills training

In order to manage the inevitable strain that a CF diagnosis places on their relationship, parents need to communicate well and work co-operatively together. Dysfunctional patterns established during the initial stages are sometimes difficult to change later, especially if the suggestion of referral to a child mental health service is perceived as a criticism and met with a defensive response. Schroder, Casadaban and Davis (1988), show how an educational format can enhance the skills couples require in a non-threatening way.

Family therapy

The impact of a CF diagnosis creates reverberations throughout the lifespan of the family, which touch each individual and their relationships. Transitions during adolescence take on additional meaning in the context of CF and can be particularly difficult for families to negotiate. A biopsychosocial systems perspective facilitating communication between family members can assist in these negotiations.

BURNOUT

CF is not only distressing to families, it also takes its toll on professionals involved with their care leaving them vulnerable to 'burnout'. Staff support groups and stress management can be employed to counteract such negative effects and strengthen staff morale.

CF is a chronic life-threatening disease with wide-reaching implications for patients and families. Most studies conclude, however, that adequate family functioning is more important for children's adjustment than illness severity. A fully integrated response therefore needs to consider interactions between physical and psychosocial factors and view the disease and its management within a family context.

REFERENCES

Bartholomew, L.K., Parcel, G.S., Seilheimer, D.K., Czyzewski, D., Spinelli, S.H. & Congdon, B. (1991). Development of a health education program to promote the self-management of cystic fibrosis. *Health Education Quarterly*, 18, 429–43.

Bluebond-Langner, M. (1991). Living with cystic fibrosis: a family affair. In J.D. Morgan (Ed) *Young people and death*, pp. 46–62, Philadelphia: Charles Press.

Geddes, D. & Hodson, M. (Eds.). (1994). *Cystic fibrosis*. London: Chapman & Hall.

Koocher, G.P., McGrath, M.L. & Gudas, L.J. (1990). Typologies of nonadherence in cystic fibrosis. *Developmental and Behavioural Pediatrics*, 11, 353–8.

Cystic fibrosis

Patterson, J.M., McCubbin, H.I. & Warwick, W.J. (1990). The Impact of family functioning on health changes in children with cystic fibrosis. *Social Science and Medicine*, **31**, 159–64.

Pearson, D.A., Pumariega, A.J. & Seilheimer, D.K. (1991). The development of psychiatric symptomatology in patients with cystic fibrosis. *Journal of the American Academy of Child and Adolescent Psychiatry*, **30**, 290–7.

Quittner, A.L., DiGirolamo, A.M., Michel, M. & Eigen, H. (1992). Parental response to cystic fibrosis: a contextual analysis of the diagnosis phase. *Journal of Pediatric Psychology*, **17**, 683–704.

Schroder, K.H., Casadaban, A.B. & Davis, B. (1988). Interpersonal skills training for parents of children with cystic fibrosis. *Family Systems Medicine*, **6**, 51–68.

Stark, L.J., Miller, S.T., Plienes, A.J. & Drabman, R.S. (1987). Behavioral contracting to increase chest physiotherapy: a study of a young cystic fibrosis patient. *Behavior Modification*, **11**, 75–86.

Stark, L.J., Bowen, A.M., Tyc, V.L., Evans, S. & Passero, M.A. (1990). A behavioral approach to increasing calorie consumption in children with cystic fibrosis. *Journal of Pediatric Psychology*, **15**, 309–26.

Thompson, R.J., Hodges, K. & Hamlett, K.W. (1990). A Matched Comparison of adjustment in children with cystic fibrosis and psychiatrically referred and nonreferred children. *Journal of Pediatric Psychology*, **15**, 745–59.

Deafness and hearing loss

LAURENCE McKENNA

Department of Clinical Psychology, Guy's Hospital, London, UK

Hearing loss which is acquired after the development of language needs to be distinguished from prelingual hearing loss. The two are quite different in their psychological and social manifestations. This chapter will focus on hearing loss which occurs after the development of language. Acquired hearing loss occurs in between 8 and 15% of the general population (Davies, 1989); it is age related and approximately one-third of people in their 60s have a hearing impairment.

Much of the work in the field has been concerned with attempts to link hearing loss with mental health problems. This literature is reviewed by Thomas (1984) and Jakes (1987). Early reports were limited to clinical observations of psychological disorder among hearing impaired people. Attempts have also been made to record the psychological impact of simulated hearing loss. While deteriorations in well-being were noted, such studies are restricted by the difficulty in achieving meaningful levels of hearing loss and by their temporary and artificial nature. A number of workers have used standardized inventories in the assessment of hearing impaired people. Elevated levels of psychopathology and maladjustment are reported among populations of hearing impaired people. Thomas and Gilhome Herbst (1980) noted that psychological disturbance among hearing impaired people was associated with poorer social life and poorer general well-being. Gilhome Herbst and Humphrey (1980) reported a high prevalence of depression among a group of elderly hearing impaired subjects. Their findings pointed to a link between hearing loss and isolation while Thomas and Gilhome Herbst (1980) suggest that, in younger groups, hearing loss is more clearly associated with loneliness. They suggested that elderly people who were either active or disengaged from society were more depressed. The majority middle group were less handicapped and less depressed.

There is a popular idea that hearing loss is particularly associated with suspiciousness or paranoid states. Thomas (1984) is critical of this idea. He reported no differences between hearing impaired patients and normal hearing controls on a scale of suspiciousness. Jakes (1987) reviewing the literature concludes that, if a person has a psychiatric breakdown, hearing loss tends to produce persecutory delusions.

Thomas (1984) criticized many studies for poor methology or other difficulties. None the less, the body of evidence does suggest a link between hearing loss and psychological disturbance. There would appear, however, to be a higher risk of psychological disturbance associated with other related audiological disorders such as tinnitus and vertigo (McKenna, Hallam & Hinchcliff (1991), Berrios and colleagues (1988)).

An alternative perspective is provided by the study of people who have had some restoration of hearing. Gildston and Gildston (1972) carried out pre- and postoperative assessments using the Guildford–Zimmerman Temperament Survey on patients undergoing surgery intended to alleviate hearing loss. They noted that patients improved postoperatively on a number of measures of psychopathology. Knutson and colleagues (1991) and McKenna and Denman (1993) reported improvements in psychological well-being among patients who had received cochlear implants.

Thomas (1984) questions whether hearing loss *per se* leads to psychological changes; he concludes that there is no evidence that hearing loss should lead to a deterioration in psychological well-being. A lack of a clear relationship between the extent of hearing loss and the extent of psychological disturbance has been a frequent observation (Thomas & Gilhome Herbst (1980); Gilhome Herbst and Humphrey (1980), Berrios and colleagues (1988)). Thomas and Gilhome Herbst (1980), however, identified psychological disturbance in a greater number of a subsample of subjects with more severe hearing loss (> 70 dB) and poor speech discrimination.

The WHO (1980) classification of impairment, disability and handicap is helpful in understanding this lack of a clear relationship between the extent of hearing loss and the level of psychological disturbance. Impairment refers to the loss of basic function measurable in the clinic or the laboratory, disability is the loss of everyday auditory ability, and handicap is the disadvantage that results. Handicap will depend upon the demands that are placed upon the individual and the extent to which the person is prevented from fulfilling particular roles. These definitions invite a behavioural perspective in the assessment and treatment of hearing problems. Little systematic work has been carried out in this context. The potential for a behavioural approach has been argued by McKenna (1987). Andersson and colleagues (1994) briefly review the literature and describe the use of functional analysis and behavioural counselling as an approach to hearing tactics training, the strategies used by a person to overcome the everyday problems associated with the hearing loss. In this controlled study, beneficial treatment effects were found.

Psychological factors are clearly involved in the illness behaviour of hearing impaired people and may disrupt the communication strategies, e.g. lip reading, used by hearing impaired people. A link between personality and vulnerability to noise induced hearing loss has been postulated. This is discussed by Jakes (1987). While links between Type A personality and noise-induced peripheral vasoconstriction, and between temporary threshold shift and vasoconstriction have been demonstrated, no clear link has been established between personality type and hearing loss. It seems unlikely that there is a psychological cause for most hearing loss.

Eriksson-Mangold (1991) discusses the likely processes involved in psychological changes related to acquired hearing loss. It may be that hearing loss has an effect through an individual's need to develop cognitive maps in order to pursue goal-orientated behaviour. The changes imposed by hearing loss may lead to inadequate or inaccurate cognitive models. The cognitive approach that points to loss of control as the central factor in producing psychological change offers an alternative perspective. Ramsdell (1962) suggested that hearing loss served three different functions. These are: symbolic, primarily concerned with communication; warning; and the perception of background noise. His contention was that the perception of background noise keeps a person in touch with the world, and that the loss of this function is the most important factor in producing depression in deafened people. Ramsdell (1962) proposed that sensory deprivation was the central factor in producing psychological disturbance. Although Ramsdell's ideas are widely quoted, they have not been systematically tested. Some early studies of simulated hearing loss lend support for his ideas. The improvements in well-being reported in cochlear implant users add to the debate. McKenna and Denman (1993) reported large improvements in people using single channel implants which offer only modest gains in acoustical ability; the most widely reported gains being in the perception of background noise. Knutson and colleagues (1993) reported significant psychological changes in implant users that were unrelated to changes in acoustical ability. In both studies, however, a number of subjects reported no psychological benefits as a result of using cochlear implants. The notion of a threshold effect is therefore questioned.

REFERENCES

Andersson, G., Melin, L., Scott, B. & Lindberg, P. (1994) Behavioural counselling for subjects with acquired hearing loss. A new approach to hearing tactivs. *Scandinavian Audiology*, 23, 49–56.

Berrios, G. Ryley, J. Garvey, T. & Moffat, D. (1988). Psychiatric morbidity in subjects with inner ear disease. *Clinical Otolaryngology*, 13, 259–66.

Dangerink, J., Dengerink, H. & Chermak, G. (1982) Personality and vascular responses as predictors of temporary threshold shifts after noise exposure. *Ear and Hearing*, 34, 196–201.

Davis, A. (1989). The prevalence of hearing impairment and reported hearing disability among adults in Great Britain. *International Journal of Epidemiology*, 18, 911–17.

Eriksson-Mangold, M. (1991). Adaptation to acquired hearing loss. Thesis. Department of Psychology, University of Goteborg, Sweden.

Gildston, H. & Gildston, P. (1972). Personality changes associated with surgically corrected hypoacusis. *Audiology*, 11, 354–67.

Gilhome Herbst, K. & Humphrey, C. (1980). Hearing impairment and mental state in the elderly living at home. *Journal of the Royal College of General Practitioners*, 31, 155–60.

Jakes, S. (1987). Psychological aspects of disorders of hearing and balance. In Stephens S.D.G. (Ed.) *Scott Brown's otolaryngology, vol 2, Adult audiology*. London: Butterworths.

Knutson, J. Schartz, H., Gantz, B., Tyler, R., Hinrichs, J. & Woodworth, G. (1991). Psychological change following 18 months of cochlear implant use. *Annals of Otology, Rhinology and Laryngology*, 100, 877–82.

McKenna, L. (1987). Goal planning in audiological rehabilitation. *British Journal of Audiology*, 21, 5–11.

McKenna, L. & Denman, C. (1993). Repertory grid technique in the assessment of cochlear implant patients. *Journal of Audiological Medicine* 2, 75–84.

McKenna, L., Hallam, R. & Hinchcliff, R. (1991). The prevalence of psychological disturbance in neuro–otology outpatients. *Clinical Otolaryngology*, 16, 452–6.

Ramsdell, D.A. (1962). The psychology of the hard of hearing and the deafened adult. In H. Davis & S.R. Silverman (Ed.). *Hearing and deafness*, pp.499–510. New York: Holt, Rinehart & Winston.

Thomas, A. (1984). *Acquired hearing loss. Psychological and psychosocial implications*. London: Academic Press.

Thomas, A. & Gilhome Herbst, K. (1980). Social and psychological effects of acquired deafness for adults of employment age. *British Journal of Audiology*, 14, 76–85.

WHO (1980). *International classification of impairments, disabilities and handicaps*. Geneva: World Health Organization.

Dementias

TONY WARD

School of Psychology, University of Luton, UK

WHAT IS DEMENTIA?

Dementia is usually defined as a global impairment of intellectual functioning, for example, in the *Diagnostic and statistical manual version three revised (DSM-3R)*. More specifically, *DSM-3R* suggests that there should be impairment of memory plus impairment in at least one other area of cognitive functioning, e.g. aphasia (see sections on memory and intelligence). Such impairment should be severe enough to interfere with work or social functioning, and be present in the absence of delirium. There should be evidence that the origin of the condition is organic in nature, or at least there should be no non-organic mental disorders apparent. Hence the term dementia does not relate to any particular aetiology but rather to a number of conditions which can lead to global intellectual impairment.

WHY IS DEMENTIA IMPORTANT?

The condition is important because of its high prevalence. Estimates vary between 1 and 9% of severe cases in the elderly. The differences are probably due to different diagnostic criteria used and different search methodologies used to find cases. There is also the problem that early cases may be hard to identify. Nevertheless, even the lowest estimate represents a sizeable problem. Figures now widely quoted for the prevalence of dementia of all severities are 10% of people over the age of 65, rising to 20% of people over 80. These figures are derived from large scale studies carried out around Newcastle (see Hart & Semple, 1990, for further discussion). Further importance is often attached to these figures because of the changing demographic make up of the western industrialized countries. Thus the proportion of the population over retirement age is set to increase as people live longer and the health of the elderly improves.

CONDITIONS LEADING TO DEMENTIA

Many conditions can give rise to dementia. Primary degenerative diseases such as Alzheimer's disease are probably the causes most readily associated with dementia by many people. In fact, Alzheimer's disease accounts for the majority of cases in the elderly, with a figure of 50% often quoted. Other, rarer conditions exist such as Pick's and Huntington's diseases. These conditions are characterized by neuronal loss, with characteristic pathology in the brain tissue.

Another large category is the vascular diseases, with multi-infarct dementia (MID) often quoted as accounting for 25% of cases.

Some dementias are thought to result from infectious agents. One widely known example is Creutzfeldt Jakob's disease, which has gained recent publicity through its similarity with bovine spongioform encephalopathy. Also, there has been recent concern that young persons infected with HIV could present with dementia following neural involvement of the virus.

Toxic substance exposure may lead to dementia, for example, in long-term chronic alcohol abuse. Also, head injury itself may lead directly to the condition or predispose to the condition at some later time.

The picture is further complicated by the fact that some functional illnesses may lead to dementia. Thus people with severe depression may appear to have global intellectual impairment. Such 'functional' dementias have been described by some as 'pseudodementia' because of the non-organic nature. Use of such terminology has been questioned, recently, for example, by Hart and Semple (1990). They suggest that such depression-induced dementias are anything but 'pseudo' and prefer the phrase 'the dementia syndrome of depression.' What is beyond dispute is that the possibility of someone having depression appearing to have dementia constitutes a potential problem which clinicians should be aware of. An attitude of therapeutic nihilism may attend a diagnosis of dementia, whereas depression is eminently treatable. Recognizing this problem, a number of researchers have attempted to find reliable ways of differentiating the dementia syndrome of depression from other causes. This issue falls within the scope of diagnosis in general, i.e. is a condition of dementia present, and if so what may be the cause? This will be discussed further in the next section.

In summary, the most common cause of dementia in the elderly is Alzheimer's disease, closely followed by Multi-infarct dementia. These two conditions are thought to account for approximately 75% of cases. Despite their different aetiologies, the conditions can be almost impossible to tell apart clinically, as will be discussed in the next section. This situation is not helped by the common co-occurrence of the two conditions.

DIAGNOSIS

Since dementia is defined by deficits in intellectual functioning, much effort has been expanded in attempts to devise instruments capable of documenting such deficits. Even a cursory glance through the literature will reveal that a substantial volume of the papers published by psychologists in this area involve evaluation of psychometric tests as diagnostic tools. Memory is often seen as a primary area of concern, with many such tests aimed at this aspect of functioning. A test which is quick to administer and simple to understand, which is capable of accurately highlighting intellectual decline, is yet to be found. The continuing publication of such papers suggests that the search for the holy grail of psychometric tests continues.

Amongst the many tests which have been put forward as able to contribute to the initial assessment of patients with possible dementia, a few have emerged with staying power. The Kendrick test battery (Kendrick, 1972) is one of the most widely known and has been in existence for over 20 years. The test consists of two simple tasks, one a memory task the other a simple digit copying task. The argument is that patients in the early stages of dementia will be impaired on these tasks compared with their age-matched peers. The battery is also said to be able to discriminate patients with organic dementia from those with the dementia syndrome of depression. The latter will have a different pattern of performance on the two tasks, with digit copying being relatively more affected.

The Clifton Assessment procedures for the elderly offer a simple and rapid evaluation of a number of areas. There is a short cognitive assessment. This involves a number of questions aimed at evaluating orientation, together with some simple motor tasks. In addition, there is a questionnaire completed by carers, to assess the extent and nature of behavioural disturbance. (Pattie & Gilleard, 1979). This test has proved very popular, and has been widely used, either as a complete test or using the individual components.

Part of the reason why these two tests have been very successful is their simplicity and speed of administration, together with their apparent face validity. Hence clinical psychologists and other professions working in this area have been able to gain quick insight into a patient's condition. This is also true of the mini-mental state examination (MMSE, Folstein, Folstein & McHugh, 1975). The MMSE consists of a short structured interview designed to assess orientation and some simple aspects of memory and attention. The test takes no more than a few minutes, and has become a universal standard for clinicians and researchers wishing to rapidly screen for dementia. A similar format has been followed in more recently developed assessments, often directly based on the MMSE. Such assessments can be rapidly completed by clinicians, serving as a useful screening instrument. A clear cut-off score (of 22 out of a possible 30 for the MMSE) enables a degree of objectivity to be introduced into the initial decision-making as to whether a particular patient is likely to be suffering from a dementia-producing condition.

Where patients are suspected of having a dementia-producing condition, then this is likely to lead to further investigations. There is agreement in the literature that one of the surest ways of enabling an accurate decision to be made regarding someone's status is to have them assessed and to have the assessment repeated after, say, six months. Ideally, the assessment should be done in some depth, to give maximum possibility of detecting change over the six-month period. Some clinical psychologists specialize in the area of neuropsychology, and are able to provide in-depth assessment of a range of intellectual functions (see section on neuropsychological assessment). Where there is decline over the six months, then the possibility arises that the person may be suffering from a progressive dementia producing condition such as Alzheimer's disease. This approach may also be one way of trying to resolve the difficult issue of whether a patient is suffering from 'pseudodementia'. This is more likely to be the case if there is no decline evident, and particularly the case if there has been improvement consequent on commencement of a course of antidepressant treatment.

An in-depth approach to assessment is also likely to be adopted in research studies. In research it may be important to try and gain an indication of underlying aetiology in order to select a homogeneous sample. Criteria for Alzheimer's disease have been widely adopted based upon the recommendations of the National Institute for Neurological, Communicative Disorders and Stroke, and the Alzheimer's Disease and Related Disorders Association (NINCDS-ADRDA, McKhann et al., 1984). These require neuropsychological evidence of impairment in two areas of intellectual functioning. Other criteria have been proposed for distinguishing Alzheimer's disease from multi-infarct dementia (Hachinski, 1975).

Besides the large amounts of literature published on assessment of dementia-producing conditions (e.g. for a review, see Morris & Kopelman, 1992), there has been an increasing amount of empirical work on the neuropsychological effects of these conditions. For a more specialized and in-depth account of the neuropsychological aspects of such conditions, see Hart and Semple (1990) or Knight (1992).

TREATMENTS

At the time of writing, the prognosis for patients with the main categories of progressive dementias is bleak. Psychopharmacological approaches explored in the past decade have centred on cognitive enhancers such as physostigmine, or choline enhancement, e.g. through oral lecithin (see section on psychopharmacology). None of these procedures has proved capable of producing clinically significant reversal or halt of decline. Future approaches are likely to involve neural transplants, possibly using cultured material to avoid the current ethical issues surrounding use of fetal brain matter. Such approaches are likely to involve retraining of patients and rehabilitation specialists (see neuropsychological rehabilitation).

There have been some psychological approaches to interventions with patients. Reality orientation attempts to keep patients orientated to their environment, through rehearsal and reinforcement of material on a daily basis (see section on reality orientation). Such approaches have had some success in maintaining orientation, but only for a limited period of time, and constant input is required. Clinical psychologists have tended to turn their attention towards caregivers, offering support and counselling (see section on counselling). Such strategies are likely to be of increasing importance with the emphasis now placed on maintaining people in their homes as long as possible. A full discussion of psychological approaches to patients with dementia producing conditions and their caregivers can be found in Woods and Britten (1985).

Inevitably, many patients will require long-stay residential care, and there has recently been some focus on the issues surrounding that care, i.e. quality of provision and type of provision. The trend towards community care has led to the development of small residential units situated within the community in some regions. This represents a move away from the provision of traditional long-stay wards within psychiatric hospitals. Also, long-stay populations are becoming the focus of more research studies. For example, Ward et al. (1993) suggest how long-stay patients can be assessed, even when they have experienced considerable deterioration. Such assessments may provide useful information for research, placement of patients, or management of resources within units. Also, long-stay patients are of interest to occupational therapists, whose interventions may improve the quality of patients' lives through stimulation. Such assessments may provide these groups of workers with the means for evaluating their impact.

CONCLUSIONS

Impairments of intellectual functioning, referred to as dementia, may result from a variety of diverse conditions. Such conditions are of increasing concern, given demographic changes resulting from a higher proportion of people living into advanced old age. The psychological contribution to our understanding of these conditions

arises largely from developments in assessment, though there is also a large body of empirical work which looks at the nature of the underlying impairments in cognitive terms. There have been some attempts to design psychological interventions with patients, though caregivers are now more frequently the target of interventions, which are designed to offer support. Treatment prospects are currently poor, with many patients requiring long-term support. Psychologists have also been involved in the evaluation of long-stay services and interventions with long-stay patients.

REFERENCES

Folstein, M.F., Folstein, S.E. & McHugh, P.R. (1975). Mini-Mental State: a practical method for grading the cognitive state for the clinician. *Journal of Psychiatric Research*, **12**, 189–98.

Hachinski, V.C., Iliff, L.D., Zilhka, E., Duboulay, G.H., McAllister, V.L., Marshall, J., Russell, R.W.R. & Symon, L. (1975). Cerebral blood flow in dementia. *Archives of Neurology*, **32**, 632–7.

Hart, S. & Semple, J.M. (1990). *Neuropsychology and the dementias*. Hove and New Jersey: Lawrence Erlbaum Associates.

Kendrick, D.C. (1972). The Kendrick battery of tests: theoretical assumptions and

clinical uses. *British Journal of Social and Clinical Psychology*, **11**, 373–86.

Knight, R.G. (1992). *The neuropsychology of degenerative brain diseases*. Hove and New Jersey: Lawrence Erlbaum Associates.

McKhann, G., Drachman, D., Folstein, M., Katzman, R., Price, D. & Stadlan, E.M. (1984). Clinical diagnosis of Alzheimer's disease: report of the NINCDS-ADRDA work group under the auspices of Department of Health and Human Services task force on Alzheimer's disease. *Neurology*, **34**, 939–44.

Morris, R.G. & Kopelman, M.D. (1992). The neuropsychological assessment of dementia. In J.R. Crawford, D.M. Parker & W.W.

McKinlay (Eds.). *A handbook of neuropsychological assessment*, Hove and New Jersey: Lawrence Erlbaum Associates.

Pattie, A.M. & Gilleard, C.J. (1979). *Manual of the Clifton assessment procedures for the elderly*. Sevenoaks, Kent: Hodder and Stoughton.

Ward, T., Dawe, B., Procter, A., Murphy, E. & Weinman, J. (1993). Assessment in advanced dementia – The Guy's advanced dementia schedule. *Age and Ageing*, **22**, 183–9.

Woods, R.T. & Britten, P.G. (1985). Clinical psychology with the elderly. London: Croom Helm.

Dental care and hygiene

GERRY HUMPHRIS

Department of Clinical Psychology, The University of Liverpool, UK

DENTAL DISEASES AND PREVENTION

Dental health is virtually unique within the sphere of health in that there is a set of behaviourally mediated procedures based upon individual action which can successfully prevent the onset of the two major diseases: dental caries and periodontal disease. Dental caries is a localized progressive decay of the tooth, marked by the demineralization of the tooth surface by organic acids. These acids develop owing to the fermentation of carbohydrates in the diet by plaque bacteria. A cavity is produced by the continued destruction of the tooth mineral and protein, resulting eventually in the tooth pulp and the surrounding tissues becoming infected. Periodontal disease is an inflammatory condition of the connective tissues which support the tooth and gums (gingivae). It is the result of toxins produced from bacterial plaque which initiate an inflammatory reaction. The tissue breakdown which ensues from this inflammatory response results, if left unchecked, in the bone supporting the tooth atrophying which leads to high tooth mobility and eventual tooth loss. Although the two diseases are not ordinarily life threatening, they do influence the public's quality of life and the economic efficiency of nations

through the loss of millions of working hours each year, costs associated with treating the diseases and debilitating pain from the diseases themselves (Miller, Elwood & Swallow, 1975).

The two dental diseases are ubiquitous. Reports from the USA and the UK show dental caries to be among the most common health problem affecting over 95% of the population. Dental caries is especially prevalent in the younger generation, whereas periodontal disease is found frequently in the middle years. However, the signs of irreversible features of periodontal disease are found in young people. Evidence for a trend in a reduction in caries is mounting, although the reasons for this are being hotly debated. Factors likely to be responsible include: water fluoridation, fluoridated toothpastes, changes in consumption of sugar-containing foods and drinks, improved oral hygiene and early treatment of cavities (Locker, 1989).

There has been a long association between behavioural scientists and dentists, due to a large degree in the proven preventability of caries and periodontal disease. The major emphasis of a great deal of this work has been to evaluate a variety of methods of changing individual preventative health behaviours. These behaviours can be divided into two main groups. First, those that help to improve oral hygiene and include toothbrushing, flossing, and resorting to a sugar-reduced diet, and, secondly, those that seek out professional advice such as attendance to oral-screening programmes and visits to the dentist for check-ups. Two sections are presented below which summarize some of the major psychological findings associated with each of the two groups of preventative health behaviours. A short section will follow noting some of the changes in dental health and how psychologists are responding.

PSYCHOLOGICAL APPROACHES TO ORAL HYGIENE

The early work by Janis and Feshbach reported in 1953 on using fear appeals adopted dental health as a model for understanding the influence of different persuasive messages on oral hygiene behaviour. Over the years, this work has been extended, with dental health being one of the first health areas to apply the Health Belief Model. Such studies have added to our understanding so that attempts to increase knowledge and change key oral health beliefs are difficult to attain and the effects may be transitory. The encouragement of new preventative health behaviours such as the use of fluoride mouthrinses, however, has demonstrated the limited positive effect of informative campaigns with young people (Kegeles & Lund, 1982). The success of these approaches may be limited as many of these behaviours are not novel. Typically, these behaviours have a strong habitual element to them, therefore previous behaviour may help to explain current behaviour (Humphris & Weinman, 1990). More recently using self-efficacy and the Theory of Reasoned Action constructs and a longitudinal design, Tedesco et al. (1993) have successfully predicted flossing and toothbrushing behaviour. Interventions which have introduced modelling and reinforcement procedures rather than concentrating solely on attitude change paradigms (for a review, see Blount, Santilli & Stokes, 1989) have shown substantial impact. These behavioural approaches have clearly demonstrated the benefit of analysing the consequences of the behaviour to the individual. However, the problems of maintenance and generalization outside the limits of the programme intervention still have to be overcome, as well as resource implications.

PSYCHOLOGICAL APPROACHES IN DENTAL CARE

There are many examples of applying psychology in the dental office or surgery, and they can be separated into understanding what is the psychological make-up of people who enter the care system, and the psychological factors responsible for individuals accepting and adhering to advice. These issues are pertinent also for continued care over extensive periods. These areas will be briefly discussed under the next three subsections.

Entrance into the care system

A large number of studies, many based upon national and regional cross-sectional surveys have investigated the variables believed to be responsible for the public's utilization of dental services. Three factors, other than the system variables associated with geographical location, supply of dental personnel, etc. include cost, perception of need for treatment, and dental anxiety or fear. A large literature now

exists on understanding the aetiology, maintenance and treatment of dental anxiety (Lindsay & Jackson, 1993). The great advantage of studying this psychological construct in the dental context is that it is common and most people are not embarrassed to discuss their worries unless their fears are very severe. Attempts to reduce dental anxiety by the use of explanatory and advisory leaflets, modelling films and introductory preparatory sessions have shown proven benefits in increased attendance especially for moderately dentally anxious people (Gatchel, 1986).

Acceptance of treatment

Avoidance of certain dental procedures such as the local anaesthetic injection and the use of the high-speed turbine drill is a common psychological phenomena which causes considerable distress to the patient and concern for the dentist. A strong finding observed with adults, children, experienced and inexperienced patients is that they expect to feel much higher levels of pain intensity than their reported levels of pain subsequent to receiving treatment (Lindsay & Jackson, 1993). This effect may explain why dental anxiety is maintained and difficult to reduce. Other explanations to account for the stability of dental anxiety and the failure of positive experiences at the dentist to habituate patient anxiety have included: cognitive models such as reconstruction of memories of traumatic experiences which involved high levels of pain, the easy imaginability of many stimuli within the dental surgery; behavioural explanations include the recognition that dental appointments are of short duration and widely spaced temporally therefore reducing the effectiveness of any habituation process. The clinician may help their patients by: attending carefully to their patients' concerns through listening, providing patients the opportunity to control aspects of the timing of their treatment (e.g. stop signals) and giving advice on pain management. Other procedures found to be effective include relaxation and distraction (Kent & Blinkhorn, 1991).

Maintenance of care

To encourage continued care over longer periods, the psychological issues discussed above for oral hygiene practices are important. The outcomes for dental visitors from utilizing screening and treatment services have been found to be important determinants for repeated appointments. Patient satisfaction scales have shown the importance of dental personnel attending not only to the technical quality of their service but also to the personal aspects of dealing with individuals, each with unique concerns and wishes. Clinicians may improve the strong associations that patients make to a particular practice by attending closely to appropriate communication skills designed to set the patient at ease, to make the dental environment predictable, and introduce a relaxed, friendly and warm personal style. Occupational stress amongst dental personnel should be recognized and procedures introduced to reduce pressures at work in order that maintenance of a high-quality and receptive service is ensured.

THE FUTURE

The trend of caries reduction, some improvements in periodontal health and increased personal longevity bring the possibility of major changes in the dental health of western industrialized populations, so that the problems experienced in the future may focus on the attrition of tooth enamel and its repair. Individuals' responses to a chronic reduction in the effectiveness and aesthetics of worn teeth will become an important area for the future. A related topic is the increasing technology of prosthetics and provision of implants to replace teeth lost through infection, traumatic accident or malignancy. The employment of psychological models of disability and distress have contributed to the careful evaluation of some of these procedures (e.g. Kent & Johns, 1993). Oral–facial cancer appears to be increasing in some subgroups of the population (e.g. people aged over 40 years in the UK), and interest is growing in attempting to prevent this particularly aggressive cancer. The field of food selection and its importance in modifying preferences to a non-cariogenic diet, the beliefs of individuals about fluoride additives in water supplies, and the public's views towards water quality, are areas to which psychologists are making increasing contributions.

REFERENCES

Blount, R.L., Santilli, L & Stokes, T.F. (1989). Promoting oral hygiene in pediatric dentistry: a critical review. *Clinical Psychology Review* 9, 737–746.

Gatchel, R.J. (1986) Impact of a videotaped dental fear-reduction program on people who avoid dental treatment. *Journal of the American Dental Association* 112, 218–1.

Humphris, G.M. & Weinman, J. (1990). Development of dental health beliefs and their relation to dental health behaviour. In LR Schmidt, P. Schwenkmezger, J. Weinman & S. Maes (Eds.). *Theoretical and applied aspects of health psychology*, pp. 227–240. London: Harwood Academic Publs.

Janis, T.L. & Feshback, S. (1953). Effects of fear-arousing communication. *Journal of Abnormal and Social Psychology*, 48, 78–92.

Kegeles, S.S & Lund, A.K. (1982). Adolescents' health beliefs and acceptance of a novel preventive dental activity. *Health Education Quarterly*, 9, 96–111.

Kent, G. & Blinkhorn, A.S. (1991). *The psychology of dental care*, pp. 77–96. London: Wright.

Kent, G. & Johns, R. (1993). Psychological effects of permanently implanted false teeth: a 2 year follow-up and comparison with dentate patients. *Psychology and Health*, 8, 213–22.

Lindsay, S.J.E. & Jackson, C. (1993). Fear of routine dental treatment in adults: its nature and management. *Psychology and Health*, 8, 135–54.

Locker, D. (1989). *An introduction to behavioural science and dentistry*. London: Tavistock/Routledge.

Miller, J. Elwood, P.C. & Swallow, J.N. (1975). Dental pain. *British Dental Journal.* 139, 327–8.

Tedesco, L.A., Keffer, M.A., Davis, E.L. & Christersson, L.A. (1993). Self-efficacy and reasoned action: predicting oral health status and behaviour at one, three and six month intervals. *Psychology and Health*, 8, 105–22.

Diabetes mellitus

CLARE BRADLEY

*Department of Psychology, Royal Holloway,
University of London, UK*[1]

INTRODUCTION

Diabetes mellitus is a chronic metabolic disorder, characterized by hyperglycaemia and glycosuria. It results from insufficient insulin production from the β cells of the pancreas or insulin resistance. Diabetes mellitus is diagnosed in approximately 2–3% of the UK population. Community studies suggest that a similar percentage have undiagnosed diabetes (Yudkin *et al.*, 1993). Prevalence rates vary markedly around the world (King & Rewers, 1993) with diabetes absent or rare in some indigenous communities in developing countries, while prevalences of 14–20% have been reported among some Arab, migrant Asian Indian, Chinese, and Hispanic American populations. The highest prevalences (41% and 50%) have been reported for Nauruans and Pima/Papago Indians. The great majority of people who have diabetes have some endogenous insulin production and are said to have non-insulin-dependent diabetes mellitus (NIDDM) or Type 2 diabetes. Insulin-dependent diabetes (IDDM), also known as Type 1 diabetes, is less common than NIDDM. Insulin injection or infusion is a vital component of treatment of IDDM along with dietary control and self-monitoring of blood glucose levels. Some individuals with NIDDM also require insulin in order to achieve good control of their diabetes. More often, however, NIDDM is treated with tablets (to stimulate endogenous insulin production or promote insulin efficiency) and/or dietary management, together with monitoring of diabetes control, with blood or urine glucose self-monitoring. Glyosylated haemoglobin (GHb or the related measures of HbA_1 or $HbA_{1}c$) provides a measure of average blood glucose over 6 to 8 weeks, while fructosamine gives an indication of average blood glucose over shorter time periods. While useful aids to diabetes management, GHb and other such measures do not provide any indication of serious episodes of hypoglycaemia, which can be damaging to psychological well-being as well as life threatening. Furthermore, GHb level does not provide any indication of the individual's quality of life which may be seriously and perhaps unnecessarily impaired, particularly by rigid treatment regimens and dietary recommendations. Complications of IDDM include the short-term complication of diabetic ketoacidosis

[1] Parts of this paper were first published in a review: Bradley, C. (1994). The contributions of psychology to diabetes management. *British Journal of Clinical Psychology*, 33, 11–21.

as well as that of hypoglycaemia. Hypoglycaemia can also be a problem with NIDDM. Longer-term complications of IDDM and NIDDM include retinopathy, nephropathy, neuropathy and the associated problems of blindness, kidney failure, foot ulcers, gangrene, and erectile impotence. Important goals of diabetes management include prevention or early detection of complications as well as avoidance of high or low blood glucose levels and associated symptoms.

Psychology is particularly important in diabetes management because the knowledge, beliefs and behaviour, both of people with diabetes and of the health-care professionals involved in diabetes management, affect diabetes control, and patients and professionals vary considerably in their beliefs, knowledge and behaviour. Evidence to suggest that chronically raised blood glucose levels are associated with increased risk of microvascular complications has been confirmed by the results of the Diabetes Control and Complications Trial (DCCT) in the United States. The DCCT had been running since 1985 comparing tight control of blood glucose levels with average control and looking at the effects on retinopathy in particular and other complications in general (Diabetes Control and Complications Trial Research Group, 1993). The DCCT group terminated the study early because the results were clear: tight control was significantly associated with reduced retinopathy and other complications. However, tight control was also associated with increased frequency of serious episodes of hypoglycaemia. Now that metabolic control has been shown to be an important determinant of long-term complications, there is increased pressure on all involved in diabetes care to improve metabolic outcomes. In order to avoid the danger that metabolic targets will be attained at the expense of psychological well-being, there is even more reason to emphasize the importance of psychological outcomes. Recent initiatives to develop methods of auditing diabetes care have recognized the importance of auditing psychological as well as metabolic and other traditional medical outcomes (e.g. Wilson *et al.*, 1993).

The measurement of psychological outcomes and processes is the first contribution of psychology to diabetes management to be addressed in more detail below. Other contributions of psychology selected here include psychological interventions to optimize blood glucose monitoring, and the use of stress management techniques to prevent the disruptive effects of stress on diabetes control. Brief mention is made of two of the many other important contributions of psychology to diabetes management; weight management and psychosexual counselling. This selection is chosen to illustrate the sometimes dramatic and often measurable ways in which patients' psychological state affects their diabetes control and vice versa, as well as the importance of the interactions between people with diabetes, their families, health-care professionals, and the treatment technology in affecting diabetes control and, hence, the risk of later complications. There are many other important contributions of psychology to diabetes and the interested reader is referred to Shillitoe (1988) and Bradley, Home and Christie (1991).

MEASUREMENT OF PSYCHOLOGICAL OUTCOMES AND PROCESSES

When the only outcomes measured are metabolic outcomes, new treatments may only be valued if they result in improved metabolic control. There is a danger that either metabolic goals are pursued at the psychological expense of miserable patients or that the patients decide to abandon the attempt for metabolic perfection in the face of unacceptable psychological costs. In some instances, particularly with older, usually tablet or diet treated, patients, doctors abandon metabolic goals on the patients' behalf. The patients may be very satisfied with their treatment and with their doctor and think that their diabetes is well controlled, yet they have high levels of GHb indicating poor diabetes control about which they have no knowledge. Typically, such patients have no feedback information from blood glucose monitoring and often the doctor has chosen not to measure GHb levels. It is hard to tell a satisfied patient that all is not well when a doctor has given inappropriate reassurances by saying 'It's just a touch of diabetes' or 'It's only mild diabetes and nothing to worry about'. Greater weight control may be needed or a change from tablets to insulin may be indicated. Blood glucose monitoring is certainly likely to be required. Patients are only likely to feel that the effort of improving their diabetes control is worthwhile if they are told about the complications of diabetes and the likely association between blood glucose control and complications. Diabetes control is just one, and not the most important one, of several important outcomes. We need to aim for the best achievable profile of outcomes where one outcome would be blood glucose control as close to non-diabetic levels as can be achieved without hypoglycaemic reactions, another outcome would be avoidance of new long-term complications. Psychological outcomes in the profile would include patients' satisfaction with the treatment regimen and their sense of positive well-being.

These psychological outcomes can be measured, but most existing generic measures are inappropriate for people with diabetes. Measures of psychological outcomes have been specifically designed and developed for diabetic populations and include measures of well-being, treatment satisfaction, quality of life, and fear of hypoglycaemia (Bradley, 1994*a*). For the most part, currently available diabetes-specific measures have been designed for research purposes rather than for routine audit of diabetes care. However, work is under way to provide short, easily scored instruments for audit purposes and the first of these, a measure of satisfaction with the diabetes care service provided (the DCSQ) and a measure of depressed well-being are now in use (Wilson *et al.*, 1993).

If satisfaction, well-being and blood glucose control are all at acceptable levels, and there are no signs of complications, then management of diabetes could be regarded as ideal. If problems are apparent in one or more outcomes, then information is needed about psychological processes, such as knowledge levels and self-care skills, in order to decide what action might be appropriate to improve outcomes. If patients with poor diabetes control are well informed about diabetes and its management, then their diabetes control would probably not be improved by giving them more information. Some patients with advanced complications might quite rationally choose to give diabetes control a low priority. If this is the patient's informed choice, that is one thing, but if poor control results from the doctor deciding what is 'best', investigation of the patient's view may reveal opportunities to improve diabetes control that have not been explored. Some patients with more recent onset of diabetes are well informed about diabetes but their blood glucose control is poor. In such cases self-management skills need investigating and enquiries made into their beliefs and priorities in life. A regimen that is more closely tailored to the individual's lifestyle may be an acceptable way of tightening up control without impairing psychological well-being or satisfaction with treatment.

Measurement of psychological processes can be highly illuminating when it comes to understanding the reasons for problems with diabetes control, reasons for patients' preferences for different technologies and for different treatment regimens. Scales to measure health beliefs and perceived control of diabetes have proved useful in understanding patients' preferences for injection treatments or continuous subcutaneous insulin infusion (CSII) pumps, useful for understanding why some patients developed diabetic ketoacidosis during pump use and useful in predicting which patients would benefit from relaxation training (see Chapters 12 and 13 in Bradley 1994a which review findings using the Diabetes-Specific Health Belief Scales and the Perceived Control of Diabetes Scales). Such measures of individual differences indicate how individual patients can be helped to choose forms of treatment that are most likely to suit them and can direct the attention of health-care professionals to the need to deal with patients' inappropriate beliefs and expectations of treatments.

Health-care professionals who acquire a good understanding of the psychological models underlying measures such as the Perceived Control of Diabetes Scales (attribution theory and social learning theory) and the Diabetes-Specific Health Belief Scales (the health belief model), will find that the ideas and concepts underpinning these scales can usefully guide their consultations with patients in routine clinical practice without requiring patients to complete questionnaires. Measures of psychological outcomes such as the Well-being Questionnaire and the Diabetes Treatment Satisfaction Questionnaire (Bradley, 1994a) are more concise and less time consuming and are recommended as more reliable and valid indicators of psychological outcomes than those gleaned informally during a routine consultation in a diabetes clinic.

Summary of expected gains from measurement of psychological outcomes and processes
- Identification and optimization of psychological benefits.
- Identification and treatment of psychological problems.
- Improved satisfaction with treatment and, hence, blood glucose control which, in turn, will reduce the risk of long-term complications.
- Less frequent clinic attendances required.

OPTIMIZING BLOOD GLUCOSE MONITORING
Most insulin-treated patients now monitor their blood glucose levels and the cost of this technology is considerable. If blood glucose control is to be maximized, all patients with diabetes, including those treated with tablets or diet alone, need to have accurate, immediate feedback about blood glucose levels. Long-term gains would be expected in terms of reduced microvascular complications but immediate financial costs would be increased substantially. However, there are a number of ways in which the cost-effectiveness of blood glucose monitoring could be improved.

Doctors often recommend times in the day when blood glucose testing should be carried out; for example, early morning fasting plus one other pre-prandial measure 6 days per week and a full profile of seven measures on one day a week. However, it is only useful

to do this if the patient can respond constructively to the results. Awaiting the comments of a doctor on a book full of results six months later is of limited value. Technologies have been developed to help process such data using computers which can be loaded with data from the memory store of a blood glucose meter and produce graphs and other summaries of the data, but this technology is only as useful as the data themselves. The problem with this kind of strategy of collecting blood glucose data is that many of the blood tests taken will indicate acceptable levels of blood glucose and require no action whereas episodes of hypo- or hyperglycaemia that occur at times other than those set times when testing has been recommended are likely to be missed. It would be far more cost effective of time, energy and health service resources to teach patients to recognize blood glucose levels outside normal levels and, once they can do this reliably, have them test when they think the blood glucose is too high or too low.

The possibility of patients being able accurately to assess their blood glucose levels has been a developing field of investigation since the early 1980s and clinical interventions are now being employed. Research findings from studies of people with IDDM, reviewed by Gillespie (in Bradley et al., 1991), can be summarized as follows:

- some people are remarkably accurate in recognizing blood glucose levels.
- some think they can tell but are not very accurate before training.
- physical symptoms and moods associated with high and low blood glucose levels are idiosyncratic but reliable.
- most, if not all, can learn to recognize their blood glucose levels.

Cox, Gonder-Frederick and their colleagues at the University of Virginia have developed a blood glucose awareness training programme and manual. Blood glucose monitoring is used, together with associated ratings of physical symptoms, mood and environmental cues, to identify those symptoms and cues predictive of high blood glucose and those predictive of low blood glucose for each individual patient. An error grid has been developed to identify those discrimination judgements that matter clinically. Efforts are then concentrated on reducing the errors that would be clinically important, e.g. the error of not detecting extremes of blood glucose.

Impressive results with blood glucose awareness training have been demonstrated. Subjects with IDDM have been shown in several studies to improve not only their estimation accuracy but also their diabetes control as indicated by GHb compared with untrained control groups. Awareness of hypoglycaemia was improved and patients trained in blood glucose awareness had significantly fewer car accidents than untrained control patients (e.g. Cox et al., 1994).

Blood glucose awareness training is likely to prove useful in helping some patients who lose their awareness of impending hypoglycaemic reaction. This can be a devastating loss leading to dangerous episodes of hypoglycaemic coma. Although such patients may have lost the symptoms that they had been accustomed to associating with low blood glucose levels, it is possible that their awareness of other cues can be developed to regain their ability to anticipate hypoglycaemia.

Summary of expected gains from blood glucose awareness training

- Improved blood glucose control resulting in reduced risk of long-term complications.
- Reduced expenditure on blood glucose reagent strips.
- Fewer hospitalizations for diabetic ketoacidosis and hypoglycaemic coma.
- Fewer accidents resulting from hypoglycaemia.

STRESS MANAGEMENT

The role of stress in the onset and course of diabetes is reviewed elsewhere (Bradley, 1988; Surwit & Schneider, 1983). There are good theoretical reasons to expect stress management to be of value in diabetes management and many diabetes centres in the USA already include some form of stress management training as part of a routine education package for people with diabetes. However, research to evaluate the effects of stress management on diabetes control has produced inconsistent findings. Although many studies have demonstrated benefits, others have shown no effects while, on occasion, hypoglycaemic episodes have followed use of relaxation techniques by individuals with previously well-controlled diabetes. Evidence from studies of responses to acute stress of people with diabetes indicates that individual differences in blood glucose response to stress are substantial and have not been adequately considered in most of the studies evaluating stress management interventions (Bradley, 1988). Individuals need to discover their own particular blood glucose responses to different stressful circumstances by using blood glucose monitoring. Relaxation techniques are unlikely to do harm except when blood glucose is already tightly controlled and the insulin dosage is not reduced to balance effects of relaxation on insulin requirements (which may well be reduced) and/or when used at a time when blood glucose is already low (>4 mmol/l). Bradley (1994b) provides more detailed recommendations. The available evidence suggests that relaxation techniques will be beneficial for some individuals with diabetes, notably for those who feel that stress disrupts their control. Benefits will be most apparent in patients with poor diabetes control who are currently experiencing considerable stress.

Summary of expected gains from stress management training

- Improved psychological well-being.
- Improved blood glucose control and hence reduced risk of long-term complications.
- Reduced insulin requirements.
- Less frequent clinic attendances.

PSYCHOLOGICAL TREATMENTS OF SEXUAL DYSFUNCTION

Men with diabetes complaining of impotence are often offered surgical or drug interventions with considerable risks of complications and unwanted consequences rather than psychosexual counselling. However, men with diabetes are at least as likely as men who have not got diabetes to have impotence of psychogenic origins. Unfortunately, the possibility of an organic component coupled with the financial interests of manufacturers of mechanical penile implants has led to a disproportionate interest in surgical solutions. Meisler *et*

al. (1989) reviewed the evidence concerning the aetiology of erectile dysfunction and offered guidelines for adopting a multidisciplinary approach to assessment. The potential contribution of psychologists in dealing with this problem has yet to be realized though the benefits are likely to include improved sexual functioning and psychological well-being, together with fewer surgical interventions and associated complications.

WEIGHT MANAGEMENT PROGRAMMES

Wing and her colleagues in Pittsburgh have conducted an impressive series of studies evaluating various weight management programmes for people with NIDDM where excessive weight is a common problem making diabetes control hard to achieve (e.g. Wing, 1993). Using programmes that include combinations of nutrition education, behaviour modification techniques, very-low-calorie diets, and exercise, the programmes evaluated so far have resulted in some dramatic weight losses, at least among some of the patients, even without individual tailoring of weight reduction strategies to suit patients' preferences. The main problem has been with maintaining the loss. It seems that it may not be enough to help people to lose weight, they also need continuing support and encouragement to maintain their lower weight. This is the challenge now being addressed.

There is good evidence that weight management programmes improve blood glucose control and will therefore reduce the risk of microvascular complications. Following reduction of excess weight, cardiovascular morbidity and mortality would be expected to be reduced and psychological well-being improved. (See also next chapter.)

OTHER CONTRIBUTIONS OF PSYCHOLOGY TO DIABETES MANAGEMENT

There are many other ways in which psychologists can make important contributions to diabetes management when they are well informed about diabetes and its management and familiar with the applications of psychology to this field. Psychologists can play a major role in individual management of patients with eating disorders including the disorder peculiar to insulin users, bingeing and omitting insulin injections in order to lose weight. Psychologists may also be able to help in improving the service by designing and evaluating education programmes, with a view to influencing beliefs and behaviour as well as increasing knowledge about diabetes.

Psychologists can be of most value when they have opportunities to share their skills, particularly their communication skills, with other health-care professionals. One approach which could be used more generally to the widespread advantage of patients is the tailoring of treatment regimens to patients' individual needs and preferences to enable each patient to follow a regimen that can be fitted in with other demands and priorities in his or her life. The importance of taking account of patients' preferences for different management regimens, including insulin delivery systems, monitoring, and educational interventions, is increasingly being recognized in the context of research as well as clinical practice. The limitations of conventional randomized controlled trials and the advantages of partially randomized patient-centred designs when evaluating treatments about which patients have preferences, have been reviewed elsewhere (Bradley, 1993).

The World Health Organization and International Diabetes Federation in 1989, launched the St Vincent Declaration Action Programme for Diabetes. The Action Programme is supported by a set of guidelines which, in the second edition, include guidelines for encouraging psychological well-being in people with diabetes and their families (Bradley and Gamsu, 1994). The well-being guidelines include practical suggestions for health-care professionals seeking to improve communication, to protect patients' self-esteem, to respond to individuals' differing needs, to help patients learn about their own individual responses, to help to motivate patients' self care, to monitor psychological well-being, and to introduce organizational changes to optimize psychosocial aspects of diabetes care. The guidelines include suggestions for further reading on these topics as well as questionnaires for measuring well-being and satisfaction with treatment which are being used in a multicentre European project, DiabCare. The DiabCare project is auditing outcomes of diabetes care in association with the St Vincent Declaration Action Programme. Implementation of the guidelines to encourage psychological well-being is expected not only to enhance well-being and reduce the occurrence of psychological problems but also to reduce metabolic problems and complications of diabetes which can be reduced, perhaps avoided, by good communication and appropriate treatment regimens tailored to suit the individual patient.

REFERENCES

Bradley, C. (1988). Stress and diabetes. In S. Fisher and J. Reason (Eds). *Handbook of life stress, cognition and health.* Chichester: John Wiley.

Bradley, C. (1993). Designing medical and educational intervention studies: a review of some alternatives to conventional randomized controlled trials. *Diabetes Care.* **16**, 509–18.

Bradley, C. (1994*a*). (ed.). *Handbook of psychology and diabetes: a guide to psychological measurement in diabetes research and practice.* Chur, Switzerland: Harwood Academic Publishers.

Bradley, C. (1994*b*). Contributions of psychology to diabetes management. *British Journal of Clinical Psychology,* **33**, 11–21.

Bradley, C & Gamsu, D.S. for members of the working group (1994). Guidelines for encouraging psychological well-being: report of a working group of the World Health Organisation Regional Office for Europe and International Diabetes Federation European Region St Vincent Declaration Action Programme for Diabetes. *Diabetic Medicine,* **11**, 510–16.

Bradley, C., Home, P. & Christie, M. (Eds.). (1991). *The technology of diabetes care: converging medical and psychosocial perspectives.* Chur, Switzerland: Harwood Academic Publishers.

Cox, D.J., Gonder-Frederick, L.A., Julian, D.M. & Clarke, W.L. (1994). Long-term follow-up evaluation of blood glucose awareness training. *Diabetes Care,* **17**, 1–5.

Diabetes Control and Complications Trial Research Group (1993). The effect of intensive treatment of diabetes on the development and progression of long-term complications in insulin dependent diabetes mellitus. *New England Journal of Medicine,* **329**, 977–86.

King, J. & Rewers, M. (1993). Global estimates for prevalence of diabetes mellitus and impaired glucose tolerance in adults. *Diabetes Care,* **16**, 157–77.

Meisler, A.W., Carey, M.P., Lantinga, L.J. & Krauss, D.J. (1989) Erectile dysfunction in diabetes mellitus: a biopsychosocial approach to etiology and assessment. *Annals of Behavioural Medicine,* **11**, 18–27.

Shillitoe, R.W. (1988). *Psychology and diabetes: psychosocial factors in management and control,* London: Chapman & Hall.

Surwit, R.S. & Schneider, M.S. (1983). Role of stress in the etiology and treatment of diabetes mellitus. *Psychosomatic Medicine,* **55**, 380–93.

Wilson, A.E. & Home, P.D. for members of the working group of the Research Unit of the Royal College of Physicians and the British Diabetic Association (1993). A data set to allow exchange of information for monitoring continuing diabetes care. *Diabetic Medicine,* **10**, 378–90.

Wing, R.R. (1993). Behavioural treatment of obesity: its application to Type II diabetes. *Diabetes Care,* **16**, 193–9.

Yudkin, J.S., Forrest, R.D., Jackson, C.A., Burnett, S.D. & Gould, M.M. (1993). The prevalence of diabetes and impaired glucose tolerance in a British population. *Diabetes Care,* **16**, 1530.

Dieting

JANE WARDLE

Health Behaviour Unit, Department of Epidemiology and Public Health, University College, London, UK

Although 'a diet' can refer to any modified food regimen (e.g. a vegetarian diet or a low-fat diet), 'dieting' usually refers specifically to modifying food intake in order to lose weight. Dieting does not denote any particular restrictive behaviours, but describes a disposition to practice some form of food restriction. The expressions 'dietary restraint' and 'restrained eating' also describe behaviours directed towards weight control, but indicate the tendency to practise weight control, rather than current actions.

THE EPIDEMIOLOGY OF DIETING

Dieting originated as 'banting', named after Dr William Banting, who, in 1864, proposed that a prescribed food plan could be used to combat 'corpulence'. Dieting continued to be predominantly a matter of medical advice to individuals with a diagnosis of obesity, until the second half of the twentieth century. Since then, however, it has become an everyday practice, associated not only with medicine, but also with a vast commercial empire providing advice on how to lose weight. The diet business in the USA is estimated to be worth over $50 billion.

National surveys in the USA suggest a dieting prevalence of around 20%, with more than 60% of adults having dieted at some point (Jeffery, Adlis & Forster, 1991). Data from the UK and Europe suggest a lower frequency; 8% of adults were currently dieting in the UK Dietary and Nutritional Survey of Adults (Gregory et al., 1990), and results from other UK surveys suggest that around 36% have tried to lose weight at some time. At all ages, dieting is almost twice as common in women as men, although there is little sex difference in overweight or obesity. Dieting is also more common among higher social status groups, while the prevalence of obesity shows the opposite distribution. Cross-sectional studies suggest that adolescence is a time of peak dieting prevalence, which causes particular concern because of the risks to growth and development. Surveys of schoolchildren indicate that 63% of American schoolgirls (Rosen & Gross, 1987) and 37% of English schoolgirls (Wardle & Marsland, 1990) are trying to lose weight at any time. It is not yet clear whether this is a cohort effect, and the current high levels of adolescent dieting will persist into adulthood, or the frequency of dieting will reduce with advancing age. Dieting has also been reported in children, among whom there now appears to be identification with the ideals of slenderness favoured by adult women (Hill, Oliver & Rogers, 1992).

DIETING AND EATING DISORDERS

The increasing popularity and commercialization of dieting has both been attributed to, and has contributed to, the growing pressure for slimness. The majority of women and a substantial minority of men want to lose weight. Ideal body shapes are increasingly discrepant from the shape of the average adult woman, promoting widespread dissatisfaction with body shape. At the same time, slimness is promoted in the popular press as a realizable goal, and prevailing cultural beliefs tend to favour attributions of personal control over weight (Brownell, 1991). Dieting is widely believed to play a significant role in the aetiology of eating disorders and the developmental course of individuals with eating disorders supports this idea, since dieting almost always precedes the appearance of the full syndrome. There is evidence that eating disorders are more common among women in occupations with an emphasis on appearance (e.g. dance), and in societies which emphasize slimness as a beauty ideal. Historical data also suggest that increases in popular dieting have paralleled increases in eating disorders. Although consistent with the idea of a sociocultural aetiology, these observations do not rule out the possibility that social factors are merely permissive of the expression of eating disorders. The fact that most young women do not develop eating disorders, despite both worrying about their weight and dieting, indicates that other factors must play an important aetiological role. However, concern about the adverse effects of dieting has led to the development of health-education programmes about the dangers and disadvantages of slimming, which are intended to reduce the prevalence of adolescent eating disorders. (See 'Anorexia Nervosa and Bulimia'.)

FOOD INTAKE AMONG DIETERS

Despite dieting being such a widespread practice, there have been comparatively few investigations of what normal dieters actually eat.

The multidimensional nature of dieting means that there are many possible ways of achieving an energy deficit, and hence it is not easy to evaluate. A number of studies using dietary diaries or 24–hour food recalls have suggested that dieters have a lower energy intake, with lower fat and sugar intakes, and a greater use of reduced fat and artificially sweetened products, than non-dieters. A low meal frequency is also common, with breakfast often being omitted. Interpretation of these results is complicated by doubts about the validity of dietary information, especially from individuals who are weight conscious, but they have been supported by evidence from studies of energy expenditure, which indicate that dieters have lower-than-average energy expenditures, and therefore by implication, lower-than-average energy needs (Tuschl et al., 1990). What is not yet clear is whether a low energy expenditure is a pre-existing characteristic of dieters or is caused by dieting, since there is evidence that effective dietary restriction reduces metabolic rate, resulting in lower energy expenditure.

DIETING AND LOSS OF CONTROL OVER EATING

Dieting has been consistently implicated in loss of control over eating, which is sometimes called disinhibition. Cross-sectional studies have found associations between scores on restrained and emotional eating scales, with restrained eaters having higher levels of emotional eating. Laboratory studies have confirmed the psychometric results, showing that restrained eaters eat more than unrestrained eaters both when they are depressed and when exposed to highly appetizing food (Polivy & Herman, 1987). That disinhibition is actually caused by dieting, is suggested by an experimental study in which women who were put on a diet experimentally, ate more under stress than women in the control treatment (Wardle & Beales 1988).

Numerous explanations have been put forward for the relationship between restraint and disinhibition, including increased hunger drive, impairments of regulation of energy intake, increased susceptibility to palatability, failure of satiety mechanisms, and the abstinence violation effect, but no definitive evidence has yet been adduced for any one process. However, the links between dieting and overeating, whatever their mechanism, point to the risk that dieting could result in a greater susceptibility to overeating, and therefore could possibly cause more weight gain in the long term than unrestricted eating. In a prospective study of weight change over a two-year period, dieting at baseline was found to be a significant predictor of weight gain (French et al., 1994).

OBESITY, DIETING AND WEIGHT CONTROL

Dieting as part of a formal weight-control programme can involve any of a range of regimens from preplanned meal schedules or calorie limits, to the use of a single food product to supply all energy and nutrient needs (e.g. the very low calorie diet). Most therapeutic dietary regimens are associated with short-term weight loss, but problems with compliance and maintenance usually compromise their effectiveness in the long term. In any cohort of overweight adults who begin a dietary regimen, only the minority will follow the plan fully for any length of time, and even among those who comply fully, longer-term follow-up usually reveals a pattern of steady regain of weight (Garner & Wooley, 1991). Despite considerable effort being directed towards developing easier regimens, booster treatment programmes, longer treatment times and relapse prevention procedures, no dieting programme has yet shown itself to be more than very modestly effective. One consequence of this is that the ethics of promoting dieting treatments in the absence of good evidence for efficacy, has been questioned (Lustig, 1991).

In effect, many dieters practise what is known as 'yo-yo' dieting – dieting successfully for a while, then stopping the diet, gaining weight, and eventually starting to diet again. There is some evidence that weight cycling, which is the inevitable consequence of yo-yo dieting, could be more hazardous to health than a high, but stable, weight. An association between weight variability and mortality has been observed in a number of studies (e.g. Lissner et al., 1991), as the reason for weight loss is not recorded in these studies, the effect may be due to confounding by underlying illness. If weight loss is the consequence of episodes of illness rather than dieting, then the associated morbidity and mortality risk is most likely to be attributable to the underlying illness. Without further empirical research, these results must be interpreted cautiously, but they emphasize the necessity for thorough investigation of dieting as a treatment for obesity.

REFERENCES

Brownell, K.D. (1991). Personal responsibility and control over our bodies: when expectation exceeds reality. *Health Psychology*, **10**, 303–10.

French, S.A., Jeffery, R.W., Forster, J.L., McGovern, P.G., Kelder, S.H. & Baxter, J.E. (1994). Predictors of weight change over two years among a population of working adults: the Healthy Worker Project. *International Journal of Obesity*, **18**, 145–54.

Garner, D.M. & Wooley, S.C. (1991). Confronting the failure of behavioral and dietary treatments for obesity. *Clinical Psychology Review*, **11**, 729–80.

Gregory, J., Foster, K., Tyler, H. & Wiseman, M. (1990). *The dietary and nutritional survey of adults.* London, HMSO.

Hill, A.J., Oliver, S. & Rogers, P.J. (1992). Eating in the adult world: the rise of dieting in childhood and adolescence. *British Journal Clinical Psychology*, **31**, 95–105.

Jeffery, R.W., Adlis, S.A. & Forster, J.L. (1991). Prevalence of dieting among working men and women: the Healthy Worker Project. *Health Psychology*, **10**, 274–81.

Lissner, L., Odell, P.M., D'Agostino, R.B., Stokes, J., III., Kreger, B.E., Belanger, A.J. & Brownell, K.D. (1991). Variability of body weight and health outcomes in the Framingham population. *The New England Journal of Medicine*, **324**, 1839–44.

Lustig, A. (1991). Weight loss programmes: failing to meet ethical standards. *Journal of the American Dietetic Association*, **91**, 1252–4.

Polivy, J. & Herman, P.C. (1987). Diagnosis and treatment of normal eating. *Journal of Consulting and Clinical Psychology*, **55**, 635–44.

Rosen, J.C. & Gross, J. (1987). Prevalence of weight reducing and weight gaining in adolescent girls and boys. *Health Psychology*, **6**, 131–47.

Tuschl, R.J., Platte, P., Laessle, R.G., Stichler, W. & Pirke, K.M. (1990). Energy expenditure and everyday eating behavior in healthy young women. *American Journal of Clinical Nutrition*, **52**, 81–6.

Wardle, J. & Beales, S. (1988). Control and loss of control over eating: an experimental investigation. *Journal of Abnormal Psychology*, **97**, 35–40

Wardle, J. & Beinart, H. (1981). Binge eating: a theoretical review. *British Journal of Clinical Psychology*, **20**, 97–109.

Wardle, J. & Marsland, L. (1990). Adolescent concerns about weight and eating: a social-developmental perspective. *Journal of Psychosomatic Research*, **34**, 377–91.

Digestive tract cancer

RUTH ALLEN

Department of Psychiatry, University College London Medical School, UK

Cancers of the digestive tract incorporate tumours of the oesophagus, stomach, small and large bowel. Eating and regular bowel habits are associated with psychological well-being in many cultures. A loss of appetite, inability to eat or to control functions can be both distressing and embarrassing. Colorectal cancer is particularly stigmatizing if an ostomy is formed during surgery with the inherent anxieties about odours, leakage, accidents and uncontrolability. There are further difficulties for individuals who place particular emphasis on physical appearance and meticulous hygiene.

CANCERS OF THE OESOPHAGUS AND STOMACH

The initial symptoms of these cancers are similar to those of indigestion, hence the diagnosis is often late and shocking. Patients usually complain of vague discomfort and difficulty in keeping food down. Treatment is generally surgery and/or radiotherapy with rapid immediate postsurgical recovery. The return to a normal routine can take some time as patients adjust to revised eating habits and attempt to gain weight. There are the usual diagnostic and recurrence anxieties common to all cancers, as well as problems with nutrition and weight loss. Psychological well-being for patients who have had the removal of part of the oesophagus and part of the stomach followed by reconstruction does improve with patients reporting less distress post surgery (Van Knippenberg et al., 1992).

CANCERS OF THE SMALL AND LARGE BOWEL

Colorectal cancer is the second largest cause of death due to cancer in the USA (Toribara & Sleisenger, 1995). In addition to genetic predisposition there are the identified behavioural risk factors of diet (high sugar and fat, not enough fibre) and smoking. There is ongoing debate as to whether personality type is a risk factor, but no conclusive research has been published (Kune et al., 1991). Elements proposed to be mediating factors are denial, avoidance of conflict, repressed anger and other negative emotions, as well as a commitment to social norms resulting in the external appearance of a nice person.

Some patients who develop colorectal cancer will have a history of chronic ulcerative colitis, and others may have had experience of colon cancer due to familial polyposis. Individuals from families with familial adenomatous polyposis may require counselling prior to genetic screening. Anxieties expressed by these individuals are fear about future health, guilt about transmitting the disease to one's children and concern about physical disfigurement resulting from surgery (Miller et al., 1987).

The initial investigation of a large bowel disorder can be an uncomfortable, painful and embarrassing procedure for patients. Although colorectal cancers that develop in the rectosigmoid could be controlled well by early screening, rigid sigmoidoscopy has had poor patient acceptance and has therefore not been successful. Research assessing rigid versus flexible sigmoidoscopy unsurprisingly found that patients reported significantly less discomfort, anxiety and embarrassment during flexible sigmoidoscopy (Winawer et al., 1987).

Widespread screening for colorectal cancer is not yet commonplace but research has assessed what predicts a person's readiness to be screened. Predicting factors identified to be of some use are sex, age, family experience with disease, smoking, recommendation for screening by a physician and the salience and coherence of testing (Myers et al., 1994). Counselling may be offered to patients prior to screening. Once diagnosed, the treatment of these cancers has an impact on bowel function regardless of whether a colostomy is formed or the bowel is re-anastomosed, careful dietary habits are essential.

Colostomies

Recent advances in surgery have led to fewer permanent colostomies. Ostomies can be sited in skin folds and at the patients' preference. Specifically trained ostomy nurses see patients prior to surgery and provide help with practical and psychological adjustment post surgery. Satisfaction with nursing care and personal control act as mediators of self-worth and aid patient's adjustment. Talking to 'cured' patients is very useful for patients undergoing ostomy surgery.

Common fears associated with ostomies are spillage, noise and odour which can lead to increased self-consciousness, feelings of decreased attractiveness, the avoidance of other people and general feelings of 'difference' (MacDonald & Anderson, 1984). These fears tend to be reported more frequently by younger patients.

Psychological morbidity associated with permanent ostomy formation has been reported in the literature. Research which assessed patients who had had stoma surgery for three different conditions (cancer, inflammatory bowel disease and diverticular disease) found that 22% of subjects had moderate or severe psychiatric disturbance at a year post surgery regardless of the initial diagnosis. Most of these patients had shown similar disturbance at a 3 month assessment. The research also highlighted that the ability to perform housework, leisure and sexual activities was impaired in a number of subjects (Thomas et al., 1987). Patients with colostomies are more likely to be severely depressed, socially isolated and stigmatized when compared to similar patients in community settings (MacDonald & Anderson, 1984). These patients also suffer more from physical problems and reduced sexual capacity, emphasising the high psychological and social costs of a colostomy.

Little research has compared ostomy patients with patients whose bowel has been re-anastomosed. Research that has compared sphincter-sacrificing (colostomy formation) or sphincter-conserving surgery (anastomosis) has highlighted differences between the two groups. Both patient groups have frequent or irregular bowel movements and diarrhoea, ostomy patients are more likely to report psychological distress as are women and younger patients. Patients with ostomies report restrictions in their social functioning, men with colostomies consistently report impaired sexual functioning and women with colostomies are more likely to suffer from dyspareunia (Sprangers et al., 1993).

REFERENCES

Kune, G.A., Kune, S., Watson, L.F. & Bahnson, C.B. (1991). Personality as a risk factor in large bowel cancer: data from the Melbourne Colorectal Cancer Study. Psychological Medicine, 21, 29–41.

MacDonald, L.D. & Anderson, H.R. (1984). Stigma in patients with rectal cancer: a community study. Journal of Epidemiology and Community Health, 38, 284–90.

Miller, H.H., Bauman, L.J., Friedman, D.R. & DeCosse, J.J. (1987). Psychosocial adjustment of familial polyposis patients and participation in a chemoprevention trial. International Journal of Psychiatry in Medicine, 16, 211–30.

Myers, R.E., Ross, E., Jepson, C., Wolf, T., Balshem, A., Millner, L. & Leventhal, H. (1994). Modelling adherence to colorectal cancer screening. Prev. Medicine an International Journal Devoted to Practice and Theory, 23, 142–51.

Sprangers, M.A.G., Te Velde, A., Aaronson, N.K. & Taal, B.G. (1993). Quality of life following surgery for colorectal cancer: a literature review. Psycho-Oncology, 2, 247–59.

Thomas, C., Madden, F. & Jehu, D. (1987). Psychological effects of stomas: I. Psychosocial morbidity one year after surgery. Journal of Psychosomatic Research, 31, 311–16.

Toribara, N.W. & Sleisenger, M.H. (1995). Screening for colorectal cancer. New England Journal of Medicine, 332, 861–7.

Van Knippenberg, F.C., Out, J.J., Tilanus, H.W. & Mud, H.J. (1992). Quality of life in patients with resected oesophageal cancer. Society Sci. Medicine, 35, 139–45.

Winawer, S.J., Miler, C., Lightdale, C., Hervert, E., Ephram, R.C., Gordon, L. & Miller, D. (1987). Patient response to sigmoidoscopy. A randomized, controlled trial of rigid and flexible sigmoidoscopy. Cancer, 60, 1905–8.

Digestive tract cancer

Drug dependence: opiates and stimulants

MICHAEL GOSSOP

National Addiction Centre, Institute of Psychiatry,
London, UK

PROBLEMS

Opiates and stimulants are among the drugs most commonly used by people presenting for treatment in recent years. (See also 'Benzodiazepine dependency'). Although the misuse of stimulant drugs is not uncommon in the UK and in other European countries, individuals approaching treatment services have most often presented with opiate problems (Strang & Gossop, 1994). In the United States attention has been directed towards the treatment of both opiate and cocaine problems. Special concern has been expressed about the problems associated with the use of crack, the smokable form of cocaine.

The classification of drug problems by specific substance can be misleading. Few drug abusers who require treatment confine themselves to the use of a single substance, and many are heavy and problematic users of more than one drug. The identification of someone as a heroin addict should not be taken to imply that the drug problem is solely that associated with the use of heroin. For example, there has been increased problematic use of cocaine and benzodiazepines by opiate users (Strang *et al.*, 1994). There are also many differences within the drug using population which are relevant to the choice of treatment intervention. Opiate misusers may include young, criminally active users of illicit heroin, medical personnel misusing opiates obtained via hospitals or pharmacies, and others whose misuse of opiates may have been initiated through a prescription originally intended for the treatment of pain or some legitimate medical disorder.

Even within drug categories (e.g. opiates or stimulants), the characteristics of the drug may vary. Some drugs are short acting, such as pethidine or cocaine. Others like methadone are long acting. Some drugs (for instance, methadone and codeine preparations) are manufactured by pharmaceutical companies and contain known ingredients. Drugs such as heroin are almost always manufactured and distributed through illegal channels and their exact ingredients are almost always unknown to the user. Other opiates which are often misused are Palfium and Diconal. However, the most important type of opiate problem in terms of drug treatment services is usually heroin addiction. Even here, there may be many different forms in which problems may be presented.

Routes of drug administration may vary. Both heroin and cocaine users may take the drug by sniffing, by inhaling the heated vapours ('chasing the dragon' for heroin, and freebasing or crack smoking for cocaine), or they may take the drug by injection. Users may, or may not, be either psychologically or physically dependent upon the drug; and they may, or may not, have experienced various sorts of physical, psychological or social harm as a result of their drug use. The decision to seek help from a treatment agency may be made voluntarily because of a sincere desire to change or it may be a decision which reflect varying degrees of influence from others (family, friends, police, etc.).

ASSESSMENT AND SETTING TREATMENT GOALS

Assessment is not an impersonal procedure to be completed prior to treatment. If carried out properly, it becomes an important first stage of treatment. The drug taker is actively involved in their own addictive behaviour and they must be actively involved in their own recovery. It is the responsibility of the therapist to use assessment as an opportunity to encourage that involvement in recovery. Indeed, it may be more appropriate to regard this first stage of treatment as reaching mutual agreement about goals rather than simply setting goals.

For all types of drug problems which require treatment, the intervention offered should be tailored to the needs and circumstances of the individual. This apparently simple and uncontentious statement turns out to have complex and far-reaching implications for policy and services if it is seriously applied in clinical practice (Gossop, 1987). There is not, nor can there be expected to be, any single best treatment for these problems. Both aetiology and outcome are influenced by a broad range of different factors. A thorough assessment should identify, for each individual case, the nature of the problem and appropriate and achievable goals for treatment. Also, the treatment process should identify as early as possible those particular factors (often outside the treatment setting) that will assist or hamper the achievement of the treatment goal(s).

It is now widely recognized that there may be a range of treatment goals. For the opiate or stimulant misusers such goals may be:

(i) reduction of psychological, social or other problems not directly related to the drug problem;

(ii) reduction of psychological, social or other problems related to the drug problem;

(iii) reduction of harmful or risky behaviour associated with the use of drugs (e.g. shared use of injecting equipment);

(iv) attainment of controlled, non-dependent, or non-problematic drug use;

(v) abstinence from the problem drug;

(vi) abstinence from all drugs.

These goals are not mutually exclusive.

Choice of treatment goals will depend upon the specific circumstances surrounding treatment. Some opiate and cocaine misusers may be at a stage of their drug taking career when they are willing to commit themselves to a determined effort to become abstinent.

Others may be unwilling to give up drugs but may still be willing to make changes in their behaviour to avoid or to reduce certain drug-related problems (e.g. avoiding infection).

It is important that both the therapist and the drug user should agree upon the goal(s) of treatment. This does not mean that the therapist cannot aspire to goals more ambitious than those set by the patient. However, it does imply that, where the therapist seeks to attain some goal beyond that which is immediately acceptable to the patient, this may create certain tensions and require careful management.

STAGES OF CHANGE

The model of change proposed by Prochaska and DiClemente (1982) describes stages of precontemplation, contemplation, decision, action and maintenance. In precontemplation, people are not intending to change their behaviour. Individuals in this stage are not aware or are not sufficiently aware that they have problems, though others (family, friends, doctors) may be acutely aware of this. When precontemplators approach treatment services it is usually because they are under pressure from others. Contemplation is the stage in which the individual shows an awareness of their problem. They begin to think about making changes but without a serious commitment to take action. People may be stuck in the contemplation stage for long periods.

After making a decision to change, the action stage involves actual attempts to modify their behaviour, experiences and/or environment in order to overcome addiction problems. People, including professionals often equate change with action and consequently overlook the important work that prepares individuals for action. During the maintenance stage the individual works to prevent relapse and consolidate their gains. It is unlikely that the actual processes of change will involve any orderly progression through the different stages.

This sort of model can be useful in drawing attention to the different processes and stages of change that may be appropriate and it can serve as an important guide to therapists. For example, patients in the precontemplation stage should be helped to recognize and develop an awareness of their problems rather than being guided directly towards behavioural change. Patients in the contemplation stage are most open to consciousness-raising interventions (such as self-monitoring procedures or educational methods) and may be resistant to the interventions of a directive action-orientated therapist. During the action stage patients are likely to require practical help with behaviour change procedures as well as encouragement and support. Preparation is required both for action and for maintenance. It is often clear that some people with addictive behaviour problems may become stuck in one or other of the stages. It is interesting that therapists as well as patients can become stuck in a favoured stage of change.

PSYCHOSOCIAL INTERVENTIONS

For many years the issue of 'motivation' has a somewhat dubious history in relation to the treatment of addictive behaviours, mainly due to the circularity in the way that the term has been used:

'The general approach is that if the drug abuser patient gets better – translated that means he gives up his drugs of choice – he was a good and motivated patient and was able to profit from our professional

expertise and skill. We cured him. If the patient continues his drug use, this is manifest evidence that he was not motivated, and a poor treatment risk who could not profit from our skill.' (Einstein & Garitano, 1972, p. 235)

This circularity has been a major factor in leading to a dissatisfaction with the concept of motivation. However, the term can be rescued from circularity by operational definition (e.g.) in terms of the strength of the addict's desire for treatment) and it can be shown to relate to treatment response (Gossop, 1978).

The recent work on motivational interviewing reflects a contemporary (and more productive) resurgence of interest in this issue. The aim of motivational interviewing is to encourage the active involvement of the client in the identification of the problem and in the cost–benefit analysis of the various available options. It is intended to enhance personal responsibility and the internal attribution of choice and control. Motivational interviewing has also been described as the supervision of a decision making process in which the client makes the decisions.

Relapse prevention has been an important form of psychosocial treatment (Marlatt & Gordon, 1985). The primary goal of relapse prevention is to teach drug users who are trying to change their drug taking behaviour how to identify, anticipate, and cope with the pressures and problems that may lead towards a relapse. Relapse prevention work involves a focus upon an awareness of high risk situations and of coping strategies to avoid or reduce the risks of relapse. In a study of former heroin addicts who had recently completed inpatient treatment, Gossop et al. (1989) found that many such individuals used opiates again in the period immediately after leaving treatment. The time immediately after leaving treatment is a critical period during which recovering addicts are at extremely high risk. This finding highlights the need for aftercare support.

Greater attention is now being paid to the clinical significance of relapse as a process in its own right. There has sometimes been a mistaken emphasis on the problem of cessation of drug use, when what is required is more emphasis on the difficulties encountered in maintenance of the change once cessation has occurred. The various factors that increase the likelihood of relapse may be associated with social, environmental or internal cognitive cues, and an important first task for the client is to develop an awareness of the way in which these relapse factors can contribute towards the development of a high risk situation. Clients may be encouraged to keep regular diaries detailing use of drugs and the extent to which they have encountered possible precipitants of relapse and a summary of their response. Structured problem-solving techniques are employed alongside rehearsal/role play. The client is warned of the dangers of the way in which covert planning may lead to relapse, and of the way in which decisions made 'by chance' may lead to high risk situations. The client must learn to spot early warning signals for these potential relapse situations. Various deconditioning ('cue exposure') treatments have been tried with addicts to help reduce relapse associated with craving. The effectiveness of such treatments with drug addicts is, as yet, unproven (Dawe et al., 1993).

PREVENTIVE MEASURES

Opiate and stimulant users may be exposed to several risks of infection. Such risks may be associated with both unsafe injection and sexual practices. HIV and hepatitis seropositivity rates are related to frequency of injection, and more specifically, to the sharing of injecting equipment (Muga *et al.*, 1990; Schoenbaum *et al.*, 1989). As a result, many countries have now adopted harm reduction policies which seek to implement prevention and treatment interventions aimed at reducing the risk of infection but without necessarily seeking to achieve abstinence from drugs.

Needle exchange schemes were established throughout in England and Wales from 1987 and within two years about one in three of all drug treatment agencies were operating some form of needle exchange. Such exchange schemes were found to be useful and increased access to injection equipment was associated with reduced levels of sharing as well as increased contact with other treatment services (Stimson *et al.*, 1990). Infection risk associated with sharing injecting equipment may be influenced by cleaning or sterilization procedures and advice on cleaning injecting equipment should be readily available to drug injectors. An outreach project in San Francisco encouraged injectors to use bleach in order to reduce infection risks and a large percentage of injectors incorporated cleaning procedures into their injecting practices (Moss & Chaisson, 1988).

Drug users may also be at risk through their sexual behaviour. Many drug users engage in unprotected sex, often with multiple partners. Rates of prostitution tend to be higher among drug users (Hart *et al.*, 1989), and prostitution may be more common among dependent drug users, since this provides a source of money to obtain drugs (Gossop *et al.*, 1993). Many drug outreach programmes provide free condoms to drug users. However, there is evidence that changing sexual behaviour is proving to be more difficult than changing drug injecting behaviour (Donoghoe, 1992). Even where drug users report regular use of condoms, the evidence is not encouraging. A study of drug using prostitutes in Amsterdam found that although 90% of the sample reported regularly using condoms, 81% had contracted a sexually transmitted disease during the 6 months prior to interview (Van den Hoek *et al.*, 1989).

Some drug users may be exposed to both drug risk and sexual risk through having a sexual partner who injects drugs. Women may be at particular risk in this way (Gossop, Griffiths & Strang 1994, a). In the United States, women infected with HIV by a drug using partner are the second largest group of women with AIDS, and HIV rates tend to be especially high among female drug injectors who had multiple sexual partners (Schoenbaum *et al.*, 1989).

Since the earliest days of the HIV epidemic it has been known that homosexual activity may carry high risks of HIV transmission. Drug users may also be exposed to this form of risk. Gossop *et al.* (1994*b*) found that the factor most strongly associated with HIV seropositive status among a sample of heroin users was men having sex with men. Conversely, the strongest predictor of hepatitis B seropositive status was a drug risk factor, the number of years injecting drugs.

PHARMACOLOGICAL TREATMENTS

Drugs may be used in the treatment of drug problems for the management of withdrawal (detoxification), or as substitute drugs. There are a number of ways in which the opiate withdrawal syndrome can be treated. These include the use of methadone, partial opiate agonists such as buprenorphine and alpha-2 agonists (such as clonidine), and various benzodiazepines. For many years, the most commonly used treatment has involved the use of gradually reducing doses of oral methadone. Methadone is also widely used as a substitute for heroin in maintenance prescribing and its effectiveness in reducing drug abuse and crime is now accepted though there is also evidence that programmes vary greatly in their efficacy (Farrell *et al.*, 1994).

Although there have been descriptions of withdrawal problems among regular stimulant users, the existence of a specific cocaine or amphetamine withdrawal syndrome is still uncertain (Lago & Kosten, 1994). Antidepressant drugs are sometimes given to counter dopamine depletion during cocaine withdrawal. Despite the theoretical rationale, the superiority of these drugs over a placebo in cocaine withdrawal has not been established (Kosten *et al.*, 1992). The use of substitute drugs for treatment of stimulant dependence is uncommon and of unknown effectiveness.

Opiate antagonist drugs such as naltrexone are also sometimes used to speed up withdrawal treatments or to help prevent relapse after detoxification. These substances bind to opiate receptors but without producing opiate type effects. They compete with opiate agonists such as heroin in such a way that opiates produce little or no effect. Antagonists appear to work well with highly motivated patients and when used under supervision (O'Brien, 1994). Because of their specific affinity for opiate receptors, such drugs have not been used or evaluated in the treatment of stimulant dependence.

TREATMENT OUTCOME

Early reviews of the effectiveness of treatments for addiction problems often reached the pessimistic conclusion that outcome for addiction was universally poor and that none of the many types of treatment being used had any impact upon outcome (e.g. Einstein, 1966; Clare, 1977). Such pessimism is no longer warranted. There is now an impressive accumulation of evidence to show that even people with severe dependence upon drugs can recover from their addictions and that treatment can play an important role in assisting recovery (Biernacki, 1986; Gossop *et al.*, 1989; Hubbard *et al.*, 1989). In many respects, it is atypical for addicts to remain addicted throughout their lives. The majority will give up at some point. Even where treated addicts do not attain abstinence, most demonstrate substantial improvement in their problem behaviours.

The Treatment Outcome Prospective Study (TOPS) involved more than 11 000 people who entered treatment for drug problems at 41 treatment programmes in the United States (Hubbard *et al.*, 1989). TOPS showed substantial decreases in the abuse of opiates and other drugs after treatment. Reductions in drug taking continued to be found even up to the longer-term three to five-year follow-up. Interestingly, in relation to the increased awareness of applying cost/benefit analysis to treatment, TOPS demonstrated the 'substantial crime-related and other costs . . . of drug abusers prior to treatment and the substantial reductions in these costs both during and following participation in treatment'. Similarly, in a study of patients receiving methadone maintenance treatment, Ball and Ross (1991) concluded that this treatment is effective in reducing drug abuse and crime.

However, a word of caution may be appropriate. For the therapist in the treatment setting it may be tempting to overestimate the impact of treatment factors. The psychology of the individual and the social setting in which the individual lives exert powerful influences upon outcome. Hubbard *et al.* (1989) note that 'The role of treatment is to change behaviours and psychological states and to direct clients to community resources during and after treatment', and that, 'Programmes have no direct control on behaviour after clients leave treatment. Rather, treatment should influence posttreatment behaviour indirectly through changes in psychological states and behaviour during treatment' (p.35). Effective treatments for drug problems should look beyond the clinic to maintaining change in the real-life social environment.

REFERENCES

Ball, J. & Ross, A. (1991). *The effectiveness of methadone maintenance treatment.* New York: Springer.

Biernacki, P. (1986). *Pathways from heroin addiction.* Philadelphia: Temple University Press.

Clare, A. (1977). How good is treatment? In G. Edwards, & M. Grant (Eds.). *Alcoholism: new knowledge and new responses.* London: Croom Helm.

Dawe, S., Powell, J., Richards, D., Gossop, M., Marks, I., Strang, J. & Gray, J. (1993). Does post-withdrawal cue exposure improve outcome in opiate addiction? A controlled trial. *Addiction*, 88, 1233–45.

Donoghoe, M. (1992). Sex, HIV and the injecting drug user, *British Journal of Addiction*, 87, 405–6.

Einstein, S. (1966). 'The narcotics dilemma: who is listening to what? *International Journal of the Addictions*, 1, 1–6.

Farrell, M., Ward, J., Mattick, R., Hall, W., Stimson, G., Des Jarlais, D., Gossop, M. & Strang, J. (1994). Methadone maintenance treatment in opiate dependence: a review. *British Medical Journal*, 309, 997–1001.

Gossop, M.R. (1987). What is the most effective way to treat opiate addiction? *British Journal of Hospital Medicine*, 38, 161.

Gossop, M., Green, L., Phillips, G. & Bradley, B. (1989). Lapse, relapse and survival among opiate addicts after treatment. *British Journal of Psychiatry*, 154, 348–53.

Gossop, M., Powis, B., Griffiths, P. & Strang, J. (1993). Sexual behaviour and its relationship to drug taking among prostitutes in south London, *Addiction*,

Gossop, M., Griffiths, P. & Strang, J. (1994a). Sex differences in patterns of drug taking behaviour: a study at a London community drug team. *British Journal of Psychiatry*, 164, 101–34.

Gossop, M., Powis, B., Griffiths, P. & Strang, J. (1994b). Multiple risks for HIV and hepatitis B infection among heroin users. *Drug and Alcohol Review*, 13, 293–300.

Hart, G., Sonnex, C., Petherick, A., Johnson, A., Feinman, C. & Adler, M. (1989). Risk behaviours for HIV infection among injecting drug users attending a drug dependency clinic. *British Medical Journal*, 298, 1081–3.

Hubbard, R., Marsden, M., Rachal, V., Harwood, H., Cavanaugh, E. & Ginzburg, H. (1989). *Drug abuse treatment: a national study of effectiveness.* Chapel Hill and London: University of North Carolina Press.

Kosten, T., Morgan, C., Falcione, J. & Schottenfeld, R. (1992). Pharmacotherapy for cocaine-abusing methadone-maintained patients using amantadine or desiprimine. *Archives of General Psychiatry*, 49, 894–8.

Lago, J. & Kosten, T. (1994). Stimulant withdrawal. *Addiction*, 89, 1477–81.

Marlatt, G.A. & Gordon, J.R. (1985). *Relapse prevention.* New York: Guilford.

Moss, A. & Chaisson, R. (1988). AIDS and intravenous drug use in San Francisco. *AIDS and Public Policy*, 3, 37–41.

Muga, R., Tor, J., Josep, M. *et al.* (1990). Risk factors for HIV-1 infection in parenteral drug users. *AIDS*, 4, 259–60.

O'Brien, C. (1994). The treatment of drug dependence. *Addiction*, 89, 1565–9.

Prochaska, J. & DiClemente, C. (1982). Transtheoretical therapy: toward a more integrative model of change. *Psychotherapy, Theory, Research and Practice*, 19, 276–8.

Schoenbaum, E., Hartel, D., Selwyn, P. et al. (1989). Risk factors for human immunodeficiency virus infection in intravenous drug users. *New England Journal of Medicine*, 321, 874–9.

Stimson, G., Donoghoe, M., Lart, R. & Dolan, K. (1990). Distributing sterile needles and syringes to people who inject drugs: the syringe exchange experiment. In Strang J. & Stimson G. (Eds.). *AIDS and drugs misuse.* London: Routledge.

Strang, J. & Gossop, M. (1994). *The British system.* Oxford University Press, Oxford.

Strang, J., Griffiths, P., Abbey, J. & Gossop, M. (1994). Survey of the use of injected benzodiazepines among drug users in Britain. *British Medical Journal*, 308, 1082.

Van Den Hoek. J., Van Haastrecht., H., Scheeringa-Troost. B., Goudsmit, J. & Coutinho, R. (1989). HIV infection and STD in drug addicted prostitutes in Amsterdam: potential for heterosexual HIV transmission, *Genitourinary Medicine*, 65, 146–50.

Dyslexia

CHRISTINE M. TEMPLE

Developmental Neuropsychology Unit, Department of Psychology, University of Essex, Colchester,

Dyslexia is a developmental disorder in the acquisition of reading skills, in children of otherwise normal intelligence, which cannot be explained on the basis of educational deprivation or sensory impairment. The child may have fluent speech and good communicative skills, yet has difficulty in mastering the formal written code employed for reading.

HISTORICAL PERSPECTIVES

At the end of the nineteenth century, the term word blindness was coined, first to refer to acquired disorders of reading resulting from brain damage, and then to refer to reading disabilities which occur developmentally. Since, the angular gyrus was damaged in many cases of acquired word blindness, there was speculation that a congenital aplasia of the angular gyrus might underlie problems in learning to read. Early discussions of congenital word blindness are given by Hinshelwood (1917).

LABELLING

Throughout the twentieth century, there has been disagreement regarding the labelling of the disorder. This continues today, with the term developmental dyslexia being accepted in most academic and medical settings but not in educational circles, where the term specific reading disabilities is employed.

INCIDENCE

Studies in the 1970s suggested an incidence of 4–6% for dyslexia. More recently, Lewis, Hitch and Walker (1994) tested the population of 9- and 10-year-olds in a single education authority district in England, finding 6.2% with specific reading disabilities. It remains unclear whether these children represent a distinct group from the main distribution, or the lower tail of a normal distribution. Lewis *et al.* (1994) also reports a male to female ratio of 3.2 : 1.

BIOLOGICAL FOUNDATIONS

Vogler, DeFries and Decker (1985) reported that the risk to a son of having an affected father was 40%, and of having an affected mother was 55%. The risk to a daughter of having an affected parent of either sex, was 17–18% In a study of dyslexic twins, Olson *et al.* (1989) found significant heritability for non-word reading accuracy. Results from linkage studies have been contradictory.

Electrophysiological studies indicate specific EEG abnormalities, which have greater focus in temporo-parietal areas in some subjects and in frontal areas in other subjects (Duffy & McAnulty, 1985). Postmortem analyses have revealed cytoarchitectonic abnormalities, in the form of foci of ectopic neurons and microgyria, constellated in the left hemisphere (Galaburda *et al.*, 1985). MRI studies reveal increased symmetry of the planum temporale (Larsen *et al.*, 1990), whilst PET studies, demonstrate abnormalities in cerebral blood flow in the left temporo-parietal region in men with dyslexia, when carrying out a rhyming task (Hagram *et al.*, 1992).

COGNITIVE NEUROPSYCHOLOGICAL ANALYSES

Surface dyslexia (see 'Dyslexia and dysgraphia: acquired')
Recent cognitive neuropsychological analyses of the developmental dyslexias have delineated several different forms of the disorder, each of which is explicable in relation to models of normal reading. In developmental surface dyslexia (e.g. Coltheart *et al.*, 1983), words that conform to spelling to sound rules (e.g. beach) are read more easily than those which are not consistent with those rules (e.g. yacht). Errors indicate the application of a rule-based system (e.g. bear → 'beer'; subtle → 'subtill'). There is also homophone confusion, affecting words with the same pronunciations but different spellings (e.g. pane defined as 'something which hurts').

Surface dyslexia can be explained in relation to stage models of normal reading development, in terms of arrestment at an alphabetic stage, within which there is emphasis upon the use of letter-sound rules, with failure to progress to later orthographic/hierarchical stages, which incorporate context sensitivity and analyses based upon meaningful subcomponents of the target word.

In relation to models of normal adult reading, surface dyslexia reflects overreliance upon a phonological reading route, which translates graphemes or letter clusters to phonological segments, and blends these to produce an integrated output. Other reading routes, usually labelled semantic and direct, are poorly established. In the normal semantic reading route, a system recognizes the whole word, causing activation of its meaning, which in turn accesses pronunciation. In the direct route, recognition of the whole word directly accesses pronunciation. The overreliance upon the phonological reading route in surface dyslexia, leads to adequate ability to read non-words, but difficulty in reading irregular words. Homophone confusions arise because meaning is activated after the activation of pronunciation.

Connectionist models, which represent relationships between orthography and phonology in a series of distributed connection weights, are able to produce parallels to elements of surface dyslexia, with emergent superiority in reading regular words. Early versions had difficulty in modelling the degree of accuracy in non-word reading. (Seidenberg & McClelland, 1989), which has been resolved in the more recent dual route connectionist model of Plaut *et al.* (1996).

Marcel (1980) suggested that reading by normal children resembled surface dyslexia, but the reaction time studies of Seymour (1986) show that surface dyslexics (whom he labels morphemic dyslexics) have response times which lie outside those of normal children.

Castles and Coltheart (1993) show that 30% of dyslexics display a surface dyslexic reading pattern.

Phonological dyslexia (see 'Dyslexia and dysgraphia: acquired'
In contrast to surface dyslexia, the major characteristic of developmental phonological dyslexia is a selective impairment of phonological reading processes. The term was first adopted by Temple and Marshall (1983), to refer to a teenage girl, who had significant difficulty in reading non-words aloud (e.g. zan → 'tan'; chait → 'chart' . . . 'trait'). Reading errors included many paralexic responses (word substitutions), including morphological paralexias (in which the base morpheme is correct but an ending is altered, e.g. image → 'imagine'; sickness → 'sicken'. Phonological dyslexia has now been described in many languages.

Phonological dyslexia cannot be explained in relation to stage models of reading development. Orthographic skills are mastered, despite failure to master alphabetic skills, yet the acquisition of alphabetic skills is supposed to precede orthographic skills. One alternative is that there are different pathways to the acquisition of reading.

Phonological dyslexia is explained with relative ease in relation to models of normal adult reading, by proposing relatively normal development of semantic and direct reading routes, but impaired development of the phonological reading route. Temple (1988) suggests the abnormality in the phonological reading route relates to an inappropriate parsing or translating mechanism, such that the units upon which the system operates are too large. This leads to responses within which whole words or morphemic subcomponents are found (e.g. laborcolator 'labor.curator'). Plaut *et al.*'s (1996) dual route connectionist model can also model phonological dyslexia.

Phonological processing

It has been suggested that a basic phonological processing deficit underlies developmental dyslexia. However, there is dispute as to whether impaired phonological awareness causes or is a consequence of dyslexia. Hatcher, Hulme and Ellis (1994) report that remediation, involving training in phonological awareness, only generalized to a significant improvement in reading when training in reading had also been involved. Cossu, Rossini and Marshall (1993) argue that phonological awareness is not a necessary prerequisite for reading development, since children who fail tests of phonological awareness nevertheless develop reading skills. Surface dyslexics are unimpaired on oral phonological tasks (Castles & Coltheart, 1996).

REFERENCES

Castles, A. & Coltheart, M. (1993). Varieties of developmental dyslexia. *Cognition*, **47**, 149–80.

Castles, A. & Coltheart, M. (1996). Cognitive correlates of developmental surface dyslexia: a single case study. *Cognitive Neuropsychology*, **13**, 25–50.

Coltheart, M., Masterson, J. Byng, S., Prior, M. & Riddoch, J. (1983). Surface dyslexia. *Quarterly Journal of Experimental Psychology*, **35**, 469–96.

Cossu, G., Rossini, F. & Marshall, J.C. (1993). When reading is acquired but phonemic awareness is not: a study of literacy in Down's Syndrome. *Cognition*, **46**, 129–38.

Duffy, F.H. & McAnulty, G.B. (1985). Brain electrical activity mapping (BEAM): the search for a physiological signature of dyslexia. In F.H. Duffy and N. Geschwind (Eds.). *Dyslexia: a neuroscientific approach to clinical evaluation*. Boston: Little, Brown and Co.

Galaburda, A.M., Sherman, G.F., Rosen, G.D., Aboitiz, F. & Geschwind, N. (1985). Developmental dyslexia: four consecutive cases with cortical anomalies. *Annals of Neurology*, **18**, 222–33.

Hagram, J.O., Wood, F., Buchsbaum, M.S., Tallal, P., Flowers, L. & Katz, W. (1992). Cerebral brain metabolism in adult dyslexic subjects assessed with positron emission tomography during performance of an auditory task. *Archives of Neurology*, **49**, 734–9.

Hatcher, P.J., Hulme, C. & Ellis, A.W. (1994). Ameliorating early reading failure by integrating the teaching of reading and phonological skills: the phonological linkage hypothesis. *Child Development*, **65**, 41–57.

Hinshelwood, J. (1917) *Congenital word blindness*. Glasgow: H.K. Lewis. Larsen, J., Hoein, T., Lundberg, I. & Odegaard, H. (1990). MRI evaluation of the size and symmetry of the planum temporale in adolescents with developmental dyslexia. *Brain and Language*, **39**, 289–301.

Larsen, J.P., Hoein, T., Lundberg, I. & Odegard, H. (1990). MRI evaluation of the size and symmetry of the planum temporale in adolescents with developmental dyslexia. *Brain and Language*, **39**, 289–301.

Lewis, C., Hitch, G.J. & Walker, P. (1994). The prevalence of specific arithmetic difficulties and specific reading difficulties in 9 – to 10-year old boys and girls. *Journal of Child Psychology and Psychiatry*, **35**, 283–92.

Marcel, T. (1980). Surface dyslexia and beginning reading: a revised hypothesis of the pronunciation of print and its impairments. In M. Coltheart. K.E. Patterson as J.C. Marshall (Eds.). *Deep dyslexia*. London: Routledge and Kegan Paul.

Olson, R., Wise, B., Conners, F. & Rack, J. (1989). Specific deficits in component reading and language skills: genetic and environmental influences. *Journal of Learning Disabilities*, **22**, 339–48.

Plaut, D.C., McClelland, J.L., Seidenberg, M.S. & Patterson, K.E. (1996). Understanding normal and impaired word reading: computational principles in quasi-regular domains. *Psychological Review*, **103**, 56–115.

Seidenberg, M. & McClelland, J. (1989). A disturbed, developmental model of word recognition and naming. *Psychological Review*, **96**, 523–68.

Seymour, P.H.K. (1986). *Cognitive analysis of dyslexia*. London: Routledge and Kegan Paul.

Temple, C.M. (1988). Developmental dyslexia and dysgraphia: persistence in middle age. *Journal of Communication Disorders*, **21**, 189–207.

Temple, C.M. & Marshall, J.C. (1983). A case study of developmental phonological dyslexia. *British Journal of Psychology*, **74**, 517–33.

Vogler, G.P., DeFries, J. & Decker, S. (1985). Family history as an indicator of risk for reading disability. *Journal of Learning Disabilities*, **18**, 419–21.

Dyslexia and dysgraphia: acquired

ELAINE FUNNELL
Royal Holloway College,
University of London, UK

INTRODUCTION

When the language processing areas of the left cerebral hemisphere are damaged, problems with reading (dyslexia) and spelling and writing (dysgraphia) typically follow. These disorders can be divided into central disorders which affect the linguistic aspects of reading and spelling and peripheral disorders which are secondary to linguistic aspects and which, in reading, may result from problems with visual or spatial processes and in writing may affect the processes involved in the selection and production of letters. This chapter will concentrate on the central disorders of reading and spelling, and will discuss only one peripheral disorder of reading (pure alexia).

[445]

There are three central disorders. Each disorder has a characteristic pattern and can be found in both reading and spelling (although not necessarily within the same individual). These disorders are (a) surface dyslexia and dysgraphia; (b) phonological dyslexia and dysgraphia; and (c) deep dyslexia and dysgraphia. These disorders will be described in more detail below; but a brief introduction may be helpful here. In surface disorders, subjects have difficulty remembering how to pronounce and spell previously familiar words and, instead, use their knowledge of associations between letters (graphemes) and sounds (phonemes) to read aloud and spell phonically; in phonological disorders, subjects can read and spell words, but have great difficulty using grapheme – phoneme mappings to pronounce novel words and non-words; and in the deep disorders, subjects are totally unable to use grapheme – phoneme mappings, and, in addition, have severe problems with reading aloud some types of words. They also misread and misspell some words as other words which are close in meaning.

A BRIEF THEORETICAL ACCOUNT OF THE CENTRAL DISORDERS

Each of these disorders can be explained by current theories of the mental lexicon which will be introduced briefly here. Although theories vary in detail (e.g. Morton & Patterson, 1987; Shallice & Warrington, 1987; Allport & Funnell, 1981), they basically agree on three points: first, familiar written and spoken words are stored in separate lexicons (or word stores); secondly, there are separate pathways between these lexicons, one passing through a further store of word meanings, the other linking written words directly with spoken word forms. Thirdly, there are sets of rules available for reading and spelling unfamiliar words. These rules convert letters into sounds or sounds into letters and are usually referred to as sublexical processes.

When reading and spelling skills are impaired following brain damage, it is necessary to investigate the contribution that each process makes to the reading and spelling pattern observed. This can be done using materials designed specifically for the purpose. It will be helpful to describe these materials next, before the disorders themselves are discussed more fully.

MATERIALS FOR ASSESSING CENTRAL DISORDERS

Familiar words, unfamiliar words and nonsense words

Previous experience with words means that some written word forms become familiar. Subjects have read and spelled familiar words before, but many real words may be unfamiliar e.g. (pegmatic) and as novel as nonsense words such as (*fol* and *bemit*). Familiar words are likely to be recorded in the lexicons of written and spoken word forms, where they can be looked up for reading and spelling. Novel stimuli have no lexical addresses, so responses to these items have to be assembled by using sublexical processes. In phonological dyslexia/dysgraphia the disorder affects unfamiliar words and nonsense words more than familiar words; in surface dyslexia the pattern is reversed.

Common and uncommon words

Some words are more common than others. Written word counts (Kucera & Francis, 1967) have shown that the most common writ-ten word is the, closely followed by of, and, to, a, in, and that. All these words occur more than ten thousand times in every million written words. Some words are much less common, words such as bacon, meek, halt, and swallow, occur only ten times in every million words, and words such as croak, deter, adverb, and plum, occur only once. The frequency of a word can affect the likelihood of the word being read and spelled correctly in both surface and phonological dyslexia and dysgraphia.

Regular and irregular words

Some words can be pronounced and spelled correctly by assembling a response using sublexical (grapheme–phoneme) processes. These words contain the most regular, or commonly used, mappings between particular graphemes and phonemes and are referred to as regular words. Examples of such words are quick, splendid, shrug, and slate. There are fewer regular words for spelling than for reading because there is a wider choice of graphemes for spelling a particular phoneme, than there is the choice of phonemes for pronouncing a particular grapheme. For example, quick, a regular word for reading, is irregular for spelling since it can be spelled phonically as *kwik*. Irregular words cannot be assembled correctly by sublexical processes. Instead, these words, which contain unusual grapheme/phoneme correspondences, have to be looked up in the lexicon. Examples of irregular words are gauge, bury, cough, blood. Regularity is an important variable for assessing surface dyslexia and dysgraphia.

Concrete words, abstract words, and imageable words

Some words are more imageable than others (Paivio, Yuille & Madigan, 1968). It is easier to conjure up a picture or sound in response to some words than others. Words such as book, chrysanthemum, dance, shiny, are highly imageable words; words such as thing, skill, do, are very low in imageability, and function words such as and, how, are not imageable at all. Concrete words are words that name objects and people (Paivio, *et al.*, 1968). All concrete words are imageable, but imageable words are not always concrete. Words such as red, shiny, tiny, shriek, are imageable but they are not concrete. Abstract words are not concrete and are usually very low in imageability. For the purposes of this chapter, concreteness and abstractness will be subsumed under differences in imageability. It is important to be clear that 'imageability' does not refer to the act of imaging the meaning of the word but refers to the properties of the word meanings; that is, some word meanings are potentially more imageable than others. Imageability is an important variable for detecting reading and spelling disorders based on the processing of word meaning. It is central to the assessment of deep dyslexia and dysgraphia and also shows up in some cases of phonological dyslexia and dysgraphia.

Homonyms

These are words that sound the same but have different meanings and different spellings. Word pairs such as berry and bury, heal and heel, fir and fur, are homonyms. Homonyms are useful when one needs to know whether an individual can understand the meaning of a written word in a reading task and whether they can use meaning to address a spelling. As we shall see, homonyms can tease apart the reading and spelling processes available in cases of surface dyslexia and some cases of phonological dyslexia.

CENTRAL DISORDERS OF READING AND SPELLING

Surface dyslexia and surface dysgraphia.

Key papers for surface dyslexia are Marshall and Newcombe (1973); Bub, Cancelliere & Kertesz (1985); Patterson, Marshall and Coltheart (1985); and surface dysgraphia: Beauvois and Derouesne (1981); Hatfield and Patterson (1983).

Surface dyslexic readers pronounce what might be expected to be familiar words as if they are no longer recognized, making errors such as listen → 'liston', island → 'izland', and phase → 'face' in which graphemes are given an alternative pronunciation or are pronounced when they should be silent. These errors have come to be called 'regularization' errors (Coltheart, 1982) and affect irregular words. Regular words are read correctly, since these use the most common grapheme–phoneme mappings. Subjects usually spell regular words correctly but make mistakes with irregular words, replacing irregular letters with more common phoneme–grapheme mappings, and missing out the letters which are not sounded.

Irregular words of low frequency are particularly vulnerable in surface dyslexia and dysgraphia. Bub et al. (1985) reported a subject who had problems in reading irregular words of low frequency such as ache and yacht. This subject could read high frequency irregular words much more successfully than low frequency irregular words. However, he could read most regular words, such as rasp and solve, even those of low frequency, because these words could be read correctly using sublexical processes.

When subjects regularize words in surface dyslexia, they are usually unable to understand the correct meaning of the written word, and base their understanding on their own pronunciation. Sometimes they misunderstand words they read aloud correctly. For example, Coltheart (1981) showed that, when surface dyslexic readers were given homonyms to define, they often gave the meaning of the wrong homonym. So, for example, the written regular word sore might be defined as 'to cut wood' and the regular word I defined as 'I have two of them'. Even irregular words, such as bury, which are sometimes read aloud correctly may be defined wrongly as, for example 'A fruit on a tree'. This last example is particularly interesting, since the word bury was pronounced correctly it must have been read lexically (that is, it must have been looked up in the lexicon) and yet it was not understood. In a spelling dictation test, subjects appear to understand the meaning of the spoken word, even though the spelling is regularized.

Neither word length or imageability affect surface dyslexia and dysgraphia: subjects read and spell short words as poorly as long, and imageable words as poorly as non-imageable words.

THEORETICAL ACCOUNT OF SURFACE DYSLEXIA AND DYSGRAPHIA

Coltheart and Funnell (1987) showed that there are at least seven different underlying disorders which can give rise to surface dyslexia and dysgraphia. These disorders affect a variety of lexical processes allowing sublexical processes to operate normally or, some-

times, near normally. Surface dyslexia and dysgraphia can be caused by a disorder affecting the lexicon of written words, the lexicon of spoken words, a disorder affecting the two lexical pathways which map written words on to spoken words, or a combination of these deficits. For attempts at computer simulations of surface dyslexia, see Patterson, Seidenberg and McClelland (1989).

PHONOLOGICAL DYSLEXIA AND DYSGRAPHIS

Key papers for phonological dyslexia are Beauvois and Derouesne (1979); Funnell (1983); Coslett (1991); and phonological dysgraphia: Shallice (1981); Bub and Kertesz (1982).

In this disorder the reading and spelling of words is greatly superior to the reading and spelling of nonsense words, indicating that reading and spelling depend upon lexical processes. This lexical effect is the hallmark of phonological dyslexia and dysgraphia. It is important to distinguish phonological dyslexia and dysgraphia from deep dyslexia and deep dysgraphia (see below) which also shows a very marked lexical effect. In general, subjects with phonological dyslexia/dysgraphia can read and spell most types of words, including words of low imageability. They fail to make semantic errors, such as reading dog as cat, which are characteristic of deep dyslexia/dysgraphia, but they may make 'visual' errors in reading, in which a visually similar word is produced instead of the correct word. For example, subjects may read smoulder as 'shoulder' and pivot as 'point'. Deep dyslexic readers make these 'visual' errors too.

Within this broad definition, rather different patterns of performance can be observed. Subjects may show an effect of word frequency by reading and spelling high frequency words more successfully than words of low frequency (although the differences can be slight and in some cases are not apparent). Generally there is little or no difference in the reading of regular and irregular words. One subject could read aloud irregular words that he did not precisely understand.

Imageable words may be read or spelled more successfully than words of low imageability, but the difference is generally fairly slight and much less marked than that observed in deep dyslexia and dysgraphia (see below). In other subjects, there is no observable effect of imageability. Unlike deep dyslexic and dysgraphic patients, subjects do not have major problems with reading and spelling non-imageable function words. In general subjects can usually comprehend the words they can read and spell. One subject could define written homophones accurately (Funnell, 1987).

THEORETICAL ACCOUNT OF PHONOLOGICAL DYSLEXIA AND DYSGRAPHIA

Since subjects cannot read or spell non-words (or can do so only poorly) it seems likely that the sublexical processes involved in assembling a pronunciation or a spelling have been damaged. Beyond this point, individual theoretical accounts are required, since the precise nature of any additional lexical disorder can vary across subjects. Most subjects appear to be able to comprehend the meanings of the words they are able to read and spell, indicating that access to word meanings is spared and may even support oral reading. However, occasional subjects appear to have lost the precise meaning of words, and here it seems that their good oral reading is carried out by the pathway linking the lexicon of written words directly to the lexicon of spoken words.

DEEP DYSLEXIA (OR PHONEMIC DYSLEXIA) AND DEEP DYSGRAPHIA

Key papers for deep dyslexia are Marshall and Newcombe (1966); Coltheart, Patterson and Marshall (1987); and deep dysgraphia: Bub and Kertesz (1982).

Subjects with deep dyslexia/dysgraphia are unable to read aloud or spell nonsense words, or match spoken non-words to written nonwords. They can read aloud and spell imageable words, such as flower and ladder more successfully than less imageable words, such as pride and depth, and fail entirely to read aloud and spell any non-imageable words, such as function words. Although a word class effect is often reported (in which nouns are read better than adjectives, which in turn are read better than verbs), this effect has been shown to be secondary to differences in imageability (Allport & Funnell, 1981).

The cardinal symptom of deep dyslexia and deep dysgraphia is the semantic error. Instead of reading or spelling the given word, the subject produces a word related in meaning. Usually it is a more imageable/concrete word than the target. For example, the written word antique may be read as 'vase' or the spoken word 'laugh' may be written as smile.

There is no effect of regularity, word frequency or word length in deep dyslexia/dysgraphia.

THEORETICAL ACCOUNTS OF DEEP DYSLEXIA AND DEEP DYSGRAPHIA

It is generally assumed that these subjects read and/or spell using the lexical–semantic: a pathway that passes from the lexicon of written words, through word meaning to the lexicon for spoken words. Only in this way could a subject produce an error in which the response is related in meaning to the target word, but bears no relationship to the sound or written pattern of the word. Thus, it appears that the ability to process words using the pathway which directly links the lexica of written and spoken words has been damaged (if this were not the case, the subjects should be able to avoid making meaning-related errors). It also appears that sublexical processes have been lost. It seems likely that the semantic system has also been damaged, preventing subjects from reliably accessing the precise meaning of the word. The range of symptoms that co-occur in deep dyslexia, has suggested that deep dyslexic reading may reflect a shift of processing to the right hemisphere (Coltheart, 1987). For computer simulations of deep dyslexia, see Plaut and Shallice (1993).

PERIPHERAL DISORDERS OF READING AND WRITING

Only the peripheral disorder, pure alexia, will be discussed here. Limits on space prevent discussion of further peripheral disorders of reading (neglect dyslexia and simultanagnosia) and of writing. For information on peripheral disorders see Ellis (1993).

PURE ALEXIA

This disorder affects reading but not spelling, and is associated with a lesion affecting the left occipital cortex and the splenium (Dejerine, 1892, cited by Walsh, 1978). Key papers are those by Warrington and Shallice (1980) and Patterson and Kay (1982).

Subjects with pure alexia can write at length without making errors of grammar or spelling, but they then have extreme difficulty in reading back their written work. Reading is more difficult with handwriting and script than with printed words, but the difficulty with print remains severe. When reading aloud, they appear unable to process the written word form as a whole, and instead seem to have to identify each letter in turn, often speaking aloud the letter names. This gives rise to the principal characteristic of pure alexia: a word length effect, in which short words are read faster than long words, since fewer letters need to be identified in short words than long words. Following identification of the letters, subjects may pronounce the word correctly. Some subjects read irregular words correctly, indicating that lexical processes must have been involved. Other subjects show a regularity effect, making regularization errors to irregular words, suggesting that the spoken letter names have not accessed lexical processes but have accessed instead the grapheme–phoneme conversion system. Some subjects do not name letters accurately, reducing the chances of accurate identification of the word.

Although it is generally assumed that the meaning of the written words cannot be accessed until the written word has been identified, usually by naming it aloud, some studies have suggested that word meaning is available at an implicit level, virtually as soon as the word is presented and a good time before the word can be named (e.g. Shallice & Saffran, 1986).

Theoretical accounts of pure alexia vary in detail. Warrington and Shallice (1980) suggest that the lexicon of written word forms is damaged, forcing the subject to identify each letter by its spoken letter name and to then use the letter names to access the spelling system. Patterson and Kay (1982) suggest that the problem lies with mapping letters in parallel on to the store of written word forms used for reading. To compensate for this difficulty, subjects use letter names to access the reading lexicon by another route. (It is important to note that these contrasting theories are based on a theory of independent lexicons for reading and spelling, a theoretical view which has not been discussed in this chapter, but is widely held.) Patterson and Kay (1982) propose that, when subjects with pure alexia produce regularization errors, the word form system is damaged also. When this occurs, knowledge of the letter identities is used to access the sublexical grapheme–phoneme conversion processes which produce regularized pronunciations of irregular words.

REMEDIATION STUDIES

Key papers for remediating deep dyslexia: de Partz (1986) and Nickels (1992); and for surface dysgraphia: de Partz, Seron and Van der Linden (1992).

Several successful attempts have been made to remediate acquired disorders of reading and spelling. A case of deep dyslexia in a French subject was successfully treated by teaching him a new set of grapheme–phoneme correspondences based on letter-sound correspondences extracted from imageable words that he could pronounce. Using this technique, the subject was able to pronounce most written words successfully and so translate written text into spoken text which he could then understand. A further French subject with surface dyslexia who spelled using phonic methods was taught to remember particular letters in irregular words by an imagery strategy. For example, the silent letter H in the French word 'pathologie' was extended into a picture of a bed with a patient lying on it. These techniques are laborious but merited by the successful restoration of reading and spelling in some individuals.

POSTSCRIPT

In this short chapter it has been impossible to do justice to the wide range of papers that have contributed to the present level of expertise in the assessment of dyslexia and dysgraphia. Nor has it been possible to do justice to the niceties of the differences between theoretical accounts of these disorders which, in most cases, have been finessed. Research in this area continues vigorously, and for those interested in pursuing this field, the following texts are recommended for further reading.

FURTHER READING

Ellis, A.W. & Young, A.W. (1996). *Human cognitive neuropsychology: a textbook with readings.* Hove: LEA.

Coltheart, M., Curtis, B., Atkins, P. & Haller, M. (1993). Models of reading aloud: dual-route and parallel-distributed-processing approaches. *Psychological Review*, **100**, 589–608.

Parkin, A. (1996). *Explorations in cognitive neuropsychology.* Oxford: Blackwells.

Plaut, D.C., McClelland, J.L, Seidenberg, M.S. & Patterson, K. (1996). Understanding normal and impaired word reading: computational principles in quasi-regular domains. *Psychological review*, **103**, 56–115.

Shallice, T. (1988). *From neuropsychology to mental structure.* New York: Cambridge University Press.

REFERENCES

Allport, D.A. & Funnell, E. (1981). Components of the mental lexicon. *Philosophical Transactions of the Royal Society of London*, **B295**, 397–410.

Beauvois, M-F. & Derouesne, J. (1979). Phonological alexia: Three dissociations. *Journal of Neurology, Neurosurgery and Psychiatry*, **42**, 1115–24.

Beauvois, M-F. & Derouesne, J. (1981). Lexical or orthographic alexia. *Brain*, **104**, 21–49.

Bub, D. & Kertesz, A. (1982). Deep agraphia. *Brain and Language*, **17**, 146–65.

Bub, D., Cancelliere, A. & Kertesz, A. (1985). Whole-word and analytic translation of spelling to sound in a non-semantic reader. In K.E. Patterson, J.C. Marshall and M. Coltheart (Eds.). *Surface dyslexia.* London: LEA.

Coltheart, M. (1982). The psycholinguistic analysis of acquired dyslexias: some illustrations. *Philosophical Transactions of the Royal Society of London*, **B298**, 151–64.

Coltheart, M. (1987). Deep dyslexia: a right hemisphere hypothesis. In M. Coltheart, K.E. Patterson & J.C. Marshall (Eds.). *Deep dyslexia.* 2nd edn. London: RKP.

Coltheart, M. & Funnell, E. (1987). Reading and writing: one lexicon or two? In A. Allport, D. MacKay, W. Prinz & E. Scheerer (Eds.). *Language perception and production.* London: AP.

Coltheart, M., Patterson, K.E. & Marshall, J.C. (1987). *Deep Dyslexia.* 2nd edn. London: Routledge and Kegan Paul.

Coslett, B. (1991). Read but not write 'idea': evidence for a third reading mechanism. *Brain and Language*, **40**, 425–43.

de Partz, M-P., (1986). Re-education of a deep dyslexic patient: rationale of the method and results. *Cognitive Neuropsychology*, **3**, 149–78.

de Partz, M-P., Seron, X. & Van der Linden, M. (1992). Re-education of a surface dysgraphic with a visual imagery strategy. *Cognitive Neuropsychology*, **9**, 369–402.

Ellis, A.W. (1993). *Reading, writing and dyslexia.* 2nd edn. Hove: LEA.

Funnell, E. (1983). Phonological processes in reading: new evidence from acquired dyslexia. *British Journal of Psychology*, **74**, 159–80.

Funnell, E. (1987). Morphological errors in acquired dyslexia: a case of mistaken identity. *Quarterly Journal of Experimental Psychology*, **39A**, 497–539.

Hatfield, F. & Patterson, K.E. (1983). Phonological spelling. *Quarterly Journal of Experimental Psychology*, **35A**, 451–68.

Kucera & Francis (1967). *Computational analysis of present-day American English.* Providence, Rhode Island: Brown University Press.

Marshall, J.C. & Newcombe, F. (1966). Syntactic and semantic errors in paralexia. *Neuropsychologia*, **4**, 169–76.

Marshall, J.C. & Newcombe, F. (1973). Patterns of paralexia: a psycholinguistic approach. *Journal of Psycholinguistic Research*, **2**, 175–99.

Morton, J. & Patterson, K.E. (1987). A new attempt at an interpretation, or, an attempt at a new interpretation. In M. Coltheart, K.E. Patterson & J.C. Marshall (Eds.). *Deep dyslexia.* 2nd edn. London: RKP.

Nickels, L. (1992). The autocue? Self-generated phonemic cues in the treatment of a disorder of reading and naming. *Cognitive Neuropsychology*, **9**, 155–82.

Paivio, A., Yuille, J.C. & Madigan, S.A. (1968). Concreteness, imagery and meaningfulness values for 925 nouns. *Journal of Experimental Psychology, Monograph Supplement*, **76**, 2–25.

Patterson, K.E. & Kay, J. (1982). Letter by letter reading: psychological descriptions of a neurological syndrome. *Quarterly Journal of Experimental Psychology*, **34A**, 411–41.

Patterson, K.E., Marshall, J.C. & Coltheart, M. (1985). *Surface dyslexia.* London: LEA.

Patterson, K.E. Seidenberg, M.S. & McClelland, J.L. (1989). Connections and disconnections: acquired dyslexia in a computational model of reading processes. In R.G.M. Morris (Ed.). *Parallel distributed processing: implications for psychology and neuroscience.* London: OUP.

Plaut, D. & Shallice. (1993). Deep dyslexia: a case study of connectionist neuropsychology. *Cognitive Neuropsychology*, **10**, 377–500.

Shallice, T. (1981). Phonological agraphia and the lexical route in writing. *Brain*, **104**, 413–29.

Shallice T. (1988). *From neuropsychology to mental structure.* New York: Cambridge University Press.

Shallice, T. & Saffran, E. (1986). Lexical processing in the absence of explicit word identification: evidence from a letter-by-letter reader. *Cognitive Neuropsychology*, **3**, 429–58.

Shallice, T. & Warrington, E.K. (1987). Single and multiple component ventral dyslexic syndromes. In M. Coltheart, K.E. Patterson & J.C. Marshall (Eds.). *Deep dyslexia.* 2nd edn. London: RKP.

Walsh, K.W. (1978). *Neuropsychology: a clinical approach.* Edinburgh: Churchill Livingstone.

Warrington, K.E. & Shallice, T. (1980). Word-form dyslexia. *Brain*, **103**, 829–53.

Dysmorphology and facial disfigurement

NICHOLA RUMSEY

Faculty of Applied Sciences, Department of Psychology, University of the West of England, Bristol, UK

DYSMORPHOLOGY

Definition and typical features

The term dysmorphobia comes from *dysmorfia*, a Greek work meaning ugliness, specifically of the face. In body dysmorphic disorder (BDD), the sufferer is considered to have a grossly exaggerated impression of a deformity. The deformity is felt to be unbearably ugly, and is regarded with loathing, repugnance and shame (Birtchnell, 1988). Typical behaviours include frequent mirror checking (though some avoid mirrors altogether), avoidance of social situations, excessive checking of appearance and the existence of severe psychological distress. The exact prevalence of BDD is unknown. Some claim it to be uncommon, though Thompson (1990) believes that numbers are on the increase due to the current emphasis in society on the body beautiful and the resulting high levels of dissatisfaction with appearance in the general population. The age of onset is typically from early adolescence though to the late 20s. It affects a ratio of three women to one man (Phillips, 1991).

Treatment decisions

Uncertainty about the aetiology of BDD is reflected in the diversity of recommendations for treatment, which include medication, psychotherapy, behavioural therapy and cosmetic surgery (Sheridan & Radmacher, 1992). In the first instance, people suffering from BDD will probably approach a plastic surgeon, oral surgeon or dermatologist for treatment. This highlights the need for collaboration and skilful assessment of psychological factors involved in requests for surgery. Expectations of outcome are often unrealistic, and surgery (if performed) is often seen as unsuccessful, leading to further requests for operations, or the shifting of dissatisfaction to another part of the body. The consensus in the literature is to avoid surgical intervention, referring sufferers instead for psychiatric assessment and treatment.

FACIAL DISFIGUREMENT

Introduction

The OPCS (1988/1989) defined a disfigured person as someone who 'suffers from a scar, blemish or deformity which severely affects (their) ability to lead a normal life'. Macgregor (1990) has described facial disfigurement as a 'psychological and social death'. The OPCS statistics suggest that 10% of the population have some kind of facial disfigurement.

The importance of the face in social interaction has long been recognized in the academic disciplines of psychology, history and anthropology. In a society which places a high premium on physical attractiveness and 'wholeness', it is not surprising that a sizeable research literature attests to the benefits of having a physically attractive facial appearance. When compared to the first impressions formed of those with an unattractive facial appearance, good-looking people are perceived to be more intelligent, popular, honest and socially desirable. Research also indicates that attractiveness is positively related to expectation of future success, happiness and marital satisfaction (Bull & Rumsey, 1988). Relatively little research and funding has been devoted to examining the effects of having an unattractive or disfigured facial appearance. However, common themes emerge from the research and writings that are available.

Problems experienced by disfigured people

Facial disfigurement can have far-reaching psychosocial consequences. The most common problems experienced by those with facial disfigurements (including cleft lip, burns, birthmarks, dermatological conditions, unattractive teeth, etc) concern difficulties in social interaction (Bull & Rumsey, 1988). First encounters are particularly problematic, and visibly disfigured people report difficulties in situations such as meeting new people, making friends, developing relationships and succeeding in job interviews. Problems are particularly apparent at times of change, for example, moving house, starting at a new school, or beginning a new job.

For children and adolescents, the majority of problems focus on teasing by others, on fear of going to new places, and on problems associated with negative feelings about the self (Bradbury, 1993). Disfigurements in children do not result in any identifiable personality pattern, in reports of delinquency, raised incidence of bad behaviour or lack of educational success. Lansdown (1990) and others believe, however, that problems in adolescence and adulthood are underreported, as most data is collected in response to questions asked in medical settings, when the atmosphere is frequently not conducive to open discussion of social and psychological issues. Life is likely to be appreciably harder for those with a face which is out of the ordinary.

Many disfigured people attribute the problems they experience to the negative reactions of others, complaining that they are avoided or rejected by the general public. Studies of the process of social interaction have shown that avoidance does occur. In addition, those people who do engage in interaction tend to stand further away from a disfigured person than from a non-disfigured one, and make less frequent eye contact during the interaction (Bull &

Rumsey, 1988). However, this avoidance is not necessarily the result of 'rejection'. A first encounter with a facially disfigured person is potentially problematic, as the normal rules of social interaction may not apply. The disfigured person's capacity to communicate may be impaired and the other party may be concerned that conventional patterns of non-verbal communication may be misconstrued (for example, that the disfigured person might interpret eye contact as staring). Avoidance may be preferable to the risk of embarrassment for either or both parties.

The behaviour of facially disfigured people themselves may play a part in the problems encountered during social interaction (Bull & Rumsey, 1988). Many disfigured people become preoccupied with their appearance and the effect it may have on others. Anticipating negative reactions from others, they may adopt a shy or defensive interaction style (Macgregor, 1990), increasing the likelihood of negative reactions from others.

Factors playing a part in adjustment

When assessing levels of psychological distress, the aetiology of the disfigurement (for example, congenital, disease, or trauma related) should be considered. Complicating factors in relation to aetiology include feelings of blame, anger, or stigmatization and whether any compensation claims are involved. Adjustment is also linked to prognosis, whether temporary (for example, acne) recurring (as in dermatological conditions), progressive, or linked to the treatment of potentially life-threatening condition such as cancer. For many, an assessment of predisfigurement levels of facial attractiveness, pre-existing repertoires of coping and skills, and levels of self-esteem are important. These factors play a part both in the initial impact of a disfigurement and in later adjustment (Partridge, 1990).

Some researchers have tried to equate the level of disfiguration (for example, mild, moderate or severe) to levels of psychological distress. Research has consistently shown that there is no relationship between these variables.

Tackling problems associated with facial disfigurement

The assumption underlying treatment offered within the NHS is that improvements in the physical appearance of disfigured people will reduce psychological distress and improve quality of life. (See also 'Plastic surgery'.) However, the problems experienced by facially disfigured people are social and psychological in nature and, although changes in appearance may be beneficial for many, they rarely provide the complete answer. Wallace and Lees (1988) found that 30–40% of adult burns patients and 75% of burned children were suffering from severe psychological problems up to two years after injury. None were receiving any professional help.

In the past, disfigured people and researchers alike have discussed the desirability of changing society's bias towards physical attractiveness and 'wholeness', removing the stigma associated with visible disfigurement. Experience in other areas (for example, racial prejudice), highlights the slow and laborious nature of attitude change. More immediate solutions are clearly needed to the problems experienced by disfigured people. The potential benefits of offering psychological interventions and support would seem to be considerable for the facially disfigured person, the family and occasionally, the staff delivering care. Interventions are likely to be particularly appropriate at key points.

The birth of a disfigured child

The reaction to the birth of a congenitally deformed child has been likened to a shock to the family system akin to a bereavement reaction. Parents typically experience a variety of emotions including grief, anxiety, frustration, guilt, hurt, resentment, and shock (Lansdown, 1990). The sensitive handling of the birth itself is essential, as is the provision of appropriate support immediately after the birth and in the weeks following discharge from hospital.

The development of disfigured children

Bradbury (1993) has advocated psychosocial interventions designed to tackle the problems faced by disfigured children (for example, play therapy; the teaching of skills to deal effectively with teasing). The family environment is of crucial importance to the well-being and support of disfigured people at all stages of development. Disfigured children (and adults) will have better prospects in a family that shows little concern for the role of physical appearance in a successful and fulfilling life. If the family is supportive and encourages expertise in other areas, then the child will be more likely to develop a positive self-image (Lansdown, 1990). Interventions may be necessary to tackle communication difficulties within families. Children may not want to hurt their parents by talking openly about their problems, and parents may feel that a cheerful exterior should be preserved at all costs. Families may need support in making treatment decisions, for example, the timing of hospitalization. Siblings may be the casualties of extra time, effort and attention devoted to the disfigured child. For many of these problems, supportive listening and empathy may suffice. Other family issues are more complex, requiring professional intervention.

Psychological interventions and dermatological conditions

Although the mechanisms are not clear, psychological distress is acknowledged to play a part in some skin diseases. In some cases, suggestion, with or without hypnosis, has been shown to produce palpable modifications of skin diseases. Grossbart and Sherman (1986) found the concept of a 'cellular battle' (in which healing forces are imagined to attack and overwhelm the skin disease) to produce beneficial results. Brown & Fromm (1987) have reviewed treatment methods for a range of diseases, including acne, psoriasis, eczema and virus-mediated diseases. Although psychological interventions have been useful in each of these, the majority of studies are case studies or small samples, with most lacking adequate controls.

Social interaction skills training

As many of the problems associated with facial disfigurement are associated with social interaction, attention has recently been focused on the technique of social interaction skills training. This has been shown to improve the quality of life for various groups with similar problems, for example, shyness and social phobia (Wlazlo et al., 1990). Evaluations of social interaction skills workshops for disfigured people currently offered by the charity 'Changing Faces' indicate that, if facially disfigured people can be taught to understand the reactions of others and can develop a repertoire of more positive social skills (for example, skills to put the other party at ease), then their social anxiety will reduce and the quality of social interaction will be markedly improved (Robinson, Rumsey & Partridge, 1996).

CONCLUSION

Facial disfigurement can have far-reaching social and psychological consequences. To date, insufficient resources have been devoted either to exploring the pressures and problems resulting from the broader social and psychological context in which the disfigured person is functioning or to the development and application of psychosocial interventions.

REFERENCES

Birtchnell, S. (1988). Dysmorphobia: a centenary discussion. *British Journal of Psychiatry*, 153, 41–3.

Bradbury, E. (1993). Psychological approaches to children and adolescents with disfigurement: a review of the literature. *ACPA Review*, 15, 1–6.

Brown, D. & Fromm, E. (1987). *Hypnosis and behavioral medicine*. Hillsdale NJ: Lawrence Erlbaum.

Bull, R. & Rumsey, N. (1988). *The social psychology of facial appearance*. New York: Springer Verlag.

Grossbart, T. & Sherman, C. (1986). *Skin deep: a mind/body program for healthy skin*. New York: William Morrow.

Lansdown, R. (1990). Psychological problems of patients with cleft lip and palate: a discussion paper. *Journal of the Royal Society of Medicine*, 83, 448–50.

Macgregor, F. (1990). Facial disfigurement: problems and management of social interaction and implications for mental health. *Aesthetic Plastic Surgery*, 14, 249–57.

Office of Population Censuses and Surveys. (1988/1989). *The disability survey*. OPCS.

Partridge, J. (1990). *Changing faces: the challenge of facial disfigurement*. Harmondsworth: Penguin.

Phillips, K. (1991). Body dysmorphic disorder: the distress of imagined ugliness. *American Journal of Psychiatry*, 148, 1138–49.

Robinson, E., Rumsey, N. & Partridge, J. (1996). An evaluation of the impact of social interaction skills training for facially disfigured people. *British Journal of Plastic Surgery*, 49, 281–9.

Sheridan, C. & Radmacher, S. (1992). *Health psychology: Challenging the biomedical model*. New York: Wiley.

Thompson, K. (1990). Refacing inmates: a critical appraisal of plastic surgery programs in prison. *Criminal Justice and Behavior*, 17, 448–66.

Wallace, L. & Lees, J. (1988). A psychological follow up study of adult patients discharged from a British burn unit. *Burns*, 14, 39–45.

Wlazlo, Z., Schroeder, H., Hand, I., Kaiser, G. & Munchau, N. (1990). Exposure *in vivo* vs. social skills training for social phobia: long-term outcome and differential effects. *Behavioural Research and Therapy*, 28, 181–93.

Encopresis

HILTON DAVIS

Bloomfield Clinic, Guy's Hospital, UK

DEFINITION

The *DSM-III-R* (1987) defines encopresis as the: 'repeated involuntary (or, much more rarely, intentional) passage of faeces into places not appropriate for that purpose'. The diagnosis requires a frequency of at least once a month for 6 months, in the absence of physical causes, and in a child more than 4 years old.

Primary and secondary enuresis are discriminated, with the latter involving a 12-month period of continence. More useful categories, however, are those of Hersov (1985): (i) adequate bowel control with voluntary defaecation in inappropriate places; (ii) inadequate control with or without awareness; and (iii) soiling because of excessive fluid, most commonly associated with diarrhoea, or constipation with overflow.

PREVALENCE

Approximately 1.5% of 7–8 year olds (Bellman, 1966) have encopresis, reducing to about 0.8% by 10–12 years (Rutter, Tizard & Whitmore, 1970). Three times as many boys as girls show the problem, which most commonly occurs during the day.

AETIOLOGY

A complex interaction of psychological, social and physical factors are likely to be operating in any particular case. Established bowel control may break down in circumstances of acute stress (e.g. separation from parents, birth of sibling), or longer-term stress (e.g. marital dysharmony or punitive child care including coersive training). Inadequate control may be associated with intellectual disability, but it may also occur with other psychological problems such as enuresis, academic difficulties, and aggressive behaviour. A disadvantaged family background and neglectful training have also been implicated in causation.

Soiling associated with excessive faecal fluid may occur because of diarrhoea induced by severe anxiety. Overflow soiling involving severe constipation may be the result of past painful defaecation (e.g. because of an anal fissure), but has also been related to parent–child conflict over toileting, coersive training, and fears of the toilet. A high rate of abnormal anal functioning is found in these children (Loening-Baucke, 1987), and is predictive of poor outcome.

Although parental behaviour is implicated in the development of encopresis, no clear pattern discriminates between the development of encitem and other symptoms, and in any single case, it is difficult to know whether psychological problems are associated, causal or secondary.

TREATMENT
Depending upon careful physical and psychological assessment, including the family context, intervention often involves counselling work with the parents and child, to defuse emotion, to institute alternative training methods, or reduce toiletting fears. Behavioural methods, including contingent reinforcement, also have a large part to play (Davis, Mitchell & Marks, 1976). Initial bowel evacuation and subsequent laxative and stool softening treatment may be needed in faecal retention. Although good results have been claimed, for example, a 78% success rate by Levine and Bakow (1976), few adequate studies are available.

REFERENCES
American Psychiatric Association (1987). *Diagnostic and statistical manual of mental disorders* (3rd ed. revised). Washington, DC: American Psychiatric Association Press.

Bellman, M. (1966). Studies on encopresis. *Acta Paediatrica Scandinavica*, Suppl. **170**.

Davis, H., Mitchell, W. & Marks, F. (1976). A behavioural programme for the modification of encopresis. *Child: Care, Health and Development*, **2**, 273–82.

Hersov, L. (1985). Faecal soiling. In M. Rutter & L. Hersov (Eds). *Child and adolescent psychiatry: modern approaches*. London: Blackwell Scientific Publications.

Levine, M. & Bakow, H. (1976). Children with encopresis: a study of treatment outcome. *Paediatrics*, **58**, 845–52.

Loening-Baucke, V. (1987). Factors responsible for persistence of childhood constipation. *Journal of Pediatric Gastroenterology and Nutrition*, **6**, 915–22.

Rutter, M., Tizard, J. & Whitmore, K. (1970). *Education, health and behaviour*. London: Longman.

Endoscopy and bronchoscopy

JEAN E. JOHNSON
School of Nursing University of Rochester
Rochester, NY, USA

Gastroendoscopy and bronchoscopy provoke negative psychological reactions in a large proportion of patients. There has been more attention, as indicated by the amount of literature, on psychological aspects of gastroendoscopy than of bronchoscopy. Because the medical management and patient's experience during the two procedures have much in common, the research on psychological reactions to endoscopy is probably applicable to bronchoscopy. With the advent of flexible instruments, there has been a large increase in the number of endoscopy procedures performed. Conscious sedation is widely used, which causes the patient to have amnaesia for the experience, but about 20% of the patients who are sedated display distress during the procedure (Thompson *et al.*, 1980). Behaviours stimulated by distress during the examination can contribute to a less than optimum examination and have been shown to be associated with cardiac complications (Segawa *et al.*, 1989).

ORIGINAL STUDIES
The first tests of psychological methods for reducing patients' reactions to endoscopy were two randomized clinical trials (Johnson & Leventhal, 1974; Johnson, Morrissey & Leventhal, 1973). It was hypothesized that reduction in discrepancy between the patient's experience during the endoscopy and prior expectations would reduce negative psychological responses. To reduce the discrepancy, patients were given a preparatory message consisting of descriptions of patients' physical sensory experience during the examination.

In the first study (Johnson & Leventhal, 1974), patients were randomly assigned to one of three preparatory groups. The groups were (i) descriptions of the sensations typically experienced, (ii) instruction in behaviours believed to facilitate the passage of the tube, (iii) a combination of the two messages, and (iv) a control condition. The information for the first three groups was audiotape recorded and patients listened to the tapes the evening prior to the endoscopy. The sensory information message focused on the patient's concrete physical sensations and experiences. For example, it included descriptions of what was felt, seen, tasted, smelled, and heard (e.g. a needle stick, drowsiness, and fullness when air was pumped into the stomach) and positions and behaviours asked of patients. The message was accompanied by a booklet of 11 photographs illustrating the environment and equipment. The instruction message instructed patients in rapid panting mouth breathing and swallowing motions to facilitate tube passage which patients practised. The control condition consisted of the usual care provided to all patients in the clinic. The physicians involved in the examination and the observer of patients' behaviour were uninformed about the content of the messages or patients' group assignment.

The sensory information was the most effective preparatory message. That group received significantly fewer milligrams of tranquillizer (for patients under 50 years of age) and fewer patients gagged during tube passage as compared to the control group. There were no significant differences between the behavioural instruction group and the control group. However, the group who received a

[453]

combination of sensory information and behavioural instruction were less apt to gag but required significantly longer time for tube passage as compared to the control group. The prolonged time for tube passage was believed to have occurred because the patients in the combined information group attended to the reflexive-like act which slowed and exaggerated the performance.

A second study was conducted in the same setting, using methods similar to those used in the first study (Johnson, et al., 1973). Because, in the first study, behavioural instruction was not effective, it was not included in the second study. A description of the procedure of the examination was used.

Consistent with the results of the first study, the sensory information group required less diazepam and displayed less tension during tube passage as compared to the control group. The patients who received the description of the examination procedure also required less diazepam than the control group. However, they were more restless during the examination than the sensory information group.

The results of these two carefully controlled clinical trials provide strong support for the conclusion that sensory preparatory information reduces the amount of diazepam required for sedation and the distress behaviours that can impede the examination.

LATER STUDIES

Shipley and colleagues have studied how the amount of exposure to preparatory information interacts with repressing and sensitizing coping style (Shipley, Butt & Horwitz, 1979; Shipley et al., 1978). Sensitizers typically seek information and repressors avoid information about a stressor. An 18-minute videotape of a male patient undergoing an endoscopy was shown to patients either not at all, one time, or three times on the evening prior to the examination. Although there were some differences in the results of the two studies, overall sensitizers displayed less distress behaviours and heart-rate increase with each exposure to the videotape. The effects for repressors were less straightforward with little evidence that they benefited from the information, and some suggestion that one exposure to the information may have increased arousal. Shipley recommended that repressors not be provided preparatory information; however, the recommendation was based on findings from exposure to a large amount of information without consideration of its content.

Wilson and colleagues (Wilson, et al., 1982) also studied the influence of coping styles on the effectiveness of information and instruction in relaxation on emotional reactions to endoscopy. The patients in the information condition listened to a audiotaped message, similar in content to that used by Johnson. The relaxation group listened to an introduction to relaxation training, followed by a 20-minute practice session.

Similar to the results of the studies by Johnson, the description of the sensory experience group had less distress during insertion of the endoscope, smaller increases in heart rate during tube insertion, and less insertion failure as compared to the control group. In addition, 71% of the patients in the sensory information group indicated that they would want to be informed in future hospital experiences as compared to 40% of the patients who did not receive the information.

Patients in the relaxation group showed less distress during tube insertion, had lower heart rate increases during tube insertion, had fewer severe problems with insertion, and reported greater positive mood after the endoscopy than did control patients.

Analysis that included individual difference variables showed several results that support the hypothesis that congruency between the patient's coping style and intervention is the most effective. For example, patients who tend to prefer avoidant-type coping exhibited low distress when they were trained in relaxation and patients who were low in avoidance showed best result when they received sensory information. Relaxation was also the most effective for patients who were high in fear prior to the examination. However, there was no evidence that patients were harmed when they received an intervention that was incongruent with their coping style.

Levy et al. (1989) reports a study of the effect of detailed explanations and descriptions of endoscopy. The information interventions were similar to those used by Shipley in that the object was to give a detailed comprehensive description of all aspects of the procedure. Consistent with the studies by Shipley, there were no direct effects of detailed explanations and descriptions of the examination on self-report of anxiety.

CONCLUSIONS

The research shows that there are two preparatory interventions that reduced amount of sedation required and/or behaviours expressing distress that can impede an endoscopy and can contribute to complications. These benefits are clinically important even though conscious sedation causing amnaesia for the experience has become a widely accepted practice. Although ideal, tailoring psychological interventions to each patient's coping style would be burdensome. A feasible alternative is to use preparatory interventions that may be especially effective for only some patients and are less effective, but not harmful, to others.

The intervention that has had the most support from research, and has been incorporated into the care routines in some endoscopy clinics, is preparatory information consisting of a description of the typical physical sensations and objective experiences. Advantages of this intervention are the short amount of time required to provide the information which makes it compatible with clinical schedules (in the original studies the tape recording was $7\frac{1}{2}$ minutes long) and that it has high patient acceptability. The effectiveness of the intervention in a number of other patient populations has been demonstrated (e.g. Johnson, Lauver & Nail, 1989), which lends further support for the usefulness of the intervention. The theory has evolved and it is no longer believed that the effect of the intervention is due to a reduction in discrepancy between expectation and experience. Rather, it is hypothesized that the intervention focuses patients' attention toward their objective experience and away from their emotional response to the experience. The intervention has been further defined as consisting of descriptions of the typical patient's objective experience which includes physical sensations, temporal dimensions, environmental characteristics including positions and behaviours expected of patients, and causes of sensations and events. Typical experience is that which at least 50% of the patients experience. Descriptions of aspects of the experience that are not likely to occur or that have no experiential reverent are not included. Descriptions of emotional responses and degree of discomforts are omitted because these descriptions focus patients attention toward those aspects of the experience and they are more likely to become emotionally aroused. Details about the characteristics of such interventions can be found in McHugh, Christman and Johnson (1982).

The other intervention that was found to be effective was instruction in systematic relaxation which also diverts attention from the emotional response. A disadvantage of that intervention is that patients must acquire some proficiency by practicing the relaxation activities. This intervention might best be used selectively for patients who are prone to focus on their emotional response and are expressing high levels of anxiety and concern about the examination.

REFERENCES

Johnson, J.E. & Leventhal, H. (1974). Effects of accurate expectations and behavioral instructions on reactions during a noxious medical examination. *Journal of Personality and Social Psychology*, **29**, 710–18.

Johnson, J.E., Morrissey, J.F. & Leventhal, H. (1973). Psychological preparation for an endoscopic examination. *Gastrointestinal Endoscopy*, **19**, 180–2.

Johnson, J.E., Lauver, D. & Nail, L.M. (1989). Process of coping with radiation therapy. *Journal of Consulting and Clinical Psychology*, **57**, 358–64.

Levy, N., Landmann, L., Stermer, E., Erdreich, M., Beny, A. & Meisels, R. (1989). Does a detailed explanation prior to gastroscopy reduce the patient's anxiety? *Endoscopy*, **21**, 263–5.

McHugh, N.G., Christman, N.J. & Johnson, J.E. (1982). Preparatory information: what helps and why. *American Journal of Nursing*, **82**, 780–2.

Segawa, K., Nakazawa, S. Yamao, K, Goto, H., Inui, K., Osada, T., Arisawa, T. & Ohta, T. (1989). Cardiac response to upper gastrointestinal endoscopy. *The American Journal of Gastroenterology*, **84**, 13–16.

Shipley, R.H., Butt, J.H., Horwitz, B. & Farbry, J.E. (1978). Preparation for a stressful medical procedure: effect of amount of stimulus preexposure and coping style. *Journal of Consulting and Clinical Psychology*, **46**, 499–507.

Shipley, R.H., Butt, J.H. & Horwitz, E.A. (1979). Preparation to reexperience a stressful medical examination: effect of repetitious videotape exposure and coping style. *Journal of Consulting and Clinical Psychology*, **47**, 485–92.

Thompson, D.G., Lennard-Jones, J.E., Evans, S.J., Cowan, R.E., Murray, R.S. & Wright, J.T. (1980). Patients appreciate premedication for endoscopy. *Lancet*, **ii**, 469–70.

Wilson, J.F., Moore, R.W., Randolph, S. & Hanson, B.J. (1982). Behavioral preparation of patients for gastrointestinal endoscopy: information, relaxation, and coping style. *Journal of Human Stress*, **8**, 13–23.

Enuresis

HILTON DAVIS

Bloomfield Clinic, Guy's Hospital, London, UK

DEFINITION

DSM-III-R (APA, 1987) defines enuresis as the 'repeated involuntary or intentional voiding of urine during the day or at night into bed or clothes, after an age at which continence is expected'. The diagnosis is not made where there are direct physical causes or before the age of 5 years, after which enuresis becomes more commonly associated with other behavioural problems. Primary and secondary enuresis are distinguished by the latter involving a significant period of continence prior to the onset of enuresis.

PREVALENCE

The prevalence of enuresis decreases with age, from about 18% at 7 years to 2.35% at 14 (Rutter, Yule & Graham, 1973). Jarvelin *et al.* (1988), using more stringent criteria, cite lower figures (9.8%) for 7 year-olds, of whom 1.8% were wet in the day, 6.4% at night, and 1.6% at both times, supporting the general finding that nocturnal enuresis is the most common. The problem is also more frequent in boys than girls in a ratio between 3 : 2 and 2 : 1.

AETIOLOGY

Whereas physical disorders (e.g. urinary tract infections) have been implicated in aetiology, only about 5% of children with enuresis have infections (Kunin, Zacha & Paquin, 1962), and the direction of causality is not clear. There is evidence of reduced functional bladder capacity, and a greater probability of developmental delay in children with enuresis (Mikkelsen, 1991). There is strong evidence for a genetic influence, with a seven times higher risk, if a parent has been enuretic (Jarvelin *et al.*, 1988). The notion that noctural enuresis results from excessively deep sleep has been disputed on the grounds that episodes are distributed through all sleep stages in proportion to the duration of each (Mikkelson *et al.*, 1980).

Enuresis is associated with other psychological disturbance in older children (Rutter, 1989), and with adverse environmental circumstances, including large, broken, impoverished or unhappy families (Shaffer, 1985).

Aetiology may be impossible to determine in individual cases, given the likelihood of a complex interaction between genetic, physical, psychological, and social factors, including the maturation and well-being of the child, the parent–child interaction, and specific training circumstances. Whatever the cause, enuresis itself may disturb the child or the parent–child interaction.

TREATMENT

Treatment should follow careful assessment of all aspects of the problem, documenting the exact nature of the disorder and associated difficulties, in the child, the family, and their interaction. Intervention should be individually tailored to address child, parent or family problems as necessary.

The most effective method for symptomatic treatment is the bell and pad (see also 'Incontinence'). Success rates in the region of 75% have been consistently found (e.g. Berg, Forsythe & McGuire, 1982). Simple reward systems (e.g. star charts) may also be effective, especially in decreasing relapse (Kaplan *et al.*, 1989). There is no evidence for the success of psychotherapy, nightlifting or fluid restriction, and retention control methods are equivocal. Drugs such as Imipramine may be effective, but the effects are short-lived, with relapse upon withdrawal (Mikkelsen, 1991).

REFERENCES

American Psychiatric Association (1987). *Diagnostic and statistical manual of mental disorders* (3rd edn. revised). Washington, DC: American Psychiatric Association Press.

Berg, I., Forsythe, I. & McGuire, R. (1982). Response of bedwetting to the enuresis alarm. *Archives of Disease in Childhood*, **57**, 394–6.

Jarvelin, M., Vikevainen-Tervonen, L., Moilanen, I., & Huttunen, N. (1988). Enuresis in seven-year-old children. *Acta Paediatrica Scandinavica*, **77**, 148–53.

Kaplan, S., Breit, M. Gauthier, B. & Busner, J. (1989). A comparison of three nocturnal enuresis treatment methods. *Journal of the American Academy of Child and Adolescent Psychiatry*, **28**, 282–6.

Kunin, C., Zacha, E. & Paquin, A. (1962). Urinary tract infections in school children: an epidemiologic, clinical and laboratory study. *New England Journal of Medicine*, **266**, 1287–96.

Mikkelsen, E. (1991). Modern approaches to enuresis and encopresis. In M. Lewis (Ed.). *Child and adolescent psychiatry: a comprehensive textbook*. Baltimore: Williams and Wilkins.

Mikkelsen, E., Rapoport, J., Nee, L., Gruenan, C., Mendelson, W. & Gillin, J. (1980). Childhood enuresis. I: sleep patterns and psychopathology. *Archives of General Psychiatry*, **37**, 1139–44.

Rutter, M. (1989). Isle of Wight revisited: twenty-five years of child psychiatric epidemiology. *Journal of the American Academy of Child and Adolescent Psychiatry*, **28**, 633–53.

Rutter, M., Yule, W. & Graham, P. (1973). Enuresis and behavioural deviance: some epidemiological considerations. In I. Kolvin, R. MacKeith & S. Meadows (Eds.). *Bladder control and enuresis. Clinics in developmental medicine*, Nos. 48/49, pp. 137–147. London: Heinemann/Spastics International Medical Publications.

Shaffer, D. (1985). Enuresis. In M. Rutter & L. Hersov (Eds.). *Child and adolescent psychiatry: modern approaches*. London: Blackwell Scientific Publications.

Epidemics

JAN STYGALL
Academic Department of Psychiatry and Behavioural Sciences, Middlesex and UCL, London, UK

An epidemic usually refers to a situation in which the incidence, generally of an infectious disease, has increased rapidly. Prior to the general acceptance of germ theory during the last century, epidemics were often regarded as the result of natural phenomena, especially astronomical mishaps. Krause (1994) suggests that epidemics usually occur because of changes in patterns of human behaviour, social organization, agriculture, and even medical practices but, most importantly, population movement.

Epidemics, which often have devastating effects, have been documented throughout history. For example, in the medieval period, the bubonic plague caused the death of a substantial proportion of the population of Europe and in the 1918–19 'Spanish flu' epidemic it was estimated that 20 million deaths occurred worldwide over a period of months. Medical advances have certainly helped the decrease in the number of epidemics, but it appears that the decline has resulted mainly from preventive measures such as improved personal hygiene and public health innovations. As most bacteria are resistant to one or more antibiotics, and some are resistant to all, prevention appears to be the key.

Hawkes and Hart (1993) argue that epidemics caused by transmissible pathogens are often seen as an imported problem. But, with the growth of international travel over the last 30 years it has become virtually impossible to prevent the spread of infectious diseases across international boundaries. Hawkes and Hart reviewed studies within the HIV/AIDS context that described or investigated risk behaviours of travellers and they highlighted the paucity of research conducted with 'holiday-makers' travelling abroad. A review of the literature found that very little research has been conducted in the area of health related behaviour and travelling in general. Coole, Wiselka and Nicholson (1989) has conducted one of the few studies, they found that people travelling to high risk areas, such as places where malaria is prevalent, have been found not to take adequate prophylaxis, some do not even seek advice. As discussed, it appears that one of the main factors in the emergence of epidemics is population movement, it is therefore extremely important that the attitudes and perceptions of travellers should be studied further.

Immunizations have been among the most successful of preventative interventions for various diseases. However, concern exists in the US that recent epidemics of vaccine preventable diseases and low rates of childhood immunizations may signal the existence of major underlying problems in immunization policy (See 'Immunization'). In the UK, in order to prevent influenza epidemics, vaccinations are offered to those at risk each year. Connolly *et al.* (1993) suggest the vaccination rate in patients at high risk of influenza is poor despite good evidence of vaccine efficacy. The reasons for low vaccination rates are thought to include a poor perception of the potential severity of influenza, concern over vaccine efficacy and possible adverse effects, and the logistics of targeting people at high risk.

AIDS has proved to be a major international epidemic, it is not a disease in the strict biomedical sense but a syndrome. In 1986, Mann (cited in Frankenberg, 1989) argued that AIDS is not one, but three separate, even though related, epidemics of (i) HIV infection, (ii) AIDS and (iii) social reaction to the syndrome. Gilmore and Somerville (1994) elaborate this argument further in suggesting that there are multiple epidemics of HIV, fear, stigmatization, scapegoating and discrimination associated with AIDS. Chliaoutakis *et al.* (1993) conducted a study in Greece among 16–49 year–olds and identified three attitudinal categories: discrimination, stigmatization and fear of those affected by AIDS.

Every epidemic arouses fear but, when the illness is life-threatening, people appear to react in extreme ways to protect themselves and those near to them. Many studies in health psychology and health promotion have shown that health-related behaviour is not based solely on knowledge but is an interplay of knowledge, attitudes and beliefs. Irrational responses to patients with AIDS and HIV have often been reported and likened to those of other historical epidemics such as plague. Wholesale segregation and blaming of selected populations was common in the Middle Ages as a consequence of the Black Death and the bubonic plague. Swenson (1988) suggests the outbreaks of the influenza epidemics occurring in the US and Western Europe in the twentieth century resulted initially in high levels of denial, which progressed to blame, among the western countries. These responses developed into derogatory exchanges among the nations. Studies have shown that, when this segregation occurs, people often feel they are not at risk of infection and, as a result, are less likely to protect themselves and others (e.g. Trezza, 1994; Elliott, Parida & Gruer, 1992). Recent studies on cross-cultural medical perspectives of AIDS (Sutherland, 1994; Feldman, 1992) suggest that global epidemics such as AIDS require both an international response and a local community understanding.

REFERENCES

Chliaoutakis, J., Socrataki, F., Darviri, C. Gousgounis, N. & Trakas, D. (1993). knowledge and attitudes about AIDS of residents of greater Athens. *Social Science and Medicine*, 37, 77–83.

Connolly, A.M., Salmon, R.L., Lervy, B. & Williams, D.H. (1993). What are the complications of influenza and can they be prevented? Lessons from the 1989 epidemic of H3N2 influenza A in general practice. *British Medical Journal*, 306, 1452–4.

Coole, L., Wiselka, M.J. & Nicholson K.G. (1989). Malaria prophylaxis in travellers from Britain. *Journal of Infections*, 18, 209–12.

Elliott, L., Parida, S, K. & Gruer, L. (1992). Differences in HIV-related knowledge and attitudes between Caucasian and 'Asian' men in Glasgow. *AIDS Care*, 4, 389–93.

Feldman, J. (1992). The French are different. French and American medicine in the context of AIDS. *Western Journal. Medicine*, 157, 345–9.

Frankenberg, R. (1989) One epidemic or three? Cultural, social and historical aspects of the AIDS pandemic. In P. Aggleton, G. Hart and P. Davies (Eds.). *AIDS: social representations, social practices.* London: Falmer Press.

Gilmore, N. & Somerville, M.A. (1994). Stigmatization, scapegoating and discrimination in sexually transmitted diseases: overcoming the 'them' and 'us'. *Social Science and Medicine*, 39, 1339–58.

Hawkes, S.J. & Hart, G.J. (1993). Travel, migration and HIV. *AIDS Care*, 5, 207–14.

Krause, R.M. (1994). Dynamics of emergence. *Journal of Infections Disease*, 170, 265–71.

Sutherland, D.C. (1994). HIV – Australasian experience. Current status of HIV infection in Australasia. *Annals of the Royal Australasian College of Dental Surgeons*, 12, 94–100.

Swenson, R.M. (1988). Plagues, history, and AIDS. *The American Scholar*, 57, 183–200.

Trezza, G.R. (1994). HIV knowledge and stigmatization of persons with AIDS: Implications for development of HIV education for young adults. *Professional Psychology Research and Practice*, 25, 141–8.

Epilepsy

GRAHAM SCAMBLER

Unit of Sociology, Department of Psychiatry and Behavioural Sciences, University College London Medical School, UK

DEFINITION AND PREVALENCE

An epileptic seizure is the product of an abnormal paroxysmal discharge of cerebral neurones, and epilepsy is sometimes defined as a continuing tendency to epileptic seizures. Seizures may take a number of different forms, depending on the site of the neuronal discharge in the brain. There are as many causes of epilepsy as there are seizure types. Rare genetic disorders like Tay–Sachs disease, congenital malformations, anoxia, trauma, brain tumours, infectious diseases, acquired metabolic diseases, degenerative disorders and chronic alcoholism can all lead to epilepsy. It also seems that a low convulsive threshold can be inherited.

If the neuronal discharge remains confined to one part of the brain, the resultant seizure is described as 'partial'. If the discharge begins in one part of the brain but subsequently spreads to all parts, the seizure is said to be 'partial with secondary generalization'. Sometimes the abnormal discharge originates in the mesodiencephalic system and spreads more or less simultaneously to all parts of the brain, in which case the reference is to a 'primary generalized' seizure. Since it is generally understood that all partial seizures arise from some focal area of structural abnormality in the brain, all partial seizures, plus those seizures which are secondarily generalized from some focal onset, can be described as 'symptomatic epilepsy'. Primary generalized epilepsy is never symptomatic of underlying structural brain damage, and can thus be described as 'idiopathic epilepsy'.

Epileptic seizures and epilepsy are more common than many realize. According to current estimates, approximately one in 40 people will experience two or more non-febrile seizures at some time, and one in 200 people will experience chronic epilepsy (Duncan, 1991). Epilepsy is the second most common reason, after headaches/migraine, for consulting a neurologist in Britain (Hopkins, Menken & Defriesse, 1989). Treatment is typically by antiepileptic drugs and early remission is achieved in 70–80% of cases (Annegers *et al.*, 1979).

SOCIAL AND PSYCHOLOGICAL SEQUELAE OF EPILEPSY

It has been estimated that approximately 1:3 people with epilepsy experience difficulties in addition to the physical impact of their epilepsy, including cognitive and psychosocial problems (McGuire & Trimble, 1990). Herman and Whitman (1986) have assessed the evidence for causal linkages between sets of 'neuroepilepsy' 'medication' and 'psychosocial' variables and psychiatric or psychological impairment. Those variables they define as 'high risk' for impairment are listed in Table 1.

Predictably, more research has been invested in the putative significance of neuroepilepsy and medication variables in this context than in that of psychosocial variables. This is ironic both because of the disappointing return to date on this investment and because of the *prima facie* plausibility of causal links between psychosocial variables and impairment. It is to the more significant of these relatively neglected variables, and to their general relevance for coping with epilepsy, that we now turn. They can be discussed under four key headings.

Professional care

It is the physician who is empowered to make the diagnosis of epilepsy and to apply the diagnostic label. But to communicate a diagnosis of epilepsy is to transform a 'normal person' into 'an epileptic' (Scambler & Hopkins, 1986). And the evidence suggests that this new, unwanted social status can be more distressing and disruptive of lives than the anticipation or fact of recurrent seizures.

However, if the communication of the diagnosis is often the most dramatic episode in relationships with physicians, it is generally but one moment in relationships beginning with the initial consultation and ending only with the cessation of antiepileptic medication or

Table 1. *Neuroepilepsy medication and psychosocial variables thought to be associated with psychiatric/psychological impairment*

Neuroepilepsy	Medication	Psycho-social
1. Age at onset	1. Polypharmacy	1. Fear of seizures
2. Seizure control	2. Serum levels of antiepileptic drugs	2. Perceived stigma
3. Duration of epilepsy	3. Type of medication	3. Perceived discrimination
4. Seizure type	4. Folic acid levels	4. Adjustment to epilepsy
5. Multiple seizure types		5. Locus of control
6. Aetiology		6. Life events
7. Type of aura		7. Social support
8. Neuropsychological status		8. Socioeconomic status
		9. Childhood home environment

death. During these relationships, people look to physicians to replace uncertainty with expert accounts of tests, aetiology, therapy and prognosis. They also aspire to be treated effectively and with consideration of the full range of psychosocial sequelae of epilepsy. Sometimes their demands may be unrealistic: for all the lapses exposed by audit, it remains the case that many of the uncertainties surrounding epilepsy cannot be alleviated given the current state of expert knowledge. But, interestingly, one common finding in Britain and the USA pertains to physicians' 'disinterest' in the day-to-day problems of coping with 'being epileptic' (Schneider & Conrad, 1983).

Personal identity

People perceive the status or identity of 'epileptic' to be discrediting through their association of epilepsy with stigma. Often it is accompanied by a sense of shame and, more saliently perhaps, a fear that 'normal people' will reject or otherwise discriminate against them solely on the grounds of their epilepsy. This fear of discrimination has been termed 'felt stigma', and actual discrimination 'enacted stigma'. And, it has been found that felt stigma predisposes most people with epilepsy to conceal their condition if they can, this being a first-choice strategy within as well as outside families. While concealment reduces the opportunities available to others to discriminate against them, paradoxically it also means that felt stigma causes more distress than enacted stigma (Scambler, 1989). Strategies other than secrecy include the minimizing of risks through avoidance of others, or even withdrawal; pragmatic or selective disclosing; or, more rarely, a determined and defiant 'avowal of normality' (West, 1985). Not surprisingly, strategies vary between social roles and over time.

Family management

Frequently epilepsy begins in childhood and children's understanding of events is conditioned by parents' explanations and behaviour. Parents may act as 'stigma coaches', training their offspring to feel ashamed and apprehensive about their epilepsy, prescribing concealment by advice or example (Schneider & Conrad, 1980). This is a form of 'over-protection'. Parental over-protection is a key source of anger and resentment among the young with epilepsy, and may be associated with behavioural and personality problems later.

In adolescence and adulthood felt stigma typically leads to concealment. Boy or girl friends tend not to be told, and even engagements may not provoke openness. Predictably, the same fear of rejection that proscribes mention of the word 'epilepsy' makes for a persistent sense of unease in case one day a seizure or other cue might lead to exposure. There is little evidence that open disclosure, even exposure, are likely to be followed by the termination of relationships, although it can happen. Uncertainty and bewilderment, and sometimes conflict, tend to be succeeded by new, 'negotiated' equilibria (Scambler, 1989).

Work opportunities

Epilepsy is associated with higher than average rates of unemployment and under-employment, although it must be remembered that epilepsy can be one symptom of conditions much more disabling in other ways. Estimates of the proportion of British adults with epilepsy experiencing employment problems vary from 25–70%, depending on the criteria used. Problems may be the consequence of enacted stigma or of discriminatory practices which even people with epilepsy may accept as 'legitimate', like driving restrictions. Felt stigma is an additional and probably under-estimated source of disadvantage: people sometimes avoid or withdraw from the labour market, or decline opportunities for advancement, through felt stigma.

A wide range of European and American studies have shown that felt stigma also leads to policies of non-disclosure to employers, at least when seizure frequency permits. While concealment reduces the prospects of encountering enacted stigma or legitimate discrimination, it can not only inhibit success in its own right, but also lead to severe daily tensions in 'information management'.

CONCLUSIONS

There are clear implications here for improved quality of epilepsy care. Many centre on the need for patients' own perspectives to be elicited and taken seriously. Typically these perspectives are characterized by: (i) 'felt stigma': the perception of epilepsy as stigmatizing and a social and psychological burden; (ii) 'rationalization': an urge to make sense of what is happening in order to restore cognitive order; and (iii) 'action strategy': a need to develop ways of coping with epilepsy and its concomitant psychosocial problems. The accumulated evidence is that physicians tend to be interested in those aspects of rationalization that promise to facilitate diagnosis or management, but not in the process *per se*. Neither felt stigma nor action strategy tend to be on the medical agenda for consultations and are generally handled inexpertly or cursorily if raised by patients (Scambler, 1989). Physicians, arguably, do not merely need to manage, inform and advise, but also to listen, which can be therapeutic in its own right.

REFERENCES

Annegers, J., Hauser, W. & Elverbalk, L. (1979). Remission of seizures and relapse in patients with epilepsy. *Epilepsia*, **20**, 729–37.

Duncan, J. (1991). Modern treatment strategies for patients with epilepsy: a review. *Journal of the Royal Society of Medicine*, **84**, 159–62.

Hopkins, A., Menken, M., DeFriesse, G. (1989). A record of patient encounters in neurological practice in the United Kingdom. *Journal of Neurological and Neurosurgical Psychiatry*, **52**, 436–8.

Hermann, B. & Whitman, S. (1986). Psychopathology in epilepsy: a multietiologic model. In S. Whitman, & B. Hermann, (Eds) *Psychopathology in epilepsy: social dimensions*. Oxford: Oxford University Press.

McGuire, A. & Trimble, M. (1990). Quality of life in patients with epilepsy: the role of cognitive factors. In D. Chadwick (Ed.). *Quality of life and quality of care in epilepsy*. London: Royal Society of Medicine.

Scambler, G. (1989). *Epilepsy*. London: Tavistock.

Scambler, G. & Hopkins, A. (1986). Being epileptic: coming to terms with stigma.

Sociology of Health and Illness, 8, 26–43.

Schneider, J. & Conrad, P. (1980). In the closet with illness: epilepsy, stigma potential and information control. *Social Problems*, 28, 32–44.

Schneider, J. & Conrad, P. (1983). *Having epilepsy: the experience and control of illness*. Philadelphia: Temple University Press.

West, P. (1985). Becoming disabled: perspectives on the labelling approach. In V. Gerhardt & M. Wadsworth (Eds). *Stress and stigma: explanation and evidence in the sociology of crime and illness*. London: Macmillan.

Epstein-Barr virus infection

RONA MOSS-MORRIS

Department of Psychiatry and Behavioural Science, School of Medicine, University of Auckland, New Zealand

The Epstein-Barr virus (EBV) is a human herpes virus known to cause infectious mononucleosis (IM). IM, commonly known as glandular fever, is an acute febrile disease characterized by generalized malaise, sore throat, enlarged lymph nodes and spleen. Reports of the incidence of IM range between 45 to 99 per 100 000 population (Evans, 1978). Primary infection with EBV typically occurs during adolescence, after which the virus latently inhabits B lymphocyte cells. Previous infection with EBV is indicated by the presence of EBV antibody titres in the serum, while lack of these antibodies indicates vulnerability to EBV infection (Kasl, Evans, & Niederman, 1979). Despite the fact that EBV infection appears to be ubiquitous in adults, only about 40% of people infected with EBV ever demonstrate the clinical signs of IM (Evans. 1978).

Whether or not people develop clinical IM and how quickly they recover from the illness may depend in part on psychosocial factors. Kasl *et al.* (1979) investigated 432 young American cadets over a 4 year period. Factors such as having a high level of motivation together with poor academic achievement, were predictive of both clinical IM and length of stay in hospital, amongst cadets recently infected with EBV. However, results from a more recent study found that experiencing stressful life events had no effect on length of time in bed, time off work, and duration of physical symptoms in IM patients (Bruce-Jones, *et al.*, 1994). The findings from these two studies suggest that differences in personality and behaviour, rather than the experience of stressful events *per se*, are associated with the onset of and recovery from IM.

A larger body of research has focused on EBV antibody titres, as a measure of immune system competence. Elevated titres of EBV antibodies, reflecting a possible reactivation of the latent EBV virus, appear to be a reliable indicator of the down regulation of cellular immunity (Van Rood *et al.*, 1993). Higher antibody levels to EBV have been associated with psychosocial stressors such as divorce, loneliness, marital dissatisfaction, caregiving for a relative with Alzheimer's disease, and university exams (Glaser *et al.*, 1993; Kiecolt-Glaser *et al.*, 1988; Kiecolt-Glaser *et al.*, 1991). Personality and coping styles including high levels of emotional suppression,

defensiveness, trait anxiety, and seeking social support have also been significantly linked to elevated EBV antibody titres (Glaser *et al.*, 1993; Esterling, Antoni & Kumar, 1990). In addition, psychological interventions designed to reduce stress have significantly decreased EBV antibody titres (Van Rood *et al.*, 1993).

Elevated antibody titres have also been implicated as causal factors in conditions such as depression and chronic fatigue syndrome (CFS). While early studies did report elevated EBV titres in these groups, subsequent well designed studies comparing depressed and CFS patients with matched healthy controls found no significant differences in EBV antibody titres (eg. Miller *et al.*, 1986, Buchwald & Komaroff, 1991). Longitudinal studies failed to find sustained evidence of EBV infection in CFS patients, and improvement in symptoms appears unrelated to changes in EBV titres (Buchwald & Komaroff, 1991). However, there is evidence that clinical IM is a risk factor for developing chronic fatigue six months after the onset of infection, whether or not the illness is caused by the EBV (White *et al.*, 1995). Pure post-IM fatigue (i.e. chronic fatigue without concurrent psychiatric illness) appears unrelated to the experience of negative life events, and may well be associated with organic causes. On the other hand, depression following IM does appear to be more closely related to the effects of negative life events than to any residual effects of infection. As such, the relationship between EBV/IM, and depression and CFS is complex. While there is little evidence that EBV is the sole cause of these conditions, it may be a relevant risk factor for the development of chronic fatigue and may interact with psychosocial factors in the onset of depression.

In conclusion, the serum antibody reaction to EBV has proved to be a valuable tool for researchers to investigate the relationship between psychological factors, intervention, and the immune system. However, the significance of elevated EBV antibody titres in the development of clinical symptoms or illness is unclear. This area of research requires further attention, as does the understanding of psychosocial risk factors in the development of clinical IM.

REFERENCES

Bruce-Jones, W.D.A., White, P.D., Thomas, J.M. & Clare, A.W. (1994). The effect of social adversity on the fatigue syndrome, psychiatric disorders, and physical recovery, following glandular fever, *Psychological Medicine*, 24, 651–9.

Buchwald, B. & Komaroff, A.L. (1991). Review of laboratory findings for patients with chronic fatigue syndrome. *Reviews of Infectious Diseases*, 13, S12–S18.

Esterling, B.A., Antoni, M.H. & Kumar, M. (1990). Emotional repression, stress disclosure response, and Epstein-Barr viral capsid antigen titres. *Psychosomatic Medicine*, 52, 397–410.

Esterling, B.A., Antoni, M.H., Kumar, M. & Schneiderman, N. (1993). Defensiveness, trait anxiety, and Epstein-Barr viral capsid antigen antibody titres in healthy college students. *Health Psychology*, 12, 132–9.

Evans, A.S. (1978). Infectious mononucleosis and related syndromes. *The American Journal of Medical Sciences*, 276, 325–39.

Glaser, R., Pearson, G.R., Bonneau, R.H., Esterling, B.A., Atkinson, C. & Kiecolt, J.K. (1993). Stress and the memory T-Cell response to the Epstein-Barr virus in healthy medical students. *Health Psychology*, **12**, 435–42.

Kasl, S.V., Evans, A.S. & Niederman, J.C. (1979). Psychosocial risk factors in the development of infectious mononucleosis. *Psychosomatic Medicine*, **41**, 445–6.

Kiecolt-Glaser, J.K., Kennedy, S., Malkoff, S., Fisher, L., Speicher, C.E. & Glaser, R. (1988). Marital discord and immunity in males. *Psychosomatic Medicine*, **50**, 213–29.

Kiecolt-Glaser, J.K., Dura J.R., Speicher, C.E., Trask, O.J. & Glaser, R. (1991). Spousal caregivers of dementia victims: longitudinal changes in immunity and health. *Psychosomatic Medicine*, **38**, 195–209.

Miller, A.H., Silberstein, C., Asnis, G.M., Munk, G., Rubinson, E., Spigland, I. & Norin, A. (1986). Epstein-Barr virus infection and depression. *Journal of Clinical Psychiatry*, **47**, 529.

Van Rood, Y.R., Bogaards, M., Goulmy, E. & van Houwelingen, H.C. (1993). The effects of stress and relaxation on the *in vitro* immune response in man: a meta-analytic study. *Journal of Behavioural Medicine*, **16**, 163–81.

White, P.D., Thomas, J.M., Amess, J., Grover, S.A., Kangro, H.O., & Clare, A.W. (1995). The existence of a fatigue syndrome after glandular fever. *Psychological Medicine*, **25**, 907–16.

Fetal alcohol syndrome

ILANA CROME

North Staffs Combined Health Care, City General Hospital, Stoke-on-Trent, UK

If diseases of so serious a nature appear in adults, from the inordinate use of vinous spirit, how much more liable must feeble infancy be to suffer from the same. I am afraid that this is no uncommon observation. It is well known that nurses, if they can deserve such a name, are in the practice of giving spirits in the form of punch to young children to make them sleep (Trotter, 1804).

In 1973 Jones reported a 'characteristic pattern of malformation' in eight children of chronic alcoholics and which is now known as fetal alcohol syndrome (FAS). This original publication described FAS as having growth deficiency of prenatal onset, characteristic facial dysmorphology and central nervous system involvement with developmental delay. By 1977, Little suggested that it was not only the high doses that were detrimental to fetal health, but moderate doses too were considered to be potentially problematic.

INCIDENCE AND IMPORTANCE

Many reports from different countries and communities endorsed the original finding that prenatal exposure to alcohol could affect the foetus. Maternal alcohol misuse within the first four weeks of conception is associated with cranofacial abnormalities, microophthalmia, flattened mid-face, small chin, thin upper lip and poorly developed philtra (ridges between mouth and nose), short upturned nose and flattened nasal bridge.

Epidemiological evidence points to a prevalence of FAS of 1–3/1000 live births and FAE of 4–6/1000 live births (Ihlen *et al.*, 1990). There are marked variations in different parts of the world but the reasons are obscure. This falls far short of the numbers of women drinking abusively as only one-third of women drinking 70 g absolute alcohol/day have babies with FAS. Genetic and maternal variables may account for this finding. Abel and Sokol (1991) have estimated that the 1200 children with FAS born annually in the USA costs $73.6 million/year to treat.

SEQUELAE

Central nervous system involvement is most significant with intellectual impairment: the average IQ slightly less than 70, but a wide range of individual scores. Microcephaly, altered muscle tone, poor co-ordination and hyperactivity lead to developmental delay. The triad of retarded growth, intellectual dysfunction or facial abnormalities defines FAS. There appears to be a correlation between severity of the signs and the amount of alcohol to which the foetus has been exposed. Six units daily for some part of the pregnancy is considered heavy.

However, the realization that there was a spectrum in the frequency and severity of problems related to maternal drinking, resulted in the term 'fetal alcohol effect' (FAE). The effects are decreased birthweight, intrauterine growth retardation, morphological abnormalities and central nervous system dysfunction. The latter include decreased muscle tone, jitteriness, tremulousness, decreased bodily vigour at birth. Infants of mothers who drank four drinks a day demonstrated compromised mental and motor development. At 4 years, decreased attentiveness, increased fidgetiness and social compliance was evident.

In addition, from perinatal mortality in very heavy drinkers, stillbirth and spontaneous abortion rates are increased in mothers who drink one to two drinks a day during pregnancy.

ASSESSMENT: CHILDREN, MOTHERS AND FAMILIES

A developmental assessment of the child affected by alcohol allows focusing on the child's potential and problem areas. Assessment must take place over time and is advised if early signs are absent. Suggested tools include Brazelton neonatal assessment, Bayley Scales of Infant Development between 2 and 30 months, i.e. at 4, 8 and 12 months. These tests should be carried out with the mother's close involvement. Older children may be assessed by a standardized intelligence test, the Reitan-Indiana Neuropsychological Test Battery and the McCarthy Scales of Children's Abnormalities. The environment in which the child is developing, including the extent of the mother's drinking problem, requires assessment and possibly treatment. Has she been abstinent and for how long? Who is the main caretaker? Is child protection an issue? Possible guilt and denial surrounding the child needs to be addressed.

Thus comprehensive assessment of substance use in pregnant women and women wishing to become pregnant is essential at the primary care level. Screening questionnaires (e.g. CAGE, T-ACE, AUDIT) can be followed by problem assessment on use of alcohol (level, pattern, history) by quantity/frequency indices, time-line methods, lifetime drinking history, drinking diaries and laboratory tests. Signs and symptoms of alcohol use can be assessed by questionnaires (SADQ) or harmful, hazardous and dependence criteria in ICD-10 or DSM IIIR. Dependence criteria are narrowing of the drinking repertoire, tolerance, withdrawal symptoms, neglect of alternative activities, subjective sense of impaired control, continuation despite consequences, relief drinking, reinstatement liability, sense of compulsion to drink. Medical, psychiatric, family, employment, legal and financial consequences of drinking are important in the context of other factors which affect the pregnancy, e.g. age, reproductive history, lifestyle, i.e. nutrition, smoking and use of other drugs.

Although many women spontaneously decrease their drinking during pregnancy, the heaviest drinkers before pregnancy appear to remain the heaviest drinkers after pregnancy.

PREVENTION

By 1981, the Surgeon General of the USA advised women who are pregnant, or considering pregnancy, to abstain from alcoholic beverages, and urged professionals who care for such women to warn them of the risks of drinking during pregnancy. The proportion of pregnant women at risk of fetal damage is difficult to determine, but prevention thus becomes a major public health concern as is the largest single preventable cause of mental retardation.

A survey in 1985 in the USA revealed that 84% of respondents identified heavy drinking with increased risk of adverse pregnancy outcomes. But, how much alcohol can be considered 'safe' during pregnancy? Controversy surrounds the methodology employed in epidemiological research in this area. Thus, it is impossible to postulate a safe threshold dose or a safe time, despite the obvious practical value to practitioners and the public.

There are questions regarding the applicability of general prevention programmes which increase awareness, modify attitudes and behaviour about drinking or the value of the specific targeting of women with special needs. Results are variable partly because of the immense difficulties of evaluating prevention programmes in the context of many confounding factors, e.g. under-reporting, additional drug use, impact of 'significant others' in altering substance use, accessibility of intervention and prevention.

REFERENCES

Abel, E.L. & Sokol, R.J. (1991). A revised conservative estimate of the incidence of FAS and its economic impact. *Alcoholism: Clinical and Experimental Research*, **15**, 514–24.

Chasnoff, I.J. (1991). Drugs alcohol pregnancy and the neonate – pay now or later. *Journal of the American Medical Association*, **266**, 1567–8.

Ihlen, B.M., Amundsen, A., Sande, H.A. & Dage, L. (1990). Changes in the use of intoxicants after onset of pregnancy. *British Journal of Addiction*, **85**, 1627–33.

Jones, K.L., Smith, D.W., Ulleland, C.N. & Streissguth, A.P. (1973). Patterns of malformation in offspring of alcoholic mothers. *Lancet*, **i**, 1267–71.

Knupfer, G. (1991). Abstaining for fetal health – the fiction that even light drinking is dangerous. *British Journal of Addiction*, **86**, 1063–74.

Masis, K.B. & May, P.A. (1991). A comprehensive local program for the prevention of fetal alcohol syndrome. *Public Health Report*, **106**, 484–9.

Plant, M.L. (1990). *Women and alcohol: a review of international literature on the use of alcohol.* Geneva: World Health Organization.

Roman, P.M. (1988). *Women and alcohol use: a review of the research literature.* Washington: National Institute of Alcohol Abuse and Alcoholism.

Rosett, H.L. & Weiner, L. (1985). Alcohol and pregnancy: a clinical perspective. *Annual Review of Medicine*, **36**, 73–80.

Streissguth, A.P., Landsman-Dwyer, S., Martin, J.C. & Smith, D.W. (1980). Teratogenic effects of alcohol in humans and laboratory animals. *Science*, **209**, 353–61.

Waterson, E.J., Evans, C. & Murray-Lyon, I.M. (1990). Is pregnancy a time of changing drinking and smoking patterns for fathers as well as mothers? *British Journal of Addiction*, **85**, 389–96.

Wilsnack, S.C. & Beckman, L.J. (1987). *Alcohol problems in women.* New York: Guilford.

Fetal well-being: monitoring and assessment

PETER G. HEPPER

and

S. SHAHIDULLAH

School of Psychology, The Queen's University of
Belfast, UK

The chief aim of obstetric practice is to achieve a healthy baby and mother at the conclusion of the pregnancy. This chapter will concentrate solely on the fetus and the methods presently available to monitor its health and well-being throughout the pregnancy.

Two general assumptions underlie the contention that monitoring of the fetus is useful: first is that these methods can detect or predict fetal compromise; and second that by interpreting and acting appropriately on these findings it may be possible to reduce the frequency and/or severity of perinatal events.

In obstetric practice various traditional techniques have been used to assess the well-being of the fetus and these are discussed below.

TRADITIONAL CLINICAL OBSTETRIC TECHNIQUES

Placental synthetic function
Since the fetus gains all of its biological requirements via the placenta the well-being of the fetus is directly related to its functioning. The endocrine function of the feto-placental unit may be monitored using biochemical tests to measure urinary oestrogens, plasma oestrogens and human placental lactogen, serum alpha-fetoprotein, human chorionic gonadotrophin (Enkin, Keirse & Chalmers, 1990).

Clinical features
Measurement of uterine size, estimation of the size of the fetus, estimation of liquor volume and estimation of fetal movement. Here, if the fetus falls outside established norms, closer monitoring is indicated to assess whether the fetus is a healthy small fetus or is indeed compromised.

Serial ultrasound measurements
A general assumption has been that if the fetus is 'growing well in size' then it must also be healthy. Therefore much importance has been placed on growth parameters of the fetus, often assessed by measuring the head, abdominal circumference, femur length and fetal weight.

Fetal heart rate monitoring
This procedure is used during both the antenatal and the intrapartum periods. It directly monitors the heart rate of the fetus in real time. Of particular interest are baseline heart rate, beat to beat variability, presence of accelerations associated with fetal movement and the presence of decelerations. Accelerations of the fetal heart rate associated with fetal movement, representing a well-oxygenated fetal central nervous system, is the most commonly used index of fetal health. Since the fetus at later gestations may exhibit four different behavioural state patterns (Nijhuis, 1986) which affect the fetal heart rate pattern, it is important that the fetal heart rate pattern is interpreted in the light of evidence of the behavioural state of the fetus (Brown & Patrick, 1981).

Biophysical profile
This is a means of assessing fetal well-being and predicting the at-risk fetus using five parameters (Manning, Platt & Sipos, 1980), fetal breathing movements, gross body movements, fetal tone, qualitative amniotic fluid volume (all assessed via ultrasound scan) and reactive fetal heart rate assessed using cardiotocography. Each parameter scores 0,1 or 2 with the maximum being 10. The score is said to be satisfactory if it is greater than 6.

FETAL BEHAVIOUR
It is accepted that the best measure of the well-being of the fetus is by assessing its neural system. The above measures only indirectly assess this and a more direct measure of central nervous system functioning is needed. One means to do this is to assess the behaviour of the fetus. As the behaviour of the fetus reflects the functioning of its nervous system this can be used in the assessment of the fetal well-being. Fetal behaviour may be defined as any action or reaction of the fetus and may be divided into two main categories: spontaneous (completely under the volition of the fetus) or elicited (response contingent to the presentation of stimulus, e.g. sound). Both may be used to assess well-being. Advances in ultrasonography have allowed the behaviour of the fetus be studied in detail. The resolution of high definition ultrasound machines enables the opening and closing of the lens of the eye to be observed accurately.

Movements of the fetus are first noticed at approximately 7 weeks of gestation, and have been described as rippling or vermicular type of movements (de Vries, 1992). The repertoire of movements increases rapidly so by 11 weeks of gestation startles, general movements, stretches, breathing movements, isolated head movements, jaw movements, hand–face contact, general rotation, yawns and tongue movements are readily observed. As the fetal neural system develops and becomes more complex, the movement repertoire of the fetus also becomes more extensive and structured.

As the normal behaviour of the fetus has been documented, the ability to detect abnormalities from observation of aberrant behaviour is possible. For example, anencephalic fetuses exhibit much grosser fetal movements than normal fetuses (Visser *et al.*, 1985), and eye movement patterns of fetuses with Trisomy 18 (Hepper and Shahidullah, 1992*a*) are reversed, compared to unaffected fetuses. The principle used here is similar to previous indirect assessments of fetal nervous system functioning, in that a picture of normal behaviour is constructed and the individual's behaviour compared to this.

Fetal behaviour may be elicited, i.e. in response to an external stimulus, e.g. a sound. One technique which has proved extremely powerful in assessing fetal neural functioning and well-being is that of habituation. Habituation is the decrement in response to repeated stimulation (Leader & Bennett, 1988). In a recent study the habituation pattern of normal fetuses was compared to those of Down syndrome fetuses (Hepper & Shahidullah, 1992*b*). The study found that not only did the Down syndrome fetuses differ from the normal

fetuses but that the habituation pattern of Down syndrome fetuses differed from one another and was predictive of outcome at birth. Thus the test discriminated both the presence of an abnormality and the severity of affect. This latter information is unavailable from the results of genetic screening tests which only detect the presence of an abnormal gene and not the severity of its effect.

Assessment of fetal behavioural abilities offers significant advances in detecting the effects of exposure to teratogens, which often affect neural functioning at doses which exert no observable structural effect. Behavioural observations of cocaine exposed fetuses, for example, indicate these individuals exhibit a number of behavioural abnormalities arising from exposure to cocaine not observed in fetuses with no exposure to cocaine (Hepper, 1995).

In summary, the well-being of the fetus is monitored by establishing norms and comparing individuals to this. Assessment of fetal behaviour, by assessing the functioning of the fetus's nervous system, offers much greater scope in assessing well-being, detecting the presence of a much wider range of abnormalities and the severity of affect.

REFERENCES

Brown, R. & Patrick, J. (1981). The non-stress test: how long is enough? *American Journal of Obstetrics and Gynecology*, **141**, 646–51.

Enkin, M., Keirse, J.N.C & Chalmers, I. (1990). Assessment of fetal well-being. In *A guide to effective care in pregnancy and childbirth*. pp. 57–67, Oxford: Oxford University Press.

Hepper, P.G. (1995). Human fetal behaviour and maternal cocaine use: a longitudinal study. *Neurotoxicology*, **16**, 139–44

Hepper, P.G. & Shahidullah, S. (1992*a*). Trisomy 18: behavioural and structural abnormalities: an ultrasonographic case

study. *Ultrasound in Obstetrics and Gynaecology*, **2**, 48–50.

Hepper, P.G. & Shahidullah, S. (1992*b*). Habituation in normal and Down syndrome fetuses. *Quarterly Journal of Experimental Psychology*, **44B**, 305–17.

Leader, L.R. & Bennett, M.J. (1988). Fetal habituation. In M.I. Levene, M.J. Bennett & J. Punt (Eds) *Fetal and neonatal neurology and neurosurgery*. pp. 59–70, Edinburgh: Churchhill Livingstone.

Manning, F.A., Platt, L.D. & Sipos L. (1986). Antepartum fetal evaluation: development of a fetal biophysical profile. *American Journal of Obstetrics and Gynecology*, **133**, 590–4.

Nijhuis, J.G. (1986). Behavioural states: concomitants, clinical implications and the assessment of the condition of the nervous system. *European Journal of Obstetrics, Gynaecology and Reproductive Biology*, **21**, 301–8.

Visser, G.H.A., Laurini, R.N., Vries, J.I.P. de, Bekedam, D.J. & Prechtl, H.F.R. (1985). Abnormal motor behaviour in anencephalic fetuses. *Early Human Development*, **12**, 173–82.

Vries, J.I.P. de (1992). The first trimester. In J.G. Nijhuis (Ed.). *Fetal behaviour: developmental and perinatal aspects*. pp. 3–16, Oxford: Oxford University Press.

Gastric and duodenal ulcers

PAUL BENNETT
Gwent Psychology Services and University of Bristol, UK

DOUGLAS CARROLL
School of Sports and Exercise Sciences, University of Birmingham, UK

Gastric and duodenal ulcers, collectively referred to as peptic ulcers, are ulcerating lesions of the stomach or duodenum. Peptic ulcers are associated with epigastric pain, usually occurring several hours after eating and relieved by food. Less typically, they may present as intestinal bleeding or obstruction of the bowel close to the stomach. Approximately 10% of the population will develop peptic ulcer disease (PUD) during their lifetime.

AETIOLOGY
Early anecdotal and epidemiological research suggested that PUD is associated with stressful events. A higher incidence of symptoms suggestive of ulcers, for example, was found within occupations thought to be particularly stressful, such as surgeons, business executives, and air traffic controllers. However, a lack of radiologically confirmed diagnoses (PUD is only confirmed in between 30 and

90% of those with presenting symptoms) renders interpretation of these data difficult. In addition, it is not clear whether the individuals with ulcers were experiencing high levels of stress. Surgeons and business executives, for example, frequently have a high degree of job latitude and control, factors which ameliorate job stress.

More substantive evidence of an association between ulceration and stress was reported by Medalie *et al.* (1992). They followed a cohort of 8458 men aged over 40 years with no history of PUD for 5 years. Multivariate logistic regression revealed a significant and independent association between confirmed duodenal ulcer incidence and baseline measures of family problems (odds ratio 1.60), low levels of intimacy and social support (odds ratio 2.06), and internalization of negative affect (1.89): the odds ratio for smoking was 1.64. Identification of participants who developed duodenal ulcers was dependent on them attending medical outpatients, and the possibility of a bias toward those who were both under stress and low in coping resources attending their doctor with PUD symptoms cannot be excluded. Nor can the possibility that stress-related increases in alcohol consumption contributed to their symptoms, although the authors describe consumption levels within the study population as 'negligible'. Clinic attendance as a biasing factor is highlighted by Sandberg and Biling's (1976) findings that clinic attenders were more anxious and depressed than non-attenders with PUD. Nevertheless, this report provides some of the strongest evidence of an association between ulceration and stress indices.

Life event studies have provided conflicting results. Nevertheless, a majority of studies have reported higher numbers of acute or chronic stressful life events preceding the development of duodenal ulcers, or that people who developed ulcers had less adequate coping resources (e.g. Ellard *et al.*, 1990) than either healthy controls or other patient comparison groups. Due to the retrospective nature of much of the life events literature, interpretation of findings is fraught with difficulties.

Prospective studies suggest life stress may prolong symptoms after onset. Hui *et al.* (1992), for example, followed a total of 122 endoscopically validated duodenal ulcer and 141 hepatitis controls either in the active or remission phase for a period of six months. Over this period, patients who remained in the active phase of disease reported less positive life events than any other group, and were the only group to report continued high levels of stress. Similar results were reported by Holtmann *et al.* (1992), who found lower 14-day healing rates and increased levels of relapse to be significantly associated with physicians' ratings of patient stress over a one- but not two-year follow-up period in a population of over 2000 duodenal ulcer patients. Although the direction of causality cannot be unequivocally determined by these findings, a direct causal link between stress and duodenal ulceration is implied. Evidence for a link between gastric ulceration and stress is less compelling; a majority of studies report no association between life events and gastric ulceration.

Although few in number and reliant on low subject numbers, psychophysiological studies have shown chronic psychological stress to be associated with hypersecretion of gastric hydrochloric acid, and, conversely, that reductions in levels of stress or relaxation can reduce such output (Peters & Richardson, 1983). In addition, early evidence (e.g. Weiner *et al.*, 1957) suggests that ulceration is most likely in patients who are both under stress and who have high rates of pepsinogen secretion.

INTERVENTION

Two intervention strategies may be identified with patients with PUD. The first involves attempts to moderate stress thought to mediate the ulcerative process, through counselling or some form of stress management. The second involves attempts to modify behaviours which may also contribute to the disease process, including smoking or alcohol consumption. Only the former has been subject to even modest amounts of empirical investigation. This probably reflects the relative cost-effectiveness of pharmacological interventions.

The primary benefit of psychological intervention may be in secondary prevention: behavioural counselling has significantly less impact on healing than treatment with an H_2-receptor antagonist (cimetidine) over a one-year follow-up period (Loof *et al.*, 1987). Nevertheless, the results of two controlled trials suggest that combined psychological and medical intervention may reduce relapse rates significantly more than pharmacological treatment alone.

Brooks and Richardson (1980) randomly allocated 22 patients with radiologically confirmed diagnoses of duodenal ulcers to either an intensive psychological intervention comprising an educative phase, relaxation training, cognitive restructuring, and the use of positive self-talk and coping imagery or an attention, placebo condition. All subjects received antacid intervention. Over a follow-up period of 60 days, patients in the intervention condition experienced significantly fewer symptomatic days and consumed less medication, although X-ray revealed similar levels of ulcer healing in both groups. It is perhaps in the long-term follow-up at $3\frac{1}{2}$ years that the strength of the active intervention was most convincing. Significantly fewer subjects in the active intervention group (one in nine) had recurrences than subjects in the placebo group (five in eight). Active intervention group subjects attended hospital less frequently, and none required surgery, whereas two in the placebo group did. Longer-term benefits were also reported by Sjodin (1983), who found significant differences in somatic complaints at 15, but not 3, month follow-up, following a combined medical and psychological intervention relative to medical treatment alone.

CONCLUSIONS

The tenor of recent review articles reflect the broad uncertainty within the literature concerning the role of stress in the aetiology of PUD. Some (e.g. Whitehead, 1992) suggest that psychological factors do play a role in the development of PUD, while others (e.g. Friedman, 1988) argue to the contrary. Such discord may stem, at least in part, from the restricted nature of much of the relevant research, which has frequently relied on retrospective and cross-sectional methods. However, prospective studies, whether in patient or healthy populations, are now identifying a modest, but significant, relationship between stress and ulceration. Whether this relationship is of sufficient clinical importance to warrant psychological intervention remains questionnable. However, the results of Peters and Richardson, if replicated in a larger sample, suggest potential benefit. In addition, psychological interventions targeted at smoking cessation or reduced alcohol intake are worthy of at least preliminary evaluation in this context.

REFERENCES

Brooks, G.R. & Richardson, F.C. (1980).
Emotional skills training: a treatment
program for duodenal ulcer. *Behavior
Therapy*, 11, 198–207.

Ellard, K., Beaurepaire, J., Jones, M., Piper,
D.W. & Tennant, C. (1990). Acute and
chronic stress in duodenal ulcer diease.
Gastroenterology, 99, 1628–32.

Friedman, G. (1988). Peptic ulcer diease.
Clinical Symptoms, 40, 1–32.

Holtmann, G., Armstrong, D., Poppel, E.
Bauerfeind, A., Goebell, H., Arnold, R.,
Classen, M., Witzel, L., Fischer, M. &
Heinisch, M. (1992). Influence of stress
on the healing and relapse of duodenal
ulcers. A prospective, multicenter trial of
2109 patients with recurrent duodenal
ulceration treated with ranitidine.
Scandinavian Journal of Gastroenterology,
27, 917–23.

Hui, W.M., Shiu, L.P., Lok, A.S.F. & Lam,
S.K. (1992). Life events and daily stress
in duodenal ulcer disease. *Digestion*, 52,
165–72.

Loof, L., Adami, H.-O., Bates, S.,
Fagerstrom, K.O., Gustausson, S.,
Nyberg, A., Nyren, O. & Brodin, U.
(1987). Psychological group counseling for
the prevention of ulcer relapses. A
controlled randomized trial in duodenal
and prepyloric ulcer disease. *Journal of
Clinical Gastroenterology*, 9, 400–7.

Medalie, J.H., Stange, K.C., Zyzanski,
S.J. & Goldbourt, U. (1992). The
importance of biopsychosocial factors in
the development of duodenal ulcer in a
cohort of middle-aged men. *American
Journal of Epidemiology*, 136, 1280–7.

Peters, M.N. & Richardson, C.T. (1983)
Stressful life events disease.
Gastroenterology, 84, 114–19.

Sandberg, B. & Biling, A. (1976). Duodenal
ulcer in army trainees during basic military
training. *Journal of Psychosomatic Research*,
20, 61–74.

Sjodin, I. (1983). Psychotherapy in peptic ulcer
disease: a controlled outcome study. *Acta
Psychiatrica Scandinavia*, 67, 307.

Weiner, H., Thaler, M., Reisner, M.F. &
Mirsky, I.A. (1957). Etiology of duodenal
ulcer 1. Relation of specific psychological
characteristics to rate of gastric secretion
(serum pepsinogen). *Psychosomatic
Medicine*, 19, 1–10.

Whitehead, W.E. (1992). Behavioral medicine
approaches to gastrointestinal disorders.
*Journal of Consulting and Clinical
Psychology*, 60, 605–12.

General cancer

BARBARA L. ANDERSEN

and

DEANNA M. GOLDEN-KREUTZ

*Department of Psychology, The Ohio State University,
Columbus, USA*

INTRODUCTION

The human cost of cancer is staggering. In many countries cancer is the second leading cause of death, only outnumbered by heart disease. In the United States, for example, over the past five years cancer diagnoses and deaths have increased by 223 000 and 44 000, respectively (American Cancer Society, 1994). Much of this increase appears to be related to advances in early detection as well as to the general ageing of the population (age is a risk factor; Garfinkel, 1994). There is, however, variability across countries. For example, age-adjusted death rates per 100 000 population for 1988–1991 ranged from 247 in Hungary to 84 in Mexico; the rate for UK and Wales is 179 (Boring *et al.*, 1994). In short, cancer is a significant medical problem that affects the health status of people worldwide.

Research on the psychological and behavioural aspects of oncology began in the early 1950s; however, significant expansion has occurred in the last 15 years. This research has clarified biobehavioural factors in illness (Andersen, Kiecolt-Glaser & Glaser, 1994), including relations between psychological responses and factors (e.g. personality, mood, coping style) and behavioural variables (e.g. compliance with treatment, diet, exercise), with more recent research incorporating biologic systems (e.g. immune and endocrine) and examining the interaction of these variables and their relationship to disease course (e.g. Fawzy *et al.*, 1993).

This chapter provides a brief overview of the central findings which have emerged on the psychological and behavioural aspects of cancer. Other chapters in this volume can be consulted for site-specific findings. By way of introduction, we will begin with data on cancer incidence, death rates, and gender differences. Where data from the US are used, we note that they represent the same general trends found in other industrialized, western countries. The remainder of the chapter organizes the findings by disease-relevant time points, from prevention to recovery and/or death. Where appropriate, specific intervention studies will be detailed. We will conclude by highlighting psychological interventions which appear to be effective in aiding cancer patients.

MAGNITUDE OF THE PROBLEM: INCIDENCE, DEATH RATES, AND GENDER DIFFERENCES

Cancers vary in their prevalence and mortality. Tables 1 and 2 display data from the USA on the incidence and death rates by specific sites and genders. These data indicate, for example, that women are more commonly diagnosed with breast cancer and men with prostate cancer, but that lung cancer is the number one killer of both sexes (American Cancer Society, 1994). Similarly, Tables 3 and 4 provide death rate data from selected countries (Boring *et al.*, 1994). These data illustrate the geographical, nationality, and sex differences which exist (e.g. lung cancer death rates of 45.1 for Australian men, but a rate of 5.0 for French women). In examining the death rates worldwide, the top killers of women include breast, colon and rectum, lung, and uterine cancers. For men, lung, colon and rectum, prostate, and stomach cancers are the common cancer killers worldwide.

Table 1. *Cancer incidence by site and gender (1994 estimates)*

	Cancer incidence		
Male (Total est. 632 000)		Female (Total est. 576 000)	
Site	Number (%)	Site	Number (%)
Prostate	200 000 (32%)	Breast	182 000 (32%)
Lung	100 000 (16%)	Colon and rectum	74 000 (13%)
Colon and rectum	75 000 (12%)	Lung	72 000 (13%)
Bladder	38 000 (6%)	Uterus	46 000 (8%)
Lymphoma	29 400 (5%)	Ovary	24 000 (4%)
Oral	19 800 (3%)	Lymphoma	23 500 (4%)
Melanoma of skin	17 000 (3%)	Melanoma of skin	15 000 (3%)
Kidney	17 000 (3%)	Pancreas	14 000 (2%)
Leukamia	16 200 (3%)	Bladder	13 200 (2%)
Stomach	15 000 (2%)	Leukamia	12 400 (2%)
Pancreas	13 000 (2%)	Kidney	10 600 (2%)
Larynx	9 800 (2%)	Oral	9 800 (2%)

Adapted from *Cancer Facts and Figures – 1994.* (1994). American Cancer Society, Inc.

Table 2. *Cancer deaths by site and gender (1994 estimates)*

	Cancer deaths		
Male (Total est. 283 000		Female (Total est. 255 000)	
Site	Number (%)	Site	Number (%)
Lung	94 000 (33%)	Lung	59 000 (23%)
Prostate	38 000 (13%)	Breast	46 000 (18%)
Colon and rectum	27 800 (10%)	Colon and rectum	28 200 (11%)
Pancreas	12 400 (4%)	Ovary	13 600 (5%)
Lymphoma	12 100 (4%)	Pancreas	13 500 (5%)
Leukaemia	10 500 (4%)	Lymphoma	10 650 (4%)
Stomach	8 400 (3%)	Uterus	10 500 (4%)
Oesophagus	7 800 (3%)	Leukaemia	8 600 (3%)
Liver	7 200 (2%)	Liver	6 000 (2%)
Bladder	7 000 (2%)	Brain	5 800 (2%)
Brain	6 800 (2%)	Stomach	5 600 (2%)
Kidney	6 800 (2%)	Multiple myeloma	4 800 (2%)

Adapted from *Cancer Facts and Figures – 1994.* (1994). American Cancer Society, Inc.

BIOBEHAVIOURAL ASPECTS

Prevention

It has been suggested that much of cancer incidence and premature death can be prevented through changes in behaviour. In the USA, for example, the National Cancer Institute (NCI) set a goal of a 50% reduction in cancer mortality by the year 2000 through prevention and control efforts focused, in large part, on lifestyle (Greenwald & Cullen, 1985). Primary prevention attempts to reduce the probability of cancer onset by decreasing exposure to risk factors. For women and men, unhealthy habits have been a behavioural research target, and smoking has been emphasized, as it is related to 30% of all cancer deaths. Cigarette smoking is directly linked to lung cancer, one of the leading causes of death for men and women, and is implicated in cancers of the larynx, head and neck, oesophagus, bladder, kidney, pancreas, and stomach.

The other major categories of lifestyle behaviours that have been linked to greater risk are diet and sun exposure (see 'Skin cancer' for extended pieces on these issues). In the area of diet, the majority of the research has dealt with diet modification (particularly reductions in fat intake and increases in complex carbohydrates and fibre and weight reduction, *per se* (Ashley, 1993; Wynder & Cohen, 1993)). These issues are salient in breast cancer prevention (see 'Skin cancer' for extended pieces of these issues), where interventions have been developed for at-risk women to reduce weight and fat intake and increase physical activity (Heber *et al.*, 1993). The available evidence suggests that restriction of fat intake will result in decreased total calorie intake and, in turn, a loss of body fat in postmenopausal women. It is the loss of fat that is hypothesized to cause a decrease in oestrogen production from adrenal androgens and thus reduce the promotion of ostrogen-dependent breast tumours.

Secondary prevention efforts have been defined as those which identify the disease at the earliest of stages (e.g. when it is preinvasive or localized and asymptomatic) so that effective treatment can be administered sooner and mortality reduced. The chances of successful early cancer detection and treatment depend upon the clinical characteristics of the disease and the screening strategy, and it is unlikely that secondary prevention can proceed effectively unless certain conditions for both are met. Behavioural scientists have focused mainly on the early detection of breast cancer. Currently,

Table 3. *Age-adjusted death rates in adult males per 100 000 for selected countries and disease sites*

Country	All sites	Colo/rectal	Lung	Prostate	Stomach
United States	164.4 (24)	16.7	57.1	16.8	5.2
Australia	164.0 (25)	21.5	45.1	17.2	8.4
Canada	170.8 (21)	17.8	57.3	16.9	8.0
Denmark	179.5 (11)	22.8	51.9	18.1	7.8
England/Wales	179.2 (12)	20.2	57.0	16.6	12.5
France	200.7 (5)	17.3	46.8	17.3	9.1
Germany (Fed)	177.9 (13)	21.1	48.7	15.9	14.9
Hungary	246.5 (1)	29.0	76.4	15.7	24.0
Ireland	174.9 (17)	23.2	47.9	17.6	12.0
Israel	115.5 (42)	14.4	24.5	8.6	7.7
Italy	192.3 (10)	15.6	58.9	11.5	18.2
Netherlands	195.3 (9)	17.9	71.2	18.3	13.1
Sweden	129.4 (40)	14.9	23.4	20.4	8.9
Switzerland	171.1 (20)	18.2	44.9	22.5	9.6
USSR	198.3 (7)	15.2	63.6	6.3	6.8

Note: Figures in parentheses are order of rank based on data from 46 countries during the years 1988–1990. Adapted from C.C. Boring, T.S. Squires, T. Tong & S. Montgomery. (1994). Cancer Statistics, 1994. CA-A *Cancer Journal for Clinicians*, **44**, 7–26.

Table 4. *Age-adjusted death rates in adult females per 100 000 for selected countries and disease sites*

Country	All sites	Breast	Colo/rectal	Lung	Uterine
United States	110.6(11)	22.4	11.4	22.4	5.2
Australia	102.2(22)	20.7	14.7	12.8	4.7
Canada	110.6(12)	23.9	12.0	20.6	4.8
Denmark	139.8(1)	27.7	17.5	23.9	8.8
England/Wales	125.7(6)	28.7	13.7	20.5	6.9
France	88.1(34)	19.7	10.3	5.0	5.8
Germany (Fed)	108.3(17)	21.9	15.2	7.8	6.8
Hungary	131.5(3)	22.6	18.1	14.9	11.8
Ireland	127.5(4)	27.8	15.1	19.2	6.1
Israel	98.7(24)	23.0	11.9	7.9	3.6
Italy	99.2(23)	20.8	10.3	7.3	6.0
Netherlands	109.8(13)	26.8	13.3	10.2	5.0
Sweden	98.1(25)	18.2	11.1	9.9	4.9
Switzerland	97.2(27)	24.3	10.9	7.2	5.9
USSR	94.5(7)	13.6	10.9	7.1	9.6

Note: Figures in parentheses are order of rank based on data from 46 countries during the years 1988–1990. Adapted from C.C. Boring, T.S. Squires. T. Tong & S. Montgomery. (1994). *Cancer Statistics*, 1994, CA-A *Cancer Journal for Clinicians*, **44**, 7–26.

there are three approaches, mammography, clinical breast examination, and breast self-examination (BSE). BSE has received considerable empirical study (for a review see Mayer & Solomon, 1992). Studies have focused on the issues which may determine the proficiency and regularity of women's BSEs. These are central issues for two reasons: (i) The medical community currently regards mammography as the most reliable means of early detection. For example, the National Cancer Institute excludes BSE as a screening technique because there are not sufficient data demonstrating its effectiveness in reducing survival. (ii) Despite this emphasis on mammography, breast cancer is usually (for upwards of 70% of women) discovered as a lump (usually in the upper outer quadrant) by the woman or her physician; a less common sign is a nipple discharge. While supporting endpoint data remain to be obtained, other health practice data would suggest that effective and regular BSE is a positive health practice.

Other investigators (e.g. Rimer, 1992) have considered the psychological, behavioural, sociodemographical, and health-care factors which appear to be related to women's usage of mammography. In many respects, this literature parallels the findings of that for BSE. Older women, poorer women, and those with weak linkages to the health-care system, for example, are less frequent users of mammography. Factors such as these result in deadly consequences for women, as poorer or older women without a history of mammography are often diagnosed with more advanced disease. Thus, to the extent that behavioural scientists can affect women's acceptance and utilization of the technique, survival may be directly improved.

There have also been efforts in the area of tertiary prevention, shortening delay to seeking a diagnosis once symptom/sign awareness has occurred. In the study of delay in seeking treatment for medical conditions, several definitions of delay have been used, but an often chosen operationalization is the number of days from the detection of the first symptom to an endpoint. This latter variable is less consistently chosen, but has included seeing a physician for symptoms (e.g. Waters *et al.*, 1983; Coates *et al.*, 1992), being diagnosed with a medical condition (Marshall, Gregorio & Walsh,

1982), or beginning treatment for the condition (e.g. Howson, 1950). According to this view, all individuals, and even some physicians, would be 'delayers'. Still, another strategy has been to designate some delay as more 'reasonable' than others (e.g. one month from symptom appearance to appearance before a physician; see early work in cancer by Pack & Gallo, 1938).

Figure 1 presents a general model of total patient delay applicable to a variety of physical disorders. This model conceives of delay as composed of a series of stages, each governed by a conceptually distinct set of decisional and appraisal processes. This model builds on work of Safer *et al.* (1979). While correlates of each stage can be studied, we have found that delay surrounding symptom interpretation (that is, the appraisal delay) accounts for most of the delay in seeking a cancer diagnosis (Andersen, Cacioppo, & Roberts, 1994). For women with gynaecological cancer, the appraisal interval was approximately 80% of the total, whereas, for women with breast symptoms, a site which has a narrower range of symptom diversity, the interval accounted for 60% of the delay.

It is likely that there are several reasons for the finding of appraisal processes accounting for the bulk of the delay time. First, the development of malignancy and the appearance of cancer symptoms are often protracted, and a complex and changing symptom picture can be typical, unlike the presentation of many other medical problems (e.g. myocardial infarction; see Matthews *et al.*, 1983). Symptoms can also vary with the site and extent of the disease. For example, ovary cancer has varied presentations (pelvic cramping, low back pain, pain or bleeding with intercourse, urinary frequency irregularities). Moreover, as cancers progress, they can involve other bodily systems (e.g. gastrointestinal, lymphatic) and the symptom picture tends to change from specific or localized complaints (e.g. vaginal discharge/bleeding) to diffuse ones (e.g. loss of appetite, nausea, 'flu' symptoms). Finally, cancer is a life-threatening and a low probability disease, and both conditions may foster distress and appraisal delay.

Briefly considering the other stages, illness delay is defined as the number of days elapsing from the time an individual concludes he or she is ill to the day s/he decides to seek medical help. At this time individuals must decide, for example, whether to seek assistance from others (e.g. physician, others with a similar condition) or to self-treat the illness. After this, the remaining delay time is spent in making two remaining decisions. One is the delay between the decision to seek medical attention and the person acting on this decision by making an appointment (behavioural delay). The other is the time that elapses between the person making an appointment and their first receiving medical attention (scheduling delay). Response-control factors such as affordability, normative factors such as family pressure, and cognitive factors such as the extent to which the decision to seek medical help is based on issue-relevant thinking, are more likely to modulate the time between a decision and an action for the behavioral delay time. In contrast, both patient characteristics (such as the manner in which the person describes their concerns and symptoms) and medical environment characteristics (such as an appointment backlog) which are not under an individual's control may modulate the delay incurred when scheduling an appointment. (See also 'Self-examination: breast, testicles.)

Diagnosis
(See also 'Breast cancer' and 'Gynaecological cancer'.)
An early clinical study suggested that the diagnosis of cancer

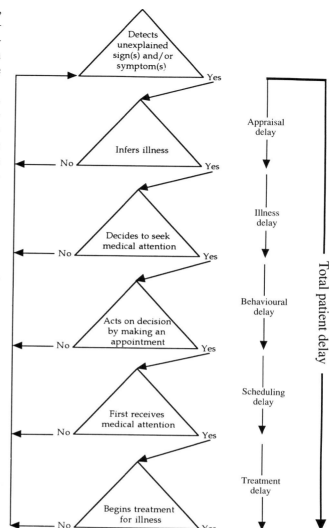

Fig. 1. A model of the course and types of patient delay.

produces an 'existential plight', meaning that the news brings shock, disbelief, and emotional turmoil (Weisman & Worden, 1976). Today, we know that individuals even become alarmed at the time of medical screening, long before a cancer diagnosis is suggested (Wardle & Pope, 1992). Perhaps because of these natural, difficult reactions, over the years there has been some variability in whether or not patients were told that their diagnosis was 'cancer'.

In the USA, as well as in most western countries, patients (including children) are now told that their diagnosis is cancer, since this is regarded as the moral, ethical, and legal procedure to follow (Woodard & Pamies, 1992). Support of this policy has documented the beneficial effects of coping successfully with an extreme stressor such as cancer (Taylor, 1983), and follow-up studies of childhood leukaemia survivors, for example, have pointed towards more favourable long-term adjustment for children when they learn of their diagnosis early, whether directly, accidentally, or through their own efforts, in comparison to children who learn late (Slavin *et al.*, 1982). Likewise, Mosconi *et al.* (1991) found that, of 1171 Italian breast cancer patients, those who were told their diagnosis was cancer, (47%) were the most satisfied with the information they had received from their physicians. Other cross-cultural research has indicated that the majority of patients want to be told their diagnosis truthfully (e.g. Japan: Mizushima *et al.*, 1990; United Kingdom: Sell *et al.*, 1993). Further, the manner in which the information is disclosed is important. Physicians who communicate hope have patients who are more hopeful, more favourable towards their cancer diagnosis, and who report more favourable overall emotional adjustment (Sardell & Trierweiler, 1993). This points to the need of physicians and other health professionals to learn more effective and thorough means of communicating information (e.g. diagnosis, treatment, prognosis) to their patients (Sell *et al.*, 1993; Woodard & Pamies, 1992).

Empirical reports clarify the specific emotions (sadness, depression, fear, anxiety, and anger) that characterize this period. It is not surprising that depression is the most common affective problem. Survey estimates for major depression are of the order of 5% to 6% (Derogatis *et al.*, 1983; Lansky *et al.*, 1985), similar to that of the general population (Locke & Regier, 1985). However, when major depression and depressed mood are considered, prevalence rates are higher (e.g. 16% in Derogatis *et al.*, 1983; 25% in a review by Massie & Holland, 1990). Lower rates have been found when specified diagnostic criteria are used and/or the patients assessed are ambulatory with good physical functioning (Levin, Jones & Sack, 1993; Massie & Holland, 1990). In general, depression is more common for those patients in active treatment rather than those on follow-up, receiving palliative rather than curative treatment, with pain or other disturbing symptoms rather than not, and/or with a history of affective disorder or alcoholism.

Study of the psychological responses which characterize the response to cancer diagnosis may shed light on the reactions of individuals to other life-threatening disease or treatment circumstances. When moods (Cassileth *et al.*, 1985; Westbrook & Viney, 1982) or coping strategies (Felton, Revenson & Hinrichsen, 1984) have been compared across disease groups (e.g. rheumatoid arthritis, diabetes, cancer, renal disease, hypertension), few differences have been found, suggesting that cancer patients may respond similarly to those with other life-threatening and/or chronic illnesses. On the other hand, patients in these studies have been heterogeneous on many disease variables (e.g. time since diagnosis, active treatment vs. follow-up status, and/or disability) that are important predictors of differential responses among cancer patients.

Differences in the patterns of emotional distress may exist. For example, it has been suggested that breast and gynaecological cancer patients are significantly less depressed, anxious, and hostile (angry) possibly due to perceptions of their illness as less serious than women with other forms of cancer (e.g. lung, gastrointestinal, head and neck; Sneed, Edlund & Dias, 1992). Similarly, a comparison of patients with limited versus extensive lung cancer and equivalent levels of physical impairment found that significantly greater mood disturbance was reported by the patients with extensive disease (and poorer prognoses; Cella *et al.*, 1987). Related findings have emerged for individuals who perceive their illness as severe (Marks *et al.*, 1986) or who have a sense of pessimism about one's life (Carver *et al.*, 1994). Carver *et al.* (1994) found that general pessimism (versus optimism) at diagnosis predicted poorer well-being (mood and life satisfaction) at one day before surgery as well as at 3-, 6-, and 12-month follow-ups. In addition, when patients are followed longitudinally, the emotional responses at recurrence are characterized by significantly higher levels of depressive and angry affect than had

been reported at the time of initial diagnosis (Andersen, Anderson, deProsse, 1989*b*).

It is encouraging that the clinical problem of diagnostic and treatment-related distress can be alleviated through psychological interventions (see Andersen, 1992 for a review) (see also 'Breast: cancer of the' and 'Gynaecological cancer'). A comprehensive example of such an effort is the study of Fawzy and colleagues (1990*a*,*b*). They attempted to reduce distress and enhance immune functioning in newly diagnosed melanoma patients via a structured group support intervention which included health education, illness related problem-solving, relaxation training, and group support. The format was weekly group treatment for six sessions. Eighty patients with early stage melanoma participated and were randomized to intervention or control conditions. The post-treatment analyses indicated that the intervention subjects reported significantly more vigour, but there were no other emotional distress differences. By six months, emotional distress had improved for the intervention subjects with significantly lower depression, confusion, and fatigue, and higher vigour. Coping data indicated that the intervention subjects reported significantly more use of active–behavioural strategies by treatment's end, a pattern which continued with the addition of active–cognitive strategies by 6 months. Regarding the immunological findings, at 6 months there was a significant difference in groups with better immunological status for the intervention subjects. These data are impressive in that they suggest that improvements in psychological status and coping are associated with changes (up-regulation) in immune responses.

Improvements such as these in mood and coping are all the more impressive because they are often achieved with brief, cost-effective interventions (e.g. 10 therapy hours with delivery in a group format; Andersen, 1992). Studies which have provided follow-up data also suggest some consolidation of intervention effects across time (upwards of 6 months post-treatment), with lowered emotional distress, enhanced coping, and/or improved sexual functioning (e.g. Capone *et al.*, 1980; Christensen, 1983).

Treatment

A certain component of the emotional distress occurring at diagnosis is due to the anticipation of treatment. Current therapies include surgery, radiotherapy and radioactive substances, chemotherapy, hormonal therapy, immunotherapy, and combination regimens and procedures (e.g. bone marrow transplantation, intraoperative radiotherapy). Some patients also undergo difficult diagnostic or treatment monitoring procedures (e.g. bone marrow aspirations), and all treatments are preceded or followed by physical examinations, tumour surveys, and/or laboratory studies. Thus, the diagnostic process of selecting the appropriate therapy and the subsequent treatment events can represent multiple occasions of medical stressors. As will be discussed below, the data are consistent in their portrayal of more distress (particularly fear and anxiety), slower rates of emotional recovery, and, perhaps, higher rates of other behavioural difficulties (e.g. food aversions, continued fatigue and malaise) than are found with healthy individuals also undergoing medical treatment. Despite the latter, the emotional crisis which characterizes the diagnostic period lessens as time passes, and longitudinal studies find that, as treatments end and recovery begins, there is an emotional rebound (e.g. Andersen, Anderson & deProsse, 1989*b*; Bloom, 1987; Devlen *et al.*, 1987; Edgar,

Rosberger & Nowlis, 1992). This lowering of emotional distress over time is found even for patients undergoing radical treatment requiring major adjustments (e.g. radical neck dissection with laryngectomy; Manuel et al., 1987). As cancer treatments (e.g. surgery, radiation, etc.) vary considerably in their intent, morbidity, and mortality, we will review each of the major modalities separately and also discuss three clinical problems (compliance, appetite and weight loss, and fatigue) which are common across therapies.

Surgery

There have been few investigations of cancer surgery, but there are numerous descriptive and intervention studies of the reactions of healthy individuals undergoing surgery for benign conditions. The latter studies are consistent in their portrayal of (a) high levels of self-reported preoperative anxiety predictive of lowered postoperative anxiety and (b) postoperative anxiety predictive of recovery (e.g. time out of bed, pain reports). What may distinguish cancer surgery patients are higher overall levels of distress and slower rates of emotional recovery. For example, Gottesman and Lewis (1982) found greater and more lasting feelings of crisis and helplessness among cancer patients in comparison to benign surgery patients for as long as two months following discharge.

Considering these data, findings on the interaction patterns of physicians and cancer patients on morning surgical rounds is disturbing. Blanchard et al. (1987) found attending physicians on a cancer unit less likely to be supportive and address patients' needs than physicians treating general medical patients. The heavier volume and more seriously ill patients common to cancer units might be sources for this unfortunate relationship. Related findings indicate that oncology nurses might find their job significantly more stressful than other assignments (e.g. cardiac, intensive care, or operating room nursing; Stewart et al., 1982), and may limit communication with cancer patients, especially those experiencing a recurrence (Wilkinson, 1991).

As noted above, there has been considerable research on the psychological and behavioural aspects of response to surgery, and many effective interventions have been tested. Components of these interventions include procedural information (i.e. how the surgery is to be performed as well as pre- and postoperative events from the perspective of the patient), sensory information on the actual physical sensations of the surgery or prepatory events, behavioural coping instructions, cognitive coping interventions, relaxation, hypnosis, and emotion-focused interventions. In a meta-analysis of this literature, Johnston & Vogele (1993) reported that procedural information and behavioural instructions show consistent and strong positive effects on postoperative recovery. Effects are significant for a broad band of measures, including ratings of negative affect and pain, amount of pain medication, length of stay, behavioural recovery, and physiological indices. (See also 'Breast cancer' for focus on lumpectomy and mastectomy.)

Radiotherapy

At least 350 000 individuals receive radiation therapy each year. Clinical descriptions have noted patients' fears (e.g. being burned, hair loss, sterility); while such outcomes do occur, they are site and dosage dependent. To understand radiation fears, the surgical anxiety studies already described above have been a paradigm. Here, again, anxiety (and sleeplessness) can often cause more overall distress than physical symptoms (Munro et al., 1989), and are pre-

dictors of treatment response (Wallace et al., 1993). If interventions to reduce distress (especially anticipatory anxiety) are not conducted, heightened post-treatment anxiety is also found (Andersen et al., 1988; Andersen & Tewfik, 1985) and might be maintained for as long as three months post-therapy, particularly when treatment symptoms linger (e.g. diarrhoea, fatigue; King et al., 1985). When acute side-effects resolve (usually by 12 months post-treatment), there appears to be no higher incidence of emotional difficulties for radiotherapy patients than for cancer surgery patients (Hughson et al., 1987).

Chemotherapy

Of all the treatment modalities, the greatest progress has been in the understanding of psychological reactions to chemotherapy and the related toxicities, particularly nausea and vomiting. Over a decade of research has revealed that approximately 60% of cancer patients will develop nausea and another 50% will develop vomiting in response to cytotoxic treatments (Morrow & Hickok, 1993). Psychological research has focused on eliminating or reducing these problems through hypnosis (e.g. Redd, Andersen & Minagawa, 1982), progressive muscle relaxation with guided imagery (e.g. Burish & Jenkins, 1992; Carey & Burish, 1988), systematic desensitization (e.g. Morrow, 1986; Morrow et al., 1992), cognitive distraction (e.g. P.G. Green, R.J. Seime & M.E. Smith, 1995, unpublished observations, Vasterling et al., 1993), and biofeedback (e.g. Burish & Jenkins, 1992; Burish, Shartner & Lyles, 1981).

The routine use of antiemetic drugs and the development of new agents has become more commonplace in recent years and this has resulted in an overall lower incidence and severity of nausea vomiting as a clinical problem. However, this change in clinical practice may have been somewhat offset by the use of more toxic regimens and the adjuvant treatment for disease types or stages which were previously not treated with chemotherapy (Andrykowski, 1993). It is clear that, in general, antiemetics need to be used from the beginning not only to control nausea and vomiting, but to reduce the likelihood of the development of anticipatory reactions. Once anticipatory nausea and vomiting develops in response to treatment, antiemetics are less effective (Morrow & Hickok, 1993), and point to the need for the use of behavioural strategies to aid patients (Andrykowski, 1993; Redd, 1993). Other research that will be helpful is that narrowing the focus on characteristics of individuals, that is individual differences (e.g. high pretreatment anxiety or autonomic activity, severity of post-treatment vomiting in the early cycles, age, susceptibility to motion sickness or gastrointestinal distress), as well as characteristics of the drugs (e.g. rated emetogenic potential of the regimen, dosages, number of agents used, etc.) that place patients at greater risk for the development of nausea and vomiting (e.g. see Carey & Burish, 1988 or Morrow, 1986 for empirical tests of variables; see Morrow & Hickok, 1993, for a review of the potential variables). (See also 'Vomiting and nausea as side-effects of drugs'.)

Bone marrow transplantation (BMT)

Over the past two decades, BMT has evolved from an experimental procedure performed as a last resort to an effective treatment routinely used for a variety of malignant conditions and solid tumours. In the past, BMT has been largely used when standard treatments have failed or have been expected to fail (Baker, Curbow &

Wingard, 1991). Initially used only for those with lymphohaemato-poietic malignancies or disorders characterized by bone marrow failure (e.g. leukaemia, Hodgkin's disease, and non-Hodgkin's lymphoma; Wingard et al., 1991), BMT is now being used with a variety of solid tumors (e.g., neuroblastomas, germ cell tumours, and cancers of the breast and ovary). The rapid acceptance and expanded use of this very toxic modality is no less than dramatic. For example, a Phase II study will soon begin in the US for BMT as an adjuvant treatment for breast cancer patients with ten or more positive lymph nodes (Winer & Sutton, 1994). If beneficial, it is possible that thousands of breast cancer patients may undergo BMT as a standard treatment for metastatic as well as regional disease in the near future (Winer & Sutton, 1994). At present, it is estimated that there are over 5000 transplants performed each year worldwide (Alby, 1991).

BMT is a complex, toxic, and potentially fatal treatment. The target of the treatment, the bone marrow, is destroyed with high dose chemotherapy, with or without whole body radiation afterwards. The transplanted bone marrow then comes from a donor (allogenic BMT) or from the patient him/herself (autologous BMT) after the marrow is removed and treated. Although allogenic BMT has a role, its expansion is limited by the need for a suitable donor and the subsequent risk of graft vs. host disease for the patient. In the case of autologous BMT, a variety of *ex vivo* procedures are used to destroy the malignant cells in the patient's marrow prior to reinfusion, including treatment with cytotoxic drugs, exposure to monoclonal antibodies which will attack tumour associated antigens, or harvesting and introducing stem cells from the patient's peripheral blood.

Patients (and their families) are faced with a number of stressors: a life-threatening illness, location of a suitable donor (for allogeneic transplants; Alby, 1991; Patenaude, 1990), toxic treatment with common and potentially fatal side-effects (e.g. liver failure; there is a 50% survival rate from the treatment). There are many other side-effects as well (e.g. hair loss, mouth and gastrointestinal mucositis, infertility, and skin breakdown, infection, pneumonia), and, of course, the treatment can fail and the disease persist or rapidly recur (Patenaude, 1990; Winer & Sutton, 1994). Hospitalization is prolonged (often 6–8 weeks or longer) and it is generally spent in isolation (Alby, 1991; Baker et al., 1991; Winer & Sutton, 1994).

The many difficulties (toxicity, uncertainty, illness and isolation, dependency, constant need for care) all contribute to patients feeling out-of-control (helplessness), alone, anxious, and/or depressed (Alby, 1991; Altmaier, Gingrich & Fyfe, 1991; Brown & Kelly, 1976). In attempting to cope, patients may be demanding, or the converse, withdrawn (Brown & Kelly, 1976; Patenaude, 1990). Psychological efforts have focused on providing support to patients, their families, and staff (Alby, 1991), and maximizing control for patients, such as making choices about the hospital environment whenever possible (Patenaude, 1990). For example, BMT rooms are often equipped with televisions/radios and weights and/or bicycles are provided for exercise as patients become stronger. Additionally, patients have been encouraged to bring personal items from home (e.g. pictures, photographs) to decorate their rooms. Increased medical complications, age, distance from home, and poorer pretransplant psychosocial adjustment are associated with the need for more intensive psychological consultation (Futterman et al., 1991).

Cross-modality problems and efforts to reduce treatment distress

Important steps have also been made towards understanding the aetiology and prevention of at least three common disease/treatment-related complications. First, appetite and weight loss are significant clinical problems for cancer patients susceptible to tumour-induced metabolism or taste changes, having tumour-related obstructions (often diagnosed as primary cachexia/anorexia), or receiving gastrointestinal–toxic chemotherapy or abdominal radiotherapy (secondary cachexia/anorexia). Malnutrition is associated with increased morbidity and mortality (Knox, 1991). Approximately 50% of the above patients will develop food aversions, averaging aversions to two or three particular foods (common aversions involve protein sources such as meats, eggs, and dairy products; for a review, see Jacobson & Schwartz, 1993. In particular, learned food aversions due to chemotherapy appear to be robust, with rapid acquisition (usually after one to three treatments) and maintenance after long delays (e.g. 48 hours) between food intake and aversive reactions (nausea) from the drugs (Bernstein, 1986; Jacobson & Schwartz, 1993). Research in this area has pointed the way, for example, to interventions employing novel tastes or 'scapegoat' foods (e.g. lemon-lime Kool-Aid, unusually flavoured hard sweets such as coconut; Jacobson & Schwartz, 1993) to 'block' conditioning to familiar diet items, reducing food and beverage intake prior to drug administration, and ingesting carbohydrate rather than protein source meals. While food aversions may not involve appetite or weight loss (e.g. patients eat other foods), patients may tend to form aversions to their favourite foods (e.g. coffee) which can affect their daily routine and perceived quality of life (Jacobson & Schwartz, 1993; Knox, 1991).

Secondly, fatigue is another dominant problem reported by the majority of patients receiving radio- or chemotherapy (Nail & King, 1987; Smets et al., 1993). Fatigue, described by patients as tiredness, lack of energy, sleepiness, confusion, poor concentration, etc., has been related to cancer morbidity and poor treatment compliance. Although a common experience, little systematic research has been conducted on the correlates of fatigue (for a review, see Irvine et al., 1991; Pickard-Holley, 1991; for a review, see Smets et al., 1993). Irvine et al. (1991) notes that research has not demonstrated consistent relationships between fatigue, anaemia, sleeplessness, and/or psychological distress (e.g. negative mood/depression), but it appears that fatigue does reduce overall functional ability. Psychological and behavioural interventions have focused on alleviating or increasing tolerance to fatigue through preparatory information on side-effects and activity/rest cycle recommendations (e.g. naps in the afternoon; Nail & King, 1987; Smets et al., 1993), as well as other coping efforts (e.g. planning/scheduling activities, decreasing non-essential activities, and relying on others for assistance as needed; Rhodes, Watson & Hanson, 1988).

The expectation and/or experience of unpleasant side-effects can comprise a patient's quality of life to the point that the patient may miss treatment appointments and/or be unwilling/unable to continue treatment, regardless if the treatment is curative or palliative (Morrow & Hickok, 1993; Richardson, Marks & Levine, 1988). Thus, if there is some non-compliance with therapy, the therapeutic dosage of treatment may be reduced which can, in turn, lower the cure rate. In short, non-compliance is a behavioural problem which can directly impact the effectiveness of cancer therapy. Non-compliance with treatment has been related to increased emotional distress (e.g. Gilbar & De-Nour, 1989; Richardson *et al.*, 1988), severity of treatment side-effects (e.g. nausea and vomiting, Lewis, Linet, & Abeloff, 1983; Richardson *et al.*, 1988), and lower income (Lebovits *et al.*, 1990). Even when patients are responsible for self-administration of therapy, such as taking their chemotherapy at home and they can reduce the number of required, but inconvenient, hospital visits, non-compliance may continue. One report of multidrug therapy with adults with haematological malignancies indicated that self-reports (versus sera reports) overestimated compliance by a factor of two (Richardson *et al.*, 1987).

Psychological interventions have focused on a variety of methods to improve patient compliance, including appointment reminders, clearly written and specific treatment communications (Anderson & Kirk, 1982), home-visits and medication-taking shaping interventions (Richardson *et al.*, 1987), and one-session interventions that include a tour of the oncology clinic, videotape presentation about the therapy, discussion/question sessions, and take-home information (Burish, Snyder & Jenkins, 1991). Burish *et al.* (1991) and others (e.g. Nail & King, 1987; Rainey, 1985) suggest that preparatory information can improve coping with treatment.

Importantly, psychological interventions can reduce distress during, and immediately following, cancer treatments. We will present the findings from two illustrative studies. Cain *et al.* (1986) compared individual and group therapy formats. The intervention had eight components including discussion of the causes of cancer at diagnosis, impact of the treatment(s) on body image and sexuality, relaxation training, emphasis on good dietary and exercise patterns, communication difficulties with medical staff and friends/family, and setting goals for the future to cope with uncertainty and fears of recurrence. The eight session programme was conducted during individual sessions conducted in the hospital or the women's home or in weekly groups of 4–6 patients conducted at the hospital. Seventy-two women with recently diagnosed or who were currently receiving therapy for gynaecological cancer participated. Outcome measures were administered pre- and post-treatment and at a 6-month follow up. Post-treatment analyses indicated all groups improved with time; however, anxiety was significantly lower for the individual therapy subjects only. Gains for the intervention subjects were more impressive with the 6 month follow-up data when there were no differences between the intervention formats, but both groups reported less depression and anxiety and better psychosocial adjustment (including health perspectives, sexual functioning, and use of leisure time) than the no treatment control group. Thus, the brief intervention, delivered either in individual or groups formats, appeared to be immediately effective, with gains enhanced during the early recovery months.

Edgar *et al.* (1992) provided a psychosocial intervention to 205 patients who were randomized into two groups: one group received the intervention soon after entering the study and the other group after a wait of four months. Both groups were assessed on depression, anxiety, illness worry, perceived personnal control, and ego strength at entry into the study, and at 4, 8, and 12-month intervals. The intervention (composed of 5 one-hour sessions) focused on coping skills and included problem-solving, goal setting, cognitive reappraisal, relaxation training, and at 4 month intervals, workshops on health-care information and available resources. The majority (*n*=159) of patients had been diagnosed with breast, colon, lung,

uterine, or head and neck cancers. While coping improved over the year for all patients, the later intervention group experienced lower levels of distress sooner than the group who had received the intervention earlier. Edgar *et al.* (1992) suggest that the delay in intervention may have been beneficial because it afforded patients the time to reduce feelings of being overwhelmed and they were, therefore, more ready to participate in the intervention. Additionally, data indicated that patients with lower ego strength and cancer diagnoses other than breast cancer appeared to experience greater distress and, therefore, particularly benefited from the intervention while patients with higher ego strength tended to cope well regardless of the intervention. These and related data (e.g. Forrester, Kornfield & Fleiss, 1985) attest to the significant distress which occurs when patients are in the midst of coping with diagnosis and treatment. Importantly, impressive gains can be achieved by the end of the intervention and often these positive effects are stronger with continued follow-up. Again, these effects have been achieved with brief interventions.

Choosing cancer treatments

Psychological and behaviour data have been (and should continue to be) important to patients and physicians alike for making choices among comparable treatments. Treatments that result in less quality of life disruption often become 'standard' treatment. The most obvious example of the importance of psychological data influencing cancer treatments was that documenting the more positive (e.g. feeling more attractive, fewer sexual difficulties) outcomes for women treated with breast saving (lumpectomy plus adjuvant radiation and/or chemotherapy) procedures rather than modified radical mastectomy (e.g. Margolis, Goodman & Rubin, 1990). Similarly, lower rates of erectile and ejaculation difficulties (e.g. 30% vs. 90%) are important reasons for some men with prostate cancer to choose supervoltage irradiation rather than surgery (radical prostatectomy; for a review see Andersen & Lamb (1995). Parallel data for women with genital cancer including treatment of women with uterine disease (Andersen, Anderson & deProsse, 1989*a*) and preinvasive vulvar disease (Andersen *et al.*, 1988) is available. Additionally, Rathmell *et al.* (1991) suggest that, unless a survival advantage is demonstrated, patients with advanced head and neck cancer may want radiotherapy alone versus surgery plus radiotherapy, as the treatment combination is associated with poorer quality of life scores (e.g. psychological well-being, speech quality, ability to eat, levels of energy and activity).

Recovery and long-term survival

The most important cancer endpoints have been treatment response rates, length of disease-free interval, and survival. Yet, as the prognosis for some sites has improved, there has been increased attention to the quality of life, particularly for long-term survivors of cancer. The term 'survivor' typically refers to individuals surviving at least five years, as the probability of late recurrence declines significantly after that time for most sites. As individuals recover and resume their life patterns, there may be residual emotional distress, other difficulties which require continued coping efforts, and even new problems (late sequelae) may occur. We will discuss each of these circumstances, and provide examples of both emotional and physical challenges which may confront the cancer survivor.

An investigation by Dunkel-Schetter *et al.* (1992) sheds light on the strategies cancer patients use as they recover and resume their life activities. They studied coping patterns of 603 cancer patients. Patient diagnoses included breast cancer, gastrointestinal, circulatory or lymph, gyneacological, and respiratory cancers, as well as others. The timing of the assessment ranged from initial diagnosis to more than 5 years post-treatment. Five coping patterns were identified: seeking or using social support, focusing on positive aspects, distancing, cognitive escape-avoidance (e.g. fantasizing or wishful thinking with fatalistic thoughts of poor outcomes), and behavioural escape-avoidance (e.g. social withdrawl, drug use). All patients used multiple coping strategies, but distancing was the most common. Unique patterns were found for subgroups. For example, individuals who viewed cancer as more stressful tended to use cognitive and behavioural escape-avoidance strategies, whereas patients reporting less distress relied on seeking or using social support, focusing on the positive, and distancing. Data such as these may have many uses; for example, they can be used to tailor psychological interventions to patient subgroups (e.g. identifying those patients who are likely to use drugs/alcohol to cope).

Lingering emotional distress from the trauma of diagnosis, treatment, and, more generally, life threat may occur for a small subset, perhaps 5–10% of cancer patients. When pronounced, such distress has been likened to post-traumatic stress disorder. (In fact, having residual distress from the diagnosis and treatment of a life-threatening illness is now included as one of the circumstances which may precipitate a DSM-IV (American Psychiatric Association, 1994) diagnosis of post-traumatic stress). In is unlikely that such extreme distress will occur for the 'average' cancer patient, and instead only occur for those who have undergone the most difficult of treatment regimens (e.g. BMT), lengthy toxic chemotherapies, as might be given to Stage III ovary patients, or for those who undergo life-altering and/or disfiguring cancer treatments (e.g. limb amputations, pelvic exenteration, larangectomies).

Secondly, some cancer survivors may need to cope with expected, but nevertheless, troubling sequelae which may be consequences of the disease or treatment and be, in large measure, permanent changes. For example, coping with body changes (e.g. loss of speech following laryngectomy) or apects of changes physical functioning (e.g. infertility) may require new behaviours/emotions and/or coping with losses (e.g. a sexual relationship that does not include intercourse). Thirdly, late side-effects of cancer treatment, for example, a bowel dysfunction which is traced to pelvic radiotherapy, can occur which changes health status as well as impact mood and coping.

Despite these possibilities, longitudinal data indicate that, if the disease is controlled, by one year post-treatment, the severe distress of diagnosis will have dissipated and emotions will have stabilized. The first longitudinal studies conducted in the United Kingdom for breast cancer patients indicated that by 12 (Maguire et al., 1978) and 24 months (Morris, Greer & White, 1977) that approximately 20% of the patients had problems with moderate to severe depression in comparison to 8% of benign disease comparison subjects. However, controlled longitudinal studies of breast (Bloom, 1987; Vinokur et al., 1989) and gynaecological (Andersen, Anderson & deProsse, 1989a, b) patients conducted in the USA and replicated with data from the Netherlands (deHaes, van Oostrom & Welvaart, 1986) have indicated no differences between the levels of emotional distress of women with cancer and either benign disease or healthy comparison subjects. Similar declines and lowered levels of distress

have been found in retrospective (Cella & Tross, 1986) and longitudinal (Devlen et al., 1987) studies of Hodgkin's disease and non-Hodgkin's lymphoma patients. The consistency of findings for the studies conducted during the 1980s is important because it represents replications across site, and, to some degree, treatment toxicity. In sum, we preface the remaining discussion by noting that global adjustment problems do not occur for the majority of cancer survivors; more likely scenarios are focused problem areas.

For example, Irvine et al. (1991) concluded, in a review of survivorship following breast cancer, that few patients experience long-term psychological distress, yet 20–30% will experience loss of roles (e.g. employment), decreased functional abilities, and problems with social relationships. Data on the adjustment of BMT survivors reveal a somewhat slower recovery (Syrjala et al. 1993). For example, comparison of BMT survivors and other cancer patients on maintenance chemotherapy indicated that psychological functioning was satisfactory when assessed 3–4 years post-diagnosis (Altmaier et al. 1991). By comparison, another study which assessed BMT patients sooner (2–4 years post-treatment) reported poorer physical functioning, greater impaired personal functioning (e.g. need for self-care assistance), and more relational problems (e.g. sexual difficulties) than individuals on maintenance chemotherapy (Altmaier et al., 1991). Also, there are data to suggest that there may be some risk of neuropsychological impairment from BMT procedures. Data from Andrykowski et al. (1992) data suggest impairments in memory and higher cognitive processing, which may be sequelae of BMT, per se, or prior cancer treatments which preceed BMT (e.g. cranial radiation, intrathecal chemotherapy). The many difficult aspects of BMT noted above (e.g. intensive chemotherapy, possible whole body irradiation, long recovery time, isolation) may account for this slowed and potentially more problematic recovery (for a review see Winer & Sutton, 1994 or Andrykowski, 1994).

Data suggest that sexuality may be one dimension that is more likely to undergo disruption than other major life areas. All cancer patients with solid tumours (approximately 85% of adult patients) are vulnerable to sexual dysfunction. Across sites, estimates range from 10% (e.g. breast cancer patients treated with lumpectomy), 70–90% (e.g. women with vulva cancer treated with modified radical vulvectomy), to 100% (e.g. men with prostate cancer treated with radical prostatectomy), with the distribution skewed towards greater levels of disruption (for a review see Andersen & Lamb, (1995)). Among the haematological malignancies, like Hodgkin's disease, estimates are in the range of 20% (Andersen & Lamb, (1995)). The data within treatment sites indicate that disease and treatment factors are the primary aetiologies for for sexual problems (e.g., gynaecological complications associated with long-term adjuvant tamoxifen therapy for breast cancer, Wolf & Jordan, 1992; female androgen deficiency syndrome resulting from cytotoxic agents and/or bilateral salpingo-oophorectomies, Kaplan & Owett, 1993). Controlled longitudinal studies of breast cancer patients (Maguire et al., 1978; Morris et al., 1977) and gynaecological cancer patients (Andersen et al., 1989a) have indicated that, if sexual problems develop, they do so as soon as intercourse resumes, and, if untreated, they are unlikely to resolve (for a discussion see Andersen & Elliott, in press). Psychological interventions such as provision of treatment side effect information and coping strategies for resuming intercourse (Capone et al. 1980. Houts et al., 1986).

The high incidence of sexual and fertility disruption has, in part, been the reason for the concern over marital disruption among adult cancer patients. For example, an early clinical study of women receiving radical mastectomy noted the realistic feelings of body disfigurement that both the women and spouses would feel – (prompting sexual retreat, emotional estrangement, and, not surprisingly, marital disruption) (Bard & Sutherland, 1952). Other concerns over the marriage originate from analyses of the interpersonal relationships, *per se*, of cancer patients (Wortman & Dunkel-Schetter, 1979). Despite the emotional distress and, for some, accompanying sexual disruption that couples experience, data from retrospective studies with comparison groups (Cella & Tross, 1986), and from the controlled longitudinal studies previously discussed, indicate that marriages remain intact and satisfactory. These data are consistent with prospective studies showing that, when health problems arise for newly married couples, they are not among those problems precipitant to divorce (Bentler & Newcomb, 1978). However, multicentre studies have indicated that young survivors are significantly less likely to marry, and once married they may be at greater risk for subfertility (Byrne *et al.*, 1985, 1988; Teeter *et al.*, 1987).

In general, the majority of cancer patients' relationships remain intact, satisfactory, and, on occasion, stronger, as found in data from single assessment (Baider & Sarell, 1984; Lichtman & Taylor, 1986) studies. Yet, the cancer experience is stressful for those closest to the patient, and the kin's distress may approach that of the patient's (Baider & De-Nour, 1988; Cassileth *et al.*, 1985). Family strain appears to be affected by illness variables (e.g. prognosis, stage/duration of illness, caregiving demands, patient's distress), family variables (e.g. age and gender of family members, socioeconomic status, other family stressors), and relational variables (e.g. quality of marriage, marital communication, family stage, and social support; for a review, see Sales, Schulz & Biegel, 1992). Young families, where the wife/mother has cancer and young children are in the home, may be at heightened risk for relational difficulties (Vess, Moreland, & Schwebel, 1985). In addition, Ell *et al.* (1988) found that those kin who were functioning poorly (e.g. lower perceived personal control, less adequate emotional support from close others, and greater stress unrelated to cancer) when the patient was diagnosed or who lost personal and social resources during the patient's treatment and recovery tended to function poorly at follow-up. In sum, a subset of partners and family members appear to be at psychosocial risk. For a review of strategies (focusing on information and support) that have been used to assist spouses of cancer patients cope with stress over the illness course, see Northouse and Peters-Golden (1993).

Finally, other, non-psychological outcomes may be disrupted following cancer, and these difficulties may have psychological concomitants (e.g. low self-esteem, perceived worthlessness). For example, it has been found that survivors of childhood or adolescent cancer are at risk for rejection from the armed services or college entrance and have difficulty obtaining health and life insurance (Teta *et al.*, 1986). Job discrimination and insurance difficulties have also been reported by survivors of bone marrow transplantation (Wingard *et al.*, 1991).

There have been few interventions targeted for cancer survivors, *per se*. One such study was that by Telch and Telch (1986). They compared the effectiveness of coping skills instruction with supportive therapy for a heterogeneous sample of cancer patients on follow-up. A novel aspect is that potential subjects were screened and only those with 'clear evidence of psychological distress' were eligible. Both interventions were offered in a group format. The coping skills instruction taught cognitive, behavioural, and affective coping strategies and included goal setting, self-monitoring, and role playing. Relaxation training and stress management skills were also included and patients provided ratings of their home practice. The group support intervention provided an environment for patients to discuss concerns but there was no specific agenda. Each group met for six weeks. Forty-one cancer patients completed the study. Analyses for the emotional distress data indicated that the coping skills group improved significantly across all measures, the support group improved on the anxiety and depression only, but the no treatment control worsened and reported significantly more mood distress.

Recurrence and death

Cancer recurrence is devastating (see 'Breast cancer' for focus on breast cancer recurrence); the magnitude of distress is even greater than that found with the initial diagnosis (Thompson, Andersen & DePetrillo, 1992), and studies contrasting cancer patients showing no evidence of disease with those receiving palliative treatment (e.g. Cassileth *et al.*, 1985) have reported the greatest distress for those with disseminated disease (Bloom, 1987). Difficult decisions (e.g. beginning a regimen that offers little chance for cure and has side effects vs. no treatment) are made in a context of extreme emotional distress and physical debilitation. The few studies of psychological interventions for adult patients have indicated that important emotional gains can be achieved during terminal stages (Linn, Linn, & Harris, 1982) and that children and adolescents, as well as adults, can make independent decisions about the continuation of therapy when death is imminent (Nitschke *et al.*, 1982).

At this time of significant emotional turmoil and physical difficulty, psychological interventions appear to enhance the quality of life. One example is an investigation of a group support intervention for women with breast cancer conducted by Spiegel, Bloom, and colleagues (Spiegel, Bloom & Yalom, 1981; Spiegel & Bloom, 1983). Women were randomized to no treatment or a group treatment intervention which included discussion of death and dying, family problems, communication problems with physicians, and living fully in the context of a terminal illness. The intervention subjects were also randomized a second time to two conditions: no additional treatment or self-hypnosis for pain problems (Spiegel & Bloom, 1983), which was incorporated into the support group format. All intervention groups met for weekly meetings for one year, for a total of 75 therapy hours. At the end of the first year the groups formally ended, but members could continue to meet as they wished or were able; some groups lasted for an additional two years. Eighty-six women, 50 intervention and 36 no treatment control, with metastatic breast cancer and referred to the intervention from her oncologist, participated. Following random assignment, there was subject loss (e.g. refusal, too weak, death) with the study beginning with 34 intervention and 24 control participants; however, the survival data is reported for the original sample of 86. Analyses indicated that the intervention group reported significantly fewer phobic responses and lower anxiety, fatigue, and confusion and higher vigour than the controls. These differences were evident at all assessments but the magnitude increased from 4 to 12 months. There was also a significant decrease in the use of maladaptive coping responses by the intervention group. Regarding the findings from the hypnosis substudy, women receiving hypnosis within the group support intervention reported no change in their pain sensations during the year, while pain sensations significantly increased for the other women in group support who did not receive hypnosis. Similar findings were reported for pain suffering a slight decrease for the women who also received hypnosis and a significant increase in suffering for the remaining intervention women). It is important to note that pain sensation scores for both groups were, however, significantly lower than those for the no intervention controls, suggesting that the hypnosis component provided an additive analgesic effect to other group treatment components. The most startling data from this project was reported in a survival analysis. A variety of follow-up analyses, controlling for initial disease stage, days of radiotherapy, or use or androgen or steroid treatments were conducted and all indicated the same survival differences favoring the intervention participants. Unlike other studies, interventions for terminal patients tend to be intensive and lengthy, such as 'several sessions', or 'until death'.

Finally, a frequent complication of disseminated disease is pain. Although it might also be one of the first symptoms of cancer or might be present when disease is only localized or spread regionally, pain is more common and less controllable for those with metastatic disease (Ahles, Ruckdeschel & Blanchard, 1984). The major cause of cancer pain, accounting for roughly 70% of the cases is due to direct tumour involvement (e.g. metastatic bone disease, nerve compression). Another 20% to 30% of cases are due to medical therapy (e.g. postoperative pain, radiation-induced pain). The remaining cases are individuals with pain problems unrelated to their cancer. The most difficult case is chronic pain associated with disease progression (e.g. patients with carcinoma of the pancreas, in which the pain escalates), where combinations of antitumour therapy, anaesthetic blocks, and behavioural approaches to pain control are considered. Behavioural research has focused on assessment strategies (Daut, Cleeland & Flanery, 1983; Keefe, Brantley, Manuel, & Crisson, 1985) and on pain reduction interventions, particularly hypnosis (Spiegel & Bloom, 1983). When palliative therapy is of little use and/or brings further debilitation, psychological interventions might provide pain control and, secondarily, prevent or treat pain sequelae, such as sleep disturbances, reduced appetite, irritability, and other behavioural difficulties.

CONCLUSION

Significant progress has been made in understanding the psychological and behavioural aspects of cancer. Contributions are significant in the areas of prevention and control. Research on smoking prevention and cessation has the potential to have an impact on the factor responsible for 30% of all cancer deaths. Similar efforts to encourage participation in screening and early-detection programmes for breast, cervix, colon and rectum cancer can help reduce cancer.

More is known about the psychological processes and reactions to the diagnosis and treatment of cancer than is known about any other chronic illness. Although most is known about the adjustment of breast cancer patients (for a review see Glanz & Lerman, 1992), other disease sites, men, and children are becoming more commonly studied. Future research will likely test the generalizability of these descriptive data and formulate general principles of adjustment to illness. While providing estimates of the magnitude of quality of life

problems, these data can be used for models which predict which patients might be at greatest risk for adjustment difficulties (see Andersen (1994) for a discussion). The latter is an important step towards designing interventions tailored to the difficulties and circumstances of cancer patients.

A growing literature on the use of psychological interventions to improve cancer patient's quality of life also exists (Andersen, 1992). The effectiveness of these interventions is robust, as they have reduced distress and enhanced the quality of life of many cancer patients differing on disease stage as well as disease site. Despite the challenges of studying these patients, well-controlled investigations have been conducted. Improvements in emotional distress are found at the end of the interventions as well with continued gains at follow-up. In addition, change in other areas (self esteem/concept, death perceptions, life satisfaction, and/or locus of control) have been found. Important for quality of life, psychological interventions could also lower or stabilize pain reports. The positive outcomes for terminal patients are notable considering their worsening pain and/or increasing debilitation.

While there appear to be unique intervention components for different phases in the disease, there are some commonalities. Therapy components have included: an emotionally supportive context to address fears and anxieties about the disease, information about the disease and treatment, behavioural coping strategies, cognitive coping strategies, and relaxation training to lower 'arousal' and/or enhance one's sense of control. The descriptive data also highlight the need for focused interventions for sexual functioning, particularly those treated for gynaecological, breast, and prostate cancer, and the intervention studies attest to the effectiveness of this specific component. These components appear more important to outcome than procedural variations. For example, therapy format, such as individual or group, appears to have little impact. Also, there were null findings for (group) interventions that included no structured content, suggesting that group support alone is insufficient to produce any measurable benefit.

How do psychological interventions achieve these effects? In large measure, the psychological mechanisms may not be different from those operative from interventions designed for coping with other stressors. That is, confronting a traumatic stressor with positive cognitive states, active behavioural strategies and, eventually, lowered emotional distress may enhance one's sense of self-efficacy, feelings of control, and provide realistic appraisals of stresses of the disease or treatment process. Similarly, for sexual interventions, information provides realistic expectations for sexuality and specific strategies to manage sexual activity when it is difficult or impossible. That the interventions produce more than situational improvement and may alter an individual's longer-term adjustment processes is suggested by the data indicating that adjustment gains continue (and often increase) during the first post-treatment year. Immediate and longer-term psychological changes may, in turn, increase the likelihood of changes in behavioural mechanisms, such as increasing the likelihood of adaptive health behaviours (e.g. complying with medical therapy; improving diet, exercise, etc.), to directly improve mental health, 'adjustment' and, possibly, medical outcomes. These data indicate that increasingly, issues of quality of life are being raised, and positive results have been achieved by behavioural sciences. But, as with most issues, further commitment and action is needed.

Ahles, T.A., Ruckdeschel, J.C. & Blanchard, E.B. (1984). Cancer related pain: I. Prevalence in an outpatient setting as a function of stage of disease and type of cancer. *Journal of Psychosomatic Research*, 28, 115–19.

Alby, N. (1991). Leukaemia: bone marrow transplantation. In M. Watson (Ed.) *Cancer patient care: psychosocial treatment methods.* Cambridge: BPS Books.

Altmaier, E.M., Gingrich, R.D. & Fyfe, M.A. (1991). Two-year adjustment of bone marrow transplant survivors. *Bone Marrow Transplantation*, 7, 311–16.

American Cancer Society. (1994). *Cancer facts and figures – 1994.* New York: Author.

Andersen, B.L. (1992). Psychological interventions for cancer patients to enhance the quality of life. *Journal of Consulting and Clinical Psychology*, 60, 552–68.

Andersen, B.L. & Elliott, M.L. (1993). Sexuality for women with cancer: assessment, theory, and treatment. *Sexuality and Disability*, 11, 7–37.

Andersen, B.L. & Lamb, M.A. (1995). Sexuality and cancer. In A.I. Holleb, D. Fink & G.P. Murphy (Eds.). *American Cancer Society textbook of clinical oncology, 2nd edition.* Atlanta: American Cancer Society, Inc.

Andersen, B.L. & Tewfik, H.H. (1985). Psychological reactions to radiation therapy: Reconsideration of the adaptive aspects of anxiety. *Journal of Personality and Social Psychology*, 48, 1024–32.

Andersen, B.L., Anderson, B. & deProsse, C. (1989a). Controlled prospective longitudinal study of women with cancer: I. Sexual functioning outcomes. *Journal of Consulting and Clinical Psychology*, 57, 683–91.

Andersen, B.L., Anderson, B. & deProsse, C. (1989b). Controlled prospective longitudinal study of women with cancer: II. Psychological outcomes. *Journal of Consulting and Clinical Psychology*, 57, 692–7.

Andersen, B.L., Cacioppo, J.T. & Roberts, D.C. (1995). Delay in seeking a cancer diagnosis: delay stages and psychophysiological comparison processes. *British Journal of Social Psychology.*

Andersen, B.L., Karlsson, J.A., Anderson, B. & Tewfik, H.H. (1985). Anxiety and cancer treatment: response to stressful radiotherapy. *Health Psychology*, 3, 535–51.

Andersen, B.L., Kiecolt-Glaser, J.K. & Glaser, R. (1994). A biobehavioral model of cancer stress and disease course. *American Psychologist*, 49, 389–404.

Andersen, B.L., Turnquist, D., LaPolla, J.P. & Turner, D. (1988). Sexual functioning after treatment of in situ vulvar cancer: preliminary report. *Obstetrics and Gynecology*, 71, 15–19.

Anderson, R.J. & Kirk, L.M. (1982). Methods of improving patient compliance in chronic disease states. *Archives of Internal Medicine*, 142, 1673–5.

Andrykowski, M.A. (1992). Neuropsychologic impairment in adult bone marrow transplant candidates. *Cancer*, 70, 2288–97.

Andrykowski, M.A. (1993). The Morrow/Hickok article reviewed: behavioral treatment of chemotherapy-induced nausea and vomiting. *Oncology*, 7, 93–4.

Andrykowski, M.A. (1994). Psychosocial factors in bone marrow transplantation: a review and recommendations for research. *Bone Marrow Transplantation*, 13, 357–75.

Ashburn, M.A. & Lipman, A.G. (1993). Management of pain in the cancer patient. *Anesthesia Analog*, 76, 402–16.

Ashley, J.M. (1993). Dietary guidelines for cancer prevention and control. *Oncology*, 7, 27–31.

Baider, L. & Sarell, M. (1984). Couples in crisis: patient–spouse differences in perception of interaction patterns and the illness situation. *Family Therapy*, 11, 115–22.

Baider, L. & De-Nour, A.K. (1988). Adjustment to cancer: who is the patient – the husband or the wife? *Israel Journal of Medicine Sciences*, 24, 631–6.

Baker, F., Curbow, B. & Wingard, J. (1991). Role retention and quality of life or bone marrow transplant survivors. *Social Science Medicine*, 32, 697–704.

Bard, M. & Sutherland, A.M. (1952). Adaptation to radical mastectomy. *Cancer*, 8, 656–71.

Bentler, P.M. & Newcomb, M.D. (1978). Longitudinal study of marital success and failure. *Journal of Consulting and Clinical Psychology*, 46, 1053–70.

Bernstein, I.L. (1986). Etiology of anorexia in cancer. *Cancer*, 58, 1881–6.

Blanchard, C.G., Ruckdeschel, J.C., Labrecque, M.S., Frisch, S. & Blanchard, E.B. (1987). The impact of a designated cancer unit on house staff behaviors toward patients. *Cancer*, 60, 2348–54.

Bloom, J.R. (1987). Psychological response to mastectomy. *Cancer*, 59, 189–96.

Boring, C.C., Squires, T.S., Tong, T. & Montgomery, S. (1994). Cancer statistics, 1994. *Cancer Journal for Clinicians*, 44, 7–26.

Brown, H.N. & Kelly, M.J. (1976). Stages of bone marrow transplantation: a psychiatric perspective. *Psychosomatic Medicine*, 38, 439–446.

Burish, T.G. & Jenkins, R.A. (1992). Effectiveness of biofeedback and relaxation training in reducing the side effects of cancer chemotherapy. *Health Psychology*, 11, 17–23.

Burish, T.G., Shartner, C.D. & Lyles, J.N. (1981). Effectiveness of multiple muscle-site EMG biofeedback and relaxation training in reducing the aversiveness of cancer chemotherapy. *Biofeedback and Self-Regulation*, 6, 523–35.

Burish, T.G., Snyder, S.L. & Jenkins, R.A. (1991). Preparing patients for cancer chemotherapy: effect of coping preparation and relaxation interventions. *Journal of Consulting and Clinical Psychology*, 39, 518–25.

Byrne, J., Mulvihill, J.J., Myers, M.H., Abbott, S.C., Connelly, R.R., Hanson, M.R., Hassinger, D.D., Naughton, M.D., Austin, D.F., Gurgin, V.A., Holmes, F.F., Holmes, G.F., Latourette, H.B., Weyer, P.J., Meigs, J.W., Teta, M.J., Strong, L.C. & Cook, J.A. (1985). Risk of infertility among survivors of childhood and adolescent cancer. *American Journal of Human Genetics*, 37, 24–48.

Byrne, J., Mulvihill, J.J., Connelly, R.R., Myers, M.H., Austin, D.F., Holmes, F.F., Holmes, G.F., Latourette, H.V., Meigs, J.W. & Strong, L.C. (1988). Reproductive problems and birth defects in survivors of Wilm's tumor and their relatives. *Medical and Pediatric Oncology*, 16, 233–40.

Cain, E.N., Kohorn, E.I., Quinlan, D.M., Latimer, K. & Schwartz, P.E. (1986). Psychosocial benefits of a cancer support group. *Cancer*, 57, 183–9.

Capone, M.A., Good, R.S., Westie, K.S. & Jacobson, A.F. (1980). Psychosocial rehabilitation of gynecologic oncology patients. *Archives of Physical Medicine and Rehabilitation*, 61, 128–32.

Carey, M.P & Burish, T.G. (1988). Etiology and treatment of the psychological side effects associated with cancerchemotherapy. *Psychological Bulletin*, 104, 307–25.

Carver, C.S., Pozo-Kaderman, C., Harris, S.D., Noriega, V., Scheier, M.F., Robinson, D.S., Ketcham, A.S., Moffat, F.L. & Clark, K.C. (1994). Optimism versus pessimism predicts the quality of women's adjustment to early stage breast cancer. *Cancer*, 73, 1213–20.

Cassileth, B.R., Lunk, E.J., Strouse, T.B., Miller, D.S., Brown, L. & Cross, P.A. (1985). A psychological analysis of cancer patients and their next-of-kin. *Cancer*, 55, 72–6.

Cella, D.F., Orofiamma, B., Holland, J.C., Silberfarb, P.M., Tross, S., Feldstein, M., Perry, M., Maurer, L.H., Cornis, R. & Orav, J. (1987). The relationship of psychological distress, extent of disease, and performance status in patients with lung cancer. *Cancer*, 60, 1661–7.

Cella, D.F. & Tross, S. (1986). Psychological adjustment to survival from Hodgkin's

General cancer

Disease. *Journal of Consulting and Clinical Psychology*, 54, 616–22.

Christensen, D.N. (1983). Postmastectomy couple counseling: an outcome study of a structured treatment protocol. *Journal of Sex and Marital Therapy*, 9, 266–74.

Coates, R.J., Bransfield, D.D., Wesley, M., Hankey, B., Eley, J.W., Greenberg, R.S., Flanders, D., Hunter, C.P., Edwards, B.K., Forman, M., Chen, V.W., Peynolds, P., Boyd, P., Austin, D., Muss, H. & Blacklow, R.S. (1992). Differences between black and white women with breast cancer in time from symptom recognition to medical consultation. *Journal of the National Cancer Institute*, 84, 938–50.

Coyle, N., Adelhardt, J., Foley, K.M. & Portenoy, R.K. (1990). Character of terminal illness in the advanced cancer patient: pain and other symptoms during the last four weeks of life. *Journal of Pain and Symptom Management*, 5, 83–93.

Daut, R.L., Cleeland, C.S. & Flanery, R.C. (1983). Development of the Wisconsin Brief Pain questionnaire to assess pain in cancer and other diseases. *Pain*, 17, 197–210.

deHaes, J.C., van Oostrom, M.A. & Welvaart, K. (1986). The effect of radical and conserving surgery on quality of life of early breast cancer patients. *European Journal of Surgical Oncology*, 12, 337–342.

Derogatis, L.R., Morrow, G.R., Fetting, J., Penman, D., Piasetsky, S., Schmale, A.M., Henricho, M. & Carnicke, C.L. (1983). The prevalence of psychiatric disorders among cancer patients. *Journal of the American Medical Association*, 249, 751–7.

Devlen, J., Maguire, P., Phillips, P., Crowther, D. & Chambers, H. (1987). Psychological problems associated with diagnosis and treatment of lymphomas. I: Retrospective study and II: Prospective study. *British Medical Journal*, 295, 953–7.

Dunkle-Schetter, C., Feinstein, L.G., Taylor, S.E. & Falke, R.L. (1992). Patterns of coping with cancer. *Health Psychology*, 11, 79–87.

Edgar, L., Rosberger, Z. & Nowlis, D. (1992). Coping with cancer during the first year after diagnosis: assessment and intervention. *Cancer*, 69, 817–28.

Ell, K., Nishimoto, R, Mantell, J. & Hamovitch, M. (1988). Longitudinal analysis of psychological adaptation among family members of patients with cancer. *Journal of Psychosomatic Research*, 32, 429–38.

Fawzy, F.I., Cousins, N., Fawzy, N., Kemeny, M.E., Elashoff, R., & Morton, D. (1990a). A structured psychiatric intervention for cancer patients: I. Changes over time in methods of coping and affective disturbance. *Archives of General Psychiatry*, 47, 720–5.

Fawzy, F.I., Kemeny, M.E., Fawzy, N., Elashoff, R., Morton, D., Cousins, N., & Fahey, J.L. (1990b). A structured psychiatric intervention for cancer patients: II. Changes over time in immunological measures. *Archives of General Psychiatry*, 47, 729–35.

Fawzy, F.I., Fawzy, N., Hyun, C.S., Gutherie, D., Fahey, J.L., & Morton, D. (1993). Malignant melanoma: effects of an early structured psychiatric intervention, coping, and affective state on recurrence and survival six years later. *Archives of General Psychiatry*, 50, 681–9.

Felton B.J., Revenson, T.A., & Hinrichsen, G.A. (1984). Stress and coping in the explanation of psychological adjustment among chronically ill adults. *Social Science Medicine*, 18, 889–98.

Foley, K.M. (1985). The treatment of cancer pain. *New England Journal of Medicine*, 313, 84–95.

Forester, B., Kornfield, D.S. & Fleiss, D.L. (1985). Psychotherapy during radiotherapy: effects on emotional and physical distress. *American Journal of Psychiatry*, 142, 22–7.

Futterman, A.D., Wellisch, D.K., Bond, G. & Carr, C.R. (1991). The psychosocial levels system: a new rating scale toidentify and assess emotional difficulties during bone marrow transplantation. *Psychosomatics*, 32, 177–186.

Garfinkel, L. (1994). Evaluating cancer statistics. *Cancer Journal for Clinicians*, 44, 5–6.

Gilbar, O. & De-Nour, A.K. (1989). Adjustment to illness and dropout of chemotherapy. *Journal of Psychosomatic Research*, 33, 1–5.

Glanz, K. & Lerman, C. (1992). Differences in crisis reactions among cancer and surgery patients. *Journal of Consulting Psychology*, 50, 381–8.

Gottesman, D. & Lewis, M. (1982). Differences in crisis reactions among cancer and surgery patients. *Journal of Consulting and Clinical Psychology*, 50, 381–8.

Greenwald, P. & Cullen, J.W. (1985). The new emphasis in cancer control. *Journal of the National Cancer Institute*, 74, 543–51.

Heber, D., Bagga, D., Ashley, J.M. & Elashloff, R.M. (1993). Nutritional strategies for breast cancer prevention. *Oncology*, 7, 43–6.

Houts, P.S., Whitney, C.W., Mortel, R. & Bartholemew, M.J. (1986). Former cancer patients as counselors of newly diagnosed cancer patients. *Journal of the National Cancer Institute*, 76, 793–6.

Howson, J.Y. (1950). The procedures and results of the Philadelphia committee for the study of pelvic cancer. *Wisconsin Medical Journal*, 49, 215–19.

Hughson, A.V., Cooper, A.F., McArdle, C.S. & Smith, D.C. (1987). Psychosocial effects of radiotherapy after mastectomy. *British Medical Journal*, 294, 1515–18.

Irvine, D., Brown, B., Crooks, D., Roberts, J. & Browne, G. (1991). Psychosocial adjustment in women with breast cancer. *Cancer*, 67, 1097–117.

Irvine, D.M., Vincent, L., Bubela, N., Thompson, L. & Graydon, J. (1991). A critical appraisal of the research literature investigating fatigue in the individual with cancer. *Cancer Nursing*, 14, 188–99.

Jacobsen, P.B. & Schwartz, M.D. (1993). Food aversions during cancer therapy: incidence, etiology, and prevention. *Oncology*, 7, 139–43.

Johnston, M. & Vogele, C. (1993). Benefits of psychological preparation for surgery: a meta-analysis. *Annals of Behavioral Medicine*, 15, 245–56.

Kaplan, H.S. & Owett, T. (1993). The female androgen deficiency syndrome. *Journal of Sex and Marital Therapy*, 19, 3–24.

Keefe, F.J., Brantley, A., Manual, S. & Crisson, J.E. (1985). Behavioral assessment of head and neck cancer pain. *Pain*, 23, 327–36.

King, K.B, Nail, L.M., Kreamer, K., Strohl, R.A. & Johnson, J.E. (1985). Patients descriptions of the experience of receiving radiation therapy. *Oncology Nursing Forum*, 12, 55–61.

Knox, L.S. (1991). Maintaining nutritional status in persons with cancer. Paper in Cancer Nursing: *Maintaining nutritional status in persons with cancer*, pp. 1–11. Atlanta, GA: American Cancer Society, Inc.

Lansky, S.B., List, M.A., Herrman, C.A., Ets-Hokin, E.G., Das Gupta, T.K., Wilbanks, G.D. & Hendrickson, F.R. (1985). Absence of major depressive disorders in female cancer patients. *Journal of Clinical Oncology*, 2, 1553–60.

Lebovits, A.H., Strain, J.J., Schleifer, S.J., Tanaka, J.S., Bhardwaj, S. & Messe, M.R. (1990). Patient noncompliance with self-administration chemotherapy. *Cancer*, 65, 17–22.

Levin, S.H., Jones, L.D. & Sack, D.A. (1993). Evaluation and treatment of depression, anxiety, and insomnia in patients with cancer. *Oncology*, 7, 119–25.

Lewis, C., Linet, M.S. & Abeloff, M.D. (1983). Compliance with cancer therapy by patients and physicians. *The American Journal of Medicine*, 74, 673–8.

Lichtman, R.R. & Taylor, S.E. (1986). Close relationships and the female cancer patient. In *Women with cancer: Psychological Perspectives*, ed. B.L. Andersen pp. 233–56. New York: Springer-Verlag.

Linn, M.W., Linn, B.S. & Harris, R. (1982). Effects of counseling for late stage cancer patients. *Cancer*, 49, 1048–55.

Locke, B.Z. & Regier, D.A. (1985). Prevalence of selected mental disorders. In C.A. Taube & S.A. Barrett (Eds.). *Mental health United States* pp. 1–6. Rockville, MD: National Institute of Mental Health.

Maguire, G.P., Lee, E.G., Bevington, D.J., Kuchemann, C.S., Crabtree, R.J. & Cornell, C.E. (1978). Psychiatric problems in the first year after mastectomy. *British Medical Journal*, 1, 963–5.

Mahon, S.M., Cella, D.F. & Donovan, M.I. (1990). Psychosocial adjustment to recurrent cancer. *Oncology Nursing Forum*, 17, 47–54.

Manuel, G.M., Roth, S., Keefe, F.J. & Brantley, B.A. (1987, Winter). Coping with cancer. *Journal of Human Stress*, pp. 149–158.

Margolis, G., Goodman, R.L. & Rubin, A. (1990). Psychological effects of breast-conserving cancer treatment and mastectomy. *Psychosomatics*, 31, 33–9.

Marks G., Richardson, J.L., Graham, J.W. & Levine, A. (1986). Role of health locus of control beliefs and expectations of treatment efficacy in adjustment to cancer. *Journal of Personality and Social Psychology*, 51, 443–50.

Marshall, J.R., Gregorio, D.I. & Walsh, D. (1982). Sex differences in illness behavior: care seeking among cancer patients. *Journal of Health and Social Behavior*, 23, 197–204.

Massie, M.J. & Holland, J.C. (1990). Depression and the cancer patient. *Journal of Clinical Psychiatry*, 51, 12–19.

Massie, M.J. & Holland, J.C. (1992). The cancer patient with pain: psychiatric complications and their management. *Journal of Pain and Symptom Management*, 7, 99–109.

Matthews, K.A., Siegel, J.M., Kuler, L.H., Thompson, M. & Varat, M. (1983). Determinants of decision to seek medical treatment by patients with acute myocardial infarction symptoms. *Journal of Personality and Social Psychology*, 44, 1144–56.

Mayer, J.A & Solomon, L.J. (1992). Breast self-examination skill and frequency: a review. *Annals of Behavioral Medicine*, 14, 189–96.

Mizushima, Y., Kashii, T., Hoshino, K., Morikage, T., Takashima, A., Hirata, H., Kawasaki, A., Konisha, K. & Yano, S. (1990). *Japanese Journal of Medicine*, 29, 146–55.

Morris, T., Greer, H.S. & White, P. (1977). Psychological and social adjustment to mastectomy: a two-year follow-up study. *Cancer*, 40, 2381–7.

Morrow, G.R. (1986). Effect of the cognitive hierarchy in the systematic desensitization treatment of anticipatory nausea in cancer patients: a component comparison with relaxation only, counseling and no treatment. *Cognitive Therapy and Research*, 10, 421–46.

Morrow, G.R. & Hickok, J.T. (1993). Behavioral treatment of chemotherapy-induced nausea and vomiting. *Oncology*, 7, 83–9.

Morrow, G.R., Asbury, R., Hammon, S., Dobkin, P., Caruso, L., Pandya, K. & Rosenthal, S. (1992). Comparing the effectiveness of behavioral treatment for chemotherapy-induced nausea and vomiting when administered by oncologists, oncology nurses, and clinical psychologists. *Health Psychology*, 11, 250–6.

Mosconi, P., Meyerowitz, B.E., Liberati, M.C. & Liberati, A. (1991). Disclosure of breast cancer diagnosis: patient and physician reports. *Annals of Oncology*, 2, 273–80.

Munro, A.J., Biruls, R., Griffin, A.V., Thomas, H. & Vallis, K.A. (1989). Distress associated with radiotherapy for malignant disease: a quantitative analysis based on patients perceptions. *British Journal of Cancer*, 60, 370–4.

Nail, L.M. & King, K.B. (1987). Fatigue. *Seminars in Oncology Nursing*, 3, 257–62.

Nitschke, R., Humphrey, G.B., Sexauer, C.L., Carton, B., Wunder, S. & Jay, S. (1982). Therapeutic choices made by patients with end-stage cancer. *Journal of Pediatrics*, 101, 471–6.

Northouse, L.L. & Peters-Golden, H. (1993). Cancer and the family: strategies to assist spouses. *Seminars in Oncology Nursing*, 9, 74–82.

Pack, G.T. & Gallo, J.S. (1938). Culpability for delay in treatment of cancer. *American Journal of Cancer*, 33, 443–62.

Patenaude, A.F. (1990). Psychological impact of bone marrow transplantation: current perspectives. *The Yale Journal of Biology and Medicine*, 63, 515–19.

Pickard-Holley, S. (1991). Fatigue in cancer patients. *Cancer Nursing*, 14, 13–19.

Rathmell, A.J., Ash, D.V., Howes, M. & Nicholls, J. (1991). Assessing quality of life in patients treated for advanced head and neck cancer. *Clinical Oncology*, 3.

Rainey, L.C. (1985). Effects of preparatory education for radiation oncology patients. *Cancer*, 56, 1056–61.

Redd, W.H. (1993). The Morrow/Hickok article reviewed: behavioral treatment of chemotherapy-induced nausea and vomiting. *Oncology*, 7, 94–5.

Redd, W.H., Andresen, G.V. & Minagawa, R.Y. (1982). Hypnotic control of anticipatory emesis in patients receiving cancer chemotherapy. *Journal of Clinical and Consulting Psychology*, 50, 14–19.

Rhodes, V.A., Watson, P.M. & Hanson, B.M. (1988). Patients' descriptions of the influence of tiredness and weakness on self-care abilities. *Cancer Nursing*, 11, 186–94.

Richardson, J.L., Marks, G., Johnson, C.A., Graham, J.W., Chan, K.K., Selser, J.N., Kishbaugh, C., Barranday, Y. & Levine, A.M. (1987). Path model of multidimensional compliance with cancer therapy. *Health Psychology*, 6, 183–207.

Richardson, J.L., Marks, G. & Levine, A. (1988). The influence of symptoms of disease and side effects of treatment on compliance with cancer therapy. *Journal of Clinical Oncology*, 6, 1746–52.

Rimer, B.K. (1992). Understanding the acceptance of mammography by women. *Annals of Behavioral Medicine*, 14, 197–203.

Safer, M.A., Tharps, Q.J., Jackson, T.C & Levanthal, H. (1979). Determinants of three stages of delay in seeking care at a medical clinic. *Medical Care*, 17, 11–29.

Sales, E., Schulz, R. & Biegel, D. (1992). Predictors of strain in families of cancer patients: a review of the literature. *Journal of Psychosocial Oncology*, 10, 1–26.

Sardell, A.N. & Trierweiler, S.J. (1993). Disclosing the cancer diagnosis. *Cancer*, 72, 3355–65.

Schonfield, J. (1972). Psychological factors related to delayed return to an earlier life-style in successfully treated cancer patients. *Journal of Psychosomatic Research*, 16, 41–6.

Sell, L, Devlin, B., Bourke, S.J., Munro, N.C., Corris, P.A. & Gibson, G.J. (1993). Communicating the diagnosis of lung cancer. *Respiratory Medicine*, 87, 61–3.

Slavin, L.A., O'Malley, J.E., Koocher, G.P. & Foster, D.J. (1982). Communication of the cancer diagnosis to pediatric patients: impact on long-term adjustment. *American Journal of Psychiatry*, 139, 179–83.

Smets, E.M., Garssen, B., Schuster-Uitterhoeve, A.L. & deHaes, J.C. (1993). Fatigue in cancer patients. *British Journal of Cancer*, 68, 220–4.

Sneed, N.V., Edlund, B. & Dias, J.K. (1992). Adjustment of gynecological and breast cancer patients to the cancer diagnosis: comparisons with males and females having other cancer sites. *Health Care for Women International*, 13, 11–22.

Spiegel, D. & Bloom, J.R. (1983). Group therapy and hypnosis reduce metastatic breast carcinoma pain. *Psychosomatic Medicine*, 45, 333–9.

Spiegel, D., Bloom, J.R. & Yalom, I. (1981). Group support for patients with metastatic cancer: a randomized outcome study. *Archives of General Psychiatry*, 38, 527–33.

Steinberg, M.D., Juliano, M.A. & Wise, L. (1985). Psychological outcome of lumpectomy versus mastectomy in the treatment of breast cancer. *American Journal of Psychiatry*, **142**, 34–9.

Stewart, B.E., Meyerowitz, B.E., Jackson, L.E., Yarkin, K.L. & Harvey, J.H. (1982, October). Psychological stress associated with outpatient oncology nursing. *Cancer Nursing*, pp. 383–387.

Strang, P. & Qvarner, H. (1990). Cancer-related pain and its influence on quality of life. *Anticancer Research*, **10**, 109–12.

Syrjala, K.L., Chapko, M.K., Vitaliano, P.P., Cummings, C. & Sullivan, K.M. (1993). Recovery after allogeneic marrow transplantation: prospective study of predictors of long-term physical and psychosocial functioning. *Bone Marrow Transplantation*, **11**, 319–27.

Taylor, S.E. (1983). Adjustment to threatening events: a theory of cognitive adaptation. *American Psychologist*, **38**, 1161–73.

Teeter, M.A., Holmes, G.E., Homes, F.F. & Baker, A.B. (1987). Decisions about marriage and family among survivors of childhood cancer. *Journal of Psychosocial Oncology*, **5**, 59–68.

Telch, C.F. & Telch, M.J. (1986). Group coping skills instruction and supportive group therapy for cancer patients: a comparison of strategies. *Journal of Consulting and Clinical Psychology*, **54**, 802–8.

Teta, M.J., Del Po, M.C., Kasl, S.V., Meigs, J.W., Myers, M.H. & Mulvihill, J.J. (1986). Psychosocial consequences of childhood and adolescent cancer survival. *Journal of Chronic Disease*, **39**, 751–9.

Thompson, L., Andersen, B.L. & DePetrillo, D. (1992). The psychological processes of recovery from gynecologic cancer. In M. Coppleson, P. Morrow & M. Tattersall (Eds.). *Gynecologic oncology* 2nd edn. Edinburgh: Churchill Livingstone.

Vasterling, J., Jenkins, R.A., Tope, D.M. & Burish, T.G. (1993). Cognitive distraction and relaxation training for the control of side effects due to cancer chemotherapy. *Journal of Behavioral Medicine*, **16**, 65–80.

Vess, J.D., Moreland, J.R. & Schwebel, A.I. (1985). A followup study of role functioning and the psychosocial environment of families of cancer patients. *Journal of Psychosocial Oncology*, **3**, 1–14.

Vinokur, A.D., Threatt, B.A., Caplan, R.D. & Zimmerman, B.L. (1989). Physical and psychosocial functioning and adjustment to breast cancer: long-term follow-up of a screening population. *Cancer*, **63**, 394–405.

Wallace, L.M., Priestman, S.G., Dunn, J.A. & Priestman, T.J. (1993). The quality of life of early breast cancer patients treated by two different radiotherapy regimens. *Clinical Oncology*, **5**, 228–33.

Wardle, J. & Pope, R. (1992). The psychological costs of screening for cancer. *Journal of Psychosomatic Research*, **36**, 609–24.

Waters, W.E., Nichols, S., Wheeler, M.J., Fraser, J. & Hayes, A.J. (1983). Evaluation of a health education campaign to reduce the delay in women presenting with breast symptoms. *Community Medicine*, **5**, 104–8.

Weisman, A.D. & Worden, J.W. (1976). The existential plight in cancer: significance of the first 100 days. *International Journal of Psychiatry in Medicine*, **7**, 1–15.

Westbrook, M.T. & Viney, L.L. (1982). Psychological reactions to the onset of chronic illness. *Social Science Medicine*, **16**, 899–905.

Wilkinson, S. (1991). Factors which influence how nurses communicate with cancer patients. *Journal of Advanced Nursing*, **16**, 677–88.

Winer, E.P. & Sutton, L.M. (1994). Quality of life after bone marrow transplantation. *Oncology*, **8**, 19–31.

Wingard, J.R., Curbow, B., Baker, F. & Piantadosi, S. (1991). Health, functional status, and employment of adult survivors of bone marrow transplantation. *Annals of Internal Medicine*, **114**, 113–18.

Wolf, D.M. & Jordan, V.C. (1992). Gynecologic complications associated with long-term adjuvant tamoxifen therapy for breast cancer. *Gynecologic Oncology*, **45**, 118–28.

Woodard, L.J. & Pamies, R.J. (1992). The disclosure of the diagnosis of cancer. *Primary Care*, **19**, 657–63.

Wortman, C.B. & Dunkel-Schetter, C. (1979). Interpersonal relationships and cancer: A theoretical analysis. *Journal of Social Issues*, **35**, 120–55.

Wynder, E.L. & Cohen, L.A. (1993). Nutritional opportunities and limitations in cancer prevention. *Oncology*, **7**, 13–16.

Genetic counselling

MAURICE BLOCH

Riverview Hospital, Port Coquitlam, BC, Canada

Genetic counselling, which developed in the first half of the twentieth Century out of the biologically based science of genetics, was little influenced by the growth and development of counselling and psychotherapy within clinical psychology and psychiatry. The reputation of genetic counselling was tainted by association with eugenics theories. The defeat of Nazi Germany as well as the infamy of the Herrenvolk principle and theories of superior races led to a decline of the eugenics movement and the rise in philosophies which value the individual above society and give precedence to individual rights and freedoms. In the post-War era, genetic counselling aligned itself with the goals of the non-directive psychological therapies (e.g. client-centred therapy) and was, in turn, influenced by their emphasis on the process of therapy, on the relationship between therapist and client and the communication between them.

The term 'genetic counselling' was first used after World War II. The most widely accepted goal at that time was to provide medical and genetic information in order to reduce the incidence of genetic disease. The process of counselling was seen generally as prescriptive with the physician or counsellor ('the expert') advising the client of the facts and of the best course of action to take. As the ethical value of autonomy gained cultural precedence, counsellors made a shift from being prescriptive to being informative. The new approach, they thought, would allow parents to make informed and 'rational' or 'appropriate' reproductive decisions. The implication was that rational decisions would lead to the elimination of, or at least reduction in, the incidence of genetic disorders.

In 1975 the report of the Ad Hoc Committee on Genetic Counselling of the American Society of Human Genetics defined genetic counselling as: 'a communication process which deals with the human problems associated with the occurrence, or risk of occurrence, of a genetic disorder in a family. This process involves an attempt by one or more appropriately trained persons to help the family (i) comprehend the medical facts, including the diagnosis, the probable course of the disorder and the available management; (ii) appreciate the way heredity contributes to the disorder and the risk of recurrence in specified relatives; (iii) understand the options for dealing with the risk of recurrence; (iv) choose the course of action which seems appropriate to them in view of their risk and the family goals, and act in accordance with that decision; and (v) make the best possible adjustment to the disorder in an affected family member and/or the risk of recurrence of that disorder.' This definition indicates a further shift away from prescribing outcomes (i.e. it does not mention reducing incidence as a goal), towards recognizing the individual or family as the ones who will determine what outcomes are desirable and what processes they wish to pursue in order to achieve their goals. Furthermore, the phrase 'a communication process' for the first time gives formal acknowledgement to the influence of 'how' counselling is done, to what happens between the counsellor and client in the session. Although this definition falls short of fully recognizing the many aspects of the counselling process, it does begin to examine process issues, such as communication.

This more psychological approach was noted by Kessler (1979). Kessler states that this approach starts with the premise that genetic counselling deals with important human concerns: health and illness, procreation, parenthood as well as life and death issues. Instead of emphasizing the transmission of information, the psychological approach emphasizes the meanings which the facts have for the clients as well as the intrapsychic and interpersonal consequences of these meanings.

Lippman-Hand and Fraser (1979) examined the influence of the communication process on the meaning of information transmitted to the client and observed that decision-making is not a straightforward and rational matter. Facts are not emotionally neutral either to the counsellor or to the client; the timing, tone and body language of the counsellor deliver non-verbal messages to the client. Following the work of Lippman-Hand and Fraser, counsellors have become increasingly aware of how the process of communication may influence the values and meaning of information and hence the decision making process. The counsellor to be effective must be familiar with the Rogerian principles of empathy, genuineness and unconditional positive regard which enhance communication and facilitate the therapeutic process.

The work of Tversky and Kahneman (1974) has further contributed to our understanding of the non-rational ways in which a decision may be reached. Most genetic decisions are based on information presented in the form of probabilities. Tversky and Kahneman have demonstrated that the interpretation of probabilities is subjective. They have demonstrated, for example, that, in the face of uncertainty, thinking is directed towards simplifying the assessment of probabilities and predicted outcomes of various choices.

In addition to the counsellor–client relationship, communication and decision-making, genetic counselling has also turned its attention to assessing the state of the client when he/she enters the counselling session. Frequently, this is at a time of crisis in the client's life. Gardner and Kugelmass (1989) point out that people respond in different ways to a crisis. They may treat it as a challenge, an ultimate defeat or as an immobilizing experience during which their decision-making capacity may be impaired and the support of family and friends needed. Crisis may also be experienced as a kind of loss. Here, and in other areas of genetic counselling, the work of Kubler-Ross (1969) has been useful. The genetic counsellor will support the client through the 'stages' of grieving until acceptance is reached. A model of stages of psychological response to the onset of Huntington's disease has been reported (Bloch et al., 1993).

Researchers have studied the impact of genetic disease on the whole family. Reports on the impact of a genetic disease indicate the profound effects diagnosis may have on the entire family. Role responsibilities, social relationships and financial status may be affected. Relationships between family members may become stressed and marriages conflictual. The burden on family caregivers may be tremendous. The family system has also been identified as contributing to a disorder's manifestations (Kessler & Bloch, 1989).

Genetic counselling in the 1990s is the domain of a counsellor who holds a graduate degree and is trained in all three of the major aspects of genetic counselling described by Emery (1984): the scientific, which is concerned with genetic mechanisms and risk of recurrence; the medical, which is concerned with diagnosis; and the psychological, which is 'concerned with understanding and appreciating the psychological effects of genetic disease. . . .' The modern genetic counsellor is firmly planted in both genetics and the social sciences.

REFERENCES

Ad Hoc Committee on Genetic Counselling (1975). Report to the American Society of Human Genetics. *American Journal of Human Genetics.*, **27**, 240–2.

Bloch, M., Adam, S., Fuller, A., Kremer, B., Welch, J.P., Wiggins, S., Whyte, P., Huggins, M., Theilmann, J. & Hayden, M.R. (1993). Diagnosis of Huntington's disease: a model for the stages of psychological response based on experience of a predictive testing program. *American Journal of Medical Genetics*, **47**, 368–74.

Emery, A.E.H. (1984). The principles of genetic counselling. In: A.E.H. Emery & I.M. Pullen, (Eds.). *Psychological aspects of genetic counselling.* pp. 1–9. London: Academic Press.

Gardner, H.A. & Kugelmass, J.S. (1989). Genetic counselling beyond Mendel. *Modern Medicine of Canada*, **44**, 378–81.

Kessler, S. (Ed.) (1979). *Genetic counseling: psychological dimensions.* New York: Academic Press.

Kessler, S. & Bloch, M. (1989). Social system responses to Huntington disease. *Family Process*, **28**, 59–68.

Kubler-Ross, E. (1969). *On death and dying.* New York: Macmillan and Co.

Lippman-Hand, A. & Fraser, F.C. (1979). Genetic counselling: provision and reception of information. *American Journal of Medical Genetics*, **3**, 113–27.

Tversky, A. & Kahneman, D. (1974) Judgement under uncertainty: heuristics and biases. *Science*, **185**, 1124–31.

Glaucoma

JOHN WEINMAN

UMDS (Guy's Campus), University of London,
UK

Glaucoma describes a range of conditions in which the intraocular pressure is raised as the result of faulty drainage of the aqueous humour. There are a number of types of glaucoma which are classified by their cause which may be primary or secondary. Whereas congenital and acute onset primary glaucoma are uncommon, the chronic simple type (primary open-angle glaucoma) is found in about 2% of 40 year-olds and is even more common in older age-groups. It affects both eyes and requires regular routine screening to assess whether treatment is needed and, if it is not treated, it can lead to blindness. Thus the primary psychological aspects of glaucoma revolve around screening, detection and treatment adherence in those without visual loss, and around the emotional and behavioural responses in those have experienced partial or total loss of vision.

Early diagnosis is vital in glaucoma and hence regular check-ups are necessary in those with raised intra-ocular pressure to check for signs of damage to the optic disc. If this occurs, then visual field defects result and, if the pressure is not controlled, then blindness can result. Treatment is not required if no adverse changes have taken place but the individual needs to attend for regular check-ups and this can be a problem since adherence rates in asymptomatic individuals are not generally very good. Moreover, since this condition runs in families, siblings and children of patients also need to be screened. Although this can result in increased anxiety and self-monitoring for possible symptoms, attendance for screening is not always regular (Marteau, 1989).

Identification of either damage to the ocular disc or visual field defects indicates the need for treatment with eye-drops and, if this is ineffective, then surgery or laser treatment may be necessary. Despite the obviously adverse consequences of non-adherence to treatment, there is evidence that this is not always very good. For example Vincent (1971) reported that, having been informed that, if they did not take their eye drops as instructed they would go blind, 58% of patients still did not adhere to their treatment. Even when these patients had begun to experience significant visual loss in one eye, adherence improved only by an additional 16%. More recently, Fingeret and Shuettenberg (1991) have recommended the use of patient dosage schedules, in which medicines are coded by bottle or cap colour, for improving levels of adherence. However, a range of factors influence adherence to any treatment (see 'Compliance in patients'), and with eye drops there is the additional problem that some patients find them difficult or unpleasant to use.

For those who do not follow or respond to treatment, then the resultant loss of vision can give rise to the same psychological consequences as are found in other types of acquired sensory loss (see 'Blindness and Visual disability'). These may include withdrawal, social isolation and negative affect, all of which are understandable reactions to the functional and social restrictions which can occur afterwards and which, in elderly patients, may be particularly disruptive. There is anecdotal evidence of mood change in people with glaucoma (Wilensky, 1981) and, although this has not been the focus of systematic research, one study has indicated quite high levels of mood disturbance (Carrieri; *et al.*, 1991). Compared with other age-matched patients with different eye disorders of comparable severity and duration and with age-matched controls without eye disorders, significantly higher levels of depression were found in the glaucoma group. However, since no association was found between the degree of depression and the extent of the visual deficit, it is not clear what the causal factors are. Nevertheless this does indicate that the loss of vision in glaucoma precipitates inevitable changes in social functioning, including losses of valued activities such as reading and possible increases in dependency on others.

REFERENCES

Carrieri, P.B., Gentile, S., Fusco, R. & Greco, G.M. (1991). Mood disorders in patients with simple glaucoma. *Psychiatry Research*, 36, 233–5.

Fingeret, M. & Shuettenberg, S.P. (1991). Patient drug schedules and compliance. *Journal of American Optometric Association*, 62, 478–80.

Marteau, T.M. (1989). Psychological costs of screening. *British Medical Journal*, 299, 527.

Vincent, P. (1971). Factors influencing patient non-compliance: a theoretical approach. *Nursing Research*, 20, 509–16.

Wilensky, J.T. (1981) Glaucoma. In G.A. Peyman, D.R. Saunders & M.F. Goldberg (Eds.). *Ophthalmology*. pp. 663–726. Philadelphia: Saunders Co.

Growth retardation

MICHAEL PREECE

Nutrition, Metabolism, Endocrinology &
Dermatology Unit, The Institute of Child Health,
London, UK

DEFINITION

Variation in the growth of children occurs in two dimensions. The easiest to understand is the simple variation in height at any given age including full maturity. Less obvious is the variation that occurs in the timing of events during the growth process such as the age at which puberty commences or adult height is reached; this is usually referred to as tempo.

In the case of boys, the average age of attaining adult height is 18 years but this may vary by as much as three years in either direction. Thus a perfectly healthy boy may not stop growing until 21 years of age and this would be an example of growth retardation (Preece, 1992). In the case of girls, the same degree of variation is seen, but, on average, adult height is achieved some two years earlier than for boys.

Once the child reaches mature height, tempo has no more effect and the variation in height amongst adults is not dependent upon it. The major influence on adult height, assuming the individuals are all healthy, is heredity with a typical correlation coefficient between the mid-parental height and the height of the subject being 0.7 (Tanner, 1966). This is in keeping with a polygenic mode of inheritance for stature. During childhood the hereditary element still applies but variation in tempo will also contribute to the total variance in height. For example, a child of parents of average height might be relatively short simply because of delayed tempo of growth; this is more commonly referred to as growth retardation. It should be clear that growth retardation should not be used to describe short stature unless there is clear evidence of delayed tempo.

Using the above strict definition, it is possible for growth retardation to be present in a child of normal height. This would apply when the child has tall parents, but the delayed tempo makes the child appear shorter than would be expected from the parents. This effect is temporary and resolves as they reach maturity and the influence of the delayed tempo ends and, unless the delay is very severe, seldom leads to clinically relevant problems.

CLINICAL INDICATORS

Short stature for a given chronological age will usually be part of the clinical picture unless the child is from a very tall family. In a child of peripubertal age there will be evidence of delay in other milestones such as the events of puberty. In many cases there will be as much concern about the latter as about the short stature. Similarly to the attainment of adult height there is a range of normal variation of about three years either side of the average age of attaining each stage of puberty. It is a convenient quirk of nature that the standard deviation of the age of attaining most pubertal events is one year (Tanner, 1962) and therefore a total range of six years around the average should include about 99% of healthy individuals.

In younger children the assessment of tempo is much more difficult on clinical grounds although dental maturation can sometimes be used. If clinically relevant, skeletal maturation can be assessed from an X-ray of the left hand and wrist and provides a useful tool. From this a 'bone-age' is calculated which is equal to the chronological age of a healthy child with the same physical appearance on the X-ray. Thus a 10-year old patient with tempo delayed two years will have a bone-age of eight 'years'.

CLINICAL RELEVANCE

Some degree of growth retardation is very common and is responsible for a large number of referrals of patients. It appears to be much more common in boys than in girls, but it is not clear whether this is due to a truly lower incidence in girls or whether it reflects social attitudes to height. It is probably a mixture of the two.

In many cases there is a combination of delayed growth and familial short stature which presumably reflects a selection bias in that children who are delayed and from short families are more likely to cause concern and present clinically. In contrast, those from tall families will only present if the delay is extreme such that they appear short compared to their peers or that the delay in puberty is sufficient to cause distress in its own right.

The importance of the condition lies in the very significant psychological distress that can result. This is not usually a great problem before the age when adolescence usually commences (about 10 years in girls and 11 years in boys) (Sandberg, Brook & Campos, 1994; Voss & Mulligan, 1994). However, adolescence is a time of much anxiety even when it proceeds uneventfully, and children with severe pubertal and growth delay experience many additional problems particularly in their relationships with their peers (Gordon *et al.*, 1982). For this reason the condition needs serious treatment and sympathy even though it is effectively an extension of normal development and by its nature, temporary. Management generally involves reassurance along with active intervention to accelerate the attainment of puberty and the adolescent growth spurt. The latter is usually achieved with a short course of low dose anabolic steroids (Stanhope & Preece, 1988).

REFERENCES

Gordon, M., Crouthamel., C., Post, E.M. & Richman, R.A. (1982). Psychosocial aspects of constitutional short stature: social competence, behaviour problems, self-esteem and family functioning. *Journal of Paediatrics*, **101**, 477–80.

Preece, M.A. (1992) Principles of normal growth: auxology and endocrinology. In A. Grossman (Ed.). *Clinical endocrinology*. pp. 801–809. Oxford: Blackwell Scientific Publications.

Sandberg, D.E., Brook, A.E. & Campos, S.P. (1994). Short stature in middle childhood: a survey of psychosocial functioning in a clinic-referred sample. In B. Stabler & L.E. Underwood (Eds.). *Growth, stature and adaptation*. pp. 19–33. University of North Carolina; Chapel Hill.

Stanhope, R. & Preece M.A. (1988) Management of constitutional delay of growth and puberty. *Archives of Diseases of Childhood*, **63**, 1104–10.

Tanner, J.M. (1962). *Growth at adolescence*. Oxford: Blackwell.

Tanner, J.M. (1966). Galtonian eugenics and the study of growth. *Eugenics Review*, **58**, 122–35.

Voss, L.D. & Mulligan, J. (1994). The short normal child in school: self-esteem, behaviour, and attainment before puberty (The Wessex Growth Study). In B. Stabler & L.E. Underwood (Eds.) *Growth, stature and adaptation*. pp. 47–64. University of North Carolina: Chapel Hill.

Gynaecological cancers

INGRID DOHERTY

Directorate of Mental Health and Adult Learning Difficulties Services Lambeth Health Care (NHS) Trust, London, UK

INTRODUCTION

A diagnosis of cancer is thought to induce in many people a dread greater than that of other diseases carrying equally serious or worse prognoses. Although many of the psychological problems of gynaecological cancer patients are similar to those of other cancer patients, research suggests that the nature of the diagnosis and treatment of gynaecological cancers can provide an added stressful burden to women. Primary gynaecological cancers occur in various sites including the endometrium, cervix, vulva and ovaries. A brief overview is provided of each of these cancers and associated medical and surgical treatments (see Andersen & Anderson, 1986 for more detailed information) together with a summary of psychological responses and interventions. Many psychological studies have grouped together patients with different gynaecological cancers (e.g. endometrial, ovarian and vulval). However, cervical cancer (together with abnormal cervical smears) is one exception with a substantial research literature pertaining to this specific condition.

OVERVIEW OF GYNAECOLOGICAL CANCERS

Ovarian cancer

Ovarian cancer has been increasing in incidence in recent years and is now the fourth commonest cause of death from cancer in women. Approximately 4500 women in England and Wales develop this cancer each year with a mortality rate as high as 70% by five years. Early symptoms include abdominal pain or swelling, weight loss, flatulence, backache, bowel dysfunction, ankle oedema and, occasionally, post-menopausal or other abnormal vaginal bleeding. Detection is difficult because these early symptoms are vague and most women present with advanced stage disease. Various studies indicate that about 90% of cases involve women aged 45 or over; risk of ovarian cancer appears to be reduced by pregnancy and is highest in infertile women. However, as there are various types of ovarian cancer (including epithelial tumours, sex chord-stromal tumours and germ cell neoplasms) it is suggested that epidemiological studies require to take account of these various disease groupings in order to establish relationships. Primary treatment is generally to remove as much of the tumour as possible and involves total hysterectomy and removal of the ovaries usually with subsequent adjuvant chemotherapy. Radiation therapy has less of a role in management as the potential benefits are questionable. As ovarian cancer is often detected at a late stage of the disease, palliation plays a major role with its emphasis on symptom reduction rather than cure.

Endometrial cancer

Endometrial cancer accounts for approximately 39% of gynaecological malignancies and occurs mainly in peri- and post-menopausal women with the average age at the time of diagnosis being 61 years. Continuous oestrogen stimulation is considered to place women at risk of developing endometrial cancer due to variables such as ovarian dysfunction, nulliparity, obesity (affecting hormonal production) and medically prescribed oestrogen therapy. Vaginal bleeding is the most common symptom in postmenopausal women whereas premenopausal women may present with menorrhagia or intermenstrual bleeding. The majority of patients are diagnosed as having early stage disease with advanced stage endometrial cancer a relatively rare occurrence. Surgery, typically involving total abdominal hysterectomy and removal of the ovaries with pelvic node sampling, is the primary treatment with whole-pelvic irradiation to counter possible disease spread.

Carcinoma of the vulva

Carcinoma of the vulva is the least common of the gynaecological cancers, accounting for 4–5% of all gynaecological tumours. The most common symptom is bleeding irregularlities. Although delays in presentation and diagnosis are common, women still tend to present with early stage disease. Reasons for delay include misinterpretation of symptomatology such as suspected vaginal infection or venereal disease or irregular bleeding associated with the menopause. Traditional treatment was total vulvectomy (which also involved removal of the clitoris and all labial tissue) and bilateral groin lymph node removal with, or without, pelvic lymph node removal. Modern management is frequently less radical and treatment for each patient more individualized. Local excision and laser therapy is used for early stage lesions with a trend toward vulvar conservation where possible.

Cancer of the cervix

The incidence of cervical cancer in the UK is approximately 4,000 new cases and about 2,200 deaths each year. These overall figures have remained steady for many years despite the introduction of cervical screening which enables cell changes in the cervix to be detected at an early stage. It should be noted that 60% of women who present with invasive disease have not been previously screened. Moreover, there has been an increase in mortality among younger women in recent years; an increase which has been thought to correspond with changes in sexual behaviour. Over three million cervical smears are taken each year with the rate of detection of abnormal cell changes (cervical intraepithelial neoplasia (CIN)) reported as approximately 3% (i.e. about 30 000 cases per year). Cervical cancer is generally considered to develop through the various stages of CIN to micro-invasive and invasive cancer. Although a debate surrounds the issue of invariable progression from mild dysplasia (CIN I) and moderate dysplasia (CIN II) to invasive disease it is generally accepted that severe dysplasia (CIN Grade III) is a high risk factor. Cervical cancer presents with local symptoms such as vaginal bleeding or discharge whereas there are no symptoms associated with CIN. The causes of the disease are not fully understood, although epidemiological studies indicate various risk factors including young age at first intercourse, multiple sexual partners, lower socioeconomic class, the presence of various strains of human papilloma virus and smoking.

The introduction of the Pap smear test has enabled the detection of early abnormal cell changes and, in this respect, has been seen as a significant breakthrough in preventative medicine. The degree of abnormality detected by cytology determines whether monitoring by further smear tests or diagnostic investigation (a colposcopy examination) and/or treatment is indicated. Treatments for non-invasive disease include CO_2 laser, cold coagulation, cryocautery, large loop excision of the transformation zone (Lletz) and cone biopsy. With the exception of the latter (which may require inpatient admission) these treatments are usually administered on an outpatient basis with a local anaesthetic.

Treatments for invasive cancer include surgery and radiation therapy (external and/or intra-cavity) which may be used alone or together. Chemotherapy is less widely used and mainly for very advanced or recurrent disease. Radical hysterectomy may or may not include removal of the ovaries and is avoided where possible in premenopausal women. Radiation therapy to the pelvis destroys ovarian functioning resulting in premature menopause in younger women with accompanying loss of fertility, hot flushes, vaginal atrophy and stenosis. Pelvic exenteration is employed for advanced and recurrent malignancy. This major surgery usually involves removal of the uterus, ovaries, tubes, bladder, rectum and vagina and in some instances part of the vulva. (For a more detailed review, see 'General cancer'.)

PSYCHOLOGICAL FACTORS AND INTERVENTIONS

Issues in detection of disease

There are frequent delays between the time when an individual first notices bodily signs and symptoms of disease and seeking medical help. Andersen and Anderson (1986) explain this delay in a sample of gynaecological cancer patients by the occurrence of an 'appraisal interval'. During this period an individual attempts to provide explanations for bodily symptoms over a period of time with an increased number of cancer explanations occurring as the interval progresses. A common explanation for delay, particularly with endometrial cancer, is misinterpreting irregular bleeding as a sign of the menopause.

An additional problem in the detection of cervical cancer is the failure of some women to avail themselves of cervical screening despite the fact that smear tests are an integral aspect of many healthcare systems (Eardley et al., 1985). Lack of understanding of the nature and progress of cervical cancer and the preventative function of cervical screening combined with the use of the term 'cancer smear test', with its inherent implication of the discovery of pathology, does not encourage participation. Postmenopausal women are less likely to attend presuming they are no longer at risk of disease of the reproductive organs and/or averse to a pelvic examination despite having had children. For those women who do attend, it may mean that they are subjected to variety of invasive procedures from the smear test itself to further diagnostic (colposcopy examination) and treatment procedures should abnormality be detected. Common to all gynaecological procedures is the pelvic examination which is generally considered to be one of the most anxiety-producing of routine medical procedures. In addition to possible physical pain (usually in connection with the insertion of the speculum) a range of negative responses have been identified including feelings of anxiety, vulnerability and humiliation.

Psychological issues and cancer

A major area of research concerns psychosocial adjustment to the diagnosis of cancer, the disease process and treatments. In the case of CIN the diagnosis is not one of invasive disease and from a medical perspective the detection and treatment of CIN can be viewed as a straightforward and minor procedure. However, the findings from a number of studies examining the psychological effects of an abnormal smear result and subsequent medical procedures indicate that many women in fact experience considerable distress (Posner & Vessey, 1988, Doherty et al., 1991). Distress is associated with a range of concerns including the causes and perceived severity of the condition, the fear of cancer and possible surgical interventions together with worries pertaining to perceived adverse effects on

[485]

childbearing (Doherty *et al.*, 1991). Lack of knowledge of both the purpose and procedural aspects of the colposcopy examination are also thought to contribute to distress (Posner & Vessey, 1988).

Weisman & Worden (cited in Andersen, 1984) use the concept of 'existential plight' to describe a frequent emotional reaction to a diagnosis of cancer whereby all aspects of the individual's current life appear fragile and continued existence is questioned. It is not surprising therefore that depression and emotional confusion are recognized as major adverse psychological responses. In addition to the potential life-threatening nature of gynaecological cancer, women are also faced with the effects of mutilating treatment. Destructive surgery of the genitalia threatens a woman's body image by assaulting body parts that help to define a woman. This, in turn can lead to relationship difficulties, decreased sexual desire and sexual dysfunction. In addition, the presumed sexually transmitted nature of cervical cancer (often stressed by the media) produces feelings of guilt. Younger women tend to experience more adverse psychological responses than older women with similar physical impairments and subsequent adjustment is poorer. Much of the research on adverse psychological effects has addressed dysfunctional sexual responses following treatment for gynaecological cancers. Although knowledge of what is normal in sexual behaviour is difficult to ascertain there is clearly a role for psychological intervention where psychosexual problems are indicated. Unfortunately, as a result of embarrassment and taboos regarding sexuality, interventions tend to focus on medical/organic aspects rather than psychological trauma (Hunter, 1989). (See also 'General cancer'.).

Psychological interventions

Psychological interventions for adverse effects of treatment for cancer and other stressful medical procedures have included relaxation and imagery, hypnosis and systematic desensitization. These have been found to reduce anxiety and in some cases severity of nausea. Research on psychological preparation for a variety of stressful medical procedures (e.g. Ludwick-Rosenthal & Neufeld, 1988) provides evidence that the provision of preparatory information can reduce patient distress and improve various aspects of recovery. Marteau (1993) reviews various techniques for improving psychological outcomes in women who have received an abnormal cervical smear, from the need to follow-up verbal information with written information, the provision of brief and simple information to looking at ways in which clinics are organized. Also discussed by Marteau (1993) is the role of individual differences in coping styles as some research suggests that the provision of information is not universally beneficial. Counselling is a generally accepted intervention for a variety of psychological traumas but as yet there has been little comparative research with this group of patients. One recent controlled study looking at the benefits of counselling with women undergoing medical procedures associated with an abnormal smear result, found that, although subjects indicated that they considered the counselling very useful, there were no differences in subsequent psychological adjustment between this group and a group of patients who received only a standard information leaflet (Raju *et al.*, 1993).

Andersen (1993) proposed a model for predicting risk for psychological and behavioural morbidity (including sexual aspects) which takes into account pre-disease factors such as sociodemographic characteristics, prior health status, existing social networks and current stressors together with disease relevant events such as diagnosis, treatment and recovery. This model was used to classify patients into low, medium and high risk categories as a systematic method of reviewing the literature on psychological interventions for gynaecological and other cancers (Andersen, 1993). The findings indicated that, for women of 'low morbidity risk' (i.e. localized disease and/or disease for which the prognosis is good) brief broad-based interventions such as crisis-oriented work, information relating to sexual issues and behavioural therapies, produced limited psychological or behavioural improvements but significant improvement in sexual functioning. For women in the 'moderate morbidity risk' category (regional disease, combination therapy and/or 50–50 chance of survival) where brief interventions also tended to be offered, stronger intervention effects were found both post-treatment and at follow-up. Findings for patients deemed to be in 'high morbidity risk' (recurrent disease or terminal disease) who not only have to face imminent death with associated extreme emotional distress but also increasing physical debilitation and/or pain indicated positive outcomes in measures of emotional distress and pain reports. The psychological interventions which included patient education and supportive group therapy, tended to be more intensive than for the other categories. The application of such a model which takes into account both pre-disease factors and disease relevant events could prove useful in determining the most appropriate type of intervention. (See also 'General cancer'.)

The above outlines some of the psychological interventions that have been used to reduce stress associated with cancer and with invasive medical procedures. However, it cannot be assumed that all women require help from professionals and it is important therefore to ascertain which women are most at risk for psychological and sexual morbidity. Other factors such as individual coping style and disease prognosis also require consideration if psychological interventions are to be beneficial.

REFERENCES:

Andersen, B.L. (1984). Psychological aspects of gynaecological cancer. In A. Broome & L. Wallace (Eds.). *Psychology and gynaecological problems*, pp. 117–141. London: Tavistock Publications.

Andersen, B.L. (1993). Predicting sexual and psychologic mobidity and improving the quality of life for women with gynecologic cancer. *Cancer Supplement*, 71, 1678–90.

Andersen, B.L. & Anderson, B. (1986). Psychosomatic aspects of gynecologic oncology: present status and future directions. *Journal of Psychosomatic Obstetrics and Gynecology*, 5, 233–44.

Doherty, I.E., Richardson, P.H., Wolfe, C.D. & Raju, K.S. (1991). The assessment of the psychological effects of an abnormal cervical smear and subsequent medical procedures. *Journal of Psychosomatic Obstetrics and Gynaecology*, 12, 319–24.

Eardley, A., Knopf Elkind, A., Spencer, B.,

Hobbs, P., Pendleton, L. & Haran D. (1985). Attendance for cervical screening – whose problem? *Social Science and Medicine*, 20, 955–62.

Hunter, M. (1989). Gynaecology. In A.K. Broome (Ed.), *Health psychology: processes and applications*, pp. 312–344. London: Chapman & Hall.

Ludwick-Rosenthal, R. & Neufeld, R.W.J. (1988). Stress management during noxious medical procedures: an evaluative review of outcome studies. *Psychological Bulletin*, **104**, 326–42.

Marteau, T.M. (1993). Psychological effects of an abnormal smear result. In W. Prendiville (Ed.). *LLETZ: a practical*

guide, pp. 99–104. London: Chapman & Hall.

Posner, T. & Vessey, M (1988). *Prevention of cervical cancer: the patient's view*. London: Kings Fund.

Raju, K.S., Richardson, P.H., Wolfe, C.D. &

Doherty, I. (1993). Controlled evaluation of the effects of information provision and counselling on the response of patients with abnormal smears. Report to the Cancer Research Campaign, London.

Haemophilia

IVANA MARKOVÁ
University of Stirling, UK

'Haemophilia' is a term referring to a group of genetically transmitted life long blood clotting disorders which are caused by a defect in the clothing mechanism in one or more of the plasma clotting factors. The most common are sex-linked recessive disorders: haemophilia A (classic haemophilia) and haemophilia B (Christmas disease), due to an isolated deficiency of the clotting activity of factor VIII or of factor IX, respectively. The mother carries a defective gene on one of her X chromosomes and there is a 50% chance that any of her sons will be affected by the disease and a 50% chance that any of her daughters will be a carrier. None of the sons of a haemophilic male will have the disease but all of his daughters will be obligatory carriers. The clinical manifestations of haemophilias A and B are identical and only blood tests can differentiate between them. Haemophilias affects approximately 1 in 5000 of the male population of all races and it also occurs in a variety of animal species. The incidence of haemophilia B is approximately 1/6 to 1/10 of that of haemophilia A. The third most common type of haemophilia, von Willebrand's disease or vascular haemophilia, is an autosomal dominant genetic disorder (it affects both men and women), due to a combination of an abnormal factor VIII molecule with abnormal platelet function.

The severity of haemophilia is related to the degree of deficiency of the relevant clotting factors(s) in the blood (mild, over 5% of the normal activity of the factor; moderate, between 2% and 5%; severe, less than 2%). People with mild haemophilia usually need special care only when having surgery, while those with severe haemophilia may bleed spontaneously, either for no obvious reason or after emotional trauma.

In the majority of families with haemophilia (approximately 70%) evidence of transmission of a defective gene can be established and family trees indicating such transmission can be constructed. In the remaining families, haemophilia could either be transmitted for generations through female carriers who themselves do not suffer the disease, or it might be due to a spontaneous mutation. If haemophilia is known to be present in a family, it can be diagnosed prenatally from a foetal blood sample. Alternatively, it will be diagnosed as a result of bruising, cutting teeth, surgery or injury. Mild haemophilia may not be diagnosed until adulthood. Until the late 1960s the main therapeutic material used in the treatment of haemophilia was plasma. The patient had to go to hospital for this treatment and, if

necessary, stay there over a period of time. Technological advancements in the late 1960s led to the production of various kinds of factor VIII concentrates. As these products became safe and stable, they could be kept in home freezers which enabled dramatic changes in the treatment of haemophilia. Programmes of home treatment were introduced enabling self-infusion or treatment to be given by a suitably trained relative or friend. Since this treatment can be administered either prophylactically or immediately after the bleeding occurs, the patient does not lose time by going to hospital, can reduce long-lasting crippling of joints and painful bleeding and can live a relatively normal life.

By the mid-1970s it was apparent that chronically treated patients had developed complications (e.g. hepatitis, chronic liver disease, inhibitors to treatment). Furthermore, in 1981 it was first reported that some patients with haemophilia had developed acquired immune deficiency syndrome (AIDS) and in 1982 the virus had been found in the factor concentrates used for their treatment. By the mid-1980s blood donors were screened for the presence of HIV, and blood products, i.e. concentrates of clotting factors used for the treatment of bleeds, were heat-treated to destroy HIV. Unfortunately, by that time, in some parts of the world as many as 90% of severely affected patients with deficient factor VIII and a small percentage of those with deficient factor IX, had become infected and many have now died.

Throughout history, haemophilia has always presented a wide spectrum of psychological and behavioural challenges to patients, carriers and to their relatives. However, the nature of these challenges keeps changing with the advances in diagnosis and treatment and with the changes due to medical complications including HIV/AIDS. The general public has many misconceptions, e.g. that a person with haemophilia can bleed to death from a needle prick. In contrast, the major dangers are internal bleedings, in particular those into the brain. People with haemophilia may suffer excruciating pain and their joints may become permanently damaged. As yet, there is no satisfactory analgesic available which does not lead to addiction.

Prospective parents must decide whether to undergo diagnostic procedures in order to discover whether the foetus is affected with haemophilia and, if it is, whether they wish to undergo a termination of the pregnancy. No matter how accurate and safe foetal diagnosis may become, the subsequent course of action is determined by the prospective parents' perception and acceptance of such procedures and their ethical beliefs.

There are several stages in bringing up a child with haemophilia that parents find particularly difficult: coping with the diagnosis, teaching the pre school child to look after himself, overcoming anxiety about the child's starting school, and solving the problem of the child's career. The main problem facing parents is to strike a balance between the necessary and unnecessary restriction of the child. With the development of factor concentrates in the last three decades, the aim for a person with haemophilia at school, at work and in the family has been 'to be as normal as possible'. However, adults with haemophilia, attempting to find employment, are faced with the problem of whether or not to tell their future employers about their disease. Getting life assurance has always been a problem for severely affected patients, and this problem has been aggravated as a result of haemophilia's association with AIDS.

People with haemophilia form approximately 1% of those who have been infected by HIV. While HIV infection in men with haemophilia is no longer due to blood products, new cases of HIV infection include women infected by their spouses and children who were infected by HIV presumably during pregnancy. In addition to the stress of being infected by HIV, psychological problems in young men include the fear of stigma and rejection by female partners mitigating against disclosing haemophilia and HIV infection.

Recently, recombinant factor VIII products have been licensed. These are produced by a human gene and they open up new prospects of treating people with haemophilia. This method provides highly purified products which are safer. In addition, there is a possibility of using human gene therapy and, eventually, of a 'cure' for haemophilia.

FURTHER READING

Bloom, A.L., Forbes, C.D., Thomas, D. & Tuddenham E.G.D. (Eds.). (1994). *Haemostasis and thrombosis*, Edinburgh: Churchill-Livingstone.

Bussing, R & Johnson, S.B. (1992). Psychosocial issues in hemophilia before and after the HIV crisis: A review of current research, *General Hospital Psychiatry*, 14, 387–403.

Lusher, J.M. & Kessler, C.M. (Eds.). (1991). *Hemophilia and von Willebrand's disease in the 1990's*, Elsevier Science Publishers.

Marková, I. (1997). The family and haemophilia. In C.D. Forbes, L. Adedort & R. Madhok (Eds.). Haemophilia. pp. 335–346. London: Chapman & Hale.

Marková, I., Wilkie, P.A., Naji, S. & Forbes, C.D. (1990). Knowledge of HIV/AIDS and behavioural change of people with haemophilia, *Psychology and Health*, 4, 125–33.

Mason, P.J. Olson, R.A. & Parish, K.L.

(1988). AIDS, hemophilia, and prevention efforts within a comprehensive care program, *American Psychologist*, 43, 971–6.

Parish, K.L. (1991). Global perspectives on HIV and hemophilia: psychosocial aspects. In J.M. Lusher & C.M. Kessler (Eds.). *Hemophilia and von Willebrand's disease in the 1990's*. Elsevier Science Publishers.

Ratnoff, O.D. & Forbes, C.D. (Eds.) (1994). *Disorders of hemostasis* 2nd ed, Philadelphia: Saunders.

Head and neck cancers

RUTH ALLEN

Department of Psychiatry, University College
London Medical School, UK

Head and neck cancers account for approximately 4% of carcinomas and include cancers of the lip, tongue, oral cavity, pharynx, nose, middle ear, sinuses and larynx (Souhami & Tobias, 1994). Common aetiological factors are tobacco consumption and alcohol intake, particularly in combination, and the management of alcohol and tobacco-related disorders may be required alongside the treatment of the cancer. The treatment itself is aggressive, with radical surgery and/or radiotherapy, resulting in facial disfigurement causing psychological morbidity.

PSYCHOLOGICAL PROBLEMS

Anxiety and depression is reported in much of the research assessing the impact of head and neck cancer on the individual. Holland and Rowland found that 50% of patients seen for psychiatric consultations had adjustment disorders with anxiety, depression or mixed mood states. Psychosocial problems reported by patients with head

and neck cancer have included coping with health problems, fears about health, communication with partner and social relationships (Rapoport *et al.*, 1993). This research also reported that, although medical problems rescind with time, psychosocial problems including anxiety and anger become worse reflecting 'patient burnout'. Research has significantly associated depression with malnutrition, weight loss, marital status (unmarried) and gender (female), but not disease extent (Westin *et al.*, 1988, Baile *et al.*, 1992).

PHYSICAL APPEARANCE

A scale has been developed to grade the severity of both disfigurement and altered functioning post radical facial surgery. The scale codes orbital extenteration resulting in the loss of an eye with radical maxillectomy as the most disfiguring procedure, and aphonia as the most severe dysfunction (Dropkin *et al.*, 1983). Research using the scale has found evidence to associate more severe disfigurement/

dysfunction with slower recovery, prolonged social isolation, lower self-esteem and severe depression. In the post-operative period it appears to be important to encourage early confrontation with physical appearance, delay of self-care beyond 5–6 days can predict poor adjustment and rehabilitation (Dropkin *et al.*, 1983).

PHYSICAL DYSFUNCTION

Functional difficulties experienced by patients include breathing, chewing, swallowing, smelling, hearing, seeing, moving and speaking. Psychological morbidity has been found to increase during radiotherapy (Browman *et al.*, 1993). Type of surgery significantly influences patients' emotional function with conservative surgical approaches enhancing quality of life (Bjordal *et al.*, 1994). Early management of communication disorders and psychiatric intervention for patients undergoing mutilating surgery has been found to be of value (Byrne *et al.*, 1993).

Psychosocial problems associated with laryngectomies are the loss of natural voice, breathing through a tracheostomy, depression, grief, anger, frustration, withdrawal and alcoholic escape or suicide (Dhooper, 1985). A sense of hopelessness, a lack of self acceptance and covert hostility have also been identified (Petrucci & Harwick, 1984). It is common and is perceived to be of value to use a multidisciplinary approach to care which involves medicine, nursing, dietary services, speech therapy, dentistry and social work. Psychologists have been employed to help patients cope with alcohol abuse, suicidal behaviours, characterological disorders, non-compliance and overall adjustment (Petrucci & Harwick, 1984).

REFERENCES

Baile, W.F., Gibertini, M., Scott, L. & Endicott, J. (1992). Depression and tumor stage in cancer of the head and neck. *Psycho-Oncology*, 1, 15–24.

Bjordal, K., Kaasa, S. & Mastekassa, A. (1994). Quality of life in patients treated for head and neck cancer: a follow-up study 7 to 11 years after radiotherapy. emotional *Journal of Radiation Oncology Biological Physics* 28, 847–56.

Browman, G.P., Levine, M.N., Hodson, D.I., Sathya, J., Russell, R., Skingley, P., Cripps, C., Eapen, L. & Girard, A. (1993). The Head and Neck Radiotherapy Questionnaire: a morbidity/quality-of-life instrument for clinical trials of radiation therapy in locally advanced head and neck cancer. *Journal of Clinical Oncology* 11, 863–72.

Byrne, A., Walsh, M., Farrelly, M. & O'Driscoll, K. (1993). Depression following laryngectomy: a pilot study. *British Journal of Psychiatry*, 163,

Dhooper, S.S. (1985). Social work with laryngectomees. *Health and Social Work* 10, 217–27.

Dropkin, M.J., Malgady, R.G., Scott, D.W., Oberst, M. & Strong, E. (1983). Scaling of disfigurement and dysfunction in postoperative head and neck patients. *Head and Neck Surgery*, 8, 559–70.

Holland, J.C. & Rowland, J.H. (Ed.). (1989). *Handbook of psychooncology, Psychological care of the patient with cancer*. New York: Oxford University Press.

Petrucci, R.J. & R.D. Harwick (1984). Role of the psychologist on a radical head and neck surgical service team. *Professional Psychology Research and Practice* 15, 538–43.

Rapoport, Y., Kreitler, S., Chaitchik, S., Algor, R. & Weissler, K. (1993). Psychosocial problems in head-and-neck cancer patients and their change with time since diagnosis. *Annals of Oncology* 4, 69–73.

Souhami, R.L. & J. Tobias (1994). *Cancer and its management*. London: Blackwell Scientific Publications.

Westin, T., Jansson, A., Zenckert, C., Hallstrom, T. & Edstrom, S. (1988). Mental depression is associated with malnutrition in patients with head and neck cancer. *Archives of Otolaryngology Head and Neck Surgery*, 114, 1449–53.

Head injury

DIANE B. HOWIESON

VA Medical Center, Portland, Oregon, USA

Brain injuries from head trauma are classified into two major types. When a head injury results in a foreign object entering the brain, such as a bullet or a bone fragment from a fractured skull, the brain injury is called a penetrating head injury. This type of injury may produce a relatively focal deficit. A closed head injury is caused by either a blunt object hitting the head or, more frequently, by a moving head hitting a stationary object, such as a windshield. Moderate to severe closed head injuries may produce widespread damage to the brain parenchyma. The majority of all head injuries in the United States are closed head injuries. Therefore, this chapter will focus on the consequences of closed head injuries.

The annual frequency of brain injuries requiring medical attention is 200 to 300 per 100 000 population in the USA and the UK. Most closed head injuries in North America occur in males ages 15 to 24 years in association with motor vehicle accidents or sporting accidents (Kraus & Sorenson, 1994) and the elderly as a result of falls (Fogel & Duffy, 1994). However, no age-group is spared. The role of psychology has been to better understand the relationship between brain injury and behavioural changes, develop assessment tools, and provide effective clinical intervention.

ASSESSMENT OF CLOSED HEAD INJURY

Approximately 80% of all head injuries brought to medical attention are mild, 10% are moderate, and 10% are severe (Kraus &

Sorenson, 1994). Head injury severity usually is assessed by the degree and duration of alteration of consciousness produced by the injury and by the duration of post-traumatic amnesia (PTA). The most commonly used instrument for assessing consciousness is the Glasgow Coma Scale (Jennett & Teasdale, 1981), which grades consciousness on a scale of 3 (no consciousness) to 15 (no impairment). Most significant head injuries will cause amnesia for the injury itself, which may represent a gap of only a few minutes. The more severe the head injury, the longer the amnesia for events preceding the head injury. This retrograde amnesia may last hours, days, weeks, or longer. Anterograde amnesia refers to the time from the injury to when the individual begins to form continuous memories. The entire duration from the beginning of retrograde amnesia until the end of anterograde amnesia is the PTA. When time has passed since the injury, PTA often is difficult to accurately reconstruct even with information from a collateral source. Other factors that affect prognosis include certain abnormal brain stem reflexes following the injury, evidence of structural damage on MRI or CT scans, age, history of previous head injury, alcohol abuse, and multiple injuries.

The disabilities associated with head injuries can be many. Potential problems may include hemiparesis, changes in vision, loss of sense of smell, problems with dizziness and balance, incoordination, and dysarthria. The psychological consequences involve a complex interaction of cognitive, emotional, and psychosocial factors. Probably the most useful data concerning the effects of head injury on cognition and behaviour have come from large, prospective studies of consecutive cases seen at medical centres. A head injured group may be compared with another accident group in which there were no head injuries in an attempt to equate for the psychological stress associated with a sudden injury and subsequent disability or time away from work. Ideally, studies are comprehensive and look at personality or behavioral changes in addition to cognitive changes. An adequate follow-up interval is desirable to track functional levels beyond the period of maximum change during the initial postinjury year. Single case study methodology has helped demonstrate unexpected outcomes in some cases. Most of what has been learned about the consequences of head trauma have come from many descriptive studies over the past several decades. The findings have been consistent with knowledge about brain–behaviour relationships.

PSYCHOLOGICAL CONSEQUENCES OF MILD HEAD INJURY

Although universal criteria do not exist, mild head injury is often defined as an initial Glasgow Coma Scale of 13–15 and post-traumatic amnesia not to exceed 24 hours. Most people will experience cognitive inefficiency following a head injury even of mild severity and complain of difficulty concentrating. Neuropsychological studies have demonstrated that the inefficiency comes from problems with attention, speed of information processes, and information processing capacity. Standardized tests used to assess these cognitive processes are presented in Table 1 (Lezak, 1995). Assessment of cognitive inefficiency is valuable in verifying or predicting problems in daily functioning. Gronwall and Sampson (1974) have shown that most persons with mild head injury usually recover fully from this inefficiency within five weeks. Other short-term consequences, referred to as the postconcussional syndrome,

Table 1. *Tests used to measure attention and speed of information processing*

Corsi-Block Tapping Test
Paced Serial Addition Test
Stroop Test
Wechsler Intelligence Scales Digit Span
Wechsler Intelligence Scales Digit Symbol

may be headache, fatigue, dizziness, sleep disturbance, irritability, distractibility, impaired memory, depression, anxiety, and impaired appetite (Levin *et al.*, 1987). Proper education and reassurance on the basis of an appropriate evaluation helps ensure recovery.

However, a minority of patients will continue to experience problems for an extended period. One of the continuing debates in the head injury field is the interpretation of persistent sequelae in some persons with mild head injury. It is likely that some individuals have occult brain lesions accounting for persistent sequelae while others appear to have affective disturbances that prolong the symptoms. Patients who are engaged in litigation are more likely to have prolonged symptoms, which raises the question in some cases of secondary gain through symptoms.

PSYCHOLOGICAL CONSEQUENCES OF MODERATE AND SEVERE CLOSED HEAD INJURY

Severe head injuries are associated with a high incidence of disability in the approximately half of those who survive them. Many survivors sustain diffuse axonal injuries, damage from excessive neuro-excitation, and focal lesions from contusions. Damage may be greater on the side opposite the traumatic impact, the contrecoup, than the site of impact or the coup. The injury caused by severe trauma also includes secondary damage from potential complications such as increased intracranial pressure, subdural hematomas, intracranial hematomas, seizures, and the development of hydrocephalus.

As severity increases beyond mild, sequelae are more likely to persist. As with mild head injury, attention is affected. An inability to effectively process more than one stimulus at a time is a robust finding in moderately to severely head injured persons. Additionally, information processing speed is slowed. Attention deficits likely result from damage to the brainstem, frontal lobes, and widespread lesions throughout the cerebral white matter. Memory impairment is another common consequence of severe head injury and appears to result from frontotemporal injuries as the brain scrapes over bony prominences in the skull's interior. As discussed above, most persons will have a PTA. In addition, memory usually is impaired for acquiring, retaining, and retrieving new information. Memory recognition, although better than free recall, may also show performance below expectation. On neuropsychological examination, the impairment usually is demonstrated in performance below expectation on tests such as those presented in Table 2 (Lezak, 1995). On the other hand, memory for old learned information may be relatively well retained.

Dikmen and her colleagues (Dikmen *et al.*, 1995) have shown that broader cognitive difficulties beyond attention and memory usually are seen in persons with coma for more than two weeks. Higher order cognitive deficits may be seen on tests presented in

Table 2. *Tests used to measure memory.*

Brown-Peterson Technique
California Verbal Learning Test
Continuous Visual Memory Test
Complex Figure Test
Rey Auditory Verbal Learning Test
Rivermead Behavioural Memory Test
Wechsler Memory Scale-Revised

Table 3. *Tests used to measure conceptualization, reasoning, and executive functions.*

Category Test
Trail Making Test
Wechsler Intelligence Scales Similarities
Wisconsin Card Sorting Test

Table 4. *Instruments for assessing emotional and psychosocial functioning*

Portland Adaptability Inventory
Patient Competency Rating Scale
Minnesota Multi Personality Inventory (MMPI-2)
Sickness Impact Profile
Symptom Check List 90 (SCL 90)

Table 3 (Lezak, 1995, which assess conceptualization, reasoning, planning, problem solving, and flexibility of thinking. In addition, head injured patients may have difficulty copying complex figures and reconstructing designs with blocks because these tasks require planning, organization, and the formulation of a strategy. These deficits comprise the frontal lobe syndrome and are associated with frontal damage often resulting from severe closed head injury. Deficits often regarded as focal in nature, such as language, occur more rarely.

The most disabling consequences of severe head injury often are changes in personality or social behaviour (Brooks, 1984; Jennett & Teasdale, 1981; Lezak, 1989), presumably from the frequent frontal and limbic injuries. Instruments for assessing the behavioural consequences of head injury are presented in Table 4. Behavioural changes that are particularly disruptive are inertia, impulsivity, disinhibiton, poor anger control, and poor self-monitoring. Research has shown that some of these behaviours, such as impulsivity or risk-taking, are more common premorbidly in persons who sustain head injury than in the general population. Therefore, behavioural problems result from interactions between premorbid characteristics and cognitive, emotional, and social impairments resulting from brain injury. To make matters worse, many severely head injured patients will lack capacity for insight regarding these problems. Unfortunately, social isolation is a frequent outcome. Depression is a common sequelae of head injury, occurring in about 42% of patients during the year following the injury (Robinson & Jorge, 1994).

Cognitive impairment usually shows the greatest improvement in the year following head injury with very gradual improvement for several years more. However, high variability exists making it impossible to predict outcome in an individual case. The effects of head injury in children must be assessed not only for previously acquired behaviours and skills, but also for effects on subsequent growth and development (Fletcher, Minor & Ewing-Cobbs, 1987). A head injury occurring early in a child's development can stifle the child's future development.

TREATMENT

The best intervention is prevention through education. However, education is not going to eliminate all head injuries. The first step in treatment is to determine when the patient is ready to engage in a treatment programme. The patient should be able to focus attention, follow directions, and have some capacity for continuous memories. The severely impaired may receive comprehensive rehabilitation that integrates treatment of cognitive, emotional, and social problems. The goal of rehabilitation is to maximize the brain-injured person's independence and productivity in society. For some, the goal may be to return to school or work. For others, the goal may be to live in supervised housing with minimal assistance in daily activities. No two patients' needs are identical, so rehabilitation efforts need to be tailored to the individual.

Early cognitive rehabilitation efforts were based on the assumption that practising domain-specific skills would result in an uninjured region of the brain taking over the impaired function through brain reorganization made possible by plasticity. However, this approach was found to be ineffective for most cognitive skills. Although practice sometimes improved performance in the rehabilitation setting, the effects rarely generalized to daily activities. When computers became readily available, computer-assisted exercises and games were employed with the belief that extensive repetition and immediate programmed feedback might improve function and be enjoyable. Computer exercises and games were found to be of little benefit in improving memory and many cognitive skills. More recent cognitive rehabilitation efforts have attempted to target practical problems and their solutions in the natural environment. Cognitive rehabilitation efforts currently used include teaching compensatory skills, reducing maladaptive behaviours, adjusting the environment to meet the individual's needs, and educating others to assist the brain-injured patient when needed. As an example, memory impairment can be compensated for with the use of daily schedules, dairies, and written reminders. Rehabilitation techniques are designed to minimize the demands on the patient in weak areas while bolstering skills that are stronger. Even with serious head injury, patients usually have some preserved skills. Few head-injured patients have impairments in such basic knowledge as old learned information, reading, and writing. An important component is instilling awareness in patients who lack insight into their acquired behavioural deficits.

The treatment of psychosocial problems following head injury focuses on helping the individual maintain interpersonal relationships. Psychotherapy is helpful in some patients. Higher functioning patients may benefit from individual psychotherapy while more severely impaired patients may profit more from group psychotherapy. Caregiver education and support are useful interventions (Gronwall, Wrightson & Waddell, 1990). Pharmacological treatment is useful in some patients. Treatment of depression may include serotonin agonists and psychostimulants. Emotional lability and dyscontrol may be treated with lithium carbonate, dopamine agonists, or anticonvulsants.

REFERENCES

Brooks, N. (1984). *Closed head injury: psychological, social, and family consequences.* Oxford: Oxford University Press.

Dikmen, S.S., Machamer, J.E., Winn, H.R. & Temkin, N.R. (1995). Neuropsychological outcome at 1-year post head injury. *Neuropsychology,* 9, 80–90.

Fletcher, J.M., Miner, M.E. & Ewing-Cobbs, L. (1987). Age and recovery from head injury in children: developmental issues. In H.S., Levin, H.M., Eisenberg, & J.E. Grafman, (Eds.). *Neurobehavioral recovery from head injury,* pp. 279–291. New York: Oxford University Press.

Fogel, B.S. & Duffy, J. (1994). Elderly patients. In J.M. Silver, S.C. Yudofsky & R.E. Hales (Eds.). *Neuropsychiatry of traumatic brain injury,* pp. 219–250. Washington, DC: American Psychiatric Press, Inc.

Gronwall, D. & Sampson, P. (1974). *Psychological effects of head injury.* Auckland: Oxford University Press.

Gronwall, D, Wrightson, P. & Waddell, P. (1990). *Head injury, the facts: a guide for families and care-givers.* Oxford: Oxford University Press.

Jennett, B. & Teasdale, G. (1981). *Management of head injury,* pp. 77–81. Philadelphia: F.A. Davis Company.

Kraus, J.F. & Sorenson, S.B. (1994). Epidemiology. In J.M. Silver, S.C., Yudofsky & R.E. Hales (Eds.). *Neuropsychiatry of traumatic brain injury,* pp. 219–250. Washington, DC: American Psychiatric Press, Inc.

Levin, H.S., Gary, H.E. Jr, High, W.M. Jr, Mattis, S., Ruff, R.M., Eisenberg, H.M., Marshall, L.F. & Tabaddor, K. (1987). Minor head injury and postconcussional syndrome: methodological issues in outcome studies. In H.S., Levin, H.M., Eisenberg, J.E., Grafman (Eds.).

Neurobehavioral recovery from head injury, pp. 262–275. New York: Oxford University Press.

Lezak, M.D. (1989). Assessment of psychosocial dysfunctions resulting from head trauma. In M.D. Lezak, (Ed.). *Assessment of the behavioral consequences of head trauma* pp. 113–143. New York: Alan R. Liss, Inc.

Lezak, M.D. (1995). *Neuropsychological assessment.* 3rd ed. New York: Oxford University Press.

Prigatano, G.P. (1985). *Neuropsychological rehabilitation after brain injury.* Baltimore: Johns Hopkins University Press.

Robinson, R.G., & Jorge, R. (1994). Mood disorders. In J.M. Silver, S.C. Yudofsky & R.E. Hales (Eds.). *Neuropsychiatry of traumatic brain injury,* pp. 219–250. Washington, DC: American Psychiatric Press, Inc.

Headache and migraine

BJØRN ELLERTSEN

*Department of Clinical Neuropsychology,
University of Bergen, Norway*

Headache is one of the most common nuisances known to man. The pain may be of secondary nature, as in fever or hypertension, or primary, as in migraine. It has been estimated that about 30% of people in the western world suffer from one or more severe headache episodes per year. In the UK, around 3 million workdays are lost per year due to headache. The majority of headache patients have migraine, tension-type headache (TTH), or combinations of these. About 65% of the patients seen in headache clinics suffer from migraine, 25% from TTH, and about 10% from other types of headache. Although such samples are selected, the relative proportions of diagnoses are probably representative of the population. The causes of headache syndromes like migraine, cluster headache and TTH are largely unknown. However, knowledge about clinical, physiological, biochemical and psychological characteristics is substantial.

The definitions of headache syndromes in the past have lacked precision (Rose, 1986), making it problematic to compare studies. Therefore, The International Headache Society (IHS) formed a Classification Committee which published diagnostic criteria in 1988 (IHS, 1988). Most research published after 1988 adheres to these criteria.

PSYCHOPHYSIOLOGY

In this field, psychological variables are manipulated while physiological variables are measured as dependent. The field has yielded important information about the pathophysiology of headache. When reviewing the literature on response characteristics of patients, it becomes evident that the earlier distinction between migraine as vascular and TTH as myalgic is oversimplified, as shown in the following. Abnormal vasomotor responses have been observed in migraine patients in a number of studies. In general, data suggest autonomic nervous system lability. In one such study, non-medicated female migraine patients showed slower habituation to strong auditory stimuli than controls. They also showed more pronounced pulse wave amplitude reduction in the temporal arteries during stressful stimulation, and a pronounced pulse wave amplitude increase while resting afterwards (Ellertsen & Hammerborg, 1982). Surface EMG levels in the frontal muscles were higher in migraine patients than controls. These findings are in agreement with the vasoconstriction (aura phase) and rebound vasodilatation (headache phase) model of migraine attacks.

In non-medicated TTH patients, significantly less pronounced heart rate responses were observed, as compared with controls. Further, TTH patients showed pulse wave amplitude increases in response to stimulation, whereas controls showed a slight decrease (Ellertsen, Nordby & Sjaastad, 1987). Thus, different vascular response patterns have been identified between migraine and TTH patients. TTH patients showed significantly higher frontal EMG levels than controls, but not higher than migraine patients. Accordingly, muscle tension may play a part in the pathogenesis of both headache syndromes and/or be secondary to the pain symptoms.

PERSONALITY AND PSYCHOPATHOLOGY

The question of psychopathology and characteristic personality traits in patients with recurring or chronic headache has been discussed in a number of publications (i.e. Philips, 1976; Adler, Adler & Packard, 1987; Ellertsen, 1992). A review of this literature on migraine and TTH shows that a main topic discussed is the question of causes and effects. Although most studies report an increased prevalence of emotional and psychological disturbances, the question of predisposing personality factors remains unanswered. Prospective studies are needed in order to shed light on these important questions, but there are few truly longitudinal studies available.

The Minnesota Multiphasic Personality Inventory (MMPI) has been used in a number of studies of headache patients. It has been discussed whether MMPI profiles obtained in pain patients actually reflect neurotic traits, since items concerning bodily symptoms contribute to the scales in question. However, affirmative responses to MMPI items concerning bodily symptoms are insufficient to drive any clinical scale into the abnormal range. Prognosis and planning of treatment is dependent on a number of variables. Some of these are undoubtedly reflected in the MMPI and other personality tests. Most MMPI studies of headache patients have demonstrated characteristic profiles in these groups. In general, the patients show 'neurotic' MMPI profiles.

Kudrow and Sutkus (1979) found that patients with 'vascular headache' (migraine and cluster headache) scored lowest, TTH and 'combination headache' intermediate, and post-traumatic and 'conversion' headache patients highest on the neurotism scales of the MMPI. One possible interpretation of these data is that a continuum of increased stress and pressures, or an interaction between stressors and predisposing personality characteristics, was reflected in the MMPI. It has been maintained that the relationship between certain personality traits and headache becomes more pronounced as the chronicity of the headache problem increases. DeDomini et al. (1983) found that MMPI elevations were more pronounced in patients with 'daily headache', as compared with patients with headache attacks. Thus, combinations of intensity, severity and duration of pain problems seem to be strongly related to the degree of neurotism, as reflected in personality tests. Zwart, Ellertsen and Bovim (in press) utilized the 1989-revision and restandardization of the MMPI (MMPI-2) and found normal profiles in migraine and cluster headache patients. Significant depression and somatization was found in TTH and cervicogenic headache patients. When all groups were analysed together, there was a strong relationship between headache duration per month and scale elevations. Comparable personality data from boys with migraine, using the Personality Inventory for Children (PIC), have yielded no significant differences between patients and controls. (Ellertsen & Troland, 1989). There was, however, a relationship between duration of headache problems and PIC factor scales indicating withdrawal and social incompetence within the patient group.

Significant lowering of MMPI scales have been reported in groups of migraine and TTH patients who responded favourably to biofeedback treatment. In one study, MMPI profiles were compared in female migraine before and after biofeedback treatment in a 2-year follow-up study (Ellertsen, Troland & Kløve, 1987). There were no differences between most and least improved patients before start of treatment. However, the least improved group showed unchanged profiles, whereas most improved patients showed significant changes on 5 MMPI scales. Decreased somatic complaints, less tension, improved interpersonal relationships and more energy was indicated. In short, the research discussed show that depression, anxiety and somatization is found in chronic headache syndromes, whereas moderate anxiety levels seem to be characteristic in recurring headache.

APPLIED PSYCHOPHYSIOLOGY

Hand temperature biofeedback has been used routinely in treatment of migraine patients since Sargent and Green (1972) first published their promising data on this method. The objective is to achieve learned control of peripheral vasomotor tonus, which in turn is assumed to contribute to normalization of autonomic lability, and hence reduced headache problems. Electromyographic (EMG) biofeedback treatment of TTH was originally described by Budzynski, Stoyva and Adler (1970). Obviously, the two different treatment approaches were inspired by the aetiological assumptions cited above.

Biofeedback treatment effects are well documented in adult and child migraine patients. In general, meta-analyses of clinical trials show that biofeedback, relaxation training and hypnosis treatment yield effects comparable to prophylactic medication, i.e. average reduction of attacks around 45%, as compared with 14% placebo effects (Holroyd & Penzien, 1990). Few studies have combined clinical trials and psychophysiological evaluation. In one study, heart rate and pulse wave amplitude response patterns predicted biofeedback treatment outcome. This points to a potential utility of psychophysiology in identifying patients who respond favourably to this type of treatment. Migraine patients showing most pronounced clinical improvement also showed a normalization of pulse wave amplitude response patterns after treatment (Ellertsen et al., 1987). In boys with migraine, normalization of hand temperature has been reported 1 year after the end of temperature biofeedback treatment group (Ellertsen & Troland, 1989).

In summary, the fields of psychophysiology, abnormal psychology and applied psychophysiology have made important contributions to our understanding of headache syndromes and contributed to improved diagnostic and treatment procedures.

REFERENCES

Adler, C.S., Adler, S.M. & Packard, R.C. (1987). *Psychiatric aspects of headache.* Baltimore: Williams & Wilkins.

Budzynski, T., Stoyva, J. & Adler, C. (1970). Feedback-induced muscle relaxation: application to tension headache. *Journal of Behavioral Therapy and Experimental Psychiatry*, 1, 205.

DeDomini, P., Del Bene, E., Gori-Savellini, S., Manzoni, G.C., Mantucci, N., Nappi, G. & Savoldi, F. (1983). Personality patterns of headache sufferers. *Cephalalgia*, **Suppl 1**, 195–220.

Ellertsen, B. (1992). Personality factors in recurring and chronic pain. *Cephalalgia*, 12, 129–32.

Ellertsen, B. & Hammerborg, D. (1982).

Psychophysiological response patterns in migraine patients. *Cephalagia*, **2**, 19–21.

Ellertsen, B. & Troland, K. (1989). Personality characteristics in childhood migraine. *Cephalalgia*, **9**, Suppl. 10, 238–9.

Ellertsen, B., Nordby, H. & Sjaastad, O. (1987). Psychophysiologic response patterns in tension headache: effects of tricyclic antidepressants. *Cephalalgia*, **7**, 55–63.

Ellertsen, B., Nordby, H., Hammerborg, D. & Thorlacius, S. (1987). Psychophysiologic response patterns in migraine before and after temperature biofeedback. *Cephalalgia*, **7**, 109–24.

Ellertsen, B., Troland, K. & Kløve, H. (1987). MMPI profiles in migraine before and after biofeedback treatment. *Cephalalgia*, **7**, 101–8.

Holroyd, K.A. & Penzien, D.B. (1990). Pharmacological versus non-pharmacological prophylaxis of recurrent migraine headache: a meta-analytic review of clinical trials. *Pain*, **42**, 1–13.

International Headache Society (1988). Classification and diagnostic criteria for headache disorders, cranial neuralgias and facial pain. *Cephalalgia*, **8**, Suppl. 7.

Kudrow, L. & Sutkus, B.J. (1979). MMPI pattern specificity in primary headache disorders. *Headache*, **19**, 18–24.

Philips, C. (1976). Headache and personality. *Journal of Psychosomatic Research*, **20**, 535–42.

Rose, F.C. (1986). Headache: definitions and classification. In F.C. Rose (Ed.). *Handbook of Clinical Neurology, vol 4 (48): Headache*. Amsterdam: Elsevier.

Sargent, J.D. & Green, E.E. (1972). The use of autogenic feedback training in a pilot study of migraine and tension headache. *Headache*, **12**, 120–4.

Zwart, J.A., Ellertsen, B. & Bovim, G. (in press). Psychosocial differences and MMPI-2 patterns in migraine, cluster headache, tension headache and cervicogenic headache. *Headache*.

Hodgkin's disease and non-Hodgkin's lymphoma

JENNIFER DEVLEN

11655 Old Mill Road, Shippensburg, PA, USA

The lymphomas are a heterogeneous group of neoplastic disorders of the lymphatic system of which there are two main types; Hodgkin's disease (HD), first described by Thomas Hodgkin in 1832, and non-Hodgkin's lymphoma (NHL). The annual incidence of Hodgkin's disease is approximately 2–3 per 100 000 population (OPCS, 1993), with bimodal peaks in early adulthood and the elderly. The incidence of non-Hodgkin's lymphoma is 9–11 cases per 100 000 per year, and tends to be more common after age 45. Both sexes are affected, with a slightly higher incidence in males. Depending on the histopathological classification and extent of disease, treatment typically consists of radiation to site of diseased lymph nodes and/or 6–8 monthly cycles of combination chemotherapy. The prognosis of these diseases has improved significantly in the past 25 years and the 5-year survival can be as high as 92% for HD and 80% for NHL.

PSYCHOLOGICAL MORBIDITY

At some time during the discovery of their disease or its treatment, as many as two-thirds of patients will be anxious, depressed or both (Devlen *et al.*, 1987a, Nerenz, Leventhal & Love, 1982). The onset of disease and referral to a specialist is associated with the highest levels of emotional distress. Using standardized psychiatric interview schedules, Lloyd *et al.* (1984) identified 37.5% and Devlen *et al.* (1987a) found 36% of patients to be suffering clinically significant anxiety or depression during this time. However, open and direct consultation with the hospital clinicians, a diagnosis and prognosis which may not be as terrible as they had feared, coupled with the commencement of treatment appears to resolve a great deal of this distress.

At any point during treatment, the overall level of psychological morbidity is never as high as during the period surrounding diagnosis of the disease. However, morbidity persists in some patients, while others are at risk of developing a depressive disorder or anxiety state. One recent prospective study examined the month by month prevalence, time of onset and duration of affective disorders in a sample of 120 patients (Devlen *et al.* 1987a). In total, 51% experienced psychiatric morbidity at some time during the 12-month postdiagnosis period. While the majority of this morbidity was found to occur in the first three months of treatment, patients were still likely to develop an affective disorder, especially depression, at any time up to one year after diagnosis.

COMPLICATIONS OF TREATMENT

Side-effects of both chemotherapy and radiotherapy are very common in HD and NHL patients. Over 70% experience hair loss, nausea and vomiting. Less prevalent but still significant complications include sore mouth, changes in perception of taste, sore skin, loss of or increase in appetite, constipation, diarrhoea, pain and peripheral neuropathy (Nerenz, Leventhal & Love, 1982; Devlen *et al.*, 1987a).

One-quarter of patients develop prechemotherapy or anticipatory nausea and vomiting (Devlen *et al.*, 1987a), a phenomenon which is commonly thought to develop as a result of classical conditioning. Previously neutral stimuli associated with the chemotherapy injection/infusion such as odours, foods and tastes, the sight of the hospital or the chemotherapy nurse have been identified as stimuli sufficient to evoke nausea or vomiting. These conditioned responses can be firmly developed by the fourth or fifth treatment cycle (Devlen *et al.*, 1987a) by which time they are particularly resistant to anti-emetic medication although there is evidence that they may be responsive to psychological treatments (Watson & Marvell, 1992).

Psychiatric morbidity is not related to disease type or stage but has been found to be correlated with treatment toxicity, particularly with side-effects involving the gastrointestinal tract: nausea, vomiting, diarrhoea, loss of appetite, sore mouth and taste changes (Devlen et al., 1987a, b). Patients often stress the importance of eating well to maintain the strength necessary to endure treatment and combat the disease, and side-effects which hinder this may explain some of this association. Patients may also misattribute treatment effects as being indicative of the recurrence of their disease, especially with vague effects such as tiredness and pain (Nerenz, Leventhal & Love, 1982) or when they occur some time after completion of treatment, as in the case of postradiation lethargy.

Chemotherapeutic agents used in the treatment of these cancers are known to affect fertility and, as such, have implications for this group which includes young adults who may be unable to start or complete a family (Fobair et al., 1986). Decreased libido and sexual activity whilst on treatment are common and, even several years after completion of therapy, the prevalence of sexual dysfunction remains high (Devlen et al., 1987b; Fobair et al., 1986).

Impairments in concentration (Cella & Tross, 1986) and memory have also been recorded. Although objective memory assessments indicate performance within the normal range, there are significant differences in test scores for those 30% of patients reporting such problems when compared with those claiming no impairment (Devlen et al., 1987a) and further investigations of cognitive difficulties are warranted

Long-term effects

Recent research indicates that some effects, such as decreased energy levels, persist long after treatment has ceased, and a significant minority experience substantial long-term physical, psychological, social and employment problems (Devlen et al. 1987b; Devlen 1987, Fobair et al. 1986, Cella & Tross 1986). Despite the impressive cure rates of these diseases, patients with Hodgkin's disease and non-Hodgkin's lymphoma pay a high price for their survival.

REFERENCES

Cella, D.F. & Tross, S. (1986). Psychological adjustment to survival from Hodgkin's disease. *Journal of Consulting and Clinical Psychology*, **54**, 616–22.

Devlen, J. (1987). The psychological and social consequences of Hodgkin's disease and its treatment. In P. Selby & T.J. McElwain (Eds.). *Hodgkin's disease*. Oxford: Blackwell Scientific Publications.

Devlen, J., Maguire, P., Phillips, P. & Crowther, D. (1987a). Psychological problems associated with diagnosis and treatment of lymphomas. II: Prospective Study. *British Medical Journal*, **295**, 955–7.

Devlen, J., Maguire, P., Phillips, P., Crowther, D. & Chambers, H. (1987b). Psychological problems associated with diagnosis and treatment of lymphomas. I: Retrospective study. *British Medical Journal*, **295**, 953–4.

Fobair, P., Hoppe, R.T., Bloom, J., Cox, R., Varghese, A. & Spiegel, D. (1986). Psychosocial problems among survivors of Hodgkin's disease. *Journal of Clinical Oncology*, **4**, 805–14.

Lloyd, G.G., Parker, A.C., Ludlam, C.A. & McGuire, R.J. (1984). Emotional impact of diagnosis and early treatment of lymphomas. *Journal of Psychosomatic Research*, **28**, 157–62.

Nerenz, D.R., Leventhal, H. & Love, R.R. (1982). Factors contributing to emotional distress during cancer chemotherapy. *Cancer*, **50**, 1020–7.

Office of Population Censuses and Surveys (1993). Cancer statistics. *Registrations of cancer diagnoses in 1987, England and Wales*. London: HMSO.

Watson, M. & Marvell, C. (1992). Anticipatory nausea and vomiting among cancer patients: a review. *Psychology and Health*, **6**, 97–106.

Huntington's disease

MAURICE BLOCH
Riverview Hospital, Port Coquitlam, BC
Canada

Huntington's disease (HD) is a genetic disease which is transmitted as an autosomal dominant trait with complete penetrance. It is a chronic degenerative disease of the central nervous system characterized by movement disorder, cognitive deterioration and personality change. While found in all parts of the world HD is most commonly found in Caucasian populations in which about 1 : 10 000 individuals are affected. Onset is subtle and insidious and occurs most frequently between 30 and 50 years of age. Juvenile onset is seen in about 10% of cases and about 20% have onset at over 50 years of age with diagnoses as late as the eighth decade reported. The disease progresses inexorably culminating in death usually 15 to 25 years after onset. Late onset HD tends to progress more slowly than early onset forms of the disease. There is thus far no effective treatment or cure for the disease.

HD, popularly called St Vitus Dance, is commonly known for its jerky, dance-like (choreic) movements. Movement may, however, also be rigid, especially in the juvenile form and the later stages of the adult form. Cognitive deficits (dementia) commonly associated with HD include difficulty with memory (primarily a retrieval problem), attention and concentration. While the dementia of HD is primarily subcortical and is non-aphasic, it includes many additional cognitive functions such as cognitive speed and fluency, verbal fluency, difficulty persisting with, or initiating, a task and with change of set.

[495]

Becoming affected with HD may have a tremendous impact on the psyche. Organic change is compounded with psychological trauma. High rates of schizophrenia, anxiety disorders, alcoholism and other psychiatric illnesses are reported. Irritability, poor impulse control, angry and hostile behaviour are observed in many sufferers of HD during circumscribed periods of the illness. While insight and orientation remain relatively intact throughout the illness, judgement is impaired in many victims of HD. This may be observed in bad business decisions, inappropriate sexual behaviour and impaired social judgement. Depression is the most common psychiatric illness seen in HD and is associated with a higher rate of suicide. An increased rate of suicide among victims of HD is well established. Harper *et al.* (1991) has surveyed the literature and has found studies reporting suicide rates which range between 0.5% and 12.7%.

It is difficult to separate out the aetiology of a mental illness when biological, psychological and social factors are all contributing, and this is the case with affective disorders associated with HD. There is, however, growing evidence that affective disorders are related to the pathophysiology of HD. In previous studies of affective disorder, a prevalence of between 9 and 44% has been reported (Harper *et al.* 1991). Peyser and Folstein (1990) found that about 10% of all HD patients have manic episodes, some have delusions and hallucinations and many respond to appropriate pharmacological treatment. Furthermore, affective disorder is more common in some families, in persons of Caucasian ancestry and in those with later onset.

Irrespective of the aetiology of the psychiatric problems or of the dyskinesia and dementia associated with HD, the impact on the individual and on the family is profound. However, recently published textbooks on HD (Folstein, 1989; Harper *et al.*, 1991) in citing over 500 publications related to HD rarely refer to any reporting on the psychosocial impact of the disease. They do cite studies on the neuropsychiatric, psychiatric and neuropsychological effects of the disease as well as papers which discuss ethical and legal issues related to HD. Although research on the psychosocial impact of the disease has been minimal, theoretical analyses, case studies and anecdotal reports of a few researchers have provided a rich source of hypothesis-generating material (Wexler, 1984; Kessler & Bloch, 1989; Bloch *et al.*, 1993). More literature is available on the psychosocial impact of predictive testing. The research team in the Department of Medical Genetics at the University of British Columbia, Vancouver, Canada is currently undertaking a study on the effects of direct mutation testing for HD on immediate family members.

The psychological adaptation of the individual to living at risk for HD and to the onset and diagnosis of the disease, is described in a Model of Psychological Response Stages (Bloch *et al.*, 1993). During the warning stage, asymptomatic individuals become aware of their risk status for HD and develop adaptive psychological defensive strategies. In response to the early signs and symptoms of HD (incipient stage) unconscious working through of this realization occurs while it is still kept out of conscious awareness. When symptoms can no longer be ignored, the possibility of the diagnosis of HD is acknowledged (breakthrough stage). After the delivery of the diagnosis during the adjustment stage, short- and long-term adaptive responses to living with HD occur.

The diagnosis of HD, however, has implications which go far beyond the affected individual alone. Living with an individual affected with HD will have serious ramifications for family members, for their roles and for the family as a system. The caregiver may have the burden of taking over the role functions of the affected person while maintaining his/her previous roles and at the same time providing care for the affected person. In the case of a genetic disease the caregiving spouse must, in addition, live with the awareness that any number of the children may have inherited the gene and go on to develop the disease. The burden is multiplied for those families in which more than one member is concurrently affected. The caregiving spouse, who has no genetic loading for the disease, is pivotal in maintaining the integrity of family functioning. The needs of the caregiver are, however, often neglected. Time taken to fulfil social and personal needs is frequently accompanied by strong guilt feelings. Attrition over the years wears the caregiver down and may culminate in family breakdown or increased vulnerability to mental health problems.

The attitude of the affected person and of the caregiver toward the disease may have a substantial influence on the attitude to the disease of any children in the family. Children are more likely to view the disease as catastrophic if the parents treat it as such. This will happen in those families where the affected individual is perceived as not accepting the disease, is rejected by the family or behaves in ways destructive and embarrassing for family members. A less threatened and more wholesome relationship to the disease is more likely to develop in those families where there is a positive attitude of challenge and struggle in a context of love and support. Nevertheless, the child too must bear a great deal. The burden of being thrust, perhaps, into a quasi-parenting role *vis à vis* the affected parent and the negative impact of the shadow of this incurable disease hanging over the at risk children may be immense. Anxiety and uncertainty must be borne and may influence important decisions about marriage, childbearing and career.

While there still is no cure for HD, advances in molecular genetics now make it possible for the at risk individual to lessen the stress of uncertainty. The discovery of a polymorphic DNA marker for the HD gene (Gusella *et al.*, 1983) lead to the availability of Predictive Testing for at risk individuals. A major goal of the research carried out on the implementation of the Predictive Test was to assess the psychosocial impact of the test results on individual candidates in order to develop guidelines for delivery of the test as a service. In surveys undertaken prior to the availability of the test the majority of at risk individuals indicated that they would participate in predictive testing programmes. In fact, a much smaller number, perhaps in the range of 15 to 20%, have come forward to take the test in the seven years that it has been available. Results from the preliminary surveys had suggested that there might be a significant negative effect on those individuals who received high risk results. In particular, a high rate of suicide or attempted suicide was predicted. This has not materialized, and, while a few individuals (including some with a decreased risk result) have had negative and difficult experiences (Huggins *et al.*, 1992; Bloch *et al.*, 1992) overall, those who have had an increased risk result and a decreased risk result show improvement at one-year follow-up (Wiggins *et al.*, 1992). The importance of preparatory and follow-up counselling in the predictive testing programme is emphasized in the guidelines published by the World Federation of Neurology: Research Group on Huntington's Chorea (1990).

More recently, the gene for HD has been isolated (HD Collaborative Research Group, 1993). The cloning of the HD gene now makes it possible for most AR individuals to be given results with 100% certainty. The protocols which evolved from the earlier linkage analysis have provided the guidelines for the new 'direct' gene testing. Pre- and postcounselling sessions are provided in which the individual is screened for psychiatric disorder, is fully informed about the science and limitations of the test, is assisted to prepare emotionally for the receipt of results, ensuring the presence of professional and social supports and of adequate follow-up to support the candidate in the post results phase. Nevertheless, this test created was new counselling challenges, ethical and moral dilemmas. Questions of the use of the test for diagnostic purposes and for the testing of minor children (Bloch & Hayden, 1990) need to be reevaluated in this new context. Issues of third-party interest, social cost and patient confidentiality will arise. (See also 'Genetic counselling'.)

REFERENCES

Bloch, M. & Hayden, M.R. (1990). Opinion: predictive testing for Huntington disease in childhood: challenges and implications. Editorial, *American Journal Medical Genetics*, 46, 1–4.

Bloch, M., Adam, S., Wiggins, S., Huggins, M. & Hayden, M.R. (1992). Predictive testing for Huntington disease in Canada: the experience of those receiving an increased risk. *American Journal Medical Genetics*, 42, 499–507.

Bloch, M., Adam, S., Fuller, A., Kremer, B., Welch, J.P., Wiggins, S., Huggins, M., Theilmann, J. & Hayden, M.R. (1993). Diagnosis of Huntington disease: a model for the stages of psychological response based on experience of a predictive testing program. *American Journal Medical Genetics* 47, 368–74.

Folstein, S.E. (1989). *Huntington's disease: a disorder of families*. Baltimore: The Johns Hopkins University Press.

Gusella, J., Wexler, N.S., Conneally, P.M., Naylor, S.L., Anderson, M.A., Tanzi, R.E., Watkins, P.C., Ottina, K., Wallace, M.R., Sakaguchi, A.Y.,

Young, A.B., Shoulson, I., Bonilla, E. & Martin, J.B. (1983). A polymorphic DNA marker genetically linked to Huntington's disease. *Nature*, 306, 234–8.

Harper, P.S., Morris, M.J., Quarrell, O. Shaw, D.J., Tyler, A. & Youngman, S. (1991). *Huntington's disease*. Philadelphia: WB Saunders.

HD Collaborative Research Group. (1993). A novel gene containing a trinucleotide repeat that is expanded and unstable on Huntington's disease chromosomes. *Cell*, 72, 971–83.

Huggins, M., Bloch, M., Wiggins, S., Adam, S., Suchowersky, O., Trew, M., Klimek, M.L., Greenberg, C.R., Eleff, M., Thompson, L., Knight, J., MacLeod, P., Girard, K., Theilmann, J., Hedrick, A. & Hayden, M.R. (1992). Predictive testing for Huntington disease in Canada: adverse effects and unexpected results in those receiving a decreased risk. *American Journal Medical Genetics*, 42, 508–15.

Kessler, S. & Bloch, M. (1989). Social system response to Huntington disease. *Family Process*, 28, 59–68.

Peyser, C.E. & Folstein, S.E. (1990). Huntington's disease as a model for mood disorders. Clues from neuropathology and neurochemistry. *Molecular and Chemical Neuropathology*, 12, 99–119.

Wexler, N. (1984). Huntington's disease and other late onset genetic disorders. In A.E.H. Emery & I. Pullen (Eds.). *Psychological aspects of genetic counselling*. New York: Academic Press (Harcourt, Brace & Jovanovich).

Wiggins, S., Whyte, P., Huggins, M., Adam, S., Theilmann, J., Bloch, M., Hayden, M.R. and members of the Canadian Collaborative Study for Predictive Testing. (1992). The psychological consequences of predictive testing for Huntington's disease. *New England Journal of Medicine*, 327, 1401–5.

World Federation of Neurology: Research Group on Huntington's Chorea. (1990). Ethical issues policy statement on Huntington's disease molecular genetics predictive test. *Journal Medical Genetics*, 27, 34–8.

Hyperactivity

HALLGRIM KLØVE
and
BJØRN ELLERTSEN
*Department of Clinical Neuropsychology,
University of Bergen, Norway*

In 1902, a paper published in *The Lancet* pointed to the fact that 'abnormal psychical conditions in children' could be caused by diseases of the central nervous system (CNS). This conclusion was based on observations of children developing hyperactive, antisocial behaviour after encephalitis (Still, 1902). The clinical picture was further discussed by Kahn and Cohen in 1934, introducing the concept 'organic driveness' (Kahn & Cohen, 1934). A few years later, clinical efficacy of CNS stimulants in hyperactive children was reported by Bradley (1937).

Recent research indicate that prenatal factors account for a large proportion of the variance with regard to learning and behavioural problems in children. This has been found in minimal brain dysfunction (MBD), attention deficit hyperactivity disorder (ADHD), low birth weight (LBW) and learning disabilities (Kløve & Hole,

[497]

1979; Sommerfelt *et al.*, 1993; Rourke, 1989). However, psychosocial factors always interact with the biological factors in question and must be taken into consideration. The MBD concept is used differently both between and within countries. Most clinicians include hyperactivity as one of several criteria for MBD, but there is no consensus about this. Accordingly, it is our recommendation that the MBD concept should be avoided both in clinical practice and research. ADHD, on the other hand, has become an internationally accepted term for the group of children described as hyperactive in earlier publications (APA, 1994).

Hyperactivity is a predominant symptom in a large proportion of ADHD children, but the relative importance of this symptom has been discussed. This point becomes clear if one study recent history of the diagnostic criteria for psychiatric disorders of infancy, childhood and adolescence. In *The Diagnostic and Statistical Manual-III* of The American Psychiatric Association (*DSM-III*), the syndrome was subdivided into attention deficit disorder with or without hyperactivity. The *DSM-III* revision broke this down into ADHD only. In the DSM-IV, the subdivision reappeared (predominantly inattentive, hyperactive–impulsive, or both). Hyperactivity may also occur as part of other clinical pictures than the typical ADHD syndrome.

Hyperactivity has been vividly described in a number of publications. The DSM-IV requires that six or more of a total of nine symptoms of hyperactivity–impulsivity have persisted for more than 6 months, and to a degree that is maladaptive and inconsistent with developmental level. The symptoms include such behaviours as fidgeting, leaving the classroom seat when inappropriate, running about or climbing in situations where this is inappropriate, difficulties in playing quietly, often 'on the go' as if 'driven by a motor', excessive talking, blurting out answers before questions are completed, difficulties in awaiting turn and interrupting or intruding on others. It is crucial to take into account the chronological and mental age level of the child when evaluating these behaviours (APA, 1994). The clinician must be trained both in normal developmental psychology and psychopathology. The incidence of ADHD range between 3 and 5% in school-age children when these criteria are adhered to. For a comprehensive review of the ADHD condition, the reader is referred to Barkley (1990).

In our opinion, an extensive evaluation comprising clinical observation, paediatric neurological examination, neuropsychological examination and personality testing is required in order to sort out the individual problem profile in ADHD. In cases where the referred child does not meet the criteria for ADHD, this extensive evaluation usually provides sufficient information to arrive at alternative diagnoses and to plan treatment accordingly. Important differential diagnoses are mental retardation, anxiety disorders, depression, coping failure, Tourettes Syndrome, psychopathology and side-effects of medication.

Data from group studies of ADHD children demonstrate that there is a relationship with dysmaturity at birth (LBW in relation to gestational age, Kløve & Hole, 1979). This relationship indicates that inattention and hyperactivity in children is related to non-optimal CNS development during pregnancy. It is, however, important to underscore that a large proportion of dysmature and LBW children show no signs of ADHD.

In 1970–71, Satterfield and coworkers found low CNS activation levels in groups of hyperactive children, as indicated by measures of activity and responsivity in the autonomic nervous system (ANS). This has later been demonstrated both in group studies and single-case studies (Kløve, 1990). Accordingly, autonomic measures are important in evaluation of ADHD children. This type of evaluation is particularly valuable when it comes to the question of pharmacological treatment. ADHD children who show a normalized arousal pattern after test-dosages of CNS stimulants are the best responders to this type of treatment (Kløve, 1990). This fact undermines the traditional view that there is a 'paradoxical' effect of central stimulants in ADHD children.

The clinical efficacy of CNS stimulant treatment of selected ADHD children is indisputable. In spite of this fact, this treatment is repeatedly and at times heavily debated. Ignorance about the pharmacological and clinical effects of the medication is one reason for this, and less than optimal diagnostic procedures leading to incorrect treatment another. In our experience, there is no doubt about the clinical effects of CNS stimulants when the indication is correct. In cases where clinicians, parents and teachers are uncertain about the clinical effect, there is always good reason to reconsider. When low CNS arousal and unequivocal pharmacologic effect are used in addition to the ADHD criteria, the incidence of candidates for this treatment approach remains uncertain, but may be below 1%. Treatment with CNS stimulants must, however, be regarded as a door-opener for other therapeutical interventions to take effect, and not as sufficient treatment in itself.

The question of prognosis in ADHD is controversial. Few prospective studies are available, but it has been reported that 30–70% of ADHD children show significant behavioural problems as adults. The term 'Residual ADHD' points to this fact. There is no question that a significant proportion of juvenile delinquents, adult criminals and substance abusers qualify for this diagnosis, and were untreated for ADHD as children. ADHD patients experience symptom relief from hard narcotics. It is, however, preferrable to obtain this relief through regulated medication. Thus, while some claim that it is unacceptable to treat children with 'narcotics', and that it may make them future abusers, the truth may be quite the opposite.

REFERENCES

American Psychiatric Association (1994). *Diagnostic and statistical manual of mental disorders*, Fourth Edition. Washington DC, American Psychiatric Association.

Barkley, R.A. (1990). *Attention Deficit Hyperactivity Disorder. a handbook for diagnosis and treatment*. New York: The Guilford Press.

Bradley, C. (1937). The behavior of children receiving benzedrine. *American Journal of Psychiatry*, **94**, 577–85.

Kahn, I. & Cohen, L.H. (1934). Organic driveness: a brainstem syndrome and an experience. *New England Journal of Medicine*, **210**, 748–56.

Kløve, H. (1990). Responders and non-responders to medication. In K. Conners and M. Kinsbourne (Eds.). *ADHD attention deficit hyperactivity disorder*. München: MMV Medizin-Verlag.

Kløve H. & Hole, K. (1979). The hyperkinetic syndrome: criteria for diagnosis. In R.L. Trites (Ed.). *Hyperactivity in children. Etiology, measurement and treatment implications*. Baltimore: University Park Press.

Rourke, B.P. (1989). *Non-verbal learning*

disabilities: the syndrome and the model. New York: Guilford Press.

Sommerfelt, K., Ellertsen, B., Markestad, T. (1993). Personality and behaviour in eight year old, non-handicapped children with birth weight under 1500 g. *Acta Paediatrica*, **82**, 723–8.

Still, G.F. (1902). Some abnormal psychical conditions in children. *The Lancet*, **i**, 1077–82.

Hyperhidrosis

GRAHAM POWELL

Department of Psychology, University of Surrey, Guildford, UK

The sympathetic nervous system innervates and controls most of the organs of the body. Malfunction of the sympathetic nervous system can cause either underactivity (e.g. postural hypotension, impotence or anhidrosis) or overactivity (e.g. paraxysmal hypertension or hyperhidrosis). Hyperhidrosis is excessive sweating, most often in the upper body, arms and hands, or of the legs and feet.

Sympathectomy is the operation whereby the appropriate nerves to the relevant part are cut. The major indication for sympathectomy is palmar hyperhidrosis (Gordon, Zechmeister & Collin, 1994), in which there is thoracoscopic ablation of the second thoracic ganglion. In a large-scale retrospective study of electrocauterization in 180 consecutive cases of palmar hyperhidrosis (Chen, Shih & Fung, 1994), there were 116 females and only 64 males, suggesting that excessive sweating is less acceptable in young women than young men (mean age of the whole sample was 21.6 years). The success rate was 98%, but 70% had a degree of compensatory sweating at other sites. However, long-term extreme satisfaction with the operation was reported by 64 of the 67 patients studied by Mares *et al.* (1994). In the Mares' study, it was found that compensatory sweating did not affect satisfaction.

In view of the high success rate of the operation and low morbidity, there is a strong argument for early surgery to save children 'many years of agony and social discomfort (Mares *et al.*, 1994)'. Koa *et al.*, (1994) report on a series of 40 children under the age of 16 years given video endoscopic laser sympathectomy, with satisfactory outcome, and Mares' own series was in fact on children and adolescents.

Pilot investigations into the psychological management of hyperhidrosis have used cued conditioning and desensitization (Moylan & Dadds, 1992), hypnosis with classical conditioning (Minichiello, 1987) and hypnosis on its own (King & Stanley, 1986).

REFERENCES

Chen, H.J., Shih, D.Y. & Fung, S.T. (1994). Transthoracic endoscopic sympathectomy in the treatment of palmar hyperhidrosis. *Archives of Surgery*, **129**, 630–3.

Gordon, A., Zechmeister, K. & Collin, J. (1994). The role of sympathectomy in current surgical practice. *European Journal of Vascular Surgery*, **8**, 129–37.

Kao, M.C., Lee, W.Y., Yip, K.M., Hsiao, Y., Lee, Y.S. & Tasai, J.C. (1994). Palmar hyperhidrosis in children: treatment with video endoscopic laser sympathectomy. *Journal of Paediatric Surgery*, **29**, 387–91.

King, M.G. & Stanley, G.V. (1986). The treatment of hyperhidrosis: a case report. *Australian Journal of Clinical and Experimental Hypnosis*, **14**, 61–4.

Mares, A.J., Steiner, Z., Cohen, Z., Finaly, R., Freud, E. & Mordehai, J. (1994). Transaxillary upper thoracic sympathectomy for primary palmar hyperhidrosis in children and adolescents. *Journal of Paediatric Surgery*, **29**, 382–6.

Moylan, A. & Dadds, M.R. (1992). Hyperhidrosis: a case study and theoretical formulation. *Behaviour Change*, **9**, 87–95.

Minichiello, W.E. (1987). Treatment of hyperhidrosis of amputation site with hypnosis and suggestions involving classical conditioning. *International Journal of Psychosomatics*, **34**, 7–8.

Hypertension

DEREK W. JOHNSTON

School of Psychology, University of St Andrews,
Fife, Scotland, UK

Primary hypertension, i.e. raised blood pressure of no clearly identified origin, is found in up to 20% of the adult population and is associated with an increased risk of cardiovascular disease. Hypertension is related to both health behaviours, such as eating too much or inappropriately and to more directly psychological factors such as stress or particular personality patterns. In this case the link with hypertension is presumably through an interaction of the central nervous system and neural and humoral factors that control blood pressure (Folkow, 1982).

PSYCHOLOGICAL AND BEHAVIOURAL FACTORS IN THE AETIOLOGY OF HYPERTENSION

It is clear from epidemiological studies that blood pressure is raised in the overweight, in those who drink excessive amounts of alcohol and in individuals with sedentary lifestyles. Salt consumption also plays a small role in pressure elevation. In animals a variety of stressful manipulations can lead to persistent elevations in pressure. Lawler *et al.* (1980) demonstrated that rats stressed by shock avoidance showed elevations in pressure only if they were genetically prone to high blood pressure. A related finding comes from Anderson, Kearns & Better's (1983) demonstration that dogs that were fed a high salt diet had persistent elevations of pressure in shock avoidant situations, but neither salt alone nor stress alone raised pressure. Such studies demonstrate a finding of fundamental importance; stress alone rarely produces hypertension rather it does so in combination with some predisposing, or sensitizing, factor.

Humans also respond to stress with large elevations in blood pressure. Brod, in a classic study, showed that tasks such as mental arithmetic raised blood pressure in normotensives as well as hypertensives (see Obrist, 1981). Blood pressure is determined by the amount of blood being pumped by the heart (cardiac output, a function of heart rate and stroke volume) and the resistance of the arterial system to the flow of that blood (peripheral resistance). High blood pressure is the result of the alteration in one of these factors without a compensating adjustment in the other. It has been accepted since Brod's time that acute stress primarily affects blood pressure by altering cardiac output. Obrist in a very influential research programme (Obrist, 1981), demonstrated that many subjects showed a large increase in cardiac output, particularly to tasks such as difficult paced choice reaction time, which involved active coping. Drug studies indicated that these effects on the heart were primarily mediated by the β-adrenergic system. The distinction between active and passive coping, the latter having little effect on the heart, has been critical to research and theorizing on the psychological precursors of hypertension although it is gradually being recognized that persistent stress can increase peripheral resistance and that the parasympathetic system is also importantly affected by stress. The work on active coping emphasized what is termed stimulus specificity, the tendency of responses to the same stimulus to be similar in different individuals. A contrary inclination in psychophysiology is to emphasize response specificity, the tendency for individuals to respond to different stimuli with similar patterns of responses. This is also seen in the cardiovascular system with a sizeable minority of subjects responding even to active stressors with increases in peripheral resistance, rather than cardiac output.

It is not yet clear if the responses seen to laboratory stress relate to blood pressure in real life, although studies using continuous, direct measures of blood pressure suggest that they may. This is a very active area of research because of its theoretical importance and the increasing used of ambulatory BP monitors in research and clinical practice (Turner *et al.*, 1994).

Cause and effect relationships cannot be determined in studies of subjects with established hypertension, although it appears that hypertensives usually respond to stress with an exaggerated increase in pressure. More convincing are studies of the offspring of hypertensives, who are known to be predisposed to hypertension. When young their blood pressure at rest is little different from subjects with no family history of hypertension but when stressed they show a greater increase in pressure (Fredrikson & Matthews, 1990). Longitudinal studies suggest, not entirely convincingly, that larger responses to stress predict future hypertension.

If stress is important in the development of hypertension, then one would expect that individuals and communities under most stress would display the greatest prevalence of hypertension. Classic studies have examined the effects of factory closure and job stress on blood pressure and have shown that pressure rises with unemployment and drops when work is found, and that subjects in stressful occupations, such as air traffic controllers, have higher blood pressure than other workers in the same airports, although the role of health behaviours, such as alcohol consumption, may also be important in such studies (DeFrank, Jenkins & Rose, 1987). One should never assume that the direct relationships between stress and blood pressure one sees in the laboratory are translated into similar relationships in other less well-controlled situations.

PSYCHOLOGICAL METHODS IN THE REDUCTION OF HYPERTENSION

There is little doubt that weight reduction is associated with a lowering of blood pressure in the grossly overweight. Even in the less obese, weight reductions of only 7 kg are associated with a greater reduction in pressure than that produced by standard pharmacological treatment for hypertension (MacMahon *et al.*, 1985). Reductions in alcohol consumption are also of value in very heavy drinkers.

Perhaps more interesting psychologically are attempts to reduce blood pressure by reducing stress. Numerous controlled trials of relaxation based stress management followed a series of pioneering studies by Patel (see Johnston, 1991). Various summary and meta-analyses reach slightly different but generally positive conclusions (see Jacob *et al.*, 1991; Johnston, 1991). However, a series of studies reported in the late 1980s and early 1990s appear to contradict these positive views. Agras and Chesney (see Johnston, 1991) found that various forms of relaxation and biofeedback-based stress management were no more effective than self-monitoring of BP in either medicated or unmedicated hypertensives, and concluded that self-monitoring was the active ingredient in stress management. Others have failed to demonstrate any effects of relaxation training on blood pressure measured continuously over a 24-hour period or found supportive psychotherapy and stress management equally effective (see Johnston, 1991). Finally Johnston *et al.* (1993) could find no difference on a wide range of measures of hypertension and its clinical consequences between relaxation and a control condition in almost 100 unmedicated hypertensives. However Schneider *et al.* (1995) found that progressive muscle relaxation and Transcendental Mediation (TM) both lowered blood pressure in elderly black Americans with mild to moderate hypertension with TM producing reliably greater reductions. Schneider *et al.*'s patients came from a disadvantaged, highly stressed group in whom hypertension may be more likely to be stress related compared to the white samples studied in most of the previous trials. Perhaps relaxation and related procedures are beneficial in subjects or populations in whom stress is more involved in the elevations in pressure observed.

On balance, the effect of stress management on blood pressure appears weak, variable and temporary. However, before dismissing it completely, it is as well to recall that heart disease is determined by the interaction of many risk factors. Stress affects most of these risk factors, and may be a risk factor in its own right. Stress management, although weak, may have pervasive effects that spread across several risk factors. These weak but wide-ranging effects may be preferable to the more powerful effects of medication which are restricted to one risk factor, or even cause an elevation in one risk factor as they reduce another.

REFERENCES

Anderson, D.E., Kearns, W.D. & Better, W.E. (1983). Progressive hypertension in dogs by avoidance conditioning and saline infusion. *Hypertension*, 5, 286–91.

DeFrank, R.S., Jenkins, C.D. & Rose, R.M. (1987). A longitudinal investigation of the relationships among alcohol consumption, psychosocial factors, and blood pressure. *Psychosomatic Medicine*, 49, 236–49.

Folkow, B. (1982). Physiological aspects of primary hypertension. *Psychological Reviews*, 62, 347–504.

Fredrikson, M. & Matthews, K.A. (1990). Cardiovascular responses to behavioral stress and hypertension: a meta-analytic review. *Annals of Behavioral Medicine*, 12, 30–9.

Jacob, R.G., Chesney, M.A., Williams, D.M., Ding, Y. & Shapiro, A.P. (1991). Relaxation therapy for hypertension: design effects and treatment effects. *Annals of behavioral Medicine*, 13, 5–17.

Johnston, D.W. (1991). Stress management in the treatment of mild primary hypertension. *Hypertension*, 17, III–63–III–68.

Johnston, D.W., Gold, A., Kentish, J., Smith, D., Vallance, P., Shah, D., Leach, G. & Robinson, B. (1993). Effect of stress management on blood pressure in mild primary hypertension. *British Medical Journal*, 306, 963–6.

Lawler, J.M., Barker, G.F., Hubbard, J.W. & Allen, M.T. (1980). The effects of conflict on tonic levels of blood pressure in the genetically borderline hypertensive rat. *Psychophysiology*, 17, 363–70.

MacMahon, S.W., MacDonald, G.J., Bernstein, D., Andrews, G. & Blackett, R.B. (1985). Comparison of weight reduction with metoprolol in treatment of hypertension in young overweight patients. *Lancet*, i, 1233–6.

Obrist, P.A. (1981). *Cardiovascular psychophysiology*. New York: Academic Press.

Schneider, R.A., Staggers, F., Alexander, C.N., Sheppard, W., Rainforth, M., Kondwani, K., Smith, S. & King, C.G. (1995). A randomized controlled trial of stress reduction for hypertension in older African Americans. *Hypertension*, 26, 820–7.

Turner, J.R., Ward, M.M., Gellman, M.D., Johnston, D.W., Light, K.C. & Van Doornen, L.J.P. (1994). The relationship between laboratory and ambulatory cardiovascular activity: current evidence and future directions. *Annals of Behavioral Medicine*, 16, 12–23.

Hyperthyroidism

NINA BUTLER

*Unit of Health Psychology, Department of
Psychiatry and Behavioural Sciences, University
College London, UK*

Hyperthyroidism almost always arises as a result of hyperactivity of the thyroid gland. Rarely it occurs as a result of other causes (such as the excessive ingestion of thyroid hormone), but a number of conditions lead to its development. Of these, Graves' disease (an organ-specific autoimmune disease with a strong familial disposition); toxic multinodular goitre (occurring in an older age group), and toxic solitary adenoma (occurring in a younger age-group) account for 95% of all cases presenting at a specialist UK clinic (McGregor, 1996). The incidence of the disorder is approximately 20 per 1000 in females and 2 per 1000 in males. The presentation of the disease is varied, but tends to be gradual rather than acute. Of the conditions' many signs, ophthalmopathy (associated with Graves' disease), weight loss in spite of increasing appetite; insomnia at night paralleled by sleepiness during the day; thinning hair, and restlessness are most commonly reported (Rockey & Griep, 1981; Werner, 1966).

TREATMENT

Treatment of hyperthyroidism is usually by chemical agents which inhibit the synthesis of thyroid hormone, although interventions to reduce the bulk of thyroid tissue (which is over-producing thyroid hormone) by either partial thyroidectomy or radioiodine administration is not uncommon. Beta-blockers are sometimes used as an adjuvant therapy to resolve peripheral manifestations such as tremor, palpitation and sweating (McGregor, 1996).

PSYCHOLOGICAL AND BEHAVIOURAL CONSEQUENCES

It has been proposed that thyroid disease has certain psychiatric manifestations (Gull, 1873; Asher, 1949; Henderson & Gillespie, 1962; Hermann & Quarton, 1965; Carney, Macleod & Sheffield 1981), although there is disagreement as to their precise nature. Impaired consciousness, depression, and a combination of paranoid & depressive features have all been implicated (Tonks, 1964; Carney *et al.*, 1981). However, while a raised incidence of thyroid disorders have been reported in female psychiatric admissions and geriatric in-patients (Nicholson, Liebling & Hall, 1976; Bahemuka & Hodkinson, 1975), there is evidence that thyroid symptomatology is at times mistaken to be the result of psychiatric caseness *per se* (Carney *et al.*, 1981). These authors point out that aches and pains, hyperkinesis and weight change are common to both psychiatric thyroid disorders, and that the manifestations of thyroid disease may take longer to become clinically apparent than those of psychiatric disorders.

Using a standardized measure of behavioural dysfunction, the Sickness Impact Profile (Bergner, Bobbitt & Kressel, 1976), Carney *et al.*, were able to demonstrate that improvements in patients' daily lives occurred with medical therapy for the thyroid condition, while Trzepacz *et al.* (1988) found that psychiatric improvements paralleled improvements in endocrine symptoms in patients treated with propranolol. The behavioural correlates of apparent psychiatric caseness already described are thus shown to be consonant with a physiological basis for the behavioural disturbance and neuropsychological deficits found in hyperthyroid patients. However, the incidence of stressful life events in the year preceding the symptoms of Graves' disease are shown to potentiate the development of hypothyroidism induced by standard therapeutic doses of radioiodine (Stewart *et al.*, 1985) during treatment.

HYPOTHYROIDISM

Whereas hyperthyroidism is caused by hyperactivity of the thyroid gland, hypothyroidism is the result of structural of functional abnormalities of the thyroid gland leading to thyroid hormone deficiency. The condition is classified according to primary and secondary causation: that resulting from thyroid disease and that resulting from disease of the hypothalamic – pituitary axis, respectively. The onset may be insidious and the symptomatology, as McGregor (1996) points out, reflects the fact 'that thyroid hormone deficiency affects every tissue in the body' (p. 1614). Clinical features associated with the condition include lethargy; weight gain; goitre; coarsening of the skin, intolerance to cold, puffy face and hands; hypersomnolence; delayed reflexes; parasthesiae, and anaemia. Aspects of mental functioning shown to be common in patients with hypothyroid syndrome are mental slowing; poor memory; inability to concentrate; depression, and psychosis.

PRIMARY HYPOTHYROIDISM AND INTELLECTUAL IMPAIRMENT

Primary hypothyroidism may be the result of previous treatment for hyperthyroidism; developmental defects in the thyroid such that there is either a failure of the gland to descend properly during embryological development or an absence of thyroid tissue altogether; a genetically determined defect in hormone biosynthesis; the presence of hypothalamic – pituitary disease; iodine deficiency or excess, or autoimmune thyroid disease (McGregor, 1996). It is most commonly the result of developmental defects and iodine deficiency. Hypothyroidism which develops in adult life is often referred to as myxoedema.

Hypothyroidism is known to present in 1 in 3500–4500 births and the consequences of it remaining clinically undetected in the newborn are disastrous: mental retardation, short stature, deaf mutism, pyramidal tract signs and a characteristic facial appearance. Neonatal screening programmes are now well established and these have gone some way to eliminating such effects (Barnes, 1985; McGregor, 1996). Research has therefore focused largely on the intellectual and neurological functioning in patients born with the condition and those who have received treatment.

Although full-blown 'cretinism' (as congenital hypothyroidism has been called) is clearly preventable given early treatment with thyroid hormone replacement, the evidence for its efficacy with regard to intellectual and motor development is equivocal (Glorieux et al., 1985; Rovet, Ehrlich & Sorboda, 1987; Heyerdahl, Kase & Lie 1991). For example, Macfaul et al. (1978) found that 77% of their sample demonstrated at least one sign of impaired brain function irrespective of very early intervention and Simons et al., (1994) showed that, although patients reached a normal IQ range, their score at age 10 was closely related to their score at age 3 and 5 and was significantly below the score of the matched controls. Also using matched controls, Murphy et al. (1990) found that, while almost all the children tested reached a normal range of intelligence, those in whom the hypothyroidism was initially most severe did less well than those with a more mild form of the condition. These authors suggest that it is the initial distinction between mild and severe hypothyroidism which explains the apparently conflicting results already noted.

THYROID-INDUCED MANIA

Patients with symptomatic hypothyroidism (which may include either primary or secondary forms of the condition) usually require treatment with thyroxin. The incidence of psychosis in association with such replacement therapy was first noted by Zeigler in 1931, and has been repeatedly observed (Josephson & Mackenzie, 1979; Easson, 1966; Browning, Atkins & Weiner, 1954; Means, 1948). It is suggested that when thyroid replacement is complicated in this way, a characteristic clinical picture unfolds. This is referred to as the PFI. It is characterized by a psychosis lasting one to two weeks which resolves without sequelae irrespective of therapeutic intervention, and seems to be distinct from the psychological changes associated with hypothyroidism (Josephson & Mackenzie, 1980). The syndrome is uncommon, but in practice may often be dismissed as a continuation of the general hypothyroid condition and consequently be under-reported. There appears to be scant clinical awareness of the psychosocial impact of the symptomatology already described. In the context both of hyper- and hypothyroidism, little or no research has addressed the psychological consequences of having been labelled erroneously with a psychiatric condition.

REFERENCES

Asher, R. (1949). Myxoedema madness. *British Medical Journal*, ii, 555–62.

Bahemuka, M. & Hodkinson, H.M. (1975). Screening for hyperthyroidism in elderly in-patients. *British Medical Journal*, ii, 601–03.

Barnes, N.D. (1985). Screening for congenital hypothyroidism : the first decade. *Archive of Disease in Childhood*, 60, 587–92.

Bergner, M., Bobbitt, R.A. & Kressel, S. (1976). The sickness impact profile: Conceptual formulation and methodology for the development of a health status measure. *International Health Services*, 3, 393–415.

Browning, T.S., Atkins, R.W. & Weiner, H. (1954). Cerebral metabolic disturbances in hypothyroidism. *Archive Internal Medicine*, 93, 938–50.

Carney, W.P., Macleod S & Sheffield, B.F. (1981). Thyroid function screening in psychiatric in-patients. *British Journal of Psychiatry*, 138, 154–6.

Easson W.M. (1966). Myxedoema with psychosis. *Archive of General Psychiatry*, 14, 277–83.

Glorieux, J, Dussault, J.H., Morisette, J. *et al.* (1985). Follow-up at ages 5 years on mental development in children with hypothyroidism detected by Quebec screening program. *Journal of Pediatrics*, 107, 913–15.

Gull, W.W. (1873). On a cretinoid state supervening in the adult life of women. *Transactions of the Clinical Society London*, 7, 180.

Henderson & Gillespie (1962). *Textbook of Psychiatry*, p. 189. London: Oxford University Press.

Hermann, H.T. & Quarton, G. (1965). Psychological changes and psychogenesis in thyroid hormone disorder. *Journal of Clinical Endocrinology*, 20, 327.

Heyerdahl, S., Kase, B.F. & Lie, S.O. (1991). Intellectual development in children with congenital hypothyroidism in relation to recommended thyroxine treatment. *Journal of Pediatrics*, 118, 850–70.

Josephson, A.M. & Mackenzie, T.B. (1979). Appearance of manic psychosis following rapid normalisation of thyroid status. *American Journal of Psychiatry*, 136, 846–7.

Josephson, A.M. & Mackenzie, T.B. (1980). Thyroid induced mania in hypothyroid patients. *British Journal of Psychiatry*, 137, 222–8

Macfaul, R, Dorner, S, Brett, E.M. & Grant, D.B. (1978). Neurological abnormalities in patients treated for hypothyroidism from early life. *Archive of Disease in Childhood*, 53, 611–19.

McGregor, A.M. (1996). The thyroid gland and disorders of thyroid function. In Weatherall, D.J., Ledingham, J.G. & Warrell D.A. (Eds.). *Oxford textbook of medicine*, 2, Sections 11–17.

Means, J.H. (1948). *Thyroid and its diseases*. Philadelphia, Lippincott.

Murphy, G.H., Hulse J.A., Smith, I. & Grant, D.B. (1990). Congenital hypothyroidism: physiological and psychological factors in early development. *Journal of Psychology and Psychiatry*, 31, 711–25.

Nicholson, G., Liebling, L.I. & Hall, R.A. (1976). Thyroid dysfunction in female psychiatric patients. *British Journal of Psychology*, 129, 236–8.

Rockey, P.H. & Griep, M.D. (1981). Behavioural disfunction in hyperthyroidism: Improvement with treatment. *Archive Internal Medicine*, 140, 1194–7.

Rovet, J. Ehrlich, R. & Sorboda, D. (1987). Intellectual outcome in children with fetal hypothyroidism. *Journal of Pediatrics*, 110, 700–4.

Simons, W.F., Fuggle, P.W. Grant, D.B. & Smith, I. (1994). Intellectual development at 10 years in early treated congenital hypothyroidism. *Archive of Disease in Childhood*, 71, 232–4.

Stewart, T., Rochon, J., Lenfesty, R. & Wise, P. (1985). Correlation of stress with outcome of radioiodine therapy for Graves' disease. *Journal of Nuclear Medicine*, 26, 592–9.

Tonks, C.M. (1964). Mental illness in hypothyroid patients. *British Journal of Psychology*, 110, 706–10.

Trzepacz, P.T., McCue, M. Klein, I. & Greenhouse, J. (1988). Psychiatric and neuropsychological response to propranolol in Graves disease. *Biological Psychiatry*, 23, 678–88.

Werner S.C. (1966). Hyperthyroidism: introduction. In *The thyroid*, 4th edn. 115, 353–366.

Zeigler, L.H. (1931). Psychosis associated with myxoedema. *Journal of Neurology and Psychopathology*, 11, 20–7.

Hyperventilation

DAVID K.B. NIAS

Department of Psychological Medicine,
St Bartholomew's Hospital Medical College,
London EC1A 7BE, UK

The definition of hyperventilation is simply 'breathing in excess of metabolic requirements', but the interesting issue concerns the clinical significance of the somatic and psychological changes it can produce. It also helps to distinguish between acute or transient overbreathing and chronic or persistent hyperventilation. While acute overbreathing can obviously occur as a consequence of distress, chronic hyperventilation has been controversially considered as a syndrome and as a causal agent in the development of somatic and psychological disorders.

Acute overbreathing can occur as part of the classic 'fight or flight' response, in which the body involuntarily prepares for action. Such breathing soon removes sufficient carbon dioxide from the lungs to lead to a measurable fall in the blood level of carbon dioxide (a state known as hypocapnia) and a loss of carbonic acid for which the body compensates leading to buffer depletion. This sets in train a number of somatic sensations which increase emotional arousal, so acting as a further stimulus to overbreathing; indeed, one of the paradoxical characteristics of hypocapnia is lack of awareness of breathlessness. The resulting chain reaction or 'vicious circle' has been seen as a mechanism by which persistent hyperventilation might lead to illness (Timmons & Ley, 1994).

Coupled with anxiety, arousal and somatic sensations, the features of hyperventilation take many forms. Respiratory signs such as rapid breathing are likely to be noted in acute rather than chronic conditions. Neurovascular signs include dizziness and headache; cardiovascular signs include palpitations and chest pain; gastrointestinal signs include nausea and dry throat; and musculoskeletal signs include aches and pains. Psychological signs include anxiety or anger and in chronic conditions, sleep loss and fatigue (Freeman & Nixon, 1985).

The dramatic effects of acute overbreathing were demonstrated to the Physiological Society in 1908, when it was reported that 'even observers became distressed'. Clinical accounts and proposed treatments appeared last century and links were made with 'effort syndrome' and exhaustion during World War I (Lewis, 1954). In the 1960s, interest in treatment was revived and reported by Lum (1976). Hyperventilation has been associated with panic disorder, in particular, and with many so-called psychosomatic conditions such as hypochondriasis, somatization disorder, and chronic fatigue syndrome. Estimates of its prevalence have varied enormously, but its status as a syndrome has been controversial and referred to as a 'grey area' (Nixon, 1993).

A widely publicized account of an overbreathing epidemic was reported by Moss and McEvedy (1966). Following a three-hour school parade in which some girls had actually fainted, many complained the next day of 'feeling dizzy and peculiar'. By the afternoon, 85 girls had been taken to hospital and the school closed; a similar pattern occurred as soon as the school was reopened. Physical examinations at the hospital were essentially negative, and detective work at the school ruled out food-poisoning and leaking gas. Because of altered sensations in the limbs (e.g. pins and needles), conversion hysteria was considered before it was concluded that hyperventilation was to blame.

Acute overbreathing, as may occur in a panic attack, is usually obvious from rapid breathing accompanied by the symptoms of hypocapnia. Chronic hyperventilation, as may occur with continuing effort and distress, is much harder to diagnose. It is usually unobtrusive, becoming clinically apparent only because of loss of performance and inability to sustain effort. Because of their various somatic complaints, patients may seek advice from many different medical specialists before tests are carried out for anxiety and hyperventilation. Presented with a list of the symptoms of hypocapnia, some patients are claimed to recognize them as applying only too well.

Because of buffer depletion, chronic hyperventilators find it difficult to hold their breath and so an obvious test is 'breath holding time'. Another is the 'voluntary hyperventilation test' in which patients are asked to overbreathe and then to rate any symptoms experienced (Lum, 1976). At the same time, levels of blood carbon dioxide can be measured by the non-invasive technique of a rapid infrared carbon dioxide analyser. A variation is the 'imagery' or 'think' test in which patients are asked to recall episodes of emotional arousal (e.g. anger) while testing for hypocapnia. Similarly, an exercise test in the form of a cycle ergometer is used to test how soon hypocapnia develops following leg ache.

It is reported that hyperventilation tests, whether conducted at rest or in response to provocation, give unreliable results (Lindsay, Saqi & Bass, 1991). The latest research has involved a double-blind trial of the 'hyperventilation provocation test' (Hornsveld *et al.*, 1996). Patients with suspected hyperventilation syndrome tended to recognize their symptoms during both this test and a placebo condition in which carbon dioxide levels were maintained by manual titration. A subgroup of patients also underwent ambulatory monitoring, and were found to overbreathe after rather than before spontaneous symptom attacks. These findings cast doubt on the validity of hyperventilation as a syndrome and suggest that it should be regarded as a consequence rather than a cause of anxiety and related disorders.

Treatment programmes have been designed to reduce overbreathing in the hope that this would ameliorate associated symptoms. One of the simplest treatments is for patients to rebreathe the air they have just breathed out from a paper bag, so restoring their blood level of carbon dioxide. Another is for patients to experience how symptoms can be created by deliberately overbreathing, and then encouraging them to reattribute the cause of these symptoms using a cognitive therapy approach (Clark, Salkovskis & Chalkley, 1985). Slow, diaphragmatic breathing exercises are then taught, usually in combination with relaxation exercises and *in vivo* expo-

sure to the circumstances that lead to overbreathing. Although promising results have been reported for panic disorder, controlled trials have indicated little more than a placebo effect (Garssen, de Ruiter & van Dyck, 1992). This is consistent with regarding hyperventilation not as a syndrome, but as another symptom of an underlying disorder. Consistent with this interpretation, treatment should be aimed at the underlying disorder before attempting to restore natural breathing patterns.

REFERENCES

Clark, D.M., Salkovskis, P.M. & Chalkley, A.J. (1985) Respiratory control as a treatment for panic attacks. *Journal of Behavior Therapy and Experimental Psychiatry*, **16**, 23–30.

Freeman, L.J. & Nixon, P.G.F. (1985) Chest pain and the hyperventilation syndrome: some etiological considerations. *Postgraduate Medical Journal*, **61**, 957–61.

Garssen, B., de Ruiter, C. & van Dyck, R. (1992). Breathing retraining: a rational placebo? *Clinical Psychology Review*, **12**, 141–53.

Hornsveld, H.K., Garssen, B., Fiedeldij

Dop, M.J.C., van Spiegel, P.I. & de Haes, J.C.J. (1996) Double-blind placebo-controlled study of the hyperventilation provocation test and the validity of the hyperventilation syndrome. *Lancet*, **348**, 154–8.

Lewis, B.I. (1954) Chronic hyperventilation syndrome. *Journal of the American Medical Association*, **155**, 1204–8.

Lindsay, S.J.E., Saqi, S. & Bass, C. (1991) The test–retest reliability of the hyperventilation provocation test. *Journal of Psychosomatic Research*, **35**, 155–162.

Lum, L.C. (1976) The syndrome of habitual

chronic hyperventilation. *Recent Advances in Psychosomatic Medicine*, 3, 196–230.

Moss, P.D. & McEvedy, C.P. (1966) An epidemic of overbreathing among schoolgirls. *British Medical Journal*, **2**, 1295–300.

Nixon, P.G.F. (1993) The grey area of effort syndrome and hyperventilation: from Thomas Lewis to today. *Journal of the Royal College of Physicians of London*, **27**, 377–83.

Timmons, B.H. and Ley, R. (Eds.). (1994) *Behavioural and psychological approaches to breathing disorders* New York: Plenum.

Hypochondriasis

LUCY RINK

and

ROBERT WEST

Psychology Department, St George's Hospital Medical School, London, UK

Hypochondriasis is a disorder characterized by a misinterpretation of physical signs that lead to the belief of having a serious disease even though repeated evaluation can elicit no indications of physical disorder.

Patients with this condition have an excessive preoccupation with the maintenance of health, a distorted perception of minor symptoms elevating them to the status of a major disease and a history of frequent medical consultations (Tyrer *et al.*, 1990). Even though they seek more medical advice than others, they also tend to distrust the physicians' judgements more (Kellner *et al.*, 1987). Hypochondriacs often have an excessive need for control, and low tolerance of uncertainty and ambiguity (Starcevic, 1990). Fear of ageing and death, greater sense of bodily vulnerability to illness and injury and the importance placed on physical appearance are also believed to play an important role in the lives of hypochondriacs (Barsky & Wyshak, 1989). Hypochondriasis also tends to be related to high levels of anxiety, depression and paranoid thinking (Gouveia *et al.*, 1986; Kellner, Abbott, Winslow & Pathak, 1987). There is also a tendency to believe that good health is symptom free, which is obviously unrealistic (Barsky *et al.*, 1993). It has been argued that

hypochondriasis is similar to panic disorder in terms of the tendency to misinterpret bodily changes as indications of catastrophic harm (Salkovskis & Clark, 1993).

It is not clear what causes hypochondriasis but there are probably several mechanisms involved. Loneliness may be one factor (Brink & Niemeyer, 1993). Worry about health may reflect a deepset personality trait and is often associated with chronic generalized anxiety and depression (Barsky, Wyshak & Klerman, 1992; Tyrer, Casey & Seivewright, 1986), and 'histrionic' personality (Starcevic *et al.*, 1992). Some evidence suggests, not unsurprisingly, that worry about health increases with age (Shimonaka, 1984) but research has failed to find an association between age and hypochondriasis (Barksy *et al.*, 1991). A study carried out by Forman and Gropper (1987) has suggested that organic brain deficits among the elderly may be linked to hypochondriacal complaints. Hypochondriasis is also sometimes observed following bereavement (Brink, 1985) and assault (Streit-Forest & Goulet, 1987).

The diagnosis of hypochondriasis obviously requires first of all ruling out any organic illness through medical examination and then taking a comprehensive psychiatric history of the patient (Fallon,

Klein & Liebowitz, 1993). Treatment may then involve general reassurance, attempting to challenge false beliefs, training patients in reinterpreting symptoms, and familiarization with disease states about which patients may have phobias, behaviour therapy and treatment for comorbid psychiatric disorders (Fallon *et al.*, 1993; Kellner, 1992; Noyes *et al.*, 1986; Visser & Bouman, 1992; Warwick, 1992).

REFERENCES

Barsky, A.J. & Wyshak, G. (1989). Hypochondriasis and related health attitudes. *Psychosomatics*, **30**, 412–20.

Barsky, A.J., Coeytaux, R.R., Sarnie, M.K. & Cleary, P.D. (1993). Hypochondriacal patient's belief about good health. *American Journal of Psychiatry*, **150**, 1085–9.

Barksy, A.J., Frank, C.B., Cleary, P.D., Wyshak, G. & Klerman, G.L. (1991). The relation between hypochondriasis and age. *American Journal for Psychiatry*, **148**, 923–8.

Barsky, A.J., Wyshak, G. & Klerman, G.L. (1992). Psychiatric co-morbidity in DSM IIIR hypochondriasis. *Archives of General Psychiatry*, **49**, 101–8.

Brink, T.L. (1985). The grieving patient in later life. *Psychotherapy Patient*, **2**, 117–27.

Brink, T.L. & Niemeyer, L (1993). Hypochondriasis, loneliness, and social functioning. *Psychological Reports*, **72**, 1241–2.

Fallon, B.A., Klein, B.W. & Liebowitz, M.R. (1993). Hypochondriasis: treatment strategies. *Psychiatrica Annals*, **23**, 374–81.

Forman, B.D. & Gropper, R.L. (1987). Hypochondriasis and organic brain syndrome in non-institutionalized elderly. *Clinical Gerontologist*, **6**, 56–8.

Hyer, L., Gouveia, I., Harrison, W.R., Warsaw, J. & Coutsouridis, D. (1987). Depression anxiety paranoid reactions hypochondriasis and cognitive decline in later life. *Patients Journal of Gerontology*, **42**, 92–4.

Kellner, R. (1992). The case for reassurance. *International Review of Psychiatry*, **4**, 71–5.

Kellner, R., Abbott, P., Winslow, W.W. & Pathak D. (1987). Fears, beliefs, and attitudes in DSM-III hypochondriasis. *Journal of Nervous and Mental Disease*, **175**, 20–5.

Noyes, R., Reich, J., Clancy, J. & O'Gorman, T.W. (1986) reduction in hypochondriasis with treatment of panic disorder. *British Journal of Psychiatry*, **149**, 631–5.

Salkovskis, P.M. & Clark, D.M. (1993) Panic disorder and hypochondriasis. *Advances in Behavior Research and Therapy*, **15**, 23–48.

Shimonaka, Y. (1984). Aging and personality. *Japanese Psychological Review*, **27**, 260–71.

Starcevic, V. (1990). Relationship between hypochondriasis and obsessive–compulsive personality disorder: close relatives separated by nosological schemes?

American Journal of Psychotherapy, **44**, 340–7.

Starcevic, V., Kellner, R., Uhlenhuth, E.H. & Pathak, D. (1992). Panic disorder and hypochondriacal fears and beliefs. *Journal of Affective Disorders*, **24**, 73–85.

Streit-Forest, U. & Goulet, M. (1987). The effects of assault six months after the attack and the factors associated with readjustment. *Canadian Journal of Psychiatry*, **32**, 43–56.

Tyrer, P., Casey, P.R. & Seivewright, N. (1986). Common personality features in neurotic disorder. *British Journal of Medical Psychology*, **59**, 289–94.

Tyrer, P., Fowler, D.R., Ferguson, B. & Kelemen, A. (1990). A plea for the diagnosis of hypochondriacal personality disorder. *Journal of Psychosomatic Research*, **34**, 637–42.

Visser, S. & Bouman, T.K. (1992). Cognitive–behavioural approaches in the treatment of hypochondriasis: six single case cross-over studies. *Behaviour Research and Therapy*, **30**, 301–6.

Warwick, H. (1992). Provision of appropriate and effective reassurance. *International Review of Psychiatry*, **4**, 76–80.

Hysterectomy

MYRA S. HUNTER

Unit of Psychology, UMDS Guy's Medical School, London, UK

Hysterectomy, surgical removal of the womb, is one of the most commonly performed operations in gynaecology. Community surveys indicate prevalence rates varying between 13 and 8% in the UK and France, respectively, to 17% in Australia and USA (Schofield *et al.*, 1991; van Keep, Wildermeersch & Lehert, 1983). The main indications for hysterectomy are abnormal menstrual bleeding, followed by fibroids and malignant disease.

Reports on the extent of psychological impact of hysterectomy have varied. The operation has been associated with sexual, emotional and physical problems and earlier retrospective studies reinforced these beliefs. More recent prospective studies, on the other hand, have found a decrease or little change in psychiatric disorder, mainly neurotic depression, and general improvements in mood following hysterectomy performed for menorrhagia (Gath, Cooper & Day, 1982). Preoperative emotional state was the best predictor of emotional problems after the operation. Similar findings emerge from studies of sexual functioning, with regard to pre and postoperative sexual functioning (Helstrom *et al.*, 1993).

Psychologists have examined knowledge, expectations and beliefs about hysterectomy, and the effects of psychologically preparing women for the operation. Misconceptions and fears about the operation and its sequelae abound, for example, whether the ovaries are also to be removed (an operation which precipitates the onset of menopause). Many women accept their doctor's opinion without a clear understanding of the reason, the alternatives available or the likely course after the hysterectomy. Fears about the impact of the operation upon sexual relationships and self-concept are common (Tsoi, Poon & Ho, 1983). In one study, negative expectations predicted poor outcome in relation to sexual problems (Dennerstein, Wood & Burrows, 1977). This work highlights the need for information and discussion before the decision to have the operation is made, especially as a proportion of women with heavy menstrual bleeding have only moderate blood loss but report high levels of psychological distress (Greenberg, 1983). The possible role of psychological interventions for some of these women could usefully be examined.

Preparatory information has tended to be provided preoperatively, on admission to hospital, with the aim of decreasing pre-and postoperative anxiety and facilitating post operative recovery. In one of the major studies, Ridgeway and Matthews (1982) compared procedural information with a booklet concentrating on cognitive coping given to women undergoing elective hysterectomy. They found that these preparations produced differential effects. Information about surgery increased knowledge and satisfaction ratings, while cognitive coping had most effect on indices of recovery, i.e. fewer analgesics and less pain. Women in the cognitive coping group also reported fewer worrying thoughts post operatively. A group format might be an efficient way of applying these results to a clinical setting. (See 'Dental Care and Hygiene' for more applications of this form of intervention.)

REFERENCES

Dennerstein, L., Wood, C. & Burrows, G.D. (1977). Sexual response following hysterectomy and oophorectomy. *Obstetrics and Gynaecology*, **49**, 92–6.

Gath, D., Cooper, P. & Day, A. (1982). Hysterectomy and psychiatric disorder. *British Journal of Psychiatry*, **140**, 335–42.

Greenberg, M. (1983). The meaning of menorrhagia: and investigation into the association between complaint of menorrhagia and depression. *Journal of Psychosomatic Research*, **27**, 209–14.

Helstrom, L., Lundberg, M.D., Sorbom, D. & Backstrom, M.D. (1993). Sexuality after hysterectomy: a factor analysis of women's sexual lives before and after subtotal hysterectomy. *Obstetrics and Gynaecology*, **81**, 357–62.

Ridgeway, V. & Matthews, A. (1982). Psychological preparation for surgery. A comparison of methods. *British Journal of Clinical Psychology*, **21**, 271–80.

Schofield, M.J., Hennrikus, D., Redman, S., Walters, W.A.W. & Sanson-Fisher, R.W. (1991). Prevalence and characteristics of women who have had a hysterectomy in a community survey. *Australian and New Zealand Journal of Obstetrics and Gynaecology*, **31**, 153–7.

Tsoi, M.M., Poon, R.S.M. & Ho, P.C. (1983). Knowledge of reproductive organs in Chinese women. *Journal of Psychomatic Obstetrics and Gynaecology*, **2**, 70–5.

Van Keep, P.A., Wildermeersch, D. & Lehert, P. (1983). Hysterectomy in six European countries. *Maturitas*, **5**, 69–77.

Iatrogenesis

PETER SLADE

Department of Clinical Psychology, School of Health Sciences, Faculty of Medicine, The University of Liverpool, UK

INTRODUCTION

The first dictum of medicine (and that of other health-care professions) is 'to do no harm' (Hippocrates). Iatrogenesis refers to the failure of doctors and other health-care professionals to satisfy this dictum, such that 'iatrogenic disorders' are those which are caused either by the implementation of medical and other treatments or by the failure to implement such treatment. Thus, iatrogenesis is caused both by errors of 'commission' and errors of 'omission'.

Iatrogenesis is a widespread fact of medical and health-care practice: one which is either openly acknowledged and discussed, or alternatively is partially disguised through the use of terms such as 'medical complications' or 'adverse drug reactions'. An example of the former is a fairly recent publication from a group of Russian Pathologists (Glumov, Gabushev & Shumikhin, 1990) who reported on the apparent level of Iatrogenesis in a sample of 2250 autopsies they carried out. They concluded that medical treatments were an immediate cause of death in 14.2% of these patients. Of these deaths, the primary cause appeared to be surgical in 70.8%, pharmacological in 18.5% and neurosurgical in 10.7% of cases. This level of fatal iatrogenesis seems high compared with what is admitted to in the west and may be influenced by the political context at the time. On the other hand, it may represent the generally true level.

Adverse drug reactions are common but not usually life threatening. Moderate reactions are found in up to 36% of hospitalized patients (D'Arcy, 1986), while the prevalence of drug-related deaths in western countries is approximately 1% (Porter & Jick, 1977). Thus, when drugs are used appropriately, adverse reactions are best viewed as problematic rather than lethal.

A good example of iatrogenic drug effects is provided by the benzodiazepines. These were introduced in the 1960s and early 1970s as non harmful minor tranquillizers and sedatives. In the 1980s it was recognized that these drugs, when used on a long-term basis, were not only ineffective but also habit forming. This has led to concerted attempts to withdraw patients from dependence on benzodiazepines, usually by training them in alternative (psychological) methods for controlling their anxiety or getting to sleep (Cormack, Owens & Dewey, 1989).

IATROGENIC DISEASE/DISORDER IN THE ELDERLY

It is generally recognized that the highest level of iatrogenic disease/disorder is to be found in the elderly. For example, in a study of 185 hospitalized patients over 75 years of age, 38% developed hospital-acquired complications (Becker *et al.*, 1987). Similarly, in another report on elderly patients admitted to hospital, 193 (39%) of 500 patients were found to suffer from iatrogenic disorders (Reichel, 1965). And, in a study specifically designed to compare the level of iatrogenic disease/disorder in the over 65s with that in the under 65s, 45% of the older group were found to have iatrogenic disease compared with only 29% of the younger group (Jahnigen, Hannon & Laxson, 1982). Thus, the most vulnerable group in society seem to be the most susceptible to Iatrogenic diseases/disorders.

A special issue of the *Journal of Gerontological Nursing*, 1991, was expressly devoted to the five, most commonly reported problems, namely: immobilization (Mobily & Kelley, 1991), adverse drug reactions (Stolley, Buckwalter & Fjordbak (1991), falls (Ross, 1991), pressure ulcers (Kelley & Mobily, 1991) and nosocomial infections (Stolley & Buckwalter, 1991). The general editors point out, however, that these problems are not independent but often interactive; such that, adverse drug reactions can cause an increase in falls, resulting in immobilization. Immobilization, in turn, may cause an increase in infection rates, especially in the respiratory and urinary tracts. This chapter will concentrate on just one of the above, namely immobilization.

The problem of immobilization (Mobily & Kelley, 1991) provides a good example of iatrogenesis due to errors of 'omission'. Bed rest is frequently prescribed for elderly persons but, if complete and protracted, produces physical and other problems. The reason for this is that muscular strength is maintained by frequent maximum tension contractions. Of muscle strength 10–15% can be lost each week that muscles are resting completely, and as much as 5.5% can be lost each day of rest and immobility. And, as muscle strength decreases, there is a concomitant decrease in endurance. The muscles most affected by immobilization are the antigravity muscles that facilitate locomotion and help maintain an upright position. These include the quadriceps, glutei, erector spinae and gastrocnemius-soleus muscles. When normal weight-bearing and movement is diminished, 'disuse osteoporosis' occurs. Bone loss increases rapidly from the third day to the third week of immobilization and peaks during the fifth or sixth week. Elderly people are especially vulnerable to the iatrogenic effects of immobilization because the consequent bone loss is compounded by bone loss resulting from age-related osteoporosis.

NOSOCOMIAL INFECTIONS

The problem of nosocomial infections is a general one, affecting all hospital patients, but particularly the elderly. It represents another example of Iatrogenesis due to errors of 'omission'.

Of every 100 patients admitted to a hospital in the western world, 5–10% will acquire an infection other than the one for which they were admitted. These hospital-acquired infections are referred to as nosocomial infections, a term not generally understood by the general public. While nosocomial infections can be acquired in a number of different ways, the most common cause is the failure of doctors and nurses to wash their hands correctly in-between their examination/contact with successive patients. Thus, nosocomial infections are usually passed on from patient to patient by the health-care professionals who have been given primary responsibility for their care. Concerted attempts to correct this situation have usually failed (Bartzokas, Williams & Slade, 1994).

PSYCHOLOGICALLY INDUCED IATROGENESIS

Psychological treatments or aspects of psychological management of patients can produce iatrogenic effects as well as physical treatments. A specific example of this is seen in relation to multiple personality disorder. A recent psychiatric review article of cases of 'multiple personality disorder' in North America (Merskey, 1992) has proposed that these are fundamentally iatrogenic disorders, caused by the use of hypnotic suggestion procedures with highly vulnerable and suggestible individuals. The writer's thesis is clearly plausible but requires further corroboration.

A much more commonly observed and widespread phenomenon is that of 'illness concern/disease conviction' stemming from the application of general and specialist medical practice (Mechanic, 1974). A good example of the latter is provided by patients with chronic low back pain. Usually, because they have no clearly demonstrable organic pathology, they are subjected to endless physical tests and referred to a countless and varied group of specialists. Behavioural scientists see the effect of all this medical activity as 'reinforcing' the patient's concern about their physical health; moreover, along the way, most chronic low back patients acquire a set of beliefs about their back problem which militates against their working with physicians to rehabilitate themselves (Rose *et al.*, 1993). Thus, chronic low back pain is an example of an acute medical problem, which is converted into a chronic one, by the nature of its medical management.

CONCLUDING STATEMENT

Iatrogenesis refers to the creation of physical and mental problems through the implementation, or failure to implement, appropriate treatments by medical, psychiatric and other health-care professionals. But, as our medical knowledge and services expand, so paradoxically do the possibilities for Iatrogenical disorders. Hence, the first dictum of medical practice, 'to do no harm', is unlikely to be an obtainable reality in the future. Perhaps the 'Hippocratic principle' should be modified, in order to reflect reality, to 'always seek to do more good than harm'!

REFERENCES

Bartzokas, C.A., Williams, E & Slade, P.D. (1994). Hospital-acquired infections: a psychological approach. New York: Edwin Mellen Press.

Becker, P.M., McVey, L.J., Saltz, C.C., Feusser, J.R. & Cohen, H.J. (1987). Hospital-acquired complications in a randomized controlled clinical trial of a geriatric consultation *Journal of the American Medical Association*, **257**, 2313–17.

Cormack, M.A., Owens, R.G. and & Dewey, M.E. (1989). Reducing benzodiazepine consumption New York: Springer Verlag.

D'Arcy, P.F. (1986) Epidemiological aspects of iatrogenic disease. In D'Arcy and Griffin (Eds.). *Iatrogenic diseases*. Oxford: Oxford University Press.

Glumov, V.I., Gabushev, P.I. & Shumikhin, K.V. (1990). Iatrogenic pathology, its role in the structure of patient morbidity and thanatogenesis. Arkh IV – Patologii, **52**, 72–4.

Hippocrates The Hippocratic Oath.

Jahnigen, D., Hannon, C. & Laxson, L. (1982). Iatrogenic disease in hospitalized elderly veterans. *Journal of the American Geriatric Society*, **30**, 387–90.

Kelley, L.S & Mobily, P.R. (1991). Iatrogenesis in the elderly – impaired skin integrity. *Journal of Gerontological Nursing*, **17**, 24–9.

Mechanic, D. (1974). *Politics, medicine and social science*. New York: John Wiley.

Merskey, H. (1992). The manufacture of personalities. The production of multiple personality disorder. *British Journal of Psychiatry*, **160**, 327–40.

Mobily, P.R. & Kelley, L.S. (1991). Iatrogenesis in the elderly – factors of Immobility. *Journal of Gerontological Nursing*, **17**, 5–10.

Porter, J. & Jick, H. (1977). Drug related deaths among medical inpatients. *Journal of the American Medical Association*, **237**, 879–81.

Reichel, W. (1965). Complications in the care of five hundred elderly hospitalized patients. *Journal of the American Geriatric Society*, **13**, 973–81.

Rose, M., Reilly, J., Pennie, B & Slade, P.D. (1993). Chronic low back pain: a consequence of misinformation? *Employee Counselling Today*, **5**, 12–15.

Ross, J.E.R. (1991). Iatrogenesis in the elderly – contributions to falls. *Journal of Gerontological Nursing*, **17**, 19–23.

Stolley, J.M. & Buckwalter, K.C. (1991). Iatrogenesis in the elderly – nosocomial infections. *Journal of Gerontological Nursing*, **17**, 30–4.

Stolley, J.M., Buckwalter, K.C. & Fjordbak, B. (1991). Iatrogenesis in the elderly – Drug-related problems. *Journal of Gerontological Nursing*, **17**, 12–17.

Immunization

NATALIE TIMBERLAKE

Academic Department of Psychiatry, Middlesex and UCL, London, UK

Immunization is one of the most important weapons in the fight against disease. It does not just protect the individual but, if enough people are immunized, there will be so few susceptible individuals in the community that the disease will not become established. In many diseases, this has not been achieved because there is still a percentage of the population who are able to be vaccinated but choose not to. Governments do not generally make vaccinations compulsory, instead, they try and educate people into accepting their value. However, the relationship between information, knowledge and behaviour, in this case vaccination, is not straightforward. The impact of information on people is influenced by a number of factors, e.g. how much and from where the information comes and the content of the information. New and Senior (1991) have reported that those parents who fully vaccinated their children received more information from health professionals than non-vaccinators but received less information from family and friends. They found that the advice full immunizers received from family and friends was more likely to be provaccination. Non-immunizers were more likely to receive provaccination advice from professional sources than partial and full immunizers. These findings suggest that the information offered by health professionals does not always have a great effect on immunization behaviour. Parental attitudes to vaccination would seem to be affected not by the amount of information they receive but from where the information comes.

The health belief model postulates that the likelihood of a behaviour being undertaken is a function of an individual's perception of the costs and benefits of the action and the cues to action. There are many different levels to this model. At a fundamental level, there is the perceived need to be vaccinated. This is related to the perceived severity and threat of a disease. Many diseases vaccinated against are considered fairly rare so the chances of catching them are thought to be minimal, e.g. tuberculosis, polio and whooping cough (Harding & O'Looney, 1984), some are considered to be relatively harmless, e.g rubella, influenza and whooping cough (Harding & O'Looney, 1984) and may even be considered a natural part of childhood conferring some benefit, such as building up resistance or increasing parent–child bonding (Haurum & Johansen, 1991; Ronne, Kaaber & Petersen, 1989). Leventhal, Singer and Jones, 1965 demonstrated that increasing the fear of a disease improves the attitude towards its vaccination. Subjects given fearful information about tetanus felt that getting a tetanus vaccination was more important and expressed greater intentions of doing so, than subjects given less fearful information.

In contrast, the perceived risks from vaccinating often exceed actual risk. One reason for this may be the tendency of the press to highlight the major side-effects from vaccines, in articles giving limited amounts of information (Harding, 1985). Appleton, 1989 report that 57% of parents who did not vaccinate their child against

Immunization

pertussis were doing so due to the adverse media reports at that time. Parental refusal is also often based on dubious contraindications or conflicting advice reported to have been ascribed by health-care professionals (Klein, Morgan & Wansbrough-Jones, 1989, Hewitt, 1989; Appleton, 1989). The cumulative effect of these factors result in the perceived benefits from vaccination to seem small compared to the perceived costs. This has been demonstrated by Bennett and Smith, 1992 who found that those parents who did not have their children vaccinated expressed more concern over side-effects due to the vaccination and saw there being less chance of the unvaccinated child contracting the disease. The vaccination was also seen as being less efficacious, with these parents expressing an increased probability of the vaccinated child still contracting the disease. Similarly, Stevens and Baker, 1989 found that parents who had not vaccinated their children against whooping cough were more anxious about the side-effects of the vaccine and less convinced about its efficacy than vaccinating parents.

Sociodemographic factors have been found to play a major role in cost – benefit analysis. A factor which is frequently cited as predictive of non-immunization is having other children (Bobo et al., 1993; Li & Taylor, 1993; Pearson et al., 1993a,b). This factor would seem to act as a barrier to immunization and there has been speculation as to how this occurs. New and Senior, 1991 found that parents who cite problems from having other young children to look after, were more frequently incomplete immunizers than complete immunizers. They suggest that having other children may restrict the ability to get to the clinic. Bennett and Smith, 1992 asked parents, who had at some point delayed or not vaccinated their children, what factors were important in this decision. 16% cited problems with getting a convenient appointment and 8% problems with getting to the surgery or clinic. However, Pearson et al., 1993a suggest that this factor may, in fact, relate to parental experience with other children, causing their views on vaccination to change. For example, previous children who had been immunised may have reacted badly to the vaccine and so the perceived dangers from vaccinating may have increased; a previous child who was not vaccinated against a disease may have not caught or only very mildly had the disease, so that the perceived benefits from vaccinating may have

diminished. Therefore, although parents may have been initially provaccination, experience with their other children may have altered this.

Other, perhaps related sociodemographic factors predictive of low immunization rates, are single parent family status (Li & Taylor, 1993; Pearson et al., 1993a,b), lower parental education (Fielding et al., 1994; Bobo et al., 1993) and living in a deprived area (Pearson et al., 1993; Li & Taylor, 1993a,b). Li and Taylor, 1993 suggest that this last factor may reflect the make-up of the population in these areas, which tends to consist of more single mothers, parents with more children and less education.

A further influence on beliefs and behaviour has been highlighted by Ritov and Baron, 1990. They have reported on the effect of omission bias in decision-making. This is the tendency to prefer potentially harmful omissions over potentially less harmful commissions. Asch et al., 1994 cite this as leading 'to a systematic failure to achieve the best outcomes'. Using simulated situations and also looking at reported behaviour, Asch et al., 1994 have been able to show that omission bias is very important in immunization behaviour. They report that some parents preferred not to vaccinate their child even when vaccinating was more likely to lead to a better outcome. It would seem that the parents considered it worse for their child to be harmed (however small the chance) due to their action rather than due to their inaction. Asch et al., 1994 demonstrate that this is not simply due to ignorance of the actual potential risks from vaccination, in that omission bias is seen in scenarios where the information on potential risks is provided. This has relevance for the cost–benefit analysis of immunization, in that some psychological factors have greater importance than the probabilites of good clinical outcome. It would seem that the reasoning behind health decisions is not always as rational as might be first thought.

Processes behind parents' decisions to vaccinate their child are highly complex. In order to understand it, we need to take into account a number of factors, from the interactions of highly complex biases in thought processes through to the physical limitations of getting to the clinic. (See also 'Rubella' and 'Tetanus' chapter for focus on immunization for a particular illness.)

REFERENCES

Appleton, R. (1989). Parents' beliefs about vaccination. British Medical Journal, 257.

Asch, D., Baron, J., Hershey, J., Kunreuther, H., Meszaros, J., Ritov, I. & Spranca, M. (1994). Omission bias and pertussis Vaccination. Medical Decision Making, 14, 118–23.

Bennett, P. & Smith, C. (1992). Parents' attitudinal and social influences on childhood vaccination. Health Education Research, 7, 341–8.

Bobo, J., Gale, J., Thapa, P. & Wassilak, S. (1993). Risk factors for delayed immunization in a random sample of 1163 children from Oregon and Washington. Pediatrics, 91, 308–13.

Fielding, J., Cumberland, W. & Pettitt, L. (1994). Immunization status of children of employees in a large corporation. Journal of

the American Medical Association, 271, 525–30.

Harding, C. (1985). Immunization as depicted by the British national press. Community Medicine, 7, 87–98.

Harding, C. & O'Looney, B. (1984). Perceptions and beliefs about nine diseases. Public Health, 98, 284–93.

Haurum, J. & Johansen, M. (1991). Attitudes and knowledge among parents who do not want their children to be vaccinated against measles, mumps and rubella (MFR-vaccination). Ugeskr-Laeger, 153, 705–9.

Hewitt, M. (1989) Incidence of contraindications to immunisation. Archive of Disease in Childhood, 64, 1052–64.

Klein, N., Morgan, K. & Wansbrough-Jones, M. (1989). Parents'

beliefs about vaccination: the continuing propagation of false contraindications. British Medical Journal, 298, 1687.

Leventhal, H., Singer, R. & Jones, S. (1965). Effects of fear and specificity of recommendation upon attitudes and behaviour. Journal of Personality and Social Psychology, 2, 20–9.

Li, J. & Taylor, B. (1993). Factors affecting uptake of measles, mumps and rubella immunisation. British Medical Journal, 307, 168–71.

New, S. & Senior, M. (1991). 'I Don't Believe in Needless': qualitative aspects of a study into the uptake of infant immunisation in two English health authorities. Social Science of Medicine, 33, 509–18.

Pearson, M., Makowiecka, K., Gregg. J., Woollard, J., Rogers, M. & West, C.

(1993a). Primary immunisations in Liverpool. 1: who withholds consent? *Archive of Disease in Childhood*, **69**, 110–14.

Pearson, M., Makowiecka, K., Gregg. J., Woollard, J., Rogers, M. & West, C. (1993b). Primary immunisations in Liverpool. 2: is there a gap between consent and completion? *Archives of Disease in Childhood*, **69**, 115–19.

Ritov, I. & Baron, J. (1990). Reluctance to vaccinate: omission bias and ambiguity. *Journal of Behavioural Decision Making*, **3**, 263–77.

Ronne, T., Kaaber, K. & Petersen, I. (1989). Knowledge of, attitudes toward and participation in the new vaccinations against measles, mumps and rubella during the first 2 Years. *Ugeskrift for Laeger*, **151**, 2418–22.

Stevens, D. & Baker, R. (1989). Parents' beliefs about vaccination. *British Medical Journal*, **299**, 257.

Incontinence

SIOBHAN HART

Essex Rivers Health Care Trust
Essex County Hospital,
Colchester, UK

Incontinence, that is the inadvertent or uncontrolled voiding of urine or faeces or of both is a common problem that is not restricted to the extremes of the lifespan. Approximately half a million children suffer from incontinence, and the condition is more common in boys. At all other ages incontinence is more prevalent in women. Widely quoted UK figures put the prevalence of urinary incontinence in the general population at about 1.6% of men and 8.5% of women in the age range 15 to 64 while the corresponding figures for those over 65 years are 6.9% and 11.6% respectively (Thomas *et al.*, 1980). However, precise figures are difficult to obtain since many cases go unreported because of embarrassment (incontinence has been dubbed 'the last taboo') or because many believe that some degree of incontinence is a normal part of ageing or an inevitable consequence of childbirth. Predictably the incidence of urinary incontinence is much higher in institutionalized populations. It has been reported that some 50% of patients in psychogeriatric wards are regularly incontinent and 20% occasionally so (Stokes, 1987).

Apart from its obvious implications for personal hygiene and general health, the psychosocial consequences of incontinence can be devastating for victims and their families causing much personal distress, as well as severely disrupting patterns of everyday living and interpersonal relationships. Psychological factors can also play a causal role, such as when emotional distress following a bereavement or some other trauma triggers incontinence which is then a cause of further distress. A vicious circle readily ensues erasing any linear relationship between cause and effect. A variety of psychological approaches have proved useful in the treatment of incontinence irrespective of its aetiology, either as primary treatments in their own right or as adjuncts to other intervention strategies.

Often the first stage is the sensitive and empathic exploration of broader psychosocial and contextual issues to establish the meaning of incontinence for affected individuals and their families as well as helping them develop realistic expectations regarding treatment procedures and their outcomes (e.g. surgical interventions). Where appropriate, stress management techniques may be taught and systemic approaches applied to explore and alter patterns of interpersonal interaction.

Successful applications of behaviour modification interventions have been documented in a wide range of client groups, including victims of head injury, degenerative diseases and those with learning difficulties (see Smith & Smith, 1987). The bell and pad method, which has often proved effective in treating enuresis, relies upon classical conditioning. An alarm triggered by urine release causes wakening and constriction of the sphincter muscle. After repeated pairings interoceptive cues of bladder distension come to be associated with the alarm and eventually come to trigger wakening prior to urination. Originally developed as an intervention with children, it has also proved effective with other client groups. Many successful interventions to promote continence have relied upon the principles of operant conditioning whereby behaviours which are positively reinforced or rewarded tend to become more frequent while those which are not reinforced are gradually extinguished (see Colling *et al.*, 1993; McAuley & McAuley, 1977; Stokes, 1987; Woods & Britten, 1985 for more detailed discussions of underlying principles and applications to various client groups). Although specific details will vary from case to case, such approaches generally share a number of common elements. First, complex sequences of behaviour, such as those involved in toileting, are broken down into their component parts. Secondly, there is a period of detailed observation to establish the frequencies of various behaviours as well as their antecedents and consequences. Thirdly, specific target behaviours are identified and are positively reinforced or non-reinforced as appropriate to change their frequency of occurrence. Fourthly the efficacy of interventions is regularly assessed with reference to pre-treatment baselines and the programme adjusted as necessary.

For a variety of theoretical and practical reasons, family members are often involved in the implementation of behaviour modification programmes. However, they sometimes find it difficult to apply reinforcement schedules with the consistency and immediacy essential for their success.

Over the last 20 or so years biofeedback techniques have been used extensively to treat incontinence (O'Donnell & Doyle, 1991; Enck, 1993), although to date there has been little in the way of standardization of treatment methods. Biofeedback provides people with continence problems with information about pressure in the bowel or bladder, or the activity of key muscle groups. This is presented as an audio and/or visual signal whose properties change as a function of changes in the physiological parameter being measured. It is particularly useful when intrinsic kinaesthetic feedback is diminished or distorted. Biofeedback can be highly effective in treating faecal incontinence with one recent study (Jorge & Wexner, 1993) claiming 90% improvement in over 60% of patients. Comparable claims have been made for its use in treating urinary incontinence (Burgio, 1990).

In dealing with incontinence, good communication between clients and health professionals is of paramount importance. However, reticence and ignorance (on both sides) are barriers to be overcome.

Health professionals must always be aware of the need to approach the topic with great sensitivity, but with openness so as to convey to clients that their incontinence is simply a problem to be dealt with. Euphemisms and sideways references to the problem such as enquiries about 'the water works' are best avoided. While they may spare patients' blushes in the short term, they will do nothing in the long term to break down the negative attitudes and nihilistic expectations that bedevil the recognition, referral and therefore prompt treatment of incontinence.

In summary, incontinence is a common and potentially serious problem that causes great misery to its victims and their families. However, while not always curable, it is always treatable and usually much can be done to improve the quality of life of those afflicted. The social taboos surrounding the topic are significant barriers to effective treatment or management and must be challenged continuously.

REFERENCES

Burgio, K.L. (1990). Behavioural training for stress and urge incontinence in the community. *Gerontology*, **36**, 27–34.

Colling, J.C., Newman, D.K., McCormick, K.A. & Pearson, B.D. (1993). Behavioural management strategies for urinary incontinence. *Journal of ET Nursing*, **20**, 9–13.

Enck, P. (1993). Biofeedback training for disordered defecation. A critical review. *Digestive Diseases Science*, **38**, 1953–60.

Jorge, J.M. & Wexner S.D. (1993). Etiology and management of fecal incontinence. *Diseases of the Colon and Rectum.* **36**, 77–97.

McAuley, R. & McAuley, P. (1977). *Child behaviour problems: an empirical approach to management.* London: The Macmillan Press.

O'Donnell, P.D. & Doyle, R. (1991). Biofeedback therapy technique for treatment of urinary incontinence. *Urology*, **37**, 432–6.

Smith, P.S. & Smith, L.J. (1987). *Continence and incontinence: psychological approaches to development and treatment.* London: Croom Helm.

Stokes, G. (1987). *Incontinence and inappropriate urinating.* Bicester: Winslow Press.

Thomas, T.M., Plymat, K.R., Balannin, J. & Meade, T.W. (1980). Prevalence of urinary incontinence. *British Medical Journal*, **281**, 1243–45.

Woods, R.T. & Britten, P.G. (1985). *Clinical psychology with the elderly.* London: Croom Helm.

Infertility

SHERYLE J. GALLANT
*Department of Psychology,
University of Kansas,
Lawrence, USA*

ANNETTE L. STANTON
*Department of Psychology,
University of Kansas,
Lawrence, USA*

INTRODUCTION

A widely accepted definition of infertility is the inability to achieve a pregnancy after 12 months of regular sexual intercourse without contraception (Mosher & Pratt, 1982). Recent national surveys estimate that infertility affects 13–14% of married couples in the US (excluding the surgically sterile) (Mosher & Pratt, 1990), with comparable rates reported for Great Britain (Greenhall & Vessey, 1990). These data indicate that infertility is a problem that many couples experience. A distinction typically is made between primary infertility, i.e. never having conceived, and secondary infertility, in which a couple experiencing infertility has at least one biological child. Although secondary infertility accounts for more than half of all infertility, rates of primary infertility have risen significantly in recent years, in part as a result of delayed childbearing and the entering into reproductive years of Baby Boom cohorts (Mosher & Pratt, 1991).

The overall rate of infertility has evidenced little change in the past 25 years. However, the number of physician visits for infertility concerns has increased dramatically, nearly tripling from 1968 to 1988 (from approximately 600 000 to 1.6 million) (US Congress, OTA, 1988). This increase reflects the rise in primary infertility for which couples are more likely to seek treatment, as well as greater awareness of advances in diagnosis and treatment of infertility, recognition of the decreased availability of adoption, and the ethical and legal issues surrounding alternatives such as surrogacy. For most couples (80–90%), a medical basis for their infertility can be determined, and the chances of achieving a viable pregnancy are about 50% (OTA, 1988).

There are no exact statistics on the percentage of cases in which problems in the male versus the female are responsible for the infertility (Taymor, 1990). It is generally estimated that approximately 30–40% of infertility can be attributed to male factors and about 40–50% to female factors. In about 10% of cases, even after a full medical evaluation, no specific cause can be identified in either partner (OTA, 1988). Sources of female infertility most commonly involve pelvic abnormalities (e.g. tubal blockage, endometriosis, uterine or peritoneal adhesions), ovulatory problems (e.g. amenorrhoea, oligomenorrhoea), and hormonal dysfunctions (e.g. luteal phase deficiency, hyperprolactinaemia), and, more rarely, immune antibodies in the cervical mucus (Davajan & Israel, 1991). Male infertility typically is due to either deficient sperm production (e.g. low volume of semen, low sperm density, poor motility or abnormal morphology) or to the impaired delivery of sperm such as results from retrograde ejaculation or impotence. Some commonly prescribed medications including antidepressants, antimalarial drugs, and antihypertensives have been shown to lower sperm quality (Taymor, 1990).

PSYCHOLOGICAL AND BEHAVIOURAL FACTORS RELATED TO INFERTILITY

Psychological factors

Until relatively recently, psychological factors were viewed as the cause of infertility in many cases, particularly those in which no medical basis could be identified (OTA, 1988). Adherents of this view focused predominantly on female infertility and hypothesized that it resulted from factors such as impaired sexual identity, maternal role conflict, or personality disturbances such as neuroticism. Research has unequivocally failed to support this view. An extensive review published more than 30 years ago (Noyes & Chapnick, 1964) cited methodological flaws and found no consistent evidence for any of the many psychological factors presumed to cause infertility. The same conclusion has been drawn in more recent reviews (e.g. Edelmann & Connolly, 1986), although the possibility remains that stress may affect spermatogenesis and ovulation (Domar & Seibel, 1990).

Although psychological factors are not a major cause of infertility, there continues to be a strong emphasis on the negative impact of infertility on psychological well-being (Stanton & Dunkel-Schetter, 1991). The clinical observational and anecdotal literature is replete with descriptions of extreme negative reactions, and there is the assumption that these may play a destructive role in dealing with infertility (Taymor, 1990). Commonly reported negative effects include reactions of grief, denial, and depression, feelings of anger, guilt, anxiety, loss of control, self-blame, personal and sexual inadequacy, threats to self-esteem, marital distress, disturbed sexual functioning, and problems in interpersonal relationships including feeling unaccepted and pressured to conceive or experiencing resentment of those who have children (Dunkel-Schetter & Lobel, 1991).

While few would disavow the importance of infertility as a life problem, this literature should be interpreted conservatively, given that empirical research examining reactions to infertility suggests that strong adverse effects are rare. The most rigorous studies find little evidence that global psychological functioning differs in infertile compared to normal couples. Although effects on sexual functioning appear common, most infertile couples report levels of negative emotions (e.g. anxiety, depression, anger, guilt) that are in the normal range, and most do not experience significant marital distress or lowered self-esteem (Dunkel-Schetter & Lobel, 1991). Whether the discrepancy in findings from the descriptive versus the empirical literature primarily reflects methodological limitations in the empirical research or the over-representation of the most distressed couples in the clinical literature is not clear at this point (Dunkel-Schetter & Lobel, 1991). It is clear that considerable variability exists in individuals' responses to infertility.

Psychological stress associated with the treatment aspects of infertility has been a focus of recent research. The rigid schedules of fertility treatments, the need for goal-directed versus pleasure-seeking sexual intercourse, and the fact that treatments are often lengthy, intrusive, time-consuming, financially costly, sometimes painful and associated with a high risk of failure, are all aspects likely to be appraised as stressful. Research reveals that both men and women experience stress in relation to aspects of treatment (Abbey, Halman & Andrews, 1992). Women with primary infertility may be especially stressed by treatment failure (Newton, Hearn & Yuzpe, 1990), and in general, the noxious aspects of treatment fall disproportionally on women, who are subjected to the most invasive and painful treatments. The potential for stress to complicate infertility treatment is suggested by a study (Harrison, Callan & Hennessey, 1987) which found that sperm quality diminished in a sample of men involved in *in vitro* fertilization.

Behavioural factors

Behavioural risk factors related to infertility have been relatively understudied. An exception is smoking. Although findings are somewhat mixed, evidence is accumulating that smoking has deleterious effects on fertility in males and females. Approximately 30% of US women of reproductive age are regular smokers. Epidemiological studies suggest that the risk of primary infertility is increased by smoking (e.g. Laurent *et al.*, 1992), and a dose–response relation has been postulated based on data indicating that the fertility of 'lighter' smokers (< a pack/day) was 75% of non-smokers, but fell to 57% for women who smoked more than a pack per day (Seibel, 1990). The effects of smoking in women appear due primarily to the effects of nicotine. Among males, a broader range of tobacco toxins may be involved since cigarette smoke, nicotine and polycyclic aromatic hydrocarbons have been found to produce testicular atrophy and alter sperm production and morphology in animal studies (Seibel, 1990). Particularly at risk may be smokers with testicular varicoceles who have been shown to have an incidence of oligospermia (low sperm density) ten times greater than non-smokers and five times greater than smokers without varicoceles (Klaiber *et al.*, 1987).

Two behavioural factors that have been infrequently studied but that may be related to female infertility are nutritional deficiencies and physical exercise. Excessive, strenuous physical exercise has been linked to ovulatory problems due to either the direct effects of endorphins on pituitary secretion of gonadotropins or indirectly through associated caloric restrictions and resultant weight loss. Societal pressures for weight control may lead some women to adopt caloric, nutrient or exercise patterns that heighten the chance of menstrual irregularities associated with infertility.

Two additional factors that have significant behavioural correlates and that affect male fertility are exposure of the testes to heat and the frequency of sexual activity. Excess heat is well known to impair sperm quality. Frequently taking hot baths, saunas or whirlpools may produce such adverse effects as may wearing tight underwear. Also it has been suggested that work which involves long hours of sitting may produce excess scrotal heat (Taymor, 1990). Regarding the frequency of sexual activity, it has been shown that frequent, even daily ejaculation has little or no effect on sperm quality in men with normal fertility. However, infertile males may experience a significant reduction in their fertility potential by such frequent ejaculations. Conversely, increased continence is associated with a rise in ejaculate volume but with a decrease in the percentage of motile sperm (Taymor, 1990).

Finally, sexually transmitted diseases, a frequent and preventable cause of infertility (OTA, 1988), are passed on through unsafe sexual practices by both men and women. Psychologists can play a valuable role through designing and implementing prevention programmes directed toward altering behavioural practices that contribute to infertility.

PSYCHOSOCIAL ASPECTS OF COPING AND ADJUSTMENT TO INFERTILITY AND THE ROLE OF THE PSYCHOLOGIST

A primary role for the psychologist who works with the infertile individual is to foster adaptive adjustment to the stresses of infertility and its treatment. The empirical literature on factors related to enhanced or problematic adjustment to infertility is instructive in this regard. At present, three factors appear promising with regard to their potential as targets for therapeutic intervention: control perceptions, coping strategies, and social support.

Although infertile individuals may participate actively in medical treatments, such participation does not guarantee a positive outcome. The experience of infertility certainly may challenge one's belief that important outcomes are under one's voluntary control. Research suggests that infertile individuals who have low perceptions of control surrounding infertility or regarding more general outcomes are likely to manifest distress (Abbey, Andrews & Halman, 1992; Campbell, Dunkel-Schetter & Peplau, 1991; Stanton, 1991). Distinguishing among relatively controllable and uncontrollable aspects of infertility and of the individual's more general experience, as well as developing mechanisms for enhancing control and productive decision-making may comprise effective intervention mechanisms (Dunkel-Schetter & Stanton, 1991).

Those who confront fertility problems initiate a variety of coping strategies to manage the associated demands (Stanton, 1991). Among these, coping through cognitive and behavioural attempts to

avoid the stressor may be particularly problematic for infertile men and women (Stanton, 1991). The association obtained between avoidant coping and greater distress in infertile couples suggests that intervention strategies designed to promote active emotional and behavioural engagement with the stressor may be productive, although this possibility awaits empirical test.

The social context in which infertility occurs also warrants attention. Research suggests that high general social support and low marital conflict are related to lower distress in infertile individuals (Abbey, Halman & Andrews, 1992; Stanton, 1991). Assessment of the quality of intimate relationships and promotion of mechanisms for obtaining support, such as participation in RESOLVE, a national infertility self-help network, are important functions of the psychologist working with the infertile individual. Further, the psychologist can assist the infertile patient in developing effective methods by which to negotiate the interpersonally and technically complex medical system designed to diagnose and treat infertility.

Although we are beginning to identify specific factors that promote or hinder adjustment of those facing infertility, very few studies of interventions designed to enhance adjustment are available. A promising programme is Domar's multimodal treatment, in which group participation in relaxation training, stress management, cognitive restructuring, and other techniques has been shown to be associated with decreased psychological symptomatology (e.g. depressed mood) in infertile women (Domar, Seibel & Benson, 1990; Domar et al., 1992). Identification of the most effective intervention components and specification of the most efficient and beneficial vehicles for treatment (e.g. group, couple, or individual approaches) await study.

In their capacities as researchers and clinicians, psychologists certainly may play a valuable role in addressing the challenges of infertility. Psychologists can aid in identifying and intervening with contributors to and consequences of infertility. In this endeavour we should remain mindful of the diversity of causes of, and responses to, infertility among those who confront it. For example, specific behavioural and psychosocial factors (e.g. smoking, unsafe sexual practices) may be important causal agents of infertility for some segment of the population, but enduring personality dispositions do not hold promise as aetiological factors. Thus, psychologists should work to target and intervene with causal agents which have empirically demonstrated associations with infertility and which are most amenable to change. Further, diversity of response to infertility implies that not every infertile individual will require psychological assessment and counselling, although psychological intervention may prove invaluable for some. Variability in reaction also reminds us that there is no single 'appropriate' way to respond to infertility, and continued work is warranted to specify risk factors for maladjustment and to tailor therapeutic interventions for promoting well-being in those who experience infertility.

REFERENCES

Abbey, A., Andrews, F.M. & Halman, L.J. (1992). Infertility and subjective well-being: the mediating roles of self-esteem, internal control, and interpersonal conflict. *Journal of Marriage and the Family,* **54,** 408–17.

Abbey, A., Halman, L.J. & Andrews, F.M. (1992). Psychosocial, treatment, and demographic predictors of the stress associated with infertility. *Fertility and Sterility,* **57,** 122–8.

Campbell, S.M., Dunkel-Schetter, C. & Peplau, L.A. (1991). Perceived control and adjustment to infertility among women undergoing *in vitro* fertilization. In A.L. Stanton & C. Dunkel-Schetter (Eds.). *Infertility: perspectives from stress and coping research,* pp. 133–156. New York: Plenum Press.

Davajan, V. & Israel, R. (1991). Diagnosis and medical treatment of infertility. In

A.L. Stanton & D. Dunkel-Schetter (Eds.). *Infertility: perspectives from stress and coping research*, pp. 17–28. New York: Plenum Press

Domar, A.D. & Seibel, M. (1990). The emotional aspects of infertility. In M. Seibel (Ed.). *Infertility: a comprehensive text*, pp. 25–35. Norwalk, CT: Appleton-Lange.

Domar, A.D., Seibel, M. & Benson, H. (1990). The mind/body program for infertility: a new behavioural treatment approach for women with infertility. *Fertility and Sterility*, 53, 246–9.

Domar, A.D., Zuttermeister, P.C., Seibel, M. & Benson, H. (1992). Psychological improvement in infertile women after behavioural treatment: a replication. *Fertility and Sterility*, 58, 144–7.

Dunkel-Schetter, C. & Lobel, M. (1991). Psychological reactions to infertility. In A.L. Stanton & C. Dunkel-Schetter (Eds.). *Infertility: perspectives from stress and coping research*, pp. 29–57. New York: Plenum Press.

Dunkel-Schetter, C. & Stanton, A.L. (1991). Psychological adjustment to infertility: Future directions in research and application. In A.L. Stanton & C. Dunkel-Schetter (Eds.). *Infertility: perspectives from stress and coping research*, pp. 197–222. New York: Plenum Press.

Edelmann, R.J. & Connolly, K.J. (1986). Psychological aspects of infertility. *British Journal of Medical Psychology*, 59, 209–19.

Greenhall, E. & Vessey, M. (1990). The prevalence of subfertility: a review of the current confusion and a report of two new studies. *Fertility and Sterility*, 54, 978–83.

Harrison, K.L., Callan, V.J. & Hennessey, J.F. (1987). Stress and semen quality in an in vitro fertilization program. *Fertility and Sterility*, 48, 633–7.

Klaiber, E.L., Broverman, D.M., Pokoly, T.B., Albert, A.J., Howard, P.J., Jr. & Sherer, J.F. (1987). Interrelationships of cigarette smoking, testicular varicocele, and seminal fluid indexes. *Fertility and Sterility*, 47, 481–6.

Laurent, S.L., Garrison, C.Z., Thompson, S.J., Moore, E.E. & Addy, C. (1992). An epidemiologic study of smoking and primary infertility in women. *Fertility and Sterility*, 57, 565–72.

Mosher, W.D. & Pratt, W.F. (1982). *Reproductive impairments among married couples: United States*. Hyattsville, MD: US Department of Health & Human Services, Office of Health Research, Statistics, and Technology, National Center for Health Statistics.

Mosher, W.D. & Pratt, W.F. (1990). Fecundity and infertility in the United States, 1965–1988. *Advance data from vital and health statistics*, No. 192, December 4, Hyattsville, MD: National Center for Health Statistics.

Mosher, W.D. & Pratt, W.F. (1991). Fecundity and infertility in the United

States: incidence and trends. *Fertility and Sterility*, 56, 192–3.

Newton, C.R., Hearn, M.T. & Yuzpe, A.A. (1990). Psychological assessment and follow-up after in vitro fertilization: assessing the impact of failure. *Fertility and Sterility*, 54, 879–86.

Noyes, R.W. & Chapnick, E.M. (1964). Literature on psychology and infertility: a critical analysis. *Fertility and Sterility*, 15, 543–58.

Seibel, M.M. (1990). Workup of the infertile couple. In M. Siebel (Ed.). *Infertility: a comprehensive text*, pp. 1–21. Norwalk, CT: Appleton & Lance.

Stanton, A.L. (1991). Cognitive appraisals, coping processes, and adjustment to infertility. In A.L. Stanton & C. Dunkel-Schetter (Eds.). *Infertility: perspectives from stress and coping research*, pp. 87–108. New York: Plenum Press.

Stanton, A.L. & Dunkel-Schetter, C. (1991). Psychological adjustment to infertility: an overview of conceptual approaches. In A.L. Stanton & C. Dunkel-Schetter (Eds.). *Infertility: perspectives from stress and coping research*, pp. 3–16. New York: Plenum Press.

Taymor, M.L. (1990). Infertility: a clinician's guide to diagnosis and treatment. New York: Plenum Medical Book Company.

US Congress, Office of Technology Assessment (1988). *Infertility: medical and social choices*, OTA-BA-358. Washington, DC: US Government Printing Office.

Inflammatory bowel disease

PAUL BENNETT

Gwent Psychology Services and University of Bristol, UK

Inflammatory bowel disease (IBD) refers to two disorders: Crohn's disease and ulcerative colitis. Both are remitting diseases, with alternating periods of exacerbation and remission with symptoms of pain, diarrhoea and anorexia. Ulcerative colitis usually affects the lower colon and results from inflammation of its inner lining. During periods of inflammation, stools are bloody and purulent. Crohn's disease results from an inflammation of the outer layers of the intestinal wall, and may occur anywhere in the gastrointestinal tract. Complications include the development of fistulas and scarring which may lead to obstruction and distension and, potentially fatal, rupture of the bowel. Both are thought to result from immune dysfunction and carry a high risk for the development of cancer.

AETIOLOGY

Initial aetiological theories suggested both ulcerative colitis and Crohn's disease to be psychosomatic in origin. Early analytical work by Alexander provided clinical evidence of this relationship, while a number of uncontrolled studies found a high percentage of IBD patients to report adverse life events prior to symptom exacerbation. However, controlled studies have shown little consistent evidence that IBD patients experience more stress preceding exacerbation than is typically encountered by healthy controls. Indeed, Mendeloff *et al.* (1970) found levels of stress reported in the previous six months by ulcerative colitis patients to be less than both those reported by patients with irritable bowel syndrome and a control group of local residents.

Such findings, however, should not be taken as suggesting stress necessarily has no role in the aetiology of IBD. The diathesis-stress model suggest only those with a biological predisposition to certain diseases will develop them in the presence of life stress. An alternative strategy to exploration of this model would be to determine whether stress is involved in the exacerbation of symptoms amongst those with the disease. Two small-scale studies have attempted to explore this relationship. Garrett *et al.*, 1988 (reported in Schwarz & Blanchard, 1991) asked 10 IBD patients to record stressful events and IBD symptoms for 28 days. They found significantly higher symptom scores on the seven days with the highest reported stress than on those with the lowest. Similar results were reported by Greene *et al.* (1989 (reported in Schwarz & Blanchard, 1991) who found correlations ranging from $r = 0.42$ and 0.68 between daily measures of stress and symptoms. Unfortunately, the simultaneous measurement of stress and symptoms in these studies means the direction of their relationship cannot be easily determined, and alternative longitudinal designs are necessary.

While the relationship between stress and symptom exacerbation remains unclear, there is unambiguous evidence that the disease impacts on patients' quality of life. Of the sample interviewed by Joachim and Milne (1985), for example, 42% reported that their illness significantly impaired their life satisfaction, 56% thought their illness contributed to feelings of low energy, while over one-third felt it contributed to feelings of depression and nervousness. Perhaps surprisingly, in view of its recurrent nature and poor prognosis, only 25% were worried about their illness. Mallett *et al.* (1982) also reported significant impairment to work and social life during periods of high symptom severity, and even when symptoms were at their lowest level, 25% of their sample reported restricted social or leisure activities. (See also next chapter.)

INTERVENTIONS

Interventions with IBD patients have been of two types: those targeted primarily at symptom reduction, and those at reducing distress resulting from symptom exacerbation. Unfortunately, few satisfactory studies of either type have been conducted, limiting the conclusions which may be drawn from this research.

A number of studies attest to the value of psychological interventions in reducing frequency of symptom exacerbation and disease progression. Karush *et al.* (1977), for example, allocated IBD patients to either medical treatment alone or in combination with supportive psychotherapy. Over the eight-year period of the study, patients in the combined treatment group experienced shorter and less severe exacerbations and longer periods of remission. However, the study was seriously compromised by non-random allocation to condition and a failure to control for the use of steroids and antibiotics. In addition, no relationship was reported between changes in psychological state and IBD symptoms. More recently, Milne, Joachim & Niedhart (1986) reported significant improvements on measures of symptomatology over a follow-up period of one year in

patients assigned to a stress management protocol relative to those assigned to a standard treatment control group. No differential changes in medication which may explain these differences occurred. However, patients in the intervention condition reported significantly more symptoms and psychological stress at baseline, and their relative improvement on both types of measure may be attributable to regression to the mean (see also previous chapter).

Schwarz and Blanchard (1991) reported the only failure of IBD patients to benefit from psychological therapy in comparison to a symptom monitoring condition. Participants in the active condition reported significant reductions in two symptoms following an intervention comprising progressive muscle relaxation, thermal biofeedback and cognitive stress management techniques. Over the same period of time, patients in the symptom monitoring group reported decreases in five of the nine symptoms being monitored. When this group subsequently received the intervention, their symptoms increased. Retrospective analyses suggested that patients with ulcerative colitis benefited more than those with Crohn's disease, and the authors suggest an uneven allocation of patients to each condition may have contributed to the apparently negative findings.

A number of studies suggest that psychological distress resulting from symptom flare up may be reduced through the use of psychological techniques. Freyberger, Kunsebeck and Lempa (1985), for example, randomly allocated 38 patients with ulcerative colitis to either a brief psychotherapy or no treatment condition. Significant improvements on measures of state anxiety, depression and mood were reported in the treatment, but not control, condition. Unfortunately, no follow-up assessments were made to assess the durability of these results. Despite the lack of symptomatic change, patients in the active intervention of Schwarz and Blanchard (1991) reported also less symptom-related stress, less depression and less anxiety than those in the control period. (See also previous chapter.)

Finally, Shaw and Ehrlich (1987) examined the impact of relaxation training on the pain associated with ulcerative colitis. Forty patients were allocated to either a relaxation training or attention control condition. Immediately following the intervention and at six week follow-up, patients in the active intervention reported significantly less frequent and intense pain, and were more able to control their pain. In addition, significantly fewer patients were taking anti-inflammatory drugs.

CONCLUSIONS

There is as yet little strong evidence to suggest a significant relationship between stress and the development of IBD, although longitudinal studies may yet provide stronger evidence for such a relationship. The majority of intervention studies suggest that psychological interventions may significantly reduce the frequency and severity of symptomatic episodes and any associated distress. Unfortunately, much of the intervention literature has been compromised by weak study designs, and few conclusions can yet be made as to the true efficacy of such interventions. (See also previous chapter.)

REFERENCES

Freyberger, H., Kunsebeck, H.-W. & Lempa, W. (1985). Psychotherapeutic interventions in alexithymic patients with special regard to ulcerative colitis and

Crohn patients. *Psychotherapy and Psychosomatics*, **44**, 72–81.

Joachim, G. & Milne, B. (1985). The effects of inflammatory bowel disease

on lifestyle. *Canadian Nurse*, **81**, 38–40.

Karush, A., Daniels, G.E., Flood, C. & O'Connor, J.F. (1977). *Psychotherapy in* *chronic ulcerative colitis*. Philadelphia: W.B. Saunders and Co.

Mallett, S., Lennard-Jones, J., Bingley, J. & Gilon, E. (1982). Colitis. *Lancet*, ii, 619–21.

Mendeloff, A.I., Monk, M., Siegel, C.I. & Lilienfeld, A. (1970). Illness experience and life stresses in patients with irritable colon and with ulcerative colitis: an epidemiological study of ulcerative colitis

and regional enteritis in Baltimore, 1960–1964. *New England Journal of Medicine*, 282, 14–17.

Milne, B., Joachim, G. & Niedhart, J. (1986). A stress management programme for inflammatory bowel disease patients. *Journal of Advanced Nursing*, 11, 561–7.

Schwarz, S.P. & Blanchard, E.B. (1990). Inflammatory bowel disease: a review of the psychological assessment and treatment

literature. *Annals of Behavioral Medicine*, 12, 95–105.

Schwarz, S.P. & Blanchard, E.B. (1991). Evaluation of a psychological treatment for inflammatory bowel disease. *Behaviour Research and Therapy*, 29, 167–77.

Shaw, L. & Ehrlich, A. (1987). Relaxation training as a treatment for chronic pain caused by ulcerative colitis. *Pain*, 29, 287–93.

Irritable bowel syndrome

PAUL BENNETT

Gwent Psychology Services and University of Bristol, UK

Irritable bowel syndrome (IBS) is a disorder of the large bowel characterized by abdominal pain and change in bowel habit (constipation or diarrhoea) in the absence of organic disease. Diagnosis depends on these symptoms lasting a minimum of three months. Until recently, IBS has been viewed as a primarily psycho-physiological disorder. Latimer (1981) even suggested that its symptoms and aetiology are synonymous with those of anxiety, with symptom choice (anxiety or IBS) being determined by social learning. A weaker 'stress' hypothesis (Whitehead & Schuster, 1985) suggests that IBS symptoms are multi-causal and result from a variety of factors which may include stress. Both models suggest that stress-related symptoms result from a hyper-reactivity of the colon, although whether this is mediated centrally, via the autonomic nervous system, or as a result of specific abnormal muscle activity in the gut (or both) is not clear.

AETIOLOGY

There is consistent evidence that patients with IBS report higher levels of distress and more negative life events, or poorer coping strategies, than normal or other patient controls (see Bennett, 1993). Unfortunately, the dependence of these studies on patients who actively sought medical treatment for their symptoms renders interpretation of their findings difficult. Up to 80% of people with IBS do not consult a physician. In addition, non-attenders visit their doctor less for other minor or vague symptoms. Accordingly, the results of patient based studies must be considered with some caution, particularly in view of the findings of three substantial studies using physician non-attenders (e.g. Drossman *et al.*, 1988) that clinic attending IBS patients report higher levels of stress than non-attenders.

Unfortunately, population studies may also distort our understanding of the relationship between stress and IBS. The diathesis–stress model suggests that stress will only cause symptoms in those who are biologically prone to them. Large-scale surveys may underestimate the significance of any idiosyncratic relationships between stress and symptoms within only a percentage of those surveyed. A

more useful methodology may be longitudinal studies of individuals who report IBS symptoms to measure the correlations between changes in stress and symptom severity.

Whitehead (1992) reported one such study, in which 39 women with clearly defined IBS were followed, with assessments of bowel symptoms and life events made every three months. The IBS group reported more life events than the control group. However, changes in life events only accounted for 10% of the variance in symptoms. The focus of this study on major life events ignored the impact of everyday stressors and may have underestimated their effect on symptom exacerbation. In a more descriptive study, Drossman *et al.* (1982) identified a group of non-clinic attending people with IBS from a large sample of hospital workers. Eighty four per cent reported that stressors caused them constipation or diarrhoea, while 69% said that stressors led to abdominal pain or discomfort. Corney *et al.* (1991) also reported a moderate dose–response relationship between changes in stress and symptom severity following a relaxation based intervention. Accordingly, there is at least some preliminary evidence to suggest that in those prone to IBS, severity of symptoms does co-vary with levels of stress (also see previous Chapter).

INTERVENTIONS

A number of psychological approaches have been used in the treatment of IBS, the majority of which have attempted to indirectly reduce symptoms through some form of stress management regime. The exception to this has been work conducted by Whitehead and colleagues who provided direct feedback on bowel motility in an attempt to teach increased bowel control. However, the procedures for this approach were rather uncomfortable and it proved no better than standard relaxation techniques. As a result, this approach has not been pursued. Three therapeutic approaches have undergone sufficient evaluation for some, tentative, conclusions to be drawn about their effectiveness: stress management training, psychotherapy, and hypnotherapy.

In a series of related studies, Blanchard and his colleagues evaluated the effectiveness of a combination of deep muscle relaxation, thermal biofeedback, and cognitive therapy in the treatment of IBS. This proved superior to no treatment in the short term, with reductions in symptoms maintained for up to four years. However, later comparison of this intervention with a placebo treatment comparing pseudomeditation in conjunction with alpha wave suppression and a symptom monitoring condition (Blanchard *et al.*, 1992) found no differences in outcome between any condition. However, the study involved only a small number of participants and those in the placebo group reported more use of relaxation and mental imagery techniques than those in the active intervention group. Accordingly, these results may be atypical and are at odds with the results of other controlled trials.

These have provided consistent evidence that stress management interventions, comprising teaching some form of relaxation techniques alone or in combination with a variety of cognitive–behavioural strategies, may prove an effective intervention in IBS. Bennett and Wilkinson (1985), for example, found similar short-term reductions in measures of pain, discomfort and diarrhoea and significantly greater reductions in anxiety among participants allocated to a stress management condition in comparison to those allocated to standard medical treatment. In a longer-term study, Voirol and Hipolito (1987) reported greater reductions in measures of pain and medical consultations in participants receiving training in relaxation methods in comparison with those receiving medical treatment over a follow-up period of 40 months.

Although later studies have provided confirmatory evidence, the most substantial study of the effectiveness of psychotherapy was reported by Svedlund (1983). He evaluated the effectiveness of medication alone or in combination with an intervention comprising up to ten hours of sessions aimed at helping participants modify maladaptive behaviour, find new solutions to problems, and to cope more effectively with stress and emotional problems. In this, it appears very close to the cognitive–behavioural interventions previously described. At one year follow-up, the combined treatment group maintained significantly greater improvements on a variety of measures of IBS symptoms, including pain and bowel dysfunction.

One group of researchers has reported on the effectiveness of hypnotherapy in IBS. Whorwell, Prior & Colgan (1987) compared a seven-week programme of hypnotherapy directed at general relaxation and control of intestinal motility with supportive psychotherapy in combination with placebo medication. Immediately following the intervention, participants in the hypnotherapy condition reported significantly greater improvements on all measures of symptoms than those in the control group, a difference which was maintained to 18 month follow-up.

CONCLUSIONS

Although the role of stress in mediating symptoms in IBS has received much attention, much has been methodologically naive and few conclusions can be drawn. Nevertheless, there is some evidence to suggest that at least some symptoms, in some people, are mediated via the stress process. In addition, although the evidence is still limited, the relatively consistent reduction of IBS symptoms following psychological intervention seems sufficient to warrant such an approach.

REFERENCES

Bennett, P. (1993). Disorders of the gut. In A. Broome & S. Llewelyn (Eds). *Health psychology: processes and applications.* London: Chapman and Hall.

Bennett, P. & Wilkinson, S. (1985). A comparison of psychological and medical treatment of the irritable bowel syndrome. *British Journal of Clinical Psychology*, **24**, 215–16.

Blanchard, E.B., Schwarz, S.P., Suls, J.M., Gerardi, M., Scharff, L., Greene, B., Taylor, A.E., Berreman, C. & Malamood, H.S. (1992). Two controlled evaluations of a multicomponent psychological treatment of irritable bowel syndrome. *Behaviour Research and Therapy*, 30, 175–89.

Corney, R.H., Stanton, R., Newell, R., Clare, A. & Fairclough, P. (1991). Behavioural psychotherapy in the treatment of irritable bowel syndrome. *Journal of Psychosomatic Research*, **35**, 461–9.

Drossman, D.A., Leserman, J., Nachman, G., Li, Z, Zagami, E.A. & Patrick, D.L. (1988). Psychosocial factors in the irritable bowel syndrome. A multivariate study of patients and non-patients with irritable bowel syndrome. *Gastroenterology*, **95**, 701–8.

Drossman, D.A., Sandler, R.S., McKee, D.C. & Lovitz, A.J. (1982). Bowel patterns among subjects not seeking medical care: use of a questionnaire to identify a population with bowel dysfunction. *Gastroenterology*, **83**, 529–34.

Latimer, P.R. (1981). Irritable bowel syndrome: a behavioural model. *Behaviour Research and Therapy*, **19**, 475–83.

Svedlund, J. (1983). Psychotherapy in irritable bowel syndrome. A controlled outcome study. *Acta Psychiatrica Scandinavica* (Suppl), **306**, 1–86.

Voirol, M.W. & Hipolito, J. (1987). Relaxation anthropoanalytique dans les syndromes de l'intestin irritable: resultats à 40 mois. *Schweizerische Medizinische Wochenschrift*, **117**, 1117–19.

Whitehead, W.E. (1992). Behavioral medicine approaches to gastrointestinal disorders. *Journal of Consulting and Clinical Psychology*, **60**, 605–12.

Whitehead, W.E. & Schuster, M.M. (1985). *Gastrointestinal disorders. Behavioral and physiological bases for treatment.* London: Academic Press.

Whorwell, P.J., Prior, A. & Colgan, S.M. (1987) Hypnotherapy in severe irritable bowel syndrome: further experience. *Gut.* 28, 423–5.

Lactose and food intolerance

MARY BANKS GREGERSON
Psychology Department,
The George Washington University,
Washington, USA

FEATURES

Intolerance to foods such as dairy products, meats, sugar, or spices can be primary (inherited) or acquired. A common intolerance, lactose is a principal carbohydrate found in milk and other dairy products. Deficient enzyme lactase in the lower intestine or other intestinal injury interferes with lactose absorption and produces unpleasant symptoms.

Lactose intolerance and maldigestion are different. Lactose malabsorption refers to the inability to digest lactose containing foods. Lactose intolerance means an adverse reaction. Maldigesters are not necessarily intolerant, and those intolerant do not necessarily have maldigestion (Escribano-Subias et al., 1993).

Lactose intolerance may have a different pathogenesis than other food intolerances (Blanco-Quiros et al., 1993). Therefore, what follows can appropriately only be considered relevant to lactose intolerance.

The clinical symptoms of lactose intolerance, apart from other food allergies, specifically produce gastrointestinal problems like flatulence, belching, diarrhoea, rectal bleeding, abdominal pain and cramping, or bloating. In addition, infants can experience colic, irritability, rashes or eczema, night awakenings, throwing up, and wheezing.

INCIDENCE

Much of the world population is lactase deficient (Gendrel et al., 1990). World-wide, all ages and races as well as both genders have demonstrated lactose intolerance. Although all newborns have lactose digesting ability, many lose it later (Thomas et al., 1990). An estimated 10% of children experience this intolerance (Bodanszky, Horvath & Horn, 1990). Different races and nationalities display a variety of prevalence rates throughout childhood (Thomas et al., 1990). Asian and African American children have the lowest rates.

Inhabitants of both third-world and industrialized nations have this problem. In the third world enteric infections related to phenomena like lactose intolerance are estimated as a primary cause of childhood illness and death.

A number of ill populations may have other complications associated with lactose intolerance. This deficiency has implications for irritable bowel syndrome, diabetes, active ulcerative colitis, Graves' disease, human immunodeficiency virus (HIV), and Crohn's disease. In some cases, such as Graves' disease, intolerance as a secondary effect can be reversed. In other diseases like HIV, the disease may directly cause the lactose intolerance.

DIAGNOSIS

Clinical history is not sufficient to diagnose lactose intolerance. Many patients do not recognize symptoms, with some even being asymptomatic. Assessment of gases, in particular, are necessary.

The main manner of diagnosing lactose intolerance is a hydrogen breath test, an easy, reliable, non-invasive, economical technique (Montes & Perman, 1991). A pocket-sized monitor has shown similar sensitivity and accuracy to the stationary system (Braden et al., 1993). End-expiratory methane production may also indicate lactose intolerance. These expiratory gas methods are time sensitive, with the most recent research indicating that at least four hours is needed between samples (Corazza et al., 1990). Sometimes a diet lactose challenge, like Lundh's test meal (Miko, Schreiner & Feher, 1990), determines intolerance. If hydrogen increases by 15–40 ppm, intolerance has been diagnosed in past research. The lactose intolerant can have hydrogen levels as high as 60 ppm compared with 7 ppm for normals (Medow et al., 1990).

TREATMENT

Many dietary restriction and supplement programmes have been developed to bypass or augment lactase deficiency. The typical programme would: (i) reduce or restrict dietary lactose; (ii) substitute alternative nutrient sources to avoid reduction in energy sources; (iii) regulate calcium intake; and (iv) use commercially available enzyme substitutes.

Besides restricting lactose-containing foods or reducing lactose in foods, changing diet fat content or calorie density can reduce symptoms (Montes & Perman, 1991). Supplemental nutrition regimens that include dairy foods or additives with lactase activity have been successful in treating children and adults alike. Lactase-based tablets also work.

Infants, in particular, are susceptible to lactose intolerance. Their diarrhoea and secondary lactase deficiency has been successfully treated with a diet maintenance of soy-protein, lactase, carbohydrate, protein, and fat-enriched formula. A powdered, fermented milk preparation has effectively countered lactose intolerance in third-world children (Gendrel et al., 1990).

BEHAVIOURAL OR PSYCHOLOGICAL ASPECTS

Since lactose intolerance is not life threatening typically, psychologists need to address its indirect effects on health and quality of life. As a health enterprise, psychologists may assist in dietary management of this disease. Action must be taken either to avoid lactose-laden foods or to add lactase enzyme or substitutes to the diet.

Education and time management may assist handling the added demands in knowledge and preparation required.

In addition to these treatment aspects, psychologists may address the socially adverse aspects of many symptoms. Educating patients and their families can decrease any unfavourable interpersonal costs associated with symptoms.

REFERENCES

Blanco-Quiros, A., Garrote-Adrados, J.A., Andion-Dapena, R., Alonso-Franch, M., CalvoRomero, C. & Bobillo-del-Amo, H. (1993). Increased serum levels of soluble IL-2 receptor in food intolerance; possible mechanism of delayed immunity in milk intolerance. *Anales Espanoles De Pediatria (Madrid)*, 38, 330–6.

Bodansky, H., Horvath, K. & Horn, G. (1990). Incidence of lactose malabsorption in the population 6–18 years of age. *Orvosi Hetilap (Budapest)* 131.

Braden, B., Braden, C.P., Klutz, M. & Lembcke, B. (1993). Analysis of breath hydrogen (H₂) in diagnosis of gastrointestinal function: validation of a pocket breath H₂ test analyzer. *Zeitschrift fur Gastroenterologie (Munchen)*, 31, 242–5.

Corazza, G.R., Sorge, M., Strocchi, A.,

Lattanzi, M.C., Benati, G. & Gasbarrini, G. (1990). Methodology of the H₂ breath test. II. Importance of the test duration in the diagnosis of carbohydrate malabsorption. *Italian Journal of Gastroenterology*, 22, 303–5.

Escribano-Subias, J., Sanz-Manrique, N., Villa-Elizaga, I. & Tomo – Carnice (1993). Relationship between primary lactose malabsorption and consumption of dairy products. *Anales Espanoles De Pediatria (Madrid)*, 38, 107–12.

Gendrel, D., Richard-Lenoble, D., Dupont, C., Gendrel, C., Nardou, M. & Chaussain, M. (1990). Use of a fermented powdered milk in malnourished or lactose intolerant children. *Presse Medicale (Paris)*, 19, 700–4.

Medow, M.S., Thek, K.D., Newman, L.J., Berezin, S., Glassman, M.S. &

Schwarz, S.M. (1990). Beta-galactosidase tablets in the treatment of lactose intolerance in pediatrics. *American Journal of Diseases in Childhood*, 144, 1261–4.

Miko, P., Schreiner, M. & Feher, J. (1990). High lactose content of the Lundh test meal adversely affects the relatibility of the ALTAB test. *Orvosi Hetilap (Budapest)*, 131, 627–9.

Montes, R.G. & Perman, J.A. (1991). Lactose intolerance. Pinpointing the source of nonspecific gastrointestinal symptoms. *Postgraduate Medicine*, 89, 175–8, 181–4.

Thomas, S., Walker-Smith, J.A., Senewiratne, B. & Hjelm, M. (1990). Age dependency of the lactase persistence and lactase restriction phenotypes among children in Sri Lanka and Britain. *Journal of Tropical Pediatrics (London)*, 36, 80–5.

Lead: health effects

MARJORIE SMITH

Thomas Coram Research Unit, Institute of Education, London, UK

Lead is a known neurotoxin, which can cause serious brain damage (including coma, and death) at high doses. The hazards of lead poisoning have been known since Roman times. Historically, lead poisoning was common in occupationally exposed adults (for example, plumbers, printers, pottery workers, workers involved in the manufacture of paint, glass, or lead acid batteries) but was rare in other adults or children. Nowadays workers exposed to lead are subject to regular blood lead monitoring and stringent health checks. Cases of lead poisoning in children were (and still are) usually due to the ingestion of leaded paint flakes.

Over 50 years ago it was noted (Byers & Lord, 1943) that children who appeared to have recovered from lead poisoning performed poorly at school, indicating some residual brain damage. This, and the finding that considerable numbers of children living in urban or near industrial areas had elevated body lead burden (measured by their blood lead level), prompted a number of epidemiological studies of the effects on children of exposure to low levels of lead. Since the pioneering study of Needleman and colleagues in 1979 (Needleman *et al.*, 1979) epidemiological studies have been conducted in Europe, including Eastern Europe, USA, Australia, New Zealand and China. These studies have been either cross-sectional, the majority using either blood or shed deciduous teeth as the indicator of lead exposure in children, or more recently prospective studies have been carried out in USA and Australia, identifying a sample of children at or before birth, and following them as they develop (reports from many of these studies are included in Smith, Grant & Sors, 1989).

The most consistently measured outcome, and the one most consistently found to be associated with lead measures, is child IQ. Tests of educational attainment, behaviour, or other specific skills, such as motor skills, or memory have been incorporated in a number of studies, but there is little consistency between studies in those that are reported as lead associated. Where lead-related associations with behavioural measures have been reported, it is usually in studies utilising short forced-choice questionnaires on child behaviour. These have been shown to be significantly related to measures of child intelligence. Observational measures of child behaviour, such as activity level, have not been found to be associated with body lead measures.

A recent systematic review of the association between full scale IQ and lead in 26 epidemiological studies published since 1979 (Pocock, Smith & Baghurst, 1994) has examined the cumulative evidence from both prospective and cross-sectional studies. It concludes that there is no evidence of an association between neonatal lead exposure and later IQ. The association of later measures of lead with IQ is evident in both prospective and cross-sectional studies. Overall, it is estimated that a typical doubling of body lead burden (from 0.48 to 0.96 μ mol/l blood lead or 5 to 10 μg/g tooth lead, is associated with a mean deficit in full-scale IQ of around 1–2 IQ points.

Despite the fact that there is now a considerable body of empirical data on the association between lead exposure and children's functioning (more than on any other toxin) the limitations of observational epidemiology mean that causal interpretations of the data are still debated. Chance can readily be ruled out as an explanation

as the association is almost always in one direction, with higher lead associated with poorer performance. It is not so easy to rule out two other possible explanations. These are reverse causality, that is, that children who are less intelligent behave in ways that increase their uptake of lead. A second possibility is that the association is due, at least in part, to uncontrolled social factors. Lead uptake by children is not random: the most disadvantaged children also have the highest body levels of lead. Although statistical control for these confounding factors reduces the strength of the association, it can never be fully satisfactory, since one can never measure or control for all the factors which contribute to the child's intellectual development.

There remains uncertainty as to the real impact that lead makes on children's neuropsychological development.

REFERENCES

Byers, R.K. & Lord, E.E. (1943). Late effects of lead poisoning on mental development. *American Journal of Diseases of Children*, 66, 471–94.

Needleman, H.L., Gunnoe, C., Leviton, A., Reed, R., Peresie, H., Maher, C. &

Barrett, P. (1979). Deficits in psychologic and classroom performance of children with elevated dentine lead levels. *New England Journal of Medicine*, 300, 689–95.

Pocock, S.J., Smith, M.A. & Baghurst, P. (1994). Environmental lead and children's intelligence: a systematic review of the

epidemiological evidence. *British Medical Journal*, 309, 1189–97.

Smith, M.A., Grant, L.D. & Sors, A.I. (Eds.). (1989). *Lead exposure and child development: an international assessment*. London: Kluwer.

Leprosy

NINA BUTLER

*Unit of Helath Psychology, Department
Psychiatry and Behavioural Sciences, University
College London (UCL), UK*

HISTORY AND BELIEFS

Leprosy is a disease which affects the body of the patient and the mind of the unaffected public. This is a concept fundamental to understanding both the disease and its social construction. It was described by Hippocrates in 460 BC, and Weymouth (1938) notes that archaeological relics found in Egypt, dating back to 4000 BC, are confirmation that leprosy existed at the time. Browne (1980) contends that around the third century BC the troops of Alexander the Great were agents of its transmission, and in the first century AD Galen provided the first scientific description of the symptomatology of the disease (Skinsnes, 1973).

Until the 1940s leprosy was incurable, uncontrollable, and synonymous with grotesque, devastating deformities (Mull *et al.*, 1989). As destructive as the physical impact of the disease, however, has been the social treatment of the leprosy sufferer: whether in Africa, Europe, Asia or the New World, leprosy victims have been feared and shunned. In antiquity people thought to have contracted leprosy were cast out of home, rejected by family, and identified as a threat to the rest of society (Goldman, Moraites & Kitzmiller, 1966; Varron, 1939), while in medieval Europe victims were burnt, drowned or buried alive (Richards, 1978; Browne, 1975a, b). Across all cultures such behaviour frequently had its origins in a belief that

the disease is a punishment from God (Brody, 1974; Skinsnes & Chang, 1985; Waxler, 1981), and in many cultures it is still the case that the moral stigma associated with leprosy adds a further burden of oppression to the one who is inflicted. As Mull *et al.* (1989) point out, in contrast to sufferers of most other diseases, the leprosy victim can be transformed into the embodiment of the disease. Indeed, the English word 'leper' has come to be synonymous with someone who is shunned on moral grounds (OED). In ancient times compulsory identification of 'lepers' was accomplished through clothing, ringing a bell in the proximity of others, and restriction to begging as the only means of survival (Volinn, 1989). Although segregated facilities for persons with leprosy are decreasing, the stigma attached to leprosy continues, overtly or covertly, to exist.

MANIFESTATION

Contrary to lay beliefs (embodied in the behavioural factors noted above), leprosy is in fact one of the least contagious of human transmissible diseases (Mull *et al.*, 1989; Skelly & Gibb, 1987). The causative agent is *Mycobacterium leprae* which is poorly adapted to man and evolved defences are thought to be present in 85–90% of human populations. Its discovery was first published by Gerhard Hansen in 1847, and it is by his name, in an attempt to ameliorate its stigma, that the disease is sometimes known (Hansen's disease). When transmitted, the bacterium is spread by open sore or nasal secretions, and malnourished peoples are thought to be most at risk (Ridley, 1987). Notwithstanding these factors, however, it is estimated that from 10 to 20 million people world-wide currently suffer from the disease. The microorganism cannot be cultured *in vitro*, and a vaccine is not yet available (Volinn, 1989).

The onset of leprosy is often insidious and its long incubation period may span up to 10 years. Five major classifications of clinical disease are thought to be determined by the host's immune response, and two extreme clinical histopathological categories are distinguished. At one pole is tuberculoid leprosy characterized by relatively few skin lesions in which the microorganism is hard to identify: at the other is lepromatous leprosy manifest by numerous skin lesions containing many bacilli (Volinn, 1989). Leprosy affects the skin, eyes, peripheral nerves, organs and mucous membranes. If untreated leprosy is progressively crippling.

TREATMENT AND PROGNOSIS

In spite of the harsh treatments accorded by society, few people die from the direct effects of the invading organism itself. In the 1990s prognosis is excellent, given early diagnosis and adherence to prescribed medication. Drugs most commonly used in the treatment on leprosy are dapsone, clofazimine, and rifampicin (Mull et al., 1989). In 1981 the World Health Organization recommended a multi-drug regimen for all leprosy patients because of the growing threat of both primary and secondary resistance. During drug treatment the disease is arrested, non-contagious, and no new symptoms will appear (Mull et al., 1989). Although the patient's life ostensibly may proceed as though there had been no leprosy encounter, adherence to treatment may be required for years. Moreover, medication may have unpleasant side-effects which can be dramatic and distressing: black patches on the face and orange-coloured urine, faeces, sputum, sweat, tears and saliva. These may be substantial and tend to be overlooked in the world literature (Mull et al., 1989). Surgery to ameliorate the symptoms of the disease is possible and is shown to have moderate results (Ramanathan et al., 1991; Ramachandra, 1968).

ADHERENCE

The World Health Organization has the global control of leprosy by the year 2000 as one of its goals (WHO, 1988). However, adherence to treatment world-wide is problematic, with some areas reporting the rate at less than 20% (Koticha & Nair, 1979). The study of the psychological processes involved in non-compliance is therefore crucial to the control of the disease in these terms. Studies of compliance have used models consonant with that of Becker et al. (1979). The probability of compliance in a given situation is regarded as a function of the patient's health beliefs; the duration and complexity of treatment; the relief of symptoms, and the doctor–patient relationship. Such formulations, however, have proved insufficiently sensitive to account for the variety of health behaviours found in the context of leprosy.

Mull et al. (1989) propose that non-compliance is, in part, due to an extremely complex interweaving of variables such as the stigma which continues to be associated with leprosy in many places. Importantly this leads in some cases to years of denial such that both

patients and their families will argue passionately that they do not have leprosy (Mull et al., 1989). It leads also to the consultation of traditional healers or inadequately trained physicians for the initial treatment of symptoms, and inadequate communication between medical personnel and patients. Studies suggest that, in the context of often close knit extended families where joint decision-making is the norm, the term 'non-compliance' is an oversimplification since it will cover a plethora of culturally constrained health-related behaviour.

PSYCHOLOGICAL ASPECTS

Depression is the main psychological feature of patients with leprosy, and anxiety, although a common feature of many clinical states, is reported to be significantly higher in inflicted patients (Ramanathan et al., 1991). It is estimated that 25% of sufferers are deformed. While many of these patients may benefit from surgical intervention and will show a significant reduction in both anxiety and depression, only 50–75% of preoperative expectations are fulfilled, and then in only 49% of patients (Dean, et al., 1983; Ramanathan et al., 1991).

Importantly, the self-concept has been shown to be impaired in a sample of children of leprosy sufferers living in an institution. It is suggested that this attributable to the parents' negative self image, to societal attitudes, and to social seclusion. This squares with the finding that leprosy patients in Indonesia and elsewhere tend to discriminate against themselves more than their healthy contacts (Elissen, 1991).

KNOWLEDGE AND ATTITUDE

Recent studies examining the world-wide knowledge of, and attitude towards, both leprosy and leprosy victims, show that the disease continues to be viewed in a way that is negative and undermining. In central Ethiopia there is a deeply entrenched belief that leprosy is both hereditary and contagious (Teckle-Haimanot et al., 1992). Cook (1982) found that 61% of her respondents in Guyana believed the disease to be incurable, while Awofeso (1992) showed that nurses in Nigeria manifest a below-average basic knowledge and a largely negative perception of the disease. In Trinidad and Tobago education about leprosy began to receive greater emphasis in the 1970s. While understanding of the symptomatology of leprosy in these countries continues to be misunderstood, Suite and Gittens (1992) were able to show a marked difference in knowledge of its cause and course when compared to respondents in Guyana. This suggests that, although the general knowledge of leprosy is deficient, educational interventions may go some way to addressing the stigma associated with the disease. This is borne out by systematic studies carried out in a formerly high endemic area in Jiangsu Province, China. Here, as a consequence of intensive educational interventions since the early 1980s, endemicity of leprosy is nearing full control (Ma et al., 1989). As such, an approach to treatment must embrace the counselling of extended families and the education of the public at large.

CONSIDERATIONS

Psychological models so far have failed to explain the complex relationship of variables associated with adherence to treatment, but studies have shown that lay perceptions of the disease are likely to mediate these to a considerable extent. Additionally, studies have highlighted the need for educational programmes which are culturally sensitive and which emphasize the bacterial causation of the disease; the efficacy of modern chemotherapy which rapidly renders the patient non-infectious, and the fact that early diagnosis and treatment is able to prevent deformity (Awofeso, 1992; Jopling, 1988; Suite & Gittings 1992). Health-care professionals have been shown to be key personnel in destigmatizing the disease (Volinn, 1983).

REFERENCES

Awofesio, N. (1992). Appraisal of the knowledge and attitude of Nigerian nurses toward leprosy. *Leprosy Review*, **63**, 169–72.

Becker, M.H., Maiman, L.A., Kirscht, J.P., Haefner, D.P., Drachman, H.C. & Taylor, D.W. (1979). Patient perceptions and compliance: recent studies of the health belief model. In R.B. Haynes, D.W. Taylor & D.L. Sackett (Eds.). *Compliance in health care*, pp. 78–109. Baltimore, MD: The Johns Hopkins University Press.

Brody, S.N. (1974). *The disease of the soul: leprosy in medieval literature*. Ithaca, NY: Cornell University Press.

Browne, S.G. (1975a). *The diagnosis and management of early leprosy*. London: The Leprosy Mission.

Browne, S.G. (1975b). Some aspects of the history of leprosy: the leprosie of yesterday. *Proceedings of the Royal Society Medicine*, **68**, 485–93.

Cook, A., (1982). An urban community's thoughts about leprosy: a survey in Guyana. *Leprosy Review*, **53**, 285–96.

Dean, D., Chetty, U.D. & Forrest, A.P.M. (1983). Effects of immediate breast reconstruction on psychosocial morbidity after mastectomy. *Lancet*, Feb, 459–62.

Elissen, M.C.C.A. (1991). Beliefs of leprosy patients about their illness: a study in the province of South Sulawesi, Indonesia. *Tropical Geographic Medicine*, **43**, 379–82.

Goldman, L. Moraites, R.S. & Kitzmiller, K. (1966). White spots in Biblical times. *Archives of Dermatology*, **93**, 744–53.

Jopling, W.H. & McDougal (1988). *Handbook of leprosy*, 4th edn, Oxford: Heinemann Professional Publishing.

Koticha, K.K. & Nair, P.R.R. (1979). Treatment of defaulters in leprosy: a reprospective study of 42,000 cases. *International Journal of Leprosy*, **47**, 50–5.

Ma, H.D., Ye, G.Y. Shu, H.W., Jiang, C. & Zhou, D.S. (1989). Studies on social medicine and leprosy in east China. *Proceedings Chinese Academy Medicine Science Peking Union Medical College*, **4**, 61–4.

Mull, J.D., Wood, C.S., Gans, L.P. & Mull, D.S. (1989). Culture and 'compliance' among leprosy patients in Pakistan. *Social Science Med*, **29**, 799–811.

Ramachandra, A.G. (1968). Reconstructive surgery as preparation for rehabilitation. *Leprosy India*, **XLI**, 210–11.

Ramanathan, U., Malaviya, G.N., Jain, N. & Husain, S. (1991). Pychosocial aspects of deformed leprosy patients undergoing surgical correction. *Leprosy Review*, **62**, 402–9.

Richards, P. (1978). *The medieval leper and his northern heirs*. Cambridge: Brewer.

Ridley, M. (1987). The parasitization of macrophages *M. Leprae. The Star*, **46**, 1–5.

Skelly, F.J. & Gibb, K. (1987). Fear of Hansen's stymies plans for clinic. *American Medical News*, **29**, 12 June.

Skinsnes, O.K. (1973). Notes from the history of leprosy. *International Journal of Leprosy*, **41**, 2.

Skinsnes, O.K. & Chang, P.H.C. (1985). Understanding of leprosy in ancient China. *International Journal of Leprosy*, **53**, 289–307.

Suite, M. & Gittens, C. (1992). Attitudes towards leprosy in the outpatient population of dermatology clinics in Trinidad. *Leprosy Review*, **63**, 151–6.

Teckle-Haimanot, R., Forsgren, L., Gebre-Mariam, A., Abebe, M., Holmgren, G., Heijbel, J. & Ekstedt, J. (1992). Attitudes of rural people in central Ethiopia towards leprosy and a brief comparison with observations on epilepsy. *Leprosy Review*, **63**, 157–68.

Varron, A.G. (1939). Fear of disease in the Middle Ages. *CIBA Symposia*, **1**, 224–9.

Volinn, I.J. (1983). Health professionals as stigmatizers and destigmatizers of disease: alcoholism and leprosy as examples. *Social Science Medicine*, **17**, 385–93.

Volinn, I.J. (1989). Issues of definition and their implications: AIDS and leprosy. *Social Science Medicine*, **29**, 1157–62.

Waxler, N.E. (1981). Learning to be a leper: a case study in the social construction on illness. In Mishler *et al.* (Eds). *Social contexts of health, illness and patient care*, pp. 169–194, Cambridge: Cambridge University Press.

Weymouth, A. (1938). Through the leper squint. *International Journal of Leprosy*, **43**, 2.

WHO (1988). *A guide to leprosy control*. Geneva: WHO.

Leukaemia

JOHN WEINMAN

UMDS (Guy's Campus), University of London, UK

Leukaemia is a disease of blood-forming tissues and acute lymphocytic leukaemia (ALL) is the commonest form of childhood cancer. Whereas most cancers grow and spread from a single focus, leukaemia is a widespread disease involving the bone marrow and other blood forming tissue. Unlike normal white blood cells which typically die and are replaced by new cells after a few days or weeks, leukaemia cells retain the ability to multiply but fail to develop to a stage where they can function as defence against infection. Moreover, if the disease progresses, leukaemia cells displace normal white cells and can then proceed to invade the central nervous system.

Children most affected by ALL are under ten years of age at diagnosis. The incidence of the disease appears to diminish after the age of five and drops fairly sharply after then. Before the 1960s the mortality rate was extremely high and less than ten percent of children survived more than five years. Death frequently resulted from progression of the disease within the central nervous system (CNS), principally involving the meninges. However, following the introduction of new treatments particularly those aimed at CNS prophylaxis, survival rates have improved dramatically and these approach 90% in most patients and approximately 70% in those identified as 'high risk' at diagnosis (Barr *et al.*, 1992). CNS prophylaxis involves the administration of cranial irradiation (usually 2400 rads) together with intrathecal chemotherapy and, although it has been very successful, is now thought to have some adverse effects on cognitive functioning (Cousens *et al.*, 1988).

There are a number of psychological aspects of leukaemia. In the early stages following diagnosis there are considerable stresses associated with the disease and treatment. For high risk children, there is still the possibility of death and the consequent demands this places on children and their parents (Maguire *et al.*, 1987) Also, for the relatively small number of patients who do not survive, there are major bereavement effects on parents and other family members. However, for the majority of children and families, the main psychological issues revolve around the immediate demands of coping with the illness and treatment, as well as the possible long-term effects of a major illness and treatment affecting the central nervous system.

Several studies have attempted to document the psychological impact on children with ALL and the picture which emerges is quite variable, depending on premorbid individual and family factors as well as patterns of coping with the illness (for a review see Madan-Swain & Brown (1991)). There is some evidence of lower self-esteem and social competence and increased isolation, but there is no strong evidence of any major psychopathology in these children. These changes may well reflect the influence of several factors including the symptoms experienced, the limited social opportunities and the effects of chemotherapy and other demanding treatments. For example, bone marrow transplantation has been found to be stressful and both social and psychological support is recommended as an integral part of this treatment (Alby, 1991).

Studies of family response to leukaemia indicate that family stress is initially high but that this generally diminishes as treatment progresses and that long-term coping is good (Kupst & Schulman, 1988). However, some studies provide evidence of more persistent distress in individual family members, even though family functioning may not be impaired (Madan-Swain & Brown, 1991). Similarly, a few studies have examined the psychosocial impact on the siblings of ALL patients and have generally found negative effects including isolation, lower self-esteem and problems in coming to terms with the parental demands and involvement with the illness and treatment. Again, there are methodological problems with many of these studies and it is clear that there is considerable variation in parental and sibling responses and that these depend on a range of factors including pre-existing family dynamics, perceptions of the child's illness and coping styles.

There are now a number of studies examining possible cognitive deficits arising from cranial irradiation treatment and the results from these are quite mixed, with some studies showing little or no effects and others showing clear adverse effects (for a review see Cousens *et al.*, 1988)). Despite this variation, the overall picture does indicate that there are often decrements in IQ and other cognitive test performance in cranially irradiated children. The effects are found more consistently in younger children and where follow-up testing is extended for longer time periods after treatment. Although some of these performance decrements are due to other psychosocial effects, including disruption of schooling and emotional reactions. it does appear that some are due directly to CNS prophylaxis. Overall, the IQ results indicate a decrement of around ten IQ points, with consistent impairments on performance tasks involving short-term memory, attention and other aspects of information-processing. Language skills are not commonly impaired, but there is some evidence that these may be found in early onset disease, particularly in children under five (Moehle & Berg, 1985). Not surprisingly, a number of studies have also shown that significantly more children with ALL experience problems in academic performance than comparison groups, such as siblings (e.g. Taylor *et al.*, 1987). It should be noted that the choice of comparison groups for these studies is sometimes questionable, particularly as such factors as school attendance and mood change were often not controlled for.

These cognitive effects are also found in the small but increasing number of long-term follow-up studies of high risk ALL patients. For example, a fairly recent study provides evidence of reduced cognitive ability in approaching 40% of survivors, between six and fifteen years after diagnosis of illness (Feeny *et al.*, 1993). However, it should be noted that this and many other studies typically involve comparisons between ALL patients and different comparison groups. Long-term prospective studies with appropriate control groups are still needed to clarify the picture.

REFERENCES

Alby, N. (1991). Leukaemia: bone marrow transplantation. In M. Watson (Ed.). *Cancer patient care: psychosocial treatment methods.* pp. 281–297, Cambridge: Cambridge University Press.

Barr, R.D., Deveber, L.L., Pai, K.M., Andrew, M., Halton, J., Cairney, A.E. & Whitton, A.C. (1992). Management of children with acute lymphoblastic leukaemia by the Dana-Fairber Cancer Institute protocols.

American Journal Pediatrics Hematology Oncology, 14, 136–9.

Cousens, P., Waters, B., Said, J. & Stevens, M. (1988). Cognitive effects of cranial irradiation in leukaemia, a survey and meta-analysis. *Journal of Child Psychology Psychiatry,* 29, 839–52.

Feeny, D. Leiper, A., Barr, R.D., Furlong, W., Torrance, G.W., Rosenbaum, P. & Weitzman, S. (1993). The comprehensive assessment of health status in survivors of childhood cancer: applications to high risk

lymphoblastic leukaemia *British Journal Cancer,* 1047–152.

Kupst, M.J. & Schulman, J.L. (1988). Long-term coping with paediatric leukaemia: a 6 year follow-up study. *Journal of Pediatric Psychology,* 13, 7–22.

Madan–Swain, A. & Brown, R.T. (1991). Cognitive and psychosocial sequelae for children with acute lymphocytic leukemia and their families *Clinical Psychology Reviews,* 11, 267–94.

Maguire, G.P., Littman, P. Fergusson, J. &

Moss, K. (1987). The psychological sequelae of childhood leukemia. *Recent Results in Cancer Research*, **88**, 47–56.

Moehle, K.A. & Berg, R.A. (1985). Academic achievement and intelligence test performance in children with cancer at diagnosis and one year later. *Developmental & Behavioural Paediatrics*, **6**, 62–4.

Taylor, H.G., Albo, V.C., Phebus, C.K.,

Sachs, B.R. & Bierl, P.G. (1987). Postirradiation treatment outcomes for children with acute lymphocytic leukaemia: clarification of risks. *Journal of Pediatric Psychology*, **12**, 395–411.

Low back pain

SVEN SVEBAK

*Division of Behavioral Medicine,
The Cancer Building, Trondheim University
Hospital, Norway*

Finneson (1980, pp. 186–187) presented a thought-compelling case of low back pain subjected to surgical 'overtreatment'. The patient had initially complained of severe pain in the lower back and extremity. He was taken through a series of three lumbar laminectomies which all increased the original pain and added serious neurological side-effects. He became a narcotics addict and still complained of his pain. Then a prefrontal lobotomy was carried out to control the addiction and alleviate the pain. A wound infection developed and necessitated removal of the entire frontal bone flap before healing occurred. On top of this unfortunate cosmetic side-effect, the patient developed severe crossed abductor spasms involving the lower extremities as well as loss of control of bladder and bowels. The treatments were conducted by outstanding and well-intentioned neurosurgeons who all wanted to help this suffering patient. None the less, the accumulated result was much worse than the original ailment, and his low back pain persisted. The idea gradually developed that the organic basis for perception of this pain involved more than the spine.

EPIDEMIOLOGY

A major proportion of low back pain is due to myalgia, myofascial pain and pain from tendons of muscles such as m. erector spinae, m. iliocostalis lumborum and m. glutaeus medius. These functional pains may not often be taken to the health care system because, in most cases, the transient disability is mild, can be treated by a day or two off work or by the consumption of over-the-counter analgesics. For these reasons, the epidemiology of low back pain is somewhat unsettled. However, surveys of musculoskeletal pain, including items on the lower back, indicate that severe episodes of low back pain may occur in less than 5% of the population, although the incidence of less severe episodes may be as high as 50% over a one year period among the adult population in western societies (Lee *et al.*, 1985; Ursin, *et al.*, 1993). Bru, Mykletun and Svebak (1993a) provided data in support of a distinction between three separate and fairly independent major factors in musculoskeletal pain: the low back area, the neck and shoulder area and the extremities. This factor structure indicates a distinction also between causal factors, and this view is supported in current research.

SURVEY AND CLINICAL ASSESSMENT OF LOW BACK PAIN

People may differ in their concept of the lower back area. Therefore, it is recommended that survey measures provide an illustration of the back where the lower back area is delineated, such as in the Standardized Nordic Questionnaire (Kourinka *et al.*, 1987; see also Westgaard & Jansen, 1992, for assessment of work-related disability). Keefe and Block (1982) presented a system for assessment of five motor behaviours in low back pain patients with good reliability and validity for use in the medical setting (guarded movement, bracing, rubbing of painful area, grimacing, sighing). A much more extensive procedure for diagnostic evaluations of sources of low back pain has been presented by Cyriax & Cyriax (1993).

THE BIOLOGY OF LOW BACK PAIN

Like all other pain, low back pain is a subjective phenomenon. It relates to spinal segments T6 or below. The psychobiological status of the central nervous system can mediate as well as moderate pain perception. This perspective on pain was presented by Melzack and Wall (1965). Since, then support has accumulated for sensitization of pain pathways that may respond with pain even to non-specific activation of the central nervous system (Cervero & Laird, 1991). These developments call upon a wider orientation to diagnostic procedures in low back pain than a search for organic changes in the lumbar area. This is not to say that surgery should be abandoned in treatment of low back pain. Rather, surgery appears to be justified provided there is (i) X-ray support to disc herniation with (ii) radicular and (iii) persistent pain along dermatome of involved extremity.

Several sources of low back pain reflect actual changes of the lower back tissue beyond those due to disc herniation. Structural changes of the spine in and of themselves seldom give rise to any symptomatic problem, although such changes can provoke pain as secondary consequences of spine-related disabilities. One example would be the muscle tension patterns to compensate a severe scoliosis. Other infrequent sources of low back pain include fractures, inflammations and tumors that affect the lumbar pain pathways.

Pain-conducting fibres reside on the outer surface of discs. The discs act as pressure-absorbing cushions located between spine segments. Spinal load can be high or low as well as acute or enduring. Some patterns of motor behaviour present cyclic rotation-related load of the spine resulting in a pumping shift of algogenic substances from the inner gel to pain fibres on the disc surface. These fibres are somatic C and A delta fibres, and they may undergo hypersensitization as well as exposure to pain-producing acid metabolites, prostaglandins and other algogenic substances that are forced out from the degenerating gel nucleus of the disc.

Surgery is grounded upon biomechanical conceptions of pathology and therapy. Despite the application of sensitive diagnostic criteria for the use of surgery in low back pain, failure rates in discectomies are around 10% and in spinal segment fusions around 15%. Major indications for artificial disc treatment should include several criteria beyond structural X-ray changes: (i) low back pain and disability for more than two years, (ii) poor response to conservative treatment, exercises and medication, (iii) moderately to severely incapacitating symptoms and (iv) a stable personal lifestyle, working as tolerated, and with motivation to get well (Ray, 1992).

THE PSYCHOLOGY OF LOW BACK PAIN

All since Taylor's (1968) pioneering report on absenteeism from work among employees in a petroleum industry in Britain, psychological factors have been increasingly more important in the study of causal factors as well as intervention procedures. This change of perspective is embedded within the multifactorial understanding of myalgia, myofascial pain and tendonitis as illustrated in Fig. 1.

The so-called psychosomatic V describes a particular response pattern to items of the Minnesota Multiphasic Personality Inventory (MMPI), and it has been proposed as a characteristic of low back pain patients. The V-pattern involves relatively high scores on hysteria and hypochondriasis in combination with a low score on items for depression. The idea of a 'psychosomatic V' personality has proven to be of little value in assessment of low back pain and prediction of treatment outcomes (Lowe & Peck, 1987; Prokop, 1986; Schmidt & Arntz, 1987). However, some findings indicate poor outcome in patients with high scores on hypochondriasis due to a general preference for chronic illness behaviour. One should keep in mind that the MMPI was established on psychiatric patients rather than on pain patients.

Patients who meet criteria for chronic low back pain (on a daily basis for 6 months or longer), have elevated scores on somatization disorder although they do not meet DSM-III criteria for this diagnosis (Bacon *et al.*, 1994). Somatization is positively correlated with incidence of lifetime major depression as well as alcohol dependence among these patients. Malingering and sickness certification depend to a large extent upon subjective statements from the patient. Around 50% of days lost due to sickness absence relate to musculoskeletal pain (Ursin *et al.*, 1993).

Personality can increase risk of low back pain in three different ways: (i) One acts upon motor behaviour patterns to mediate effortful coping with ergonomic load. An example would be heavy lifting at work where the lumbar load can be more severe in employees who score high on motivational measures of habitual impatience and the willingness to respond with high motor effort in coping with ergonomic load (Bru, Mykletun & Svebak, 1993b). This over-responsiveness to ergonomic load presents a risk of pain both from

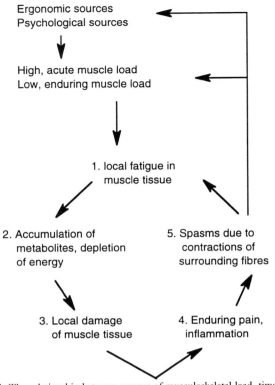

Fig. 1. The relationship between sources of musculoskeletal load, time parameters and tissue tolerance. The arrows indicate hypothesized patterns of nested 'vicious circles' in musculoskeletal pain.

(a) lumbar spine load as well as from (b) lower back soft tissue load. (i) The other acts upon sensory processing to (a) mediate or (b) moderate the experience of pain. One example of mediation of pain is unemployment where the attention upon body states is facilitated in lack of extrinsic attentional demands (Pennebaker, 1982). An example of moderation is the old use of hypnotic suggestibility to facilitate a focus of attention away from pain (Mumford, 1962). (iii) More indirect psychological sources of load to the spine are due to (a) dysfunctional habitual body postures that cause enduring muscle strain and (b) obesity due to eating habits that cause accumulated body weight.

Low back pain is sometimes part of a more generalized pattern of musculoskeletal pain, such as in fibromyalgia (Masi & Yunus, 1990) and long-standing hypothyroidism resulting in proximal myopathy (Krupsky *et al.*, 1987). In such cases, muscle tension and spinal load appear to have little causal importance in the direct sense (e.g. Svebak, Anjia & Kårstad, 1993), and psychological changes such as depression and apathy may be consequences of pain rather than causal.

PSYCHOLOGICAL INTERVENTION

It is increasingly more obvious from modern research that mental passivity and physical inactivity can make pain worse as well as increase illness behaviour. Inactivity should therefore, be discouraged in most cases of functional low back pain, and appropriate mental and physical activity levels should be encouraged (e.g. Fordyce *et al.*, 1986). Load tolerance can be increased by physical training under expert supervision to avoid additional strain. The first successful behavioural programme for low back pain intervention was reported by Fordyce (1976) and focused upon the extinction of pain behaviours and increase of well behaviours. This approach has later been combined with gradual increases in guided exercise (Anderson et al., 1977; Turner & Clancy, 1988). Turner et al. (1990) compared the effectiveness of behavioural therapy with that of aerobic exercise in 96 mildly disabled low back pain patients. They concluded that no significant difference emerged between programmes including also a group of combined behavioural and exercise treatment, and that all groups remained significantly improved over a follow-up period of 12 months. However, the efficacy of guided strength-enhancing isometric exercise in low back pain intervention remains unsettled.

Bru and colleagues (1994) compared the efficacy of different interventions across areas of the back (neck/shoulder versus lower back). One hundred and nineteen hospital staff volunteered on the basis that they reported pain in neck, shoulders and/or low back (i) over the last seven days, (ii) that had caused leave of absence for some period over the last twelve months and (iii) pain for at least two periods over the last six months. A new approach to interventions was offered to one group in a ten-week cognitive stress management training programme of two hours per week. A contrasting programme of relaxation training was offered to another group, whereas a third group was given a combined cognitive plus relaxation pro-gramme. A waiting list control group was also included. Results showed a significant interaction between type of intervention and area of pain due to superior efficacy for cognitive intervention in neck and shoulder pain, whereas relaxation was superior in low back pain. All these subjects were actively employed as hospital staff throughout intervention.

CONCLUSIONS

Low back pain has emerged as a genuinely biopsychosocial problem where surgery is justified only in cases that meet a set of strictly defined diagnostic criteria. Personality risk factors for low back pain reflect high sensitivity to ergonomical demands combined with impatience and effortful ways of motor coping. These factors appear as different from those in neck and shoulder pain where sensitivity to high emotional load seems to be more involved. Behaviour modification and cognitive coping skills training have proven to be successful in low back pain intervention, and so has physical exercise. A combination of aerobic and low-intensity isometric exercise with relaxation training may prove to be a superior intervention in low back pain among employed staff although it remains to be firmly tested in future research. Enduring physical inactivity is strongly discouraged and should be of particular concern in cases of unemployment or long-term sick leave.

REFERENCES

Anderson, T.P., Cole, T.M., Gullickson, G., Hudgens, A. & Roberts, A.H. (1977). Behavior modification of chronic pain: a treatment program by a multidiciplinary team. *Clinical Orthopaedics and Related Research*, 129, 96–100.

Bacon, N.M.K., Bacon, S.F., Atkinson, J.H., Slater, M.A., Patterson, T.L., Grant, I. & Garfin, S.R. (1994). Somatization symptoms in chronic low back pain patients. *Psychosomatic Medicine*, 56, 118–27.

Bru, E., Mykletun, R. & Svebak, S. (1993a). Assessment of musculo-skeletal and other health complaints in female hospital staff. *Applied Ergonomics*, 25, 101–5.

Bru, E., Mykletun, R. & Svebak, S. (1993b). Neuroticism, extraversion, anxiety and Type A behaviour as mediators of neck, shoulder and lower back pain in female hospital staff. *Personality and Individual Differences*, 15, 485–92.

Bru, E., Mykletun, R., Berge, W.T. & Svebak, S. (1994). Effects of different psychological interventions on neck, shoulder and low back pain in female hospital staff. *Psychology and Health*, 9, 371–82.

Cervero, F. & Laird, J.M.A. (1991). One pain or many pains? A new look at pain mechanisms. *News in Physiological Sciences*, 6, 268–73.

Cyriax, J.H. & Cyriax, P.J. (1993). *Cyriax's illustrated manual of orthopedic medicine* 2nd edn. Oxford: Butterworth-Heinemann.

Finneson, B.E. (1980). Psychology of low back dysfunction. In B.E. Finneson (Ed.). *Low back pain*, pp. 179–197. Philadelphia: Lippincott.

Fordyce, W.E. (1976). *Behavioral methods in chronic pain and illness*. St Louis: Mosby.

Fordyce, W.E., Brockway, J.A., Bergman, J.A. & Spengler, D. (1986). Acute back pain: a control-group comparison of behavioral vs. traditional management methods. *Journal of Behavioral Medicine*, 9, 127–40.

Keefe, F.J. & Block, A.R. (1982). Development of an observation method for assessing pain behavior in chronic low back pain patients. *Behavior Therapy*, 13, 363–75.

Kourinka, I., Jonsson, B., Kilbom, A., Vinterberg, H., Biering-Sorensen, F., Andersson, G. & Jorgensen, K. (1987). Standardized Nordic Questionnaires for the analysis of musculo-skeletal symptoms. *Applied Ergonomics*, 18, 233–7.

Krupsky, M., Flatau, E., Yarom, R. & Resnitzky, P. (1987). Musculoskeletal symptoms as a presenting sign of long-standing hypothyroidism. *Israel Journal of Medical Sciences*, 23, 1110–13.

Lee, P., Helewa, A., Smythe, H.A., Bombardier, C. & Goldsmith, C.H. (1985). Epidemiology of musculoskeletal disorders (complaints) and related disability in Canada. *Journal of Rheumatology*, 12, 1169–73.

Lowe, A.W. & Peck, C.L. (1987). The MMPI and psychological factors in chronic low back pain: a review. *Pain*, 28, 1–12.

Masi, A.T. & Yunus, M.B. (1990). Fibromyalgia – which is the best treatment? A personalized, comprehensive, ambulatory, patient-involved management programme. *Baillière's Clinical Rheumatology*, 4, 333–69.

Melzack, R. & Wall, P.D. (1965). Pain mechanism: a new theory. *Science*, 150, 971–9.

Mumford, J. (1962). *Psychosomatic yoga*. London: Thorsons Publishers.

Pennebaker, J.W. (1982). *The psychology of physical symptoms*. New York: Springer-Verlag.

Prokop, C.K. (1986). Hysteria scale elevations in low back pain patients: a risk factor for misdiagnosis? *Journal of Consulting and Clinical Psychology*, 54, 558–62.

Ray, C.D. (1992). The artificial disk: introduction, history and socioeconomics. In J.N. Weinstein (Ed.). *Clinical efficacy and outcome in the diagnosis and treatment of low back pain*. pp. 205–225. New York: Raven Press.

Schmidt, A.J.M. & Arntz, A. (1987). Psychological research and chronic low back pain: a stand-still or breakthrough? *Social Science in Medicine*, 25, 1095–104.

Svebak, S., Anjia, R. & Kårstad, S.I. (1993). Task-induced electromyographic activation in fibromyalgia subjects and controls. *Scandinavian Journal of Rheumatology*, 22, 124–30.

Low back pain

Taylor, P.J. (1968). Personal factors associated with sickness absence: a study of 194 men with contrasting sickness absence experience in a refinery population. *British Journal of Industrial Medicine*, **25**, 106–18.

Turner, J.A. & Clancy, S. (1988). Comparison of operant behavioral and cognitive – behavioral group treatment for chronic low back pain. *Journal of Consulting and Clinical Psychology*, **56**, 261–6.

Turner, J.A., Clancy, S., McQuada, K.J. & Cardenas, D.D. (1990). Effectiveness of behavioral therapy for chronic low back pain: a component analysis. *Journal of Consulting and Clinical Psychology*, **58**, 573–9.

Ursin, H., Endresen, I.M., Svebak, S., Tellnes, G. & Mykletun, R. (1993). Muscle pain and coping with working life in Norway: a review. *Work and Stress*, **7**, 247–58.

Westgaard, R. & Jansen, T. (1992). Individual and work-related factors associated with symptoms of musculoskeletal complaints. 1: a quantitative registration system. *British Journal of Industrial Medicine*, **49**, 147–53.

Lung cancer

ROBERT WEST

and

LUCY RINK

Psychology Department,
St George's Hospital Medical School,
London, UK

Cancer of the lung is an almost wholly preventable disease that claims more than a million lives each year world-wide. Survival rates following diagnosis are around 1 in 10. Cigarette smoking is believed to account for at least 85% of cases (e.g. Bartecchi, Mackenzie & Schrier, 1994). Giving up smoking after diagnosis of lung cancer improves the prospects of survival (Johnston-Early *et al.*, 1980), although many smokers continue smoking after treatment (Davison & Duffu, 1982). Environmental tobacco smoke may also be responsible for cases of lung cancer in non-smokers (Environmental Protection Agency, 1992; Wang *et al.*, 1994). There is some evidence to suggest that there is an increased risk of developing lung cancer when smoking is combined with eating a large amount of cholesterol in the diet (Goodman *et al.*, 1988). Prolonged exposure to radon gas, which accumulates in basements of houses situated in granite areas, also appears to increase risk of lung cancer (Ennever, 1990). Genetic factors probably influence susceptibility to environmental carcinogens (Bernhardt & Rauch, 1993). It has also been suggested that exposure to stressful life events may increase susceptibility (Bandyopadhyay *et al.*, 1986).

The psychological distress caused by lung cancer is probably a function of fear of death, discomfort and disability caused by the disease and the side-effects of treatment. A study carried out on the quality of life of women suffering from lung cancer showed that they suffered from fatigue, difficulty with household chores, worry about their ability to care for themselves, and worry about progression of the disease (Sarna, 1993).

As would be expected, level of emotional support appears to help mitigate psychological distress in sufferers (Ell *et al.*, 1988; Quinn, Fontana & Reznikoff, 1986). It may also prolong survival (Ell *et al.*, 1992).

Some coping strategies which have been observed are wish-fulfilling fantasy, self-blaming, denial, and emotional expression (Quinn, Fontana & Reznikoff, 1986). There is some evidence that greater postdiagnosis distress is linked with lower survival rates (Kukull, McCorkle & Driever, 1986) and that greater anxiety at the start of treatment is linked with poorer functioning post-treatment (Graydon, 1988). This suggests that psychological help for patients diagnosed with lung cancer should involve helping to establish and reinforce emotional support networks and counselling to reduce anxiety. It would also be worthwhile providing assistance with smoking cessation.

REFERENCES

Bandyopadhyay, S., Ghosh, K.K., Chattopadhyay, P.K. & Majumdar, A. (1986). Hormone correlates of life stress events in lung and oral cancer patients. *Social Science International*, **2**, 1–10.

Bartecchi, C., Mackenzie, T. & Schrier, R. (1994). The human cost of tobacco use. *The New England Journal of Medicine*, **330**, 907–13.

Bernhardt, B. & Rauch, J.B. (1993). Genetic family histories: an aid to social work assessment. *Families in Society*, **74**, 195–206.

Davison, G. & Duffu, M. (1982). Smoking habits of long term survivors of surgery for lung cancer. *Thorax*, **37**, 331–3.

Ell, K.O., Nishimoto, R.H., Mantell, J.E. & Hamovitch, M.B. (1988). Psychological adaptation to cancer: a comparison among patients, spouses, and nonspouses. *Family Systems Medicine*, **6**, 335–48.

Ell, K., Nishimoto, R., Mediansky, L., Mantell, J & Hamovitch, M. (1992). Social relations, social support and survival among patients with cancer. *Journal of Psychosomatic Research*, **36**, 531–41.

Ennever, F.K. (1990). Predicted reduction in lung cancer risk following cessation of smoking and radon exposure. *Epidemiology*, 1, 134–40.

Environmental Protection Agency. (1992). *Respiratory health effects of passive smoking: lung cancer and other disorders.* Washington

DC: Office of Health and Environmental Assessment.

Goodman, M.T., Kolonel, L.N., Yoshizawa, C.N. & Hankin, J.H. (1988). The effect of dietary cholesterol and fat on the risk of lung cancer in Hawaii. *American Journal of Epidemiology*, **128**, 1241–55.

Graydon, J.E. (1988). Factors that predict patients' functioning following treatment for cancer. *International Journal of Nursing Studies*, **25**, 117–24.

Johnston-Early, A., Cohen, M.H., Minna, J.D., Paxton, L.M., Fossieck, B.E. Jr., Ihde, D.C.,

Kukull, W.A., McCorkle, R. & Driever, M. (1986). Symptom distress, psychosocial variables, and survival from lung cancer. *Journal of Psychosocial Oncology*, **4**, 91–104.

Quinn, M.E., Fontana, A.F. & Reznikoff, M. (1986). Psychological distress in reaction to lung cancer as a function of spousal support and coping strategy. *Journal of Psychosocial Oncology*, **4**, 79–90.

Sarna, L. (1993). Women with lung cancer: impact on quality of life. *Quality of life Research. An International Journal of Quality of Life, Aspects of Treatment, Care and Rehabilitation*, **2**, 13–22.

Wang, F., Love, E., Liu, N. & Dai, X. (1994). Childhood and adolescent passive smoking and the risk of female lung cancer. *International Journal of Epidemiology*, **23**, 223–30.

Malaria

JAN STYGALL

*Academic Department of Psychiatry and
Behavioural Sciences, Middlesex and UCL,
London, UK*

Malaria is one of the commonest parasitic diseases. It is estimated that over half the world's population live in endemic areas. The disease is transmitted by the bite of an infected female mosquito. The clinical picture is one of recurring rigors, anaemia, toxaemia and enlargement of the spleen, and in its most virulent form the disease can be life threatening.

In the 1950s the World Health Organization supported moves to eradicate the disease worldwide. Unfortunately, financial constraints, poorly developed basic health services and resistance to commonly used insecticides and drugs have prevented the elimination of the disease therefore, efforts now concentrate on control. But, the implementation of these control programmes has also proved problematic. The failure of control programmes has often been attributed to lack of co-operation and poor compliance of the indigenous population. Although there has been extensive evaluation of environmental control methods, very little attention has been directed towards the psychological factors which may influence adherence.

The studies that have been conducted have shown that health and illness behaviour of people in malarious areas are related not only to socioeconomic and demographic characteristics, but also indigenous knowledge, beliefs and perceptions about the disease (Fungladda, 1991). Knowledge regarding the causation of the disease varies widely, area by area, with some studies indicating that the indigenous population have a good knowledge of disease causation and others show that various communities are often not aware of the causes of malaria (Okunmekan 1983), or do not believe that the disease is caused by a mosquito (Barnes, 1968; Agyepong, 1992; Aikins *et al.*, 1993). In certain areas diseases are believed to be invoked by the spirits of the dead, anger of local deities and black magic. These, often firmly held, beliefs have proved to be a barrier to the effectiveness of control programmes. Barnes (1968) found that appropriate beliefs regarding causation were related to adherence of mosquito net use. Rauyajin conducted a study in Thailand (cited in a review by Rauyajin, (1991) and found that, although 98.7% of his study population believed that mosquitos could cause malaria, 73.6% believed that other factors (eg dirty water, spirits) were also vectors of the disease. It is common, in many developing countries, for traditional beliefs to exist side by side with orthodox medicine in this manner. It has been argued that traditional theories and practices can remain fairly dominant. This is particularly likely with a disease as old and familiar to communities in endemic areas as malaria. Agyepong (1992) has shown that ethnomedical perceptions and practices relating to malaria are different from the biomedical ones on which malaria control is based.

Perceived susceptibility and severity of malaria has been found to be associated with malaria-related preventative and illness behaviours. One of the main reasons given for the failure of health education in malaria control in Nepal was that no threat of malaria by the rural people was perceived (Dhillon & Kar, 1965; Gramicca, 1981). For centuries people in malarious areas have considered malaria to be part of their everyday lives and, as such, cannot see the reason for concern.

Studies have reported (Rauyajin, 1991) that, even in high endemic areas, a significant proportion of the community did not perceive any threat of malaria to themselves, and 82% of the villagers felt that malaria was so common that it was not frightening. Interestingly, she also found that perceived susceptibility and severity of malaria was not related to mosquito net use and that perceived severity was negatively associated with mosquito repellent use, it was suggested that the villagers may protect themselves by more traditional methods.

Conversely, a study conducted in rural Ghana by Belcher, Nicholas and Blumenfeld in 1975 found a positive relationship between mothers' perception of the severity of malaria and their co-operation with the malaria prophylaxis programme.

Malaria

Ager (1992) interviewed 120 individuals from the rural Malawian population, where malaria is highly prevalent. Malaria was commonly perceived as both an unpredictable and uncontrollable health risk. Adherence to malaria preventative practices was not predicted by judgements of the likelihood, seriousness, predictability or controllability of infection, but more likely to be determined by other factors such as requests from the village headman. These studies indicate that social and traditional mechanisms play an important part in the community's health behaviour, therefore such factors must be well researched before embarking on a prevention programme.

Although malaria occurs naturally in many parts of the tropics and subtropics, it is increasingly seen outside these areas due to air transport of infected mosquitoes or asymptomatic individuals already infected, entering the country. The number of reported cases of malaria in the UK has progressively increased. Data suggest that the groups who are importing malaria are already resident in Britain and travel for short visits to malarious areas (Phillips-Howard et al., 1988). Coole, Wiselka and Nicholson (1989) revealed that many people who travel to places where malaria is prevalent do not take adequate prophylaxis, some do not even seek advice. This was particularly so of people, now established in the UK, returning to their country of origin for a holiday, who often consider that they are still immune to malaria.

Malaria is likely to become a growing problem with more frequent travel and increasingly resistant strains of the parasite.

REFERENCES

Ager, A. (1992). Perception of risk for malaria and schistosomiasis in rural Malawi. *Tropical Medicine and Parasitology*, **43**, 234–8.

Agyepong, I.A. (1992). Malaria: ethnomedical perceptions and practice in an Adangbe farming community and implications for control. *Social Science Medicine* **35**, 131–7.

Aikins, M.K., Pickering, H., Alonso P.L. D'Alessandro, V., Lindsay, S.W., Todd, J. & Greenwood, B.M. (1993). A malaria control trial using insecticide-treated bed nets and targeted chemoprophylaxis in a rural area of The Gambia, West Africa. 4. Perceptions of the causes of malaria and of its treatment and prevention in the study area. *Transitions of the Royal Society of Tropical Medicine and Hygienic* **87**, Suppl 2, 25–30.

Barnes, S.T. (1968). Malaria eradication in Surinam: prospects of success after five years of health education. *International Journal of Health Education*, **11**, 20–31.

Belcher, W.D., Nicholas, D.D. & Blumenfeld, S.N. (1975). Factors influencing utilization of malaria prophylaxis programme in Ghana. *Social Science Medicine*, **9**, 241–8.

Coole, L., Wiselka M.J. & Nicholson, K.G. (1989). Malaria prophylaxis in travellers from Britain. *Journal of Infection*, **18**, 209–12.

Dhillon, H.S. & Kar, S.B. (1965) Malaria eradication – an investigation of cultural patterns and beliefs among tribal populations in India. *International Journal of Health Education* **8**, 31–40.

Fungladda, W. (1991). Health behaviour and illness behaviour of malaria: a review. In S. Sornmani & W. Fungladda (Eds.). *Social and economic aspects of malaria Control.* Bangkok: MRC Propmed.

Gramicca, G. (1981). Health education in malaria control – why has it failed? *World Health Forum.* **2**, 285–93.

Okunmekan, D.A. (1983). Control of malaria with special reference to socioeconomic factors. *Tropical Doctor*, 185–6.

Phillips-Howard, P.A., Bradley, D.J., Blaze, M. & Hum, M. (1988). Malaria in Britain 1977–86. British Medical Journal **296**, 245–8.

Rauyajin, O. (1991). Factors affecting malaria related behavior: a literature review of behavioral theories and relevant research. In S. Sornmani and W. Fungladda (Eds.). *Social and economic aspects of malaria control.* Bangkok: MRC Propmed.

Mastalgia

CAROL A. MORSE

Faculty of Nursing Royal Melbourne Institute of Technology, Victoria, Australia

Mastalgia (benign breast disease) regarded as an aberration of the normal rather than a disease process (Gateley *et al.*, 1992), refers to pain and swelling in the breasts that may be related or unrelated to phases of the menstrual cycle particularly the luteal phase. It is reported commonly by pre menopausal women and the peak incidence occurs around 34 years of age. Women may seek medical advice for breast 'lumps' with or without shooting pains through the breast tissue, or generalized 'soreness' or tenderness. Up to 70% of well women report mastalgia occurring every two to three months (Leinster, Whitehouse & Walsh, 1987), with 60% of employed women reporting cyclical breast pains, although less than 4% actually use treatments for relief.

Typically, mastalgia is characterized by multiple small nodules rather than the development of any particular dominant lump, and on histological biopsy or ultrasonography no cellular changes are detectable. The main reason for investigation is to exclude sub clinical cancer through palpation, inspection of any visible changes, and mammography which should be carried out on any woman with a family history of breast cancer among first-degree female relatives, or those aged over the age of 30 years. Differential diagnostics should seek to exclude confounding of primary mastalgia from that associated with premenstrual syndrome, caffeinism, and stressful lifestyles. Women may seek help because of worry about their breast problem or because of secondary effects arising from increased tension, irritability, disturbed sleep, uncomfortable sexual relations, and general interference with their preferred lifestyle.

ASSESSMENT

A detailed history should include precise information of site, spread, onset, timing of pain, relationship to menstrual cycle phase and any other symptoms that may suggest a cancer. Any milk-like fluid from a nipple suggests the need to measure serum prolactin levels for possible prolactinoma. A daily breast and menstrual chart, completed for at least two consecutive months, will provide information on presence and severity of breast pain, presence of nodules, and their relationship to the timing and heaviness of the menstrual flow.

Women using the oral contraceptive pill should be advised to try non-hormonal means of contraception during a comparative assessment phase, as cyclical mastalgia in oral contraceptive users has been associated with an increased relative risk of breast cancer (Plu-Bureau *et al.*, 1992).

MANAGEMENT

Treatments include Danazol, the drug of choice, Bromocriptine, Evening Primrose Oil or luteinizing hormone releasing hormone (LHRH) (Mansel, 1988).

Danazol, an anti-gonadotropin agent, is effective on local breast tissue and the pituitary–ovarian axis. Initial use promoted high doses of over 400 mg daily that produced side-effects of acne, facial hirsutism and deepened voice. Dosage is now recommended at 100 mg twice daily, and, reduced to a maintenance level of 50–100 mg daily, fewer side-effects have been reported.

Bromocriptine, a dopamine receptor agonist that inhibits prolactin secretion has been shown to be most suitable for cyclical breast pain when taken across the whole cycle. Doses are usually 2.5–5 mg daily, although side-effects of nausea, vomiting, postural hypotension and headache have been reported at levels over 2.5 mg.

Evening Primrose Oil reduces the elevated saturated fatty acids commonly found in mastalgia sufferers using western diets and overcomes the hypothesized deficiency in essential fatty acids. There have been fewer instances of side-effects, but efficacy is also lower and slower. However, no controlled studies of evening primrose oil have been conducted, so claims must be regarded with caution. Effective nutritional management including reduction of caffeine intake could also be of use in reducing the severity of breast symptoms. High caffeine consumption has been linked to fibrocystic breast disorders by Minton and colleagues (1979) and to human fertility problems (James & Paull, 1985).

LHRH agonists have been utilized for tumours dependent on steroid sex hormones, contraception, menorrhagia and endometriosis in particular. Agonists may be delivered by intranasal spray, intramuscular injection or subcutaneous implant. Relief of breast symptoms must be weighed against the likelihood of induced reduction of oestradiol release in premenopausal women. Over time, this could result in undesirable bone demineralization, the development of osteoporosis and possibly increased risks for heart disease.

Treatment-resistant mastalgia has been noted in up to 40% of women attending breast disorders clinics (Jenkins *et al.*, 1993). Psychological morbidity of major depression, anxiety or panic disorder may be revealed on psychiatric evaluation that is amenable to psychotropic medication before relief of the mastalgia is attempted.

Psychological therapies have not been specifically evaluated for symptom relief of mastalgia. A recent controlled study in England (Cooper & Garagher, 1992) compared the coping strategies of 1596 women referred to a breast screening clinic for breast disease. Women identified with either no disease or benign disease used more effective positive coping strategies than did other subjects. This suggests that cognitive–behavioural strategies to promote and enhance coping skills may have a prophylactic role to play, particularly if stress management is learned that can positively influence a woman's total lifestyle. Thus, behavioural management strategies could have a considerable, if not major, role to play in the relief of breast problems.

REFERENCES

Cooper C.L. & Garagher E.B. (1992). Coping strategies and breast disorders/cancer. *Pschological Med.* **22**, 447–55.

Gateley, C.A. Maddox, P.R. Pritchard, G.A. & Hughes, L.E. (1992). Plasma fatty acid profiles in benign breast disorders. *British Journal of Surgery*, **79**, 407–9.

James, J. & Paull, I. (1985). Caffeine and human reproduction. *Review of Environmental Health*, **5**, 151–62.

Jenkins P.L. Jamil, N. Gateley, C.A. & Mansel, R.E. (1993). Psychiatric illness in patients with severe treatment-resistant mastalgia. *General Hospital Psychiatry*, **15**, 55–7.

Leinster, S.J., Whitehouse, G.H. & Walsh P.V. (1987). Cyclical mastalgia: clinical and mammographic observations in a screened population. *British Journal of Surgery*, **74**, 220–22.

Mansel R.E. (1988). Investigation and treatment of benign cyclical breast disease. In M.G. Brush & E.M. Goudsmit (Eds.). *Functional Disorders of the menstrual cycle.* pp. 191–198. London: John Wiley & Sons Ltd.

Minton, J.P., Foecking M.K., Webster, D.J. & Matthews R.H. (1979). Caffeine, cyclic nucleotides and breast disease. *Surgery*, **135**, 157–8.

Plu–Bureau, G., Thalabard J.C., Sitruk-Ware, R, Asselain & Mauvais-Jarvis, P. (1992). Cyclical mastalga as a marker of breast cancer. *British Journal of Surgery*, **65**, 945–9.

Meningitis

JAN STYGALL

Academic Department of Psychiatry and
Behavioural Sciences, Middlesex and UCL,
London, UK

Infection of the central nervous system (CNS) can affect the membranes surrounding the brain and spinal cord (meninges), giving rise to meningitis. The disease develops rapidly. There are various forms of meningitis, some life-threatening, especially if diagnosis is delayed. With most forms, the patient suffers headache, vomiting and neck stiffness. Children and young adults are the most vulnerable, although childhood meningitis from Haemophilus influenzae type b (Hib) is disappearing as widespread vaccination programmes are being implemented.

Recovery may be associated with long-term CNS damage manifesting in neurological disorders. Taylor (1987) found that the greatest impairments were on tasks of visuomotor skill, problem-solving, memory and learning, and psychomotor and mental efficiency. The nature and extent of the morbidity associated with meningitis varies with disease type.

For example, Gade *et al.* (1992) suggested that detectable and sometimes serious cognitive impairment does occur in survivors from pneumococcal meningitis, although it is probably infrequent. Bergman *et al.* (1992), however found no impairments of neurological function or development in their study of survivors of enteroviral meningitis.

Many neuropsychological studies have been conducted into the consequences of meningitis but there is a dearth of literature regarding health-related behaviour or psychosocial aspects of the disease. Family's socioeconomic status has been shown to have an effect on the aftermath of the disease. Taylor *et al.* (1990) found that the consequences of Haemophilus influenzae type b meningitis affects multiple aspects of child development. They found Index subjects had poorer reading skills than their siblings and were more likely to be receiving special education. Age at time of testing, sex and family's socioeconomic status influenced the sequelae of the disease.

A study by Feldman and Michaels (1988) included among its measures family and school support, i.e. interest in, and help with, school work. They found their group of children, who had recovered from meningitis due to Haemophilus influenzae, where achieving as well at school as their siblings. They argued that this differing result from other studies could be due to the fact that their subject group appeared to receive more school and family support than the siblings. The parents did not attribute their increased support directly to the child's previous illness or to fears of brain damage, but suggested that their children solicited more help.

Ramachandran and Prabhaker (1992) report a study of children receiving chemotherapy for tuberculosis meningitis. They found a high rate of compliance and punctuality was achieved which they attributed to initial and periodic motivation from the staff.

Since 1987 when Taylor suggested that more studies should be directed to examine the psychosocial aspects of the disease, very little research has been conducted into the psychological factors that may contribute to risk of meningitis or those that may influence recovery.

REFERENCES

Bergman, I., Painter, M., Wald, E., Chiponis, D. Holland, A.L. & Taylor H. G. (1992). Outcome in children with enteroviral meningitis during the first year of life. *Journal of Pediatrics*, 110, 705–9.

Feldman, H.M. & Michaels R.H. (1988). Academic achievement in children ten to 12 years after *Haemophilus influenzae* meningitis. *Pediatrics*, 81, 339–44.

Gade, A., Bohr, V., Bjerrum, J., Udesen &

Mortensen, E.L. (1992). Neuropsychological sequelae in 91 cases of pneumococcal meningitis. *Developmental Neuropsychology*, 8, 447–57.

Ramachandran, P. & Prabhakar, R. (1992). Defaults, defaulter action and retrieval of patients during studies on tuberculous meningitis in children. *Tuberculous Lung Disease*, 73, 170–3.

Taylor, H.G. (1987). Childhood sequelae of early neurological disorders: a contemporary perspective. *Developmental Neuropsychology*, 3, 153–64.

Taylor, H.G., Mills, E.L. Du Berger, R., Walters, G.V., Gold, R. MacDonald, N., & Michaels, R.H. (1990). The sequelae of *Haemophilus influenzae* meningitis in school-age children. *New England Journal of Medicine*, 323, 1657–63.

Menopause and postmenopause

MYRA S. HUNTER

*Unit of Psychology, UMDS (Campus) University
of London, Guy's, London, UK*

The menopause literally refers to a woman's last menstrual period occurring, on average, between 50 and 51 years of age. Cessation of menstruation is preceded by a gradual reduction in output of oestrogen by the ovaries and fewer ovulatory cycles (see Richardson, 1993). The menopause transition is characterized by hot flushes and night sweats, or vasomotor symptoms, which are experienced by between 50 and 70% of women in western cultures. For the majority of women these are not seen as problematic. It is estimated that between 10 and 15% find them difficult to cope with, mainly because of their frequency or their disruptive effects upon sleep. The average duration of the menopause transition, assessed by menstrual changes and hot flushes, is estimated to be four years but there is considerable variation between women (McKinlay, Brambrilla & Posner, 1992).

The menopause has for centuries been associated with emotional and physical pathology, and myths about its impact upon sexual life, femininity, ageing and women's sanity abound. Although once thought to cause psychosis (involutional melancholia), there is no evidence to suggest that psychiatric disorder is caused by the menopause. The commonly used term 'change of life' reflects the view that the menopause is closely associated with general emotional and social adaptations of mid-life.

It was the development of hormone replacement or oestrogen therapy (HRT) that has had major impact upon definitions of the menopause and medical practice. The menopause is seen as a cluster of physical and emotional symptoms that is caused by deficiency in reproductive hormones. The symptoms are then treated with HRT. While initially recommended for the treatment of hot flushes, HRT has, during the past 10 to 15 years, been advocated for the alleviation of emotional and physical symptoms, as well as the prevention of osteoporosis and cardiovascular disease in postmenopausal women. Nevertheless, uptake and adherence to HRT regimes is relatively low, particularly in the UK where it is estimated that it is used by 9% of menopausal women. Moreover, studies of the effects of HRT for psychological symptoms have not provided adequate evidence to support this use of the treatment (Hunter, 1993a). (See 'Osteoporosis' for more on HRT.)

Psychologists and other social scientists have attempted to understand the nature of changes across the menopause transition: in particular, to clarify the relationship between menopause and depressed mood. Early studies suffered from methodological problems, such as reliance upon clinical samples, use of unstandardized measures, and failure to control for age effects and cohort differences when comparing groups of women of differing menopausal status. Cross-sectional studies produced mixed results, but several prospective studies carried out in the 1980s together provide fairly strong evidence that the menopause does not have a negative effect upon mood or well-being for the majority of mid-aged women (see Greene & Visser, 1992). In contrast, those seeking help from menopause clinics report higher levels of distress and psychosocial problems.

Studies comparing the experience of the menopause in different cultures tend to reveal a diversity of experience, suggesting that the meaning ascribed to it and women's reactions to it are, in part, culturally determined (Lock, 1986). Psychologists have examined the influence of psychosocial factors such as life stresses, beliefs and expectations, as well as sociodemographic variables as predictors of menopausal experience. In general, psychosocial factors have been found to account for a greater proportion of the variation in measures of mood and psychological symptoms than stage of menopause.

Predictors of depressed mood during the menopause include a history of depressed mood, low socioeconomic status, life stress (particularly that involving losses or exits of people from the social network), and negative beliefs, for example, that the menopause is likely to bring emotional and physical problems. Women who have an early menopause, those who have severe hot flushes and those who have undergone surgical menopause have been found to be more likely to experience emotional reactions (see Hunter, 1993b). Correlational studies have failed to find a significant relationship between oestrogen levels and depressed mood. However, it is possible that the rapid withdrawal of hormones, as occurs with removal of the ovaries, might have impact upon mood.

The implications of this research have been an increased awareness of the need to provide balanced information and to counter negative beliefs about the menopause and postmenopause, as well as the need to develop clinical interventions for those women who do experience problems during this time of life.

A recent study has evaluated the effects of workshops preparing 45 year-old women for the menopause upon knowledge and attitudes of premenopausal women (Liao & Hunter, 1994), and significant increases in knowledge and reductions in negative beliefs were evident following the workshops.

Given that women who do seek help for menopausal problems tend to have higher levels of distress than non-attenders at clinics, it has been suggested that they may be attributing distress resulting from life problems to the menopause. Problem clarification using a biopsychosocial framework might enable a range of possible influences to be considered. There is some evidence to suggest that psychological therapies might be beneficial in helping these women to find appropriate solutions to their problems (Greene & Hart, 1987).

Psychological treatments for menopausal hot flushes using forms of relaxation and counselling have also been developed with promising results (see, for example, Freedman & Woodward, 1992).

REFERENCES

Freedman, R.R. & Woodward, S. (1992). Behavioral treatment of menopausal hot flushes: evaluation by ambulatory monitoring. *American Journal of Obstetrics and Gynecology*, **167**, 436–9.

Greene, J.G. & Hart, P.M. (1987). The evaluation of a psychological treatment programme for menopausal women. *Maturitas*, **9**, 41–8.

Greene, J.G. & Visser, A. (1992). Longitudinal studies of the menopause. Special Issue. *Maturitas*, **14**, 117–26.

Hunter, M.S. (1993*a*). The effects of oestrogen therapy on mood and well-being. In G.

Berg & M. Hammar (Eds.). *The modern management of the menopause*, pp. 177–184. London: Parthenon.

Hunter, M.S. (1993*b*). Predictors of menopausal symptoms – psychological aspects. In H.G. Burger (Ed.). *The menopause. clinical endocrinology and metabolism*, pp. 33–46. London: Baillière Tindall.

Liao, K.L.M. & Hunter, M.S. (1994). The women's midlife project: an evaluation of psychological services for mid-aged women in general practice. *Clinical Psychology Forum*, **65**, 19–22.

Lock, M. (1986). Ambiguities of ageing: Japanese experience and perceptions of the menopause. *Culture, Menopause and Psychiatry*, **10**, 23–46.

McKinlay, S.M., Brambrilla, D.J. & Posner, J. (1992). The normal menopause transition. *Maturitas*, **14**, 103–16.

Richardson, S. (1993). The biological basis of the menopause. In H.G. Burger (Ed.). *The menopause, clinical endocrinology and metabolism*, pp. 1–16. London: Baillière Tindall.

Menstrual abnormalities

CAROL A. MORSE

Faculty of Nursing, Royal Melbourne Institute of Technology, Victoria, Australia

Menstrual abnormalities are defined as conditions from unusual bleeding patterns (heavy bleeding, reduced or absent bleeding – (amenorrhoea)); conditions arising from abnormal neurotransmitter activity (dysmenorrhoea); and clusters of subjectively experienced complaints (premenstrual syndrome).

BLEEDING DISORDERS

Menorrhagia

Menorrhagia (heavy bleeding) is diagnosed when menstrual bleeding exceeds 80 ml per menstruation or 'period' in any one cycle. Women may experience bleeding that is prolonged beyond a five-day span; or bleeding that over time exceeds their past usual pattern; or that occurs more frequently than every three to four weeks. Such blood losses over time will lead to iron deficiency anaemia characterized by fatigue, low mental and physical energy, shortness of breath, palpitations, skin paleness, swelling of hands, feet and even of the face in prolonged cases.

Aetiology

Evidence during the last decade implicates abnormal prostaglandin levels in endometrium showing increased $PGF_{2\alpha}$ and PGE_2 production during the menstrual flow of women suffering heavy bleeding (Rees *et al.*, 1984). Alternatively, benign growths (fibroids) of the myometrium may contribute to an enlarged surface area that produces a greater bleeding loss.

Assessment and Treatment

Many studies have relied on women's subjective reports of heavy and increased blood loss. Blood loss should be assessed objectively through weighing collected tampons and pads used each bleeding period for at least two consecutive cycles and again during medical treatment to accurately evaluate changes in blood loss.

If fibroids are discovered, simple myectomy or surgical removal of the total uterus may be advocated. Excessive prostaglandin levels in menorrhagia respond well to the use of prostaglandin synthetase inhibitors. Mefenamic acid reduces both $PGF_{2\alpha}$ and PGE_2 endometrial concentrations (Fraser, 1983) and, if women wish to conceive, may be given only during menstruation. Additional advice can be given about improved nutrition of iron-rich foods or systemic iron therapy to reverse the symptoms of anaemia.

Amenorrhoea

Amenorrhoea is absent menstruation. Primary amenorrhoea refers to failure of the menstrual process beyond the age of 16 years in adolescent girls (delayed menarche). This may be due to sex-linked genetic disorder, pituitary tumour or eating disorders. Secondary amenorrhoea refers to loss of menstruation once the cycle is established and may be due to organic disease, eating disorders, excessive mental and/or physical stress, or pregnancy.

Delayed menarche can be directly related to interaction between body weight, psychological and physical stress. Warren (1980) reported a significant delay in menarche in girls training for ballet dancing and long distance endurance sports. Menstrual irregularities such as reduced menstrual flow (oligomenorrhoea) or lack of menstrual flow (amenorrhoea) have been commonly reported to occur in teenaged female athletes when involved in intense training and participation in major competitions. These menstrual abnormalities have been attributed to failures to attain a critical body weight particularly of adipose tissue composition. Reversal of the secular trend for menarche of a steady earlier timing of puberty, with a reduction of about one year every generation from about 1830 until the late 1960s has occurred during the last two decades. This is attributed to the contemporary commitment of girls and women in western societies to dieting, stereotypic slimness and small body size. The secular trend began to slow during the 1970s until now, the mean age of menarche in white Australian girls is about 12.8–13 years of age. This accords with historical estimates of the first menstruation during ancient Greek and Roman times, and in medieval Europe of close to the thirteenth birthday. Some recent studies do not support body weight as the major factor responsible for menstrual abnormalities in girls and women with eating disorders (Weltman *et al.*, 1990), while other studies (e.g. Kreipe *et al.*, 1989) propose a strong relationship between disordered eating, menstrual dysfunction and fertility. In addition, women with chronic alcoholism also report a higher variability in menstrual cycle length and bleeding flow although, as indicated by a higher number of pregnancies, fertility is not altered.

Assessment and Treatment

These complex disorders clearly warrant a multimodal assessment approach to evaluate the young woman's psychological profile of development, anxiety, anger, depression and ego strength as well as the neurohormonal functions of menstrual cycle mechanisms. In addition, behavioural analyses should be carried out of related nutrition behaviours and intakes, substance use (e.g. alcohol) and abuse, exercise levels and lifestyle stresses.

Treatment requires a team approach, clearly structured and developed to appropriately address all the issues. Psychological management will provide the central focus through a variety of cognitive–behavioural strategies to address the young woman's emotional and psychological problems of negative self concept, internal conflicts, social difficulties, and learned patterns of maladaptive behaviours. With young teenagers, a family systems framework may be adopted to address issues of faulty family dynamics. With older women, assistance in dealing with destructive relationships or absence of supportive social networks may be required. Not uncommonly, issues of past or present incestuous, sexually abusive and violent domestic relationships, are uncovered when women present with menstrual problems. However, management of the menstrual abnormalities alone may deal with only the surface problem.

ABNORMAL NEUROTRANSMITTER ACTIVITY

Dysmenorrhoea

Painful menstruation occurs as primary dysmenorrhoea with no identifiable pelvic pathology, or as secondary dysmenorrhoea in the presence of other pelvic pathology such as endometriosis, benign uterine tumours (fibroids), or pelvic inflammatory disease.

Primary dysmennorhoea is believed to affect up to 50% of nulliparous women in ovulatory cycles, and affects young women particularly during teenage years within a year or two of menarche. Symptom experiences are typically of spasmodic lower abdominal and pelvic cramp pains and backache during the menstrual phase, frequently associated with gastrointestinal disturbances of nausea, vomiting and diarrhoea, headache, and vasovagal induction of faintness and dizziness. Some writers (e.g. Dalton, 1969) have described a second subtype, congestive dysmenorrhoea, characterized by premenstrual pelvic heaviness, with dull, aching pain in the lower abdomen spreading to the lumbar spine. Primary dysmenor-

rhoea is now generally attributed to excess prostaglandin production with abnormal vasopressin levels, and is characterized by excessive amplitude and frequency of uterine contractions with a higher than usual refractory 'resting' tone between contractions. Endometrial contractions constrict the uterine blood vessels so there is a close inter-relationship between intense pelvic pains and minimal blood flow (Lumsden, 1985).

Young women prone to primary dysmenorrhoea quickly develop a learned anticipatory fear response to the approach and onset of menstruation. Research studies have suggested that regular physical exercise is associated with fewer premenstrual and menstrual symptoms but findings are equivocal. Sustained aerobic activities are likely to enhance blood perfusion that could reduce the sensations of pelvic heaviness and congestion of congestive dysmenorrhoea. It is more likely that regular vigorous exercise stimulates the release of endogenous opiates, beta-endorphins, that diminish the effects of dysphoric moods and stress and function as non-specific pain relief. However, women would have to be committed exercisers to persist in the presence of strong cramps and gastrointestinal disturbances.

An evaluation of the relationships between exercise, stress, moods and menstrual cycle symptoms (Metheny & Smith, 1989) found, paradoxically, that self-reported symptom severity increased in regular exercisers compared with low exercisers or sedentary women. This may be attributed to exercisers being more attuned to their bodies and aware of changed sensations. The study also reported that life stress and negative moods were related to reports of severe dysmenorrhoea, with the pronounced symptom reporters also scoring high on tests of pessimism, loss of well-being, stress and feeling overwhelmed.

The proposed distinctions between congestive and spasmodic dysmenorrhoea have not been supported in a recent study of Amodei and Nelson-Gray (1989). Responses to experimentally induced pain revealed no menstrual cycle phase differences by dysmenorrhoeics confirmed as congestive or spasmodic subtypes. Both categories of dysmenorrhoea sufferers compared to non-sufferers reported higher levels of pain and distress in both the premenstrual and menstrual phases compared to the intermenstrual phase (days 12–16) where there were no group differences.

Treatment

In the long term, severity of dysmenorrhoea frequently diminishes with age, oral contraceptive use and childbirth. Symptomatic relief may be obtained through use of aspirin, paracetamol or codeine, but use of prostaglandin synthetase inhibitors is now the treatment of choice and advocated once menstruation ensues (Rees, 1988).

Psychological management has a role to play in helping women reduce and overcome more global issues of felt stress, low well-being and negative moods, and anticipatory fearfulness of the menstrual process. Chesney and Tasto (1975) found behaviour modification and relaxing visual imagery effective in reducing symptom severity in spasmodic dysmenorrhoeics. Increased regular aerobic exercise can help to improve well-being, general body fitness and reduce body weight. Dealing with underlying psychoemotional problems can reduce muscular tension and fatigue that exacerbate pain experiences. Given the current lack of clear support for two subcategories of dysmenorrhoea there would appear to be no case for different procedures.

[535]

REFERENCES

Amodei, N. & Nelson-Gray, R.O. (1989). Reactions of dysmenorrheic and non-dysmenorrheic women to experimentally induced pain throughout the menstrual cycle. *Journal of Behavioural Medicine*, 373–85.

Chesney, M.A. & Tasto, D.L. (1975). The effectiveness of behaviour modification with spasmodic and congestive dysmenorrhoea. *Behavioural Research and Therapy* 13, 245–53.

Coyne, J.C. & Holroyd, K. (1982). Stress, coping and health: a transactional perspective. In T. Millon, G. Green & R. Meagher (Eds). *Handbook of clinical psychology*. pp.103–127, Plenum Press.

Dalton, K. (1969). *The menstrual cycle*. New York: Pantheon Books.

Fraser, I.S. (1983). The treatment of menorrhagia with mefanemic acid. *Research Clinics Forums*, 5, 93–9.

Kreipe, R.E. Strauss, J., Hodgman, C.H. & Ryan, R.M. (1989). Menstrual abnormalities and subclinical eating disorders: a preliminary report. *Psychosomatic Medicine*, 51, 81–6.

Lumsden, M.A. (1985). Dysmenorrhoea. In Studd, J. (ed). *Progress in obstetrics and gynaecology*, vol.5. pp.276–92 Edinburgh: Churchill Livingstone.

Metheny W.P. & Smith R.P. (1989). The relationship among exercise, stress and primary dysmenorrhea. *Behavioural Medicine*. 12, 569–86.

Morse, C.A. & Dennerstein, L. (1988). Cognitive therapy for PMS. In M.J. Brush & E. Goudsmit, (Eds). *Functional disorders of the menstrual cycle*. pp.177–190, London: John Wiley & Sons.

Mullen, F.G. (1968). Treatment of dysmenorrhoea by behaviour therapy techniques. *Journal of Nervous and Mental Diseases*, 147, 371–6.

Rees, M.C.P., (1988). Recent progress in the aetiology of dysmenorrhoea and menorrhagia. In M.J., Brush & E. Goudsmit, (Eds). *Functional disorders of the menstrual cycle*. pp.239–250, London: John Wiley & Sons.

Rees, M.C.P., Anderson, A.B.M., Demers, L.M. & Turnbull, A.C. (1984). Prostaglandins in menstrual fluid in menorrhagia and dysmenorrhoea. *British Journal of Obstetrics and Gynaecology*, 91, 673–80.

Warren, M.P. (1980). The effects of exercise on pubertal progression and reproductive function in girls. *Journal of Clinical Endocrinology and Metabolism*, 51, 1150–7.

Weltman, E.A., Stern, R.C., Doershuk, C.F., Moir, R.J., Palmer, K. & Jaffe, A.C. (1990). Weight and menstrual function in patients with eating disorders and cystic fibrosis. *Pediatrics* 85, 282–7.

Motor neurone disease

LOUISE EARLL
*Health Psychology Department,
Gloucestershire Royal Hospital,
Gloucester, UK*

MARIE JOHNSTON
*School of Psychology, St Andrews
University, Fife, UK*

THE CONDITION

Motor neurone disease (MND), or amyotrohpic lateral sclerosis (ALS), is the name given in the British medical literature to a progressive, non-inflammatory, degenerative and fatal disease of the central nervous system. The disease affects the motor neurones in the brain and spinal cord. Motor neurones are those nerve cells that control muscles, hence degeneration causes weakness and wasting in the muscles supplying the limbs, face and throat, with the consequent problems of thick speech and difficulty chewing and swallowing. MND is progressive over a variable time period, with death usually resulting from respiratory failure. The overall mean survival from diagnosis is approximately four years, with about 10% surviving for over ten years (Mulder & Howard, 1976). The disease may commence at any age in adult life, but it has a peak age of onset at 55 to 60 years. The cause of the disease is unknown. Many theories have been proposed, the ones receiving the most attention being viral infection, heavy metal poisoning, metabolic disturbance and immunological defects. Between 5% and 10% of MND cases in most countries are familial, with an autosomal dominant pattern of inheritance. MND is a clinical syndrome dependent for its diagnosis on clinical history, examination and electromyography. There is as yet no single confirmatory diagnostic test. Thus the syndrome is primarily identified clinically, yet the diagnosis is one that is made with considerable agreement among independent examiners.

Approximately 1 : 50 000 adults will develop MND in any one year, with 5 000 patients in the UK at any one time with some degree of regional variation. Almost twice as many men as women are diagnosed with MND. As yet there is no specific treatment that will arrest or slow down the progress of the disease.

PSYCHOLOGICAL APPROACHES

Like other conditions studied by psychologists, MND was first examined using personality theory and stress and coping models. More recently, Earll and Johnston (1993) and Johnston *et al.* (1996) have used self-regulation theory as developed by Leventhal and colleagues to understand how people respond to chronic illness.

As with other chronic diseases, a number of studies examined the personality characteristics of people with MND. On the whole, the most consistent finding to arise from this research paradigm has been that people with chronic illness tended to be more depressed than healthy people. Friedman and Booth-Kewley (1985) have referred to this as the 'disease prone personality', depression preceding not resulting from disease. However, many of the studies they reviewed used cross-sectional or retrospective designs, measuring personality after the onset of disease, and it seems plausible that at least some part of the depression was the result, rather than the cause of the disease.

The findings on chronic disease and distress can be interpreted within the framework of models of coping with chronic disease. Theories of stress and coping and the evidence that major life events may trigger stress would lead to the prediction that illness should result in distress. Being ill and having MND can be seen as a stressful, major life event, involving loss of functional abilities and eventually life, having an unpredictable course and being as yet uncontrollable by medical means. Work in this area has concentrated on two aspects: first, the perception of stressors and the role of appraisal in determining whether a given person perceives an event to be stressful, and secondly, having judged the event as stressful, an appraisal of the resources the person has available to cope with the event and the likelihood of a successful outcome (Folkman & Lazarus, 1985).

In a longitudinal study by McDonald *et al.* (1994). Patients with ALS were classified as having a positive or negative psychological profile. A positive profile was defined following a factor analysis and consisted of: 'low hopelessness, depression and perceived stress; expressive of anger; well-defined purpose; internal control; and high satisfaction with life'. When followed up over 18 months, those with a positive psychological profile had a lower risk of dying and a longer survival time than those with a negative profile, even allowing for length of illness, disease severity and age. It is possible that those with a positive psychological profile cope with their condition differently from those with a negative profile.

Leventhal and colleagues (Leventhal & Diefenbach, 1991; Leventhal, Nerenz & Steele, 1984; Nerenz & Leventhal, 1983) have proposed that coping with chronic disease can be examined within the framework of self-regulation theory, where events such as the onset of disease can be seen in the context of the individual's attempts to control and cope with objective problems and emotional reactions to them. The critical elements of this theory are first, that people develop a representation of their condition which may or may not match the medical representation; components of the representation found in previous studies include the identity of the illness (both label and symptoms), perceived cause, perceived consequences, perceived time line and perceived cure. Secondly, coping efforts are directed at the person's own objective assessment of it. Thirdly, people make their own evaluations of their coping efforts and this may be different from other people's evaluations.

Earll and Johnston (1993) in a cross-sectional study of 50 people with MND and their carers used this theoretical framework to investigate how people with MND coped with the disease. They found that individual representations varied and did not relate to overall severity or to the speech and swallowing problems which are distinctive features of MND; instead, they related to objective problems in daily living. This group of people were more likely to have expended effort in trying to understand their condition than in trying alternative remedies. In a condition without any effective cure, one might have expected more attempts to seek alternative cures. There has been considerable discussion in the coping literature about which forms of coping are adaptive. There was no evidence in this study of some coping styles being associated with better emotional outcomes than others. Emotional outcomes did not indicate high rates of emotional disorder, and did not relate to overall objective severity. However, 'activities of daily living and mobility' were associated with depression, more active individuals being less depressed.

Findings from this study together with those from a series of cross-sectional and longitudinal studies of MS and MND, Earll (PhD thesis, 1994) suggests that self-regulation theory is a useful framework within which to understand how people cope with chronic neurological illness. In MND where there is neither cure nor effective palliative treatments people's representations of their condition and evaluation of their coping efforts predicted outcome. The low level of psychological distress found in these studies suggests that, while no particular coping actions are associated with better outcomes, it may be that taking some kind of action, rather than taking no action, in a situation where there is nothing the medical profession can do is sufficient to minimize subsequent depression. Prior to this research, intervention would have focused on the actions people took to manage their condition. Using this framework has suggested that interventions aimed at changing representations and enhancing people's own evaluations of how well they have managed may be more appropriate targets and have more influence on outcome.

REFERENCES

Earll, L. (1994). Coping with chronic neurological illness: An analysis using self-regulation theory. Unpublished PhD thesis. London University.

Earll, L. & Johnston, M. (1993). Coping with motor neurone disease – an analysis using self-regulation theory. *Palliative Medicine*, 7, 21–30.

Folkman, S. & Lazarus, R.S. (1985). If it changes it must be a process: Study of emotion and coping during three stages of a college examination. *Journal of Personality and Social Psychology*, 48, 150–70.

Friedman, H.S. & Booth-Kewley, S. (1985). The 'disease-prone personality': a meta-analytic view of the construct. *American Psychologist*, 42, 539–55.

Johnston, M., Earll, L., Mitchell, E. & Morrison, V. (1996). Communicating the diagnosis of motor neurone disease. *Palliative Medicine*, 10, 23–34.

Leventhal, H. & Diefenbach, M. (1991). The active side of illness cognition. In J.A. Skelton & R.T. Croyle (Eds). *Mental representation in health and illness*. pp.247–272, Springer-Verlag.

Leventhal, H., Nerenz, D. & Steele, D.J. (1984). Illness representations and coping with health threats. In A. Baum, S.E. Taylor & J.E. Singer (Eds). *Handbook of psychology and health vol IV: Social psychological aspects of health*. pp.2219–252, Lawrence Erlbaum Associates.

McDonald, E.R., Weidenfeld, S.A., Hillel, A., Carpenter, C.L. & Walter, R.A. (1994). Survival in amyotrophic lateral sclerosis: the role of psychological factors. *Archives in Neurology*, 51, 17–23.

Mulder, D.W. & Howard, F.M. (1976). Patient resistance and prognosis in amyotrophic lateral sclerosis. *Mayo Clinic Proceedings*, 51, 537–41.

Nerenz, D. & Leventhal, H. (1983). Self-regulation theory in chronic illness. In: T. Burish & L.A. Bradley (Eds). *Coping with chronic disease: research and applications*. pp.13–37, London: Academic Press.

Multiple sclerosis

SIMON DUPONT

Department of Clinical Psychology, Guy's
Hospital, London, UK

INTRODUCTION

Multiple sclerosis (MS) is an inflammatory disease of the central nervous system, especially affecting white matter, brainstem, spinal cord and optic nerves. MS is characterized by multifocal demyelination (destruction of myelin sheaths with preservation of axons) and death of oligodendrocytes (myelin-producing cells), resulting in areas called plaques or sclerosis. Sclerosis disrupts the transmission of nerve impulses and symptoms may include spasticity, bladder disturbance, cognitive changes, ataxia, loss of sensation, paraesthesiae, fatigability, visual impairment and sexual dysfunction (Matthews, 1990).

Aetiology of MS is still very much in debate. There is a genetic susceptibility to acquiring MS that exists most frequently in persons of Northern European ancestry. There may also be a genetically determined protective factor that plays a role in lessening the risk of acquisition. An environmental factor may be a dormant childhood virus infection which provokes vigorous antibody reaction following a secondary infection. The blood–brain barrier is altered, permitting fluid, lymphocytes and macrophages to penetrate into the nervous system with the resultant production of MS symptoms (Posner, 1992).

Around 80 000 people in Britain are known to have MS with females being more commonly afflicted than males in a ratio of three to two. Incidence peaks between 20 and 40 years old and can affect all social classes. Prognosis varies from asymptomatic throughout the course to a fulminant, rapid progression to death. Most patients have a course somewhere between these two extremes.

There are two patterns of MS, relapse-remitting and chronic progressive. In the former, which occurs in 90% of patients, the initial symptoms diminish over a period of weeks or months and either disappear completely or leave behind some residual disability. When a relapse occurs the symptoms return and the process continues. Chronic progressive MS involves a slow, steady deterioration in function over months or years. About 60% of relapse-remitting cases will switch to a chronic progressive pattern at some stage in the disease.

There is currently no cure for MS, although symptomatic treatment of fatigue, spasticity, bladder disturbance and ataxia is available. Present treatment for relapses is with steroids (ACTH or methylprednisolone). Immunosuppressives such as azathioprine are used to help prevent the progression of MS. The usefulness of beta-interferon is currently being tested (Hughes, 1994).

Due to the diversity of neurological symptoms, unknown aetiology, lack of specific treatment, and varied behavioural consequences, there has been much interest in the psychological aspects of the disease.

EUPHORIA

When MS was first described in detail by Charcot in 1877, euphoria was considered one of the more salient symptoms. It was characterized by a marked sense of well-being out of proportion with the patients physical condition. Lack of reliable and standardized methods of diagnosis resulted in prevalence rates ranging from 63% to 0%. The present consensus is that it occurs in about 10% of patients, that it is a neurologically based emotional state, produced by demyelination, and not a psychological process. It is found primarily in patients with severe disability, long duration of symptoms, chronic progressive pattern of MS, enlarged ventricles on CT scan, and cognitive impairment. There is no known treatment of euphoria (Minden & Schiffer, 1990).

PATHOLOGICAL LAUGHING AND CRYING

This is another rare neurological condition characterized by the abnormal display of emotion only and not accompanied by the subjective emotional state. Accurate prevalence rates are unknown but estimates range between 7 and 10%. It has been reported to be associated with the presence of pontine, brain stem and periventricular lesions probably causing a frontal disconnection syndrome. It can be treated either with low-dose amitriptyline or levodopa (Ron & Feinstein 1992).

DEPRESSION

The first studies to focus primarily on depression did not appear until the 1950s. Depression may appear before or after MS diagnosis. Prevalence rates for the latter case vary between 27 and 54%. Typically, depression is moderately severe and patients are angry, irritable, worried and discouraged, rather than self-critical, withdrawn and uninterested. The unanswered question is whether depression is a neurologically based disorder or a psychological response to MS. Evidence to support the former view includes the following: MS patients have more depressive disturbances than do patients with other medical and neurological illnesses, and patients with non-central nervous system disabling disorders such as spinal cord injury. Evidence for the reactivity hypothesis is that depression is unrelated to neurological features such as severity and type of disability, type of MS and duration of symptoms. It is a common view that both organic and psychogenic mechanisms are in operation: vulnerability created by the presence of brain damage greatly enhances the effect of environmental factors in producing depression.

Scant attention has been paid to the management of depression in MS. Psychotherapy and antidepressant medication have not been systematically tested to produce reliable results (Berrios & Quemada, 1990).

BIPOLAR AFFECTIVE DISORDER

Bipolar disorder has an unexpectedly high prevalence rate of 13% in MS patients. There are preliminary reports of familial clustering of MS and bipolar disorder. Hypomania and mania may also occur with treatment with some steroids; patients at risk appear to be those with a history of previous depressive episodes and a family history of depression and alcoholism. Good therapeutic studies are not available for bipolar disorder in MS patients, although lithium carbonate has been shown to have a beneficial effect (Minden & Schiffer, 1990).

COGNITIVE IMPAIRMENT

The prevalence rate of cognitive impairment in MS patients attending hospital is about 50–60% and slightly fewer for community-based patients (McIntosh-Michaelis et al., 1991). Recent memory, sustained attention and conceptual/abstract reasoning are commonly impaired, with relative sparing of language function and immediate memory (Rao et al., 1991). Patients with chronic progressive MS show greater cognitive impairment than those with relapse-remitting course. Physical disability and duration of illness are also associated with cognitive impairment, although not exclusively. Severity of cognitive dysfunction correlates with the extent of brain pathology shown by MRI, although correlation of specific lesions and cognitive impairment is difficult (Ron & Feinstein, 1992). The wide range of cognitive test procedures on disparate and relatively small patient samples and control groups has led to the preparation of guidelines for future research (Peyser et al., 1990). Patients with cognitive impairment have significantly more difficulties in their work, social contact, sexual lives and activities of daily living, than those without (Rao et al., 1991). Treatment options are minimal.

SEXUAL CHANGES AND PREGNANCY

Sexual dysfunction affects between 50 and 90% of MS patients. Typical difficulties for women include anorgasmia, decreased sensation and libido, dyspareunia, vaginal dryness and dyseasthesia. Men report erectile dysfunction, reduced libido, ejaculation problems and fatigue. The aetiology of sexual dysfunction is at present unresolved. The same sacral segments of the spinal cord control bladder, bowel and sexual response. Organic damage to the sacral region may, though not inevitably, lead to bladder and bowel incontinence as well as altered sexual responses. Psychological issues may also play an important part in the aetiology and/or maintenance of sexual dysfunction. A combination of both organic and psychological causes may exist: sexual changes caused by neurological damage may affect the individual's psychological state and heighten dysfunction. The influence of MS on sexual satisfaction in the spouse is unknown. Treatment options include conjoint therapy, penile implants, vacuum constriction devises or intracorporeal injections of papaverine to induce transient erections (Barrett, 1991).

Pregnancy and MS is relatively understudied as a possible source of treatment development to suppress disease activity. Most investigations show a reduction of the relapse rate during pregnancy with an increase in the rate in the first three months of the puerperium (Hutchinson, 1993). An explanation for the protective effect of pregnancy is elusive.

ROLE OF FAMILY AND FRIENDS

As with any chronic illness, MS has an enormous impact on an individual's view of self, the world and the future. It can impinge on all areas of a person's life; social, vocational, marital and sexual. The family and friends of MS patients often exert a major influence on the patient's ability to cope, yet may not be aware or informed of their importance in the adaptation process. Concerns about disease fluctuations, lifestyle changes, increased dependency, marital disharmony, physical deterioration and feelings of obligation or embarrassment may disrupt relationships within the family and present obstacles to effective coping. Particular points of vulnerability include: the initial MS diagnosis, any exacerbation, loss of mobility, bladder, bowel or 'normal' sexual function, loss of job status at the time of severe physical dependency, and possible loss of spouse or significant other (Simons, 1984). Research into the most effective coping strategies is ongoing and includes accepting the diagnosis, minimizing the impact of physical symptoms and fighting to gain control of psychological problems. Ineffective ways of coping include attempting to equal able-bodied people, rejecting help, and avoiding discussions on disability (Simons, 1984).

It is the responsibility of the primary health professional to inquire about the patient's or carer's concerns and to utilize the support team who include the care assistant, local MS society, district nurse, physiotherapist, occupational therapist, speech therapist, day centre staff, respite care (hospital nurses), social worker, clinical psychologist, GP and neurologist.

REFERENCES

Barrett, M. (Ed.). (1991). Sexuality and multiple sclerosis. Ontaria: Multiple Sclerosis Society of Canada.

Berrios, G.E. & Quemada, J.I. (1990). Depressive illness in multiple sclerosis. Clinical and theoretical aspects of the association. British Journal of Psychiatry, 156, 10–16.

Charcot, J.M. (1877). Lectures on the diseases of the nervous system (trans G Sigerson). First series, lecture 6. London: The New Sydenham Society.

Hughes, R.A.C. (1994). Immunotherapy for multiple sclerosis. Journal of Neurology, Neurosurgery and Psychiatry, 57, 3–6.

Hutchinson, M. (1993). Pregnancy in multiple sclerosis. Journal of Neurology, Neurosurgery and Psychiatry, 56, 1043–5.

McIntosh-Michaelis, S.A., Wilkinson, S.M., Diamond, I.D., McLellan, D.L., Martin, J.P. & Spackman, A.J. (1991). The prevalence of cognitive impairment in a community survey of multiple sclerosis. British Journal of Clinical Psychology, 30, 333–48.

Matthews, W.B. (1990). McAlpine's multiple sclerosis (2nd edn.). Edinburgh: Churchill Livingstone.

Minden, S.L. & Schiffer, R.B. (1990). Affective disorders in multiple sclerosis.

Review and recommendations for clinical research. Archives of Neurology, 47, 98–104.

Peyser, J.M., Rao, S.M., LaRocca, N.G. & Kaplan, E. (1990). Guidelines for neuropsychological research in multiple sclerosis. Archives of Neurology, 47, 94–7.

Posner, C.M. (1992). Multiple sclerosis. Observations and reflections – a personal memoir. Journal of the Neurological Sciences, 107, 127–40.

Rao, S.M., Leo, G.J., Bernardin, L., Ellington, L., Nauertz, T. & Unverzagt, F. (1991). Cognitive dysfunction in multiple sclerosis. Neurology, 41, 685–96.

Multiple sclerosis

Ron, M.A. & Feinstein, A. (1992). Multiple sclerosis and the mind. *Journal of Neurology, Neurosurgery and Psychiatry*, **55**, 1–3.

Simons, A.F. (1984). Problems of providing support for people with multiple sclerosis and their families. In A.F. Simons (Ed.).

Multiple sclerosis – psychological and social aspects London: Heinemann.

Munchausen's syndrome

ROBERT WEST
and
LUCY RINK
*Psychology Department, St George's Hospital
Medical School, London, UK*

Munchausen's syndrome is a chronic disorder with physical symptoms that are of such a degree as to require multiple hospitalizations, even though no organic basis for the symptoms can ever be determined. Munchausen's syndrome by proxy is an emotional disorder in which the parent, almost always the mother, induces or fabricates illness in her child in order to gain medical attention (Yorker & Kahan, 1990). It has in some cases been considered to be a variety of child abuse.

Munchausen's syndrome has been noted to coincide with multiple personality disorders. Common traits which can be seen in both Munchausen's syndrome and multiple personality disorder are, self-mutilating behaviours, multiple somatic symptoms, having been accused of lying, use of many different names, and fugue-like disappearances (Goodwin, 1988). There is also evidence of aggressive behaviour, leaving the hospital against medical advice, multiple hospitalizations while travelling, and absence of any obvious secondary gain (Ludviksson, Griffin & Graziano, 1993). Sufferers of the syndrome can receive a large amount of treatment (e.g. Baer, 1987).

There are several reported cases of factitious anaemia due to self-inflicted phlebotomy which result in patients requiring numerous transfusions (Price & Giannini, 1986), and a case of factitious arthritis after the self-insertion of needles and fragments of metallic paper clips into the knee joint area (Samaniah *et al.*, 1991).

Munchausen's syndrome by proxy can put the child in great danger. The child may present with many conditions, including bleeding problems, seizures and failure to thrive (Ayass, Bussing & Mehta, 1993) and can involve a foetus. One reported case involved self-induced preterm delivery by rupturing the membranes at 26 weeks gestation (Goss & McDougall, 1992). Another involved chronic illicit insulin administration to a 1 year-old girl, and even after treatment the factitious illnesses continued, with urine specimen contamination, laxative-induced diarrhoea, suspected bladder catheterization, and suspected poisoning (Mehl, Coble, Johnson, 1990).

Studies of many single cases suggest many different causes of Munchausen's syndrome. One case was thought to be due to brain damage (Lawrie, Goodwin & Masterson, 1993); another patient was believed to resort to frequent hospitalization to avoid economic hardship (Arya, 1993). The psychological state of one patient was noted as the contributing factor; his developmental history was notable for dyslexia and pathological lying from early childhood. He later developed Munchausen's syndrome following a sudden separation from his terminally ill father (Geracioti *et al.*, 1987). Possible co-morbidity with personality disorder has been noted (Larsen, 1991). Some cases of the syndrome arise in high-risk groups for the presenting disease. For example, some cases of factitious AIDS have been found in members of a group who are, in fact, at high risk for human immunodeficiency virus (Zuger & O'Dowd, 1992).

Treatment of Munchausen's syndrome can be extremely frustrating, as the patients appear to have a desire not to respond to medical intervention (Leland, 1993). Diagnosis itself is also difficult because clinical presentations of the illness are variable. Therefore approaches to treatment vary greatly and success remains elusive (Leland, 1993). However, to attempt to proceed with diagnosis and successful treatment, a careful personality study of the patient and family members is believed to be important (Rinaldi *et al.*, 1993). Early diagnosis is also considered to be important in Munchausen patients because it could forestall the unnecessary complications of medical and surgical procedures to which patients are attempting to expose themselves (Gattaz, Dressing & Hewer, 1990). It is advised that patients who display the characteristics of Munchausen's syndrome should be carefully observed and an attempt to clarify both the medical and the psychiatric diagnosis should be made before any invasive procedure is undertaken (Gattaz *et al.*, 1990).

REFERENCES

Arya, D.K. (1993). Psychiatric hospitalisation in Munchausen's syndrome: is it an answer? *Irish Journal of Psychological Medicine*, **10**, 20–1.

Ayass, M., Bussing, R. & Mehta, P. (1993). Munchausen syndrome presenting as haemophilia: a convenient and economical 'steal' of disease treatment, *Pediatric Hematology and Oncology*, **10**, 241–4.

Baer, J.W. (1987). Case report: Munchausen's/AIDS. *General Hospital Psychiatry*, **9**, 75–6.

Gattaz, W.F., Dressing, H. & Hewer, W. (1990). Munchausen syndrome: psychopathology and management. *Psychopathology*, **23**, 33–9.

Geracioti, T.D., Van-Dyke, C., Mueller, J. & Merrin, E. (1987). The onset of

Munchausen's syndrome. *General Hospital Psychiatry*, **9**, 405–9.

Goodwin, J. (1988). Munchausen's syndrome as a dissociative disorder. *Dissociation Progress in the Dissociative Disorders*, **1**, 54–60.

Goss, P.W. & McDougall, P.N. (1992). Munchausen syndrome by proxy – a cause of preterm delivery. *Medical Journal of Australia*, **157**, 814–7.

Iarsen, F. (1991). Munchausen syndrome. A rare condition requiring many resources. *Munchausen syndromet. En sjelden, men svaert ressurskrevende tilstand, Nordisk Medicin*, **106**, 330–2.

Lawrie, S.M., Goodwin, G. & Masterson, G. (1993). Munchausen's syndrome and organic brain disorder. *British Journal of Psychiatry*, **162**, 545–9.

Leland, D.G. (1993). Munchausen's syndrome: a brief review. *South Dakota Journal of Medicine*, **46**, 109–12.

Ludviksson, B.R., Griffin, J. & Graziano, F.M. (1993). Munchausen's syndrome: the importance of a comprehensive medical history. *Wisconsin Medical Journal*, **92**, 128–9.

Mehl, A.L., Coble, L. & Johnson, S. (1990). Munchausen syndrome by proxy: a family affair. *Child Abuse and Neglect*, **14**, 577–85.

Price, W.A. & Giannini, A.J. (1986). Factitious anemia: case reports and literature review. *Psychiatric Forum*, **13**, 60–4.

Rinaldi, S., Dello Strologo, L. Montecchi, F. & Rizzoni, G. (1993). Relapsing gross haematuria in Munchausen's syndrome. *Pediatric Nephrology*, **7**, 202–3.

Samaniah, N., Horowitz, J., Buskila, D. & Sukenik, S. (1991). An unusual case of factitious arthritis. *Journal of Rheumatology*, **18**, 1424–6.

Toth, E.L. & Baggaley, A. (1991). Coexistence of Munchausen's syndrome and multiple personality disorder: detailed report of a case and theoretical discussion. *Psychiatry*, **54**, 176–83.

Yorker, B.C. & Kahan, B.B. (1990). Munchausen's syndrome by Proxy as a form of child abuse. *Archives of Psychiatric Nursing*, **4**, 313–18.

Zuger, A. & O'Dowd, M.A. (1992). The baron has AIDS: a case of factitious human immunodeficiency virus infection and review. *Clinical Infectious Diseases*, **14**, 211–6.

Myasthenia gravis

RUTH EPSTEIN

Ferens Institute, The Middlesex Hospital, London, UK

Myasthenia gravis is a neurological disease which is characterized by abnormal muscle fatigability. It may affect any group of muscles; head and neck muscles are initially most affected, with extraocular muscles most commonly involved (Stell, 1987). This condition occurs in all ages, but is usually seen in young adults and is twice as common in women as men.

Aetiology is unknown, but current evidence suggests that it is an autoimmune disease attributed to a decrease in the number of acetylcholine receptors in the motor end plate (Fritze *et al.*, 1974).

Symptoms typically appear in the evening when the patient is tired. Initial symptoms in approximately 50% of patients are ocular. If it is restricted to the bulbar muscles, they report dysarthria characterized by hypernasality, reduced loudness, increased breathiness and articulatory imprecision (Aronson, 1990). Other associated problems may include swallowing difficulties and reduced movements of the tongue, palate and pharynx.

Diagnosis depends on the typical clinical picture and can be confirmed by intravenous administration of edrophonium (Tensilon Test), electromyographic measurements or detection of anti-acetylcholine receptor antibodies in the blood. If the patient is asked to count aloud, the voice gets progressively less distinct and more nasal.

A common clinical diagnostic pitfall is the interpretation of symptoms of myasthenia gravis as being psychogenic, especially if the patient has a history of psychiatric illness. Furthermore, physical signs in early myasthenia gravis are often precipitated by emotional stress, accounting for the possibility of mistaking this disease for a conversion reaction (Ball & Lloyd, 1971).

Medical management of myasthenia gravis consists of administration of neostigmine or pyridostigmine with steadily increased dosage, until the desirable effect is obtained. The effectiveness of thymectomy (removal of the thymus gland), remains debatable.

Most remissions occur in the first few years of the disease, but relapses are common. Neonatal myasthenia is occasionally seen in infants of affected mothers, but usually resolves in a few weeks. (See also 'Voice disorders, 'Stuttering', 'Dyslexia'.)

REFERENCES

Aronson, A.E. (1990). *Clinical voice disorders* 3rd ed. New York: Thieme Medical.

Ball, J.R.B. & Lloyd, J.H. (1971). Myasthenia gravis as hysteria. *Medical Journal of Australia*, **1**, 1018–20.

Fritze, D., Hermann, C., Naiem, F., Smith, G.S. & Walford, R.L. (1974). HL–A antigens in myasthenia gravis. *The Lancet*, **1**, 240.

Stell, P.M. (Ed.) (1987). *Scott-Brown's otolaryngology* 5th ed. London: Butterworth & Co.

Neurofibromatosis 1

ROSALIE E. FERNER

*Department of Neurology, United Medical and
Dental Schools of Guy's and St Thomas'
Hospitals, London, UK*

Neurofibromatosis 1 (NF1) is a common autosomal dominant disease with a minimum prevalence of 1 in 5 000 (Huson, Harper & Compston, 1988). The principal and defining features of the disorder are café au lait spots and peripheral nerve neurofibromas (National Institutes of Health Consensus Development Conference 1988), (Table 1). The complications are legion and vary even within families (Riccardi, 1992). The gene for NF1 has been cloned on chromosome 17 q 11.2 and the gene product called neurofibromin, is thought to act as a tumour suppressor by downregulating the protooncogene ras P21 and thereby controlling cell growth and proliferation (Viskochil *et al.*, 1990, Wallace *et al.*, 1990). Neurofibromatosis 1 is clinically and genetically distinct from Neurofibromatosis 2, a rare condition characterized by vestibular schwannomas (Evans *et al.*, 1992).

The neurological manifestations of NF1 include both optic nerve and parenchymal gliomas. (Hughes, 1993) Intellectual problems are a common and clinically important complication, but the cause is unknown Ferner *et al.*, 1996. Recent research has established that patients with NF1 may present with low IQ, specific learning problems, behavioural difficulties or a combination of these.

The majority of NF1 patients have an IQ which is in the low average range, and the mean IQ is between 89 and 94 (Riccardi, 1992; North *et al.*, 1994, Legius *et al.*, 1995, Ferner *et al.*, 1996). Profound cognitive deficit is rare and only 4–8% of NF1 sufferers have an IQ less than 70 (Riccardi, 1992; North *et al.*, 1994, Ferner *et al.* 1996). Early paediatric studies showed that children with NF1 have lower performance than verbal IQs, although this discrepancy is not evident in recent studies on children or adults (Eliason, 1988, North *et al.*, 1994; Ferner *et al.*, 1996).

Specific learning difficulties occur in between 30% and 65% of children with NFI and include poor reading, spelling, visual spatial problems and incoordination (North *et al.*, 1994; Hofman *et al.*, 1994; Legius *et al.*, 1995; Ferner *et al.*, 1996). NF1 patients have slower reaction times and higher error rates on continuous attention and divided attention tasks compared with matched controls (Riccardi, 1992; Ferner, 1993).

Children with NF1 may exhibit impulsive behaviour and distractibility and are socially imperceptive. Psychiatric problems including depression, psychosis, alcoholism and anorexia nervosa

Table 1. *Diagnostic criteria for neurofibromatosis 1*

1. Café au lait spots
2. Two or more neurofibromas or one plexiform neurofibroma
3. Axillary or groin freckling
4. Lisch nodules
5. Optic nerve glioma
6. A first-degree relative with NF1
7. A distinctive osseous lesion such as sphenoid wing dysplasia or thinning of the long bone cortex with or without pseudarthrosis

   Two or more criteria are required for diagnosis.

have been noted but do not occur more frequently than in the general population. However patients with unsightly facial and truncal neurofibromas suffer more anxiety than those without (North *et al.*, 1994; Ferner *et al.*, 1996).

There have been few neuropathological studies which have considered the anatomical basis on intellectual impairment in NF1. Rosman and Pearce (1967), hypothesized that migrational problems in the brain of the developing foetus were responsible for the intellectual problems encountered in NF1. Increased intensity lesions on T2-weighted magnetic resonance images are a common feature of the brains of children and young adults with NF1, and are not found in the general population. They might be hamartomas aberrant nyelination or slow growing gliomas (DiPaolo *et al.*, 1995). There has been no consensus as to whether or not these lesions are associated with intellectual impairment in NF1. Some studies have found no relation between the presence, number, size and sites of T2 weighted lesions and cognitive deficit (Ferner *et al.*, 1993; Legius *et al.*, 1995) but others have noted a significant association between the presence T2 weighted brain MRI lesions and mild intellectual problems in NF1 (North *et al.*, 1994; Hofman *et al.*, 1994).

These discrepancies indicate that if any such relationship exists, it is not uniform and may depend on selection of the subjects tested by criteria which are not yet clear and further study is needed.

Sociodemographic factors, age, sex differences and the presence of macrocephaly do not contribute to intellectual impairment in NF1. The presence of neurological and/or medical complications is weakly associated with a lower mean full-scale IQ in NF1 patients. The recent discovery of the NF1 gene will permit a molecular gen-

REFERENCES

Di Paolo, D.P., Zimmerman, R.A., Rorke, L.B., Zackai, E.H., Bilaniuk, L.T., Yachnis, A.T. (1995). Neurofibromatosis type 1: pathologic substrate of high

intensity foci in the brain. *Radiology*, **195**, 721–4.

Eliason, M.J. (1988). Neuropsychological patterns: neurofibromatosis compared to

developmental learning disorders. *Neurofibromatosis*, **1**, 17–25.

Evans, D.G.R., Huson, S.M., Donnai, D., Neary, W., Blair, V., Teare, D. *et al.*

(1992). A genetic study of type 2 neurofibromatosis in the United Kingdom. 1. Prevalence, mutation rate, fitness, and confirmation of maternal transmission effect on severity. *Journal of Medical Genetics*, 29, 841–6.

Ferner, R.E. (1993). Intellectual impairment in Neurofibromatosis 1. In S.M. Huson & R.A.C. Hughes (Eds.). *The neurofibromatoses: a pathogenetic and clinical overview*. London: Chapman and Hall.

Ferner, R.E., Chaudhuri, R., Bingham, J., Cox, T. & Hughes, R.A.C. (1993). MRI in neurofibromatosis 1. The nature and evolution of increased intensity T2 weighted lesions and their relationship to intellectual impairment. *Journal of Neurology, Neurosurgery and Psychiatry*, 56, 492–5.

Ferner, R.E., Hughes, R.A.C., Weinmar, J. (1996). Intellectual impairment in neurofibromatosis I. *Journal of the neurological sciences*, 138, 125–33.

Hofman, K.J., Harris, E.L., Bryan, R.N., Denckla, M.B. (1994). Neurofibromatosis

type 1: the cognitive phenotype. *Journal of Paediatrics*, 124, 51–58.

Hughes, R.A.C. (1993). Neurological complications. In S.M. Huson & R.A.C. Hughes (Eds.). The *neurofibromatoses: a pathogenetic and clinical overview*. London: Chapman and Hall.

Huson, S.M., Harper, P.S. & Compston, D.A.S. (1988). Von Recklinghausen Neurofibromatosis: a clinical and population study in South East Wales. *Brain*, 111, 1355–81.

Legius, E., Descheemaeker, M.J., Steyaert, J., Spaepen, A., Vlietnick, R., Casaer, P. *et al.* (1995). Neurofibromatosis I in childhood: correlation of MRI findings with intelligence. *Journal of Neurology, Neurosurgery and Psychiatry*, 59, 638–40.

National Institutes of Health Consensus Development Conference (1988). Neurofibromatosis. *Archives of Neurology, Chicago*, 45, 575–8.

North, K., Joy, P., Yuille, D. Cocks, N., Mobbs, E., Hutchins, P. *et al.*, (1994).

Specific learning disability in children with neurofibromatosis type 1: significance of MRI abnormalities. *Neurology*. 44, 878–83.

Riccardi, V.M. (1992). *Neurofibromatosis: phenotype natural history and pathogenesis*. Baltimore: Johns Hopkins University Press.

Rosman, N.P. & Pearce, J. (1967). The brain in multiple neurofibromatosis (von Recklinghausen's disease): a suggested neuropathological basis for the associated mental defect. *Brain*, 90, 829–38.

Viskochil, D., Buchberg, A.M., Xu, G., Cawthon, R.M., Stevens, J., Wolff, R.K. *et al.* (1990). Deletions and a translocation interrupt a cloned gene at the neurofibromatosis type 1 locus. *Cell*, 62, 187–92.

Wallace, M.R., Marchuk, D.A., Anderson, L.B., Letcher, R., Oden, H.M., Saulino, A. *et al.* (1990). Type 1 neurofibromatosis gene: Identification of a larger transcript disrupted in three NF1 patients. *Science*, 249, 181–6.

Osteoarthritis

ROBERT WEST

and

LUCY RINK

Psychology Department, St George's Hospital Medical School, London, UK

Osteoarthritis (OA) is a term given to a group of joint disorders characterized by cartilage degradation, inflammation, pain and loss of joint mobility. It usually occurs in the elderly or in individuals whose joints have been deformed. The most commonly affected joint is the knee, followed by the hip. OA is probably the single largest cause of pain and disability in the general population.

Obesity has been linked, though not consistently nor equally for men and women, with the development of OA of the hip, knee and extremities (eg Carman *et al.*, 1994; Hart & Spector, 1993; Tepper & Hochberg, 1993). Regular participation in vigorous sporting activities or other activities that place stress on joints appears also to be linked with OA (Vingard *et al.*, 1993). For example, Lindberg, Roos & Gardsell (1993) reported that OA of the hip was more common in former soccer players than in controls. Joint trauma can also lead to OA (Slemenda, 1992; Tepper & Hochberg, 1993). Although regular, long-term participation in a wide range of sports is associated with increased rate of hospital admissions for OA, the age of admission is higher for individuals engaging in endurance sports rather than power sports and mixed sports (Kujala, Kaprio & Sarna, 1994).

It is possible to distinguish between the physical pain of OA, the level of physical disability and the psychological impact of the disease. Exposure to stressors appears to have a have an adverse effect on all these dimensions (Weinberger *et al.*, 1990). Increased age is positively associated with greater physical disability but negatively associated with pain and psychological distress (Weinberger *et al.*, 1990). As would be expected, pain and disability are associated with extent of cartilage and bone degeneration, muscle weakness and joint immobility (Dekker *et al.*, 1993). Anxiety, coping style and tendency to focus on symptoms are also linked with level of pain and disability (Dekker *et al.*, 1993). It is widely believed that once OA has begun to develop, it is important to maintain activity levels and avoid a downward spiral of inactivity, joint stiffness, pain and depression. There is some evidence that training in pain–coping skills can help reduce the impact of OA (Keefe *et al.*, 1990). Evidence on the effectiveness of educational and behavioural programmes to reduce the impact of arthritis is mixed (Bill *et al.*, 1989; Calfas, Kaplan & Ingram, 1992).

REFERENCES

Bill, H., Rippey, R., Abeles, M., Donald, M. et al., (1989) Outcome of an osteoarthritis education program for low-literacy patients

taught by indigenous instructors. *Patient Education and Counselling*, 13, 133–42.

Calfas, K.J., Kaplan, R.M. & Ingram, R.E.

(1992). One year evaluation of cognitive–behavioural intervention in osteoarthritis. *Arthritis Care and Research*, 5, 202–9.

Carman, W.J., Sowers, M., Hawthorne, V.M. & Weissfeld, L.A. (1994). Obesity as a risk factor for osteoarthritis of the hand and wrist: a prospective study. *American Journal of Epidemiology*, **139**, 119–29.

Dekker, J., Tola, P., Aufdemkampe, G. & Winckers, M. (1993). Negative affect, pain and disability in osteoarthritis patients: the mediating role of muscle weakness. *Behaviour Research and Therapy*, **31**, 203–6.

Hart, D.J. & Spector, T.D. (1993). The relationship of obesity, fat distribution and osteoarthritis in women in the general population: the Chingford study. *Journal of Rheumatology*, **20**, 331–5.

Keefe, F.J., Caldwell, D.S., Williams, D.A., Gil, K.M. et al. (1990). Pain coping skills training in the management of osteoarthritic knee pain: a comparative study. *Behaviour Therapy*, **21**, 49–62.

Kujala, U.M., Kaprio, J. & Sarna, S. (1994) Osteoarthritis of weight bearing joints of lower limbs in former elite male athletes. *British Medical Journal*, **308**, 231–4.

Lindberg, H., Roos, H. & Gardsell, P. (1993). Prevalence of coxarthrosis in former soccer players. *Acta Orthopedica Scandinavica*, **64**, 165–7.

Slemenda, C.W. (1992). The epidemiology of osteoarthritis of the knee. *Current Opinion in Rheumatology*, **4**, 546–51.

Tepper, S. & Hochberg, M.C. (1993). factors associated with hip osteoarthritis: data from the First National and Nutrition Examination Survey. *American Journal of Epidemiology*, **137**, 1081–8.

Vingard, E., Alfredsson, L., Goldie, I. & Hogstedt, C. (1993). Sports and osteoarthritis of the hip. An epidemiologic study. *American Journal of Sports Medicine*, **21**, 195–200.

Weinberger, M., Tierney, W.M., Booher, P. & Hiner, S.L. (1990). Social support, stress and functional status in patients with osteoarthrtis. *Social Science and Medicine*, **30**, 503–8.

Osteoporosis

MYRA S. HUNTER

Unit of Psychology, UMDS (Guy's Campus)
Univ of London, UK

Osteoporosis is an age-related condition characterized by decreased bone mass and increased susceptibility to fractures. It does affect men but is more common in women after the menopause, predisposing older women particularly to fractures of the wrist, spine and hip. Osteoporosis is considered a major health problem and is increasing in prevalence due to changes in lifestyle, increasing longevity and the greater proportion of older people in the population. It is estimated that one in four women over the age of 65 have, or are at risk of developing, osteoporosis, with over 50 000 hip fractures occurring annually in Britain: fractures which are associated with reduced quality of life and mortality (see Smith, 1990).

Osteoporosis is usually defined, somewhat arbitrarily, by bone density measures of bone mass lower than aged-matched norms; fractures may not develop until the seventieth decade. Peak bone mass occurs at the age of 35, after which time bone repair becomes gradually less efficient, and after the menopause bone is lost more rapidly for about 3 to 5 years, and then slows down again. Genetics, exercise, hormones and diet throughout life play complex roles in bone formation.

Prevention and treatment of osteoporosis include: (i) primary prevention, which aims to increase bone mass during years of bone maturation in the general population, (ii) secondary prevention, refers to efforts to minimize bone loss due to ageing and post-menopausal changes, while (iii) treatment refers to efforts to maintain and prevent further loss, as well as orthopaedic interventions and rehabilitation, in those suffering from osteoporosis. Because an ideal treatment for osteoporosis has yet to emerge, strong emphasis is placed on the need for prevention. Psychologists, and social scientists have been slow to develop research in these areas. However, the potential for health promotion interventions is considerable.

The main focus of medical research has been on the use of oestrogen, or hormone replacement therapy (HRT), which if taken for five years at the onset of menopause can reduce the rate of bone loss by approximately 50% while the treatment is taken (Cummings *et al.*, 1990). However, bone density measures are limited in their ability to predict who should be recommended preventative HRT, only a small proportion of women are prepared to take HRT long term, and more research is needed to evaluate the long-term effects of HRT upon fracture rates (Freemantle, 1992). (See 'Menopause' and 'Post-menopause' for more on HRT.)

Possible targets for primary prevention include adequate calcium intake (800–1000 mg per day), regular weight-bearing exercise (e.g. brisk walks) and reduction in tobacco, alcohol and caffeine use, in order to maximize peak bone mass. Increasing knowledge amongst young people and producing life style changes for a condition that may, or may not, develop in the future is a problem for primary prevention. Klohn and Rogers (1991) examined young women's intentions to prevent osteoporosis by increasing calcium intake and exercise. They manipulated descriptions of osteoporosis along dimensions of visibility, time of onset and rate of onset. Their results indicated that persuading young women that osteoporosis can result in visible or disfiguring consequences increased the appraisal of severity of the condition and also increased intentions to comply with a regimen of increased calcium and exercise. Further prospective research is needed to examine the relationships between intentions and behavioural change in younger women.

Secondary prevention includes assessment of risk and advice, mainly about diet, exercise and hormone use, for mid-aged women. Although there are conflicting reports, it is generally considered that increasing calcium alone has minimal impact upon reducing bone loss, unless levels are unduly low initially. However, adequate calcium is essential for benefits to be gained from exercise (Smith, 1987).

Exercise, and physical activity, has been associated with a positive influence on bone mass in a range of cross-sectional studies. The effects of exercise interventions have been less consistent. Exercise regimes have been variable between studies, as has the duration of the intervention (Smith & Gilligan, 1991). In one of a series of studies, Notelovitz (1988) compared the effects of three types of exercise on the bone density of postmenopausal women who exercised under supervision three times a week. After one year, treadmill walkers gained 0.4% bone mass, while bicycle and muscle strengthening groups and the control groups lost 0.5%, 3.8%, and 9.9%, respectively. In a recent randomized trial of weight-bearing exercise among women treated with HRT after a surgical menopause, the addition of exercise was associated with a highly significant 8% increase in spinal bone density in one year, compared with HRT alone, which maintained bone density (Notelovitz et al., 1991).

In addition, cessation of smoking and reductions in excessive alcohol and caffeine use is recommended. Smoking is associated with an earlier menopause, which increases women's exposure to lower levels of oestrogen. Preliminary results from a community health promotion study suggest that two 2-hour workshops for 45 year-old women can increase knowledge about the menopause and HRT (Liao & Hunter, 1994). After one year women who had attended the workshops had reduced cigarette smoking by approximately 50%, compared with no change in the control group.

Further intervention studies are needed, as well as investigation of factors that might increase adherence to hormonal, exercise and dietary regimes. Another approach which warrants attention in the prevention of osteoporotic fractures, particularly hip fracture, is the avoidance of falls. Strategies to reduce the incidence of falls in the elderly, for example, elimination of environmental hazards and avoidance of drugs which impair balance, need prospective evaluation. For those who develop fractures which cause pain and reduced mobility, research could usefully explore ways of improving the quality of life of these men and women (Cook et al., 1993).

REFERENCES

Cook, D.J., Guyatt, G.H., Adachi, J., Clifton, J., Griffith, L.E., Epstein, R.S. & Juniper, E.F. (1993). Quality of life issues in women with vertebral fractures due to osteoporosis. *Arthritis and Rheumatism*, 36, 750–6.

Cummings, S.R., Kelsey, J.L. & Nevitt, M.C. (1990). Appendicular bone density and age predict hip fracture in women. *Journal of American Medical Association*, 263, 665–8.

Freemantle, N. (1992). Screening for osteoporosis to prevent fractures. *Effective Health Care*, 1, 1–11.

Klohn, L.S. & Rogers, R.W. (1991). Dimensions of the severity of a health threat: the persuasive effects of visibility, time of onset and rate of onset on young women's intentions to prevent osteoporosis. *Health Psychology*, 10, 323–9.

Liao, K.L.M. & Hunter, M.S. (1994). The women's midlife project: an evaluation of psychological services for mid-aged women in general practice. *Clinical Psychology Forum*, 65, 19–22.

Notelovitz, M. (1988). Non-hormonal management of the menopause. In J.J. Studd & M.I. Whitehead (Eds.). *The menopause*, pp. 107. London: Blackwell.

Notelovitz, M., Martin, D., Tesar, R., Khan, F.Y., Probart, C., Fields, C. & McKenzie, L. (1991). Estrogen therapy and variable resistance weight training increase bone mineral in surgically menopausal women. *Journal of Bone Mineral Research*, 6, 583–90.

Smith, R. (1987). Osteoporosis: cause and management. *British Medical Journal*, 294, 329–32.

Smith, R. (1990). *Osteoporosis 1990*. London: Royal College of Physicians.

Smith, E.L. & Gilligan, C. (1991). Physical activity effects on bone metabolism. *Calcified Tissue International*, 49, 50–4.

Parkinson's disease

MARJAN JAHANSHAHI

Department of Clinical Neurology, Institute of Neurology, and Medical Research Council, Human Movement and Balance Unit, The National Hospital for Neurology and Neurosurgery, London, UK

This progressive neurological disorder is named after James Parkinson who first described it in 1817 under the label of 'shaking palsy'. The major symptoms are resting tremor, slowness of movement initiation and execution, muscular rigidity and postural abnormality. About 1 in 1000 of the population suffer from it. It is a disorder of old age, with the average age of onset in the 60s, although in hospital-based series 10 to 20% of cases started before the age of 40. The disorder is related to degeneration of dopamine-producing cells in the substantia nigra resulting in depletion of striatal dopamine. Dopamine replacement therapy is the main medical treatment. Parkinson's disease provides a model of basal ganglia dysfunction, through which the contribution of the striatum to cognitive and motor function can be studied.

PSYCHOLOGICAL FEATURES

Cognitive impairment

Dementia, that is a loss of intellectual abilities and memory impairment of sufficient severity to interfere with social or occupational functioning, when present develops late in the course of the illness. The rate of dementia in Parkinson's disease has been estimated to be 15–20% (Brown & Marsden, 1984). It has been suggested that the nature of dementia in Parkinson's disease and other subcortical disorders such as Huntington's disease and Progressive Supranuclear Palsy may be different from the cortical dementia of Alzheimer's disease (Albert, Feldman & Willis, 1974). Instead of the amnesic, aphasic, apraxic and agnosic features of cortical dementia, subcortical dementia is characterized by forgetfulness, slowing of thought processes, alterations in personality and mood and a reduced ability to manipulate acquired knowledge. However, the validity of the distinction between cortical and subcortical dementia has been questioned on the basis of the neuropathological and neuropsychological evidence (Whitehouse, 1986; Brown & Marsden, 1988).

Cognitive impairment in non-demented patients with Parkinson's disease is more prevalent, affecting about 40% of patients (Cummings, 1988). Impairment on cognitive tasks requiring effortful processing, internal control of attention, self-directed planning, sequencing and temporal ordering have been described in these patients. The basal ganglia are intimately linked with the prefrontal cortex and since the general picture of cognitive dysfunction in non-demented patients with Parkinson's disease has similarities to that shown by patients with damage to the prefrontal cortex, many refer to the 'frontal deficit' in Parkinson's disease (see Brown & Jahanshahi, 1991).

Depression and sexual dysfunction

The rate of depression in Parkinson's disease is estimated to be between 30 and 50% (Cummings, 1992). Depression in Parkinson's disease may be a result of the alteration of brain monoamines that are implicated in the aetiology of both Parkinson's disease and depression. Alternatively, depression may be a reaction to the onset and experience of living with the progressive illness which entails disability in daily activities, alteration of social and occupational roles, financial worries and hardship, and dependence on others. Although physical disability is a major contributor to depression, psychological factors such as low self-esteem and use of maladaptive coping strategies are also important determinants of depression in Parkinson's disease. Certain subgroups of Parkinson's disease patients may be more vulnerable to depression: patients in the earliest as well as those in the most advanced stages of illness, those with an early age of onset, and those with rapid progression (see Brown & Jahanshahi, 1994).

Sexual problems are relatively common but often overlooked in Parkinson's disease because of the advanced age of most sufferers. For the male patients, disorders of arousal (erectile dysfunction) and orgasm (premature ejaculation), and for the female patients diminished desire, are the major complaints. Besides depression and the stress of the chronic illness, some of the other factors that may contribute to the development of sexual problems are: the interfering effect of the motor symptoms on sexual behaviour, autonomic dysfunction present in some cases, antiparkinsonian medication reportedly producing hypersexuality (levodopa) or erectile dysfunction (bromocriptine) in some sufferers (see Brown et al., 1990).

Sleep disturbance and pain are two other common complaints in Parkinson's disease, both with multiple causes, but often secondary to the motor symptoms such as rigidity that can make turning in bed difficult or result in aching of the neck and back.

MANAGEMENT

The course of this progressive disorder varies across patients, with some showing little disability, cognitive impairment or depression after many years, while others becoming severely disabled, demented or depressed. The approach to management should therefore, be tailored to the needs of the individual patient.

Neuropsychological assessment may aid in differential diagnosis of idiopathic Parkinson's disease from other akineto-rigid parkinsonian syndromes. Behavioural techniques can be used to manage the behavioural problems associated with dementia, and the carer/family's need for support should not be ignored.

The natural history of depression in Parkinson's disease is not linear or parallel to the progression of the physical illness. Therefore, it can not be assumed that symptomatic improvement of Parkinson's disease would result in a parallel improvement of depression. Depression in Parkinson's disease needs to be treated directly and independently of the neurological illness. Evidence suggests that depression in Parkinson's disease is undertreated (Cummings, 1992). One reason for this may be a failure to detect depression because of the similarity of some of the symptoms of the two disorders (e.g. psychomotor retardation, lack of facial expression). Another reason for a failure to detect and treat depression in Parkinson's disease may relate to the fact that adaptation to chronic illness is a dynamic process which shows many variations across time and individuals. Thus, the peak time of psychological distress and depression may differ across sufferers: for some it may be early on in relation to accepting the diagnosis, for others it may be later in the course of illness as it becomes more disabling or when dopaminergic medications lose some of their efficacy and medication-related complications such as on–off fluctuations, end-of-dose akinesia, and dyskinesias develop. Individually tailored therapeutic programmes should be on offer throughout the course of the disease from the point of diagnosis to allow the patient and the family to adjust to the changing demands of the disease. Cognitive–behavioural techniques are useful in the management of these patients (Ellgring et al., 1990). Antidepressant medications are effective in the treatment of depression in Parkinson's disease (Cummings, 1992).

Given their multifactorial nature, it cannot be assumed that sexual problems, sleep disturbances or pain in Parkinson's disease can be 'cured' simply by treating the motor symptoms. Sex therapy taking account of the added stresses of chronic illness and the interfering effect of the motor symptoms and medication may be appropriate. Similarly, direct management of the sleep problems and pain may be necessary.

REFERENCES

Albert, M.L., Feldman, R.G. & Willis, A.L. (1974). The 'subcortical dementia' of progressive supranuclear palsy. *Journal of Neurology, Neurosurgery and Psychiatry*, 37, 121–30.

Brown, R.G. & Jahanshahi, M., (1991). Neuropsychology of Parkinsonian syndromes. In T. Caraceni & G. Nappi

(Eds.). *Focus on Parkinson's disease*, pp.121–1330. Milan: Masson.

Brown, R.G. & Jahanshahi, M. (1994). Depression in Parkinson's disease – A psychosocial viewpoint. In W.J. Weiner & A.E. Lang (Eds.). *Behavioural neurology of movement disorders. Advances in Neurology*, vol. 65, New York: Raven Press.

Brown, R.G., Jahanshahi, M., Quinn, N. & Marsden, C.D. (1990). Sexual function in patients with Parkinson's disease and their partners. *Journal of Neurology, Neurosurgery and Psychiatry*, **53**, 480–6.

Brown, R.G. & Marsden, C.D. (1984). How common is dementia in Parkinson's disease? *Lancet*, **ii**, 1262–5.

Brown, R.G. & Marsden, C.D. (1988). 'Subcortical dementia': the neuropsychological evidence. *Neuroscience*, **25**, 363–87.

Cummings, J.L (1988). Intellectual impairment in Parkinson's disease: clinical, pathologic, and biochemical correlates. *Journal of Geriatric Psychiatry and Neurology*, **1**, 24–36.

Cummings, J.L. (1992). Depression in Parkinson's disease: a review. *American Journal of Psychiatry*, **149**, 443–54.

Ellgring, H., Seiler, S., Nagel, U., Perleth, B., Gasser, T. & Oertel, W.H. (1990). Psychosocial problems of Parkinson patients: approaches to assessment and treatment. In M.B. Streifler, A.D. Korcyzn, E. Melamed & M.H.H. Youdim (Eds.). *Parkinson's disease: anatomy, pathology and therapy, Advances in Neurology*, vol 53, pp.349–353. New York: Raven Press.

Whitehouse, P.J. (1986). The concept of subcortical dementia: another look. *Annals in Neurology*, **19**, 1–6.

Pelvic pain

SHIRLEY PEARCE

School of Health Policy and Practice Unit,
University of East Anglia, Norwich, UK

INTRODUCTION

Pelvic pain is one of the most common problems among women presenting to gynaecologists (Beard & Pearce, 1989) and has been estimated to cost the NHS £163 million (0.6% of total expenditure) per year. It may arise from a number of benign causes, and medical and surgical interventions are often either not appropriate or even counter-productive. Beard & Pearce (1989) quote a number of studies showing that less than half the women presenting with pelvic pain have any obvious identifiable pathology. Recent debates concerning the physical component of pelvic pain surround the role of venous congestion following the studies by Beard *et al.* (1984), which suggest that a significant proportion of women with unexplained pain may have pelvic venous congestion (engorgement of pelvic veins with blood).

PSYCHOLOGICAL FACTORS IN THE EXPERIENCE OF PELVIC PAIN

The relationship between the extent of pathology and the experience of pelvic pain is complex. Where pelvic abnormalities can be found, they are not necessarily causal. Likewise, the demonstration of psychological abnormalities does not mean that these cause the pain problem. Considerable research energies have, however, been directed towards identifying the psychological characteristics of women with chronic pelvic pain. Typically, studies in this area compare patients with undiagnosed chronic pelvic pain with those without pain, using psychometric tests or psychiatric interviews, discrepant findings have resulted. Gidro-Frank, Gordon and Taylor (1960) report a high incidence of psychiatric problems in women with unexplained pelvic pain, while others (e.g. Castelnuovo-Tedesco & Krout, 1970) fail to find such relationships. Similarly, Pearce (1989) found no difference on measures of mood and personality when comparing women with pain in the presence or absence of organic pathology. Some differences on other psychological measures did, however, emerge. Women experiencing pain in the absence of observed pathology were found to have higher disease conviction scores on the modified Illness Behaviour Scale. There was also a trend for the no-pathology group to have higher hypochondriasis scores than a pathology group. This suggests that women in the no-pathology group may be more concerned about their physical state, and hence they may be monitoring bodily sensations more closely than the pathology group. It was also noted that women in the no-pathology group reported higher rates of serious illness and death of family members. Such exposure is not sufficient to cause unexplained pelvic pain, but it suggests that exposure to serious illness may influence attitudes, causing closer monitoring of bodily sensations and well-being. A similar finding comes from Kellner (1988) who found that a significant proportion of women with unexplained pelvic pain believed they has a serious illness and had been misdiagnosed.

Some studies have suggested that attitudes to sex may influence the likelihood of reporting pelvic pain. Gross *et al.* (1980) identified early traumatic sexual experiences (incest) in 9 out of 25 patients with chronic pelvic pain. Walker *et al.* (1988) found a higher prevalence of sexual dysfunction and sexual abuse in women with chronic pelvic pain in comparison to women without gynaecological conditions. The generality of these findings is unclear, and in the absence of reliable estimates of population norms for child sexual abuse, the identification of a particular incidence of abuse in any particular clinical group must be treated with some caution. Erskine and Pearce (1991).

PSYCHOLOGICAL TREATMENT FOR CHRONIC PELVIC PAIN

Practical details of psychological interventions for pelvic pain are described in detail by Pearce and De Haro (1993). Unfortunately, few of the numerous studies evaluating the efficacy of psychological treatments for chronic pain (see 'Pain management') have focused on the specific problem of chronic pelvic pain in women. Farquar *et al.* (1989) report a study evaluating the integration of psychological treatment with pharmacological control of vascular congestion. This study was a randomized controlled investigation of psychological intervention and Provera, a drug which suppresses ovarian activity. Psychological and pharmacological treatments were provided both alone and in combination. In the short term, clear benefits of Provera, either alone, or with psychotherapy, emerged. At nine months, however, although all groups had improved, the Provera plus psychotherapy group showed significantly more pain free days

than any of the other treatment groups. This suggests an interaction between psychological and pharmacological treatments. It appeared that patients for whom reductions in pain were effected by Provera early in treatment were better able to learn the cognitive pain management strategies which formed part of the psychological treatment. This observation provides further support for the view that pain should be both assessed and treated at psychological and physical levels.

REFERENCES

Beard, R.W. & Pearce, S. (1989). Gynaecological pain. In P.D. Wall & R. Melzack (Eds.). *The textbook of pain*, 2nd edn., Chap. 33, pp. 466–481. London: Churchill Livingstone.

Beard, R.W., Reginald, P., Pearce, S. & Highman, R. (1984). Diagnosis of pelvic varicosities in women with chronic pelvic pain. *Lancet*, ii, 946.

Castelnuovo-Tedesco, P. & Krout, B.M. (1970). Psychosomatic aspects of chronic pelvic pain. *International Journal of Psychiatric Medicine*, 1, 109–26.

Erskine, A. & Pearce, S. (1991). Pain in gynaecology. In H. Davis & L. Fallowfield (Eds.). *Counselling and communication in health care*. Chap. 11, pp. 177–191. Chichester: John Wiley.

Farquar, C.M., Rogers, V., Franks, S., Pearce, S., Wadsworth, J. & Beard, R.W. (1989). A randomized controlled trial of medroxyprogesterone acetate and psychotherapy for the treatment of pelvic congestion. *British Journal of Obstetrics and Gynaecology*, 96, 1153–62.

Gidro-Frank, L., Gordon, T. & Taylor, H.C. (1960). Pelvic pain and female identity. *American Journal of Obstetrics and Gynaecology*, 79, 1184–202.

Gross, R.J., Doer, H., Caldirola, P., Guzinski, G. & Ripley, H.S. (1980). Borderline syndrome and incest in chronic pain patients. *International Journal of Psychiatry in Medicine*, 10, 79–86.

Kellner, R. (1988). Fears and beliefs in patients

with the pelvic pain syndrome. *Journal of Psychosomatic Research*, 32, 303–10.

Pearce, S. (1989). The concept of psychogenic pain. An investigation of psychological factors in chronic pelvic pain. *Current Psychological Research and Reviews*, 6, 16–21.

Pearce, S. & De Haro, L. (1993). Assessment and treatment of pelvic pain. In A. Kuczmierczyk & A. Reading (Eds.). *Handbook of behavioural obstetrics and gynaecology*. Chap. 32, pp. 365–374. New York: Guilford.

Walker, E., Katon, W., Harrop-Griffiths, J., Holm, L., Russo, J. & Hickok, L.R. (1988). Relationship of chronic pain and childhood sexual abuse. *American Journal of Psychiatry*, 145, 75–80.

Plastic and cosmetic surgery

NICHOLA RUMSEY

Department of Psychology, University of the West of England, Bristol, UK

INTRODUCTION

Until relatively recently, plastic surgery was often sought covertly (Macgregor, 1979). Currently, however, plastic surgery is considered a boom industry. Studies of the outcome of plastic surgery report mainly positive findings. The majority of patients are satisfied postsurgery, and findings demonstrate decreases in depression, self-consciousness and social anxiety, and increases in self-esteem, (Sheridan & Radmacher, 1992). It has recently been argued by Pruzinsky (1988) that psychological factors are important at every stage of treatment, including the decision to seek surgery, the assessment of suitability for treatment, preparation for surgery, postoperative coping and in long-term adjustments to changes in appearance. Pruzinsky and others have emphasized the potential value of psychological assessment and, if appropriate, intervention at all of these stages.

PREOPERATIVE ASSESSMENT

Research has indicated that there are relationships between several factors identifiable preoperatively and postoperative adjustment,

thus routine preoperative assessment is advisable in order to maximize the chances of a successful outcome. The older research literature tended to suggest that people seeking cosmetic surgery were frequently neurotic, with a substantial proportion suffering from a discernible psychiatric diagnosis (for example, disturbances of body image such as body dysmorphic disorder). More recent research suggests that the proportion of these patients is relatively small. Most writers in the field recommend that this minority should be referred for psychiatric assessment and treatment rather than be accepted for plastic surgery. However, Edgerton, Langman and Pruzinsky, (1991) concluded that combined surgical–psychological rehabilitation provided relief for 83% of a sample of 67 cases, who were judged preoperatively to have moderate or severe psychological disorders. For the majority, decisions to consult are influenced by multiple factors, predominantly social and psychological in nature (Bull & Rumsey, 1988). A common complaint is that the person's social life has been impaired because of distress relating to their appearance. Feelings of social anxiety and evidence of behavioural avoidance are common. Many experience self-consciousness and suffer from a lowered self-esteem as a result of problems encountered in social interaction. On-going speculation about the existence of a relationship between the extent of the deformity and the degree of preoperative distress has consistently proved to be unfounded.

Many prospective patients will feel very anxious at the initial consultation and will need to be put at their ease. They may be embarrassed to ask for surgical intervention, and may experience guilt about wishing to change their appearance (especially if this is related to a familial or cultural feature). Careful exploration of the motivation to seek surgery is appropriate. The decision to seek surgery should be a personal one and not the result of pressure from family or friends (Bull & Rumsey, 1988). It is likely that the majority of prospective patients will have been experiencing distress for some time. It is therefore relevant to explore the timing of the decision to seek surgery as there is likely to be some kind of precipitating factor.

Care should be taken that expectations of outcome are realistic. In particular, there should be a realization that, despite messages to the contrary in media articles and advertising, surgical intervention will not provide a 'magical' cure for all the problems experienced presurgery. Having made the decision to proceed with surgery, it is important that the surgeon makes the change that the patient wants, and resists any temptation to choose instead a procedure which will produce a technically more beautiful face (Macgregor, 1979).

The timing of surgery may be critical. In a preoperative assessment of readiness for surgery, the psychologist should decide whether another intervention, for example, counselling, psychotherapy or social skills training would be appropriate either as a forerunner (to increase suitability), an adjunct, or as an alternative to surgery. If the person is experiencing significant additional life stressors, it may be appropriate to delay surgery in case the disfigurement has become a 'hook' on which to hang other problems. If surgery is planned on the NHS, in particular if the defect does not involve any functional impairment, there may be an enforced wait for surgery. In such cases it would be appropriate to offer interventions to improve the person's quality of life in the meantime (for example, to offer coping strategies designed to reduce the person's avoidance of social situations).

For children and adolescents with very visible disfigurements, the balance between waiting for physical growth to be completed and the psychological problems associated with waiting, is a precarious one (Bull & Rumsey, 1988). There are suggestions in the literature that, the longer a person has to accommodate to a malformation, the greater the dependence on that malformation, and the greater the problems of adjustment on its removal (Bradbury, 1993).

PREPARATION FOR SURGERY
Once the decision to proceed with surgical intervention has been made, psychologists can usefully play a part in preparation for surgery. Prospective patients are likely to benefit from the provision of accurate information about the procedures they will undergo. Realistic expectations about the likely results should be established, in order to minimize disappointment from a discrepancy between expectations and outcome, whether successful or less than ideal (Sheridan & Radmacher, 1992). Information should be provided to ensure that patients' expectations of the postoperative period are realistic (for example, in relation to bruising, swelling and the initial

appearance of surgical wounds). This is particularly important in procedures that require an unusual level of postsurgical discomfort. In orthognathic surgery for example, patients may be required to endure mechanical restraint of the jaw for a period of several weeks and may be restricted to a liquid diet. Not surprisingly, many patients experience distress postoperatively, with some experiencing feelings of panic resulting from the restriction. Buffone (1989) has suggested that patients with a history of compliance problems in other treatment regimes may find this type of procedure particularly hard to endure.

Presurgically, patients tend to be anxious. As highly anxious patients may tend towards longer recovery periods, the psychologist could usefully provide relaxation training and/or cognitive-behavioural interventions to help them cope. Those patients who have demonstrated a good repertoire of coping skills in response to previous stressors are more likely to do well (Buffone, 1989). Outcome research in the areas of plastic and orthognathic surgery have suggested that other predictors of positive adaptation include good overall body image, good social support and a positive relationship with the treatment team.

THE POSTOPERATIVE PERIOD
Pruzinsky (1988) has pointed out that, in the immediate postoperative period, patients often experience depression, anxiety and doubts concerning the eventual outcome of the surgical procedure. Buffone (1989) has estimated that 30% of patients undergoing orthognathic procedures will experience a reactive depression. Preparation for surgery may reduce levels of psychological morbidity. However, reassurance and empathy are also appropriate postoperatively and are likely to be well received from a psychologist or healthcare professional who has established rapport with the patient in the preoperative stage.

EMERGENCY ADMISSIONS
Many psychological factors are relevant in the acute and postoperative phases for plastic surgery patients admitted as emergencies. Chedekel (1983) and others have highlighted the potential of psychological interventions to relieve the distress experienced by burns patients, their families and by the staff treating them. In the acute phase, distress frequently relates to the experience of pain, to sleep deprivation, to anxiety associated with unplanned hospitalization and emotions relating to the cause of the injury. Distress can be alleviated through the provision of support, reassurance and understanding. In the reconstructive phase, intervention may be required in order to establish realistic expectations of the outcome of surgery (for example the relationship of likely outcomes to a person's original appearance and function). Interventions can be provided in the form of play therapy for children, or individual treatment or support groups for adolescents and adults. In the later phases of treatment, liaison with schools or the workplace has been shown to be beneficial, both in terms of preparing the patients for a return to school or the workplace, but also for peers or colleagues who may be uncertain of how to behave towards the patient (Chedekel, 1983).

LONG-TERM FOLLOW-UP
Although it is normal procedure to discharge patients once their scarring has settled, many experience problems adjusting to altera-

tions in appearance in the longer term, whether or not a 'good' surgical outcome has been achieved. In these cases psychological support and appropriate intervention have the potential to improve adjustment. Some people experience unwelcome feelings of change to their 'identity'. Some experience difficulties in dealing with increased attention from other people, others have problems coping with the lack of attention afforded to anyone with an unremarkable appearance. Others express disappointment as their expectations of change are not fulfilled. A few patients may display an insatiable desire for further surgery. For the majority of these, a psychiatric referral is widely considered more appropriate than offers of further surgery.

CONCLUSION

Psychological factors play a part in all stages of elective and reconstructive surgery. The participation of psychologists in the evaluation, treatment and follow-up of plastic surgery patients has the potential to significantly improve the quality of care provided for these people.

REFERENCES

Bradbury, E. (1993). Psychological approaches to children and adolescents with disfigurement: a review of the literature. *ACPA Review*, **15**, 1–6.

Buffone, G. (1989). Consultations with oral surgeons: new roles for medical psychotherapists. *Medical Psychotherapy: An International Journal*, **2**, 33–48.

Bull, R. & Rumsey, N. (1988). *The social psychology of facial appearance*. New York: Springer Verlag.

Chedekel, D. (1983). The psychologist's role in comprehensive burn care. N. Bernstein & M. Robson (Eds). *Comprehensive approaches to the burned person*. Chapter 13, New York: Medical Examination Publishing Co Inc.

Edgerton, M., Langman, M. & Pruzinsky, T. (1991). Plastic surgery and psychotherapy in the treatment of one hundred psychologically disturbed patients. *Plastic and Reconstructive Surgery*, **88**, 594–608.

Macgregor, F. (1979). *After plastic surgery: adaptation and adjustment*. New York: Praeger.

Macgregor, F. (1979). Facial disfigurement: problems & management of social interactions and implications for mental health. *Aesthetic Plastic Surgery*, **14**, 249–57.

Pruzinsky, T. (1988). Collaboration of plastic surgeon and medical psychotherapist. *Medical Psychotherapy*, **1**, 1–13.

Sheridan, C. & Radmacher S. (1992). *Health psychology: challenging the biomedical model*. New York: Wiley.

Post-traumatic stress disorder

ANDREW BAUM

and

STACIE SPENCER

University of Pittsburgh, USA

In general, psychological reactions to extreme adversity have not been well understood. The history of medicine, occupational health, and psychiatry is punctuated by recurring themes related to what is now called post-traumatic stress disorder (PTSD). For several centuries, aversions to, and maladies from, extremely stressful events have been described, but clues to their causes have only recently been discovered. Prior to the current PTSD diagnosis, several accounts described 'railway spine', 'battle fatigue', and 'shellshock' following traumatic events. Over the past 20 years, investigation of traumatic stress has exploded and a substantial mass of research evidence has been gathered. Initially, this was primarily due to an interest in the uniquely pervasive symptoms of Vietnam veterans. However, tragedy is not limited to war and the development of PTSD is not limited to soldiers. The recent proliferation of PTSD research in diverse populations has added to the understanding of PTSD as a mental health disorder, to our understanding of human reactions to stress, and to knowledge about possible links between mental and physical health.

While a review of the evolution of the PTSD diagnosis is described elsewhere (see McFarlane, 1990; Tomb, 1994), several notable advances will be described. As a diagnostic label, PTSD first appeared in the third version of the *Diagnostic and Statistical Manual* of the American Psychiatric Association (*DSM-III*, 1980) and was clarified in *DSM-IIIR* (1987). Prior to this time, it was believed that prolonged reaction to a traumatic event was due to pre-existing personal weakness (McFarlane, 1990; Tomb, 1994). However, with the accumulation of data indicating a consistency in reactions to combat and non-combat traumatic events, it became apparent that the nature of the traumatic event plays an important role in the reaction to that event. Thus, the severity of the event was one of the criteria for a diagnosis of PTSD and was defined as that which would be 'markedly distressing to almost anyone'. This tautological definition was challenging to operationalize. In DSM-IV, the focus shifted from the severity of the event to exposure and reaction to the event.

PTSD is best described as an anxiety disorder that often follows exposure to an extreme stressor that causes injury, threatens life, or threatens physical integrity (*DSM-IV*, 1994). Characteristics of PTSD include persistent re-experiencing of the event through intrusive distressing thoughts and dreams, acting or feeling like the event is recurring, and intense psychological and physiological reactions to cues that are associated with the event. Also characteristic of

PTSD are the avoidance of thoughts, feelings, people, places, and activities related to the event, difficulty remembering important aspects of the event, restricted range of affect, feeling detached, and a sense of a shortened life-expectancy. The signs and symptoms of PTSD can be either acute, lasting for less than three months, or more chronic, lasting for several years. In some cases, the onset of symptoms is delayed for six months or more.

INCIDENCE OF PTSD

PTSD has most commonly been associated with Vietnam combat veterans over the past 20 years and a great deal of data have come from studying this group. Family and relationship abuse, criminal assault, rape, motor vehicle accidents, airplane crashes, natural disasters (e.g. floods, earthquakes, and hurricanes), human-caused disasters (e.g. the Buffalo Creek Dam collapse), exposure to noxious agents (e.g. Three Mile Island) or pathogens (e.g. HIV) have also been associated with PTSD symptoms. Though studies and stressors vary, approximately 10–30% of people who are exposed to an extreme stressor appear to develop PTSD and 9% of the population in the United States, overall, experience symptoms of PTSD in their lifetime (Breslau et al., 1991; Tomb, 1994). Incidence rates vary with the event: incidence of PTSD following rape is estimated at 80%, after tragic death at 30%, after motor vehicle accidents with injury at 23%, following childhood molestation at 23%, and after serious accidents at 13% (Breslau et al., 1991; Green, 1994). PTSD rates in firefighters following a serious bushfire were as high as 36% (McFarlane, 1992), and PTSD rates for male and female Vietnam veterans are as high as 31% and 27%, respectively (Fairbanks et al., 1994 as cited in Green, 1994; Kulka et al., 1990).

These rates reflect *lifetime* rates for PTSD and are considerably larger than *current* rates. For example, as noted above, the lifetime rate of PTSD among Vietnam veterans has been estimated at 31% for males and 27% for females. However, the current rate from 1990 to 1994 was approximately 15% for males and 9% for females (Fairbanks et al., 1994 as cited in Green, 1994; Kulka et al., 1990). In approximately 50% of combat veterans diagnosed with PTSD, symptoms diminish within the first few years (Mellman et al., 1992). Because PTSD symptoms subside in many people over time, and emergence of symptoms may wax and wane, it is important to examine long-term experience. For example, longitudinal data indicate a drop in PTSD symptoms in rape victims from 94% two weeks following the event to 65% two months later (Rothbaum & Foa, 1993; Rothbaum et al., 1992). Rates dropped to 47% at three months and stayed at this level at nine months. In contrast, 65% of criminal assault victims experienced PTSD symptoms following the assault, but none of them experienced symptoms nine months later (Rothbaum et al., 1992).

PTSD FOLLOWING SPECIFIC TRAUMATIC EVENTS

As suggested above, a number of highly stressful events have been identified that can cause people to experience symptoms of PTSD. Typically, these events involve life threat or otherwise compromise victims' sense of safety and control. While there are many other situations associated with PTSD, we will briefly consider a few major areas of investigation focused on well-established causes of the disorder.

Criminal Assault and Rape

As noted above, rates of PTSD are high immediately following rape (e.g. Rothbaum et al., 1992). In about half of these cases, symptoms gradually improve and cease to exist by the end of three months. However, PTSD symptoms tend to persist beyond the third month if they do not improve by the end of the first month following rape (Rothbaum et al., 1992). In addition, specific crime features have been associated with the onset of PTSD symptoms in rape victims. If the rape was by a stranger, involved use of weapons, was perceived as life threatening, or resulted in actual injury or completed rape, victims appear to be more likely to develop symptoms of PTSD (Bownes, O'Gorman & Sayers, 1991; Resnick et al., 1992).

Evidence suggests that perceptions of control are important in the development of PTSD following criminal assault, and general perception of control over aversive events is predictive of PTSD symptom severity (Kushner et al., 1993). In contrast to perceived control during assault or over future assaults, which do not predict PTSD symptom severity, a more generalized view of world order or one's ability to control his or her experiences is related to PTSD (Kushner et al., 1993). Evidence also suggests that intrusive thoughts play a significant role in maintaining PTSD symptoms following rape. Victims with PTSD symptoms take longer to process or respond to high-threat words than do rape victims without PTSD and no-rape controls (Cassidy, McNally & Zeitlin, 1992; Foa et al., 1991). Interference on this task has been correlated with scores on the intrusive thoughts scale from Horowitz's Impact of Event Scale (Cassidy et al., 1992).

Disasters

Research on disaster-related PTSD covers a wide range of events including earthquakes (Ahearn, 1981; Popovic & Petronic, 1964), tornadoes (Bolin & Klenow, 1982–1983; North et al., 1989), cyclones (Parker, 1977; Patrick & Patrick, 1981), volcanic eruptions (Adams & Adams, 1984), bushfires (McFarlane, 1986), floods (Green et al., 1990a; Lifton & Olson, 1976 Miller, Turner & Kimball, 1981; Smith et al., 1989, Smith et al., 1986), airplane crashes (Perlberg, 1979; Smith et al., 1989), and nuclear accidents (Baum, Fleming & Davidson, 1983; Wert, 1979). It is difficult to summarize findings regarding PTSD across these disasters because of methodological differences in research on them. For example, studies vary with regard to which symptoms and reactions were measured, the assessment devices that were used for a specific symptom, and how long after the disaster event assessments were made (Smith & North, 1993). The variability in methodology across studies may help explain why symptom rates reported in disaster studies range from 2–100% and why there is no apparent pattern of symptoms by disaster event (Smith & North, 1993).

As in the case of rape, there are specific features of disasters that are related to PTSD. One distinguishing characteristic is whether the disaster is 'natural' or 'technological'. Results indicate that natural disasters are often associated with more acute stress and technological disasters are often associated with more chronic stress (e.g., Baum et al., 1983). For example, symptoms of PTSD persisted for as long as 6 years following the radioactive gas leak at Three Mile Island and for as long as 14 years following the Buffalo Creak Dam collapse (Baum, Cohen & Hall, 1993; Green et al., 1990b. Symptoms of stress appear to be more prevalent and to last longer following technological disasters, although exposure to both kinds of disasters is often brief (Smith *et al.*, 1989).

An important difference between natural and technological disasters has been described in terms of perceptions of control (Baum *et al.*, 1993; Davidson, Baum & Collins, 1982). Though we may be able to improve our predictive abilities, people do not perceive that they have control over natural disasters. There is nothing we can do to prevent hurricanes, volcanic eruptions, or earthquakes. On the other hand, we assume that there are systems in place to check and maintain the safety of what we have built. As a result, we should be able to prevent failures of these systems and subsequent disasters from occurring. Natural disasters are distressing, but human-made disasters threaten our assumptions about order and control. For example, one study compared flood victims and a no-disaster control group to a group of neighbours of a leaking hazardous waste dump and found that the latter were more alienated, physiologically aroused, and performed less well on challenging tasks nine months after finding out about the leak (Baum *et al.*, 1992).

Vietnam Veterans

Research on PTSD in Vietnam veterans is different from studies of non-combat-related PTSD. First, while the experience of other traumas may be similar (i.e. threat to body and life) (Cameron, 1994), the stimuli that provoke anxiety or fear are specific to the traumatic experience (McNew & Abell, 1995). Secondly, in contrast to victims of rape, disasters, or accidents, Vietnam veterans experienced stressors repeatedly over weeks and months. Thirdly, studies of Vietnam veterans differ methodologically; while studies of PTSD in rape and disaster victims take place near the time of the event, studies of PTSD in Vietnam veterans have been undertaken many years (even decades) after the original event(s).

Issues of time delay and memory are important to consider when interpreting self-report data that may change from assessment to assessment. For example, estimates of combat activity differ over time (Reaves, Callen & Maxwell, 1993). These changes may be due to normal changes in memories of a distant event. However, neuropsychological evidence suggests that Vietnam combat veterans with PTSD experience memory deficits and a sensitivity to proactive interference (Bremner *et al.*, 1993; Uddo *et al.*, 1993). While memories for combat experience and exposure to traumatic events may change in content or quality across time, this does not mean that they become fewer or less powerful. The persistence of PTSD symptoms is associated with intrusive memories of combat events (Davidson & Baum, 1993). Like rape victims in studies described above, Vietnam combat veterans demonstrated interference for combat-trauma related stimuli but not for neutral, positive, or other threat stimuli (McNally, English & Lipke, 1993).

War-related PTSD is not unique to Vietnam veterans. There is evidence of PTSD among World War II and Korean War veterans, but more cases have been reported from the Vietnam War. The most obvious reason for the difference in reported rates may simply be that researchers were alerted to, and looking for, PTSD in Vietnam veterans. At the same time, there appear to have been characteristics of the Vietnam conflict that may have contributed to unexpectedly high rates of distress. Scurfield (1993) described many of the unique features of the Vietnam War including the involvement of non-military people in combat, the use of body count rather than

occupation of area as a measure of military success, the abandonment of the Vietnam people, rejection and betrayal faced upon return to the US, post-war employment problems, and uncertainties regarding exposure to toxic chemicals. Together with unit rotation policies and the hazy purpose of the conflict, these factors may have contributed to sustained distress and PTSD.

PREDICTORS OF PTSD

Not all of those exposed to traumatic stressors develop PTSD afterwards. In fact, most do not. Other variables, including childhood trauma, early separation from parents, abnormal adolescent development, preexisting personality disorders (e.g. depression and anxiety disorders), or family history of anxiety may make some people more susceptible to developing PTSD (Astin *et al.*, 1995; Brady *et al.*, 1994; Green *et al.*, 1990a). Women appear to be more likely to develop PTSD following exposure to a traumatic event, as are people high in neuroticism (Breslau *et al.*, 1991). Factors that precede exposure to traumatic factors and interactions among past, present, and anticipated events appear to be important as well (Breslau *et al.*, 1991; Hendin *et al.*, 1983; Holloway & Ursano, 1984). However, evidence does not support the notion that premorbid factors alone determine development of the disorder (e.g. Boman, 1986; Foy *et al.*, 1984; Green *et al.*, 1990a; Green & Berlin, 1987; Ursano *et al.*, 1981). It may be that pre-exposure variables may only predict PTSD in extreme cases (Allodi, 1994).

While these factors may make someone more vulnerable to PTSD, the persistence of stress beyond the existence of the stressor is likely to be due to the continued appraisal of threat and response to that appraisal (Baum *et al.*, 1992). The perception of control and memories of the event influence this appraisal. Memories of the event are highly predictive of chronic stress symptoms (Baum *et al.*, 1993). Horowitz (1986) described an information-processing model of the reaction to a traumatic event and the ways in which 'normal' reactions become symptoms of PTSD. According to Horowitz, the immediate reaction to a traumatic event or to the receipt of tragic information is outcry. This is quite literal in some situations when a person cries out, 'watch out', 'oh no', or 'help'. In other cases crying out is non-verbal in the form of a sob, stare, or grimace. The outcry reaction does not always occur at the time of the traumatic event, and delays of hours, days, or months are not uncommon.

Following exposure to the traumatic event, victims often experience intrusive and avoidant thoughts, emotions, and behaviours. Unbidden ideas, emotions, and compulsive acts turn to denial of the implications of the event, emotional numbing, and/or withdrawal of interest in life. The cycling back and forth from intrusive to avoidant thoughts, emotions, and behaviours occurs in most individuals following a traumatic event and subsides as the implications of the event are worked through. However, if the individual is overwhelmed by the event, or experiences extreme avoidance, intrusive thoughts, or psychosomatic responses, he/she may fail to work through the implications of the event (Horowitz, 1993). PTSD may then develop when an individual is unable to find meaning in the event given his or her cognitive schema of the world (Green *et al.*, 1985).

It is also possible that the more powerful, sensual, and evocative the event, the more likely the survivor will be to develop PTSD. This is consistent with data that indicate that higher rates of PTSD are observed following severe, horrific, and grotesque events (e.g. Green, 1990; Green *et al.*, 1990*a*). While evidence from WWII POWs suggests that the severity of the trauma (e.g. amount of weight lost, amount of torture) can predict PTSD (Speed *et al.*, 1989), for most traumatic events PTSD is predicted by the individual's appraisal of the event as severe rather than the objective severity of the stressor (Perry *et al.*, 1992). In fact, intrusive thoughts about combat in Vietnam was a better predictor of current distress than was severity of combat exposure (Davidson & Baum, 1993).

In a longitudinal study of burn survivors, Perry *et al.* (1992) measured PTSD symptoms at 2, 6, and 12 months following the traumatic event. Rates of PTSD at 2 months were predicted by lower perceptions of social support and greater emotional distress the first week following the event. At 6 months, PTSD was predicted by negative affect and intrusive thoughts experienced at 2 months, and at 12 months PTSD was predicted by negative affect and avoidant thoughts experienced at 6 months. Neither intrusive nor avoidant thoughts predicted PTSD at 2 months, consistent with the theory that intrusive and avoidant thoughts are normal reactions in the immediate aftermath of traumatic events and are associated with PTSD if they do not diminish over time.

COMORBIDITY

One of the most striking characteristics of PTSD is the high rate of associated major psychological disorders. It has been estimated that PTSD patients are twice as likely to meet the diagnostic criteria for another disorder than are non-PTSD patients (Helzer, Robins & McEvoy, 1987). In many cases, patients average three to four diagnoses, including the diagnosis of PTSD (Keane & Wolfe, 1990; Mellman *et al.*, 1992). The rate of PTSD patients in the VA system meeting diagnostic criteria for another disorder is as high as 84% (Sierles *et al.*, 1983; Sierles *et al.*, 1986). Studies have indicated that approximately 84% of VA inpatients and outpatients with PTSD are diagnosed with substance abuse problems, 68% with lifetime major depression, 53% with panic disorder, 53% with generalized anxiety disorder, 34% dysthymic disorder, and 26% with personality disorder (Keane & Wolfe, 1990, Mellman *et al.*, 1992).

The rates of comorbid psychological disorders is high among non-combat PTSD as well. Crime victims with PTSD are also diagnosed with sexual dysfunction (41%), major depression (32%), and obsessive–compulsive disorder (27%) (Kilpatrick *et al.*, 1987). High rates of obsessive–compulsive disorder, agoraphobia, dysthymia, mania, and panic disorders have been reported for rape survivors with PTSD (Breslau *et al.*, 1991). Comorbidity in disaster patients with PTSD includes depression and anxiety disorders (Green *et al.*, 1992).

The nature of the relationship between PTSD and these other disorders is difficult to disentangle. While it is possible that exposure to a traumatic event causes PTSD and other disorders, it is also possible that vulnerability to these disorders makes a person more likely to develop PTSD when a traumatic event is encountered (Keane & Wolfe, 1990). Although symptoms of PTSD and other diagnoses tend to appear within six months of the event, symptoms of PTSD precede other symptoms (Mellman *et al.*, 1992). In the case of substance abuse, the abuse may be secondary to the diagnosis of PTSD if alcohol and/or drugs are used to reduce intrusive thoughts or physiological reactivity (Keane *et al.*, 1985).

BIOBEHAVIOURAL FACTORS

While the extent to which PTSD and more common forms of distress share common pathways and origins is not clear, some have argued that PTSD can be considered an extreme consequence of stress (e.g. Davidson & Baum, 1986). As such, several biological substrates for the disorder have been proposed, and research has begun to identify important links between systems and hormones long thought to be important in stress as possible causes of PTSD. Some have investigated 'trauma centres' in the brain, focusing on noradrenergic activity. This research has centred on the locus coeruleus as a centre for sympathetic activity in the brain (e.g. Krystal, 1990). Noradrenergic activity has been implicated as a key component of stress responding, and inhibition of central noradrenergic activity with drugs decreases the stress response (Redmond & Krystal, 1984). Manipulation of norepinephrine and other catecholamines also affects fear-enhanced startle responses, and enhanced startle reactions are symptomatic of PTSD (Davis, 1980; Orr, 1990). Alternatively, some have argued that helplessness is an important aspect of PTSD and the biological effects of inescapable shock in animals have been used as the basis for a model of the profound changes associated with PTSD (e.g. van der Kolk *et al.*, 1985). Such stressors cause helpless-like states and also deplete central norepinephrine and serotonin, and this has been linked to reductions in activity, motivation, and increased depression in humans (Goodwin & Bunney, 1971).

More recently, investigators have drawn clear links between PTSD and hormonal changes often associated with stress. Unlike results in other areas, post-traumatic stress syndromes appear to reflect decreases in some hormones while increasing others; in one study mean urinary cortisol in male inpatients with PTSD were comparable to those of paranoid schizophrenics but lower than those exhibited by other schizophrenics or patients with bipolar or major depressive disorders (Kosten *et al.*, 1987). At the same time, PTSD patients showed norepinephrine levels that were greater than those of the other patient groups and more epinephrine than all but bipolar (manic) patients. These findings have been replicated and extended and the norepinephrine/cortisol ratio has been used as a diagnostic tool for PTSD (Mason *et al.*, 1988). Irregularities in the cortisol-producing hypothalamic–pituitary–adrenal cortical axis have been investigated in more detail and appear to be a likely factor in the development and/or maintenance of PTSD (e.g. Yehuda, Southwick, Perry, Mason, & Giller, 1990).

REFERENCES

Adams, P.R., & Adams, G.R. (1984). Mount St Helens's ashfall: evidence for a disaster stress reaction. *American Psychologist*, **39**, 252–60.

Adler, A. (1943). Neuropsychiatric complications in victims of Boston's Cocoanut-Grove disaster. *Journal of the American Medical Association*, **123**, 1098–101.

Ahearn, F.L. (1981). Disaster mental health: a pre- and post-earthquake comparison of psychiatric admission rates. *Urban and Social Change Review*, **14**, 22–8.

Allodi, F.A. (1994). Post-traumatic stress disorder in hostages and victims of torture.

Psychiatric Clinics of North America, **17**, 279–88.

American Psychiatric Association. (1980). *Diagnostic and statistical manual of mental disorders, 3rd edition*. Washington, DC: American Psychiatric Association.

American Psychiatric Association. (1987). *Diagnostic and statistical manual of mental disorders, 3rd Edition, Revised*. Washington, DC: American Psychiatric Association.

American Psychiatric Association. (1994). *Diagnostic and statistical manual of mental disorders, 4th edition*. Washington, DC: American Psychiatric Association.

Astin, M.C., Ogland-Hand, S.M., Coleman, E.M. & Foy, D.W. (1995). Posttraumatic stress disorder and childhood abuse in battered women: comparisons with mentally distressed women. *Journal of Consulting and Clinical Psychology*, **63**, 308–12.

Baum, A., Cohen, L. & Hall, M. (1993). Control and intrusive memories as possible determinants of chronic stress. *Psychosomatic Medicine*, **55**, 274–86.

Baum, A., Fleming, R. & Davidson, L.M. (1983). Natural disaster and technological catastrophe. *Environment and Behavior*, **15**, 333–5.

Baum, A., Fleming, I., Israel, A. & O'Keefe, M.K. (1992). Symptoms of chronic stress following a natural disaster and discovery of a human-made hazard. *Environment and Behavior*, **24**, 347–65.

Bolin, R. & Klenow, D. (1982–1983). Response of the elderly to disaster: an age-stratified analysis. *International Journal of Aging and Human Development*, **16**, 283–96.

Boman, B. (1986). Combat stress, post-traumatic stress disorder, and associated psychiatric disturbance. *Psychosomatics*, **27**, 567–73.

Bownes, I.T., O'Gorman, E.C. & Sayers, A. (1991). Psychiatric symptoms, behavioural responses and post-traumatic stress disorder in rape victims. *Issues in Criminological and Legal Psychology*, **1**, 25–33.

Brady, K.T., Killeen, T., Saladin, M.S. & Dansky, B. (1994). Comorbid substance abuse and posttraumatic stress disorder: characteristics of women in treatment. *American Journal on Addictions*, 3, 160–4.

Bremner, J.D., Scott, T.M., Delaney, R.C. & Southwick, S.M. (1993). Deficits in short-term memory in posttraumatic stress disorder. *American Journal of Psychiatry*, **150**, 1015–19.

Breslau, N., Davis, G., Andreski, P. & Peterson, E. (1991). Traumatic events and post-traumatic stress disorder in an urban population of young adults. *Archives of General Psychiatry*, **48**, 216–22.

Cameron, C. (1994). Veterans of a secret war: survivors of childhood sexual trauma compared to Vietnam war veterans with PTSD. *Journal of Interpersonal Violence*, **9**, 117–32.

Cassidy, K.L., McNally, R.J. & Zeitlin, S.B. (1992). Cognitive processing of trauma cues in rape victims with posttraumatic stress disorder. *Cognitive Therapy and Research*, **16**, 283–95.

Davidson, L.M. & Baum, A. (1986). Chronic stress and posttraumtic stress disorders. *Journal of Consulting and Clinical Psychology*, **54**, 303–8.

Davidson, L.M. & Baum, A. (1993). Predictors of chronic stress among Vietnam veterans: Stress exposure and intrusive recall. *Journal of Traumatic Stress*, **6**, 195–212.

Davidson, L.M., Baum, A. & Collins, D.L. (1982). Stress and control-related problems at Three Mile Island. *Journal of Applied Social Psychology*, **12**, 349–59.

Davis, M. (1980). Neurochemical modulation of sensory–motor reactivity: acoustic and tactile startle reflexes. *Neuroscience Biobehavioral Review*, **4**, 241–63.

Foa, E.B., Feske, U., Murdock, T.B. & Kozak, M.J. (1991). Processing of threat-related information in rape victims. *Journal of Abnormal Psychology*, **100**, 156–62.

Foy, D.W., Sipprelle, R.C., Rueger, D.B. & Carroll, E.M. (1984). Etiology of posttraumatic stress disorder in Vietnam veterans: analysis of premilitary, military, and combat exposure influences. *Journal of Consulting and Clinical Psychology*, **52**, 79–87.

Goodwin, F. & Bunney, W.E. (1971). Depression following reserpine: a reevaluation. *Seminars in Psychiatry*, **3**, 435–48.

Green, B.L. (1990). Defining trauma: terminology and generic stressor dimensions. *Journal of Applied Social Psychology*, **20**, 1632–42.

Green, B.L. (1994). Psychosocial research in traumatic stress: An update. *Journal of Traumatic Stress*, **7**, 341–62.

Green, B.L. & Berlin, M.A. (1987). Five psychosocial variables related to the existence of post-traumatic stress disorder symptoms. *Journal of Clinical Psychology*, **43**, 643–9.

Green, B.L., Grace, M.C., Lindy, J.D., Gleser, G.C. & Leonard, A. (1990*a*). Risk factors for PTSD and other diagnoses in a general sample of Vietnam veterans. *American Journal of Psychiatry*, **147**, 729–33.

Green, B.L., Lindy, J.D., & Grace, M.C. (1985). Posttraumatic stress disorder. *Journal of Nervous and Mental Disease*, **173**, 406–11.

Green, B.L., Lindy, J.D., Grace, M.C. & Gleser, G.C. (1990*b*). Buffalo Creek survivors in the second decade: stability of stress symptoms. *American Journal of Orthopsychiatry*, **60**, 43–54.

Green, B.L., Lindy, J.D., Grace, M.C. & Leonard, A.C. (1992). Chronic posttraumatic stress disorder and diagnostic comorbidity in a disaster sample. *Journal of Nervous and Mental Disease*, **180**, 760–6.

Helzer, J.E., Robins, L.M. & McEvoy, L. (1987). Post-traumatic stress disorder in the general population: findings of the epidemiologic catchment area survey. *New England Journal of Medicine*, **317**, 1630–4.

Hendin, H., Hass, A.P., Singer, P., Gold, F. & Trigos, G.G. (1983). The influence of precombat personality on posttraumatic stress disorder. *Comprehensive Psychiatry*, **24**, 530–4.

Holloway, H.C. & Ursano, R.J. (1984). The Viet Nam veteran: memory, social context, and metaphor. *Psychiatry*, **47** 103–8.

Horowitz, M.J. (1986). Stress-response syndromes: a review of posttraumatic and adjustment disorders. *Hospital and Community Psychiatry*, **37**, 241–9.

Horowitz, M.J. (1993). Stress-response syndromes: a review of posttraumatic stress and adjustment disorder. In J.P. Wilson & B. Raphael (Eds.). *International handbook of traumatic stress syndrome* pp. 49–60. New York: Plenum Press.

Keane, T.M. & Wolfe, J. (1990). Comorbidity in post-traumatic stress disorder: an analysis of community and clinical studies. *Journal of Applied Social Psychology*, **20**, 1776–88.

Keane, T.M., Fairbank, J.A., Caddell, J.M., Zimering, R.T. & Bender, M.E. (1985). A behavioral approach to assessing and treating posttraumatic stress disorder in Vietnam veterans. In C.R. Figley (Ed.). *Trauma and its wake*, pp. 257–294. New York: Brunner/Mazel.

Kilpatrick, D.G., Best, C.L., Saunders, B.E. & Veronen, L.J. (1987). Rape in marriage and in dating relationships: how bad is it for mental health? *Annals of the New York Academy of Sciences*, **528**, 335–4.

Kosten, T.R., Mason, J.W., Giller, E.L., Ostroff, R.B. & Harkness, L. (1987). Sustained urinary norepinephrine and epinephrine elevation in posttraumatic stress disorder. *Psychoneuroendocrinology*, **12**, 13–20.

Krystal, J.H. (1990). Animal models for post-traumatic stress disorder. In E. Giller (Ed.). *Biological assessment and treatment of P.T.S.D.* pp. 3–26. Washington DC: APA Press, Inc.

Kulka, R.A., Schlenger, W.E., Fairbank, J.A., Jordan, B.K., Hough, R. L.K., Marmar, C.R. & Weiss, D.S. (1990).

Trauma and the Vietnam war generation. New York: Brunner/Mazel.

Kushner, M.G., Riggs, D.S., Foa, E.B. & Miller, S.M. (1993). Perceived controllability and the development of posttraumatic stress disorder (PTSD) in crime victims. *Behaviour Research and Therapy*, **31**, 105–10.

Lifton, R.J. & Olson, E. (1976). The human meaning of total disaster: the Buffalo Creek experience. *Psychiatry*, **39**, 1–18.

McFarlane, A.C. (1986). Posttraumatic morbidity of a disaster: a study of cases presenting for psychiatric treatment. *Journal of Nervous and Mental Disease*, **174**, 4–13.

McFarlane, A.C. (1990). Vulnerability to posttraumatic stress disorder. In M.E. Wolf & A.D. Mosnaim (Eds.). *Posttraumatic stress disorder: etiology, phenomenology, and treatment.* Washington, DC: American Psychiatric Press, Inc.

McFarlane, A.C. (1992). Avoidance and intrusion in posttraumatic stress disorder. *Journal of Nervous and Mental Disease*, **180**, 439–45.

Maida, C.A., Gordon, N.S., Steinberg, A. & Gordon, G. (1989). Psychosocial impact of disasters: victims of the Baldwin Hills fire. *Journal of Traumatic Stress*, 37–48.

Mason, J.W., Giller, E.L., Kosten, T.R. & Harkness, L. (1988). Elevation of urinary norepinephrine/cortisol ratio in posttraumatic stress disorder. *Journal of Nervous and Mental Disease*, **176**, 498–502.

McNally, R.J., English, G.E. & Lipke, H.J. (1993). Assessment of intrusive cognition in PTSD: use of the modified Stroop paradigm. *Journal of Traumatic Stress*, **6**, 33–41.

McNew, J.A. & Abell, N. (1995). Posttraumatic stress symptomatology: similarities and differences between Vietnam veterans and adult survivors of childhood sexual abuse. *Social Work*, **40**, 115–26.

Mellman, T.A., Randolph, C.A., Brawman-Mintzer, O., Flores, L.P. & Milanes, F.J. (1992). Pheonomenology and course of psychiatric disorders associated with combat-related posttraumatic stress disorder. *American Journal of Psychiatry*, **149**, 1568–4.

Miller, J.A., Turner, J.G. & Kimball, E. (1981). Big Thompson Flood victims: one year later. *Family Relations*, **30**, 111–16.

North, C.S., Smith, E.M., McCool, R.E. & Lightcap, P.E. (1989). Acute postdisaster coping and adjustment. *Journal of Traumatic Stress*, **2**, 353–60.

Orr, S.P. (1990). Psychophysiologic studies of posttraumatic stress disorder in E.L. Giller, Jr. (Ed). *Biological assessment and treatment of posttraumatic stress disorder.* Washington, DC: American Psychiatric Press.

Parker, G. (1977). Cyclone Tracy and Darwin evacuees: on the restoration of the species. *British Journal of Psychiatry*, **130**, 548–55.

Patrick, V. & Patrick, W.R. (1981). Cyclone '78 in Sri Lanka: the mental health trail. *British Journal of Psychiatry*, **138**, 210–16.

Perlberg, M. (1979). Trauma at Tenerife: the psychic aftershocks of a jet disaster. *Human Behavior*, 49–50.

Perry, S., Difede, J., Musngi, G., Frances, A.J. & Jacobsberg, L. (1992). Predictors of posttraumatic stress disorder after burn injury. *American Journal of Psychiatry*, **149**, 931–5.

Popovic, M. & Petrovic, D. (1964). After the earthquake. *Lancet*, **ii**, 1169–71.

Reaves, M.E., Callen, K.E. & Maxwell, M.J. (1993). Vietnam veterans in the general hospital: seven years later. *Journal of Traumatic Stress*, **6**, 343–50.

Redmond, E.D. & Krystal, J.H. (1984). Multiple mechanisms of withdrawal from opioid drugs. *Annual Review of Neuroscience*, **7**, 443–78.

Resnick, H.S., Kilpatrick, D.G., Best, C.L. & Kramer, T.L. (1992). Vulnerability-stress factors in development of posttraumatic stress disorder. *Journal of Nervous and Mental Disease*, **180**, 424–30.

Rothbaum, B.O. & Foa, E.B. (1993). Subtypes of posttraumatic stress disorder. In J.R.T. Davidson & E.B. Foa (Eds.). *Post-traumatic stress disorder: DSM IV and beyond.* Washington, DC: American Psychiatric Press.

Rothbaum, B.O., Foa, E.B., Riggs, D.S., Murdock, T. & Walsh, W. (1992). A prospective examination of post-traumatic stress disorder in rape victims. *Journal of Traumatic Stress*, **5**, 455–75.

Scurfield, R.M. (1993). Posttraumatic stress disorder in Vietnam Veterans. In J.P. Wilson & B. Raphael (Eds.). *International handbook of traumatic stress syndromes*, pp.285–295. New York: Plenum Press.

Sierles, F.S., Chen, J., McFarland, R.E. & Taylor, M.A. (1983). Posttraumatic stress disorder and concurrent psychiatric illness: a preliminary report. *American Journal of Psychiatry*, **140**, 1177–9.

Sierles, F.S., Chen, J., Messing, M.L., Besyner, J.K. & Taylor, M.A. (1986). Concurrent psychiatric illness in non-Hispanic outpatients diagnosed as having posttraumatic stress disorder. *Journal of Nervous and Mental Disease*, **174**, 171–3.

Smith, E.M. & North, C.S. (1993). Post traumatic stress disorder in natural disasters and technological accidents. In J.P. Wilson & B. Raphael (Eds.) *International handbook of traumatic stress syndromes*, pp. 405–419. New York: Plenum Press.

Smith, E.M., North, C.S., McCool, R.E. & Shea, J.M. (1989). Acute post-disaster psychiatric disorders: identification of those at risk. *American Journal of Psychiatry*, **146**, 202–6.

Smith, E.M., Robins, L.N., Przybeck, T.R., Goldring, E. & Solomon, S.D. (1986). Psychosocial consequences of a disaster. In J.H. Shore (Ed.). *Disaster stress studies: new methods and findings*, pp. 50–76. Washington, DC: American Psychiatric Press.

Speed, N., Engdahl, B., Schwartz, J. & Eberly, R. (1989). Posttraumatic stress disorder as a consequence of the POW experience. *Journal of Nervous and Mental Disease*, **177**, 147–53.

Tomb, D.A. (1994). The phenomenology of post-traumatic stress disorder. *Psychiatric Clinics of North America*, **17**, 237–50.

Uddo, M., Vasterling, J.J., Brailey, K. & Sutker, P.B. (1993). Memory and attention in combat-related post-traumatic stress disorder (PTSD). *Journal of Psychopathology and Behavioral Assessment*, **15**, 43–52.

Ursano, R.J., Boydstan, J.A. & Wheatly, R.P. (1981). Psychiatric illness in U.S. Air Force Vietnam prisoners of war: a five-year follow-up. *American Journal of Psychiatry*, **138**, 310–13.

van der Kolk, B., Greenberg, M., Boyd, J. & Krystal, J. (1985). Inescapable shock, neurotransmitters and addiction to trauma: towards a psychobiology of post traumatic stress. *Biological Psychiatry*, **20**, 314–25.

Wert, B.J. (1979). Stress due to nuclear accident: a survey of an employee population. *Occupational Health Nursing*, **27**, 16–24.

Yehuda, R., Southwick, S.M., Perry, B.D., Mason, J.W. & Giller, E.L. (1990). Interactions of the hypothalamic – pituitary – adrenal axis and the catecholaminergic system in posttraumatic stress disorder. In E.L. Giller, Jr. (Ed.). *Biological assessment and treatment of posttraumatic stress disorder.* Washington DC: American Psychiatric Press.

Postpartum depression

SANDRA A. ELLIOTT

University of Greenwich School of Social Sciences,
Avery Hill Road, London SE9 2UE, UK

Postpartum Depression, known in Britain as Postnatal Depression, is one of the commonest complications of childbirth. Studies of depressive symptomatology report figures up to 30%. Research employing standardized psychiatric interviews 2 or 3 months postnatal to identify Depression as a syndrome or diagnosis, characterized by persistent depressed mood in combination with one or more other symptoms, consistently report prevalence figures of around 10% (O'Hara & Zekoski, 1988). These figures do not include the Blues (emotional lability for a day or two around days 3 to 5) or Puerperal Psychoses (severe, but rare, disorders with onset typically within 14 days and usually requiring hospitalization). These two postnatal disorders are sometimes included under the term Postnatal Depression. However, they are explicitly excluded from the term in this text since they have been shown to differ in prevalence, presentation, prognosis and preferred treatment. In this text the psychiatric diagnosis of non-psychotic depression, i.e. the syndrome of Postnatal Depression, is indicated by the use of capitals. Depressive symptomatology to which a diagnosis has not been applied is referred to as postnatal depression.

THE EXPERIENCE AND CONSEQUENCES

Controlled studies have demonstrated marked differences in prevalence between postnatal women and appropriate controls for both Blues and Puerperal Psychoses but not for the diagnosis of Postnatal Depression. However, postnatal women do report higher levels of depressive symptomatology and social maladjustment, particularly marital adjustment, than their matched non-childbearing controls (O'Hara et al., 1990). The research is therefore consistent with clinical experience that depression in the puerperium has a greater psychosocial impact than depression at other times. Many women are very distressed about the depression itself when it occurs at this critical time in their life and relationships. They remember postnatal depression many years on and talk of 'missing' the first months of their baby's life.

Physical health outcomes for mother and child have yet to be assessed. Research could look for a relationship with immunization rates and accidental injury. (Non-accidental injury is rarely reported though fears of neglecting or harming the child are expressed since, in depressed women, low self-esteem often focuses on their mothering skills.) In contrast, there is an increasing body of evidence for an association with long-term psychological outcomes for mother (Philipps & O'Hara, 1991) and child (Murray et al., 1993). Despite the fact that, in the majority of cases, the depressive episode had remitted by three to four months postpartum, at 18 months of age infants of mothers who experienced Postnatal Depression were more likely to be insecurely attached to their mothers, to have beha-viourial problems and deficits in cognitive functioning. Studies employing detailed ratings of video taped mother–infant interactions at 2 months postpartum are beginning to reveal specific differences enabling psychologists to test hypotheses regarding the mechanisms by which Postnatal Depression influences subsequent infant development. The characteristics of interaction which are typical of parent–child communication, and which attract infant attention, are the very characteristics most disrupted by depression. For example, not only do depressed women express more negative emotions but also their speech is less focused on infant experience and tends to show less acknowledgement of infant agency (Murray et al., 1993).

VULNERABILITY FACTORS AND PRECIPITANTS

Almost every conceivable factor has been postulated as a cause for Postnatal Depression and submitted as a test of association with it. Few have proved consistently positive (O'Hara & Zekoski, 1988). The biggest surprise may be the absence of any evidence for an association with progesterone level or other hormonal factors. Whilst hormones show dramatic change with childbirth (and may make some contribution to the blues), no hormone has yet been identified which distinguishes those who become depressed.

Not all methodological problems have been solved so it is not possible to state with confidence that hormonal dysfunction plays no part in the aetiology (O' Hara et al., 1991). Claims that Postnatal Depression has been proved to be caused by the hormonal changes at birth are however, much exaggerated.

Research which consistently fails to provide support for medical models is broadly consistent with psychosocial models which view childbirth as a significant life event at a time of increased physical and emotional vulnerability, with the same potential for precipitating depression in women with preexisting vulnerability as other major events. Though many academic disputes remain (e.g. Elliott, 1990) researchers agree that Postnatal Depression is related to: a previous psychiatric history, previous consultation with a doctor for depression, anxiety or 'nerves', depression or anxiety during pregnancy, a poor marital relationship and inadequate social support.

Most psychological models of depression propose a vulnerability – stress aetiology which predicts that the combination of pre-existing vulnerability and the occurrence of stressful events is particularly devastating. Research findings for both Postnatal Depression diagnosis and for postnatal depressive symptomatology are consistent with such models (O'Hara et al., 1991).

Leverton devised questions to assess such vulnerability factors antenatally and embedded them in a questionnaire for use at the first antenatal clinic visit. Psychiatric interviews and self-rating questionnaires used at 3 months postnatal with first and second time mothers established that the questionnaire could meaningfully identify more and less vulnerable groups (though not 'high risk' individuals). Such instruments are very valuable for research purposes. However, ethical and practical difficulties seriously limit their use in clinical practice (Elliott, 1989).

DETECTION

Women are reluctant to report depressive symptomatology for fear of damage to their public image through illness labelling or even because they believe (incorrectly) that postnatal depression can lead to the removal of their baby by health or social workers. Many health workers are reluctant to 'see' depression because of their own sense of impotence in the face of it. Many hidden depressions improve with time and the help of family or friends. However, some do not, and untreated can last past the babies first birthday. Cox and colleagues therefore developed a screening questionnaire which is short, quick and acceptable for use at the 6 week postnatal check and at specified intervals thereafter. The positive predictive value of this questionnaire, known as the Edinburgh Postnatal Depression Scale (or EPDS) is surprisingly high, though it varies with the population under test and the type of criterion psychiatric interview (Cox & Holden, 1993). Screening questionnaires share the ethical dilemmas of invasion of privacy, labelling and practical problems for large-scale administration with vulnerability questionnaires. However, when used by properly trained health professionals they can form part of valuable treatment interventions.

PREVENTION AND TREATMENT

Multilevel, multidisciplinary systems are required to make the most effective use of the high levels of health professional contact in pregnancy and the puerperium. Psychologists have worked with psychiatric, obstetric and primary care staff to develop and evaluate programmes for prevention (Elliott, Sanjack & Leverton, 1988) and treatment (Brierley 1988; Holden, Sagovsky & Cox, 1989). In accordance with the research on aetiology, these programmes focus on psychological vulnerability and psychosocial stress rather than the biological changes after delivery. A common theme to these programmes is demystifying the experience of depression (Elliott, 1990). Unhappy feelings are expected, accepted and understood. Previously 'invisible' stresses in women's lives become visible, enabling women to come to terms with or change the aspects of their lives which depress them. Cognitive models are particularly useful in this therapeutic context (Brierley, 1988; Elliott, 1989) though non-directive counselling can achieve the same results for many women (Holden *et al.*, 1989).

Preventive programmes in this model include challenges to Madonna and Child fantasies of the puerperium. They discourage 'superwoman' ambitions whilst acknowledging womens need to feel respected and valued in their maternal role. Women are warned that both physical and emotional coping resources will be reduced after childbirth and encouraged to build up their networks for social support and practical help. When depression does occur, early detection should ensure that non-directive counselling intervention (active listening) by a primary-care professional will be sufficient to halt and reverse the spiral towards Postnatal Depression (with the possible exception of women with personal or family history of Psychoses or Endogenous Depression requiring psychiatric admission). Occasionally counselling in primary care reveals a complex relevant past history such as of abuse in childhood, neglect or difficult relationship with mother, previous pregnancy loss or cot death, bereavement (particularly problematic if it occurred before the birth) or marital problems. Referral on to more skilled cognitive or psychodynamic psychotherapy from a clinical psychologist or other mental health professional should then be suggested to the mother.

REFERENCES

Brierley, E. (1988). A cognitive–behavioural approach to the treatment of post-natal distress. *Marce Society Bulletin*, 1, 27–41.

Cox, J.L. & Holden, J. (Eds.) (1993). *Prevention of depression after childbirth: use and misuse of the Edinburgh Postnatal Depression Scale*. London: Gaskell Press.

Elliott, S.A. (1989). Psychological strategies in the prevention and treatment of Postnatal Depression. *Baillière's Clinical Obstetrics and Gynaecology*, 3, 879–903.

Elliott, S.A. (1990). Commentary on 'childbirth as a life event'. *Journal of Reproductive and Infant Psychology*, 8, 147–59.

Elliott, S.A., Sanjack, M. & Leverton, T.J. (1988). Parents' group in pregnancy: a preventive intervention for postnatal depression? In B.J. Gottlieb (Ed.). *Marshalling social support; formats, process and effects*. California: Sage.

Holden, J.M., Sagovsky, R. & Cox, J.L. (1989). Counselling in a general practice setting: controlled study of health visitors' intervention in treatment of postnatal depression. *British Medical Journal*, 298, 223–6.

Murray, L., Kempton, C., Woolgar, M. & Hooper, R. (1993). Depressed mother's speech to their infants and its relation to infant gender and cognitive development. *Journal of Child Psychology and Psychiatry*, 34, 1083–2001.

O'Hara, M.W. & Zekoski, E.M. (1988). Postpartum depression: a comprehensive review. In R. Kumar & F. Brockington (Eds.). *Motherhood and mental illness; vol 2. causes and consequences*, pp. 17–63. London: Wright.

O'Hara, M.W., Zekoski, E.M., Philipps, L.H. & Wright, E.S. (1990). Controlled prospective study of postpartum mood disorders; comparison of childbearing and non-childbearing women. *Journal of Abnormal Psychology*, 99, 3–15.

O'Hara, M.W., Schlechte, J.A., Lewis, D.A. & Varner, M.W. (1991). Controlled prospective study of postpartum mood disorders. Psychological, environmental and hormonal variables. *Journal of Abnormal Psychology*, 100, 63–73.

Philipps, L.H.C. & O'Hara, M.W. (1991). Prospective study of Postpartum Depression: 4½-year follow-up of women and children. *Journal of Abnormal Psychology*, 100, 151–5.

Premenstrual syndrome/Late luteal phase disorder

JANE M. USSHER

Women's Health Research Unit, Psychology
Department, University College London, UK

DIAGNOSTIC CRITERIA AND INCIDENCE

Following the first description of premenstrual tension in the 1930s, a considerable amount of medical and psychological research has been devoted to discerning both the underlying causes of premenstrual symptomatology and the most effective forms of treatment. Renamed premenstrual syndrome (PMS) in 1953, because of the wide array of symptoms, and more recently 'late luteal disphoric phase disorder' (LLPD) in the *DSMIV*, PMS includes a range of up to 150 different physical and psychological symptoms, including irritability, depression, tiredness, lack of concentration, hostility, aches and pains, diarrhoea and constipation. National Institute of Mental Health guidelines published in 1983 suggested that PMS should be assessed using prospective (daily) rating of symptoms over at least two cycles, and that diagnosis depends on finding at least a 30% increase two or more symptoms during the five days prior to menses in each cycle, compared with the follicular phase of the cycle.

Recent community surveys have reported that 50% of women experience premenstrual symptoms in all or the majority of cycles, and that between 10 and 40% of women experience serious disruption to their lives premenstrually because of physical or psychological symptoms (Mortola, 1992).

AETIOLOGICAL THEORIES AND TREATMENTS FOR PMS

Medical theories and therapies

A range of aetiological theories and treatments have been proposed to explain the multiple symptom complex of PMS. Much of the research to date has focused on biological or hormonal treatments, and over 50 different treatments have been suggested (Ussher, 1992). These can be differentiated on the basis of those which operate on a hormonal level (i.e. progesterone; oestradiol implants), those which attempt to alter the menstrual cycle (i.e. GnRH agonists which induce 'medical castration' through down regulation of the pituitary–ovarian axis), nutritional agents (i.e. vitamin B6), psychotropic intervention (i.e. fluoxetine), and those which aim at altering fluid or electrolyte imbalance (i.e. diuretics). However, a number of recent reviews of the literature come to the same conclusion: there is no simple biological or hormonal substrate for PMS, and, whilst many medical treatments are effective in symptom reduction, methodological difficulties such as retrospective assessment of symptoms, or absence of placebo control groups, mean that positive results of many treatment trials must be interpreted with caution (Bancroft, 1994).

Psychological theories and therapies

The inconsistencies and contradictions between the biological theories and therapies, the inability of researchers to clearly identify an hormonal substrate, and the high placebo response, have lent strength to the view that psychosocial factors are implicated in the aetiology of PMS, and that psychological interventions may be appropriate, either in addition to or instead of medical treatments.

Stress has been implicated as a major influence on reporting of premenstrual mood or behavioural disturbance. It has been argued that menstrual and premenstrual distress are significantly correlated with undesirable life events, with increases in life stress resulting in increases in menstrual cycle complaints. This may be explained within a vulnerability model, as it has been reported that reactivity to stressors varies throughout the cycle (Hastrup & Light, 1984), with the greatest response being recorded in the premenstrual phase. This has led to the suggestion that the premenstrual phase of the cycle acts as a stressor for some women, because of negative attitudes and expectations associated with menstruation, resulting in life events being perceived or experienced as more stressful when experienced in the perimenstrual period. The evidence that attribution of arousal or negative symptomatology varies during the cycle, with negative symptoms being attributed to the menstrual cycle premenstrually yet attributed to environmental factors intermenstrually, has led to the suggestion that women may be more vulnerable to external stressors in the perimenstrual period because of the perception and differential attribution of symptoms (Koeske, 1980). A recent study which found poor marital satisfaction to be the best predictor of PMS after life events had been controlled for (Coughlin, 1990), suggests that coping with symptomatology is also related to social support. These theories provide an explanation for the fact that women do not report premenstrual symptoms in every cycle, as there are monthly changes in social circumstances and life stress.

One other explanation offered for the apparent anomalies in the literature, and the apparent high rates of individual differences between women, is the influence of cognitive–personality factors. It has been found that women who report PMS score more highly on measures of neurotic and A type personality than non-sufferers: personality types associated with greater reactions to stress. Thus stress and personality factors may combine to 'sensitize premenstrual symptoms in women', and contribute to a diagnosis of PMS (Heilbrun & Frank, 1989).

However, the growing interest in psychosocial explanations for PMS has not as yet resulted in the widespread development of psychological interventions. For, as Slade has noted 'in comparison

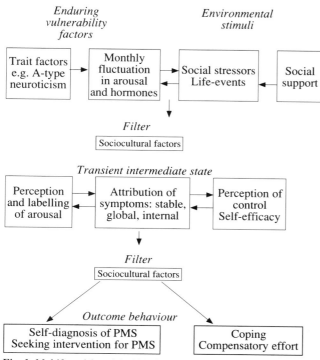

Enduring vulnerability factors

Environmental stimuli

Trait factors e.g. A-type neuroticism → Monthly fluctuation in arousal and hormones → Social stressors Life-events ← Social support

Filter

Sociocultural factors

Transient intermediate state

Perception and labelling of arousal → Attribution of symptoms: stable, global, internal → Perception of control Self-efficacy

Filter

Sociocultural factors

Outcome behaviour

Self-diagnosis of PMS Seeking intervention for PMS

Coping Compensatory effort

Fig. 1. Multifactorial model of PMS.

measures such as exercise or diet. There have been to date ten published studies using cognitive or behavioural therapies to treat PMS (Kirkby, 1994), all showing positive results in treating both psychological and behavioural symptoms for the majority of cases. However, firm conclusions cannot be reached regarding the relative efficacy of these different approaches, owing to the paucity of controlled trials of psychological therapy in comparison with other treatments for PMS.

Multifactorial models

Given the contradictions in the research, it is becoming increasingly common for multifactorial approaches to be adopted for assessment and treatment of PMS, where biological and psychosocial factors can be addressed within a framework that does not privilege one or the other. Figure 1 is an example of such a model developed by Ussher (1992). These models suggest a movement away from the existing dichotomy of medical and psychological treatments, advocating a combination of treatments within a symptom based approach, taking account of the fact that symptom profiles vary greatly between women. One suggestion (O'Brien, 1993) is that counselling is offered as an initial treatment, succeeded by one of the medical treatments which have been shown to be effective in placebo-controlled trials: fluoxetine, progestogens, oral contraceptives, or danazol and oestradiol patches (plus cyclic progestogen), prescribed in an hierarchical manner, depending on severity of symptoms and the woman's response to treatment. If a woman's presenting symptoms are primarily psychological, psychological therapy may be most appropriate, in addition to, or instead of, medical intervention (Kirkby, 1994). (See also 'Menstrual abnormalities'.)

with the extensive trials of medication, specific psychological interventions have been scarce' (1989, p. 135). Psychological interventions which have been advocated for PMS have included stress management, behaviour therapy, cognitive–behavioural therapy, and rational emotive therapy. Others have advocated more practical

REFERENCES

Bancroft, J. (1994). The premenstrual Syndrome: a reappraisal of the concept and the evidence. *Psychological Medicine*, Suppl. 24 1–47.

Coughlin, P.C. (1990). Premenstrual syndrome: How marital satisfaction and role choice affect symptom severity. *Social Work*, 35, 351–5.

Hastrup, J. & Light, K. (1984). Sex differences in the cardiovascular stress response: modulation as a function of menstrual cycle phases. *Journal of Psychosomatic Research* 28, 275–83.

Heilbrun, A.B. & Frank, M.E. (1989). Self-preoccupation and general stress level

as sensitizing factors in premenstrual and menstrual distress. *Journal of Psychosomatic Research*, 33, 571–7.

Kirkby, R.J. (1994). Changes in premenstrual symptoms and irrational thinking following cognitive–behavioural coping skills training. *Journal of Consulting and Clinical Psychology*, 62, 1026–32.

Koeske, R. (1980). Theoretical perspectives on menstrual cycle research: the relevance of attributional approaches for the perception and explanation of premenstrual emotionality. In A.J. Dan, E. Graham & C. Beecher (Eds.). *The menstrual cycle*, vol I, New York: Springer.

Mortola, J. (1992). Assessment and management of premenstrual syndrome. *Current Opinion in Obstetrics and Gynaecology*, 4, 877–85.

O'Brien, P.M.S. (1993). Helping women with premenstrual syndrome. *British Medical Journal*, 307, 1474–8.

Slade, P. (1989). Psychological therapy for premenstrual emotional symptoms. *Behavioural Psychotherapy*, 17, 135–50.

Ussher, J.M. (1992). Research and theory related to female reproduction: implications for clinical psychology. *British Journal of Clinical Psychology*, 31, 129–51.

Pregnancy and childbirth

LYN QUINE

Centre for Research in Health Behaviour,
Department of Psychology, University of Kent at
Canterbury, UK

Almost three-quarters of a million children will be born in England and Wales this year. While the huge majority of these will be healthy, some 6000 will die before their first birthday and some 45 000 will be of low birthweight, placing them at risk. Still others will be disabled as a result of complications during the pregnancy or birth. For some mothers the quality of the birth experience will be poor and their satisfaction with antenatal services low. In this review we examine the principal social and psychological variables that may affect these outcomes and consider the contribution that psychological theory has made to understanding the epidemiological facts of pregnancy and childbirth.

There are three sections. First, we present the published data on pregnancy outcome. For the sake of brevity we shall highlight only three outcomes: early childhood mortality, low birthweight, and complications of pregnancy, though our argument also applies to perceptions of the birth and satisfaction with services. Secondly, we examine psychosocial and behavioural risk factors for poor outcome. The principal risk factors discussed are psychosocial factors, including negative life events and social support; emotional factors, including distress, anxiety, self-esteem, and depression; cognitive factors, including knowledge, beliefs, and attitudes to pregnancy; coping resources and strategies; and behavioural factors, for which we take one example, that of smoking. We argue that the risk factors are not distributed randomly in society and independent of working and living conditions, but are disproportionately prevalent among lower socioeconomic groups. In the third section we suggest a model which draws out the pathways by which risk factors may mediate social inputs and outcomes, and may help to guide future research.

EARLY CHILDHOOD MORTALITY

Infant mortality in England and Wales has fallen by 64%, from 17.5 per 1000 live births in 1971 to 6.3 per 1000 in 1993. Improvements in absolute social conditions have played a major role in reducing mortality, along with increased medical knowledge and improved services, but marked effects of relative social and economic disadvantage are present. For example, there are noticeable regional differences across the country, and large differences between district authorities within the same region, associated with their prevailing social and economic conditions.

The significance of social class is extremely marked. Although the greatest risk at birth is to children of mothers who are older or have had several children already (Macfarlane & Mugford, 1984), mortality rates during the first year are strongly class related even when age and parity are controlled. The Office of Population Censuses and Surveys publishes data based on the father's occupation, and for each of the indices there is a steady gradient from low mor-

tality in Social Class I to high mortality in Social Class V. Social Class V has twice the rate of Social Class I in the figures for 1992 and over the last decade. The steepest gradient, however, occurs for the postneonatal period: 2.7 : 1 for postneonatal mortality against 1.6 : 1 for neonatal mortality. Postneonatal mortality is of particular importance because the child who dies after the first month of life will normally have been discharged from hospital and therefore domestic, social, and environmental factors are more likely to be implicated than quality of neonatal medical care. This is supported by the fact that, unlike the overall mortality rates, the causes of postneonatal mortality are distributed evenly across the classes, which indicates that children at the bottom of the social scale have an overall vulnerability and run the highest risk of poor outcomes in general. Middle-class circumstances offer overall, non-specific protection. Biomedical risk factors in poor pregnancy outcome are now reasonably well understood, and an important challenge is to understand the role of social and psychological factors.

LOW BIRTHWEIGHT

Another index of pregnancy outcome is low birthweight, now normally defined as 2499 g or less. As with early childhood mortality, there is a sharp difference between the top and bottom of the social scale in England and Wales, with ratios for Class V to Class I of 1.4 : 1 in 1990. The pattern is repeated for low birthweight children who die early in childhood, though the ratios this time are less marked and have shown greater signs of improvement with a sharp decline in both perinatal and infant mortality among low birthweight children over the years (OPCS Series DH3 and Monitors). Low birthweight children who survive have high rates of medical and developmental problems (see the recent work of, for example, Lloyd, 1984; Marlow, D'Souza & Chiswick, 1987), though whether these too are class related is not known.

COMPLICATIONS OF PREGNANCY

It is more difficult to obtain recent national figures for complications of pregnancy, labour and delivery. Since the most useful source, the Hospital In-Patient Enquiry (HIPE), was discontinued in 1985, the 1982–1985 HIPE maternity tables (OPCS, 1988) provide the most recent figures available. The most important measure is the estimated total maternity discharges (of delivered women only) by complications. This includes a very wide range of complications: those related mainly to pregnancy such as antepartum haemorrhage, hypertension and early or threatened labour; those that indicate the need for greater care in pregnancy, labour and delivery, such as multiple gestation, malpresentation of the foetus or suspected fetal abnormality; complications occurring mainly in the course of labour, such as long labour or postpartum haemorrhage; and complications of the puerperium, such as puerperal infection or obstetrical pulmonary embolism.

The figures indicate a trend towards a higher number of reported complications. In 1985, only 37.9% of deliveries were considered uncomplicated, compared with 45% in 1975 and 45% in 1980. Estimated total complications for 1984 were 641 780. Hypertension constituted 8.3% of the total complications reported in 1984, early or threatened labour 4%, long labour 5.7% and obstetrical trauma 12.3%. Women who experience complications during pregnancy and labour are more likely to give birth to a baby with complications than women who do not, 22% in 1985, for example, against 7% (OPCS, 1988, Series MB4, No 28, Table 7.5). Although the figures are not broken down by social class, the literature indicates that some pregnancy complications, notably pre-term delivery, are class-related (for example, Sanjose, Roman & Beral, 1991). (See 'Abortion' chapter for miscarriage figures.)

SOCIAL AND PSYCHOLOGICAL FACTORS AFFECTING PREGNANCY AND CHILDBIRTH

The preceding review of epidemiological data has shown that one of the most important social inputs affecting pregnancy outcome is social class. There is a downward trend towards adverse pregnancy outcomes through the social classes, a pattern that has been reported many times throughout the health literature on children and adults alike. Our next concern is to examine whether social and psychological risk factors are disproportionately prevalent among lower socioeconomic groups and whether such factors might act as mediators between social class and outcome, thus providing a psychological explanation for some of the statistics.

Psychosocial factors: life events and social support

Studies have found that a high frequency of life events during pregnancy is associated with pre-term births and other adverse pregnancy outcomes (Williamson, Lefevre & Hector, 1989), and that working-class women have significantly more life events during their pregnancies than middle-class women (Newton & Hunt, 1984). Newton and Hunt found that low birthweight was predicted by life events and, even more strongly, by smoking during pregnancy, which they suggested was a mediator of stress (as Graham, 1976, 1984 has also argued). Many other studies have reported similar findings (for reviews see Oakley, 1985; Levin & DeFrank, 1988).

The literature also suggests that a woman can be protected or buffered from the effects of severe life events if she has good support networks (Collins et al., 1993). In a study of army wives, Nuckolls, Cassel and Kaplan (1972) examined the relationship of stressful life events and 'psychosocial assets' (such as social support and self-esteem) to pregnancy complications. It was found that neither was related to increased risk when examined alone, but that life events were associated with complications of both pregnancy and delivery when social supports were absent. A subsequent re-analysis splitting stress and social support at the median found that 91% of women with high stress but low social support had complications, against only 33% with high stress and high social support, a highly significant difference.

The problems in disentangling the effects of social support and life events are well documented. Many life events, such as bereavement, also involve loss of social support. In addition, there are problems in disentangling the effects of personality variables such as neuroticism and self-esteem. Intervention studies that have manip-

ulated social support are therefore instructive. Social support throughout the pregnancy has been shown in some studies to reduce the incidence of low birthweight and pregnancy complications, hospital admission in pregnancy, and use of neonatal intensive care. Some of the beneficial effects are still apparent over one year after the birth (for reviews see Oakley, 1985; 1988; and the intervention study by Oakley and her colleagues, Oakley, Rajan & Grant, 1990). Though this study reports successful results, a recent randomized trial in Switzerland in which social support was provided to women at risk of having a low birthweight baby failed to find an effect (Villar et al., 1992).

Simply having another woman present at the birth has been shown to reduce length of labour, complications during labour and delivery, and admissions to neonatal intensive care, and to increase mother–infant interaction in the first minutes after the birth (Klaus et al., 1986; Hofmeyr et al., 1991). Support immediately after the birth, especially from health professionals, may also lead to a reduction in maternal anxiety during the first year of the child's life (Parker & Barnett, 1987).

Emotional factors: maternal distress, anxiety, and depression

A number of authors have found a significant relationship between emotional factors and a variety of pregnancy outcomes from low birthweight to complications of pregnancy and satisfaction with the birth experience (for example, Levin & DeFrank, 1988). Lederman et al. (1978, 1979) found a correlation between anxiety and uterine contractions and length of labour. The most recent literature, however, has concentrated on the role of psychological rather than physiological processes. A longitudinal study on pregnancy and mothering in the East End of London carried out by Wolkind and Zajicek (1981), for example, found that the average weight of children born to mothers with a diagnosed psychiatric condition was significantly lower than for children with psychiatrically healthy mothers. The disturbed mothers were on average younger, attended antenatal classes less frequently, and smoked more; and it was smoking that predicted low birthweight best of all. The evidence thus begins to suggest a complex pattern of relationships between social class and outcome, with psychosocial risk factors acting as mediators.

An important study by Norbeck and Tilden (1983) investigated the effects upon pregnancy outcome of life stress, social support, and 'emotional disequilibrium', a construct made up of state anxiety, depression, and low self-esteem. Although inter-related, life stress, social support, and emotional disequilibrium were found to have separate effects: life stress was associated with difficulties in pregnancy, emotional disequilibrium with complications in the health of the child. As in the earlier study by Nuckolls et al., when life stress was present but social support was absent, a higher number of complications were noted in a whole range of outcomes, including pregnancy, delivery, and the condition of the child, thus confirming the stress-buffering role of social support.

Other studies have explored a variety of related concepts, including trait and state anxiety, psychodynamic defences, maternal distress, and emotional state. Some writers argue that psychological and life stress variables do not function independently but work in synergy. A useful review of the entire area is to be found in Reading (1983).

Cognitive factors: knowledge, beliefs, and attitudes to pregnancy

Two main approaches have been adopted in research on the role of knowledge as a mediator of health behaviours and outcomes. The first is descriptive, and the most influential model here has been that of Ley (1988), who has been concerned primarily with describing the relationships between cognitive variables and patients' satisfaction, particularly their satisfaction with medical communications. The model argues that the most important predictors of satisfaction with medical communications are comprehension and memory, and that satisfaction in turn leads to compliance. In the absence of knowledge, comprehension and memory, and consequently satisfaction, will be low, leading to a low level of compliance.

The second approach is the use of intervention studies, and almost all the research on pregnancy has been of this type. The main interest has been to test whether increasing knowledge, for example through antenatal classes, leads to more appropriate behaviours and more positive outcomes. The effects of antenatal classes on behaviour have been reviewed by Nelson (1982), and effects on outcome by Bakketeig, Hoffman and Oakley (1984). The evidence is not entirely consistent in either area, but the overall trend is towards positive relationships.

According to the Health Belief Model of Becker and his colleagues (Janz & Becker, 1984), whether a woman takes action to avoid complications in pregnancy, by making full use of antenatal services, smoking less, and changing her diet, for example, is predicted by three main variables: how vulnerable she perceives herself to be to the complications; how severe or important she believes them to be; and her evaluation of the benefits and costs of taking action.

It has been suggested by Becker that, in order for health beliefs to be translated into action, a trigger is necessary to reinforce their personal relevance. In a study by Reading *et al.* (1982), this idea was applied to the role of ultrasound scanning. Of two groups of women who were scanned at their first antenatal visit, one group were given high feedback, in which they were shown the size and shape of the foetus and its movements were pointed out, and the other group were given no picture and no specific verbal description or comments. Both groups were given advice about smoking and drinking. At follow-up, compliance with this advice was significantly higher in the women who had been given feedback than in those who had not. Two other studies have used the Health Belief Model successfully in research into pregnancy outcomes, one to predict those women who would choose amniocentesis (French *et al.*, 1992) and one to predict attendance for antenatal care (Zweig, Lefevre & Kruse, 1988).

Three other studies of beliefs during pregnancy have used Fishbein and Ajzen's Theory of Reasoned Action (Fishbein & Ajzen, 1975). Manstead, Proffitt and Smart (1983) used the model to predict which of a group of mothers-to-be would choose to breastfeed, Godin and LePage (1988) to predict the intentions of first-time mothers to smoke cigarettes after the birth of their child, and Lowe and Frey (1983) to predict intentions to use the Lamaze method of childbirth. In each case, the model showed that beliefs played an important role.

Findings concerning the relationship between women's attitudes towards pregnancy and pregnancy outcome are by no means clear (Chalmers, 1982). It has been argued that attitudes may influence a woman's behaviour during pregnancy, posture, diet, smoking, drinking, how early she visits a doctor for antenatal care, how well she takes care of herself, and so on, all of which, in turn, may affect the outcome of the pregnancy. Negative attitudes towards pregnancy and motherhood have been found to be related to vomiting during pregnancy (Chertok, 1972), prolonged labour (Yang *et al.*, 1976), pain during labour (Beck *et al.*, 1980) and high levels of medication (Doering & Entwisle, 1975; Yang *et al.*, 1976), toxaemia (Ringrose, 1972), and prematurity (Blau *et al.*, 1963). However, other research has led to rather different conclusions. Chalmers (1983) and Zajicek (1981), for example, could find no relationship between attitudes to pregnancy and motherhood and either length of labour or drug dosage.

Coping resources and strategies

It is in the way that women cope with their pregnancy that many of the psychosocial mediators are drawn together. Coping has been defined as the problem-solving efforts made by an individual when the demands of a given situation tax adaptive resources (Lazarus, Averill & Opton, 1974; Pearlin & Schooler, 1978). The central process is cognitive appraisal, which is a mental process by which people assess whether a demand threatens their well-being (primary appraisal), appraise their resources for meeting the demand, formulate solutions, and select strategies (secondary appraisal). For a number of women, lack of material resources may reduce their choice of coping strategies; lack of physical resources may mean that pre-existing physical or psychological ill-health will impede the process of coping; lack of social resources may mean that fewer people can be called upon to help; lack of psychological and intellectual resources may produce cognitive problems including an inability to respond to difficulties in optimistic, persistent and flexible ways, an explanatory style that focuses on the internal, stable and global factors of negative events, and low self-efficacy. Pregnancy care will be seen as the responsibility of outside professionals, and internal locus of control will be weak. This may lead, in turn, to the selection and use of ineffectual coping strategies, and the likely result will be an increased willingness to take dangerous behavioural risks, whether failing to carry out positive measures, such as taking up antenatal services, or continuing to pursue negative behaviours, such as smoking and drinking in pregnancy. The central issue is whether such women can be identified and classified, and the answer appears to be that many are from lower socioeconomic groups where material deprivation is prevalent (Blaxter, 1987; Pill & Stott, 1985).

A prospective study by Doering, Entwisle and Quinlan (1980), based on Janis's theory of stress and coping, offers interesting findings on the role of antenatal education in reducing stress and increasing coping behaviour. Women who were more informed about childbirth, whether their information came from classes, books, television, or any other source, were found to need less medication and anaesthesia during the birth of their child than other women. This meant that they were able to retain awareness and control, which in turn resulted in a more enjoyable birth. The husband's support and presence emerged as an important second factor and, together, preparation and support accounted for more than half the variance in the dependent measures. Other research into the factors predicting successful coping has been reported by Leventhal *et al.* (1989), and Byrne-Lynch (1991).

Behavioural factors: smoking

As an example of behavioural factors associated with pregnancy outcome we select just one, that of smoking. An excellent summary of research on smoking and pregnancy outcome appeared in the Fourth Report of the Independent Scientific Committee on Smoking and Health (Froggatt, 1988). Smoking during pregnancy has been shown many times to be associated with foetal and neonatal mortality, low birthweight, and developmental retardation and indeed the first evidence appeared as early as 1957. For mothers who smoke, the increase in perinatal mortality is estimated at 28%, the reduction in birthweight is 150 g to 250 g on average, and the risk of having a low birthweight baby is doubled (see the references to the work of Bakketeig *et al.* (1994) and Simpson and Smith in Froggatt, 1988). Simpson and Smith go so far as to say that smoking is responsible for 20% of all low weight births in this country. All the reported effects increase with the number of cigarettes smoked but, if the mother changes her behaviour before the end of the fourth month of pregnancy, the risk to the baby is determined by the new pattern of behaviour and not the original one. Recent evidence suggests that so-called 'passive smoking', exposure to environmental tobacco smoke produced by other people, may also be associated with reduced birthweight.

Although these studies provide evidence that the association is causal and serious, some researchers have claimed that the correlation may be spurious (Oakley, 1989). Oakley, for example, argues that smoking in pregnancy is linked to various aspects of women's maternal and social position. Working class women experience poorer material conditions and lower social support, which makes negative life events and chronic long term difficulties more likely. These, in turn, lead to stress. Smoking is a coping strategy used in response both to stress and to impoverished material and social conditions.

An important point to emerge from Froggatt (1988), in contrast, is that the effects of smoking during pregnancy appear to operate independently of potentially confounding factors, such as social class, parity, the mother's age and height, and the sex of the child, though there are, of course, marked differences in the incidence of smoking by social group. For example, more than twice as many women smoke in Class V as Class I, 36% against 16% according to OPCS data for 1990 (OPCS, 1991). Data from the British Perinatal Mortality Survey and the British Births Survey indicate that 41.3% of pregnant women smoked in 1970 against 29.5% in 1958 (Peters *et* *al.*, 1983), and the equivalent estimate made by Simpson and Smith for their 1984 data based on the General Household Survey was 29%, ranging from 13% in Class I to 31.5% in Class V. The implication is that most women who smoke continue to do so during pregnancy: pregnancy does not stop them.

Further evidence against non-causal explanations of the association between smoking and low birthweight come from the results of randomized intervention trials, in which mothers-to-be were encouraged to stop smoking during pregnancy. Froggatt reviews three. The first, by Donovan, was inconclusive but produced some indication of an increase in birthweight in comparison with a control group whose mothers continued to smoke. The second, by Sexton and Habel, showed that, among singletons 'experimental' babies were born an average of 92 g heavier and 0.6 cm longer than 'control' babies, and the third, by MacArthur, Newton and Knox, produced figures of 68 g and 0.75 cm. Intervention studies offer the best evidence so far of a causal link, but whether the link is a direct physiological one or is mediated through the effects of stress buffering and support, for example, has yet to be determined.

PREGNANCY OUTCOME: A SUMMARY

In this review we have seen that social class has marked effects on pregnancy outcome. We have examined the psychosocial and behavioural risk factors for poor outcome and concluded that they, also, are distributed disproportionately among the lower socio-economic groups. Now we suggest a model to try to piece together some of the relationships (see Fig. 1). The most important aspect of lower social class appears to be impoverished material and social conditions and resources, which lead, we argue, to two principal effects. On the one hand, they produce an increase in negative life events and chronic long-term difficulties, often with an absence of social support. On the other, they lead to a reduction in the level of access to information, in part through lack of education. Life events and lack of support may lead in turn to emotional problems, including lowered self-esteem, stress, anxiety, and depression, while poor education and lack of access to information produce a corresponding range of cognitive problems, including a lack of knowledge and a set of beliefs and attitudes that lead the woman to see herself as vulnerable to illness and complications but helpless to prevent them. The emotional and cognitive effects combine to produce a set of coping styles and strategies that are characterized by hopelessness and a willingness to

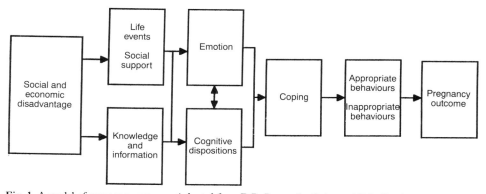

Fig. 1. A model of pregnancy outcome. (adapted from D.R. Rutter, L. Quine and D.J. Chesham (1993). *Social Psychological Approaches To Health* Harvester-Wheatsheaf).

take potentially serious risks. From there, it is a short step to inappropriate behaviours, poor uptake of maternity services and attendance at antenatal care, smoking, drinking, poor diet and self-care, and thence to negative outcomes. A fuller review of psychosocial and behavioural factors that may affect pregnancy outcome is to be found in Rutter, Quine and Chesham (1993).

The model presented here is, at present, essentially a framework for integrating past findings and guiding future research. There are many gaps to be filled in the existing body of knowledge and much to be done to establish the strengths and weights of the proposed links and causal pathways. Not all links between class and poor pregnancy outcome will be mediated by psychosocial and behavioural variables. However, as the review makes clear, further examination of psychosocial and behavioural factors offers great promise for understanding the underlying processes that link deprivation to pregnancy outcome.

REFERENCES

Bakketeig, L.S., Hoffman, H.J. & Oakley, A.R. (1984). Perinatal mortality. In M.B. Bracken (Ed.). *Perinatal epidemiology.* Oxford: Oxford University Press.

Beck, N.C., Siegel, L.J., Davidson, N.P., Kormeier, S., Breitenstein, A. & Hall, D.G. (1980). The prediction of pregnancy outcome: maternal preparation, anxiety and attitudinal sets. *Journal of Psychosomatic Research*, **24**, 343–51.

Blau, A., Slaff, B., Easton, K., Welkowitz, J., Springarn J. & Cohen, J. (1963). The psychogenic etiology of premature births, *Psychosomatic Medicine*, **25**, 201.

Blaxter, M. (1987). Evidence of inequality in health from a national survey, *The Lancet*, July 4 30–3.

Byrne-Lynch, A. (1991). Coping strategies, personal control and childbirth. *International Journal of Psychology*, **12**, 145–52.

Chalmers, B. (1982). Psychological aspects of pregnancy: some thoughts for the eighties. *Social Science and Medicine*, **16**, 323–31.

Chalmers. B. (1983). Psychosocial factors and obstetric complications. *Psychosomatic Medicine*, **13**, 333–9.

Chertok, L. (1972). The psychopathology of vomiting of pregnancy. In J. Howells (Ed.). *Modern perspectives in psycho-obstetrics.* pp. 269–282, Edinburgh: Oliver and Boyd.

Collins, N., Dunkel-Schetter, C. Lobel, M. & Scrimshaw, W. (1993). Social support in pregnancy: psychosocial correlates of birth outcomes and postpartum depression. *Journal of Personality and Social Psychology*, **56**, 1243–58.

Doering, S.G. & Entwisle, D.R. (1975). Preparation during pregnancy and ability to cope with labour and delivery. *American Journal of Orthopsychiatry*, **45**, 825–37.

Doering, S.G., Entwisle, D.R. & Quinlan, D. (1980). Modeling the quality of women's birth experience. *Journal of Health and Social Behaviour*, **21**, 12–21.

Fishbein, M. & Ajzen, J. (1975). *Belief, attitude, intention and behaviour: an introduction to theory and research.* Reading, Mass: Addison-Wesley.

French, B., Kurczynski, T., Weaver, M. & Pituch, M. (1992). Evaluation of the Health Belief Model and decision-making regarding amniocentesis and women of advanced maternal age. *Health Education Quarterly*, **19**, 177–86.

Froggatt, P. (1988). *Fourth report of the independent scientific committee on smoking and health.* London: HMSO.

Godin, G. & LePage, L. (1988). Understanding the intentions of pregnant nullipara not to smoke cigarettes after childbirth. *Journal of Drug Education*, **18**, 115–24.

Graham, H. (1976). Smoking in pregnancy: the attitudes of expectant mothers. *Social Science and Medicine*, **10**, 399.

Graham, H. (1984). *Women, health and the family.* Brighton: Wheatsheaf.

Hofmeyr, G.I., Nikodem, V.C., Wolman, W.L., Chalmers, B.E. & Kramer, T. (1991). Companionship to modify the clinical birth environment: effects on progress and perceptions of labour and breast feeding. *British Journal of Obstetrics and Gynaecology*, **98**, 756–64.

Janz, N.K. & Becker, M.H. (1984). The Health Belief Model: a decade later. *Health Education Quarterly*, **11**, 1–47.

Klaus, M.H., Kennell, J.H., Robertson, S.S. & Sosa, R. (1986). Effects of social support during parturition on maternal and infant morbidity. *British Medical Journal*, **293**, 585–7.

Lazarus, R.S., Averill, J.R. & Opton, E.M. (1974). The psychology of coping: issues of research and assessment. In G.V. Coehio, D.A. Hamburg & J.E. Adams (Eds.). *Coping and adaptation.* New York: Basic Books.

Lederman, R., Lederman, E., Work, B. & McCann, D.A. (1978). The relationship of maternal anxiety, plasma catecholamines and plasma cortisol to progress in labour. *American Journal of Obstetrics and Gynecology*, **132**, 495–500.

Lederman, R.P., Lederman, R., Work, B.A. & McCann, D.S. (1979). Relationship of psychological factors in pregnancy to progress in labour. *Nursing Research*, **28**, 94–102.

Leventhal, E., Leventhal, A., Schacham, S. & Easterling, D. (1989). Active coping reduces reports of pain from childbirth. *Journal of Consulting and Clinical Psychology*, **57**, 365–1.

Levin, J.S. & DeFrank, R.S. (1988). Maternal stress and pregnancy outcomes: a review of the psychological literature. *Review of Psychosomatic Obstetrics and Gynaecology*, **9**, 3–16.

Ley, P. (1988). *Communicating with patients.* London: Chapman and Hall.

Lloyd, B.W. (1984). Outcome of very-low-birthweight babies from Wolverhampton. *The Lancet*, September 29, 739–41.

Lowe, R. & Frey, J. (1983). Predicting Lamaze childbirth intentions and outcomes: an Extension of the Theory of Reasoned Action to a joint outcome. *Basic and Applied Social Psychology*, **4**, 353–72.

Macfarlane, A. & Mugford, M. (1984). *Birth counts: statistics of pregnancy and childbirth.* National Perinatal Epidemiological Unit (in collaboration with OPCS). London: HMSO.

Manstead, A.S.R., Proffitt, C. & Smart, J.L. (1983). Predicting and understanding mothers' infant-feeding intentions and behaviour: testing the theory of reasoned action. *Journal of Personality and Social Psychology*, **44**, 657–71.

Marlow, N., D'Souza, S.W. & Chiswick, M.L. (1987). Neurodevelopmental outcome in babies weighing less than 2001 g at birth, *British Medical Journal*, **294**, 1582–6.

Nelson, M.K. (1982). The effect of childbirth preparation on women of different social classes. *Journal of Health and Social Behaviour*, **23**, 339–52.

Newton, R.W. & Hunt, L.P. (1984). Psychosocial stress in pregnancy and its relation to low birthweight. *British Medical Journal*, **288**, 1191–4.

Norbeck, J.S. & Tilden, V.P. (1983). Life stress, social support and emotional disequilibrium in complications of pregnancy: a prospective multivariate study. *Journal of Health Social Behaviour*, **24**, 30.

Nuckolls, K.B., Cassel, J. & Kaplan, B.H. (1972). Psychosocial assets, life crisis and the prognosis of pregnancy. *American Journal of Epidemiology*, **95**, 431–41.

Oakley, A. (1985). Social support in pregnancy: the 'soft' way to increase birthweight? *Social Science and Medicine*, **21**, 1259–68.

Oakley, A. (1988). Is social support good for the health of mothers and babies? *Journal of Infant and Reproductive Psychology*, **6**, 3–21.

Oakley, A. (1989). Smoking in pregnancy: smokescreen or risk factor? Towards a materialist analysis. *Sociology of Health and Illness*, **11**, 311–35.

Oakley, A., Rajan, L. & Grant, A. (1990). Social support and pregnancy outcome. *British Journal of Obstetrics and Gynaecology*, **97**, 155–62.

OPCS: Office of Population Censuses and Surveys (1988). *Hospital in-patient enquiry maternity tables 1982–1985, Series MB4 No 28*. London: HMSO.

OPCS: Office of Population Censuses and Surveys (1991). General household survey: cigarette smoking 1972 to 1990. *OPCS Monitor*, SS 91/3.

Parker, G. & Barnett, B. (1987). A test of the social support hypothesis. *British Journal of Psychiatry*, **150**, 72–7.

Pearlin, L.I. & Schooler, C. (1978). The structure of coping. *Journal of Health and Social Behaviour*, **22**, 337–56.

Peters, T.J., Golding, J., Butler, N.R., Fryer, J.E., Lawrence, C.J. & Chamberlain, E.V.P. (1983). Plus ça change: predictors of birthweight in two national studies. *British Journal of Obstetrics and Gynaecology*, **90**, 1040–5.

Pill, R. & Stott, N.C.H. (1985). Choice or chance: further evidence on ideas of illness and responsibility for health. *Social Science and Medicine*, **20**, 981–91.

Reading, A.E. (1983). The influence of maternal anxiety on the course and outcome of pregnancy: a review. *Health Psychology*, **2**, 187–202.

Reading, A.E., Campbell, S., Cox, D.M. & Sledmere, C.M. (1982). Health beliefs and health care behaviour in pregnancy. *Psychological Medicine*, **12**, 379–83.

Ringrose, C.A. (1972). Psychopathology of toxaemia of pregnancy. In J. Howells (Ed.). *Modern perspectives in psycho-obstetrics*. pp. 283–291, Edinburgh: Oliver and Boyd.

Rutter, D.R., Quine, L. & Chesham, D.J. (1993). *Social psychological approaches to health*. Hemel Hempstead: Harvester Wheatsheaf.

Sanjose, S., Roman, E. & Beral, V. (1991). Low birthweight and preterm delivery, Scotland, 1981–84: effect of parents' occupation, *The Lancet*, **338**, 428–31.

Villar, J., Farnot, U., Barros, F. & Victora, C. (1992). A randomized trial of

psychosocial support during high risk pregnancies. *New England Journal of Medicine*, **327**, 1266–71.

Williamson, H., Lefevre, M. & Hector, M. (1989). Association between life stress and serious perinatal complications, *Journal of Family Practice*, **22**, 489–94.

Wolkind, S. & Zajicek, E. (Eds.). (1981). *Pregnancy: a psychosocial and social study*. London: Academic Press.

Yang, R., Zweig, A., Ponthitt, T. & Federman, E. (1976). Successive relationships between maternal attitudes during pregnancy, analgesic medication during labour and delivery and newborn behaviour. *Developmental Psychology*, **12**, 6–14.

Zajicek, E. (1981). The experience of being pregnant. In S. Wolkind & E. Zajicek (Eds.). *Pregnancy: a psycho-social and social study*. London: Academic Press.

Zweig, S., Lefevre, M. & Kruse, J. (1988). The Health Belief Model and attendance for prenatal care. *Family Practice Research Journal*, **8**, 32–41.

Premature babies

DEBORAH ROSENBLATT

Psychology Department,
Reading University, UK

Prematurity refers to infants born preterm (before 37 weeks gestation). Although maturity is the best predictor of the severity of neonatal illness and long-term outcome, gestation is not always reliable so studies often refer to birthweight categories: extremely low birthweight (ELBW ≤ 1000 g; approximately 23–27 weeks gestation), very low birthweight (VLBW 1001–1500; 28–31 weeks), low birthweight (LBW 1501–2500; 32–36 weeks). Infants may also be small-for-gestational age (SGA, sometimes referred to as SFD 'small-for-dates'), indicating poor intra-uterine growth. Across developed countries preterm births account for 5–8% of deliveries, representing about 40 000 in the UK and 350 000 in the USA. An infant born at less than 28 weeks is likely to need intensive care (including artificial ventilation) for at least a month, whereas at 34 weeks he or she may only need warmth and supplementary tube feeding and can remain with the mother in a specialized postnatal ward. Infants less than 1000 g represent only 2% of deliveries, but half of infants weighing as little as 750 g now survive and more than 95% of those weighing more than 1500 g.

'HIGH-RISK' PREGNANCY AND DELIVERY

A mother-to-be expects a trouble-free pregnancy, normal delivery and a short hospital stay in which she will develop skills and affections that are rewarding to the baby, herself and her wider family. Only one-third of women who deliver early have identifiable risk factors so the diagnosis of threatened preterm labour, or problems which necessitate a planned early delivery, is likely to be unexpected and disturbing. Her new high-risk label implies interventions and changes in lifestyle, and reliance on professional caretakers rather than family and friends. She may become emotionally dependent on demanding treatments (many without proven benefit) and blame herself if her inability to comply seems to result in a poor outcome. Feelings of loss of control, shame and learned helplessness can lead to continued vulnerability and dependence. Prolonged antenatal admission can further deplete emotional resources because of separation from her family and worry about financial matters.

PSYCHOSOCIAL PREDICTORS OF PRETERM LABOUR

Recent prospective studies in Denmark (Hedegaard *et al.*, 1993) and the USA (Wadhwa *et al.*, 1993) confirm that maternal stress around 30 weeks of pregnancy is associated with decreased birthweight and gestation at delivery. Unfortunately, the implication that providing social support to high-risk women can improve the perinatal outcome has not been confirmed although mothers report that such intervention had enhanced a potentially traumatic experience (Oakley, 1992) (see previous chapter). Preterm delivery has a high recurrence rate. During subsequent pregnancy these mothers are likely to remain anxious beyond their period of medical risk, to express uncertainty about the outcome and maintain a more negative attitude toward the pregnancy and fetus. However, postpartum feelings and behaviours in relation to the new infant are positive and do not differ from those of low-risk women (van den Akker & Rosenblatt, 1993).

PRETERM BIRTH AND ATTACHMENT

Early delivery cuts short the emotional and practical preparation for birth and is likely to reduce autonomy and choice because of the increased need for operative delivery and medical attendance. The baby's 'high-tech' birth and transfer to a neonatal unit can trigger a range of emotional response: (i) fears about his, or her, survival and outcome, (ii) guilt about personal behaviours (e.g. working, smoking) which might have compromised his health, (iii) anger that professional staff were unable to diagnose and prevent the early delivery, (iv) feelings of helplessness in relation to the skilled staff and the more experienced parents in the neonatal unit (Rosenblatt & Redshaw, 1984). Seminal observations 30 years ago described this as a crisis for parents, involving unforeseen and unexpected events, unfamiliar settings and personnel, an inescapable set of demands and an uncertain outcome. Parental behaviour is likely to be determined by features of the situation itself, pre-existing personality, cultural factors and the parents' interactions with significant others (Caplan, Mason & Kaplan, 1965). Soon after this, Klaus and Kennel (1970) drew attention to a higher incidence of failure-to-thrive and abuse in preterm infants and suggested that this may be due to a lack of 'bonding' as a result of separation. It is more likely, however, that the maternal factors associated with infrequent visiting also determine later childcare practices. In a sample of 'high-risk' women, parent–infant attachment at 1 week and 8 months was predicted by parental competence but not by early parent–infant contact (Mercer & Ferketich, 1990). In addition, preterm infants may show increased irritability during the first year because of low sensory thresholds, gastroesophageal sensitivity leading to discomfort and inadequate caloric intake, and learned aversion. Persistent, seemingly inexplicable crying can further undermine parental confidence and lead to fears of an underlying cerebral problem.

DEVELOPMENTAL OUTCOME

The majority of preterm infants are born after 32 weeks and show few major problems, but infants less than 28 weeks have a disability rate of 20%. However, this still represents fewer than 1% of the total of disabled children in the community and has remained constant over the last 25 years. Outcome studies are confounded by different sampling methods (varying birthweight bands, uncertain gestations), age at testing (no standard screening age, few cohorts over 10 years of age, use of real vs. 'corrected' age), selection of controls, definition of good vs. poor outcome and diversity of outcome measures (usually academic achievement or cognitive measures only). Common findings are lower IQ scores, language and reading problems and poor visual–motor co-ordination, all of which have implications for educational resourcing (Pharoah et al., 1994). Both parent and teacher ratings of LBW children indicate a higher incid-ence of behaviour disorder in the preschool and school years, with the prevalence of clinically significant problems increasing with age. Lower SES and (stress as measured by negative life events) are associated with behaviour problems at school age, and it is also possible that parental expectation, anxieties and childcare patterns contribute to the development and management of difficult behaviour (Rose et al., 1992). Mothers of preterm infants also view their 3–8 year-old child as more 'vulnerable' even in the absence of defined problems. This may lead to an unwillingness to set limits on behaviours, to encourage autonomy and to expand the child's physical and social horizons (Culley, Perrin & Chaberski 1989). The continuing sophistication of neonatal care techniques in preventing cerebral haemorrhage, respiratory compromise and metabolic imbalance may improve the developmental outcome of infants born now.

MEETING FAMILY NEEDS

Psychosocial ward rounds enable the multidisciplinary team (e.g. paediatricians, neonatal nurses, social workers, occupational and physiotherapists, psychologists) to share information and address existing or potential problems associated with difficulties (e.g. social isolation, marital problems, personality disorder, poor self-esteem).

Most neonatal units in the UK and the USA provide social work, psychological or counselling services but unfortunately these are usually crisis led and receive low priority in hospital and community budgets. The use of interviews or standardized psychological assessment of parents prior to discharge may reveal depression which is often masked by the excitement of homecoming and dismissed as transient anxiety. Most parents do develop successful coping strategies during their infant's hospitalization and early years, especially if staff provide opportunities where positive feedback is likely, both from the infant and the hospital staff. The emergence of parent-to-parent networks represents egalitarian support systems in which families can share difficult feelings, encourage self-respect and autonomy and find common solutions to their challenging situations.

ENHANCING DEVELOPMENTAL OUTCOME

Since the mechanisms which account for developmental problems are not fully understood and prediction of which individual infants are 'at risk' is imprecise, varied approaches have been utilized. In hospital the provision of life-saving technology results in an inappropriate developmental environment, including sensory deprivation, overstimulation and nursing and social intervention, which is not related to the infant's physiological and behavioural cues. The NIDCAP (Neonatal Individualized Developmental Care and Assessment Programme) (Als et al., 1986) enables staff to observe, quantify and enhance the infant's behaviour as he/she progresses from physiological organization to behavioural responsiveness to reciprocity with caregivers. In the USA, developmental specialists are key workers in hospital and federally mandated programmes provide screening and intervention from birth to 3 years for preterm infants and others with special needs. Programmes combining structured home and centre developmental services plus parent-to-parent support result in enhanced cognitive performance and fewer behaviour problems (IHDP, 1990). However, effects are greatest in families of the least educated mothers and the predictive value of the individual elements is unclear (Brooks-Gunn et al., 1992). In designing and implementing interventions, it is important that parents do not feel overburdened with the responsibility of providing constant teaching and stimulation, with the consequence that other family needs remain unmet and they then feel doubly guilty if their child does not progress.

PERINATAL BEREAVEMENT
Success stories in the media and an optimistic prognosis from the medical staff may mislead parents into believing that even the smallest, sickest baby will survive. Some very immature infants will develop chronic lung disease and die after many months in hospital. And, because of the higher incidence of Sudden Infant Death Syndrome (SIDS) in preterm infants, even a low-risk baby may survive months of hospital care only to die unexpectedly a few weeks after discharge.

Fertility treatments have increased the number of very immature multiple births. Parents whose triplets or quads do not all survive may feel angry that they were not made aware of such risks and guilty that they compromised pregnancy outcome by asking for or allowing multiple egg implantation.

Every Neonatal Unit should have a set of procedures to be followed when an infant is dying, including a checklist to document the information, advice, services and support offered to, and taken up by, parents. Attention should be paid to factors that affect parents' reactions and their interaction with neonatal staff, including religious and cultural beliefs about pregnancy 'failure', 'imperfect' infants, and the parents' role in decision-making. Parents praise staff who show respect for their own autonomy, ensure good communication, reassure them that all appropriate treatments were tried, and who provide time and space for decision-making while continuing to cherish the baby. Follow-up counselling and support should be available but may not be taken up until a subsequent pregnancy or crisis occurs.

STAFF NEEDS AND RESPONSES
Neonatal staff perform highly skilled tasks in a crowded and complex environment, in which their responsibility includes both infant and family. Their long hours in artificial light and high temperatures may be associated with the increased levels of sick leave, anxiety and depression in neonatal nurses (Redshaw, Harris & Ingram, 1994). Reported stressors seem to be similar in frequency for nurses and doctors, and include understaffing, decisions on prioritizing care and interpersonal conflicts. However, when decisions are made to discontinue care, nurses bear the brunt of parental anger and frustration, while doctors may worry about personal prosecution, loss of attending privileges, departmental status and medical budgets (Astbury & Yu, 1982). Common coping strategies include cognitive processing or distancing (information seeking, search for meaning), revision and rehearsal for difficult situations, use of personal–social skills, and escape or avoidance (Jacobson, 1988). Staff support groups are often underutilized because of time pressures, the existence of informal support networks and a reluctance to reveal personal inadequacies to colleagues.

PSYCHOLOGICAL SERVICES
It is clear that the birth of an infant weeks or months before term has psychosocial implications for the child and his family, professional caretakers, and hospital and community services. Although psychologists may play only a small part in the direct care of an individual family, they can make a major contribution to:

(i) Education and training of staff (e.g. in developmental profiles, therapeutic approaches, assessment of anxiety, depression and family relationships).
(ii) Liaison between service providers (e.g. referrals for special needs assessment, decisions about placement in early intervention or educational programmes).
(iii) Facilitating a supportive climate and innovative psychological services (e.g. involvement in parent-to-parent organizations and help-lines, staff support groups and interdisciplinary forums).

REFERENCES
Als, H., Lawhorn, G., Brown, E., Gibes, R., Duffy, F.H., McAnulty, G. & Blickman, J.G. (1986). Individualized behavioral and environmental care for the very-low-birth-weight preterm infant at high risk for broncopulmonary dysplasia: neonatal intensive care unit and developmental outcome. *Pediatrics*, 78, 1123–32.
Astbury, J. & Yu, V.H.Y. (1982). Determinants of stress for staff in a NICU. *Archives of Disease in Childhood*, 57, 108–11.
Brooks-Gunn, H., Gross, R.T., Kraemer, H.C., Spiker, D. & Shapiro, S. (1992). Enhancing the cognitive outcome of low birth weight, premature infants: for whom is the intervention most effective? *Pediatrics*, 89, 1209–15.
Caplan, G., Mason, E. & Kaplan, D. (1965). Four studies of crisis in parents of prematures. *Community Mental Health Journal*, 1, 149–61.
Culley, B.S., Perrin, E.C. & Chaberski, M.J. (1989). Parental perceptions of vulnerability of formerly premature infants. *Journal of Pediatric Health Care*, 3, 237–45.
Hedegaard, M., Henricksen, T.B., Sabroe, S. & Secher, N.J. (1993) Psychological distress in pregnancy and preterm delivery. *British Medical Journal*, 37, 234–9.
Infant Health and Development Program (1990). Enhancing the outcomes of low-birth-weight, premature infants. *Journal of the American Medical Association*, 263, 3035–2.
Jacobson, S.F. (1988). Coping skills for neonatal nurses. Neonatal Nurses Conference, Nottingham (24 September 1988).
Klaus, M.H. & Kennel, J.H. (1970). Mothers separated from their newborn infants. *Pediatric Clinics of North America*, 17, 1015–1037.
Mercer, R.T. & Ferketich, S.L. (1990). Predictors of parental attachment during early parenthood. *Journal of Advanced Nursing*, 15, 268–80.
Oakley, A. (1992). Social support in pregnancy: methodology and findings of a 1-year follow-up study. *Journal of Reproductive and Infant Psychology*, 10, 219–31.
Pharoah, P.O.D., Stevenson, C.J., Cooke, R.W.I. & Stevenson, R.J. (1994). Clinical and subclinical deficits at 8 years in a geographically defined cohort of low birthweight infants. *Archives of Disease in Childhood*, 70, 264–70.
Redshaw, M.E., Harris, A. & Ingram, J.C. (1994). The neonatal unit as a working environment: a survey of neonatal nursing. *MIDIRS Midwifery Digest*, 4, 213–16.
Rose, S.A., Feldman, J.F., Rose, S.L.,

Wallace, I.F. & McCarton, C. (1992). Behavior problems at 3 and 6 years: prevalence and continuity in full-terms and preterms. *Development and Psychopathology*, 4, 361–74.

Rosenblatt, D.B. & Redshaw, M.E. (1984). Factors influencing the psychological adjustment of mothers to the birth of a preterm infant. In J.D. Call, E.

Galenson, & R.L. Tyson (Eds.). *Frontiers of infant psychiatry*, pp. 239–245. New York: Basic Books.

van den Akker, O. & Rosenblatt, D. (1993). Factors associated with pregnancy and the post-natal period in women at risk for pre-term delivery. In *Targeting health promotion: reaching those in need*. Vol. 3,

pp. 24–37. Cambridge: Trust. The Health Promotion Research.

Wadhwa, P.D., Sandman, C.A., Porto, M., Dunkel-Schetter, C. & Garite, T.J. (1993). The association between prenatal stress and infant birth weight and gestational age at birth: a prospective investigation. *American Journal of Obstetrics and Gynaecology*, vol. 858–865.

Radiation

DEANNA BUICK

Department of Psychiatry and Behavioural Science, School of Medicine, The University of Auckland, New Zealand

The majority of present cancer treatments consist of various combinations of surgery, radiation, chemotherapy, and hormone therapy. Radiation is therefore, an integral part of the management of patients with cancer. Radiation is often curative for certain types of malignancies, notably skin cancers, early-stage head and neck cancers and early-stage Hodgkin's disease. When combined with surgery and chemotherapy, radiation is used as an adjuvant treatment in many paediatric tumours, head and neck tumours, and soft tissue sarcoma. Radiation has come to play an important role in the treatment of early breast cancer, permitting more conservative surgical procedures to be used, followed by radiation. In addition, the terminal patient may obtain significant palliation of symptoms and some prolongation of life from appropriate radiation treatment.

Radiation affects both normal and malignant cells. Side-effects occur when radiation damages normal tissue and its tolerance to withstand the radiation is surpassed. The systemic reactions of fatigue and weakness are commonly reported by patients. Local reactions in the treated area include skin irritation, peeling, burns, and hair loss. Approximately 79% of patients receiving radiation to the abdomen, pelvic, and spine regions report some degree of nausea and vomiting, resulting in anorexia and weight loss (Welch, 1980). The side-effects usually begin after the first treatment and increase in severity with successive treatments, although this is dependent upon the type of cells irradiated, tissue-volume, dose-rate and time-fractionation.

Vast individual differences among patients in their psychological reaction to radiation have been found (Andersen & Tewfik, 1985). Research suggests that psychological distress associated with radiation is characterized by anxiety rather than depression (Andersen, Karlson, Andersen and Tewfik, 1984; Forester, Kornfeld & Fleiss, 1978), and men appear to experience more distress than women (Forester *et al.*, 1978). Patients who experience high levels of tension-anxiety when they begin radiation are likely to have poorer functioning following the course of treatment, than those who are not distressed when radiation commences (Graydon, 1988). However, moderate and realistic anxiety may be adaptive in cancer

patients and may apply to the adjustment of patients to radiation. Clinical descriptions of patients' reactions are available (for example, Peck & Boland, 1977; Rotman *et al.*, 1977; Welch, 1980).

High levels of anxiety directly after treatment may be related to the cumulative effect of side-effects during radiation. Symptoms like fatigue, sore throat, anorexia, and skin irritation have been reported at three months post-treatment (King *et al.*, 1985). The termination of treatment may raise a number of issues for the patient, including loss of medical support and monitoring, and vulnerability to recurrence without active treatment. These issues may contribute to the higher post-treatment anxiety responses in cancer patients in contrast with reports from other patients receiving surgical or diagnostic procedures, who generally report a reduction in anxiety. Medical personnel may require additional training to recognize common psychological problems presented by radiation patients.

Patients may hold a number of misconceptions about the nature of radiation, and the equipment used to deliver the treatment (Peck & Boland, 1977; Rotman *et al.*, 1977). For example, some patients fear that radiation may cause individuals to become radioactive (Rotman *et al.*, 1977). Mitchell and Glicksman (1977) found that 52% of patients felt that the referring physician had been of no help in preparing them for treatment. Patients who have completed radiation treatment report still feeling imperfectly informed about treatment procedures and side-effects (Cassileth, Volckmar & Goodman, 1980). In addition, patients appear hesitant to approach physicians and other medical staff with complaints or questions (Mitchell & Glicksman, 1977; Welch, 1980). Low levels of knowledge regarding radiation have been shown to correlate with patients engaging in minimal self-care activities during treatment (Dodd, 1984).

Radiation demands a high level of co-operation from patients. Descriptions of the treatment and side-effects that must be tolerated to achieve the desired effects are required. The anxiety and confusion characteristic of many radiation patients may be reduced if adequate educational preparation is provided. Effective, clear communication which is understood by the patient, reduces anxiety (Rainey, 1985), and the amount of disruption in patients' usual activities during and following radiation (Johnson, Lauvier & Nail, 1989). Contrary to medical practitioners' concerns, there is no relationship between forewarning patients of possible side-effects and the incidence of later symptoms (Peck & Boland, 1977; Welch, 1980). Patients' need for information appears to include intensified support for their beliefs, concern for them as a person, and confirmation of the validity of what the person thinks he or she knows (Cassileth *et al.*, 1980). An adequate explanation of treatment may facilitate the patient's sense of control in a relatively powerless situation. Patients who use denial as a defence mechanism may prefer to avoid information; preferences not to receive information about radiation therapy may play a role for some individuals.

The total care of the radiation patient goes beyond the technical aspects of treatment and encompasses multiple facets of support. The current state of research strongly suggests the need for more psycho-educational intervention built into the pre- and post-treatment clinical management of patients undergoing radiation.

REFERENCES

Andersen, B.J. & Tewfik, H.H. (1985). Individual differences in psychological response to radiation treatment: a reconsideration of the adaptive aspects of anxiety. *Journal of Personality and Social Psychology*, 48, 1024–32.

Anderson, B.L., Karlson, J.A., Anderson, B. & Tewfik, H.H. (1984). Anxiety and cancer treatment: response to stressful radiotherapy. *Health Psychology*, 3, 553–51.

Cassileth, B.R., Volckmar, D. & Goodman, R.L. (1980). The effect of experience on radiation therapy patients' desire for information. *International Journal of Radiation Oncology, Biology and Physics*, 6, 493–6.

Dodd, M.J. (1984). Patterns of self-care in patients receiving radiation therapy. *Oncology Nursing Forum*, 11, 23–7.

Forester, B.M., Kornfeld, D.S. & Fleiss, J. (1978). Psychiatric aspects of radiotherapy. *American Journal of Psychiatry*, 135, 960–3.

Graydon, J.E. (1988). Factors that predict patients' functioning following cancer treatment. *International Journal of Nursing Studies*, 25, 117–24.

Johnson, J.E., Lauvier, D.R. & Nail, L.M. (1989). Process of coping with radiation therapy. *Journal of Consulting and Clinical Psychology*, 57, 358–64.

King, K.B., Nail, L.M., Kreamer, K., Strohl, R.A. & Johnson, J.A. (1985). Patients descriptions of the experience of receiving radiation therapy. *Oncology Nursing Forum*, 12, 55–61.

Mitchell, G.W. & Glicksman, A.S. (1977). Cancer patients: knowledge and attitudes. *Cancer*, 40, 61–6.

Peck, A. & Boland, J. (1977). Emotional reactions to radiation treatment. *Cancer*, 40, 180–4.

Rainey, L.C. (1985). Effects of preparatory patient education for radiation oncology patients. *Cancer*, 56, 1056–61.

Rotman, M., Rogow, L., DeLeon, G. & Heskel, N. (1977). Supportive therapy in radiation oncology. *Cancer*, 39, 744–50.

Welch, D.A. (1980). Assessment of nausea and vomiting in cancer patients undergoing external beam radiotherapy. *Cancer Nursing*, 3, 365–71.

Radiotherapy

RUTH ALLEN

Department of Psychiatry, University College London Medical School, UK

Historically, medicine used radiotherapy to treat conditions such as eczema and ankylosing spondylitis. It is now used virtually exclusively in the treatment of patients with cancer. At least 40% of patients diagnosed with cancer will receive radiotherapy at some point during their treatment (Souhami & Tobias, 1994). Radiotherapy has a number of advantages over other treatments for cancer as it is a localized treatment customarily lasting a few weeks with limited toxicity and immediate effect. Radiotherapy is used with various treatment intents: curative, adjuvant, palliative and prophylaxis (brain metastases). Limited disease basal cell carcinomas, thyroid cancer, Hodgkin's lymphomas, seminomas and some head and neck cancers can be cured by radiotherapy alone. Radiotherapy is frequently used adjuvantly for locally resected tumours, e.g. breast, cervical, soft tissue/bone sarcomas, melanoma, etc. Palliative radiotherapy is effective in the symptomatic relief of bone and brain metastases, spinal cord compression, pathological fractures and superior vena cava obstruction. Radioactive implants are used in some cancers such as cervix, prostate and thyroid. Although little research has assessed the psychological impact of receiving radiotherapy, evidence suggests that, for the patient, there are significant negative aspects to radiation treatment. Four research areas have been considered in some detail: beliefs and anxieties towards receiving radiotherapy, the amount of information required by patients, immediate and long-term side-effects of radiotherapy, and psychological intervention studies.

BELIEFS AND ANXIETY ABOUT RECEIVING RADIOTHERAPY

Two fears are commonly reported by patients receiving radiotherapy. First, that radiation treatment can cause cancer and secondly that radiotherapy is a palliative not curative treatment (Holland & Rowland, 1989). The fear that radiation causes cancer is also associated with diagnostic X-ray procedures. In both diagnostic X-rays and radiotherapy treatment patients are treated alone in a bare room and when the machine is switched on there is a whirring sound while staff take refuge behind protective screens. These procedures are likely to engender anxiety and it is important to provide appropriate information.

Research has identified varying levels of anxiety in patients attending radiotherapy departments. In one study, 44% of newly referred patients had above normal anxiety scores, in another, assessing women with breast cancer at the start of adjuvant radiotherapy, 14% had scores indicating morbid anxiety (Young & Maher, 1992). However, the reason for raised anxiety levels may be more than the treatment itself. For example, many patients may have only recently received a cancer diagnosis or may have relapsed after previous cancer treatment. They will be concerned about the outcome of the radiotherapy, whether the treatment intent is curative or palliative. Patients may be anxious about a deterioration in their physical health or about particular side effects that they have been told could occur during radiotherapy. Cancer patients have high levels of anxiety and depression at times other than during, or at the end of, radiotherapy. Up to 30% of patients find the end of treatment itself upsetting (Holland & Rowland, 1989). In addition, although a large proportion of patients receiving palliative radiotherapy report high levels of psychological distress, those in pain and of reduced mobility are more likely to be distressed (Kaasa et al., 1993).

Patients also have difficulty confiding their anxieties to the radiotherapist or referring physician. In one study 82% of patients having radiotherapy would not have confided in their radiotherapist or their referring physician. A particular dilemma for radiotherapy patients is that it is often unclear who their primary doctor is. Patients generally remain under the care of their referring clinician unless they have problems specifically associated with radiotherapy.

INFORMATION

Some patients feel poorly informed about the radiotherapy they are about to receive and would prefer more information. Rainey (1985) demonstrated that, regardless of coping style, patients receiving more information are less anxious and have lower mood disturbance than those who have received limited information. In another study a booklet about radiotherapy was sent with admission letters to 200 patients who were later compared to 215 control patients. Although there were no differences in terms of overall worry between the two groups, patients who were given the booklet were twice as likely to be satisfied with the amount of information they had received about radiotherapy.

Holland et al. have suggested that information given to patients should include aims of the treatment, scheduling and duration details and an outline of possible side-effects. In particular, patients need to be prepared for possible side-effects that could lead to them feeling worse at the end of radiotherapy than when they began (Holland & Rowland, 1989). This level of information helps patients both to change their beliefs about radiotherapy and reduce anxiety.

SIDE-EFFECTS OF RADIOTHERAPY

Side-effects generally appear during the second and third week of radiotherapy and can continue for a while after treatment has fin-

ished (e.g. fatigue). Patients receiving cranial irradiation will experience alopecia, upper abdominal treatment often leads to nausea and vomiting and lower abdominal radiotherapy can cause diarrhoea. Patients can find the skin marking for radiotherapy frightening as the site marked is usually larger then expected and the tattoo is very obvious. They are warned not to wash the marks off and to be careful of the skin within the treated area which can become very sore, red and noticeable. Complaint about not being able to wash within the radiotherapy site frequently occurs.

FATIGUE

Fatigue is often reported during and after radiotherapy treatment. The number of patients experiencing fatigue is dependant upon the site of radiotherapy. For example, 65% of male genitourinary patients as compared to 93% of patients receiving chest radiotherapy reported fatigue (Smets et al., 1993). Other factors associated with fatigue in cancer are malnutrition, anaemia, drugs with a sedative effect (anti-emetics, analgesics), insomnia, pain, immobilization and depression (Hayes, 1991). Radiation fatigue with cumulative radiotherapy appears to drop from the first to second week of treatment, levels out during the fourth week and falls off within three weeks of treatment cessation (Greenberg et al., 1992).

MENTAL FUNCTION

Cranial irradiation produces particular problems and a somnolence syndrome in adult patients post cranial radiotherapy has been described. The syndrome involves excessive sleep, drowsiness, lethargy and anorexia. This may frighten patients if they have not been given sufficient information pre-radiotherapy.

LONG-TERM INTELLECTUAL FUNCTIONING

Intellectual functioning can be harmed by radiotherapy. Research involving children who had been treated for primary intercranial tumours between 3 and 20 years previously found that, although the average IQ for the total series was within normal limits, 23% of the patients were functioning at an educationally subnormal level. There were also significant correlations between intelligence, age at treatment ($\uparrow$ or $\downarrow$ 5yrs.) and site of primary tumour. A prospective study found that children demonstrated deficits in fine motor, visual–motor, and visual–spatial skills and memory difficulties, and had an increased need for special help at school postcranial radiotherapy. In younger children the impairment was more pronounced in non-verbal than in verbal intellectual abilities. Those who had had cranial irradiation at less than 36 months demonstrated below age-based normative means in intellectual, memory, attention, motor and visual–spatial tasks.

Radiotherapists need to be aware of the long-term implications of using prophylactic cranial radiation in children with acute lymphoblastic leukaemia, especially infants, when the immature brain is extremely susceptible to treatment related changes. It has been demonstrated that children who have received radiation to their brain have lower intellectual functioning than those children treated without cranial irradiation.

Neuropsychological research in adults has also indicated damage post radiotherapy. Patients treated for nasopharyngeal cancer demonstrated poorer overall IQ and non-verbal memory in addition to reporting a greater number of memory-related complaints.

SEXUAL BEHAVIOUR & INTEREST IN SEX

Studies of patients who receive radiation have shown reduced frequency or difficulties with sexual intercourse in both men and women. Women treated for cervical cancer have reported lower self-esteem, sexual desirability and attractiveness. Research involving men who had received radiotherapy for seminoma found that 19% reported low rates of sexual activity and 12% had a decreased interest in sex. Physically 15% had erectile dysfunction, 14% premature ejaculation and 10% had difficulty reaching orgasm. Men treated for prostate cancer are more likely to have erection problems if the quality of erections before radiotherapy was borderline. In women receiving total body irradiation for leukaemia anxieties regarding sterility, femininity, and appearance were reported and resulted in reduced self-confidence (Cust *et al.*, 1989). Women receiving pelvic irradiation were found to have been given little specific information preparing them for treatment and toxicity. Gynaecological cancer patients receiving internal radiotherapy application can be particularly anxious and distressed both pre- and post-treatment.

Although important, the incidence and psychological impact of sterility post radiotherapy has rarely been investigated. Women and teenage girls who have received pelvic irradiation to both ovaries are likely to be sterile. Men and teenage boys who have received testicular irradiation have lowered sperm counts but can procreate. Research has reported that 30% of men who received radiotherapy for seminoma worried at least occasionally about their fertility.

INTERVENTIONS

Other than increased information, here have been few studies evaluating interventions to reduce distress associated with radiotherapy. A recent study demonstrated that group psychotherapy reduced patients' psychological and physical distress during radiotherapy. Relaxation training has been used in the radiation oncology department leading to reductions in tension, depression, anxiety and fatigue. However, research has also indicated that, for some patients, radiotherapy has little impact on quality of life (Wallace *et al.*, 1993).

Holland has suggested a number of ways to reducing anxiety associated with receiving radiotherapy (Holland & Rowland, 1989):

- Psychological aspects of patient care should be part of the training of radiotherapists, radiographers and radiotherapy technicians.
- Orientation sessions for new patients to the radiotherapy department, e.g. videotapes, a tour of the department including the treatment machines.
- Weekly multi-disciplinary team meetings to discuss and pass on information concerning the patients currently receiving treatment.
- A relaxed ambience: small waiting areas which do not mix acutely ill patients with those receiving radiotherapy as an outpatient.

REFERENCES

Cust, M.P., Whitehead, M.I., Powtes, R., Hunter, M. & Milliken, S. (1989). Consequences and treatment of ovarian failure after total body irradiation for leukaemia. *British Medical Journal*, 299, 1494–7.

Greenberg, D.B., Sawicka, J., Eisenthal, S. & Ross, D. (1992). Fatigue syndrome due to localized radiation. *Journal of Pain Symptom Management* 7, 38–45.

Hayes, J.R. (1991). Depression and chronic fatigue in cancer patients. *Primary Care*, 18, 327–39.

Holland, J.C. & Rowland, J.H. (Eds). (1989). *Handbook of psychooncology. Psychological care of the patient with cancer*. New York: Oxford University Press.

Kaasa, S., Malt, U., Hagen, S., Wist, E., Moum, I. & Kvitstad, A. (1993). Psychological distress in cancer patients with advanced disease. *Radiotherapy and Oncology*, 27, 193–7.

Rainey, L.C. (1985). Effects of preparatory patient education for radiation oncology patients. *Cancer*, 56, 1056–61.

Smets, E.M., Garssen, B., Schuster-Uitterhoeve, A.I. & de Haes J.C. (1993). Fatigue in cancer patients. *British Journal of Cancer*, 68, 220–4.

Souhami, R.L. & Tobias, J. (1994). *Cancer and its management*. London: Blackwell Scientific Publications.

Wallace, L.M., Priestman, S.G., Dunn, J.A. & Priestman, T.J. (1993). The quality of life of early breast cancer patients treated by two different radiotherapy regimens. *Clinical Oncology Royal College of Radiology*, 5, 228–33.

Young, J. & Maher, E.J. (1992). The role of a radiographer counsellor in a large centre for cancer treatment: a discussion paper based on an audit of the work of a radiographer counsellor. *Clinical Oncology Royal College of Radiology*, 4, 232–5.

Rape and sexual assault

IRENE HANSON FRIEZE
*Department of Psychology,
University of Pittsburgh, USA*

MAUREEN C. McHUGH
*Women's Studies, Indiana University
of Pennsylvania, USA*

Rape is defined in various ways by different legal codes, but basically involves forced sexual contact. The most common form of rape involves a male perpetrator and a female victim, but other forms also exist. The rapist may be a complete stranger, someone who casually knows the victim, or someone who is well known. Marital rape is increasingly being recognized as a crime.

Studies attempting to determine the prevalence of rape provide widely varying estimates, depending on the methodologies used.

Acts that are legally defined as rape may not be perceived as such by the victim. And, many rapes are never reported to authorities. Given these qualifications, it is estimated that 15 to 22% of women in the USA have been raped at some point in their lives (Koss & Burkhart, 1989). Many of these involve acquaintance rapes. Younger women and adolescents and African American women are the most common victims of rape in the USA. Rates vary greatly across the world. Rape is used during wartime as a form of aggression.

Researchers have debated whether rape is primarily a sexual crime or an aggressive crime. It is generally believed that both can be true, and that some rapists are more motivated by sex and others by aggressive feelings. Some rapists appear to believe that their victims enjoy being forced to have sex and may even seek out the same victim again. Others clearly intend to physically injure or even kill their victims (Groth, 1979).

Those who have been raped may show reactions to that event for many years. Typical reactions do vary over time and a number of stage models have been proposed to describe these changing reactions (e.g. Burgess & Holmstrom, 1985). The victim of rape, similar to victims of other traumatic events, typically has an immediate emotional reaction which may take the form of denial, disbelief, numbness or disorientation (Frieze, Hymer & Greenberg, 1987). The specific reactions of rape victims have been labelled as 'Rape Trauma Syndrome' (Burgess & Holmstrom, 1985). After the initial shock, rape victims might experience any of a variety of emotions including anger, anxiety, helplessness, and psychosomatic and other physical symptoms. Unlike other crime victims, rape victims often experience difficulties in sexual functioning. There may also be difficulties in relating to men in general, and to a husband or boyfriend, for the female who has been raped. These short-term reactions are followed by more long-term effects which may include nervous breakdown, attempted suicide, and other effects labelled as post-traumatic stress disorder (American Psychiatric Association, 1980; Kilpatrick et al., 1985).

The strong psychological reactions of rape victims appear to be greater than one might expect by analysing only the physical injury resulting from the rape (Frieze et al., 1987). One reason for this is that rape and other forms of victimization lead the victim to question or reassess basic assumptions about the world. People generally believe that they are safe and are not potential rape victims. Even those women who do fear rape attempt to live their lives in ways that they feel will protect them. When someone does become a rape victim, they must cope not only with the direct consequences of whatever happened to them, but also with the violation of their belief in a safe world. The fear and anxiety so commonly found in rape victims results from a fear of what could happen again even more than from what has already happened.

A number of coping mechanisms have been identified that characterize rape victim responses. These include redefining what happened so that it provides a sense of meaning to the victim. Reactions such as self-blame can be dysfunctional if they add to guilt feelings in the victim or cause her to withdraw from normal activities (Burt & Katz, 1987). It is not uncommon for rape victims to move their residences and to stop seeing old friends. This may be done to protect themselves from the possibility of another rape or because previous social interactions have become uncomfortable.

Rape victims may hesitate in seeking help from the medical or therapeutic communities, police, or even from friends, because they have found that other people have negative beliefs about victims generally, and rape victims in particular. A set of stereotypic beliefs ('rape myths') that blame women for tempting men or being in the wrong place at the wrong time are widely held (Burt, 1980). Such feelings may be communicated to the help-seeking victim, resulting in a 'second injury' of a psychological nature (Symonds, 1976).

The first form of treatment for rape victims is often medical. The physician must look for signs of physical injury and for signs of sexually transmitted disease or pregnancy. Once these medical needs are taken care of, the rape victim may then seek psychological counselling (Allison & Wrightsman, 1993). Although this may be one-to-one therapy, treatment often occurs in self-help groups. Many clinicians and others working with women who have been raped feel that they should be labelled as 'rape survivors' rather than 'rape victims' once they have begun to cope with their trauma.

Other forms of sexual assault tend to have similar consequences for their victims, but are generally less traumatic. These include exhibitionism, voyeurism, and forced touching.

REFERENCES

Allison, J.A. & Wrightsman, L.S. (1993). *Rape: the misunderstood crime.* Newbury Park, CA: Sage.

American Psychiatric Association (1990). *Diagnostic and statistical manual of mental disorders.* 3rd edn. Washington, DC.

Burgess, A.W. & Holmstrom, L.L. (1985). Rape trauma syndrome and post-traumatic stress response. In A.W. Burgess (Ed.). *Research handbook on rape and sexual assault.* pp. 46–61. New York: Garland.

Burt, M.R. (1980). Cultural myths and supports for rape. *Journal of Personality and Social Psychology*, 38, 217–30.

Burt, M.R. & Katz, B.L. (1987). Dimensions of recovery from rape: Focus on growth outcomes. *Journal of Interpersonal Violence*, 2, 57–81.

Frieze, I.H., Hymer, S. & Greenberg, M.S. (1987). Describing the crime victim: psychological reactions to victimization. *Professional Psychology: Research and Practice*, 18, 299–315.

Groth, N. (1979). *Men who rape: the psychology of the offender.* New York: Plenum.

Kilpatrick, D.C., Best, C.L., Veronen, L.J.,

Maick, A.E., Villeponteaux, L.A. & Ruff, G.A. (1985). Mental health correlates of criminal victimization: a random community survey. *Journal of Consulting and Clinical Psychology*, 53, 866–73.

Koss, M.P. & Burkhart, B.R. (1989). A conceptual analysis of rape victimization. *Psychology of Women Quarterly*, 13, 27–40.

Symonds, M. (1976). The rape victim: psychological patterns of response. *American Journal of Psychoanalysis*, 35, 27–34.

Renal failure, dialysis and transplantation

KEITH PETRIE

*Department of Psychiatry and Behavioural
Science, Auckland University School of Medicine,
New Zealand*

THE TREATMENT OF CHRONIC RENAL FAILURE

A chronic loss of kidney function may be caused by a number of factors, these commonly include diabetes, glomerulonephritis, chronic hypertension and familial polycystic renal disease. A decline in renal function causes a gradual accumulation of the body's waste products and this is indicated by increasing levels of urea and creatinine in the blood. The metabolic disturbance accompanying renal failure leads to a number of physical symptoms, most notably lethargy and drowsiness, nausea and vomiting, as well as anorexia.

The point at which patients are offered dialysis as a treatment for renal failure can vary according to the different policies of renal units, but treatment is typically instituted when the patient's renal symptoms reach a level that interferes with their ability to carry out their work or normal daily functions. Earlier treatment is associated with better survival and a preservation of nutrition. Some patients with a particularly poor medical prognosis, or with other major health problems that interfere with successful adaptation to a life on dialysis, may be advised against, or even not be offered, treatment. The current rate of patients on dialysis in Australia and New Zealand is 192 patients per million of population.

Haemodialysis and continuous ambulatory peritoneal dialysis (CAPD) are the two types of dialysis treatment used to correct the on-going effects of kidney failure. In haemodialysis, the patient's blood is passed through an artificial kidney machine that removes waste products by passing the blood across a semi-permeable membrane. Most patients on haemodialysis must dialyse three times a week for between four and six hours. Often this can be done independently by the patient in their own home or through coming in to a dedicated hospital haemodialysis unit.

CAPD works according to the same general principle as haemodialysis but the whole process is conducted inside the body. In CAPD, dialysis fluid is run into the peritoneal cavity via a surgically implanted catheter. The peritoneum is a large semi-permeable membrane that lines the cavity, and once the dialysis fluid has been run in, it is left to exchange substances with the patient's blood. The fluid is drained after about 4–6 hours and the whole cycle is repeated each day, on three or four occasions. Improved rates of survival and correction of anaemia, as well as a more liberal diet, are features of CAPD. The choice between haemodialysis and CAPD is an important one for patients with each treatment having both advantages and disadvantages that have to be set against the patient's social, and occupational circumstances.

The transplantation of a kidney from a cadaver or a living relative is the other treatment option for renal failure patients. The introduction of a new generation of immunosuppressive drugs has resulted in improved rates of graft function with now 80% successful after one year (cadaver donor). Transplantation is generally recognized as the best treatment available for end-stage renal failure. Freed from the drudgery of dialysis and the symptoms of kidney failure, transplant patients report significantly higher quality of life and have lower rates of psychological problems (Evans *et al.*, 1985). However, there are some disadvantages to transplantation in terms of the need to take long-term medication and increased rates of malignancy. The possibility of coping with a failed graft for patients is a significant psychological blow, and one some patients do not want to risk facing again. A failed graft is often particularly traumatic when the kidney has been donated by a relative. Unfortunately, the demand for kidneys is outstripped by their availability, which consigns a sizeable proportion of patients to long-term dialysis. The impending arrival of successful xenografts will overcome the current shortage of kidneys but will undoubtedly bring with it additional psychological adjustment problems.

PSYCHOLOGICAL PROBLEMS AND QUALITY OF LIFE

The difficulties inherent in renal disease are a function of the physiological consequences of kidney failure, the restrictions imposed by a relentless dialysis regimen and the on-going psychological adjustments required by a chronic illness. One of the most disabling effects of end-stage renal disease (ESRD) is lethargy and tiredness. This interferes not only with daily work function, but also with family relationships, as the patient often lacks the energy to engage in previously enjoyed social activities. A reduction in sexual activity is also common in ESRD. Patients on dialysis also complain of a variety of other physical symptoms such as itchy skin and sleep problems that interfere with their daily life. The recent development of recombinant human erythropoietin that acts to raise the oxygen–carrying capacity of the blood has had a major impact on treatment of ESRD by reducing tiredness and other symptoms due to anaemia (Evans *et al.*, 1990).

The process of dialysis treatment also creates difficulties that compromise well-being. Most common among these are problems with the fluid and diet restrictions required, the development of needle stick fears in haemodialysis patients, and trouble with dialysis technique that can result in periodic infections. Often patients' frustrations with their condition and on-going dialysis show themselves in compliance problems with the treatment, diet and fluid restrictions. Non-compliance is a major problem in patients on dialysis as the regimen has many of the characteristics that work to decrease compliance. The treatment is complex, long-lasting, and directly impacts on the patient's lifestyle. Non-compliance can also lead to conflict between staff and patients. Staff may become aggravated with patients who are perceived as not doing their share in managing their condition and, conversely, patients can come to see staff as representing an enforcement rather than a therapeutic role. This can result in patients feeling unable to bring up their personal difficulties and problems with staff.

Given this combination of physiological and psychological problems it is not surprising to find higher rates of psychiatric problems and impaired well-being in dialysis groups when compared to renal transplant patients and general population groups (Evans *et al.*, 1985; Simmons, Anderson & Kamstra, 1984). This seems to be predominately due to a significant increase in the negative component of their subjective mental health, characterized by higher levels of depression and a loss of emotional control (Petrie, 1989). Despite the difficulties in assessing depression in dialysis patients because of the overlap in somatic symptomotology, high levels of depression have been consistently found in dialysis patients (see Levenson & Glocheski, 1991).

ADJUSTMENT TO TREATMENT

The adjustment to treatment for renal failure shares similar characteristics to other chronic illnesses. The first part of this process involves coping with a loss of body function and an awareness of the need for long-term treatment. The next phase is learning the techniques associated with dialysis and dealing with the restrictions that this routine places on daily life and relationships. The final phase is an incorporation of the changes in appearance, function and lifestyle necessary with treatment into a new self-image and identity. The ability of patients to deal with each of these stages varies quite significantly depending on their own psychological resources. Difficulties in the early stages can have considerable impact on eventual adjustment to dialysis. A common emotional reaction is that of denial. This may range from a reluctance to accept that dialysis is really necessary to a casualness in using proper dialysis technique, or frequent breaking of dietary and fluid restrictions later in the treatment process.

Studies looking at predictors of adjustment and survival on renal dialysis have often failed to control for health status (in particular, the co-existence of other diseases requiring on-going treatment) and the type of dialysis. Results of many of the studies are contradictory for age, level of education, marital status, locus of control and intelligence (see Maher *et al.*, 1983). However, some psychosocial factors have been found more consistently to predict adjustment to dialysis, although the overall effects do not tend to be strong. Social support and a coping spouse, continuing involvement in employment and leisure activities, as well as a history of effective coping with life stressors have all been found to predict subsequent adjustment (Burton *et al.*, 1988; Devins *et al.*, 1990; Farmer *et al.*, 1979).

The treatment of renal failure creates considerable difficulties for patients and their families. They must adapt to the loss of a bodily function and the accompanying energy-sapping symptoms. Given the demands and restrictions of life on dialysis as well as the psychological issues of dependency and an uncertain future, the surprising aspect is perhaps not how many patients become depressed but how resilient the majority are to the demands and restrictions of renal disease.

REFERENCES

Burton, H.J., Kline, S.A., Lindsay, R.M. & Heidenheim, P. (1988). The role of support in influencing outcome of end-stage renal disease. *General Hospital Psychiatry*, **10**, 260–6.

Devins, G.M., Mann, J., Mandin, H., Paul, L.C., Hons, R.B., Burgess, E.D., Taub, K., Schorr, S., Letourneau, P.K. & Buckle, S. (1990). Psychological predictors of survival in end-stage renal disease. *Journal of Nervous and Mental Disease*, **178**, 127–33.

Evans, R.W., Manninen, D.L., Garrison, L.P., Hart, L.G., Blagg, C.R., Gutman, R.A., Hull, A.R. & Lowrie, E.G. (1985). The quality of life of patients with end-stage renal disease. *New England Journal of Medicine*, **312**, 553–9.

Evans, R.W., Rader, B., Manninen, D.L. and the Cooperative Multicentre EPO Clinical Trial Group. (1990). The quality of life of hemodialysis recipients treated with recombinant human erythropoietin. *Journal of the American Medical Association*, **263**, 825–30.

Farmer, C.J., Bewick, M., Parsons, V. & Snowden, S.A. (1979). Survival on home haemodialysis: its relationship with physical symptomotology, psychosocial background and psychiatric morbidity. *Psychological Medicine*, **9**, 515–23.

Levenson, J.L. & Glocheski, S. (1991). Psychological factors affecting end-stage renal disease: a review. *Psychosomatics*, **32**, 382–9.

Maher, B.A., Lamping, D.L., Dickinson, C.A., Murawski, B.J., Olivier, D.C. & Santiago, G.C. (1983). Psychosocial aspects of chronic hemodialysis: the national co-operative dialysis study. *Kidney International*, **23**, S50–7.

Petrie, K.J. (1989). Psychological well-being and psychiatric disturbance in dialysis and renal transplant patients. *British Journal of Medical Psychology*, **62**, 91–6.

Simmons, R.G., Anderson, C. & Kamstra, L. (1984). Comparison of quality of life of patients on continuous ambulatory peritoneal dialysis, hemodialysis, and after transplantation. *American Journal of Kidney Diseases*, **4**, 253–5.

Repetitive strain injury

SUSAN H. SPENCE

Department of Psychology, University of
Queensland, Australia

BACKGROUND

Repetition Strain Injury (RSI) is a summary term used to describe a range of musculoskeletal pain conditions resulting from repetitive or forceful body movements, sustained or constrained postures, or vibration. Such problems are also described in the literature under the terms occupational cervico-brachial disorder, cumulative trauma disorder and occupational overuse syndrome. Although most studies have focused upon upper extremity problems resulting from work activities, RSI may also occur in the lower limbs and in response to recreational pursuits. The term RSI encompasses a wide range of musculoskeletal disorders, including tenosynovitis, bursitis, epicondylitis, and carpal tunnel syndrome to mention just a few. As such, the symptoms are variable and the term RSI stresses the causal role of physical activities in the development of the disorders.

There is now overwhelming evidence that certain forms of repetitive movements and postures may lead to the development of musculoskeletal pain disorders for some individuals. Certain occupational groups whose work involves high levels of repetitive motion are particularly prone to RSI problems, such as assembly line workers, meat cutters, poultry processors, meat packers, musicians and keyboard workers (Fredrick, 1992). Females also appear to be at greater risk than males, even when engaged in the same occupational task (e.g. Hadler, 1992). Exact figures regarding the prevalence of these disorders across different occupational groups are lacking, but evidence is gradually accumulating to enable us to identify those occupations at particular risk. Prevalence figures vary, depending upon how severe and long lasting the symptoms must be for the disorder to be viewed as present. Data from the USA suggest that the prevalence of RSI problems increased markedly during the 1980s and currently form around 50% of occupational illness (OSHA, 1990).

PSYCHOLOGICAL CONSIDERATIONS

From a psychological perspective, one of the fascinating features of RSI problems concerns the epidemics that have been reported across the world. It has been proposed by some authors that the sudden increases in reported cases that occurred in some industries during the 1980s, both in the USA and Australia, may reflect psychosocial in addition to physical influences. Such psychosocial influences include fear-generating media reports that espoused the dangers of repetitive tasks, workers' compensation systems that reinforce sick rather than well behaviour, and medical practices, such as surgical interventions, that serve to confirm the patients beliefs about problem severity (Hadler, 1992). Hadler demonstrated how the rate of cases of RSI amongst telecommunications worker in the same company differed markedly across four US states, even though the workers were using the same equipment and engaging what appeared to be the same work practices. What differed was the therapeutic response of those involved in the management of reported cases. Hadler acknowledged that occupational tasks can generate musculoskeletal problems, but proposed that psychosocial factors such as medical practices may play a role in the development of RSI epidemics.

The psychosocial features of RSI vary according to the severity and duration of the problem. Fortunately, most individuals who develop RSI pain problems recover relatively quickly following periods of rest and careful attention to work practices, and there is little evidence to suggest psychopathology amongst these acute cases (Spence, 1990). There remains, however, a small proportion of patients whose pain persists and does not respond to traditional medical and physiotherapy interventions. Chronic RSI of this type has many of the psychological features characteristic of other chronic, musculoskeletal–skeletal pain disorders, including depression, anxiety, fear, guilt, pain behaviours, avoidance of activity and severe interference in daily living skills. Thus, assessment and treatment needs to take into account the psychological components of these conditions, in addition to the biological aspects.

ASSESSMENT AND TREATMENT

Psychological interventions have a role to play in the prevention of RSI problems, dealing with individuals at the point of first presentation and also in the rehabilitation of chronic cases. It is clear that education concerning appropriate work practices (such as taking regular rest breaks, even pacing of work loads and attention to ergonomic features of postures and movements involved in work tasks) may go a long way towards reducing the prevalence of new cases (e.g. Chaterjee, 1992). Organizational psychologists may also contribute towards job redesign to enhance job satisfaction and reduce work-related stress, given that these factors have been linked to high rates of RSI reporting (Hopkins, 1990). Electromyograph (EMG) biofeedback training to enhance the performance of movements in a manner which generates minimal levels of muscular tension may also be beneficial amongst occupational groups in which RSI is linked with excessive muscular tension responses. For example, Moulton and Spence (1992) found that musicians with RSI pain showed an unusual pattern of muscle reactivity to stress situations compared to musicians who did not experience such pain.

The treatment of long-term RSI problems generally involves a multidisciplinary approach which considers ergonomic and work practice factors, medical and physiotherapy treatment of musculoskeletal and neurological symptoms, in addition to dealing with the psychosocial features of the disorders (Feuerstein *et al.*, 1993).

Studies with chronic RSI patients have shown that a cognitive–behaviour therapy (CBT) approach can be beneficial in reducing symptoms of pain, psychological distress and interference in daily living (Spence, 1991; Spence & Sharpe, 1993). The CBT approach included relaxation training, goal setting to increase activity levels, attention diversion methods for dealing with pain, and cognitive challenging of maladaptive thoughts. Spence (1991) followed up two groups of RSI patients and found that the vast majority were still experiencing debilitating pain problems two years after CBT, and to some extent had lost some of the benefits produced by treatment. Most patients had continued with other medical and physiotherapy treatments. Thus, it seems that once RSI problems become chronic, the goal of psychological treatment for many patients becomes one of learning to cope with, and adjust to, the pain problem, rather than expecting a 'cure' for the disorder. Attempts to develop a self-help intervention for chronic RSI sufferers were only partially successful in that many patients were not able to cope with a self-help approach and failed to complete the programme (Spence & Sharpe, 1993). Those patients who did complete the self-help intervention, however, reported equivalent benefits to those patients who complete the same programme through clinic attendance with a therapist. A recent examination of the effects of EMG biofeedback or applied relaxation training in the treatment of chronic RSI patients also found short-term benefits in terms of reductions in pain, psychological distress and disability, but these effects were relatively short lasting and dissipated once treatment ended (Spence, 1992). Thus, although EMG biofeedback or applied relaxation training may be a useful component of psychological intervention for chronic RSI problems, these techniques are insufficient if used in isolation.

FUTURE DIRECTIONS

Future developments for psychological research in the area of RSI include the generation of more effective methods in the rehabilitation of chronic RSI. To a large extent this is likely to mirror developments in the treatment of other forms of chronic pain condition. There is also a strong need to identify the characteristics of those individuals who are most likely to develop RSI problems given the same work practices and equipment. These factors may then be tackled in prevention programmes, along with ergonomic and work practice changes. Similarly, we need to know why some individuals recover relatively quickly once they first experience pain from an occupational task. The identification of those features that predict chronicity may enable the design of early intervention programmes, to prevent progression to chronic status.

REFERENCES

Chaterjee, D.S. (1992). Workplace upper limb disorders: a prospective study with intervention. *Occupational Medicine*, **42**, 129–36.

Feuerstein, M., Callan, H., Hickey, P., Dyer, D., Armbruster, W. & Carolsella, A.M. (1993). Multidisciplinary rehabilitation of chronic work-related upper extremity disorders: long term effects. *Journal of Occupational Medicine*, **35**, 396–403.

Fredrick, L.J. (1992). Cumulative trauma disorders: an overview. *AAOHN Journal*, **40**, 113–16.

Hadler, H.M. (1992). Arm pain in the workplace: a small area analysis. *Journal of Occupational Medicine*, **34**, 113–19.

Hopkins, A. (1990). Stress, the quality of work and repetition strain injury in Australia. *Work and Stress*, **4**, 129–38.

Moulton, B. & Spence, S.H. (1992). Site-specific muscle hyper-reactivity in musicians with occupational upper limb pain. *Behaviour Research and Therapy*, **30**, 375–86.

OSHA (Occupational Safety and Health Administration). (1990). *Ergonomics program management guidelines for meatpacking plants*. Washington DC: OSHA 3123.

Spence, S.H. (1990). Psychopathology amongst acute and chronic patients with occupationally related upper limb pain versus accident injuries of the upper limbs. *Australian Psychologist*, **25**, 293–305.

Spence, S.H. (1991). Long term outcome of cognitive-behaviour therapy in the treatment of chronic, occupational pain of the upper limbs: a two year follow-up. *Behaviour Research and Therapy*, **29**, 503–9.

Spence, S.H. (1992). Effectiveness of EMG biofeedback in the rehabilitation of chronic RSI. Paper presented at the World Congress on Behaviour Therapy, Gold Coast.

Spence, S.H. & Sharpe, L. (1993). Problems of drop-out in the self-help treatment of chronic, occupational pain of the upper limbs. *Behavioural and Cognitive Psychotherapy*, **21**, 311–28.

Rheumatoid arthritis

STANTON NEWMAN

Unit of Health Psychology, Department of Psychiatry and Behavioural Sciences, University College London Medical School, UK

Rheumatoid arthritis (RA) is a chronic inflammatory disease that affects the synovial tissue surrounding the joints. This inflammation is associated with swelling and pain. As the disease progresses, joint tissue may become permanently damaged. The combined effects of inflammation and joint damage result in progressive disability. The causes of RA are, as yet, unknown but it is generally considered an autoimmune disease, although there is no clear evidence of what factors trigger this destructive response of the body's immune system.

The onset of symptoms is gradual and insidious in most instances, although a small proportion of individuals (10–15%) may have a more rapid progression. Joint pain, swelling and stiffness are the main symptoms of the disease, but individuals also report fatigue and general malaise (Liang, Logigian & Sledge, 1992). Fatigue is greater during flare-ups, during periods of emotional distress, or unusual levels of activity, and requires substantial adjustment on the part of the individual to preserve energy (Tack, 1990). Recent in-depth, qualitative research also suggests that patients with RA are able to recognize and describe a number of different 'types' of fatigue which require different coping strategies (Papageorgiou, 1994).

The impact of RA on individuals' lives is considerable. Amongst individuals in the community reporting self-defined arthritis, between 30% and 60% report some limitation arising from arthritis, depending on the precise measures of limitations used in the survey (Verbrugge, Gates & Ike, 1991). These limitations are most likely to involve problems of mobility around the house, ability to walk distances outside or use of public transport. A small minority of people with RA are wheelchair or bed-bound. For the rest, walking may be both difficult and tiring. Individuals with RA also report being constantly concerned about falling when they do move around, so that they may further restrict their mobility. The net effect of RA on individuals' quality of life is considerable and it reduces capacity to work (Locker, 1983), which results generally in reduced income (Mitchell, Burkhauser & Pincus, 1988). It also reduces social and leisure activities, ability to perform domestic roles (Reisine, Goodenow & Grady, 1987) and contact with friends and acquaintances, and results in less satisfaction with these relationships (Fitzpatrick et al., 1988).

Studies which have compared individuals with RA to the general population have found raised levels of depression in individuals with RA (DeVellis, 1993). It is important, however, that RA, although it is frequently accompanied by chronic pain does not lead to higher levels of depression than other clinical conditions (DeVellis, 1993). Studies have, however, failed to find a direct relationship between the physical markers of the extent or activity of the disease and clinical depression or depressed mood (Newman et al., 1989). Evidence has been accumulating that the impact of RA is mediated through a number of psychological and social factors. Notable amongst these are coping responses and social supports.

Pain and stiffness as the dominant features of RA have been singled out for detailed examination. Individuals with RA describe their pain as throbbing and burning, but never as scalding, drilling or cutting (Wagstaff, Smith & Wood, 1985). Their description of their pain is different to individuals with osteoarthritis, in particular they were are likely to refer to 'heat'. Stiffness has always been more difficult to define and individuals with RA refer to resistance to movement (31%), limited range (31%) and lack of movement (20%) to define their stiffness (Helliwell & Wright, 1991).

Research regarding the way in which individuals cope with the demands of rheumatoid arthritis has been growing in recent years (see Newman & Revenson, 1993). Studies may be divided into those which have focused on coping with specific symptoms of RA, such as pain, and those which consider coping with rheumatoid arthritis in general.

Studies on coping with pain in RA have assessed whether particular coping strategies lead to better psychological well-being. Rosenstiel and Keefe (1983) used the Coping Strategies Question-naire (CSQ) and demonstrated that perceptions of control over the pain and the absence of catastrophizing resulted in higher levels of psychological well-being and lower levels of disability. In a longitudinal study, Keefe et al. (1989) examined the Catastrophizing Sub-Scale of the CSQ in 233 RA patients. High scores on catastrophizing at Time 1 were associated with poorer outcome on measures of disability and psychological well-being six months later. They also established that individuals tended to be consistent in their use of catastrophizing over time.

Many studies that have examined how individuals cope with RA have used a general questionnaire to assess coping (Ways of Coping Scale or its derivatives, Lazarus, 1993). A number of these studies have found that the coping strategy of cognitive restructuring (rethinking the cognitions around the illness and its implications) tends to be associated with better psychological well-being, and the strategy of wishful thinking is associated with poorer well-being (Newman & Revenson, 1993). In addition, information seeking has been found in one study to be associated with improved outcome (Manne & Zautra, 1990).

Other studies have used questionnaires specifically developed to encompass the specific coping strategies that individuals use to deal with the stresses of RA. Newman et al. (1989) examined a group of 158 RA patients, and used a cluster analytic technique to divide them into four groups who differed in how they attempted to deal with the stresses of arthritis. The findings showed that, although the four groups did not differ on any medical or clinical assessments, one had higher levels of psychological well-being, lower levels of symptom reports and disability.

These studies established that what one does to confront RA has an impact and have spawned a number of approaches to intervention which aim to alter how individuals cope with RA in order to improve psychological well-being and reduce disability.

PSYCHOLOGICAL INTERVENTIONS

The interventions developed and applied to individuals with RA have involved a variety of components. These have included education, such as the provision of information, training in self-management skills, biofeedback, relaxation training, restructuring coping strategies and social support. It is difficult to evaluate the efficacy of each component because most interventions involve a mixture of interventions and the studies have used different outcomes such as psychological well-being, reductions in pain, disability, knowledge, etc. (DeVellis & Blalock, 1993). Consequently, it has proved difficult to ascertain which component has had an important effect on the outcome variable under study.

An additional complication in interventions in RA is that chronic pain may be accompanied by depression. This raises questions about whether the depression should be treated concurrently with the pain or whether it is best to treat it before or after the pain is relieved. Recent studies of individuals with RA suggest that it is more likely that depression has an effect on pain than vice versa (Parker et al., 1992). Skevington (1994) argues that pain and depression should be treated together as a unit to provide relief from both.

One of the most widely used psychological interventions in RA and other chronic painful disorders is cognitive – behaviour therapy (CBT). CBT includes a number of components such as relaxation training, cognitive coping strategies, goal-setting with self-reinforcement, communications training, assertiveness training, problem-solving (Parker *et al.*, 1993). One of the objectives of cognitive – behaviour therapy is to enable individuals with RA to perceive themselves to have more personal control over symptoms like pain (Skevington, 1983) and over the course of their disease as increased perceptions of control have been found to have a positive effect on mood and other aspects of well-being (Affleck *et al.*, 1987).

Relaxation training has been used as a component in cognitive–behaviour therapy for some time. Some results have shown that, when progressive muscular relaxation, meditative deep breathing exercises and training to generate images of warmth and warm colours are practised twice daily, they lead to significant relief of pain for periods of up to 14 months (Varni, 1981). Other studies have shown the value of a once per day use of relaxation training (Affleck *et al.*, 1992). Other components of CBT that have been successfully applied to individuals with RA with some success include biofeedback and mental imagery (DeVellis & Blalock 1993).

The most widely used intervention in RA is the Arthritis Self-management Programme (Lorig, 1986). This multicomponent intervention involves training with a lay person, where individuals with RA receive a combination of education and self-management training with the aim of increasing control and improving individuals' responses to their illness. This intervention has had moderate success in increasing knowledge, self-management skills and reducing pain (DeVellis & Blalock, 1993). More interesting perhaps is the difficulty of establishing a relationship between self-management practices and pain reduction. Further research has suggested that the changes observed in this intervention are unrelated to behaviour and that the improvements observed were more associated with individuals' perceptions of self-efficacy (that they are able to carry out the activities that they wish to).

REFERENCES

Affleck, G., Tennen, H., Pfieffer, C. & Fifield, J. (1987). Appraisals of control and predictability in adapting to a chronic disease. *Journal of Personality and Social Psychology*, **53**, 273–9.

Affleck, G., Tennan, H., Urrows, S. & Higgins, P. (1992). Neuroticism and the pain-mood relation in Rheumatoid Arthritis: insights from a prospective daily study. *Journal of Consulting and Clinical Psychology*, **60**, 119–26.

DeVellis, B.M. (1993). Depression in rheumatological diseases. In S. Newman & M. Shipley (Eds.) *Psychological aspects of rheumatic disease. Ballière's Clinical Rheumatology*, vol. 7, pp. 241–258. London: Baillière-Tindall.

DeVellis, R. & Blalock, S.J. (1993). Psychological and educational interventions to reduce arthritis disability. In S. Newman & M. Shipley (Eds.). *Psychological aspects of rheumatic disease. Ballière's Clinical Rheumatology*, vol. 7, pp. 397–416. London: Baillière-Tindall.

Fitzpatrick, R., Newman, S., Lamb, R. & Shipley, M. (1988). Social relationships and psychological well-being in rheumatoid arthritis. *Social Science and Medicine*, **27**, 399–403.

Helliwell, P.S. & Wright, V. (1991). Stiffness – a useful symptom but an elusive quality. *Proceedings of the Royal Society*, **84**, 95–8.

Keefe, F.J., Brown G.K., Gregory, K., Wallston, K.A. & Caldwell, D.S. (1989). Coping with rheumatoid Arthritis pain: catastrophising as a maladaptive strategy. *Pain*, **37**, 51–6.

Lazarus, R.S. (1993). Coping theory and research: past, present, and future. *Psychosomatic Medicine*, **55**, 234–47.

Liang, M.H., Logigian, M.A. & Sledge, C.B.

(1992). *Rehabilitation of early rheumatoid arthritis*. Boston: Little Brown and Co.

Locker, D. (1983). *Disability and disadvantage: the consequences of chronic illness*, London: Tavistock.

Lorig, K. (1986). Development and dissemination of an arthritis patient education course. *Family and Community Health*, **9**, 207–52.

Manne, S. & Zautra, A. (1990). Couples coping with chronic illness: women with rheumatoid arthritis and their healthy husbands. *Journal of Behavioural Medicine*, **13**, 327–43.

Mitchell, J., Burkhauser, R. & Pincus, T. (1988). The importance of age, education and comorbidity in the substantial earnings losses of individuals with symmetric polyarthritis. *Arthritis and Rheumatism*, **31**, 348–57.

Newman, S.P. Fitzpatrick, R., Lamb, R. & Shipley, M. (1989). The origins of depressed mood in rheumatoid arthritis. *Journal of Rheumatology*, **16**, 740–4.

Newman, S. & Revenson, T.A. (1993). Coping with rheumatoid arthritis. In S. Newman & M. Shipley (Eds.). *Psychological aspects of rheumatic disease. Ballière's Clinical Rheumatology*, **vol. 7** pp. 259–280. London: Baillière-Tindall.

Newman, S.P., Fitzpatrick, R., Lamb, R. & Shipley, M. (1900) Patterns of coping in rheumatoid arthritis and *Psychology Health*, **4**, 187–200.

Papageorgiou, A. (1994). Fatigue in Rheumatoid Arthritis. Unpublished MSc Dissertation, Faculty of Medicine, University of Manchester.

Parker, J.C., Smarr, K.L., Angelone, E.O., Mothersead, P.K., Lee, B.S., Walker, S.E., Bridges, A.J. & Caldwell, C.W. (1992). Psychological factors, immunologic activation and disease activity in

rheumatoid arthritis. *Arthritis Care and Research*, **5**, 196–201.

Parker, J.C., Iverson, G.L., Smarr, K.L. & Stucky-Ropp, R.C. (1993). Cognitive-behavioural approaches to pain management in rhematoid arthritis. *Arthritis Care and Research*, **6**, 207–12.

Reisine, S., Goodenow, C. & Grady, K. (1987). The impact of rheumatoid arthritis on the homemaker. *Social Science and Medicine*, **25**, 89–96.

Rosenstiel, A.K. & Keefe, F.J. (1983). The use of coping strategies in chronic low back pain patients: relationship to patients characteristics and current adjustment. *Pain*, **17**, 33–40.

Skevington, S.M. (1983). Chronic pain and depression: universal or personal helplessness? *Pain*, **15**, 309–17.

Skevington, S.M. (1994). The relationship between pain and depression: a longitudinal study of early synovitis. In G.F. Gebhart, D.L. Hammond & T.S. Jensen (Eds.). *Proceedings of the 7th World Congress on pain. Progress in pain research and management*, vol 2, pp. 201–210, Seattle: IASP Press.

Tack, B. (1990). Fatigue in rheumatoid arthritis. *Arthritis Care and Research*, **3**, 65–70.

Varni, J.W. (1981). Self-regulation techniques in the management of chronic arthritic pain in haemophilia. *Behaviour Therapy*, **12**, 185–94.

Verbrugge, L., Gates, D. & Ike, R. (1991). Risk factors for disability among US adults with arthritis. *Journal of Clinical Epidemiology*, **44**, 167–82.

Wagstaff, S., Smith, O.V. & Wood, P.H.N. (1985). Verbal pain descriptors used by patients with arthritis. *Annals of the Rheumatic Diseases*, **44**, 262–5.

Road traffic accidents

JAMES ELANDER
*MRC Child Psychiatry Unit,
Institute of Psychiatry, London,
UK*

ROBERT WEST
*Psychology Department, St George's
Hospital Medical School, London,
UK*

Road traffic accidents (RTAs) killed 44,529 people in the USA in 1990 and 4568 people in the UK in 1991 (Department of Transport, 1992), and these are countries with relatively good safety records. Worldwide fatalities have been estimated at over half a million per year, with around 70 times as many injuries (Evans, 1991). Cancer and heart disease kill more people but those deaths tend to occur much later in life, whereas RTAs account for nearly half of deaths among 19 year-olds and are a much more serious health problem in terms of person–years, or working years, lost annually (Evans, 1991).

Behavioural factors, in the form of habitual risky styles of driving and ineffective responses to developing hazards, play a role in the causation of up to 90% of RTAs. The concept of 'accident proneness' is rarely used nowadays in road safety research, but drivers who have been involved in accidents during one period are significantly more likely to be involved during a subsequent period, especially if they could be judged to have been responsible in some way for the accidents. Relatively stable characteristics of drivers therefore play an important role in accident causation, often in interaction with temporary or local risk factors. The most important risk-related driving behaviour is probably excess speed, followed by readiness to violate driving regulations and failure to recognize situations as potentially hazardous, and all of these factors go some way towards explaining the over-representation of young and inexperienced drivers in RTA involvement. The main impact of RTAs on health services is in emergency medicine, but many accident victims also suffer less urgent chronic and acute physical injuries, and some go on to suffer psychological problems as a result of the trauma of RTA involvement.

THE ROLE OF DRIVING SKILL IN RTA CAUSATION

It is well established that most drivers overestimate their own driving skill and underestimate their relative risk of accident. However, the evidence that greater driving skill alone can reduce the risk of accident is not conclusive. Learner driver and defensive driver training have not been convincingly shown to be effective (Lund & Williams, 1985; Robertson, 1980), and, in a study of presumably very highly skilled drivers, accident rates were actually higher among racing club license holders than matched control groups of drivers (Williams & O'Neill, 1974).

Very closely defined skills, such as detecting and responding to driving hazards, have been shown to play an important role in the acquisition and development of driving ability, but have rarely been related directly to criteria of accident involvement (but see Quimby

et al., 1986). A range of studies using driving simulators and in-car ratings and observations have shown that visual scanning patterns, hazard detection, and perceived risk all differed between drivers of different ages and experience, with better performance among lower risk groups.

Skills of this type might be expected to relate to more basic cognitive abilities such as reaction time and visuo-motor co-ordination, and to higher order skills such as field dependence and attention switching. There is, however, almost no evidence for a relationship between very basic cognitive abilities and RTA involvement except in elderly drivers, where impaired visual function has been shown to be an important cause of accidents (Owsley *et al.*, 1991). Field independence (the ability to identify visual patterns among complex backgrounds) has been related to performance measures of response to hazard in driving simulators, but has not always correlated significantly with accident involvement. Attention switching ability (measured typically in dichotic listening tasks) has been more reliably associated with accident frequency, but it is unclear as yet what aspects of driving behaviour mediate the relationship.

MOTIVATIONAL FACTORS

The reason why measures of driving skill are not more closely related to on-the-road accident involvement is probably that driving is a 'self-paced' task that can be made more or less demanding by the behaviour of the driver. Many risk-related driving behaviours reflect underlying motives and attitudes rather than driving ability.

By far the most important driving behaviour from a safety point of view is excess speed, which has been shown to be a consistent aspect of individual driving style and has been reliably associated with RTA involvement by studies using a range of different techniques including roadside observations, questionnaire surveys, and analyses of performance in instrumented cars and driving simulators. Young people have been shown to drive faster, and faster driving has been related to more general traits such as Type-A behaviour and social deviance.

The next most important class of driving behaviours relate to the violation of driving regulations, which have been shown to be more closely related to RTA involvement than driving errors (Parker *et al.*, 1992). In that study violators were also more likely to be male, to have a higher than average opinion of their own skill, and to be less constrained by the opinions of others and the consequences of their own behaviour. Accident risk can be modelled as a problem behaviour arising from inconsiderate, self-serving attitudes that generalize beyond the driving domain (West, Elander & French, 1993).

TRANSIENT FACTORS

Motivational and skill factors also influence the extent to which alcohol, fatigue, weather conditions, and problems related to road and vehicle design lead to accidents, because riskier driving styles and behaviours reduce the margin for error in potentially hazardous situations. The role of alcohol is more complicated because it not only impairs judgement and responsiveness but also disinhibits the drinker, releasing potentially risky impulses and motives. Alcohol has differential effects on younger drivers, so that the risk of accident is increased at lower blood-alcohol levels than in older drivers (Mayhew *et al.*, 1986). This may be because of the disinhibiting effects of alcohol in younger drivers, but may also be because over-learned and highly practised skills are less disrupted by alcohol than more newly acquired ones. One temporary human factor that has been examined in relation to RTA involvement is life events, where there was evidence that high proportions of accident involved drivers had recently experienced stressful or disturbing events (Selzer & Vinokur, 1974). Again, more stable driver characteristics may affect the extent to which road safety is compromised by stressful experiences on the part of the driver.

Estimation of the extent to which different behavioural characteristics of drivers contribute to RTA causation, and identification of the mechanisms involved in each case, is therefore far from straightforward (Elander, West & French, 1993). Many human risk factors overlap, so that multivariate statistical methods are needed to assess the roles played by each. Account also needs to be taken of the extent to which individuals are exposed to risk of RTA through the behaviour of other drivers, and of the fact that particular types of driver error and driver behaviour differentially increase risk for specific categories of accident.

EFFECTS OF RTAs ON SURVIVORS

Non-fatal casualties of RTAs are much more difficult to quantify than fatalities because physical injuries vary greatly in severity and many accidents are not reported. However, RTA involvement can clearly constitute a disturbing life event, and may have significant psychological consequences. Research on the psychological consequences of RTAs is much more limited than that on their causes, however, and the conclusions that can be drawn from existing findings are constrained by factors including the possibility of litigation arising from the RTA concerned and absence of information about psychological status prior to the accident.

One study which followed up the victims of serious RTAs found that around 10% showed signs of post traumatic stress six months after their accident (Brom, Kleber & Hofman, 1993), although the measures used were of intrusion and avoidance symptoms rather than a formal psychiatric diagnosis of PTSD. In a study of RTA victims presenting for psychiatric consultations following RTAs, Goldberg and Gara (1990) found that a depressive syndrome (including anhedonia, insomnia and self-blame) was most common, with only one-third as many patients showing features of PTSD.

REFERENCES

Brom, D., Kleber, R.J. & Hofman, M.C. (1993). Victims of traffic accidents: Incidence and prevention of post-traumatic stress disorder. *Journal of Clinical Psychology*, **49**, 131–40.

Department of Transport (1992). *Road accidents Great Britain 1991*. London: HMSO.

Elander, J., West, R. & French, D. (1993). Behavioural correlates of individual differences in road-traffic crash risk: an examination of methods and findings. *Psychological Bulletin*, **113**, 279–94.

Evans, L. (1991). *Traffic safety and the driver*. New York: Van Nostrand Reinhold.

Goldberg, L. & Gara, M. (1990). A typology of psychiatric reactions to motor vehicle accidents. *Psychopathology*, **23**, 15–20.

Lund, A.K. & Williams, A.F. (1985). A review of the literature evaluating the defensive driving course. *Accident Analysis and Prevention*, **17**, 449–60.

Mayhew, D.R., Donelson, A.C., Beirness, D.J. & Simpson, H.M. (1986). Youth, alcohol and relative risk of accident involvement. *Accident Analysis and Prevention*, **18**, 273–87.

Owsley, C., Ball, K., Sloane, M.E., Roenker, D.L. & Bruni, J.R. (1991). Visual/ cognitive correlates of vehicle accidents in older drivers. *Psychology and Ageing*, **6**, 403–15.

Parker, P., Manstead, A.S.R., Stradling, S.G., Reason, J.T. & Baxter, J.S. (1992). Intention to commit driving violations: an application of the theory of planned behaviour. *Journal of Applied Psychology*, **77**, 94–101.

Quimby, A.R., Maycock, G., Carter, I., Dixon, R. & Wall, J. (1986). *Perceptual abilities of accident involved drivers*. Rep. No. 27. Crowthorne, England: Transport and Road Research Laboratory.

Robertson, L.S. (1980). Crash involvement of teenaged drivers when driver education is eliminated from high school. *American Journal of Public Health*, **70**, 599–603.

Selzer, M.L. & Vinokur, A. (1974). Life events, subjective stress and traffic accidents. *American Journal of Psychiatry*, **13**, 903–6.

West, R., Elander, J. & French, D. (1993). Mild social deviance, Type-A personality and decision-making style as predictors of self-reported driving style and traffic accident risk. *British Journal of Psychology*, **84**, 207–19.

Williams, A.F. & O'Neill, B. (1974). On-the-road driving records of licensed race drivers. *Accident Analysis and Prevention*, **6**, 263–70.

Rubella

NATALIE TIMBERLAKE

*Academic Department of Psychiatry, Middlesex
and UCL, London, UK*

Rubella is a relatively mild infectious disease, which rarely gives rise to complications in those infected. However, one serious consequence of rubella infection is that, if it is contracted by mothers during gestation, it can result in miscarriages, stillbirths and infants born with congenital rubella syndrome (CRS). Therefore, rubella is different from most preventable diseases in that its main threat is to pregnant women.

The vaccination for rubella is normally given to children between the ages of 1 and 2 years, in combination with the measles and mumps vaccine (MMR). In Europe and Britain, there is a target uptake rate of 90% (Begg & Noah, 1985). Similarly, in the USA, the Healthy People 2000 report sets a minimum vaccination level of 90% of children (US Department of Health and Human Services, 1990). Although this is achieved in some areas of the USA and the UK, there is wide variation between localities. Uptake rates are generally reported to range from 69–91% (Li & Taylor, 1993). Research on the reasons why some people do not vaccinate for rubella has found that are a number of important issues involved. (See also 'Immunization'.)

(a) *Ethnicity*. Children from ethnic minorities have an increased risk of non-vaccination (Kaplan *et al.*, 1990; Peckham *et al.*, 1983; Miller *et al.*, 1987).

(b) *Primary immunization status*. Children who have not received their primary vaccinations, especially pertussis, are less likely to have MMR (Li & Taylor, 1993).

(c) *Birth order/size of family*. As the number of siblings in a family increases, there is a decreasing probability of the youngest child being vaccinated (Li & Taylor, 1993; Pearson *et al.*, 1993*b*).

(d) *Area of residence*. In highly deprived areas, there is a lower rate of vaccination (Li & Taylor, 1993; Pearson *et al.*, 1993*a*).

(e) *Single parent family status*. There is an increased risk of lower vaccination rates in families with only one parent at home. (Li & Taylor, 1993; Pearson *et al.*, 1993*b*).

(f) *Place of registration for immunization*. Vaccination levels in health clinics are lower than in general practices (Li & Taylor, 1993).

(g) *Postnatal migration*. Moving into a new area shortly after birth is associated with a lower vaccination rate. (Pearson *et al.*, 1993*a,b*).

Some of these factors are related to immunization in general (see 'Immunization'); however, some are more specific to rubella. The issue of ethnicity seems to have a special relevance for rubella vaccination. It has been reported that the incidence of congenital rubella syndrome is 2.3 times higher in Asian (immigrants from India, Pakistan, Bangladesh or Sri Lanka or east African Asians) in than non-Asian births in England and Wales (Miller *et al.*, 1987). Similarly, in the USA, Kaplan *et al.* (1990) have reported that the risk for black women of giving birth to a child with congenital rubella syndrome is 2.5 times higher than for white women. It would seem that Asian women are not only less likely to test for the disease or have abortions but also have a decreased level of immunization (Peckham *et al.*, 1983; Miller *et al.*, 1987). The barriers to immunization for ethnic minorities are probably multifaceted with many of the sociodemographic factors mentioned previously playing a large part. However, a barrier which seems particular to Indian cultures is lack of knowledge of the disease and its teratogenic effects (Sim, 1983; Morgan *et al.*, 1987). Morgan *et al.* (1987) suggest that this reflects the relatively mild nature of the disease in India where infectious diseases are responsible for a high proportion of child mortalities. Morgan *et al.* (1987) and Sim (1983) found no specific term for rubella in some Asian languages. Morgan *et al.* (1987) found only one word which referred to a number of illnesses involving a minor rash. This highlights the level of importance given to the disease in Indian cultures and the difficulties in promoting the vaccine to this group.

Perceiving rubella as a harmless disease may not just be restricted to Asian cultures. Harding and O'Looney (1984) report that, although the disease is seen as very common, it is not seen as dangerous. Therefore, if the perceived threat from the disease is not very high, the perceived benefits gained from vaccinating against it will be low. Efforts in the USA to raise the perceived benefits have been achieved by some states necessitating blood tests for immunization level, for marriage and for entry into school/college. This has gone some way to capturing those at risk; however, many still slip through the net (Lee *et al.*, 1992).

Women of childbearing age may perceive potential costs in vaccinating. The teratogenic potential of the vaccine has acted as a deterrent for some doctors and women due to the concern that they may become pregnant (Kaplan *et al.*, 1990). This is a demonstration of omission bias in that health carers and women prefer omissions rather than commissions in situations when either one may cause harm (Ritov & Baron, 1990). It has been reported that omission bias is particularly marked in situations where there is a degree of ambiguity (Ritov & Baron, 1990). As there is uncertainty over whether the women will become pregnant and the chances of the vaccine affecting the foetus, this situation is especially prone to omission bias. However, although pregnancy is treated as a contraindication to immunization, the actual risk is very low as there have been no reported cases of a child being born with CRS as a result of a mother being vaccinated whilst pregnant (Bakshi & Cooper, 1990).

Therefore, it would seem that, in order to increase the rate of vaccination, more information on the effects of rubella and the con-traindications to vaccination needs to be publicized. A further aid to improving vaccination levels would be to highlight the threat posed by rubella. This could be achieved by promoting the link between rubella and CRS. This and, more generally, information needs to be especially aimed at vulnerable groups.

REFERENCES

Bakshi, S. & Cooper, L. (1990). Rubella and mumps vaccines. *Pediatric Clinics of North America*, **37**, 651–68.

Begg, N.T. & Noah, N.D. (1985). Immunisation targets in Europe and Britain. *British Medical Journal*, **291**, 1370–1.

Harding, C. & O'Looney, B. (1984). Perceptions and beliefs about nine diseases. *Public Health*, **98**, 284–93.

Kaplan, K., Cochi, S., Edmonds, L., Zell, E. & Preblud, S. (1990). A profile of mothers giving birth to infants with congenital rubella syndrome. *American Journal of Diseases Children*, **144**, 118–23.

Lee, S., Ewert, D., Frederick, P. & Mascola, L. (1992). Resurgence of congenital rubella syndrome in the 1990s. *Journal of the American Medical Association*, **267**, 2616–20.

Li, J. & Taylor, B. (1993). Factors affecting uptake of measles, mumps and rubella immunisation. *British Medical Journal*, **307**, 168–71.

Miller, E., Nicoll, A., Rousseau, S., Sequeira, P., Hambling, M., Smithells, R. & Holzel, H. (1987). Congenital rubella in babies of South Asian women in England and Wales: an excess and its cause. *BMJ*, **294**, 737–9.

Morgan, S., Aslam, M., Dove, R., Nicoll, A. & Stanford, R. (1987). Knowledge of infectious diseases and immunisation among Asian and white parents. *Health Education Journal*, **46**, 177–9.

Pearson, M., Makowiecka, K., Gregg. J., Woollard, J., Rogers, M. & West, C. (1993a). Primary immunisations in Liverpool. 1: Who withholds consent? *Archives of Diseases in Childhood*, **69**, 110–14.

Pearson, M., Makowiecka, K., Gregg. J., Woollard, J., Rogers, M. & West, C. (1993b). Primary immunisations in Liverpool. 2: Is there a gap between consent and completion? *Archives of Disease of Childhood*, **69**, 115–19.

Peckham, C., Tookey, P., Nelson, D., Coleman, J. & Morris, N. (1983). Ethnic minority women and congenital rubella. *British Medical Journal*, **287**, 129–30.

Ritov, I. & Baron, J. (1990). Reluctance to vaccinate: omission bias and ambiguity. *Journal of Behavioural Decision Making*, **3**, 263–77.

Sim, F. (1983). Ethnic minority women and congenital rubella. *British Medical Journal*, **287**, 130.

US Department of Health and Human Services, Public Health Service. (1990). *Healthy People 2000: National health promotion and disease prevention objectives*. US. Government Printing Office.

Self-examination: breast, testicles

R. GLYNN OWENS

Department of Psychology, University of Auckland
(Tamaki Campus), New Zealand

Although there exist technological approaches to screening for certain cancers (e.g. breast, cervix) there remains, nevertheless, a potential role for these to be supplemented by self-examination procedures. Reasons for this include (a) the absence of systematic technological screening procedures for many cancers (b) the limited frequency with which, for reasons of cost and/or safety, technological procedures can be applied and (c) the limited range of individuals to whom such procedures can be made available.

For example, in Britain some 1 in 12 women will have breast cancer at some point in their lives. Many of these women will fall outside the 50–64 age group currently receiving regular mammograms by invitation; some will have a clear mammogram on one occasion but have grown a large and dangerous tumour during the three-year interval before the next. For most cancers no routine screening programme exists for example, testicular cancer, the commonest malignancy in young men in the European Community, and malignant melanoma, whose incidence in Britain is rising faster than any other cancer. Survival in both of these is a function of early detection and treatment, yet neither has a routine screening programme, and self-reporting of symptoms remains the major reason for presentation.

However, for a self-examination programme to be effective it needs to fulfil certain conditions including:

(i) It needs to be capable of detecting tumours at a sufficiently early stage to influence prognosis, whilst at the same time minimizing the number of false positives.

(ii) It needs to be practised appropriately by those who are potentially susceptible to the disease.

(iii) Any abnormalities detected by the process need to be presented without delay, and treated quickly if malignant.

Such problems indicate a number of respects in which a better understanding of psychological processes may increase the effectiveness of self-examination procedures.

[582]

SELF-EXAMINATION IN PRACTICE

In the field of self-examination, overwhelmingly the greatest attention has been paid to breast self-examination (BSE), with increasing attention in recent years being paid to testicular self-examination. There is surprisingly little evidence for the effectiveness of either procedure; such lack of evidence may, however, reflect not a lack of value, but rather a failure of the techniques used to evaluate them.

With respect to both breast and testicular self-examination, a common recommendation is that the procedures should be carried out once per month; in practice, studies show only a tiny minority of individuals performing regular self-examination. Studies of BSE report, usually, only around 10% of women performing monthly self-examination (Duffy & Owens, 1984) and, for testicular self-examination, the figure is around 2% for those self-examining at the regular time and with the proper method (Sheley *et al.*, 1991); around 90% of men report never performing testicular self-examination (Reno, 1988). It should be noted, moreover, that studies of this kind inevitably rely on the self-report of the individual, with the concomitant risk that the figures given are inflated by social desirability effects.

In the field of breast cancer a number of studies have failed to show benefits of BSE in terms of the staging of tumours presented by women. For example, Philip *et al.* (1984) in a longitudinal study failed to show any significant difference in the staging of tumours presented by women who had been taught BSE from those who had not, although those presented by the former were significantly smaller.

In addition, self-examination, besides having all the evaluative problems of other screening procedures (e.g. lead-time bias) has a distinctive problem of its own; that of delay. Clearly, any benefit of early detection of a tumour will be lost if the patient then delays presenting this for diagnosis and treatment. Research suggests that around 15–20% of women delay three months or longer before presenting symptoms. Whilst it might be expected that those who take the trouble to self-examine would then be unlikely to delay, research shows no correlation between promptness of reporting and practice of BSE (Duffy & Owens, 1984). To date, there have been few substantial studies of delay in testicular cancer, although improvements in treatment since the end of the 1970s may mean that delay is less important than previously (Moul *et al.*, 1990). Again, it should be noted that estimates of delay based on self-report may be subject to social desirability biases, although a study using a guided-recall procedure supports the notion that such reports show little bias (Owens & Heron, 1990). (See also 'General cancer'.)

PSYCHOLOGICAL CONTRIBUTIONS

Clearly, there is the potential for psychological contributions to each of the three areas outlined above. Whilst there are physical limits to the possible sensitivity and specificity of the procedures used, it is unlikely that most practitioners are operating at these limits. It may therefore be possible to increase the effectiveness of individuals' technique by providing systematic feedback and knowledge of results; an unpublished study by Clarke (1988) showed higher levels of confidence in BSE amongst women who had been taught using a synthetic module in which the texture and feel of different-sized tumours could be represented. A considerable amount of research has examined psychological differences between those who do and do not practise regular self-examination, commonly drawing on models such as Becker's (1974) Health Belief Model or Fishbein & Ajzen's (1975) Theory of Reasoned Action and its later development, the Theory of Planned Behaviour (Ajzen & Fishbein, 1980). Whilst these models have been considered with respect to both BSE (e.g. Duffy & Owens, 1984) and TSE (e.g. Brubaker & Wickersham, 1990) results have not always been consistent; for example Reno (1988) found significant correlations between TSE and the Perceived Benefits and Perceived Susceptibility dimensions of the Health Belief Model, whilst an unpublished doctoral dissertation by O'Connell (1989) reported no relationship between Health Belief Model dimensions and TSE. Actual knowledge of the disease has been reported as a significant predictor of behaviour by a number of workers, both with respect to both testicular cancer (e.g. Rudolf, 1988) and breast cancer (e.g. Owens, Duffy & Ashcroft, 1985).

CONCLUSIONS

The limitations of existing technological screening methods indicate the desirability of effective self-examination procedures. Such procedures need to show adequate sensitivity and specificity, to be used appropriately by those at risk and any findings need to be responded to promptly. To date, evaluations of self-examination procedures have shown disappointing results, but this may result, at least in part, from the problems of obtaining reliable data through self-report and from patient delay, a problem specific to self-screening. There is a great need for psychological strategies to be developed which will enhance take-up of effective self-examination in conjunction with prompt responding to any abnormalities detected.

REFERENCES

Ajzen, I. & Fishbein, M. (1980). *Understanding attitudes and predicting behavior*. Englewood Cliffs: Prentice-Hall.

Becker, M.H. (1974). The Health Belief Model and sick role behavior. *Health Education Monographs*, **2**, 409–19.

Brubaker, R.G. & Wickersham, D. (1990). Encouraging the practice of testicular self-examination: a field application of the theory of reasoned action. *Health Psychology*, **9**, 154–63.

Clarke, H. (1988). Unpublished MClin Psychol thesis, University of Liverpool.

Duffy, J.E. & Owens, R.G. (1984). Factors affecting promptness of reporting in breast cancer patients. *Hygie: International Journal of Health Education*, **2**, 29–32.

Fishbein, M. & Ajzen, I. (1975). *Belief, attitude, intention and behavior*. Reading, MA: Addison-Wesley.

Moul, J.W., Paulson, D.F., Dodge, R.K. & Walther, P.J. (1990). Delay in diagnosis and survival in testicular cancer: impact of effective therapy and changes during 18 years. *Journal of Urology*, **143**, 520–3.

Owens, R.G. & Heron, K. (1990). Accuracy of estimates of delay by women seeking breast cancer treatment. *Journal of Psychosocial Oncology*,

Owens, R.G., Duffy, J.E. & Ashcroft, J.J. (1985). Women's responses to detection of breast lumps: a British study. *Health Education Journal*, **44**, 69–70.

O'Connell, L.G. (1989). The influence of knowledge, self-concept, and health beliefs on young men's practice of testicular self-examination. Unpublished Doctoral Dissertation, Catholic University of America.

Philip, J., Harris, W.G., Flaherty, C., Joslin, C.A.F., Rustage, J.H. & Wijesinghe,

D.P. (1984). Breast self-examination; clinical results from a population-based prospective study. *British Journal of Cancer*, **50**, 7–12.

Reno, D.R. (1988). Men's knowledge and health beliefs about testicular cancer and testicular self-examination. *Cancer Nursing*, **11**, 112–17.

Rudolf, V.M. (1988). The practice of TSE among college men: effectiveness of an educational program. *Oncology Nursing Forum*, **15**, 45–8.

Sheley, J.F., Kinchen, E.W., Morgan, D.H. & Gordon, D.F. (1991). Limited impact of testicular self-examination promotion. *Journal of Community Health*, **16**, 117–24.

Sexually transmitted diseases

BARBARA HEDGE

Andrewes Unit, St Bartholomew's Hospital,
London, UK

INTRODUCTION

Sexually transmitted diseases (STDs) rank among the most common infectious illnesses with over 333 million new STD infections per year being reported world-wide plus 30 million new infections with genital papilloma virus, 20 million new infections of genital herpes and 7 million new infections of chancroid (Adler, 1996). In recent decades there has been a change in the spectrum of STDs away from those associated with bacterial (e.g. gonorrhoea) or spirochaetal infections (e.g. syphilis) which respond well to antibiotic treatments, towards those caused by viral infections such as genital warts and herpes simplex.

STDs frequently give rise to local symptoms such as painful, burning or itching lesions or discharge in the genital, anal and oral regions. They may also result in systemic disease with potentially serious consequences. Gonorrhoea can result in sterility, syphilis can damage the cardiovascular and central nervous systems, chlamydia can cause pelvic inflammatory disease and subsequent ectopic pregnancy or infertility, and genital warts have been linked with cervical carcinoma. There is also strong evidence that the transmission of HIV which can lead to AIDS is increased by the presence of STDs. As STD infection implies sexual activity, which historically carries connotations of illicit, casual, sexual encounters, acquiring a STD is frequently associated with embarrassment and social stigma.

PSYCHOLOGICAL DISTURBANCE

Psychological distress in people attending genitourinary medicine (GUM) clinics is common. A survey by Ikkos *et al.* (1987) reported significant psychiatric symptomatology in 20–40% of clinic attenders with more frequent symptoms in females, in those with social and marital difficulties and in those with sexual dysfunction.

The psychological and psychiatric disturbance encountered in GUM clinics is not a unitary phenomena. It can relate to the distress associated with illness, but a similar high rate of psychiatric disturbance is found in the significant proportion of STD clinic attenders who have no physical symptoms (Barczak *et al.*, 1988; Catalan *et al.*, 1981). The distress in those without physical illness cannot be explained by associated social stigma, severity of symptoms or fears of physical illness progression. Rather, it appears to be related to abnormal illness concern and behaviour, such as nosophobia, hypochondriasis or the persistent pursuit of medical care in response to the belief of infection, for which there is no supporting clinical or serological evidence (Ikkos *et al.*, 1987). Sexual dysfunction is another common presentation in STD clinics (Catalan *et al.*, 1981). Dysfunction may be associated with STD infection or the belief of infection, but presentation in an STD clinic may simply be because the clinic is perceived as an empathic, confidential setting in which to discuss sexual matters.

PSYCHOLOGICAL ASPECTS OF STDS

Most of the studies investigating the psychological effects of having a STD have been carried out with respect to genital herpes, a common, recurrent and often painful infection, especially in the primary attack. Responses to diagnosis can include depression, anxiety, anger, a desire to withdraw and feelings of loneliness (Drob, Loemer & Lifshutz, 1985). Sexual enjoyment and activity can also be negatively affected.

Recurrence of genital herpes has been noted to coincide with psychiatric illness, stress and menstruation. There is an ongoing debate (Goldmeier & Johnson, 1982; Carney *et al.*, 1993) as to the direction of causation between stress and recurrent episodes. A causal role for stress is not supported; it appears that it is the physical reality of blisters and sores which leads to emotional problems. Frequency of recurrence and the discomfort experienced appear to be related to the strategies used to cope with the stress. The highest frequency of recurrence appears to be in those who view their fate as beyond personal control and who show emotion focused, avoidance thought patterns.

Genital warts are associated with carcinoma of the cervix. This relationship increases the distress of diagnosis and often leads to fears of transmitting the disease to partners during sexual intercourse, which in turn can adversely affect sexual enjoyment.

A population at risk for STDs is those who are sexually assaulted, when safer sexual practices are rarely adopted. It has been reported that 29% women reporting rape in a GUM clinic have a STD. This population frequently requires psychological support as well as STD management.

PSYCHOLOGICAL INTERVENTIONS

The aims of psychological interventions within a STD clinic are to:

- increase coping with infection
- reduce the probability of future infection
- maintain compliance with medication regimes
- reduce somatic symptoms misattributed to a STD
- treat sexual dysfunction

Coping with Infection

Cognitive behavioural strategies which equip people to reduce emotional and physical distress by increasing their cognitive control of the situation, e.g. positive thought control, pre-event planning and decatastrophization (Hawton et al., 1989) can be useful. Addressing any loss of self-esteem associated with the social stigma of having a STD can improve mood state.

Training in anxiety management techniques, such as relaxation and breath control, can enable individuals to develop methods of reducing stress, for example, that associated with a recurrence of genital herpes, and thus minimize its negative impact on their lives.

Prevention of Infection

In order to prevent the spread of infection, it is necessary that individuals can communicate their desire for sexual abstinence, or for safer sex and that they have sufficient self-esteem and motivation to do so. Training in communication, social and assertiveness skills can be useful in increasing people's control of sexual situations.

Compliance

Many bacterial STDs can be controlled with appropriate antibiotic therapy. However, patient compliance with medication regimes is often poor because of either a lack of understanding of the need for completion of a course of treatment, or because the instructions have been forgotten within minutes of leaving the consultation, or because of specific fears concerning the medication (Ley, 1988). Adherence with recommended medical interventions and protocols can be enhanced by the provision of information (e.g. by leaflets), which clearly and simply explain what investigations involve and the recommended medication regimes, together with opportunities for discussion (e.g. with a counsellor) of fears and concerns.

Somatic Symptoms

High rates of hypochondriasis and veneroneurosis (a strong conviction of having a venereal disease) are found in STD clinics and are frequently associated with psychiatric morbidity. The health preoccupation model of Salkovskis and Warwick (1986) suggests that reassurance of the absence of infection only results in short-term relief from symptoms. It suggests that rather than providing further reassurance, therapy can assist people to reinterpret their somatic symptoms in terms of anxiety rather than as STDs. Stress inoculation training can further enable people to cope with the situations which triggered the initial ruminations and compulsive behaviours and prevent relapse.

Sexual dysfunction

Sexual dysfunction may occur in people with STDs secondary to the pain, trauma or relationship difficulties associated with their infections. Relationship and sexual difficulties may stem from fears of rejection, fears of infecting others or fears of being reinfected. Necessary psychological input thus ranges from the provision of information explaining the link between STDs and sexual dysfunction to behavioural and cognitive therapeutic interventions which deal with the dysfunction directly, or are aimed at increasing self-esteem, communication skills and the better management of stress (Hawton et al., 1989).

CONCLUSION

A diverse range of psychological symptomatology is associated with STDs. Provision of psychological support can effectively reduce the distress associated with disease, contribute to the control of infection, increase compliance with medication regimes and investigations, reduce somatic symptoms and enhance the sexual health of the STD clinic population.

REFERENCES

Adler, M. (1996). Sexually transmitted disease control in developing countries. *Genitourinary Medicine*, **72**, 83–8.

Barczak, P., Kane, N., Andrews, S., Congdon, A., Clay, J. & Betts, T. (1988). Patterns of psychiatric morbidity in a genitourinary clinic. *British Journal of Psychiatry*, **152**, 700–2.

Carney, O., Ross, E., Ikkos, G. & Mindel, A. (1993). The effect of suppressive oral acyclovir on the psychological morbidity associated with recurrent genital herpes. *Genitourinary Medicine*, **69**, 457–9.

Catalan, J., Bradley, M., Gallwey, J. & Hawton, K. (1981). Sexual dysfunction and psychiatric morbidity in patients attending a clinic for sexually transmitted diseases. *British Journal of Psychiatry*, **138**, 292–6.

Drob, S., Loemer, M. & Lifshutz, H. (1985). Genital herpes: the psychological consequences. *British Journal Medical of Psychology*, **58**, 307–15.

Goldmeier, D. & Johnson, A. (1982). Does psychiatric illness affect the recurrence rate of genital herpes? *British Journal of Venereal Diseases*, **58**, 40–3.

Hawton, K., Salkovskis, P., Kirk, J. & Clark, D. (1989). *Cognitive behaviour therapy for psychiatric problems: a practical guide*. Oxford: Oxford University Press.

Ikkos, G., Fitzpatrick, R., Frost, D. & Nazeer, S. (1987). Psychological disturbance and illness behaviour in a clinic for sexually transmitted diseases. *British Journal of Medical Psychology*, **60**, 121–6.

Ley, P. (1988). *Communicating with patients*. London: Chapman & Hall.

Salkovskis, P. & Warwick, H. (1986). Morbid preoccupation, health anxiety and reassurance: a cognitive–behavioural approach to hypochondriasis. *Behaviour Research and Therapy*, **24**, 597–602.

Sexually transmitted diseases

Sickle cell disease

JAMES ELANDER

MRC Child Psychiatry Unit,
Institute of Psychiatry, London, UK

Sickle cell disease (SCD) is a group of inherited blood disorders in which an abnormal form of haemoglobin (sickle haemoglobin, or HbS) polymerizes under conditions of low oxygen tension, making the red cells stiffen and elongate into a characteristic crescent or sickle shape. The deformed cells can disrupt blood supply in the micro-vasculature, causing episodic vaso-occlusive crises in which oxygen deprivation causes severe pain and damage to affected tissue and organs.

The cause of the illness is Mendelian inheritance of the recessive sickle β globin gene. When this is inherited from both parents, the result is sickle cell anaemia. SC disease and sickle β thalassaemia (the other most common forms of SCD) are caused by co-inheritance with the structural globin variant C or with a β thalassaemia gene.

SCD is encountered in all parts of the world where malaria has been endemic and where people have migrated from these areas, predominantly northern Europe and the USA, where over 50 000 people are affected. In the UK there are around 5,000 sufferers. Severity is highly variable between individuals, but most live with intermittent pain and occasional serious complications, and risk early and sudden death related to the condition. Carriers of the sickle trait are usually symptom-free under all but the most extreme conditions.

In the absence of reliably effective anti-sickling agents, treatment is predominantly supportive and symptomatic, aiming to relieve pain, prevent infections, and combat complications as they occur (Davies & Brozovic, 1989).

PSYCHOLOGICAL EFFECTS OF SCD

Vaso-occlusive episodes in the central nervous system can cause strokes, and sickling in the brain might be responsible for cognitive deficits even in the absence of overt neurological damage. However, most of the psychological effects of the condition stem from the experience of episodic pain and from the disruption of education, work and family life caused by periodic acute illness and measures taken to prevent sickling.

Most of the evidence on levels of maladjustment and psychiatric symptomatology in relation to SCD comes from studies of children and adolescents. This is mixed, with the better controlled studies generally failing to show poorer outcomes among young people with SCD (Midence, Fuggle & Davies, 1993). Demographic and family factors have been related more consistently than measures of illness severity to adjustment and development, with greater problems experienced by older male children, those in poorer socioeconomic circumstances, and those in less cohesive families. A smaller number of more consistent findings have shown adults with SCD to have higher levels of psychiatric morbidity, most commonly depression, than those with chronic illnesses such as diabetes. Perceived stress associated with daily hassles, rather than measures of illness severity, has been found to predict poorer adjustment (Thompson *et al.*, 1992).

In several studies, children with SCD performed at lower levels than matched controls on tests of cognitive ability (Brown, Armstrong & Eckman, 1993). This may be because subtle neurological defects caused by sickling can affect cognitive functioning even in the absence of overt neurological complications. However, there is little evidence of a relationship between test performance and illness severity, and it is unclear to what extent the former could be affected by factors like reduced access to schooling due to illness and hospital attendance in children with SCD.

TREATMENT IMPLICATIONS

Improved treatment for the most serious complications of sickling crises and preventive measures against infections have raised the life expectancy of sufferers, and many now survive into late middle age and beyond. However, there is considerable scope for improving the management of painful crises, which account for over 90% of hospital admissions in SCD (Brozovic, Davies & Brownell, 1987). Interview data from patients indicates high levels of dissatisfaction with service provision, and studies of knowledge and attitudes among medical staff suggest that much sickling pain may be undertreated or inappropriately treated with analgesia (Midence & Elander, 1994). Risk of dependence and abuse is often overestimated by doctors, many of whom have little expertise in pain relief or management of SCD, and there is no systematic evidence for a raised risk of drug misuse among people with SCD. Various behavioural methods for pain control, most involving combinations of biofeedback, self-hypnosis and relaxation, have been examined with broadly encouraging results, but few have been properly evaluated. Specific non-pharmacological techniques may be effective only for milder pain, whereas interventions to integrate and coordinate the delivery of existing medical and psychosocial services for SCD have been shown to be effective in reducing requirements for emergency medical attention (Vichinski, Johnson & Lubin, 1982).

A small number of bone marrow transplants have been performed for children with SCD (Kirkpatrick, Barrios & Humbert, 1991). The operation can cure the illness but carries a significant risk of mortality, and the decision to proceed for any individual means making an assessment of the long-term severity and manageability of the condition and the extent to which it would compromise quality of life, both of which are difficult to estimate in early life.

Because the majority of those affected by SCD are African or

Afro-Caribbean in origin, there is a need to take greater account of ethnic factors in research on the psychological effects of the condition and patients' responses to treatment, for cultural influences on the perception and management of pain and illness, along with racial inequalities in access to services, have the potential to moderate outcomes in ways that may go undetected by standard research designs.

REFERENCES

Brown, R.T., Armstrong, F.D. & Eckman, J.R. (1993). Neurocognitive aspects of pediatric sickle cell disease. *Journal of Learning Disabilities*, **26**, 33–45.

Brozovic, M., Davies, S.C. & Brownell, A.I. (1987). Acute admissions of patients with sickle cell disease who live in Britain. *British Medical Journal*, **294**, 1206–8.

Davies, S.C. & Brozovic, M. (1989). The presentation, management and prophylaxis of sickle cell disease. *Blood Reviews*, **3**, 29–44.

Kirkpatrick, D.V., Barrios, N.J. & Humbert, J.H. (1991). Bone marrow transplantation for sickle cell anemia. *Seminars in Hematology*, **28**, 240–3.

Midence, K. & Elander, J. (1994). *Sickle cell disease: a psychosocial approach*. Oxford: Radcliffe Medical Press.

Midence, K., Fuggle, P. & Davies, S.C. (1993). Psychosocial aspects of sickle cell disease (SCD) in childhood and adolescence: a review. *British Journal of Clinical Psychology*, **32**, 271–80.

Thompson, R.J., Gil, K.M., Abrams, M.R. & Phillips, G. (1992). Stress, coping, and psychological adjustment of adults with SCD. *Journal of Consulting and Clinical Psychology*, **60**, 433–40.

Vichinski, E.P., Johnson, R. & Lubin, B.H. (1982). Multi-disciplinary approach to pain management in SCD. *American Journal of Pediatric Hematology and Oncology*, **4**, 328–33.

Skin cancer

RON BORLAND

*Centre for Behavioural Research in Cancer,
Anti-Cancer Council of Victoria, Australia*

EPIDEMIOLOGY OF SKIN CANCER

Skin cancers can be broadly classified into two types, melanomas and non-melanomas. Melanomas are cancers of the melanocytes which lie in the basal layer of the epidermis. Melanomas, unless detected at an early stage have a high fatality rate. Non-melanocytic skin cancers, include two major types, basal cell carcinomas and squamous cell carcinomas. Both of these forms of skin cancer are relatively benign; however, if neglected they can result in significant morbidity and, in some cases, death (especially from squamous cell carcinoma).

The incidence of skin cancer is rising among fair-skinned populations throughout the world with the highest rates in Australia. People whose skin burns easily are at the highest risk. The principle aetiological factor for skin cancer is ultraviolet (UV) radiation, the main source of which comes from the sun's rays (Marks & Hill, 1992). Around two-thirds of daily UV radiation is transmitted in the two hours each side of true midday. In tropical areas, UV levels are high all year round. In temperate zones, UV levels only reach high levels in the summer months, except at high altitudes, or in reflecting environments where the levels can be much higher than normal.

There is no clear consensus on the mechanisms by which UV radiation leads to skin cancers. One of the major problems is the difficulty of measuring UV exposure across the lifespan. There is some evidence that melanoma may be a result of both acute episodic overexposure, best indexed by sunburn and very high levels of cumulative exposure (such as is achieved in tropical and subtropical climates). By contrast, non-melanoma skin cancers may be more closely linked to total UV exposure. Exposure in childhood and adolescence may be more important than adult exposure for later development of skin cancer. Regular use of sunscreen (which reduces UV exposure) can reduce both the prevalence and incidence of solar keratoses, which are precursor lesions for cancer (Thompson, Jolley & Marks, 1993).

PREVENTION

To reduce skin cancer risk involves reducing UV exposure, particularly acute over-exposure (or sunburn) and to focus these preventative activities on young people, while not neglecting the benefits that may come from reduced exposure at all ages.

The most effective ways of reducing UV exposure are staying out of the sun when UV levels are high by staying indoors or seeking shade, covering up with clothing, wearing hats, and using sunscreens. The sunscreens recommended vary from country to country, but generally a broad spectrum sun protection factor (SPF) 15 or greater is considered adequate, that is, sunscreens that block out around 94% of all UV radiation.

The linchpin for the systematic scientific approach to melanoma control is good data: epidemiological data on the incidence and mortality from the disease, data on identified behavioural risk factors, data on the value of the risk behaviour to 'at risk' groups, and data from the systematic evaluation of interventions.

Measuring sun protection

Strategies to measure sun protection fall into four broad categories: observation, diaries, recall of specific events, and reports of overall behaviour.

Measuring sun protection behaviour is difficult because the need for it varies as a function of time of day, season of the year, time outside and prevailing weather conditions. Further, the extent to which extra protective action is required will vary as a function of the normal dress for the activities engaged in, eg swimmers need to rely more on sunscreen than golfers. This means that it is difficult for people to estimate what is usual across all kinds of activities and situations. People tend to over-estimate the extent to which they take protective actions (at least in the context of a population who are well informed of the need to take such actions). This has been most clearly demonstrated in children. Estimates of sun protection based on overall reports should be treated with caution.

Direct observation, using observers or photographs can provide an accurate and potentially unbiased estimate of behaviour. However, it is restricted to visibly observable sun protection (thus excluding sunscreen use) and to public places (for practical and ethical reasons). It is also not practical to observe individuals over extensive periods, so data may not be representative of the people observed, though it can be of the situations observed.

Diaries of sun protective actions and outdoor experiences can be kept reliably (Girgis et al., 1993) and thus they have the potential to accurately describe individual behaviour. However, there are limits on how long people will keep them for, and demand characteristics associated with keeping them may lead to changes in sun protection behaviour, either for social desirability reasons or to minimize the amount of recording necessary.

Recall of specific events can only reasonably be done for a relatively short period (days). Measurement cannot change the actual behaviour, but recall can be selectively influenced by demand characteristics and may also vary with the salience of the activities. Attempts to validate specific recall with observational strategies suggest they are reasonably accurate, at least for behaviours in public places. Specific recall is likely to be representative for situations, although it may not be for individuals. It is probably the best method for monitoring population-wide trends.

The Challenge

Risk of UV exposure is related to aspects of lifestyle. Exposure can be incidental to outdoor activity or can be actively sought, as in sunbathing. There is limited capacity for getting people to spend less time outside, although it is possible to get people to schedule more of that time outside peak UV periods. The major focus needs to be on getting people to take suitable precautions when they are outside. Both qualitative and quantitative research has identified a desire for a suntan as a major barrier to sun protection. Suntans are related to a self-image of being active, healthy and attractive, and others see suntanned individuals in a similar way (Miller et al., 1990). Other factors inhibiting sun protection are the perceived unfashionability of clothes and protective hats and, especially among men and older people, a reluctance to use sunscreen.

Hill et al. (1992) using specific recall in representative population samples in Australia have shown that the above barriers are most prevalent in younger people. They also found that young people are more likely to get sunburnt than older people, and men are more likely to get burnt than women. Young people, especially young males, spend more time out in the sun and expose more of their skin to the sun. Young people, especially young women, are more likely to rely on sunscreens for sun protection. Men are more likely to

wear sunhats than women, but women are more likely to avoid the sun or use sunscreens as protective measures. Such data provides a baseline understanding of community behaviour, from which planning for behaviour change can proceed.

Behaviour change

The first stage of a prevention campaign involves informing the public about the risk; about strategies to reduce risk, and that risk reduction is worth considering. Health education programmes in schools and workplaces have been shown to produce improvements in sun protection, especially where they have used programmes that actively engaged participants. In many countries most, or all, of the population are at risk, so comprehensive mass-reach, population-based behaviour change strategies are required (Marks & Hill, 1992). These should include education and other activity directed at personal behaviour change, combined with activity directed at changing aspects of the physical or social context to make sun protection easier and/or more desirable.

One of the most extensive skin cancer prevention programmes has occurred in Victoria, Australia. In 1980, a small scale campaign called 'Slip! Slop! Slap!' (Slip on a shirt!, Slop on sunscreen! and Slap on a hat!) was launched. By 1987 there was virtually total community awareness of the need for sun protection, but inadequate levels of behaviour change. In 1988, with funds from a hypothicated levy on tobacco a more extensive campaign called SunSmart was launched. At its peak it had a budget of about 30 ¢ US per person per year (for a population of around 4 million). The campaign aimed to change public perceptions of the acceptability of sun protection by linking it with fashionable images in TV and other advertising. The advertising also helped put skin cancer on the public agenda, which was important in encouraging community involvement both in education and in fostering appropriate structural change to support sun-protection behaviour. For example, availability of fashionable sun protective hats and clothes, cheaper sunscreens, more appropriate outdoor policies in schools and workplaces, and increased provision of shade.

The first two years of this campaign were associated with a marked increase in sun protection behaviour: hat use and sunscreen use increased markedly, as did the proportion of the population avoiding at least part of the peak UV radiation period of 11am – 3pm (Hill et al., 1993). Furthermore, reported desire for a suntan fell as did personal beliefs about the desirability of a tan and beliefs that others preferred tans. It is likely that much of this change was either directly or indirectly due to the campaign. Keeping the public aware of the reasons why sun-protection is important provides a strong basis for sustained attitudinal and behaviour change (see Accidents for more on population intervention).

EARLY DETECTION

Because skin cancers grow in the skin, they are readily observable, particularly if they grow in easy to see areas. Thus it is potentially easy to detect them at an early stage of development when treatment is almost always successful. A variety of strategies have been used to encourage one-off self-screening. These can lead to an increase in melanoma detection through more people presenting to doctors with suspicious lesions (e.g. Doherty & MacKie, 1988). Similar effects have occurred through increased community awareness of skin cancer. There is still room to improve people's understanding of what to look for. For example, most Australians believe melanomas are raised lesions even though virtually all early melanoma are flat (Borland, Marks & Noy, 1992). This may be leading to some melanomas being ignored. Educational resources are needed that enable people to accurately distinguish potentially dangerous spots from those that are clearly benign.

There is increasing medical interest in instituting systematic programmes of self-screening or screening by professionals where all or most of the body could be checked on a regular basis. As yet there is no evidence about whether this would increase detection sufficiently to justify its adoption, even for high-risk groups. Behavioural research is needed to determine levels and frequencies of self-screening people can be encouraged to persist with. Efforts to maximize screening will involve developing strategies to minimize embarrassment, provide the skills to do the self-examination properly, ensure appropriate confidence in decisions to engender

appropriate action, and ensure that people perform self-examinations regularly. A balance will need to be found between the potential benefits to health and the what people are willing or able to do.

When people have identified spots which are of concern, it is crucial that they seek medical advice as quickly as possible. There is no good data available on the extent of delay in presenting, but some people do delay enough to affect their prognosis. Research is needed to identify modifiable determinants of delay.

A self-detection programme depends on more than an educated and willing public. It also requires doctors and other health practitioners who have the necessary knowledge and skills in accurate diagnosis and management, and who encourage the public to engage in appropriate self-screening. Regardless of whether systematic self-screening proves effective and practical, better informing the public about the risk of skin cancer, and of what to look for, can reduce skin cancer morbidity and mortality.

REFERENCES

Borland, R., Marks, R. & Noy, S. (1992). Public knowledge about characteristics of moles and melanomas. *Australian Journal of Public Health*, **16**, 370–5.

Doherty, V.R. & MacKie, R.M. (1988). Experience of a public education programme on early detection of cutaneous malignant melanomas. *British Medical Journal*, **297**, 388–91.

Girgis, A., Sanson-Fisher, R.W., Tripodi, D.A. & Golding, T. (1993). Evaluation of interventions to improve solar protection in primary schools. *Health Education Quarterly*, **20**, 275–87.

Hill, D., White, V., Marks, R., Theobald, T., Borland, R. & Roy, C. (1992). Melanoma prevention: behavioural and non-behavioural factors in sunburn among an Australian urban population. *Preventive Medicine*, **21**, 654–9.

Hill, D., White, V., Marks, R. & Borland, R. (1993). Changes in sun-related attitudes and behaviours, and reduced sunburn prevalence in a population at high risk of melanoma. *European Journal of Cancer Prevention*, **2**, 447–56.

Marks, R. & Hill, D. (1992) (Eds.). *The public*

health approach to melanoma control: prevention and early detection. Geneva: International Union Against Cancer (UICC).

Miller, A.G., Ashton, W.A., McHoskey, J.W. & Gimbel, J. (1990). What price attractiveness? Stereotype and risk factors in suntanning behavior. *Journal of Applied Social Psychology*, **20**, 1272–300.

Thompson, S.C., Jolley, D. & Marks, R. (1993). Reduction of solar keratoses by regular sunscreen use. *New England Journal of Medicine*, **329**, 1147–51.

Spina bifida

TRUDY HAVERMANS

Veldhoven, The Netherlands

Spina Bifida is a spinal deformity caused by an incomplete closure of one or more vertebrae (the bones which form the backbone), with an incidence of approximately one affected infant per 1000 live births. There are three main types of Spina Bifida, namely (i) Spina Bifida Occulta, which is a mild and common form that rarely causes disability, (ii) Spina Bifida Cystica, in which the visible signs are a sac or cyst, like a large blister on the back, covered by a thin layer of skin (two forms: Meningocele and Myelomeningocele) and (iii) Cranium Bifida, where the bones of the skull fail to develop properly. Most babies born with Spina Bifida also have hydrocephalus (an accumulation of cerebro-spinal fluid).

Modern medicine has resulted in greatly improved life expectancy, but children still suffer from a range of problems, including incontinence, chronic renal infections, lower extremity deformities

or scoliosis (Association for Spina Bifida and Hydrocephalus, 1991).

Spina Bifida can be diagnosed immediately after birth, and the baby is typically removed directly for medical attention. The amount of stress will partly depend on the physical condition of the child, the medical treatment, how parents are told the diagnosis, what they already know about Spina Bifida and how they are helped in further decision-making processes. A major problem confronting parents is how to care for the baby.

As the child gets older, the physical handicaps, if present, are primary stressors. For example, impaired mobility can cause stigma, limit social opportunities and burden family members as they need to provide for the Spina Bifida child's activities of daily living. Major predictors of greater impact include the number of restrictions in the child's activities, parental perceptions of the child's

Spina bifida

health, low maternal education, low family income, number of adults in the family and parental unemployment status. Furthermore, the quality and duration of the marital relationship before the birth of the child has been reported to be an important factor explaining parental adaptation. Wallander *et al.* (1988) found that the mother's perception of current marital satisfaction was the single best predictor of their mental, physical and social adaptation.

Because Spina Bifida involves an abnormality of the CNS, there is a concern for its impact on intellectual functioning and academic performance (Varni and Wallander, 1988). School placement may be problematic. For example, Lord *et al.* (1990) found that, although children in normal schools achieved greater success academically, they were more likely to perceive themselves as isolated and lonely in comparison with those attending specialist units. In addition,

there are many indicators of psychological consequences for the children themselves (Lavigne *et al.*, 1988; Kazak & Clark, 1988).

Most attention in terms of research and intervention has been directed towards increasing self-help skills (e.g. dressing, grooming, feeding and hygiene), ambulation, obesity, chronic incontinence and pressure sores.

While acknowledging the potential adversities that confront families of children with Spina Bifida, it is increasingly clear that families demonstrate enormous resilience and coping resources (Spaulding & Morgan, 1986). It is important to realize that families with a child with a chronic condition like Spina Bifida, are very much 'normal' families coping with exceptional circumstances (Perrin & MacLean, 1988). Providing help should therefore be matched with the needs of each individual family.

REFERENCES

Association for Spina Bifida and Hydrocephalus (1991). Information sheet 1, Peterborough.

Kazak, A.E. & Clark, M.W. (1988). Stress in families of children with Myelomeningocele. *Developmental Medicine and Child Neurology*, 28, 220–8.

Lavigne, J.V., Nolan, D. & McLone, D.G. (1988). Temperament, coping, and psychological adjustment in young children with myelomeningocele. *Journal of Pediatric Psychology*, 13, 363–78.

Lord, J., Varzos, N., Behrman, B., Wicks, J. & Wicks, D., (1990). Implications of mainstream classrooms for adolescents with spina bifida, *Developmental Medicine and Child Neurology*, 32, 20–9.

Perrin, J.M. & MacLean, W.E. (1988). Children with chronic illness: the prevention of dysfunction. *Pediatric Clinics of North America*, 35, 1325–37.

Spaulding, B.R. & Morgan, S.B. (1986). Spina Bifida and their parents: a population prone to family dysfunction? *Journal of Pediatric Psychology*, 11, 159–374.

Varni, J.W. & Wallander, J.L. (1988). Pediatric chronic disabilities: haemophilia and Spina Bifida as examples. In D.K. Routh (Ed.). *Handbook of pediatric psychology*. New York: Guilford.

Wallander, J.L., Varni, J.W., Babani, L., Banis, H.T. & Wilcox, K.T. (1988). Children with chronic physical disorders: maternal reports of their psychological adjustment. *Journal of Pediatric Psychology*, 13, 197–212.

Spinal cord injury

PAUL KENNEDY

Department of Clinical Psychology, National Spinal Injuries Centre, Stoke Mandeville Hospital, Aylesbury, Bucks, UK

AETIOLOGY, INCIDENCE AND PREVALENCE

The successful rehabilitation and community reintegration of people with spinal cord injury (SCI) has only occurred in the past 50 years. Until rehabilitation was pioneered by Guttmann at Stoke Mandeville, in 1944, 90% of persons with a spinal cord injury died within the first year. Now, most industrialized economies provide comprehensive treatment and rehabilitation care for people with traumatic and non-traumatic injuries. Almost half (47%) of traumatic spinal cord injuries are caused by road traffic accidents. Domestic and industrial falls are the cause of 27%, and between 15 and 20% are from sporting injuries. In the UK, 5% are caused by self-harm and 0.5% from acts of violence. In the USA, 15% of injuries are caused by criminal assault (Kennedy, 1995; Stover & Fine, 1986). Causes of non-traumatic injuries include infective diseases, ischaemic insults, neoplastic disorders and multiple sclerosis.

There are four males for every female spinal cord injury. The

mean age is 28 and the mode is 19. The annual incidence of spinal cord injury in the UK, like most other European countries, is between 10 and 15 per million; in the USA it is thought to be nearer 30, and in Japan, 27 per million. There are an estimated 40 000 people in the UK and 200 000 in the USA. Life expectancy estimates vary: for a young, incomplete person, the relative survival is 96%, but for complete tetraplegics over 50, it is estimated to be 33%. A reasonably good life expectancy is probable for most people. Primary causes of early mortality include pneumonia, septicaemia, heart disease and pulmonary emboli.

THE PHYSICAL IMPACT

An injury to the spinal cord occurs when sufficient force causes the cord to be compressed, lacerated, or stretched and may be associated with a fracture or fracture–dislocation of the vertebral column and displacement of the inter-vertebral discs. These hyper-extension injuries are often the consequence of sudden impact as with car accidents and falls. The neurological losses will depend upon completeness of the injury. Cervical (neck) injury may result in tetraplegia (quadriplegia). Injuries to the thoracic, lumbar and sacral levels (upper, middle and lower back) may result in paraplegia. Of injuries 53% are neck injuries and 47% are back injuries. A complete injury is one in which all motor and sensory functions are lost below the level of the injury, as well as the loss of control of visceral functions, such as bladder, bowel and sexual function. In paraplegia, lower trunk muscles are impaired whilst cervical injuries result in loss of function in the hands, arms, shoulder, diaphragm as well as the lower thorax. Complete injuries above the seventh cervical segment may preclude the possibility of independent living. Sensory losses are similar to the areas of motor loss, and include loss of touch, pressure, temperature regulation and position. The loss of sexual sensation and responsivity, control of bladder and bowel function are common to all complete lesions above the sacral roots. Incomplete injuries may result in partial damage of the cord. Complications post-discharge include pressure sores, urinary tract infections, muscular spasm and chronic pain.

REHABILITATION

Most people are transferred to a specialist spinal cord injury treatment and rehabilitation centre shortly after the onset of the disorder. Once any fracture is stabilized, either through internal of external fixation, or postural reduction, the person begins a period of rehabilitation which can last between three months and one year, depending on the level of the injury and social circumstances. Rehabilitation enables the person to acquire new skills to address their needs and adjust physically, socially and psychologically to their physical disability. This includes learning to manage bladder and bowel functions, wheelchair use, and the maintenance and development of functional independence skills. Exploring adaptations to accommodation, financial independence and personal assistant needs may also be necessary. People also require information about their new needs and emotional support in maintaining general psychosocial well-being.

PSYCHOLOGICAL REACTIONS

A spinal cord injury requires major adjustments to physical, psychological and social domains. The extent to which people manage the consequences of the disability will depend on internal psychological factors, such as self-efficacy and coping styles, and external factors, such as prevailing social attitudes and social support. The cultural beliefs that underpin social policy are important, given that it is not the specific disability that causes most of the difficulties but existing within physical, psychological and socially disabling environments.

The immediate psychological impact of the injury may be compounded by severe pain and disturbed consciousness because of brain injury, medication or sensory deprivation. Trieschmann (1988) points out that, in the acute phase, psychological disturbances may result from sensory responses to injury, the hospital environment and procedures utilized in the survival of the person, rather than consideration of the spinal cord injury itself. Almost 60% of patients interviewed wished to have been told their prognosis within two weeks of injury. Once the patient is medically stable, clear, and accurate information should be given about their

prognosis, and the nature of the resources available to help them cope with the consequences of the injury.

PSYCHOLOGICAL IMPACT

Many studies have explored both the psychological impact and psychological adjustment factors. Early researchers explored psychological adjustment to spinal cord injury in the form of a variety of stages. Whilst these models may have had some utility in recognizing and normalizing emotional reactions, there is little empirical evidence that they exist or, indeed, are helpful in fostering adjustment, Morris (1992). Current models that are helpful in conceptualizing the process of adjustment and the management of psychological impact include the behaviour environment–person interaction model, proposed by Trieschmann (1988), the Stress and Coping Paradigm developed by Lazarus and Folkman (1984) and Becks' Cognitive Behavioural Model as applied to this client group by Kennedy (1991) and Crewe and Krause (1987).

The emotional impact is typified by increased levels of depression, anxiety (and associated avoidance behaviours), indirect self-destructive behaviour, increased suicidal ideation, communication problems and social isolation. However, negative emotional responses are neither universal nor necessary for successful rehabilitation. Estimates of the prevalence of depression, using clinical interview and standardized measures, indicate that between 20 and 34% of people during the acute rehabilitation phase are depressed (Kennedy, 1995; Judd et al., 1989). Despite psychological function improving with time since injury, Krause and Crewe (1991) found that significant levels of psychological distress do persist in some individuals. In a study of 9000 people injured between 1974 and 1984, DeVivo et al. (1991), found that 50 people had committed suicide, producing a standard mortality ratio of 4.9. They concluded that, whilst it occurred more often in a spinal injured population, in an absolute sense it is a rare event. Suicidal ideation is more common and 34% of spinal cord injured persons engage potentially harmful forms of self-neglect.

Spinal cord injury also has an impact on family members and the social context. Recent studies suggest that there are fewer marriages and more divorces than the able-bodied population, although people who marry after injury are generally happier, more independent and sexually active than those who were married before their injury (Crewe, Athelstan & Krumberger, 1979).

In people with complete spinal cord injury, sexual function is usually impaired. Males and females lose their ability to experience orgasm and general neurophysiological sexual responsivity. However, some males retain the capacity for reflex erections, and some people report 'phantom' orgasms. Despite these losses, many people engage in sexual activity and 57% rated post-injury sexual relations as satisfying, or at least as satisfying (Siosteen et al., 1990).

PSYCHOLOGICAL ADJUSTMENT AND QUALITY OF LIFE

Factors which influence adjustment, such as personality characteristics, level of injury and social supports have been investigated. There is no evidence (Trieschmann, 1988) that any personality pattern is associated with having a spinal cord injury. Frank and Elliott (1989) administered the Multi-dimensional Health Locus of Control Scale (MDHLC) and the Beck Depression Inventory (BDI) to

53 spinal cord injured people post-discharge and found that those with more fatalistic beliefs about their health tended to be more depressed. Morris (1992) reviewed studies of attributional style and found that acceptance of disability was unrelated to any attributional tendency. Whilst counter-intuitive, there is a general consensus that the severity of injury does not predict positive adjustment (Kennedy, 1995; Trieschmann, 1988). Krause and Crewe (1990) followed a cohort from 1974 until 1984, and their results confirm research findings that quality of life improves with time. Positive levels of satisfaction and psychological status were maintained with increases in marriage rates and hours spent working. Social support is beneficial to long-term adjustment, even at six weeks post-injury, Kennedy (1995) found that social support was negatively correlated with depression, anxiety and intrusive thoughts.

COPING

Reidy, Caplan and Shawaryn (1991) explored coping strategies among 54 individuals with recently acquired traumatic spinal cord injury using the Ways of Coping Questionnaire (Folkman & Lazarus, 1980). They report that patients rely most strongly on the strategies of social support, positive re-appraisal and planful problem-solving. In a two-year follow-up, they noted a decrease in seeking social support. Depression was found to a have strong correlation with the use of the escape/avoidance strategies. They conclude that pro-active problem-focused coping strategies are associated with positive mood and little psychological distress. Bombardier (1992), using a multiple assessment longitudinal design, found that emotion-focused coping styles are associated with poorer outcomes following spinal cord injury. Kennedy (1995), followed a cohort of 84 people with spinal cord injury during the first 6 months post-injury. Using the COPE (Carver, Scheier & Weintraub, 1989) and various measures of psychological impact, he found that planning was the only coping strategy that increased over time. Acceptance was more likely to be used by those who were not depressed or anxious and those who were more distressed tended to use denial, disengagement, venting emotions and alcohol/drug use ideation. Using a series of stepwise multiple regression analyses, patterns of coping styles associated with positive psychological well-being were identified.

At six weeks post-injury, 55% of the variance in anxiety scores were accounted for through the use of two coping strategies, i.e. behavioural disengagement and low acceptance. At 18 weeks post-injury 60% of the variance in depression was predicted through the use of behavioural disengagement and denial. Using the coping styles at six weeks, 30% of the variance in depression at 24 weeks was accounted for by the use of alcohol/drug use ideation and behavioural disengagement. The high level of active coping observed in this group suggested that people perceive that many aspects of their difficulties are controllable and this associated with the widespread use of acceptance for those factors which cannot change may form the basis of an effective coping pattern.

PSYCHOLOGICAL INTERVENTIONS

The main aims of psychological intervention with spinal cord injured people are to foster coping and adaptation, preserve social value and maximize the rehabilitation potential. This is achieved by individual and group psychotherapy, working with relationships and underpinning rehabilitation programmes with behavioural principles. Counselling helps people express their concerns, consider coping strategies and accept the consequences of the illness or injury. During rehabilitation, many people are confronted with change and experience a sense of loss. Whilst depression may emerge as part of a normal response, it can precipitate distorted modes of thinking which generate negative beliefs about disability. Cognitive behaviour therapy is used to identify and challenge such negative beliefs (Kennedy, 1991; Crewe & Krause 1987). Thoughts like 'I'm just going through the motions of life' and 'I can't do anything any more' and associated negative assumptions can be challenged effectively using techniques of self-observation, problem-solving and graded exposure. In the early stages, many people over-estimate the negative aspects of the injury and under-estimate their skills, resources and competence levels.

Group counselling and educational approaches have also developed as part of rehabilitation programmes, Treischmann (1988). The most effective group approaches embrace information-giving with basic problem-solving skills. Patient education manuals, audiovisual materials and access to peer counsellors are other essential components.

Individuals and couples also require access to sexual counsellors. The PLISSIT model developed by Annon (1974) is one of the most useful. This approach allows counsellors to structure an intervention according to the counsellors level of competence. It begins with 'permission giving' which refers to a general responsiveness to the discussion of sexual concerns. This is followed by the provision of 'limited information' such as through teaching sessions, education materials and videos. 'Specific suggestions' may then be offered to individuals or couples which highlight changes in sexual function and techniques for maintaining activity. This may be followed by 'intensive therapy' whereby techniques such as Masters and Johnsons' sensate focus may be required.

Treischmann describes rehabilitation as a lifelong process but Norris-Baker et al. (1981) proposed that long-term adjustment could be predicted by engagement and rehabilitation. Developing this theme, Kennedy and Pearce (1993) used goal planning successfully to identify individual needs and increase engagement in rehabilitation. This involved the development of a Needs Assessment checklist of basic behavioural indicators, the training of key workers and regular progress review meetings. Goal planning provides a forum for the provision of regular positive feedback on mastery of specific issues, thereby minimizing helplessness and fostering self-efficacy.

REFERENCES

Anon, J.S. (1974). *The behavioural treatment of sexual problems.* vol.1. Honolulu: Enabling Systems Inc.

Bombardier, C.H. (1992). Coping with spinal cord injury: a longitudinal pilot study.

Paper presented at the American Psychological Association Convention in Toronto.

Carver, C.S., Scheier, M.F. & Weintraub, J.K. (1989). Assessing coping strategies: a

theoretically based approach. *Journal of Personality and Social Psychology*, **56**, 267–83.

Crewe, N.M. & Krause, J.S. (1987). Spinal cord injury: psychological aspects. In

B.Caplan (Ed.). *Rehabilitation psychology*, pp.3–33. Baltimore: Aspen.

Crewe, N.M., Athelston, G.P. & Krumberger, J. (1979). Spinal cord injury: a comparison of pre-injury and post-injury marriages: *Archives of Physical Medicine and Rehabilitation*, **60**, 252–6.

DeVivo, M.J., Black, K.J., Richards, J. & Stover, S.L. (1991). Suicide following a spinal cord Injury. *Paraplegia*, **29**, 620–7.

Folkman, S. & Lazarus, R.S. (1980). An analysis of coping in a middle-aged community sample. *Journal of Health and Social Behaviour*, **21**, 219–39.

Frank, R.G. & Elliott, T.R. (1989). Spinal cord injury and health locus of control beliefs. *Paraplegia*, **27**, 250–6.

Judd, S.K., Stone, J., Webber, J., Brown, D.J. & Burrows, G.D. (1989). Depression following spinal cord injury: a prospective in-patient study. *British Journal of Psychiatry*, **154**, 668–71.

Kennedy, P. (1991). Counselling with spinal cord injured people. In H. Davis & L. Fallowfield (Ed.). *Counselling and communication in healthcare*. Chichester: John Wiley & Sons.

Kennedy, P. (1995). Psychological aspects of spinal cord injury: behavioural approaches, emotional impact and coping strategies. Unpublished Doctoral Dissertation, University of Ulster.

Kennedy, P. & Pearce, N. (1993). Goal planning, needs assessment and advocacy. *Journal of Health Services Management*, **89**, 17–24.

Krause, J.S. & Crewe, N.M. (1990). Long term prediction of self-reported problems following spinal cord injury. *Paraplegia*, **28**, 186–202.

Krause, J.S. & Crewe, N.M. (1991). Chronological age, time since injury and time of measurement: effect on adjustment after spinal cord injury. *Archives of Physical Medicine and Rehabilitation*, **72**, 91–100.

Lazarus, R.S. & Folkman, S. (1984). *Stress, appraisal and coping*. New York: Springer.

Morris, J. (1992). Psychological and sociological aspects of patients with spinal injuries. In H.L. Frankel (Ed.). *Handbook of clinical neurology: spinal cord trauma*, vol.61, London: Elsevier Science.

Norris-Baker, C., Stephens, M.A., Rintala, M.A. & Willens, E.P. (1981). Patient behaviour as a predictor of outcomes in spinal cord injury. *Archives of Physical Medicine and Rehabilitation*, **62**, 602–8.

Reidy, K., Caplan, B. & Shawaryn, M. (1991). Coping strategies following spinal cord injury: accommodation to trauma and disability. Presented at the 68th Annual Meeting of the American Congress of Rehabilitation Medicine, Washington, DC.

Siosteen, A., Lundqvist, C., Blomstrand, C., Sullivan, L. & Sullivan, M. (1990). Sexual ability, activity, attitudes and satisfaction as part of adjustment in spinal cord injured subjects. *Paraplegia*, **28**, 285–95.

Stover, S. & Fine, R. (1986). *Spinal cord injury: the facts and figures*. Birmingham, Alabama: University of Alabama.

Trieschmann, R.B. (1988). *Spinal cord injuries: psychological, social and vocational rehabilitation*. Scottsdale, Arizona: Demos.

Sterilization and vasectomy

ROBERT J. EDELMANN

Department of Psychology, University of Surrey, Guildford, UK

Sterilization, either in the form of tubal sterilization for women or vasectomy for men is a widely used method of contraception. There has been a steady increase in the use of such methods so that, by 1987 sterilization was used by 51% of married couples in the USA who were using some form of contraception; the proportion of couples using female versus male sterilization being about equal (28% and 24%) (Forrest & Fordyce, 1988). Similar increases in the in the use of sterilization have been reported in the UK (Wellings, 1986). As might be expected, these high levels of protection by sterilization increase considerably among older couples. Even though it is possible to reverse both tubal sterilization and vasectomy with microsurgical techniques the chances of an attempted reversal actually resulting in a subsequent pregnancy are so uncertain that it is generally treated as an irreversible course of action.

Numerous studies from many countries have examined the social and psychological correlates of voluntary sterilization. However, it is worth noting that, as recently as 1985, Philliber & Philliber concluded from a comprehensive review of such studies that most were merely descriptive and many lacked methodological rigour. More rigorous research studies conducted over the last decade have enabled more substantive conclusions to be drawn. Two broad sets of psychosocial issues have been explored in relation to sterilization:

(i) factors influencing the couple's decision about contraceptive method and (ii) outcome after sterilization in relation to (a) the couple's marital and sexual relationship, (b) the incidence of psychological/psychiatric problems and (c) post-sterilization regret and the consequent wish for reversal of sterilization.

FACTORS INFLUENCING THE COUPLE'S DECISION ABOUT CONTRACEPTIVE METHOD

Although the evidence is equivocal, research findings tend to suggest that women who are sterilized are slightly more at a disadvantage socially than those who opt for other methods of contraception, that they tend to have more children and that they are more likely to have given birth before the age of 20 years. However, the most important factor determining use of sterilization rather than an alternative method of contraception is a decision by the couple that their family is complete (Hunt & Annandale, 1990). Relatively few studies have been conducted to examine psychosocial factors predictive of choice of sterilization method. However, there is some evidence to suggest that, while vasectomy is chosen because it is perceived as easier and tubal sterilization because of its convenience (frequently being conducted at the time of delivery), it is the spouse who most wants to stop childbearing who is most influential in the decision about which method of sterilization to use (Miller, Shain & Pasta, 1991a).

OUTCOME AFTER STERILIZATION

The couple's marital and sexual relationship

In their review, Philliber & Philliber (1985) note that, in the majority of studies worldwide, 'no change' is the most frequently endorsed reponse to questions relating to sexual desire, sexual functioning and the couple's marital and sexual relations irrespective of the sterilization method used. A similar conclusion is reached in a more recent review of research on the effects of vasectomy on the male's sexual relationship (Thonneau & D'Isle, 1990). As both sets of authors note though, the lack of good studies in this area makes the interpretation of results uncertain. However, a recent carefully designed longitudinal study investigating the impact of tubal sterilization or vasectomy on female sexuality concluded that there are no detrimental effects and some short-term benefits of both procedures (Shain et al., 1991)

The incidence of psychological/psychiatric problems

There is a large and conflicting literature on the incidence of psychological problems and/or psychiatric disorder subsequent to sterilization. In the case of tubal sterilization, estimates of psychiatric morbidity after surgery have varied widely from a high of 60% to a low of 8.8% (Philliber & Philliber, 1985). Figures have tended to be lower in more recent research, which no doubt partly reflects the increased use of standardized and more accurate methods of psychiatric assessment. Gath & Cooper (1983) concluded from their own findings that 'the operation seldom leads to psychiatric disorder' (p.235). Psychological or psychiatric problems which do occur tend to be associated with pre-operative psychological or psychiatric disturbance (Cooper et al., 1985). It seems reasonable to conclude that, for a small minority of women, sterilization will act as a precipitating factor for psychiatric disturbance while, for the majority, there seem to be no ill effects.

A recent review of ten years of research on the somatic and psychological consequences of vasectomy also suggests that there is no evidence that the procedure is associated with physical or mental health problems (Thonneau & D'Isle, 1990).

Post-sterilization regret

There is evidence that post-sterilization regret, particularly in the case of women, may be a problem of considerable magnitude. In Europe and North America reported rates of regret for women range from less than 10% to as high as 43%, with reported rates of regret amongst men tending to be less than 5% (Philliber & Philliber, 1985). A recent longitudinal study conducted over a 5-year period indicated that the major pre-sterilization predictors of regret for women included being relatively young, being ambivalent about future childbearing, holding negative attitudes towards sterilization, the woman's husband being dominant in the decision making process during which time she was in conflict with her husband (Miller, Shain & Pasta, 1991b). These authors further suggest that post-sterilization regret is not a simple psychological state but a complex process which begins with a renewed interest in having a baby, proceeds to the development of negative feelings about the set of decisions that led to sterilization (i.e. the decision to terminate childbearing, to use sterilization as opposed to other contraceptive methods and which member of the couple was to be sterilized) and concluded with a desire to reverse the surgery.

Those requesting a reversal are, however, far fewer than those who voice regret (Philliber & Philliber, 1985). The most frequently cited reason for a reversal of both tubal sterilization and vasectomy is a change in marital status, that is, a desire to have a child with a new partner. In this context, a number of authors (e.g. Miller, Shain & Pasta, 1991b) have argued that the best prevention of regret lies in adequate pre-sterilization counselling and information provision.

REFERENCES

Cooper, P., Bledin, K.D., Brice, B. & Mackenzie, S. (1985). Effects of female sterilization: one year follow-up in a prospective controlled study of psychological and psychiatric outcome. *Journal of Psychosomatic Research*, 29, 13–22.

Forrest, J.D. & Fordyce, R.R. (1988). U.S. women's contraceptive attitudes and practice: how have they changed in the 1980s? *Family Planning Perspetives*, 20, 112–18.

Gath, D. & Cooper, P.J. (1983). Psychiatric aspects of hysterectomy and female sterilization. *Recent Advances in Clinical Psychiatry*, 5, 75–100.

Hunt, K. & Annandale, E. (1990). Predicting contraceptive method usage among women in West Scotland. *Journal of Biosocial Science*, 22, 405–21.

Miller, W.B., Shain, R.N. & Pasta, D.J. (1991a). Tubal sterilization or vasectomy: how do married couples make the choice. *Fertility and Sterility*, 56, 278–84.

Miller, W.B., Shain, R.N. & Pasta, D.J. (1991b). The predictors of post-sterilization regret in married women. *Journal of Applied Social Psychology*, 21, 1083–10.

Philliber, S.D. & Philliber, W.W. (1985). Social and psychological perspectives in voluntary sterilization: a review. *Studies in Family Planning*, 16, 1–29.

Shain, R.N., Miller, W.B., Holden, A.E.C. & Rosenthal, M. (1991). Impact of tubal sterilization and vasectomy on female marital sexuality: results of a controlled longitudinal study. *American Journal of Obstetrics and Gynecology*, 64, 763–71.

Thonneau, P. & D'Isle, B. (1990). Does vasectomy have long-term effects on somatic and psychological health status? *International Journal of Andrology*, 13, 419–32.

Wellings, K. (1986). Trends in contraceptive method usage since 1970. *British Journal of Family Planning*, 12, 15.

Steroids

JAMES ELANDER
*MRC Child Psychiatry Unit,
Institute of Psychiatry, London,
UK*

SALLY PORTER
*Department of Mental Health
Sciences, St George's Hospital
Medical School, London, UK*

Steroids are a family of natural and synthetic compounds derived from the non-glyceride portion of fats, mainly cholesterol. They include the corticosteroids, produced in the adrenal cortex, which regulate carbohydrate metabolism and mediate physiological responses to stress, and anabolic steroids, usually synthetic derivatives of testosterone, which increase nitrogen retention and promote protein synthesis. The male and female sex hormones, also steroid compounds, are considered elsewhere in this handbook.

CORTICOSTEROIDS

Glucocorticoids (e.g. cortisone) and ACTH are frequently used in the treatment of shock, severe asthma, acute lymphoblastic leukaemia, and inflammatory disorders such as rheumatoid arthritis, ulcerative colitis and systemic lupus erythematosus (SLE), and have been associated with a range of psychological side-effects. In studies reviewed by Lewis and Smith (1983), the average incidence of severe psychiatric symptoms was 5.7%, with between 13% and 62% of patients suffering mild to moderate alterations in mood. Depression was the most common disturbance (40% of cases), followed by mania (28%), psychosis (14%), delirium (10%), and mixed affective disorder (8%).

The mechanisms underlying these affective and psychotic reactions are not yet understood (Ling, Perry & Tsuang, 1981) and may include physical changes in the condition for which steroids were prescribed, but patients treated with corticosteroids are affected to a greater extent than those who are not. Disturbances usually subside when the steroid therapy is stopped or changed, and short courses of psychotropic medication or electroconvulsive therapy may be needed in a few cases. Disturbances of mood and behaviour have also been noted following withdrawal of medication, and euphoric effects can lead to psychological dependence. Higher doses increase the likelihood of mental disturbance, but neither dose levels nor duration of corticosteroid therapy predict the time of onset, duration, severity or type of response. Risk factors for adverse psychological reactions include gender (with females at greater risk) and treatment for SLE (which is itself associated with psychiatric disturbance), but not age or previous adverse psychological reaction to corticosteroid therapy. It is still unclear to what extent, and in what ways, pre-existing psychological factors act to promote adverse reactions.

Cushing's syndrome usually involves raised levels of endogenous cortisol (it can also result from treatment with corticosteroids), and is frequently associated with psychiatric symptoms. Depression is the most common, followed by disturbed cognition and psychotic illness, but euphoria is rare by contrast with reactions to exogenous corticosteroids. A full recovery is usually made when the underlying endocrine disorder is treated, but psychiatric symptoms sometimes precede physical signs, and Cohen (1980) noted a high incidence of factors predisposing to depression among patients with Cushing's syndrome, raising the possibility that the former may play a role in precipitating the latter.

In Addison's disease all adrenal steroid levels are reduced, causing weakness, loss of appetite and loss of weight. Psychiatric abnormalities, most commonly apathy and negativism, are almost always present but psychotic reactions are much less common than in Cushing's disease, and most symptoms respond well to hormone replacement therapy. Increased irritability and apprehension sometimes precede Addisonian 'crises', in which acute organic reactions can cause clouding of consciousness, delirium, and convulsions.

ANABOLIC STEROIDS

Anabolic steroids have limited medical uses (including the treatment of certain anaemias and breast cancers), and are more commonly self-administered to increase body mass and improve athletic performance (Haupte & Rovere, 1984). Controlled trials of therapeutic doses rarely show psychological side-effects, but behavioural alterations, notably increased aggression and psychiatric symptomatology leading in some cases to violent crime, are common in descriptive reports (Williamson & Young, 1992). This may be because very high doses of combinations of anabolic substances are sometimes used in cycles lasting several weeks, or because user groups include relatively high proportions of people with violent tendencies and a predisposition to psychiatric illness. Baseline measures of psychopathology are rarely available in such studies, and the samples are probably not representative of the much larger population of anabolic steroid users, which, according to one US survey, included one senior male student in 15 (Buckley *et al.*, 1988). Pope and Katz (1988) looked at psychiatric symptomatology among anabolic steroid users recruited at gymnasia in the US. Criteria for a psychotic episode during periods of steroid use were met by 12% of the sample, with another 10% reporting milder psychotic symptoms. The same proportion (12%) reported a manic episode while using steroids, with a further 19% meeting all but one of the criteria. Nearly one-third of the group had a history of substance abuse or dependence, but past psychiatric history was otherwise unremarkable, and no psychotic or manic symptoms were reported before or between periods of steroid use. Those who had a first-degree relative with major affective disorder (17% of the sample) were apparently at no greater risk of affective or psychotic symptoms during periods of steroid use than those without such a history.

Steroids

More recently, attention has focused on the addictive properties of anabolic steroids, which, by altering mood and behaviour during intoxication, and inducing symptoms of withdrawal and craving during periods of abstinence, have the potential to produce a compulsive pattern of use in the same way as substances traditionally regarded as drugs of dependence (Kashkin & Kleber, 1989). Brower *et al.* (1991) reported that over a half of a sample of steroid-using weight lifters met criteria for a classification of substance dependence, the most commonly reported feature of which was a withdrawal syndrome including fatigue (reported by 43% of the sample), depressed mood (41%), desire to take more steroids (52%), and dissatisfaction with body size (42%). Severity of dependence was most closely related to the level of dose used, the number of cycles of use reported, and levels of dissatisfaction with body size. About 80% of the sample had injected steroids, and although none reported sharing injecting equipment, HIV has been transmitted apparently by non-sterile injection of anabolic steroids (Scott & Scott, 1989).

REFERENCES

Brower, K.J., Blow, F.C., Young, J.P. & Hill, E.M. (1991). The symptoms and correlates of anabolic–androgenic steroid dependence. *British Journal of Addiction*, 86, 759–68.

Buckley, W.E., Yesalis, C., Friedl, K.E., Anderson, W.A., Streit, A.L. & Wright, J.E. (1988). Estimated prevalence of anabolic steroid use among male high school seniors. *Journal of the American Medical Association*, 260, 3441–5.

Cohen, S.I. (1980). Cushing's syndrome: a psychiatric study of 29 patients. *British Journal of Psychiatry*, 136, 120–4.

Haupte, H.A. & Rovere, G.D. (1984). Anabolic steroids: a review of the literature. *American Journal of Sports Medicine*, 12, 469–84.

Kashkin, K.B. & Kleber, H.D. (1989). Hooked on hormones? An anabolic steroid addiction hypothesis. *Journal of the American Medical Association*, 262, 3166–70.

Lewis, D.A. & Smith, R.E. (1983). Steroid-induced psychiatric syndromes: a report of 14 cases and a review of the literature. *Journal of Affective Disorders*, 5, 319–32.

Ling, M.H.M., Perry, P.J. & Tsuang, M.T. (1981). Side effects of corticosteroid therapy: psychiatric aspects. *Archives of General Psychiatry*, 38, 471–7.

Pope, H.G. & Katz, D.L. (1988). Affective and psychotic symptoms associated with anabolic steroid use. *American Journal of Psychiatry*, 145, 487–90.

Scott, M.J. & Scott, M.J. (1989). HIV infection associated with injections of anabolic steroids (letter). *Journal of the American Medical Association*, 262, 207–8.

Williamson, D.J. & Young, A.H. (1992). Psychiatric effects of androgenic and anabolic–androgenic steroid abuse in men: a brief review of the literature. *Psychopharmacology*, 6, 20–6.

Stigma

ELIZABETH BURRIN

and

ROBERT WEST

Psychology Department, St George's Hospital Medical School, London, UK

Some illnesses lead to negative evaluations of the sufferers by others, including pity, disgust, disapprobation and denigration (Goffman, 1963). These can result in unfair treatment or overt hostility. Negative evaluations and their consequences have been referred to as 'enacted stigma' (Scambler & Hopkins, 1986). Even when there is no evidence of negative evaluations as a result of an illness, the sufferer may feel loss of self-esteem, 'damaged' or worry that others hold a negative evaluation of him or her. This has been referred to as 'felt stigma' (Scambler & Hopkins, 1986). Part of the problem of stigma may be due to the stigmatizing condition or its label dominating perception of the individual and obscuring the sufferer's positive attributes (see Link, Mirotznik & Cullen, 1991).

Several factors influence whether a medical condition attracts stigma. Stigma is associated with an 'abnormal' appearance (e.g. facial disfigurement, obesity, baldness), behaviours that appear bizarre (e.g. tics), frightening (e.g. epileptic fits), annoying or dangerous (e.g. delusional behaviour), and conditions that are considered to have been brought about in part as a result of actions that are considered immoral (e.g. AIDS) or reflect adversely on a patient's strength of character (e.g. hypochondriasis).

Stigma can result in low self-esteem, depressed mood, and anxiety. These may be sufficiently severe that they require treatment. Stigma can also lead to isolation and a restriction of activities. Clinicians' negative evaluations of patients with particular conditions may adversely affect treatment (e.g. Hall, 1992). Not surprisingly, stigmatized conditions that are perceived as being controllable are more likely to induce hostility in others, while those that are viewed as outside the sufferer's control tend to elicit pity (Weiner, Perry & Magnusson, 1988).

Obviously the most effective method of reducing stigma is to cure the medical condition. There appears to be little that can be done psychologically and indeed coping strategies such as defensive hostility and avoidance of contact with others can exacerbate the problem (see Link *et al.*, 1991). In cases of purely 'felt stigma' there may be scope to educate patients to realize that others do not view them the way that they think. Otherwise the most effective strategy may be to increase exposure of society at large to cases of stigmatiz-ing conditions so that they understand them better (Levy, 1993). Self-help groups and support groups may also help in some cases. Where mood disturbance is severe, psychological symptomatic treatment may be warranted.

REFERENCES

Goffman, E. (1963). *Stigma: notes on the management of spoiled identity.* New York: Simon and Schuster.

Hall, B. (1992). Overcoming stigmatization: social and personal implications of the human immunodeficiency virus diagnosis. *Archives of Psychiatric Nursing*, 6, 189–94.

Levy, A.J. (1993). Stigma management: a new clinical service. *Families in Society*, 74, 226–31.

Link, B.G., Mirotznik, J. & Cullen, F.T. (1991). The effectiveness of stigma coping orientations: can negative consequences of mental illness labelling be avoided? *Journal of Health and Social Behavior*, 32, 302–20.

Scambler, G. & Hopkins, A. (1986). Being epileptic: coming to terms with stigma. *Sociology, Health and Illness*, 8, 26–43.

Weiner, B., Perry, R.P. & Magnusson, J. (1988). An attributional analysis of reactions to stigma. *Journal of Personality and Social Psychology*, 55, 738–48.

Stroke

THEO JOHN PIMM

Rayners Hedge, Croft Road, Aylesbury, Buckinghamshire, UK

INTRODUCTION

Stroke is an abrupt focal neurological disorder lasting more than 24 hours caused by either haemorrhage or infarction of the cerebral vascular vessels. It is the third highest cause of death in the UK and US and also results in chronic disability requiring major expenditure of health and social care resources. The annual incidence of stroke is estimated to be 150–200 per 100 000. The incidence rises with age, but 25% are under the age of 65 years. The prevalence of stroke is estimated to be 550 per 100 000 (Weddell, 1980), representing a substantial proportion of those with disability living in the community. The mortality rate is approximately 35–40% in the first month, but survivors live on average for seven years and 30–50% will have some residual neurological deficit (Halligan & Cockburn, 1993).

PSYCHOLOGICAL EFFECTS OF STROKE

Awareness of the psychosocial consequences of stroke has increased because of the improved survival rates for people suffering devastating strokes. Studies of rehabilitation outcomes have shown that despite reasonable physical recovery many stroke survivors suffer emotional distress and social restrictions. These psychosocial consequences impede coping and adaptation to stroke.

Stroke can lead to marked changes in cognitive, emotional, and behavioural function. Neurological damage may directly affect neuropsychological processes including perception, thinking, feeling, and communication. The impairments and disabilities associated with stroke, e.g. paralysis, visual impairment, epilepsy, and impotence can have a devastating impact on the person's emotional state. They can also have widespread repercussions for their family, and social relationships, work and leisure.

Cognitive effects

Stroke can lead to cognitive deficits in: perception, memory, language, attention, speed of information processing and general intellectual skills. Cognitive deficits after stroke can severely disrupt rehabilitation and impair recovery but are frequently overlooked.

After the initial clouding of consciousness has cleared, cognitive deficits tend to be focal, and depend on the size and location of the lesion. Hemispheric specialization is an important determinant of the effects of stroke. Lesions in the left hemisphere lead to hemiparesis and visual field deficit on the right side of the body, and may produce difficulties in speech, the ability to understand written and spoken language, praxic, and calculation disorders.

Dysphasia is found in 10–16% of community samples and may vary from mild naming difficulties to severe expressive language problems. Expressive dysphasia may be fluent, characterized by non-words (jargon), or non-fluent, where the main feature is poverty of speech. Comprehension difficulties are particularly associated with fluent dysphasia. Most of the improvement in dysphasia occurs during the first ten weeks after stroke (Ebrahim, 1990).

Lesions of the right hemisphere lead to hemiparesis and visual field deficits on the left side of the body and may cause perceptual and spatial deficits, difficulties in emotional expression and anosognosia (denial of neurological impairment). Disorders of visual attention, e.g. left visual neglect, severely affect ability to function in everyday tasks, e.g. dressing, which may account for the poor prognosis of right hemisphere patients shown in some studies.

Many stroke patients report subjective memory problems including difficulty remembering names, appointments and messages. Wade, Parker and Hewer (1986) showed that, on memory tests at 3 months, 29% of stroke patients had verbal memory deficits and

14% visual memory deficits. There were some signs of improvement by 6 months. Other studies have suggested that memory impairment may be more common and enduring, and occurs in the absence of general intellectual impairment (Halligan & Cockburn, 1993).

General intellectual impairment is common in stroke patients and has a major impact on recovery and re-integration. It is characterized by impaired memory, orientation, and deficits in other cognitive domains, e.g. language and attention. Tatemichi *et al.* (1993) found dementia in 26% of older patients 3 months after ischaemic stroke. They suggest that it results from a number of independent factors including multiple small subcortical and large cortical infarcts.

Emotional and behavioural effects

Stroke is a frightening experience, raising fears of death, disability, and disfigurement, which leads to significant losses. A wide range of emotional and behavioural reactions have been reported including: depression, anxiety, pathological emotionalism, apathy, and anosagnosia.

Depression is the most commonly reported emotional reaction to stroke. It can be a major barrier to rehabilitation, impeding recovery in functional ability. Prevalence estimates vary considerably from 11–60%. This probably reflects differences between studies in the definition of depression, types of assessment measure used and time since stroke.

In a 3-year prospective longitudinal study Astrom, Adolfsson and Asplund (1993) found the prevalence of depression was 25% in the acute phase, 31% at 3 months, 16% at 1 year, 19% at 2 years, and 29% at three years. Although 60% of people with acute onset depression recovered by 1 year, those remaining were at high risk of chronic depression.

It seems likely that biological and psychosocial factors interact in the development and maintenance of depression. For example, Astrom *et al.* (1993) found depression was predicted in the acute phase by left anterior lesions, dysphasia, and living alone; at three months by dependence in activities of daily living; from 1–3 years by few social contacts outside the family; and at 3 years cerebral atrophy made a contribution. It has been suggested that depression in the acute phase is related primarily to biological factors, e.g. lesion location, in the recovery phase to the patient's increased awareness of the neurological, cognitive, and functional disability, and in the chronic phase to restrictions on their ability to integrate into established social roles.

Anxiety disorders, e.g. agoraphobia and generalized anxiety disorder are commonly reported, and hinder community re-integration. For example, generalized anxiety disorder was found in 11% of stroke patients when those with depression were excluded and 27% when they were not (Castillo *et al.*, 1993).

Pathological emotionalism, uncontrolled crying or laughing occurs frequently, e.g. 11% of stroke patients at one year (Anderson, Vestergaard & Riis, 1993). It is distressing and socially embarrassing. The symptoms come on suddenly and include facial grimaces and uncontrolled crying or laughing in response to stimuli with little or no emotional content. Catastrophic reactions, i.e. extreme emotional outbursts with physical and verbal aggression, are rare and usually occur in response to physical or cognitive challenge associated with aphasia.

Apathy, a lack of emotion or indifference is a common sequelae of stroke. Starkstein *et al.* (1993) found apathy in 23% of acute stroke patients. It was associated with major depression, cognitive impairment, older age, reduced ability in activities of daily living, and lesions of the posterior limb of the internal capsule. Apathy combined with anosagnosia may lead to frustration, unrealistic expectations, refusal of treatment, and demanding behaviour.

Behaviour problems include: distractibility, irritability, impulsiveness, somnolence, and anosagnosia. It is unclear whether these problems reflect underlying cognitive or emotional deficits. For example, anosagnosia has been described as a form of denial, a coping mechanism for protection of self-image, or a multimodal sensory perceptual deficit due to somatic and visual inattention. These behavioural problems interfere with rehabilitation. Identification and behavioural management strategies may lead to improved rehabilitation outcomes.

Social effects

The majority of stroke patients are discharged home. However, community re-integration may be limited with marked effects on work, leisure, and social relationships. Gresham *et al.* (1975) found that, of 119 stroke survivors, 80% were living at home, 67% were independent for activities of daily living, but only 29% were gainfully employed, and 62% reported reduced social activity. Contact with the family is often maintained, but interaction with friends is restricted. A supportive family can be beneficial, maintaining treatment gains and providing care at home. However, some families can be over-protective, restricting the person's independence. Factors associated with limited socialization include: female sex, higher educational level, being cared for at home by spouse, environmental barriers, cognitive impairment, depression, agoraphobia and fear of falling.

Sexual problems are reported by men and women and include loss of sexual interest, erectile, and orgasmic dysfunction, and feelings of unattractiveness. Psychosocial factors associated with sexual problems include: depression, anxiety, e.g. of having another stroke, altered body image, loss of self-esteem, role conflicts, and relationship with spouse.

After the neurological and functional recovery of the first few months some people may be able to return to their previous job or re-train for alternative employment. Younger patients with less residual disability, and those working in management rather than manual occupations are more likely to return to work. Psychosocial factors, especially aphasia, perceptual and spatial difficulties, low self confidence, and lack of family support, influence return to work. Many younger stroke survivors lack suitable occupation as opportunities for sheltered work are limited and younger people may find day centres unstimulating.

Family effects

After the shock of the stroke, and the anxious wait for signs of recovery, the family share in the long struggle to regain lost skills. The family is a vital source of support. However, adopting the role of carer or therapist in home-based treatment for the disabled person may place stress on family members. In particular, spouses may feel that this role is incompatible with that of a sexual partner.

Studies of the impact of stroke on family members have been reviewed by Tyerman, Hobbs and Measures (1994). The most commonly reported problems are in the carer's physical and emotional health, e.g. worry, fatigue, irritability, sleep problems, headaches. Emotional distress has been reported in between 12 and 39% of spouses depending on time since stroke and type of assessment used, but occurs even when the level of physical disability is minimal. Emotional and health problems are reported more frequently in spouses when dysphasia is present.

Spouses also report loss of freedom and social activity, e.g. always looking out for the partner, less vacations and social outings, lack of private time, and fewer visits by friends.

Problems in family relationships, especially marital discord, are frequently found, with reports of impatience, anger, guilt, poor communication, loneliness, and embarrassment, that may increase over time. These problems may be particularly severe for spouses of people with dysphasia. Family functioning, e.g. problem-solving and family roles, may also be affected.

Coughlan and Humphrey (1982) report that, of 87 couples with children living at home, 53% of spouses felt that the children had suffered adverse long-term effects, which were often attributed to their disrupted relationship with the parent with the stroke. However, others commented on a rapid maturing and growth in tolerance. The impact on children is therefore unclear.

PSYCHOLOGICAL ASSESSMENT

Cognitive impairments, e.g. visual neglect and comprehension problems, are frequently missed in hospital settings. Screening for cognitive impairment has been recommended, using tests such as the Mini Mental State Examination (Falstein, Falstein & McHugh 1975). However, cognitive screening instruments are of little use with aphasic patients, do not discriminate well between depression and dementia, and omit important areas of cognitive function. Assessment for cognitive impairment should also include a careful clinical history and observation over time. Neuropsychological assessment is very useful for the detection and description of cognitive deficits. It is critical when cognitive deficits interfere with rehabilitation, when people with cognitive impairments wish to return to work, and to discriminate between depression and dementia. Speech therapy assessment is essential to clarify the nature of language impairment. Recently cognitive tests with better ecological validity have been developed, e.g. the Behavioural Inattention Test (Halligan & Cockburn 1993), that may be more appropriate for cognitive assessment in rehabilitation settings.

Emotional problems are often missed, so screening, with self-report questionnaires, e.g. Beck Depression Inventory and Hospital Anxiety and Depression Scale, has been recommended. Self report questionnaires may be difficult for people with aphasia to complete, omit common emotional problems, e.g. lability, and may be difficult to interpret as items may be confounded by physical problems, e.g. fatigue. A more detailed psychological assessment is essential for those identified as experiencing significant emotional distress or those who are unable to complete self report questionnaires. It is also important to assess family function, and the availability of social support and community resources.

PSYCHOSOCIAL INTERVENTION

Stroke rehabilitation aims to produce optimum recovery of function and ensure a good quality of life. Psychosocial factors have a major influence on stroke outcome. Cognitive impairment, depression, and family functioning affect rehabilitation and community re-integration. There is also evidence that a person's beliefs about their stroke, e.g. perceived control over recovery (Partridge & Johnston, 1989), and the coping strategies they use to manage the stroke, e.g. problem-solving, finding meaning in the experience, may influence adaptation to stroke. In addition, the psychosocial impact has a major effect on the person's quality of life. Inadequate intervention may lead to the failure to achieve or maintain recovery of physical and cognitive function, depression, and poor community integration, leading to longer hospital stay, more hospital re-admissions, and increased institutionalization. Therefore, intervention to prevent and ameliorate psychosocial consequences of stroke should be a major priority. Intervention may be helpful before the stroke, during acute care, rehabilitation, and long-term management.

Primary prevention

Psychological principals and methods may be helpful in the primary prevention of stroke. Ebrahim (1990) suggests that risk factors for stroke with high attributable risk should be primary targets for intervention. In stroke, these include raised blood pressure, smoking, and low physical activity. Health promotion programmes incorporating cognitive–behavioural strategies, e.g. goal setting and relaxation are likely to be effective in helping people in high-risk groups, e.g. hypertension, transient ischaemic attacks, to make behaviour changes.

Acute care

As people regain consciousness, they may experience a period of disorientation and confusion. Staff need advice in the management of behaviour and the promotion of cognitive recovery. People may need repeated explanation of what has happened to them. A major need at this stage is the support and counselling of family members. They also need repeated and sensitive discussions about the stroke, the likely course, and when the immediate danger to the person's life is over, the extent of recovery. It is important to avoid giving unrealistic short-term reassurance about recovery. This may cause problems later in rehabilitation, when relatives may cling to early assurances of a full recovery. It is best to be honest about the seriousness of current problems and the prospects for recovery. This can allow for optimism about marked improvements but doubt about the extent of recovery.

Rehabilitation

Rehabilitation that addresses cognitive, emotional, family and social needs will improve motivation, foster adherence to treatment, and enhance long-term management of residual disabilities and handicaps by the person and family. Some aspects of good psychological care apply to most patients, e.g. providing feedback on progress. However, psychological care may need to be tailored to meet individual needs, e.g. providing reassurance for an anxious person or minimizing distraction for a person with cognitive impairment.

Cognitive rehabilitation is a developing field which seems likely to make a significant contribution to stroke rehabilitation. Clinical psychologists can provide advice to patients and families on the management of cognitive problems. They can develop and implement individual and group cognitive rehabilitation programmes to ameliorate impairments, e.g. perceptual re-training for left visual neglect, and introduce compensatory strategies, e.g. external memory aids (diaries, calendars and note-pads) (Riddoch & Humphreys, 1994). Speech therapists can provide: advice to patients, carers, and staff, communication aids, and groups for dysphasia sufferers and their relatives (Ebrahim, 1990).

With respect to emotional problems, given the multiple causal factors, several intervention methods should be considered, e.g. anti-depressant medication, cognitive – behaviour therapy, counselling, education and support groups. Anti-depressant treatment is effective in reducing depression and improves rehabilitation outcomes. Brief psychological interventions, e.g. cognitive – behaviour therapy, are very effective for emotional problems but there are few studies conducted specifically with stroke. For emotional lability, the patient and carer should be reassured that this is a consequence of stroke and that symptoms tend to diminish over time. When progress in rehabilitation is affected, or the person is socially handicapped by the symptoms, anti-depressant treatment especially with specific serotonin re-uptake inhibitors (SSRI) may be effective in reducing the frequency of crying episodes (Anderson *et al.*, 1993). Emotional, instrumental and informational support enhance recovery (Glass & Maddocks, 1992). Education and counselling interventions can improve family functioning after stroke and should be included in comprehensive rehabilitation programmes.

Long-term management

Case conferences, discharge planning, home assessment, and referral to community services facilitate re-integration. Many of the psychosocial consequences of stroke may not be obvious until the person has returned home, and therefore follow-up by hospital teams, GPs, and community rehabilitation services is important to assess and meet these needs. Community rehabilitation services can help with encouraging adherence to treatment recommendations, long-term adjustment, leisure and work rehabilitation. Such community-based education and counselling programmes can help stroke survivors to find meaning in the experience, develop a sense of purpose, and invest energy in new life goals. Day centres, stroke clubs, and support groups for family/carers provide opportunities for education, social support, and respite.

CONCLUSION

In recent years there have been considerable advances in knowledge about the psychological effects of stroke. The detection and exploration of these problems has been facilitated by the development of instruments to assess cognitive and emotional difficulties. Progress in cognitive rehabilitation and cognitive – behaviour therapy have the potential to make major contributions to stroke rehabilitation. Further work is needed to evaluate the benefits of intervention.

REFERENCES

Andersen, G., Vestergaard, K. & Riis, J. (1993). Citalopram for post-stroke pathological crying. *The Lancet*, **342**, 37–9.

Astrom, M., Adolfsson, R. & Asplund, K. (1993). Major depression in stroke patients a three year longitudinal study. *Stroke*, **24**, 976–82.

Castillo, C.S., Starkstein, S.E., Fedoroff, J.P., Price, P.R. & Robinson, R.G. (1993). Generalized anxiety disorder after stroke. *Journal of Nervous and Mental Disease*, **181**, 100–5.

Coughlan, A.K. & Humphrey, M.E. (1982). Presenile stroke: long-term outcome for patients and their families. *Rheum. Rehabilitation*, **21**, 115–22.

Ebrahim, S. (1990). *Clinical epidemiology of stroke*. New York: Oxford University Press.

Falstein, M.F., Falstein, S.E. & McHugh, P.R. (1975). Mini-mental state a practical method for grading the cognitive state of patients for the clinician. *Journal of Psychiatric Research*, **12**, 189–98.

Glass, T.A. & Maddocks, G.L. (1992). The quality and quantity of social support: stroke recovery as psychosocial transition. *Social Science and Medicine*, **34**, 1249–61.

Gresham, G.E., Fitzpatrick, T.E., Wolf, P.A. *et al.* (1975). Residual disability in survivors of stroke: the Framingham Study. *New England Journal of Medicine*, **293**, 954.

Halligan, P.W. & Cockburn, J. (1993). Cognitive sequelae of stroke: visuo-spatial and memory disorders. *Critical Reviews in Physical and Rehabilitation Medicine*, **5**, 57–81.

Partridge, C. & Johnston, M. (1989). Perceived control of recovery from physical disability: measurement and prediction. *British Journal of Clinical Psychology*, **28**, 53–9.

Riddoch, J. & Humphreys, G. (1994). *Cognitive neuropsychology and cognitive rehabilitation*, Hove:LEA.

Starkstein, S.E., Fedoroff, J.P., Price, T.R.,

Leiguarda, R. & Robinson, R.G. (1993). Apathy following cerebral vascular lesion. *Stroke*, **24**, 1625–30.

Tatemichi, T.K., Desmond, D.W., Paik, M., Figueroa, M., Gropen, T.I., Stern, Y., Sano, M., Remien, R., Williams, J.V. & Mohr, J.P. (1993). Clinical determinants of dementia related to stroke. *Annals Neurology*, **33**, 568–75.

Tyerman, A.D., Hobbs, L. & Measures, A.C. (1994). Quality of life in family members of persons with chronic neurological disability. In M.R. Trimble & W.E. Dodson (Eds) *Epilepsy and quality of life*, pp. 33–48. New York: Raven Press.

Wade, D.T., Parker, V. & Hewer, R.L. (1986). Memory disturbance after stroke: frequency and associated losses. *International Disability Studies*, **8**, 60–4.

Weddell, J.M. (1980). Applications of a stroke register in planning. In F. Clifford-Rose (Ed.). *Clinical neuroepidemiology*, Tunbridge Wells, UK:Opitman Medical.

Stuttering

PEGGY DALTON

20 Cleveland Avenue, London W4, UK

Stuttering (often termed 'stammering' in the UK) is a disorder of speech rhythm or fluency. Speakers are prevented from saying what they wish to say by involuntary repetition, prolongation or cessation of speech sound or syllable. In its more severe forms, breathing irregularities, facial contortions and bodily movements may accompany the act of speaking. Stuttering normally begins in childhood, in some cases from the time the child begins to speak, in others after a period of normal fluency. A later onset of dysfluency after some years of normal speech may also occur in relation to a disturbing event or set of circumstances.

DIAGNOSING STUTTERING

In order for a diagnosis of stuttering to be made in the speech of young children, the dysfluency patterns described above need to be distinguished from normal non-fluencies, such as the repetition of whole words and phrases and the use of interjections, where there is no sign of struggle or abnormal tension. Due to cases of late onset and early remission, the prevalence of stuttering is not easy to assess, but it is said that just under 5% of all children will experience a period of stuttering lasting for three months or more, three times as many more of them being boys than girls (Andrews, 1987, p. xvii). Four out of five such children will have recovered by the age of 16.

A considerable body of research exists showing inheritance to be a major determinant in many cases, although the severity and type of dysfluency does not appear to be governed genetically. It can be caused by brain disturbances in children and adults, and there is increased prevalence associated with a number of neurological conditions. Contrary to popular belief, tests of neurological functioning have shown there to be no differences between those who stutter and those who do not in terms of laterality as measured by handedness, dichotic word tests or the intracarotid sodium amytal test. People who stutter do, however, perform less well on tests of central auditory function, auditory and visual voice reaction times and in auditory – motor tracking tasks. The search for constitutional differences, in particular in hemispheric functioning, continues. But it is unlikely that any one factor will be found to be common to all cases of stuttering.

THE DEVELOPMENT OF STUTTERING

The development of stuttering is related not only to the constitutional risk factors referred to but also precipitating and perpetuating factors to be found within the environment and within the speakers themselves. A young child still developing speech and language skills, who is either constantly interrupted by highly articulate older siblings or continually questioned and asked to express themselves

verbally, will be under considerable pressure. Beginning school brings with it added demands for general adaptation and a specific increase in focus on communication.

Although the origins of stuttering can rarely be shown to be emotional, there is no doubt that, where dysfluency continues, psychological factors play their part in perpetuating the disorder and can have damaging effects on the person's sense of self. Teasing or impatience from others and the experience of anxiety in an increasing range of communication situations can lead to loss of confidence and feelings of general inadequacy. At worst, speaking situations will be avoided, relationships with others no longer sought and the person's life may become severely restricted.

THE TREATMENT OF STUTTERING

Currently, the main division amongst clinicians is between those who focus largely on the speech itself, seeking to modify stuttering through the use of fluency techniques (e.g. Ingham, 1984) and those who see the psychological aspects of the experience of dysfluency, especially in older children and adults, as the primary concern of therapy (e.g. Dalton, 1994). Many speech and language therapists will attempt to teach speech modification procedures and, at the same time, seek change in the attitudes of parents of young children and of older dysfluent people towards themselves and towards communication (see Rustin *et al.*, 1987 in Andrews (1987)).

Most are agreed on the need for prevention both of an increase in dysfluent behaviour in young children and the development of frustration and anxiety in their experience of communication. Work with the parents is aimed at reducing disruption, allowing these vulnerable children the time and space to express themselves and providing them with models of more relaxed speech patterns.

With older children and adults, while speech modification procedures such as prolonged speech (Ryan, 1986) have proved useful in reducing dysfluency, such improvement is seldom maintained without considerable work on the person's anxieties with regard to particular speech situations and, above all, on their perceptions of themselves as a whole. Lack of confidence in themselves as communicators will often bring with it a deep sense of failure and poor self-esteem.

PSYCHOLOGICAL APPROACHES

Counselling as an aspect of the treatment of stuttering is widely practiced. Approaches such as cognitive–behaviour therapy (Butcher, Elias & Raven, 1993) and Adlerian therapy (Clifford & Watson, 1987) have also been developed in this area. The most widely used psychotherapeutic approach to stuttering in the UK is, however, Kelly's personal construct psychology (1955), introduced by Fransella (1972). Here, the aim is, first, to explore with the client the personal meaning of stuttering, in order to discover how it governs expectations of him or herself and others. On this basis, change or reconstruction may be brought about through challenging such

anticipations which are often limited to issues of speech and fluency alone. At the same time, by elaborating perceptions of the self on other dimensions, the client is enabled to approach life as 'a person' rather than simply 'a stutterer'. (See also 'Voice disorders'.)

REFERENCES

Andrews, G. (1987). 'A tutorial on stuttering'. In L. Rustin, H. Purser & D. Rowley (Eds.). *Progress in the treatment of fluency disorders.* London, New York and Philidelphia: Taylor Francis.

Butcher, P., Elias, A. & Raven, R. (1993.) *Psychogenic voice disorders and cognitive – behaviour therapy.* London: Whurr.

Clifford, J. & Watson, P. (1987). Family counselling with children who stutter: an Adlerian approach. In C. Levy (Ed.). *Stuttering therapies: practical approaches.* London, New York, Sydney: Croom Helm.

Dalton, P. (1994). *Counselling people with communication problems.* London, Thousand Oaks, New Delhi: Sage.

Fransella, F. (1972). *Personal change and reconstruction.* London, New York: Academic Press.

Ingham, R.J. (1984). *Stuttering and behaviour therapy: current status and experimental foundations.* San Diego: College-Hill Press.

Kelly, G.A. (1955). *The psychology of personal constructs.* New York: Norton.

Ryan, B.P. (1986). Postscript: operant therapy for children. in G.H. Shames & H. Rubin (Eds.). *Stuttering then and now.* Colombus, OH: Merrill.

Suicide

DAVID LESTER

Center for the Study of Suicide, Blackwood, New Jersey, USA

Suicide refers to a range of self-destructive behaviours ranging from non-lethal acts which have been called suicidal gestures, attempted suicide, parasuicide, and more recently self-injury or, if poisoning in used, self-poisoning, to lethal acts in which the person dies, commonly called completed suicide.

THE EPIDEMIOLOGY OF SUICIDE

Rates of completed suicide range from 3.8 per 100 000 people per year in Greece (in 1989), according to latest WHO figures, to 39.9 in Hungary (in 1990). The rate in the USA was 12.4 (in 1988) and in the UK 8.1 (in 1990). It is estimated that perhaps there are ten suicidal attempts for every completed suicide, indicating that rates of attempted suicide may range from 40 to 400 per 100 000 per year.

Official rates of completed suicide have been criticized for their inaccuracy, especially because of the reluctance of some coroners, medical examiners, and police officers to certify deaths as suicide. However, although official rates of completed suicide may be lower than the actual incidence, studies have shown that completed suicide rates among immigrant groups to a nation are in roughly the same rank order as the rates in their home nations, indicating some degree of validity.

In most nations, completed suicide is more common in men whereas attempted suicide is more common in women. In developed nations, completed suicide rates rise with age, sometimes peaking in middle age (especially for women) and sometimes in old age. In less developed nations and among aboriginals, completed suicide rates are often higher in young adults. Islamic nations appear to have low rates of completed suicide.

THE PHYSIOLOGY OF SUICIDE

There is no evidence that the tendency to suicide *per se* is inherited. However, since suicide is more common in those who have a psychiatric disorder, and since there is evidence that psychiatric disorder has a genetic component, suicide may appear to have a genetic component.

Studies of the biochemistry have failed to reveal unique characteristics of suicidal individuals. Since the majority of suicides are depressed, and many have a depressive disorder, biochemical studies of the blood, cerebral spinal fluid and brain typically find features characteristic of depressed individuals, such as abnormalities in the serotonergic neural pathways.

PSYCHIATRIC DISORDER

Suicide is found to be more common among patients diagnosed with depressive disorders, schizophrenia, and substance abuse. Recently there has been interest in the high rate of lethal and non-lethal suicidal behaviour in those diagnosed with a borderline personality disorder.

However, retrospective diagnoses (using psychological autopsies) reveal that some suicides show no signs of psychiatric disorder. Increasingly, suicide in those with terminal illness and with other extreme trauma is being viewed as rational.

The single most powerful predictor of past, present and future suicidality is depression as measured by a standardized scale. Many of these scales cover a variety of symptoms, and Aaron Beck (Freeman & Reinecke, 1993) has found that hopelessness, a cognitive component of depression, is the most useful symptom for predicting suicidality.

Other personality traits associated with suicidal behaviour include low self-esteem, anger (and aggression), deficient problem-solving skills, and rigid and dichotomous thinking.

LIFE EXPERIENCES OF SUICIDAL INDIVIDUALS

A number of early experiences are associated with subsequent suicidal behaviour, including loss of parents (through death or divorce), physical and sexual abuse, suicidal behaviour in relatives and friends, and dysfunctional families. Suicidal individuals have experienced high levels of stressors in the year prior to their suicidal behaviour, and they differ from depressed non-suicidal people in experiencing a further increase in stressors in the weeks prior to the suicidal act. Media publicity of suicides by celebrities seems to provoke suicides in the following week.

Younger suicidal individuals appear to be more motivated in their suicidal behaviour by interpersonal problems, while older suicidal individuals are more motivated by intrapsychic problems.

Medical illness is often a precipitant of suicide, especially in older individuals. Illnesses especially associated with suicide include AIDS, epilepsy, Huntington's disease, renal disease (especially among those on dialysis), spinal cord injuries, transplants and possibly cancer.

PREVENTING SUICIDE

The detection and appropriate treatment of depressed individuals is useful for the successful prevention of suicide. In Sweden, the physicians in one region were given educational programmes for this purpose, and the suicide rate dropped in that region compared to the rest of Sweden.

However, the medications used to treat depressed patients can also be used for suicide. In recent years, several authorities have calculated rates of death (per 1000 prescriptions) for various antidepressants, and some (especially the newer ones) do appear to be safer than others, though the reasons for this are obscure. Careful monitoring of the medications given depressed patients is important.

Suicide prevention centres exist in many nations, and some nations have comprehensive coverage so that almost everyone can call a suicide prevention or crisis intervention service. It has been difficult to show that these services do prevent suicide, yet no one denies that the services give excellent crisis counselling and serve as effective referral agencies for the communities they serve.

In recent years, a third technique for suicide prevention has been suggested, namely restricting access to lethal methods of suicide. Some of this has occurred incidentally, such as the switch from very toxic coal gas to less toxic natural gas for domestic use and the removal of carbon monoxide from car exhaust as a means of pollution control. However, measures focused on suicide prevention can be proposed, such as fencing in the places from which people jump to their death (such as bridges), mixing emetics in medications or prescribing medications in suppository form, and passing stricter gun control laws. Available evidence suggests that the majority of people denied access to their preferred method for suicide will not switch to alternative methods. The detoxification of domestic gas in England and Wales resulted in a lower total suicide rate.

Finally, the trauma experienced by those surviving the suicide of a loved one has spurred the growth of groups to help survivors cope with their loss. Since having a loved one complete suicide is a factor which increases the risk of subsequent suicide, these groups may be useful for preventing suicide.

FURTHER READING

Bongar, B. (1991). *The suicidal patient: clinical and legal standards of care.* Washington, DC: American Psychological Association.

Freeman, A. & Reinecke, M.A. (1993) *Cognitive therapy of suicidal behavior.* New York: Springer.

Fremouw, W.J., de Perczel, M. & Ellis, T.E.

(1990). *Suicide risk: assessment and response guidelines.* Oxford: Pergamon.

Jacobs, D. (Ed.). (1992). *Suicide and clinical practice.* Washington, DC: American Psychiatric Press.

Lester, D. (1989). *Questions and answers about suicide.* Philadelphia, PA: Charles Press.

Lester, D. (1992). *Why people kill themselves: a 1990s summary of research findings on suicidal behavior.* 3rd edn. Springfield, IL: Charles Thomas.

Lukas, C. & Seiden, H.M. (1987). *Silent grief.* New York: Scribners.

Tetanus

NATALIE TIMBERLAKE

Academic Department of Psychiatry, Middlesex and University College London, UK

Tetanus is an acute infectious disease now relatively rare in the developed world. It is caused by the introduction to the body, via a penetrating injury, of the tetanus bacillus. The individual then develops painful muscular contractions initially affecting the facial and neck muscles and later the muscles in the trunk. Involvement of

the respiratory muscles leads to compromised breathing. In untreated cases, mortality is high (approximately 60%).

The vaccination against tetanus is part of a combined injection which vaccinates for diphtheria, tetanus and pertussis (DTP), although it can be given singularly. The generally accepted schedule is a course of three or four vaccinations for DTP when children are under two years old, with further boosters as they grow up. Uptake rate of tetanus immunization alone or combined with diphtheria is generally reported in the UK to be between 83% and 98% (Appleton, 1989; Klein, Morgan & Wansbrough Jones, 1989; Pearson et al., 1993a; Hewitt, 1989). This is one of the highest rates for vaccines and probably reflects the acceptability of the vaccination amongst parents and health-care professionals, due to its few contraindications. In a study by Klein et al. (1989) of 173 children, only one had true contraindications to diphtheria, tetanus and polio and only 3% had not been vaccinated due to parents' belief in false contraindications. This is compared to pertussis vaccination where 6% had true contraindications and 14% false contraindications. Similarly Hewitt (1989) found that, out of 522 children, not one had a recognized contraindication to tetanus, and parents refused vaccination for tetanus, diphtheria and polio in only 2.6% of cases, none of which was due to false contraindications. Therefore, it would seem that, in contrast to pertussis, parents are generally very accepting of the tetanus vaccine and do not see vaccinating as a risky action.

Although uptake rates are generally reported as high, this may not be so in certain pockets of the population. A study by Barrett and Ramsay (1993) in a deprived inner city area of London (UK) reported that the uptake of the third dose of diphtheria–tetanus vaccine was 71%. They found that living in temporary housing was associated with reduced uptake. This led them to suggest that it is increased mobility in these deprived areas which is important in lowering uptake. Similarly, Pearson et al. (1993a,b) report that the factor which best predicts non-vaccination for diphtheria, tetanus and polio is postnatal migration. Pearson et al. (1993a) also comment on the importance of differentiating between initial consent and the completion of the full course of vaccination. They found that the rate of consent to initial tetanus vaccination was 98% but that only 87% were fully vaccinated by their second birthday. It would seem that, for some children, although they start the vaccination programmes they often fail to complete the course. They suggest that one factor that may be important in lowering the rate of completion is the mobility of their parents. Similarly, Feder, Vaclavik and Streetley (1993) report that children of travellers are significantly more likely to start, but not complete, immunization. This reduction in completion rates may reflect problems in continuity of care when changing health districts. Barrett and Ramsay (1993) suggest that children from mobile families should be immunized promptly and that 'mechanisms should exist to ensure that children who move district are notified to the next child health service'. The accelerated vaccination schedule now in use was started in 1990 in the hope of reducing the drop-out rate between the first and the third dose. It was thought that, by providing uniformity across different health districts, the completion rate would be increased in highly mobile families (Davies & Davies, 1993). (See also 'Immunization' chapter.)

REFERENCES

Appleton, R. (1989). Parents' beliefs about vaccination. *British Medical Journal*, **299**, 257.

Barrett, G. & Ramsay, M. (1993). Improving uptake of immunisation: mobile children miss out. *British Medical Journal*, **307**, 681–2.

Davies, B. & Davies, T. (1993). *Community health, preventive medicine and social services*. Baillière-Tindall.

Feder, G., Vaclavik, T. & Streetly, A. (1993). Traveller gypsies and childhood immunisation: a study in East London. *British Journal of General Practice*, **43**, 281–4.

Hewitt, M. (1989). Incidence of contraindications to Immunisation. *Archives of Diseases of Childhood*, **64**, 1052–64.

Klein, N., Morgan, K. & Wansbrough-Jones, M. (1989). Parents' beliefs about vaccination: the continuing propagation of false contraindications. *British Medical Journal*, **298**, 1687.

Pearson, M., Makowiecka, K., Gregg, J., Woollard, J., Rogers, M. & West, C. (1993a). Primary immunisations in Liverpool. 1: who withholds consent? *Archives of Diseases Childhood*, **69**, 110–14.

Pearson, M., Makowiecka, K., Gregg, J., Woollard, J., Rogers, M. & West, C. (1993b). Primary immunisations in Liverpool. 2: is There a gap between consent and completion? *Archives of Disease in Childhood*, **69**, 115–19.

Tinnitus

LUCY YARDLEY

Department of Psychology, University College, London, UK

Sounds which apparently emanate from the ear(s) or head of the perceiver are referred to as 'tinnitus'. Spontaneous tinnitus is a very common phenomenon, between 15 and 20% of the population report having experienced tinnitus which lasted more than five minutes and did not occur immediately after exposure to loud noise. The nature of the tinnitus can vary widely, and may be uni- or bilateral, intermittent, pulsatile or continuous. Depending on the tonal quality, pitch and loudness of the tinnitus, it may be described as a whistling, hissing, buzzing or roaring sound. It is often possible to gain an impression of the tinnitus by asking the individual concerned to 'match' their tinnitus to an external sound with similar pitch and loudness characteristics, which many people are able to do with a reasonable degree of consistency.

The principal practical difficulties reported by people with troublesome tinnitus are disturbed sleep, inability to concentrate or relax, headache, and difficulty understanding speech or listening to music. Psychosocial consequences include fatigue, irritation and depression, which can result in disruption to family and other social relationships (Tyler & Baker, 1983). The hearing-related problems are often actually attributable to hearing loss, which commonly accompanies tinnitus but is frequently unrecognized; about three out of every four individuals with tinnitus have hearing impairment, and a similar proportion of those with hearing loss have tinnitus.

Only around a quarter of people with tinnitus describe it as severe or distressing. The reported severity and annoyance of tinnitus is not closely or reliably related to hearing loss, age, general health, sleep disturbance, the loudness of a sound matched to the tinnitus, or whether the tinnitus is continuous or intermittent (although infrequent tinnitus is seldom troubling). Hence, it seems probable that predisposing psychological factors contribute to complaints and distress associated with tinnitus, which have been shown to correlate with trait anxiety, depression and poor coping (Halford & Anderson, 1991; Kirsch, Blanchard & Parnes, 1989). Nevertheless, there is evidence that the uniquely intrusive and inescapable nature of tinnitus can lead to a degree of psychological disturbance even in people who do not complain of their tinnitus (e.g. Attias et al., 1992).

Since there is no safe and effective medical treatment for tinnitus, a psychoacoustic approach to management has been popular, based on the application of external sound to 'mask' the tinnitus. A small proportion of sufferers report temporary relief from tinnitus following a period of masking, and others state that it is helpful simply to have some control over, and alternative to, the interminable noise that they endure. However, controlled trials suggest that masking generally adds little benefit to that gained from enthusiastic counselling (Hazell et al., 1985).

Analysis of the neuropsychological aspects of tinnitus perception (Hallam, 1987; Jastreboff & Hazell, 1993) has provided the rationale for treatments which promote relaxation, distraction, and attitude change. Excessive awareness of tinnitus can be conceptualized as a failure of the normal habituation process, which should ensure that attention is diverted from a repetitive but insignificant sound. Tinnitus does not have the same auditory perceptual properties as an external sound, and it is possible that the inability to habituate to tinnitus is related to defective central auditory processing, which may mediate the generation or continued detection of some types of tinnitus. Although these central defects may not themselves be remediable, several factors which can be manipulated are known to affect habituation.

First, attention to a sound is influenced by competing demands for auditory attention. Logically, awareness of tinnitus should therefore be reduced if external noise is introduced as a distractor, even if it does not actually mask the tinnitus. Some therapists recommend listening to the radio, music, or white noise if the tinnitus is disturbing in quiet surroundings or when trying to sleep. Hearing aids can be utilized not only to restore the background environmental noise which normally masks and distracts from internally generated sound, but also to overcome the hearing difficulties commonly associated with tinnitus. Specific training in switching attention away from the tinnitus may prove helpful (Hallam, 1987).

A second factor which may affect tinnitus perception is the individual's level of arousal, since heightened arousal is known to retard habituation. Relaxation might consequently be expected to reduce the perceived loudness of the tinnitus, as well as alleviating the accompanying stress and fatigue. House (1991) notes that the use of biofeedback for relaxation training is particularly beneficial for individuals who are reluctant to acknowledge any psychological aspect to their problem.

The meaning attached to the tinnitus represents a third factor likely to influence both the amount of attention it attracts and the distress that it provokes. Signals perceived as significant or threatening elicit continuous monitoring, as well as heightened anxiety and arousal. People who complain of severe tinnitus tend to also report negative attitudes, such as a belief that the tinnitus is an unfair and intolerable affliction (Hiller & Goebel, 1992). If less pessimistic evaluations of the tinnitus can be encouraged by means of cognitive therapy, both psychological adjustment and psychoacoustic habituation to the tinnitus may be enhanced. Controlled clinical trials (Henry & Wilson, 1992; Jakes et al., 1992) have provided promising evidence that cognitive therapy can help to reduce the distress of people with tinnitus.

REFERENCES

Attias, J., Shemesh, Z., Sohmer, H., Zinger, J. & Bliech, A. (1992). Psychological profile of help and non-help seeking chronic tinnitus patients. In J.-M. Aran & R. Dauman (Eds.). *Tinnitus 91*. Kugler: Amsterdam.

Halford, J.B.S. & Anderson, S.D. (1991). Anxiety and depression in tinnitus sufferers. *Journal of Psychosomatic Research*, 35, 383–90.

Hallam, R.S. (1987). Psychological approaches to the evaluation and management of tinnitus distress. In Hazell, J. (Ed.). *Tinnitus*. Churchill Livingstone: Edinburgh.

Hazell, J.W.P., Wood, S.M., Cooper, H.R., Stephens, S.D.G., Corcoran, A.L.,

Coless, R.R.A., Baskill, J.L. & Sheldrake, J.B. (1985). A clinical study of tinnitus maskers. *British Journal of Audiology*, 19, 65–146.

Henry, J.L. & Wilson, P.H. (1992). Psychological management of tinnitus: an evaluation of cognitive interventions. In J.-M. Aran & R. Dauman (Eds.). *Tinnitus 91*. Kugler: Amsterdam.

Hiller, W. & Goebel, G. (1992). A psychometric study of complaints in chronic tinnitus. *Journal of Psychosomatic Research*, 36, 337–48.

House, P.R. (1991). Psychological issues of tinnitus. In A. Shulman (Ed.). *Tinnitus*. Lea & Febiger: Philadelphia.

Jakes, S.C., Hallam, R.S., McKenna, L. & Hinchcliffe, R. (1992). Group cognitive therapy for medical patients: an application to tinnitus. *Cognitive Therapy and Research*, 16, 67–82.

Jastreboff, P.J. & Hazell, J.W.P. (1993). A neurophysiological approach to tinnitus: clinical implications. *British Journal of Audiology*, 27, 2–17.

Kirsch, C.A., Blanchard, E.B. & Parnes, S.M. (1989). Psychological characteristics of individuals high and low in their ability to cope with tinnitus. *Psychosomatic Medicine*, 51, 209–17.

Tyler, R.S. & Baker, L.J. (1983). Difficulties experienced by tinnitus sufferers. *Journal of Speech and Hearing Disorders*, 48, 150–4.

Tinnitus

Tobacco smoking

NEIL E. GRUNBERG,*
KELLY J. BROWN
and
LAURA COUSINO KLEIN
*Department of Medical and Clinical Psychology,
Uniformed Services University of the Health
Sciences, Bethesda, Maryland, USA*

INTRODUCTION

Of all topics at the nexus of psychology and medicine, tobacco smoking probably is the most important. Cigarette smoking is the single most preventable cause of death and illness in the USA and in much of the world. In the USA alone, approximately 400 000 people a year die from smoking-related illnesses, killing more Americans than AIDS, alcohol, car accidents, murders, suicides, drugs, and fires combined (Lynch & Bonnie, 1994). It is estimated that roughly 3 million people die each year from tobacco use in the world. Current worldwide projections are that there will be 10 million deaths a year from smoking by 2020. Roughly half a billion people living in the world today will die from tobacco use (Peto & Lopez, 1990). These staggering numbers are particularly tragic because the causal relationships between this behaviour and serious physical illnesses are well established and well known, and because this self-destructive behaviour can be stopped and can be prevented.

To effectively treat and prevent cigarette smoking, it is critical to understand the underlying psychological and biological principles and mechanisms that contribute to the initiation, maintenance, and relapse to smoking behaviour. This chapter presents the major issues and information about tobacco smoking. The chapter begins with information about smoking prevalence in adults and children. Next, the health hazards of smoking are listed. Then, the discussion turns to the central question: why do people smoke and why is it so hard to quit? In this section, psychological, behavioural, social, and biological factors are presented. Finally, the important topics of smoking cessation techniques, prevention strategies, and effects of cessation are discussed.

PREVALENCE

Table 1 presents cigarette smoking prevalence among adults in the USA by sex and by race from 1955–1991. Forty years ago, there was a dramatic difference in smoking by men and women. Currently, 25% of American adults smoke cigarettes with roughly comparable prevalence among men and women, whites and blacks. In the USA, over 50 million Americans continue to smoke but, happily, the over-

all proportion and total number of Americans who currently smoke has decreased over the past 30 years (USDHHS, 1989). The overall prevalence data and trends about smoking behaviour, however, mask some of the most important variables relevant to smoking cessation and prevention. The dramatic decreases in smoking in the USA over the past few decades have occurred in the upper social economic status (SES) groups (see Table 2) and by men (see Table 1). Lower SES groups continue to smoke at alarmingly high prevalence rates. In addition, women are now roughly comparable to men in smoking prevalence. These changes in the demographics of typical smokers reflect changes in culture, societies, perceptions of the effects of smoking, and advertising (Grunberg, Winders & Wewers, 1991).

Table 3 presents smoking status of high school seniors (17–18 years of age) in the USA between 1976 and 1993. Despite the optimistic view suggested by overall prevalence rates, the distressing news is that smoking among minors is not decreasing and that roughly 3000 adolescents, in the USA alone, start to smoke each day (USDHHS, 1989). According to the latest US Surgeon General's Report (USDHHS, 1994), at least 3.1 million adolescents are current smokers and tobacco is often the first drug used by young people who use alcohol and illegal drugs. It is important to note, however, that self-reported smoking status among African–American youth is decreasing dramatically, whereas smoking among white youth is markedly higher and on the increase.

HEALTH HAZARDS

The overall premature mortality of cigarette smoking is estimated to be 2.0. This means that smokers have a 100% greater chance of dying prematurely than do non-smokers. Smoking is responsible for roughly one-third of all cases of cancer, one-third of all cases of coronary heart disease, and the majority of cases of pulmonary dysfunction or disease (USDHHS, 1988). The major causes of death from smoking are: cardiovascular diseases, cancers, and chronic obstructive pulmonary diseases (COPDs). In addition, smoking causes non-neoplastic bronchopulmonary diseases, foetal health problems, peptic ulcer disease, and allergic reactions and immunosuppression. Smoking-related cardiovascular diseases include: sudden cardiac death, cerebral vascular disease, aortic aneurysms, atherosclerosis, and hypertension. Smoking-related cancers include: lung, larynx, oral cavity, oesophagus, bladder, kidney, and pancreas. COPDs

* The opinions or assertions contained herein are the private ones of the authors and are not to be construed as official or reflecting the views of the Department of Defense or the Uniformed Services University of the Health Sciences.

Table 1. *Trends[a] in cigarette smoking prevalence (%) by sex and by race 1955–1991*

| Year | United States, ages 18+ | | | | |
| | Overall population | Sex | | Race | |
		Males	Females	Whites	Blacks
1955	41.7	56.9	28.4	—	—
1965	42.4	51.9	33.9	42.1	45.8
1966	42.6	52.5	33.9	42.4	45.9
1970	37.4	44.1	31.5	37.0	41.4
1974	37.1	43.1	32.1	36.4	44.0
1976[b]	36.4	41.9	32.0	36.0	41.5
1977[b]	36.0	40.9	32.1	35.5	42.2
1978	34.1	38.1	30.7	33.9	37.7
1979	33.5	37.5	29.9	33.3	36.9
1980	33.2	37.6	29.3	32.9	36.9
1983	32.1	35.1	29.5	31.8	35.9
1985	30.1	32.6	27.9	29.6	34.9
1987	28.8	31.2	26.5	28.5	32.9
1988	28.1	30.8	25.7	27.8	31.7
1990	25.5	28.4	22.8	25.6	26.2
1991	25.7	28.1	23.5	25.5	29.1

[a] All numbers represent the percentages of the total US population.
[b] Ages 20+.
Source: Current Population Survey, 1955, National Health Interview Surveys, 1965–1991; data compiled by the Office on Smoking and Health, National Center for Chronic Disease Prevention and Health Promotion, Centers for Disease Control and Prevention.

Table 2. *Percentage of adults who were current cigarette smokers[a] by sex and by education and poverty status United States, National Health Interview Survey, 1991[b]*

	% Men	% Women	Total
Education (years)			
<12	37.4	27.4	32.0
12	33.5	27.1	30.0
13–15	25.1	22.0	23.4
≥16	14.5	12.5	13.6
Poverty Status[c]			
At/above poverty level	26.8	22.8	24.7
Below poverty level	39.3	29.3	33.1
Unknown	31.0	22.4	26.0

[a] Persons aged ≥18 years who reported having smoked at least 100 cigarettes and who were currently smoking.
[b] Sample size = 43,154; excludes 578 respondents with unknown smoking status.
[c] Poverty statistics are based on definitions developed by the Social Security. Administration that includes a set of income thresholds that vary by family size and composition.

include emphysema and asthma. It is important to note that smoking also interacts with other ingested drugs to potentiate health hazards. Perhaps the most striking and serious example is that smoking and oral contraceptive use increase the risk of heart attack by tenfold. It is a tragic fact that a remarkably small percentage of women are aware of this interaction. In addition, smoking and alcohol interact to exacerbate smoking-related health hazards, such as cancer of the oral cavity, oesophagus, and larynx (USDHHS, 1979, 1982).

Passive smoking, environmental tobacco smoke (ETS), or involuntary smoking also is a serious problem, particularly for children. ETS is estimated to cause 3000 lung cancer deaths annually in the USA. For Greece (2.00), Hong Kong (1.61), and Japan (1.44), the estimated relative cancer risks are even higher than in the USA (1.19). It is most noteworthy that ETS is a major cause of respiratory problems in children, including pneumonia and bronchitis, and is estimated to cause 150 000 to 300 000 cases a year in infants and children up to the age of 18 months in the USA. In addition, more than 700 US infants die each year from Sudden Infant Death Syndrome attributable to maternal smoking. Furthermore, ETS in the USA is causally associated with increased severity of asthmatic symptoms in 200 000 to 1 000 000 children a year and is a risk factor for new cases of asthma in children with no previous conditions (NIH, 1993).

Prenatal exposure to smoking results in increased risk of spontaneous abortion, foetal death, and neonatal death. The pattern of foetal growth retardation that occurs with maternal smoking includes a decrease in body length, chest circumference, and head circumference. Studies of long-term growth and development suggest that smoking during pregnancy also affects offspring's physical growth, mental development, and behavioural characteristics at least up to the age of 11. In addition, maternal smoking during pregnancy increases the probability that female adolescents will smoke and will persist in their smoking habit (Kandel, Wu & Davies, 1994). Recent animal research indicates that exposure of pregnant rats to nicotine results in offspring with changes in activity and sensory gating (Popke *et al.*, 1995; Richardson & Tizabi, 1994) and therefore, suggests that smoking may result in hyperactivity and attention deficit disorders in children of smoking, pregnant mothers.

Tobacco smoking

Table 3. *Smoking status^a of high school seniors in the USA: Monitoring the future project 1976–1993*

Year^b	Total	Sex		Race	
		Males	Females	Whites	Blacks
1976	28.8	28.0	28.8	28.8	26.8
1977	28.9	27.2	30.1	29.0	23.7
1978	27.5	25.9	28.3	27.8	22.2
1979	25.4	22.3	27.9	25.8	19.3
1980	21.4	18.5	23.5	21.8	15.7
1981	20.3	18.1	21.7	20.9	13.6
1982	21.0	18.2	23.2	22.4	12.4
1983	21.1	19.2	22.1	21.9	12.6
1984	18.7	16.0	20.5	20.1	9.0
1985	19.5	17.8	20.6	20.7	10.8
1986	18.7	16.9	19.8	20.4	7.8
1987	18.7	16.4	20.6	20.6	8.1
1988	18.1	17.4	18.1	20.5	6.7
1989	18.9	17.9	19.4	21.7	6.0
1990	19.1	18.7	19.3	21.8	5.4
1991	18.4	18.8	17.9	21.1	4.9
1992	17.2	17.2	16.7	19.9	3.7
1993	19.0	19.4	18.2	22.9	4.4

^a Percentage who smoked 1 or more cigarettes per day during the previous 30 days.

^b 95% confidence intervals, for any year, do not exceed: ± 1.3% for the total population, ± 1.6% for males, ± 1.6% for females, ± 1.4% for whites, ± 3.5% for blacks.

Source: Institute for Social Research, University of Michigan, Monitoring the Future Project.

WHY PEOPLE SMOKE

Tobacco smoking is a result of psychological, behavioural, social, and pharmacological variables. These variables are best conceptualized within the major stages of smoking initiation, maintenance, cessation, and relapse.

Initiation

Reasons for initiation include social pressures and psychological variables. Role modelling and peer smoking behaviour are powerful influences on smoking initiation by youth. Rock stars and athletes, for example, pictured in magazines with a cigarette in hand have strong effects on adolescent attitudes and behaviours about smoking. Moreover, smoking behaviour is often associated with attractiveness, sociability, and sexual activity. In addition, rebelliousness, immediate reward with delayed consequences, attitudes toward mortality, perceptions of health risks, perceptions of benefits (e.g. weight control, stress management, increased attention), and perceptions of ability to stop smoking as easily as starting smoking all contribute to smoking initiation.

Sadly, tobacco advertising can have a profound effect on the attitudes and beliefs of children and adults with regard to smoking behaviour, the risks of smoking, the benefits of smoking, and the effects of smoking on other aspects of life (Aitken *et al.*, 1991; Pierce, Lee & Gilpin, 1994). Cigarettes are one of the most heavily advertised products in the print media (USDHHS, 1994) with expenditures in this advertising medium alone approaching one-half billion dollars per year in the USA. Moreover, minors are the target of much of tobacco advertising. In the USA, for example, Joe Camel has been rated as second only to Mickey Mouse in face recognition among American children. Consequently, 37% of adolescent smokers begin with Camels or

Camel Lights, quite a tribute to the effectiveness of Madison Avenue. For adults, images of beauty, athletic prowess, sexual encounters, and material wealth, permeate print advertisements and billboards. Coupons, athletic event promotions, duffel bags, baseball caps, jean jackets, and so on, surround us with images of cigarettes, fun, sex, and adult status.

In addition to these psychological and social variables, psychobiological effects contribute to the likelihood of smoking initiation after initial experimentation. Specifically, the relative unpleasantness of early experimentation with smoking is related to the likelihood of subsequent use. Although this point may seem obvious, it is relevant to recognize that well-intentioned public health campaigns, including reduced tar and nicotine yields of cigarettes, actually can result in increased likelihood of transition from smoking experimentation to use if the initial experience is with a low nicotine cigarette that causes minimal nausea and dizziness.

Maintenance

Once an individual begins to smoke tobacco products, psychological and biological processes are important in the maintenance of this behaviour. The same psychological, social, and behavioural variables relevant to initiation, also are relevant to maintenance. In addition, nicotine addiction and other psychopharmacological effects of tobacco smoking become critical. Also, psychobiological interactions contribute to smoking behaviour.

Tobacco smoke includes more than 4000 chemicals, many of which are bioactive and contribute to the health hazards of smoking. It is now firmly established that: (i) cigarettes and other forms of tobacco are addicting; (ii) nicotine is the drug in tobacco that causes addiction; and (iii) the pharmacological and behavioural processes that determine addiction are similar to those that determine addiction to drugs such as heroin and cocaine (USDHHS, 1988). Nicotine acts via positive reinforcement and negative reinforcement to increase the likelihood of continued smoking behaviour. In addition to classical drug-reward mechanisms, nicotine is a positive reinforcer because it suppresses appetite for specific foods, controls body weight, and enhances attention. Nicotine acts as a negative reinforcer by attenuating unpleasant withdrawal effects of smoking cessation (USDHHS, 1988; West & Grunberg, 1991).

As information has accumulated regarding the role of nicotine in tobacco use, laboratory investigations of nicotine have exploded. We now know that nicotine acts at nicotinic cholinergic receptors (nAChR) in the periphery at neuromuscular junctions and end-plates and that nicotine acts in the brain and central nervous system at several different receptor sites. The principal central cholinergic receptor appears to be the $\alpha 4\beta 2$ Torpedo receptor but there also are nicotinic receptors that include $\alpha 3\beta 2$ and $\alpha 7$. Nicotine administration stimulates the sympathetic nervous system and releases catecholamines, serotonin, corticosteroids, neuropeptides, and pituitary hormones. In addition to these endocrine effects, nicotine administration results in electrocortical activation and skeletal muscle relaxation (USDHHS, 1988). All of these effects contribute to the reinforcing actions of nicotine self-administration.

The psychological and pharmacological effects of tobacco and nicotine that contribute to maintenance of smoking behaviour become intertwined. For example, environmental stimuli (such as a bar filled with smokers or the smell of smoke) and cues associated with smoking (such as an ashtray, coffee mug, or a particular location) come to elicit smoking behaviour because these stimuli have been previously reinforced by subsequent self-administration of nicotine. As a result, the psychological and situational cues actually can produce, via classical conditioning, operant conditioning, or paired associations, similar behavioural and biological responses as do nicotine and nicotine cessation. These phenomena contribute to the powerful connection among psychological, situational, and pharmacological effects of tobacco. The repetitive reinforcement of these relationships (hundreds of thousands of events for a pack a day smoker after just 20 years) make smoking cessation that much more difficult.

Relapse

Today, it is estimated that more than 30 million Americans are ex-smokers. However, among smokers who successfully abstain from tobacco smoking for a week or more, approximately 75% relapse within one year of smoking cessation (Shumaker & Grunberg, 1986). This discouraging statistic is tempered a bit by the fact that many smokers abstain on their own and therefore, may be under-represented in relapse statistics. Also it is important to understand that patterns of relapse behaviour vary considerably among individuals. Relapse episodes vary in the degree of: (i) length of abstinence; (ii) number of behavioural slips prior to the relapse episode; and (iii) time from the relapse episode to the recommencement of habitual tobacco smoking either at or below baseline smoking levels (Lichtenstein et al., 1986). Understanding these individual difference variables enables the health-care professional to plan, and to implement, smoking cessation interventions and relapse prevention programmes.

CESSATION TECHNIQUES

On a societal or community level, mass methods of getting people to quit smoking include: public health education campaigns; education of medical students, physicians, and health-care professionals; role modelling by health-care providers; posters, billboards, and electronic media spots. Success of each of these specific programmes is difficult to assess, yet it is estimated that it takes five to seven repeated attempts to quit smoking before the smoker no longer relapses. Therefore, salience of broad-scale cessation programmes or reasons to quit certainly may help to motivate some smokers to give up tobacco and to avoid relapse. Although these large-scale methods have cost-effective and time-efficient appeal, many smokers need or prefer the attention and focus of small group or individualized cessation programmes.

With regard to effective small group or individualized smoking cessation, it is important that the smoker is motivated to quit. This motivation can be encouraged by determining the reasons why the smoker smoked, why s/he wants to quit, and then by accentuating those factors that the smoker identified as important reasons to quit and by providing additional information to reinforce motivation to quit.

Individualized smoking cessation programmes should be based on the relative psychological and pharmacological contributions to the maintenance of smoking behaviour. The same principles that promote smoking initiation and maintenance play a critical role in the cessation of the smoking habit. The health-care professional should consider previously unsuccessful methods, techniques that are acceptable to the individual, and cessation approaches that are easily integrated into the individual's daily routine. Appropriate behavioural modifications should be used to replace the reward of smoking and to help the individual cope with psychological and pharmacological abstinence. Based on the analysis of the initial information, the health-care professional should encourage the smoker to decide the specifics of an individualized plan based on the following principles: (i) choose target dates to begin and to achieve cessation goal; (ii) decide whether or not to use pharmacological adjunct therapy (e.g. nicotine replacement products [NRP] such as nicotine polacrilex gum or nicotine patches; other medications such as clonidine, anxiolytics, or antidepressants); (iii) select specific behavioural and cognitive coping strategies (e.g. counting cigarettes, counting puffs, guided imagery, restricting places where smoking can occur, nicotine fading, rapid smoking); (iv) select coping strategies to deal with cessation withdrawal symptoms (e.g. relaxation training, exercise); (v) make a salient list of reasons for quitting smoking; (vi) enlist support of significant others; (vii) select and use rewards and punishments for reaching reduction and cessation targets; and (viii) select relapse prevention strategies (Grunberg, 1995; Schwartz, 1987).

EFFECTS OF CESSATION

Smoking cessation has major health benefits for men and women of all ages and some of these benefits (e.g. pulmonary function) occur soon after cessation. These benefits apply to individuals with and without smoking-related diseases. Smoking cessation decreases the risk of lung cancer, other neoplastic diseases, heart attack, stroke, and COPDs; former smokers live longer than persistent smokers; and women who quit smoking prior to, or during, the first trimester of pregnancy significantly reduce the risk of having a low birthweight baby. Smoking cessation also has some unpleasant effects including: irritability, sleep disturbances, inability to concentrate, and weight gain. The health benefits of smoking cessation far exceed the risks from the average post-smoking weight gain or any adverse psychological effects that may follow quitting, but it is important for health-care practitioners to prepare smokers for the sequelae of smoking cessation so that they can best cope with these effects and avoid relapse (Grunberg & Bowen, 1985; USDHHS, 1990).

PREVENTION

Ideally, tobacco smoking should be prevented before it begins. It is estimated that, in the USA, the tobacco industry needs to recruit 2 million new smokers each year to replace former smokers who die or quit each year (Lynch & Bonnie, 1994). It is no wonder therefore, that tobacco marketing and advertising are focused on recruitment of new smokers. Educational programmes in schools, public health messages through the media, and bans of tobacco advertising can help to impact the tobacco industry. In addition, increasing tobacco taxes and increasing the saliency of health-warning labels can aid in the deterrence of the initiation of tobacco smoking. Furthermore, individual comments and information from physicians and health-care professionals can be effective to deter tobacco use. More, however, can and should be done. Health-care professionals (including psychologists, physicians, nurses, dentists) should more actively address the danger of tobacco use in patients and clients who do not smoke but who might start. In addition, counter-advertising that accurately portrays the harmful effects of tobacco use and that off-sets the glamorous and seductive images associated with tobacco use should be prominent on billboards, print media, and electronic media. Moreover, low-priced tobacco products should not be allowed to flood the markets of developing nations. The health hazards of tobacco smoking are unequivocal and tobacco use should be prevented.

CONCLUSION

Tobacco smoking is a behaviour that affects hundreds of millions of people around the world. It causes premature deaths, results in debilitating diseases, and pollutes the environment. This preventable, life-threatening behaviour, however, also is a multi-billion dollar industry that affects the livelihoods of millions of people. The clash between health promotion and free market practices is deafening with regard to tobacco smoking.

Tobacco smoking involves the interaction of powerful psychological, social, and biological forces. Once begun, it is difficult to quit smoking, but it certainly is possible. From a perspective of health, tobacco smoking should be prevented and cessation should be encouraged. Current knowledge allows success on both fronts.

REFERENCES

Aitken, P.P., Eadie, D.R., Hastings, G.B. & Haywood, A.J. (1991). Predisposing effects of cigarette advertising on children's intentions to smoke when older. *British Journal of Addiction*, 86, 383–90.

Grunberg, N.E. (1995). A custom-tailored approach to smoking cessation. *International Journal of Smoking Cessation*, 4, 2–5.

Grunberg, N.E. & Bowen, D.J. (1985). Coping with the sequelae of smoking cessation. *Journal of Cardiopulmonary Rehabilitation*, 5, 285–9.

Grunberg, N.E., Winders, S.E. & Wewers, M.E. (1991). Gender differences in tobacco use. *Health Psychology*, 10, 143–53.

Kandel, D.B., Wu, P. & Davies, M. (1994). Maternal smoking during pregnancy and smoking by adolescent daughters. *American Journal of Public Health*, 84, 1407–13.

Lichtenstein, E., Weiss, S.M., Hitchcock, J.L., Leveton, L.B., O'Connell, K. & Prochaska, J.O. (1986). Task force 3: patterns of smoking relapse. *Health Psychology*, 29–40.

Lynch, B.S. & Bonnie, R.J. (Eds.). (1994). *Growing up tobacco free: preventing nicotine addiction in children and youths.* Washington, DC: National Academy Press.

National Institutes of Health. (1993). *Respiratory health effects of passive smoking: lung cancer and other disorders. The Report of the US Environmental Protection Agency.* (NIH Publication No. 93–3605).

Washington, DC: US Government Printing Office.

Peto, R. & Lopez, A.D. (1990). Worldwide mortality from current smoking patterns. In B. Durston & K. Jamrozik (Eds.). *Tobacco and health 1990: the global war Proceedings of the Seventh World Conference on Tobacco and Health*, pp. 66–68. World Conference on Tobacco and Health, Australia.

Pierce, J.P., Lee, L. & Gilpin, E.A. (1994). Smoking initiation by adolescent girls, 1944 through 1988: an association with targeted advertising. *Journal of the American Medical Association*, 271, 608–11.

Popke, E.J., Tizabi, Y., Rahman, M.A & Grunberg, N.E. (1995). Effects of prenatal nicotine exposure on pre-pulse inhibition in male and in female rats. Presented at the annual meeting of the Society for Research on Nicotine and Tobacco, San Diego, California.

Richardson, S.A. & Tizabi, Y. (1994). Hyperactivity in the offspring of nicotine-treated rats: role of the mesolimbic and nigrostriatal dopaminergic pathways. *Pharmacology, Biochemistry and Behavior*, 47, 331–7.

Schwartz, J.L. (1987). *Review and evaluation of smoking cessation methods: the United States and Canada, 1978–1985.* (NIH Publication No. 87–2940). Washington, DC: US Government Printing Office.

Shumaker, S.A. & Grunberg, N.E. (1986).

Introduction to proceedings of the National Working Conference on Smoking Relapse. *Health Psychology*, 5, 1–2.

US Department of Health, Education & Welfare. (1979). *Smoking and health: a report of the Surgeon General.* DHEW Publication No. 79–50066. Washington, DC: US Government Printing Office.

US Department of Health & Human Services. (1982). *The health consequences of smoking: nicotine addiction. A report of the Surgeon General.* (DHHS Publication No. 82–50179). Washington, DC: US Government Printing Office.

US Department of Health & Human Services. (1988). *The health consequences of smoking: nicotine addiction. A report of the Surgeon General.* (DHHS Publication No. 88–8406). Washington, DC: US Government Printing Office.

US Department of Health & Human Services. (1989). *Reducing the health consequences of smoking: 25 years of progress. A report of the Surgeon General.* (DHHS Publication No. 89–8411). Washington, DC: US Government Printing Office.

US Department of Health & Human Services. (1990). *The health benefits of smoking cessation: a report of the Surgeon General.* (DHHS Publication No. 90–8416). Washington, DC: US Government Printing Office.

US Department of Health & Human Services. (1994). *Preventing tobacco use* among young people: a report of the Surgeon General. Atlanta, Georgia: US Department of Health & Human Services, Public Health Service, Centers for Disease Control and Prevention, National Center for Chronic Disease Prevention and Health Promotion, Office on Smoking and Health. Washington, DC: US Government Printing Office.

West, R. & Grunberg, N.E. (1991). Implications of tobacco use as an addiction: introduction. British Journal of Addiction, 86, 485–8.

Torticollis

GRAHAM POWELL

Department of Psychology University of Surrey,
Guildford, Surrey GU2 5XH, UK

Torticollis or Spasmodic Torticollis (ST) is an involuntary contraction of the muscles of the neck which rotates the head to the left or right, resulting in an abnormal posture, sometimes with abnormal movements (Rondot, Marchand & Dellatrolas, 1989; Jahanshahi & Marden, 1989). There may also be an abnormality of tilt (laterocollis) or backwards or forwards extension (retrocollis and antecollis).

Findings are conflicting regarding sex ratio but several studies do show a female preponderance. For example, Rondot et al. (1989) and Duane (1988) both find a male : female ratio of 1.0 : 1.6. Age of onset is fairly consistent across studies, with a median in the early 40s.

There is a longstanding, unresolved debate over whether it is an organic or psychogenic condition. In the Rondot study, a large-scale retrospective analysis of 220 cases, 38.5% noted extrapyramidal symptoms before the onset of ST, particularly postural tremor, and such a tremor was also common in their families (first-degree relatives). On the other hand, 58% of cases had an antecedent psychological disorder (33% of a moderate nature, including dysthymia, somatoform disorder and personality disorder; 25% of a severe nature including schizophrenia and major depressive illness).

The mode of onset is typically progressive (83% of cases in the Rondot study) often with an initial head tremor (34% of cases).

Information about prognostic factors is limited, but Jahanshahi, Marion and Marsden (1990) found those that spontaneously remitted tended to have an earlier onset.

Treatment seems to benefit only about half the patients (e.g. Lal, 1979). Most are tried on anticholinergic drugs (e.g. procyclidin), often in combination with physiotherapy and alcohol injections, and there has been some recent work on the use of botulinum toxin injections by Jahanshihi and Marsden (1992), in which 85% of 26 patients and 88% of relatives thought the torticollis improved.

Psychological treatments centre on EMG feedback (e.g. Korein & Brudney, 1976; Jahanshahi, Sartory & Marsden 1991; Soga, 1989), sometimes in conjunction with curtaneous shock (Russ, 1975) or heart rate feedback (Williams, 1975).

REFERENCES

Duane, D. (1988). Spasmodic torticollis: clinical and biological features and their implications for focal dystonia. In S. Fahn et al. (Ed.). Advances in neurology, vol 50, New York: Raven Press.

Jahanshahi, M. & Marsden, C.D. (1989). Motor disorders. In G. Turpin (Ed.) Handbook of clinical psychophysiology Chichester: John Wiley Jahanshahi et al.

Jahanshahi, M. & Marsden, C.D. (1992). Psychological functioning before and after treatment of torticollis with botulinum toxin. Journal of Neurology, Neurosurgery and Psychiatry, 55, 229–31.

Jahanshahi, M., Marion, P.H. & Marsden, C.D. (1990). Natural history of adult onset idiopathic torticollis. Archives of Neurology, 47, 548–52.

Jahanshahi, M., Sartory, G. & Marsden, C.D. (1991). EMG biofeedback treatment of torticollis: a controlled outcome study. Biofeedback and Self Regulation, 16, 413–48.

Korein, J. & Brudny, J. (1976). Integrated EMG feedback in the management of spasmodic torticollis and focal dystonia: a prospective study of 80 patients. In M.D. Yahr (Ed.). The basal ganglia New York: Raven Press.

Lal, S. (1979). Pathophysiology and pharmacotherapy of spasmodic torticollis: a review. Canadian Journal of Neurological Sciences, 6, 427–35.

Rondot,. P, Marchand, M.P. & Dellatrolas, G. (1989). Spasmodic torticollis – review of 220 patients. Canadian Journal of Neurological Sciences, 18, 143–51.

Russ, K.L. (1975). EMG biofeedback of spasmodic torticollis: a case study. Annual proceedings of the Biofeedback Research Society

Soga M (1989) Treatment of 27 patients with spasmodic torticollis by EMG biofeedback and self-monitoring. Japanese Journal of Behaviour Therapy, 15, 1–10

Williams, R.B. (1975). H.R. feedback in the treatment of torticollis: a case report. Psychophysiology, 12, 237.

Torticollis

Transplantation

STANTON NEWMAN

Unit of Health Psychology, Department of
Psychiatry and Behavioural Sciences, University
College London Medical School, UK

Organ transplantation has become an important tool in the armoury of medicine. It is customarily used as the intervention of last resort and has become increasingly popular partly out of its increased success. For example, over 26 000 heart transplants have been performed worldwide since 1982, and the five-year survival rate exceeds 60% (Hosenpud *et al.*, 1994). From the patients perspective, organ transplantation has the prospect of transforming their lives often after years of chronic illness and disability. The one cost for most patients is that they are expected to adhere to what is often a complex regime of medicine and diet. The likelihood of following a complex regimen has been found to be related to the expectations that patients have prior to the transplant. Leedham *et al.* (1995) found that positive expectations prior to surgery were associated with an increased likelihood of heart transplant patients following their regimen.

The psychological issues around transplantation begin with the decision for an organ to be used. This may be on the basis of a donor card and or a family decision to accept that an organ may be removed for transplantation. There is vast cultural diversity in these attitudes. For example, in Japan, despite possessing the requisite training and technology, surgeons have performed only one heart transplant in the quarter century since the procedure was developed. Mistrust of the medical profession, traditional outlooks on death, and the primacy placed on consensual decision, as well as the lack of a brain death standard, have limited the availability of transplantable organs (Feldman, 1994).

A number of proposals have been made with regard to the selection of candidates for organ transplantation. This has been felt to be of particular importance in that, following transplantation, patients are on a complicated medication regimen, and the need to adhere as closely as possible to the regimen is considered important. In cardiac surgery, preoperative personality disorders have been found to be associated with non-compliance but presurgery depression and anxiety have not (Shapiro, 1992). The issues regarding selection of patients on the basis of psychological features remains controversial.

Quality of life has been examined in many studies of transplantation. In renal transplantation, these have produced equivocal results. In some studies, patients may experience less fatigue, less time spent on medical care, higher income and less emotional problems (Morris, 1988; Piehlmeier *et al.*, 1991; Russell *et al.*, 1992; Gouge *et al.*, 1990, Gorlen *et al.*, 1993). Other studies have shown that changes in personal appearance as a result of immunosuppressive drugs may be a source of emotional difficulties (Kalman, Wilson & Kalman, 1983; Kutner, 1993). The integration of the new organ is another source of difficulties, the organ may be seen as foreign, or an enemy and may be a source of fantasies (House & Thompson, 1988). As a result of these difficulties, quality of life and emotional adjustment have not been found to improve following renal transplantation in other studies, even though physical well-being may have improved (Parfrey *et al.*, 1987; Kalman *et al.*, 1983).

In cardiac transplantation both benign side-effects such as acne and hirsutism and more life-threatening problems such as infections combine to result in a variable response with regard to quality of life. In general, however, the more physical symptoms and disability the worse the reported quality of life (Lough *et al.*, 1987). Because of the appearance altering side-effects in some heart transplant patients' body image has been found to be an important issue, in particular with children (Shapiro, 1992).

Leedham *et al.* (1995) studied factors predictive of psychological well being following heart transplantation and found that patients' self-reported positive expectations were generally associated with good mood, adjustment to the illness, and quality of life, even in patients who experienced health setbacks. Internal health locus of control has also been found to predict good emotional adjustment following heart transplantation (Kugler *et al.*, 1994). One of the biggest concerns in the early phase following transplantation revolves around possible rejection. It constitutes a major source of anxiety and when it occurs, anger (House, Dubovsky & Penn, 1983; House & Thompson, 1988).

Cognitive deficits have frequently been reported in patients with kidney disease. The impact of renal transplantation on the cognitive functioning of patients previously maintained on dialysis has indicated a reversal of the cognitive dysfunction along with the reversal of uraemic symptoms (Teschan *et al.*, 1979). The reversal of hepatic encephalopathy has been documented following liver transplantation (Powell *et al.*, 1990). Using neuropsychological assessment, improvements were found in visual–motor co-ordination, perceptual organization and attention.

Tarter *et al.* (1990) conducted a similar study, and found a significant improvement in cognitive functioning posttransplantation as opposed to pretransplantation in heart patients. Similar results have been reported by Bornstein, Starling and Myerowitz (1992).

Studies of children who undergo cardiac, renal, and liver transplantation have indicated that deficits ranging from gross IQ deficits to subtle neuropsychological dysfunction are present in some of these children both before, and after, transplantation, but the factors associated with these declines remain unclear (Stewart *et al.*, 1994).

REFERENCES

Bornstein, R., Starling, R., & Myerowitz, P. (1992). Neuropsychological function before and after cardiac transplantation. In P.J. Walter (Ed.). *Quality of life after open heart surgery*, pp. 419–424, Netherlands: Kluwer Academic Publishers.

Feldman, E.A. (1994). Culture, conflict, and cost. Perspectives on brain death in Japan. *International Journal of Technological Assess Health Care*, 10, 447–63.

Gouge, F., Moore, J., Bremer, B.A., McCauly, C.R. & Johnson, J.P. (1990). The quality of life of donors, potential donors, and recipients of living-related donor renal transplantation. *Transplantation Proceedings*, 22, 2409–13.

Gorlen, T., Abdelnoor, M., Enger, E. & Aarseth, H.P. (1993). Quality of life after kidney transplantation, a 10–22 years follow-up. *Scandinavian Journal of Urology and Nephrology*, 27, 89–92.

Hosenpud, J.D., Novick, R.J., Breen, T.J. & Daily, O.P. (1994). The Registry of the International Society for Heart and Lung Transplantation: eleventh official report, 1994. *Journal of Heart and Lung Transport*, 13, 561–70.

House, R.M. & Thompson, T.L. (1988). Psychiatric aspects of organ transplantation. *Journal of the American Medical Association*, 260, 535–9.

House, R.M., Dubovsky, S.L. & Penn, I. (1983). Psychiatric aspects of hepatic transplantation. *Transplantation*, 36, 146–50.

Kalman, T.P., Wilson, P.G. & Kalman, C.M. (1983). Psychiatric morbidity in long-term renal transplant recipients and patients undergoing haemodialysis. *Journal of the American Medical Association*, 250, 55–8.

Kugler, J., Tenderich, G., Stahlhut, P., Posival, H., Korner, M.H., Korfer, R. & Kruskemper, G.M. (1994). Emotional adjustment and perceived locus of control in heart transplant patients *Journal of Psychosomatic Research*, 38, 403–8.

Kutner, N.G. (1993). Rehabilitation revisited. *Transplantation Proceedings*, 25, 2506–7.

Leedham, B., Meyerowitz, B.E., Muirhead, J. & Frist, W.H. (1995). Positive expectations predict health after heart transplantation. *Health Psychology*, 14, 74–9.

Lough, M., Lindsay, A.M., Shinn, J.A. & Stotts, N.A. (1987). Impact of symptom frequency and symptom distress on self reported quality of life in heart transplant recipients. *Heart and Lung*, 16, 193–200.

Morris, P.J. (1988). *Kidney transplantation*. Philadelphia, USA: W.B. Saunders.

Parfrey, P.S., Vavasour, H., Bullock, M., Henry, S., Harnett, J.D. & Gault, M.H. (1987). Symptoms in end-stage renal disease. *Transplantation Proceedings*, 19, 3407–9.

Piehlmeier, W., Bullinger, M., Nusser, J., Konig, A., Illner, W.D., Abendroth, D., Land, W. & Landgraf, R. (1991). Quality of life in Type I diabetic patients prior to and after pancreas and kidney transplantation in relation to organ function. *Diabetologia*, 34, s150–7.

Powell, E.E., Pender, M.P., Chalk, J.B., Parkin, P.J., Strong, R., Lynch, S., Kerlin, P., Cooksley, W.G., Cheng, W. & Powell, L. (1990). Improvement in chronic hepatocerebral degeneration following liver transplantation. *Gastroenterology*, 98, 1079–82.

Russell, J.D., Beecroft, M.L., Ludwin, D. & Churchill, D.N. (1992). The quality of life in renal transplantation – a prospective study. *Transplantation*, 54, 656–60.

Shapiro, P. (1992). Quality of life after open heart surgery: strategies to improve quality of life after heart transplantation. In P.J. Walter (Ed.). *Quality of life after open heart surgery*, pp. 507–515. Netherlands: Kluwer Academic Publishers.

Stewart, S.M., Kennard, B.D., Waller, D.A. & Fixler, D. (1994). Cognitive function in children who receive organ transplantation. *Health Psychology*, 13, 3–13.

Tarter, R.E., Switala, J., Arria, A., Plail, J. & Van Thiel, D.H. (1990). Subclinical hepatic encephalopathy. *Transplantation*, 50, 632–7.

Teschan, P.E., Ginn, H.E., Bourne, J.R., Ward, J.W., Hamel, B., Nunnally, J.C., Musso, M. & Vaughn, W.K. (1979). Quantitative indices of clinical uraemia. *Kidney International*, 15, 676–97.

Transsexual surgery

GEORGE HIGGINS

Counseling Center, Trinity College, Hartford, USA

Transsexualism is a condition marked by 'strong and persistent cross-gender identification . . . [and] . . . persistent discomfort with his or her sex or sense of inappropriateness in the gender role of that sex (*DSM-IV*, 1994).' The condition is diagnosed as occurring in adults, *DSM-IV* 302.85, or in children, *DSM-IV* 302.6.

The incidence of gender identity disorders, including transsexualism, has been estimated at fewer than 3 per 100 000 in males and under 1 per 100 000 in females (Walinder, 1986). The desire for transsexual surgery varies among persons with gender identity disorders from being an attractive but rejected idea to a procedure that is urgently sought out (Benjamin, 1966).

Male-to-female surgery involves the creation of a neo-vagina which can provide sexual pleasure, although many experience problems with narrowing, and the neo-vagina requires considerable post-operative self-care. Female-to-male surgery involves chest reconstruction, and less frequently, the creation of a neo-phallus. The procedures for creating a neo-phallus are variable; some are not aesthetically pleasing, many do not permit the neo-phallus to be used for urination or for intercourse, although new procedures are being developed which allow for both functions. A psychologist may use the general information services listed below to remain abreast of available procedures and where they are performed. The Web sites are particularly useful for current information.

Psychologists may make significant contributions in three areas

[613]

with respect to transsexual surgery. The first is to help persons with gender identity questions to determine whether surgery is desirable for their particular condition and life circumstances. The second is to help the gender dysphoric person who chooses to live as the opposite sex to make the transition as successfully as possible. Finally, the psychologist can be particularly helpful postsurgically since many transsexuals have expectations about surgery which are not realized.

A clear differential diagnostic determination among transvestite, transsexual, and transvestite homosexuality must be made. Only transsexuals are aided by surgery, and even among transsexuals the importance of surgery varies. The psychologist should facilitate weighing the value of surgery in each case, and not indicate that all transsexual persons automatically need surgery.

All transsexual persons wish to appear in public as the opposite sex, and the Standards of Care (Benjamin Association, 1990) require transsexual persons to live for at least one year before surgery as a person of the sex to which they will be assigned. Public presentation exacerbates existing characterological traits and defensive behaviours with which psychologists should deal therapeutically. Many transsexuals have complex psychological pathology in addition to their transsexuality (Lothstein, 1982a, b), and satisfactory postsurgical adjustment is enhanced if therapy is begun before surgery.

Transsexual persons often know that some psychological difficulties are related to their transsexuality, and unfortunately many of them have the unjustified expectation that these problems will be solved by surgery. Transsexual persons are very prone to depression and suicide, and this can become a particular problem when unwanted characterological traits remain after surgery. Transsexuals are often socially withdrawn during childhood and adolescence because of the awkwardness they feel about being the wrong sex. They therefore, do not develop the social skills a normal child does during the routine give and take of growing up. Many transsexuals expect surgery to result in their feeling socially comfortable and skilled. When this does not occur, severe depression can result, thus postoperative psychological attention is essential.

INFORMATION SERVICES

American Educational Gender Information Service, PO Box 33724, Decatur GA 30033 USA: Voice: 770–939–2128; Fax: 770–939–1770; Email: aegis@mindspring.com; www.ren.org/rafi/AEGIS.html

Harry Benjamin International Gender Dysphoria Association, Inc., 3790 El Camino Real, #251, Palo Alto CA 94306 USA; Voice 415–322–2335; Fax 415–322–3260; Email thbigda@aol.com

Ingersoll Gender Center, 1812 East Madison, Suite 106, Seattle WA 98122 USA; Voice 206–329–6651; Email: ingersol@halcyon.com; www.halcyon.com/ingersol/iiihome.html

Intelligence Engineering Transgender Information, www.pcnet.com/elspeth/tg1.html

International Foundation for Gender Education, PO Box 229, Waltham, MA 02154–0229 USA; Voice: 617–894–8340 or 617–899–2212; Fax: 617–899–5703; Email: ifge@world.std.com; www.transgender, org/tg/ifge/index.html

Sex Change Indigo Pages, www.servtech.com/public/perette/Sc/sexchange.html

REFERENCES

Benjamin, H.S., International Gender Dysphoria Association, Inc. (1990). *Standards of care*, Palo Alto: Harry S. Benjamin Gender Dysphoria Association, Inc.

Benjamin, H.S. (1966). *The transsexual phenomenon*. New York: Warner Books.

DSM-IV. (1994). *Diagnostic and statistical manual of mental disorders*. (4th ed.). Washington: The American Psychiatric Association.

Lothstein, L.M. (1982a) Sex reassignment surgery: historical, bioethical, and theoretical issues. *American Journal Psychiatry*, **139**, 417–26.

Lothstein, L.M. (1982b). *Female-to-male transsexualism: historical, ethical, and theoretical issues*. Boston: Routledge & Kegan Paul.

Walinder, J. (1986). Transsexualism: Definition, prevalence, and sex distribution. *Acta Psychiatrica Scandinavica*, **203**, 255–8.

Vertigo and dizziness

LUCY YARDLEY

Department of Psychology, University College London, London, UK

Although in lay usage the term vertigo denotes a fear of heights, the medical meaning is an illusion of movement caused by balance system (usually vestibular) dysfunction. The sensations that characterize vertigo range from vague giddiness or unsteadiness to a feeling that oneself or the environment is spinning rapidly, accompanied by partial loss of postural control and a range of autonomic symptoms such as pallor, cold sweating, nausea, and vomiting. More than five people per thousand at risk consult their doctor each year on account of classic vertigo, and a further ten complain of non-specific dizziness, although the incidence of balance system dysfunction within the latter group remains uncertain since a multitude of medical conditions can give rise to dizziness. Most people recover from an attack of vertigo within a few weeks or months by a natural process of neurophysiological habituation, but a significant proportion suffer from repeated spontaneous attacks or residual movement-provoked dizziness.

Complaints of vertigo are frequently accompanied by elevated levels of anxiety and signs of emotional disturbance, and a number of possible psychosomatic mechanisms have been proposed to account for this relationship. There is currently no reliable evidence for a causal link between either personality or stress and the onset of episodes of acute vertigo (for a review and thorough longitudinal study, see Crary & Wexler, 1977). However, anxious individuals may be more likely to monitor and report mild sensations of disorientation (Stephens, Hogan & Meredith, 1991), whether induced by minor perceptual deficits, anxiety, or perceptually complex environments (Jacob et al., 1989). Dizziness may also result from the heightened physiological arousal or hyperventilation associated with anxiety or panic (Jacob et al., 1992).

Somatopsychic explanations for the association between anxiety and vertigo highlight the intrinsically frightening nature of vertigo attacks, which can lead to panic and agoraphobic behaviour in people with a previously normal psychiatric history (Pratt & McKenzie, 1958). However, studies of hospital outpatients indicate that psychological and behavioural responses to dizziness may play an important role in determining the handicap and distress arising from a given degree of impairment (Hallam & Stephens, 1985). Yardley has developed a model of the relationship between vertigo, anxiety and handicap which describes how fear of provoking vertigo, and concern about potential stigmatization, can motivate withdrawal from valued activities and functions (Yardley et al., 1992; Yardley, 1994a,b). A cycle of escalating disability and distress may result; handicap can lead to a general loss of confidence which is likely to augment the specific fears which give rise to voluntary limitation of activity, while deliberate restriction of movement may indefinitely retard the process of neurophysiological habituation. Reactions to vertigo may also be aggravated by a predisposition to anxiety (Eagger et al., 1992) or preoccupation with physical symptoms (Yardley, 1994a,b), and it is possible that, as in panic, negative perceptions of the autonomic symptoms initially triggered by vertigo may themselves give rise to further anxiety and arousal. Effective rehabilitation therefore requires a programme of exercises to promote both habituation and confidence in movement, supplemented by discussion of the significance of symptoms and training in techniques to reduce arousal (Beyts, 1987).

REFERENCES

Beyts, P. (1987). Vestibular rehabilitation. In S.D.G. Stephens (Ed.). *Adult audiology, Scott-Brown's otolaryngology* (5th edn) vol. 2. London: Butterworths.

Crary, W.G. & Wexter, M. (1977). Menière's disease – a psychosomatic disorder? *Psychological Reports*, 41, 603–45.

Eagger, S., Luxon, L.M., Davies, R.A., Coelho, A. & Ron, M.A. (1992). Psychiatric morbidity in patients with peripheral vestibular disorder: a clinical and neuro-otological study. *Journal of Neurology, Neurosurgery and Psychiatry*, 55, 383–7.

Hallam, R.S. & Stephens, S.D.G. (1985). Vestibular disorder and emotional distress.

Journal of Psychosomatic Research, 29, 407–13.

Jacob, R.G., Lilienfeld, S.O., Furman, J.M.R., Durrant, J.D. & Turner, S.M. (1989). Panic disorder with vestibular dysfunction: further clinical observations and description of space and motion phobic stimuli. *Journal of Anxiety Disorders*, 3, 117–30.

Jacob, R.G., Furman, J.M.R., Clark, D.B. & Durrant, J.D. (1992). Vestibular symptoms, panic and phobia: overlap and possible relationships. *Annals of Clinical Psychiatry*, 4, 163–74.

Pratt, R.T.C. & McKenzie, W. (1958). Anxiety states following vestibular disorders. *Lancet*, ii, 347–9.

Stephens, S.D.G., Hogan, S. & Meredith, R. (1991). The desynchrony between complaints and signs of vestibular disorders. *Acta Otolayngologica*, 111, 188–92.

Yardley, L. (1994a). Contribution of symptoms and beliefs to handicap in people with vertigo: a longitudinal study. *British Journal of Clinical Psychology*, 33, 101–13.

Yardley, L. (1994b). *Vertigo and dizziness.* Routledge: London.

Yardley, L., Todd, A.M., Lacoudraye-Harter, M.M. & Ingham, R. (1992). Psychosocial consequences of vertigo. *Psychology and Health*, 6, 85–96.

Voice disorders

RUTH EPSTEIN

Speech and Language Therapy Department, The Middlesex Hospital, London, UK

Voice disorders represent an area of communication dysfunctions which affects a large population of people. People with voice disorders range from a simple case of laryngitis that usually resolves spontaneously to more physical or organic conditions such as laryngeal malignancy.

The main symptom in people with voice disorders is hoarseness or dysphonia which describes an alteration in voice quality. It is difficult to define a normal or an abnormal voice quality in the absence of a fixed, uniform standard of abnormal voice but according to Aronson (1990) 'a voice disorder exists when quality, pitch, loudness or flexibility differs from the voices of others of similar age, sex and cultural group'. In medical practice, hoarseness is described as a symptom of disease of the larynx which is often the first and only signal of dangerous disease, local or systemic, involving this area.

The differential diagnosis is important since many different medical and surgical conditions may result in hoarseness. Voice disorders can be aetiologically classified into organic types and non-organic types, that are often referred to as functional or psychogenic types.

In organic voice disorders, the faulty voice is caused by structural or physical disease which can be a disease of the larynx itself, or by systemic illnesses which alter laryngeal structure (Boone & McFarlane, 1988).

Organic disorders of vocal mechanisms that may result in voice problems include keratosis, granulomas, leucoplakia, papillomas, carcinoma and other malignancies. Voice problems associated with nervous system involvement are technically considered dysarthrias. They also include: spasmodic dysphonia, myasthenia gravis and vocal fold paralysis.

Functional or psychogenic voice disorders are caused by a non-physical cause or faulty habits of voice use. The voice sounds abnormal despite normal laryngeal anatomy and physiology. Non-organic disorders or functional voice disorders can be divided into habitual vocal problems, secondary to vocal misuse/abuse, and psychogenic vocal problems. Habitual dysphonias include nodules, polyps, cysts, oedema, ventricular dysphonia, laryngitis and contact ulcer. Psychogenic voice disorders include musculoskeletal tension disorders and conversion voice disorders: muteness, aphonia and dysphonia which can be traced to the anxiety or depression produced by life stress, psychoneuroses or personality disorders.

The incidence of voice disorders in school-age children, mostly caused by vocal abuse, is 6 to 9% (Wilson, 1979). Other studies, however, claim that the incidence is possibly higher (Yairi et al., 1974; Silverman & Zimmer, 1975). Statistics on the incidence of voice disorders in adults are not well documented. In one representative study, investigating 1262 patients drawn from several otolaryngological practices, it was found that the most common disorders reported were vocal nodules, oedema, polyps, carcinoma, vocal fold paralysis and dysphonia without laryngeal pathology. Laryngeal pathologies were most common in middle age-groups (45 years of age and over) and in people diagnosed as having psychogenic voice disorders, 85% were females, 35% of them housewives (Herrington-Hall et al., 1988).

Mirror laryngoscopy is the most common method used by otolaryngologists, of viewing the interior of the larynx. For more specialized studies direct laryngoscopy, laryngography, radiology, video stroboscopy and videofluoroscopy are used. The voice evaluation is performed in order to assist the laryngologist in differential diagnosis of the voice disorder and to recommend appropriate treatment.

The differential diagnosis begins with categorizing the abnormal voice based on laryngological, physiological and neurological evidence. Assessment of the voice disordered patient is enhanced by input from various disciplines (otolaryngologist, speech and language therapist, voice scientist, radiologist) through a team approach.

There are three general approaches to the management of voice problems: surgical, medical and behavioural (Colton & Casper, 1990). It is often the case, however, that optimal treatment requires the use of combined treatment modalities. Surgical management is considered the more radical form of intervention and is referred to as phonosurgery – surgical techniques aimed at improving voice quality.

The medical approach to the treatment of voice disorders refers to non-invasive techniques which do not involve surgical removal of tissue, reconstruction or alteration.

The behavioural approach consists of voice therapy which aims at restoring the best voice possible within the patient's anatomical, physiological and psychological capacity.

The diagnosis of the voice disorder will determine the treatment. Some organic voice disorders will be improved by phonosurgery. In laryngeal carcinoma, surgery will be used to eradicate cancer.

Acute laryngeal problems in which the vocal folds demonstrate redness, swelling or irritation will be medically treated. When vocal abuse appears to be the cause of the laryngeal problem, voice therapy will be carried out, using principles of vocal re-education, and reduction of stress factors that drive the patient into patterns of vocal misuse. The treatment of conversion voice disorders, where the patient has a need to be partially or completely without voice is based on re-establishment of the patient's conscious awareness of greater phonatory capability, and discussing the emotional conflicts that have generated the voice disorder, while monitoring the possibility of referral for psychotherapy.

Progression from abnormal to normal voice occurs as a product of the patient's conscious, voluntary response to the clinician's instruction and encouragement. In organic disorders, the main principle of therapy is either muscle strengthening or adaptation to the mechanical problems through compensatory phonatory and respiratory manoeuvres.

In non-organic voice disorders involving excess musculoskeletal tension, treatment is based on the principle that, when the muscular tension is reduced, the larynx will return to its normal phonatory ability. This is achieved by mechanical relaxation of musculature and psychological release of the anxiety causing the tension.

Knowledge of the principles and skills of psychological interviewing and counselling are essential in the diagnosis and treatment of voice disorders. Virtually all patients with voice disorders, organic or psychogenic, have some degree of emotional imbalance, either as a cause or effect of the voice disorder. Many functional voice disorders disappear or improve during discussion of life stresses responsible for those disorders.

In voice therapy in particular, the association between stress, emotional states and voice has led to a very strong emphasis on psychodynamic theory in the explanation of the causes of some types of voice disorders. Awareness of more serious emotional problems in patients who have voice disorders can facilitate referrals to professional mental health specialists. (see also 'Stuttering'.)

REFERENCES

Aronson, A.E. (1990) *Clinical voice disorders.* 3rd Edn. New York: Thieme Medical, 1990.

Boone, D.R. & McFarlane S.C. (1988) *The voice and voice therapy* 4th Edn. New Jersey: Prentice Hall.

Colton, R.H. & Casper J.K. (1990) *Understanding voice problems.* Baltimore: Williams & Williams.

Herrington-Hall, B.L., Lee L., Stemple, J.C., Viemi, K.R. & McHone, M.H.M. (1988). Description of laryngeal pathologies by age, sex and occupation in a treatment-seeking sample. *Journal of Speech and Hearing Disorders*, **53**, 57–64.

Silverman, E.M. & Zimmer, C.H. (1975) Incidence of chronic hoarseness among school-age children. *Journal of Speech and Hearing Disorders*, **40** 211–15.

Wilson, K. (1979) *Voice and problems of children*, 2nd edn. Baltimore: Williams & Williams, Co.

Yairi, E., Currin, L.H., Bulian, N. & Yairi, J. (1974) Incidence of hoarseness in school children over one year period. *Journal of Communication Disorders*, **7**, 321–8.

Volatile substance abuse

MICHAEL GOSSOP

*National Addiction Centre, Institute of Psychiatry,
London, UK*

Volatile substance abuse is often, though inaccurately, referred to as glue sniffing. It differs from other types of drug abuse in that it is primarily a problem of children and adolescents. Although reliable prevalence estimates are difficult to obtain, it has been suggested that between 3.5% and 10% of adolescents may have at least experimented with volatile substances, and that between 0.5% and 1% of the secondary school population may be current users (Ashton, 1990). Solvent abuse is often very localized and in these circumstances the percentage of young people using these substances may be considerably higher. The majority of volatile substance abusers are aged between 12 and 19.

The possibility of making solvent abuse an offence in Britain was considered in 1983 in consultation with a wide range of statutory and voluntary agencies. The majority view was opposed to it on the grounds that young people would be deterred from seeking help from adults or from helping agencies, that it would increase the likelihood of such behaviour becoming more deeply hidden, thereby increasing the risk of accidents in circumstances in which help would be unavailable, and that it would lead to an unnecessary criminalization of juveniles.

One factor underlying volatile substance abuse is the ready availability of these substances. The average home is likely to contain dozens of substances which are capable of being abused, including aerosols (paints, lubricant sprays, and deodorants), as well as lighter fuel, petrochemicals, glues, thinners, and other solvents. The almost universal availability of volatile substances creates a special problem since it is impractical to prevent the abuse of these substances through restricting access to them. In England and Wales, the Intoxicating Substances (Supply) Act of 1985 makes it an offence to supply or offer to supply any volatile substance to a person under the age of 18 if the substance is likely to be misused for the purpose of causing intoxication.

There are differences in the degree of risk associated with different types of volatile substances. Two of the more risky forms of volatile substance abuse appear to be the inhalation of cigarette lighter fuel and inhaling the contents of fire extinguishers (Gossop, 1993). Both have been linked to fatalities. The level of risk to the user may also differ with the precise method of administration. Methods that involve putting plastic bags over the head of the user are risky and may lead to asphyxiation.

Because volatile substance abusers tend to be so young, concern can sometimes take the form of excessive reactions. The strength of these reactions, often coupled with demands for instant response, may complicate the ability of those concerned to identify and provide the most appropriate interventions. Only a minority of those who experiment with these substances go on to become regular users, and only a minority of regular users are likely to experience serious problems or harm as a result of their use.

Family doctors, social workers and other carers sometimes acknowledge their own lack of expertise in this area and refer the young person to another agency which is assumed to have greater knowledge or skills. This may be psychiatrist or a drug treatment service. Such referral may be neither necessary nor desirable. Many useful interventions can be delivered at the primary health-care level or by non-specialists working with young people such as teachers, counsellors or social workers.

Volatile substance abuse may reflect underlying psychiatric problems but this is not always the case. Some cases involve 'experimental' behaviour by otherwise well-adjusted individuals. Some cases reflect 'subcultural' patterns of abuse in which the individual has been socialised in the abuse of volatile substances by their peers. This is not to deny the risks that may be involved. But it should raise questions about how most effectively to intervene in such cases. Although volatile substance abuse clearly is a type of drug problem, it should not automatically be assumed that referral to a specialist drug dependence treatment service is the most appropriate response. Such services are often geared to the needs of adult (and young adult) users of drugs such as heroin, cocaine or amphetamine. Many of these drug takers will be severely dependent (addicted), and many will be drug injectors. In contrast, comparatively few volatile substance abusers will be addicted in the sense of being either physically or psychologically dependent upon their drugs. There is an obvious risk of exposing 15 year old solvent abusers to an environment where they could be expected to be influenced by adult heroin injectors.

It can be useful to interpret the behaviour and problems of volatile substance abusers in terms of other more familiar adjustment problems that affect young people. The factors that lead to volatile substance abuse may be similar to those that lead to stealing, bullying, persistent misbehaviour or general 'naughtiness'. Volatile substance abuse may be accompanied by behaviour problems of this sort and, although volatile substance abuse may be the presenting problem, it may be only one of a number of problems, and not necessarily the most important. When viewed in a broader perspective, the types of interventions that are used with other adolescent problems may appear more applicable with volatile substance abusers. There is no simple or established treatment that can be applied specifically to those involved in volatile substance abuse.

The risk of accidental injury is always a problem for the volatile substance abuser. Acute effects like drunkenness, may be accompanied by confusional or hallucinatory states. One of the most worrying features of volatile substance abuse is that the risk is not proportionate to the degree or the duration of involvement. First-time users may be at high risk. The number of young people who die as a consequence of volatile substance abuse is relatively small in comparison to the number of users but it is a matter for serious concern that over the past decade or so, there has been a steady increase in the number of deaths associated with these substances (Pottier *et al.*, 1992). Tragically, many of these have involved children and young people (deaths have been recorded for 10 and 11 years-olds, and 60% of deaths are among people aged 17 or less).

Volatile substances act like general anaesthetics with a similar picture of acute intoxication. These substances are generally highly fat soluble and diffusely toxic to the nervous system. The toxicology of each of the volatile substances may carry different risks for the user, and persistent volatile substance abuse may create medical problems that require attention (Sharp & Rosenberg, 1992). Chronic abuse may lead to weight loss, muscle weakness, disorientation and lack of co-ordination. Chronic exposure to some organic solvents may cause polyneuropathy. Volatile substances affect brain function in many ways, though most of these effects appear to be reversible. Exceptions can generally be attributed to cerebral hypoxia or a metabolic acidosis. There is also concern about the toxic effects of volatile substance abuse upon other organ systems, including kidney, liver, heart and blood. Death is rare but may occur as a result of asphyxia, ventricular fibrillation, or induced cardiac arrhythmia.

REFERENCES

Ashton, C.H. (1990). Solvent abuse. *British Medical Journal*, **300**, 135–6.

Gossop, M. (1993). Volatile substances and the law. *Addiction*, **88**, 311–4.

Pottier, A., Taylor, J., Norman, C., Meyer, L., Anderson, H. & Ramsey, J. (1992). *Trends in deaths associated with abuse of volatile substances 1971–1990*. Report No.5, London: Department of Public Health Sciences.

Sharp, C. & Rosenberg, N. (1992). Volatile Substances In J. Lowinson, P. Ruiz, R. Millman & J. Langrod (Eds.). *Substance abuse: a comprehensive textbook*. Baltimore: Williams and Wilkins.

Vomiting and nausea as side-effects of drugs

DAVID JAMES DE LANCY HORNE

*Department of Psychology, University of
Melbourne, Royal Melbourne Hospital, Victoria,
Australia*

Nausea and vomiting occur when a specialized part of the brain called the vomiting centre is stimulated by signals which can arise from various points in both the brain and body, e.g. the digestive system; the parts of the brain responsible for consciousness; the inner ear. Signals may also arise from an area of the brain called the chemoreceptor trigger zone which stimulates the vomiting centre if it detects any harmful substances present in the blood. Antiemetic drugs may act at any one or more of these locations.

Nausea is a common side-effect of many drugs including some antidepressants and anti-inflammatory medication, but vomiting rarely occurs and the nausea usually subsides after a period. However, it is the nausea and vomiting from chemotherapy for various forms of cancer that has received most psychological attention, since these can be so severe as to lead to patients refusing chemotherapy treatment even when it is known to be beneficial. Uncontrolled vomiting is also very dangerous because it can cause dehydration, electrolyte abnormalities and weight loss. Also, in the treatment of cancer by chemotherapy, nausea and vomiting are the most feared side-effects.

Some chemotherapy drugs, such as high dose cisplatin, can result in 100% of recipients developing serious vomiting if effective antiemetics are not administered (Sagar, 1991). Without antiemetics, adjuvant chemotherapy used for treating breast cancer can result in severe nausea in 65–83% and vomiting in 52–78% of patients. Refusal to receive further highly emetogenic chemotherapy can be as high as 30% in these patients, and an additional 20% may delay treatment due to anxieties regarding nausea and vomiting (Lindley, Bernard & Fields, 1989).

Patient factors may also influence the incidence and degree of emesis. Alcohol consumption of more than 100 grams per day for several years results in better control, as does a history of marijuana abuse when cannabinoid antiemetics are used (Pollera & Gianarelli, 1989).

Nausea and vomiting responses to chemotherapy are also associated with anticipatory nausea and vomiting (ANV). ANV is generally less well controlled by antiemetic medication than post-chemotherapy NV, with AN occurring in up to 35% of patients and AV in 16%, with refusal to continue therapy in up to 10% (Bakowski, 1984).

Thus, symptoms of nausea and vomiting are of such major concern when treating cancer patients that there has been an intensive search for ever more effective antiemetic medication.

However, even with the development of powerful new antiemetic drugs for use in association with chemotherapy, such as odansetron, total control over NV is by no means assured. Even when vomiting is eliminated, many patients may still experience unpleasant, prolonged nausea, anxiety and general discomfort, not to mention distressing physical side-effects of chemotherapy such as electrolyte imbalance, oesophageal tears, hair loss and skeletal fractures (Sagar, 1991).

By contrast, the research into psychological factors associated with the causes of N and V and their management remains relatively limited.

For example, in reviewing the literature for characteristics associated with the development of ANV, it is evident that an important goal remains to isolate psychological traits or certain clinical characteristics that increase the likelihood of early detection of those patients who will experience ANV. Psychological screening procedures may well be developed that would permit targeting patients who would most benefit from some psychological intervention prior to, or early on in, the course of chemotherapy.

Various factors are believed to increase the likelihood of patients exhibiting ANV. Some of these include: greater postchemotherapy nausea and/or vomiting, higher dosages and more emetogenic chemotherapy drugs, lengthier infusions, greater state and/or trait anxiety, tastes and smells associated with chemotherapy, being younger, a history of motion sickness, gastrointestinal susceptibility and being treated in a large group room rather than a small private room (e.g. Andrykowski, Redd & Hatfield, 1985; Morrow & Dobkin, 1988; van Komen & Redd, 1985).

Much of the phenomenology of ANV is readily accounted for by a classical conditioning paradigm. For example, various incidental features of the chemotherapy process itself, such as the sight of the clinic entrance, the odour of the clinic, nurses' or doctors' uniforms, or even the mere thought of chemotherapy, are enough on their own to produce nausea and vomiting in some patients after two or three chemotherapy treatments.

However, a classical conditioning explanation alone may be an oversimplification (Morrow & Dobkin, 1988); and, as indicated above, a range of factors appear to be associated with a propensity to develop ANV.

From the evidence briefly reviewed so far, it is possible to come to some conclusions about how psychological assessment and intervention can be used in combating the extremely unpleasant effects of nausea and vomiting.

For straightforward postchemotherapy nausea and vomiting, the most effective treatment is by antiemetic medication and new drugs, such as odansetron, seem to be particularly effective. However, well-designed studies of the effects of odansetron, and similar drugs, on ANV have not been carried out. In any case, patients who are highly anxious about chemotherapy could all probably benefit from

relaxation training prior to chemotherapy commencing. In addition, the preparation of patients for chemotherapy rarely systematically utilizes the findings from psychology about preparation of patients for invasive medical and surgical procedures (Horne, Vatmanidis & Careri, 1994a, b).

It may be useful, and further research is certainly warranted, to assess all patients about to undergo chemotherapy for their levels of anxiety and 'conditionability' and, in addition, to pay particular attention to the environment in which chemotherapy takes place so that exposure to cues likely to become conditioned trigger stimuli and reminders of chemotherapy, eliciting nausea and vomiting in their own right, is reduced to a minimum. The more comfortable, less institutional and personal the setting for chemotherapy, the less likely is the occurrence of adverse psychological reactions to treatment, including ANV.

As far as ANV is concerned, it would be helpful to detect those at risk prior to the first chemotherapy infusion because the ANV symptoms usually do not emerge until the third or subsequent chemotherapy treatment, by which time much associative learning (conditioning) may have occurred. Some very recent data from work currently in progress at the Royal Melbourne Hospital, shows that AN can emerge after a single high dose chemotherapy treatment in up to 50% of cases. There is some evidence that directly measuring heart-rate arousal and conditionability in the laboratory can allow prediction of those patients who will subsequently develop ANV or, more commonly, AN alone. (Ligdopoulos, 1991; Horne et al., 1996). The use of behavioural therapies for treating ANV has been reported as successful (e.g. Morrow & Dobkin, 1988).

The psychological assessment of patients about to undergo chemotherapy should specifically inquire about depression and phobic anxiety. If there is a pre-existing medical phobia (e.g. of blood and/or injections) then appropriate preparation of the patient prior to commencing chemotherapy may be crucial to the patient completing the course. It is the author's experience that this kind of assessment and psychological preparation is not routinely done by oncologists and surgeons.

A programme that this author has found helpful in treating phobic anxiety and ANV involves a combination of training in relaxation using guided imagery, systematic desensitization to a medical phobic hierarchy combined with exposure to video modelling of having a needle or catheter inserted (Horne et al., 1986). The use of video modelling is particularly useful because it allows patients to play the modelling videotape as often as they like whilst retaining control over exposure by using the pause and on/off switches. This is consistent with general evidence that modelling is an effective means of preparation for invasive procedures (Horne, Vatmanidis & Careri, 1994a, b).

Thus, to conclude it is clear that nausea and vomiting side-effects of drugs occur with a variety of drugs but most worrying is their presence in cancer chemotherapy. New antiemetic drugs are appearing which are more effective than previous antiemetics. However, for some patients nausea and vomiting remain a problem, particularly when, through conditioning, they become ANV. Measuring psychological factors such as anxiety, physiological arousal and conditionability could be useful in detecting those patients at risk of developing ANV and cognitive – behavioural therapies can be effective in ameliorating these distressing and dangerous side-effects. In any case, given existing knowledge, proper psychological preparation of all cancer chemotherapy patients is likely to significantly reduce unpleasant side-effects, enhance coping with chemotherapy and improve quality of life.

ACKNOWLEDGEMENTS

I am greatly indebted to Katerina Ligdopoulos, formerly at the University of Melbourne, Australia, and now a clinical psychologist at Guy's Hospital, London, UK, for help in preparing this chapter.

REFERENCES

Andrykowski, M.A., Redd, W.H. & Hatfield, A.K. (1985). Development of anticipatory nausea: a prospective analysis. *Journal of Consulting and Clinical Psychology*, 53, 447–54.

Bakowski, M.T. (1984). Advances in antiemetic therapy. *Cancer Treatment Reviews*, 11, 237–56.

Horne, D.J. de L., McCormack, H.M., Collins, J.P., Forbes, J.F. & Russell, I.S. (1986). Psychological treatment of phobic anxiety associated with adjuvant chemotherapy, *The Medical Journal of Australia*, 145, 346–8.

Horne, D.J. de L., Vatmanidis, P. & Careri, A. (1994a). Preparing patients for invasive medical and surgical procedures 1: adding behavioural and cognitive interventions. *Behavioural Medicine*, 20, 5–13.

Horne, D.J. de L., Vatmanidis, P. & Careri, A. (1994b). Preparing patients for invasive medical and surgical procedures 2: using psychological interventions with adults and children. *Behavioural Medicine*, 20, 15–21.

Horne, D.J. de L., Shardey, V., Green, M., Allen, N. & Madden, C. (1996). Anxiety and conditionability in the prediction of anticipatory nausea and vomiting in chemotherapy. *Conference Abstract in Psycho-Oncology*, 5, 169–70.

Ligdopoulos, K. (1991). Psychological aspects of anticipatory nausea and vomiting in cancer chemotherapy patients. MA (Clinical Psychology) thesis, University of Melbourne, Australia.

Lindley, C.M., Bernard, S. & Fields, S.M. (1989) Incidence and duration of chemotherapy-induced nausea and vomiting in the outpatient oncology population. *Journal of Clinical Oncology*, 7, 1142–9.

Morrow, G.R. & Dobkin, P.L. (1988) Anticipatory nausea and vomiting in cancer patients undergoing chemotherapy treatment: prevalence, aetiology and behavioural interventions. *Clinical Psychology Review*, 8, 517–56.

Pollera, C.F. & Gianarelli, D. (1989) Prognostic factors influencing cisplatin-induced emesis. *Cancer*, 64, 1117–22.

Sagar, S.M. (1991). The current role of antiemetic drugs in oncology: a recent revelation in patient symptom control. *Cancer Treatment Reviews*, 18, 95–133.

Van Komen, R.W. & Redd, W.H. (1985). Personality factors associated with anticipatory nausea/vomiting in patients receiving cancer chemotherapy. *Health Psychology*, 4, 189–202.

Well woman/Well man clinics: the Australian context

CAROL A. MORSE

Faculty of Nursing, Royal Melbourne Institute of Technology, Victoria, Australia

Establishing a special clinic has several benefits. The clinic's name provides identification of its major focus to potential users and referral sources. Centralization can enable interdisciplinary specialists to work together on common themes and issues. A total assessment of each user leads to the development of a clear, comprehensive and balanced picture of their descriptive and proscriptive needs. Different management and treatment modalities can be controlled and evaluated at various time points and strategies can be increasingly tailored to meet expressed wants. This process facilitates the formation of a database so that experiences can be shared, knowledge and expertise can be generalized. Within the clinic, clients can obtain accurate information and increase their awareness of care options of health concerns. Externally, outreach education initiatives increase the knowledge, awareness and sensitivity of the community.

Well Woman Clinics aim to promote the health of the total woman rather than attending to a specific site of pathology. The focus is on wellness rather than only disease and total wellness means giving attention also to the active promotion of health and well-being. A social model of health is woven into the philosophy of these units so that problems of psychosocial origin and significance are validated equally with biomedical disorders (Pearson, Spencer & McKenna, 1991).

These clinics for women tend to be provided by women professionals. The expectation of women seeking help is that women health professionals provide a greater intuitive and experiential similarity that enhances the quality of care provided (Waller, 1988). This assumption of shared life experiences of both social and physiological origin overcomes some of the many potential barriers that often exist in cross-gendered consultation settings.

In Australia, the National Women's Health Program is the major component of the National Women's Health Policy, which was launched in April 1989 following an extensive consultation process with women's groups, professional and lay public, State and Territory Governments. The prime aim of the Program is to encourage the health system to be more responsive to women's health and well-being needs (OSW, 1991).

Combined funding from the Commonwealth and States for a period of four years, 1990–1994, of $33.5 million was allocated to promote primary health-care initiatives. The main foci were women's reproductive health and sexuality, emotional and mental health, violence against women, occupational health and safety, health needs of women carers, and the health effects of sex role stereotyping. Projects have been promoted to examine inequalities due to economic disadvantage, low cultural relativity, geographic or linguistic isolation. Information processes and education strategies to inform women on the above health issues have been examined and developed, training and education on women's health issues for health-care providers have also been initiated. Since 1991, Well Women Clinics have appeared throughout the country through funding grants obtained from the National Women's Health Program.

As yet, no comprehensive evaluation of their national utility, cost-effectiveness or popularity has been carried out. A sample of six centres randomly selected included one from a major metropolitan city (Sydney); one from a regional city in South Australia (Mount Gambier); one from a rural centre 200 km from the major metropolitan city of Adelaide in South Australia (Southern Yorke Peninsula); one from a rural centre in Western Australia (Hedland); and three from remote centres in far north Western Australia (Nintirri, Tom Price and Paraburdoo). Each of these serves different populations of women including Anglo-Australians, Aboriginal Australians, and migrant women from non-English speaking backgrounds (NESB). The age range of women who attend these clinics is from early teen years to postmenopause.

The focus of the centres' activities is on wellness, assessment, and non-medical management of personal problems, and family stress problems. Problems identified as requiring medical intervention are referred back to the women's own general practitioner who may refer on to a medical specialist. Some centres provide regular sessions by a medical practitioner at times separate from the Clinic's main health-care provider, who is always likely to be a nurse practitioner. Most clinic services are free except those of medical practitioners who provide services through bulk billing.

All the Clinics provide information on women's reproductive functions including the menstrual cycle. Breast examination and cervical smears are available everywhere together with training in breast self-examination. At some Clinics, pregnancy testing is provided and information given on menopause and hormone replacement therapies. All centres utilize a variety of delivery methods of individual, small and large group discussions, workshops, seminars and programmes running weekly on particular themes (e.g. lifestyle improvement, nutrition, weight control and body image). Some Clinics concentrate on the issues most relevant to young adults to mid-aged women, while others also provide services for teenagers on drug and alcohol-related problems, sexuality and safe sex practices. The type of population served by the Clinic determines the inclusion or exclusion of particular services or topics. The rural and remote Clinics also provide for socializing through Orientation Programmes for New Families, New Mothers Support Groups, and the formation of discussion groups on domestic violence, stress management and alternative therapies.

All the Clinics are staffed by nurse practitioners who usually work in isolation from other health professionals and often without clerical assistance. Some of these nurses have undergone short courses of training in women's health provided by the Royal College of Nursing Continuing Education Programme or the Family Plan-ning Association, others have no specialist training or education in women's health other than their basic nurse education and their own life experiences.

Problems experienced by them all include the need for tireless public relations exercises and advertising on minimal budgets coupled with community and/or health professionals' resistance to the Well Women Clinics' initiatives. Some innovative measures have been introduced. South Australia have provided a 'mammography bus' to bus women 200 km to the metropolitan city of Adelaide for breast examinations. South Hedland Well Women's Centre obtained a receptionist/secretary for six months, funded by monies from the local lotteries. These Clinics have filled a significant gap in women's health services and have managed to survive till the present time under increasingly tenuous political and economic support.

Within the last few years, the appearance of the National Mental Health Policy (1993) has prompted greater attention being given to mental illness and wellbeing in the community. Several Area Health Services provided some funding for additional staff to work specifically with mentally distressed and ill women through the Women's Health Centres. Simultaneously, repeated restructuring of services within States and Territories has resulted in changes to the situation, personnel and structure of the Clinics. Some have been subsumed into other units, i.e., within hospital clinics (e.g. Adelaide's Women's Health Centre). Others have continued to adopt increasingly innovative methods to spread their services even further than initially offered. For example, the Southern Yorke Peninsula Health Service utilized a small sum of money to equip and mobilize a caravan into a Mobile Clinic that travelled the length and breadth of the Peninsula to take health care and education to the people.

To the present time, these innovative programmes are still hanging on to slender grants from the National Women's Health Program but have received no CPI increases since their initial funding four years ago. The National Women's Health Program is currently under review and its continuation, and those of its funded projects, cannot be guaranteed beyond January 31st 1997. Clearly, the community needs exist. The critical question is whether other services would be able and willing to take over these activities in the current climate of economic rationalist user-pays ideologies.

WELL MAN'S CLINICS

There has been no comparable development or provision of holistic health services for men even though a widely publicized National conference on Men's Health took place in 1994 that was meant to result in the production of a Men's Health Policy. Since then, some initiatives have appeared in sporadic fashion in Western Australia, Melbourne, and South Australia.

In Western Australia, a Health Department grant provided for the development of a review of men's health issues, prevalence rates and needs (Huggins, 1996). An academic stream of postgraduate study and research in Men's Health has been developed by the Department of Public Health at Curtin University, Perth. The curriculum focuses on the main aspects of health risk behaviour patterns and socialization effects in adulthood. Attention is particularly directed to identifying the socio-cultural influences that determine stereotyped male behaviours of health neglect and stoicism, healthcare utilization patterns, emotional denial and suppression, and the factors leading to domestic violence. While many of these aspects are commonly viewed as typifying the Australian male, clearly they have a western universalism. Two self-help groups have also appeared in Western Australia: the Male Support Group, and the Men's Health and Wellbeing Association.

In South Australia, at Southern Yorke Peninsula, no distinctive Men's Health activities have occurred on a regular basis. A one-off Men's Health Night in recent times attracted over two hundred and fifty men who sought information and help on cardiovascular illnesses, stress in men's lives, genito-urinary problems, and issues of farm-based occupational safety. In that State and nationally, health promotion and education has also targeted the schools down to the preschool kindergarten level. Using colourful cartoon characters like 'Giddy Goanna', issues of farm safety, emotional and physical well-being, healthful nutrition have been addressed and promoted to raise awareness through the total family.

In Melbourne, Men's Clinics have operated only out of the private health sector, provided by interested general practitioners on a free-for-service basis. The range of issues addressed tend to focus on traditional aspects of physical illnesses, sexual health and problems rather than on holistic and social models of health.

At this time, in late 1996, many perplexities abound. The continuation of the National Women's Health Program beyond January 1997 is uncertain. If it disappears, a small but significant pool of funding will go and will take some innovative though constrained programmes of community health services with it. If the Women's Health initiative loses its significant individual identity, it is unlikely that resources would be re-allocated to fund Men's Health except in covert ways. A loud public outcry from women and women's groups would be anticipated. At the present time when increasing cost-and service-shifting is occurring away from formal services out into the community and back on to families and consumers themselves, it would appear that holistic health and well-being services for women and for men represent a growing need not a lesser one.

REFERENCES

Commonwealth of Australia. (1993). *The National Mental Health Policy.* Canberra: Australian Government Publishing Service.

Huggins, A. (1996). Report on Men's Health. Perth: Western Australia Department of Health and Human Services.

Office of the Status of Women (1991). *National Agenda for Women: implementation report.* Canberra: Australian Government Publishing Service.

Pearson, M., Spencer, M. & McKenna, M. (1991). Patterns of uptake and problems presented at Well Woman Clinics in Liverpool. *Journal of Public Health Medicine,* **13**, 7.

Waller, K. (1988). Women doctors for women patients? *British Journal of Medical Psychology,* **61**, 125–35.

AUTHOR INDEX

[629]

SUBJECT INDEX

economic factors
  and health, 107–9
  quality of life assessment costs, 313
  socioeconomic status, 171–3
  unemployment, 186–9
  Whitehall studies, 107, 171–2
education see health education
educators, training, 328–30
effect, theories of, 170
efficacy beliefs see self-efficacy concept
elaboration-likelihood model, 6
elderly people
  health behaviours, 143–6
  hospitalization, 128–1
  iatrogenic disorders, 508
electromyogram (EMG), 47
elimination diets, food allergies, 352–3
emotion
  atopic dermatitis, 373
  breaking bad news, 273–5
  burnout in health-care professionals, 275–8
  cerebral representation, 369
  and coping strategies, 104–5
  expression and health, 103–6; evaluation, 103;
    short-term investigation, 104
  laboratory setting, 46
emphysema, 392–4
encopresis, 452–3
endometrial cancer, 484
endorphins, 416
  and alcoholism, 348
endoscopy and bronchoscopy, 453–5
enuresis, 455–6
epidemics, 456–7
epilepsy, 457–9
Epstein–Barr virus infection, 460–1
ethnic factors in health, 98–103
exercise, see also physical activity
exercise counselling, 156
experiments and research, 57–9
  archival research, 58–9
  surveys, 59–60
extraversion, 33

facial disfigurement, 450–2
  cleft lip and palate, 409–10
family
  alcohol abuse and alcoholism, 349–50
  health influences of, 107–9
  impact of HIV infection and AIDS, 345
  risk factors, distribution, 107–9
  violence: battering, against women, 375–6; child
    abuse, 400–3
fear, laboratory setting, 46
fear arousal and appraisal, 6
fetal alcohol syndrome, 461–2
fetus, monitoring and assessment, 463–4
field experiment, 57–8
field theory, 56
Flesch Reading Ease Score, 332
fluoxetine, alcoholism treatment, 349
folklore, cure procedures, 133
food allergies, 352–3
  atopic dermatitis, 373
food intolerance, 519–20
fragile X syndrome, 405

G-proteins, 40–1
GABA receptors, 40–1
gastric ulcers, 464–6
gender issues
  and health, 110–12
  labelling theory, 111
general practitioners
  burnout, 275–8
  communication, 284–7; teaching skills, 322–5

consultation, communication, 284–7
  diagnostic accuracy, 305–6
  doctor–patient relationship: HIV infected patients,
    346; patient satisfaction, 301–4
  stress levels, 319–20
genetic counselling, 480–1
Gestalt theory, 56
glaucoma, 482
glucose monitoring, 434–5
glutamate receptors, 41
grid techniques, 251–4
grief, 83
  breaking bad news, 273–5
  see also bereavement
group therapy, 213–15
  applications, 215
  efficacy, 214–15
  therapeutic factors, 214
growth retardation, 483–4
gynaecological disorders
  cancers, 484–7
  hysterectomy, 506–7
  pelvic pain, 547–8

Haddon Matrix, 341
haemophilia, 487–8
handicap, defined, 209
head injury, 227–8, 489–92
  rehabilitation, 230–3
head and neck cancers, 488–9
headache and migraine, 492–4
health
  childhood influences, 78–80
  defined by WHO, 141
  economic factors, 107–8
  family influence, 107–9
  gender issues, 110–12
  health belief model (HBM), 5
  lay beliefs, 131–5
  and life events, 136–9
  noise, effects, 139–43
  and physical activity, 154–7
  social support, 168–70
  and socioeconomic status, 171–3
  workplace factors, 107
  workplace interventions, 264–8
health behaviours, 117–21
  attitude–behaviour relationship, 4–5
  behaviour change, 155–6; processes, 181–2;
    stage-matched interventions, 182; stages, 180–1
  and beliefs about health, 5, 131–5
  common dimensions, 117–18
  determinants, 118–19
  elderly people, 143–6; health issues, 143–6
  locus of control, 151
  perceived control, 151–3
  risk-taking, 157–60; in adolescence, 78–9, 108;
    Behavioural Risk Factor Surveillance System, 117;
    mental models, 159; qualitative assessment, 158–9;
    quantitative assessment, 157–8; road traffic
    accidents, 53, 108
  self-efficacy concept, 114, 152, 160–2
  sexual behaviour, 162–5
  social factors, 118–19
  theories, 119; criticism of theories, 179–80;
    meta-analysis, 179; Theory of Planned Behaviour,
    5, 152–3, 177, 178–9; Theory of Reasoned Action,
    4–5, 177–8; transtheoretical model of change,
    180–2
  type A (coronary-prone), 183–5; beta-blockers,
    effects, 381
  see also coping strategies
Health Belief Model (HBM), 113–17, 153
  evidence for/against, 114–15
  implications for practice, 116
  origins and components, 113–14

health-care practice, 269–335
health-care professionals
  attitudes, 271–2
  burnout, 275–8
  compliance, 278–80
  imparting bad news, 273–5
  psychological support, 307–10
  social support, 307–10
  socialization, 326
  stressors, 288–90
  training and development, 325–8; partnership
    model, 327–8
  work environment, 288–901
health education, 216–19
  compliance promotion: patients, 281–4;
    professionals, 280
  health messages, recall, 316–17
  injury prevention, 341–3
  planning, 216–17
  Precede–Proceed model, 217
  social skills training, 261
  teaching communication skills, 322–5
  theories, implementation, 218–19
  training educators, 328–30
  training and professional development, 325–8
Health-Promoting Lifestyle Profile (HPLP), 117
health status
  assessment, 220–3
  HSA indexes, 222
  measurement, 221–3
  SF-36, 222
hearing loss, 426–7
herbalism, 414, 416
heuristics and biases, 23–4
histamine, IgE, immediate immune hypersensitivity
  type I, 353
HIV infection and AIDS, 343–7
  epidemiology, 457
  and haemophilia, 487–8
  health-care staff, 346
  impact on family, 345
  testing, reactions, 345–6
Hodgkin's disease, 494–5
homeopathy, 414, 416
hormones, and mental health, 111
hospitalization
  adults, 121–3
  children, 124–7
  elderly people, 128–1
hostility
  Cook–Medley scale, 184
  modification, 185
Huntington's disease, 495–7
hyperactivity, 497–9
hypercalcaemia, idiopathic (Williams syndrome), 405–6
hyperhidrosis, 499
hypertension, 500–1
hyperthyroidism, 502–3
hyperventilation, 504–5
hypnosis, 224–7
hyponotics see benzodiazepines
hypochondriasis, 505–6
hypothermia, preoperative (CABG), 397
hysterectomy, 506–7

iatrogenesis, 507–9
iatrogenic and medical accidents, 291–4
IgE
  atopy, 353
  food allergies, 352–3
  immediate immune hypersensitivity type I, 353
illness
  attributions and adjustment, 75–6
  coping strategies, 84–7, 131–5
  and death, perception by children, 81–2
  lay beliefs, 131–5, 131–5